# Skin Lymphoma

# Skin Lymphoma

## The Illustrated Guide

**Lorenzo Cerroni, MD**

Director, Dermatopathology Research Center
Medical University of Graz
Graz, Austria

**Sixth Edition**

WILEY

This edition first published 2026


*Edition History*
John Wiley & Sons, Ltd (1e, 1998); (2e, 2004); (3e, 2009); (4e, 2014); (5e, 2020)



*Registered Offices*
John Wiley & Sons, Inc., 111 River Street, Hoboken, NJ 07030, USA
John Wiley & Sons Ltd, New Era House, 8 Oldlands Way, Bognor Regis, West Sussex, PO22 9NQ, UK

For details of our global editorial offices, customer services, and more information about Wiley products visit us at www.wiley.com.

The manufacturer's authorized representative according to the EU General Product Safety Regulation is Wiley-VCH GmbH, Boschstr. 12, 69469 Weinheim, Germany, e-mail: Product_Safety@wiley.com.

Wiley also publishes its books in a variety of electronic formats and by print-on-demand. Some content that appears in standard print versions of this book may not be available in other formats.



*Library of Congress Cataloging-in-Publication Data*
Names: Cerroni, Lorenzo author
Title: Skin lymphoma : the illustrated guide / Lorenzo Cerroni, MD, Director, Dermatopathology Research Center, Medical University of Graz, Graz, Austria.
Description: Sixth edition. | Hoboken, NJ, USA : Wiley, 2026. | Includes index.
Identifiers: LCCN 2025043736 (print) | LCCN 2025043737 (ebook) | ISBN 9781394235483 cloth | ISBN 9781394235506 adobe pdf | ISBN 9781394235490 epub
Subjects: LCSH: Skin–Cancer | Lymphomas
Classification: LCC RC280.S5 C47 2026 (print) | LCC RC280.S5 (ebook)
LC record available at https://lccn.loc.gov/2025043736
LC ebook record available at https://lccn.loc.gov/2025043737

Cover Design: Wiley
Cover Images: © yuansdrt/Shutterstock, Courtesy of Lorenzo Cerroni

Set in 9.5/12pt Minion Pro by Straive, Pondicherry, India

Printed in Singapore
M127674241125

*To Heinz Kutzner, Phil LeBoit, and Luis Requena, the three musketeers of dermatopathology.*

*Your knowledge, curiosity, and passion are a continuous source of inspiration in my professional career; your friendship is a blessing in my life.*

# Contents

## Section 4: Specific cutaneous manifestations of leukemias and of precursor hematologic neoplasms



## Section 5: Cutaneous manifestations of other lymphomas and non-neoplastic cutaneous signs of systemic lymphomas



## Section 6: Cutaneous lymphomas and lymphoproliferative disorders in children and adolescents



## Section 7: Pseudolymphomas of the skin

# Preface

Five years have elapsed since the publication of the last edition of this book, and many things have changed in the field of cutaneous lymphoproliferative disorders. Most important of all, and most disappointing, we are back to the confused situation of the past when different classifications of lymphomas and leukemias were published by different groups. Two classification schemes are currently in use: the first is the International Consensus Classification (ICC) of Myeloid and Lymphoid Neoplasms prepared by the Society for Hematopathology and the European Association for Haematopathology together with hematologists, oncologists, and scientists through a joint Clinical Advisory Committee; and the second is the fifth edition of the World Health Organization (WHO) Classification of Haematolymphoid Tumours. Although for the most part the two classifications overlap, they differ in some definition and even in listing, or not listing, some entities, thus causing confusion. A different problem, found in both classifications, is the large number of "molecular entities," particularly among the leukemias and precursor lymphomas. Although this is the expected result of continuous progress in the field of lymphomas and leukemias, at the same time it renders the use of the adopted terminology problematic for many of the laboratories that process and report biopsies, even in public hospitals. Contrary to what John Lennon sang in the beautiful song "Watching the wheels" ("I tell them there's no problem, only solutions"), this is a problem, and there's no solution, as on the one hand we strive for and welcome progress, but on the other one many laboratories face budget limitations, and in many countries reimbursement for molecular investigations by the national health system is still limited. Notwithstanding these problems and limitations, for what concerns cutaneous lymphoproliferative disorders the ICC and WHO classifications have only minimal differences, and mostly semantic rather than substantial.

In the field of cutaneous lymphomas, many progresses have been made thanks to the efforts of the European Organization for Research and Treatment of Cancer – Cutaneous Lymphoma Tumour Group (EORTC-CLTG), the International Society for Cutaneous Lymphomas (ISCL), and the United States Cutaneous Lymphoma Consortium (USCLC). In addition to these groups, several national societies have published guidelines for diagnosis and treatment of cutaneous lymphomas, particularly for mycosis fungoides and Sézary syndrome, aiming at facilitating and standardizing the work of physicians in this complex medical field. However, besides excellent publications, many articles are still being published with what, judging from the pictures and data provided, seem to be incorrect diagnoses, representing dangerous pitfalls because of the potential for misleading those reading them. This problem is not new, yet the incredible increase in the number of low-quality, though "Science Citation Index (SCI) listed," journals, most of which working on a "pay-per-publish" basis, has dramatically amplified it. It was never as important as it is today to read critically any given publication (including, of course, this book) and to form one's own opinion. It is my advice to the many young physicians coming to Graz for variably long fellowships to never *believe* anything they read or hear, but to filter every information with their own experience, and compare it to other sources before reaching a conclusion. This is becoming of paramount importance in times when unfiltered Internet-based knowledge is constantly sought by the new (and old) generations of doctors.

Speaking of Graz, although officially I retired in October 2024, I still work part-time in the Dermatopathology Unit of the Department of Dermatology. I have the privilege to be surrounded by competent colleagues who, at the same time, are extraordinary human beings. Being (by far) the oldest member of the group, sometimes I feel like a Jurassic animal, yet they manage to transmit me freshness and motivations that I couldn't get by myself alone. I am very grateful to them for providing a friendly, relaxed, and funny atmosphere that greatly facilitates a difficult work – difficult because of the complexity of some of the cases, of the human implications of many of our diagnoses, and unfortunately sometimes also because of the bureaucratic hurdles that all those working in medicine have to face.

My family, too, has been paramount during all these years, as I couldn't do anything without the love, affection, and support of my wife, Ricarda, and my children, Livia and Luca. Luca finished brilliantly his studies in mechanic engineering and started to work in a company (while keeping playing piano on a semi-professional level), while Livia is a successful fifth-year student of medicine, already starting to work in hospitals and to attend patients. Although she doesn't want to pursue a career in dermatology or dermatopathology, discussing with her non-dermatological medical problems is stimulating, albeit at the same time showing me how much of general medicine I forgot during all these years (a tribute that many of us, I guess, have to pay to the yearlong focus on a narrow field).

I also clearly realize that I have reached an age when I no longer have the mental and physical strength to set the bar ever higher. In the last chapter of the book *A philosophy of practice of surgical pathology*, Bernie Ackerman wrote: "Then, out of nowhere, it suddenly became obvious to me that other, younger eyes were not only faster than mine; some, I am pleased to record, were even better.", thus realizing that the time had arrived for him to shift the emphasis of his professional life. Bernie Ackerman has been a continuous source of inspiration for me. When he was still alive, he taught me dermatopathology and helped me to build my professional career: without him, I would have never been able to accomplish what I did. Even after his death, he represents for me the model of what I am striving for as a teacher and as a mentor. Besides Bernie, I have had the unique privilege of working with giants in the fields of dermatology, dermatopathology, and cutaneous lymphoproliferative disorders, learning from them and at the same time enjoying their unique friendship. Neil Smith, Walter Burgdorf, Jean Bolognia, Rein Willemze, Chris Meijer, Andreas Chott, Werner Kempf, Wolfram Sterry, Emilio Berti, Nicola Pimpinelli, Marco Santucci, Janine Wechsler, Phil LeBoit, Heinz Kutzner, and Luis Requena among many others have been key to my achievements over the years, as well as Helmut Kerl and Kevin Gatter, of course, who have also been essential for the birth of this book. Sadly, some of them passed away, and I miss them much more than words can say.

It was fun to prepare this edition of the book, and I really enjoyed it, and learned much. But I am not planning a new edition after this one. The years spent working on this book, from the first edition in 1998 until today, have been rich of professional satisfactions, ways beyond what I would have ever dreamed of as a young medical student, with medical problems that have stimulated my interest and curiosity, and human relations that have deeply enriched my life. It has been a fantastic journey: fascinating and inspiring, with much fun and some sorrows, yet for the most part delighting, gratifying, and rewarding, and I am deeply grateful to all those who have accompanied me on it during so many years.

Today, I feel that the promise of medicine as a call rather than a job, as a profession full of interests, humanity, and compassion has been kept, and I can look back at more than forty years of professional life with amazement, and some pride.

Graz, October 2025

**CHAPTER 1**

# Introduction

Primary cutaneous lymphomas represent distinct clinical and histopathologic subtypes of extranodal lymphomas. They can be defined as neoplasms of the immune system, characterized by a proliferation of either T, natural killer (NK), or B lymphocytes, which show a particular tropism for the skin. By definition, primary cutaneous lymphomas show no evidence of extracutaneous manifestations at presentation. Besides malignant lymphomas, the skin may be the primary site of onset of other hematological malignancies such as myeloid leukemia ("aleukemic leukemia cutis") and blastic plasmacytoid dendritic cell neoplasm; although staging investigations may be negative at presentation, these disorders should be better regarded as a secondary cutaneous manifestation of an undiscovered malignant hematological disease, and treated accordingly.

Primary cutaneous lymphomas should be separated from secondary skin manifestations of extracutaneous (usually nodal) lymphomas and leukemias, which represent metastatic disease characterized usually by a worse prognosis, and requiring different treatments. Since the histopathology of primary and secondary cutaneous lymphomas may be similar or identical, in many cases complete staging investigations are needed to establish this distinction (early mycosis fungoides representing the most important, but not the only exception to this rule).

Besides cutaneous lymphomas, many diseases that simulate them either clinically, histopathologically, or both, are a daily source of diagnostic problems (cutaneous pseudolymphomas). Criteria for diagnosis and differential diagnosis of these benign lymphoproliferative conditions are discussed in Chapter 31 of this book.

Finally, besides infiltration by neoplastic lymphocytes, the skin may present with several specific or nonspecific signs and symptoms related to extracutaneous lymphomas, some of which are highly suggestive of specific conditions. A discussion of non-neoplastic cutaneous manifestations of systemic lymphomas and leukemias is provided in Chapter 29.

## Classification of cutaneous lymphomas

Regrettably, as in past times, different classifications for lymphomas and leukemias are again in use. A Clinical Advisory Committee (CAC) together with world leading hematopathologists published the International Consensus Classification (ICC) *of Myeloid and Lymphoid Neoplasms* in 2022 [1] (the ICC book has been subsequently published in 2025) [2]. On the other hand, the World Health Organization (WHO), prepared in 2022 the 5th revision of the *Classification of Haematolymphoid Tumours* [3, 4] (the WHO book has been subsequently published in two volumes in 2024) [5]. However, the ICC and WHO schemes differ only in some parts, and there is no major discrepancy for what concerns skin lymphomas; the entities relevant for the skin are listed in Table 1.1. For what concerns cutaneous lymphomas, the ICC and WHO schemes are based on the seminal work made by the European Organization for Research and Treatment of Cancer (EORTC) – Cutaneous Lymphomas Task Force, which in 1997 published the first comprehensive classification of cutaneous lymphomas [6], subsequently revised together with a WHO panel in 2005 and 2018, and updated in 2024 (Table 1.1) [7]. In fact, in contrast to previous editions, in the last edition of the WHO *Classification of Haematolymphoid Tumours* published in 2024, primary cutaneous T-cell lymphomas are listed as a distinct group (most primary cutaneous B-cell lymphomas are referred to as specific entities in the context of other extracutaneous B-cell lymphomas) [3]. Curiously enough, however, Sézary syndrome has not been included in the group of cutaneous T-cell lymphomas in the WHO classification. The recognition of cutaneous lymphomas as a distinct group (after decades of disregard by most hematopathologists) is mainly due to the work done in the past by the Dutch and Austrian groups, particularly by Rein Willemze and Helmut Kerl.

Despite the presence of an accepted frame for classification of primary cutaneous lymphomas, in many publications obsolete terminology such as "cutaneous T-cell lymphoma" is still used. Under this term cases of mycosis fungoides and Sézary syndrome (and sometimes of other T-cell lymphomas arising in the skin as well) are lumped together, thus hindering any meaningful analysis of the published data. In order to compare data, it is paramount that physicians in different countries and centers classify cutaneous lymphomas in a repeatable way.

*Skin Lymphoma: The Illustrated Guide*, Sixth Edition. Lorenzo Cerroni.

**Table 1.1** Comparison of the International Consensus Classification *of Myeloid and Lymphoid Neoplasms* and the 5th edition of the WHO *Classification of Haematolymphoid Tumours* for entities relevant to the skin, and corresponding entities in the 2018 WHO-EORTC Classification of Cutaneous Lymphomas

| International consensus classification | WHO 5ed | 2018 WHO-EORTC classification of cutaneous Ly. |
|---|---|---|
| Mycosis fungoides and variants | Mycosis fungoides and variants | Mycosis fungoides and variants |
| *Folliculotropic mycosis fungoides* | *Folliculotropic mycosis fungoides* | *Folliculotropic mycosis fungoides* |
| *Pagetoid reticulosis* | *Pagetoid reticulosis* | *Pagetoid reticulosis* |
| *Granulomatous slack skin* | *Granulomatous slack skin* | *Granulomatous slack skin* |
| Sézary syndrome | Sézary syndrome | Sézary syndrome |
| Adult T-cell leukemia/lymphoma | Adult T-cell leukemia/lymphoma | Adult T-cell leukemia/lymphoma |
| Cutaneous CD30$^+$ lymphoproliferative disorders | Cutaneous CD30$^+$ lymphoproliferative disorders | Cutaneous CD30$^+$ lymphoproliferative disorders |
| *Cutaneous anaplastic large cell lymphoma* | *Cutaneous anaplastic large cell lymphoma* | *Cutaneous anaplastic large cell lymphoma* |
| *Lymphomatoid papulosis* | *Lymphomatoid papulosis* | *Lymphomatoid papulosis* |
| Subcutaneous panniculitis-like T-cell lymphoma | Subcutaneous panniculitis-like T-cell lymphoma | Subcutaneous panniculitis-like T-cell lymphoma |
| Extranodal NK/T-lymphoma, nasal-type | Extranodal NK/T-lymphoma, nasal-type | Extranodal NK/T-lymphoma, nasal-type |
| Cutaneous γ/δ T-cell lymphoma | Cutaneous γ/δ T-cell lymphoma | Cutaneous γ/δ T-cell lymphoma |
| Cutaneous aggressive epidermotropic CD8+ CTCL | Cutaneous aggressive epidermotropic CD8+ CTCL | Cutaneous aggressive epidermotropic CD8+ CTCL *(provisional)* |
| pCSMPCD4$^+$ T-cell lymphoproliferative disorder | pCSMPCD4$^+$ T-cell lymphoproliferative disorder | pCSMPCD4$^+$ T-cell lymphoproliferative disorder *(provisional)* |
| Acral CD8$^+$ T-cell lymphoproliferative disorder | Acral CD8$^+$ T-cell lymphoproliferative disorder | Acral CD8$^+$ T-cell lymphoma *(provisional)* |
| EBV$^+$ T/NK-cell lymphoproliferative disorders of childhood | EBV$^+$ T/NK-cell LPs and lymphomas of childhood | Chronic active EBV infection |
| Peripheral T-cell lymphoma, NOS | Cutaneous peripheral T-cell lymphoma, NOS | Cutaneous peripheral T-cell lymphoma, NOS |
| Cutaneous marginal zone lymphoproliferative disorder | Cutaneous marginal zone lymphoma | Cutaneous marginal zone lymphoma |
| Cutaneous follicle center lymphoma | Cutaneous follicle center lymphoma | Cutaneous follicle center lymphoma |
| Cutaneous diffuse large B-cell lymphoma, leg-type | Cutaneous diffuse large B-cell lymphoma, leg-type | Cutaneous diffuse large B-cell lymphoma, leg-type |
| Intravascular large B-cell lymphoma | Intravascular large B-cell lymphoma | Intravascular large B-cell lymphoma |
| EBV$^+$ mucocutaneous ulcer | EBV$^+$ mucocutaneous ulcer | EBV$^+$ mucocutaneous ulcer *(provisional)* |

*NK: natural killer; CTCL: cutaneous T-cell lymphoma; pCSMPCD4$^+$: primary cutaneous small/medium pleomorphic CD4-positive; NOS; not otherwise specified; LPs: lymphoid proliferations.*

## Examination of patients

Primary cutaneous lymphomas represent a heterogeneous group of diseases with different clinicopathologic presentations and prognostic features. In order to classify patients correctly, it is crucial that a complete clinical history is obtained and integrated with histopathologic, immunophenotypical, and molecular data. To take but one example, some lesions of lymphomatoid papulosis show histopathologic features that may be indistinguishable from those observed in mycosis fungoides, anaplastic large cell lymphoma, or cutaneous CD8$^+$ aggressive epidermotropic cytotoxic T-cell lymphoma, and differentiation can only be achieved by correlation with the clinical picture.

## Staging investigations

As a general rule, complete staging investigations at presentation include physical examination, laboratory investigations, ultrasound of lymph nodes and visceral organs, computed tomography (CT) scans and/or positron emission tomography (PET), and bone marrow biopsy. In most centers, PET has replaced CT as the first choice for radiological staging. Patients with several types of low-grade cutaneous lymphoma (e.g., mycosis fungoides, lymphomatoid papulosis, and subcutaneous panniculitis-like T-cell lymphoma among others) do not require extensive investigations. Patients with cutaneous CD4$^+$ small–medium T-cell lymphoproliferative disorder, too, do not require staging investigations. The necessity of staging investigations in patients with primary cutaneous marginal zone lymphoproliferative disorder is also questionable [8], and many centers do not suggest to perform it in otherwise asymptomatic patients.

A staging classification system for mycosis fungoides, Sézary syndrome, and other cutaneous T- and B-cell lymphomas was proposed by a joint working group of the International Society of Cutaneous Lymphoma (ISCL) and the EORTC Cutaneous Lymphoma Task Force [9]. This system has been subsequently slightly modified in conjunction with the United States Cutaneous Lymphoma Consortium (USCLC) (Tables 1.2 and 1.3) [11, 12].

## Surgical techniques

In general, when dealing with cutaneous lymphomas shave biopsies must be avoided (Fig. 1.1). A possible exception may be represented by early lesions of mycosis fungoides, in which a

**Table 1.2** Staging of mycosis fungoides and Sézary syndrome according to the ISCL–EORTC–USCLC

| **Skin** | |
|---|---|
| $T_0$ | Absence of clinically suspicious lesions |
| $T_1$ | Limited patches*, papules, and/or plaques† covering <10% of the skin surface. May be further stratified into $T_{1a}$ (patches only) versus $T_{1b}$ (plaques ± patches) |
| $T_2$ | Patches, papules, or plaques covering >10% of the skin surface. May be further stratified into $T_{2a}$ (patches only) versus $T_{2b}$ (plaques ± patches) |
| $T_3$ | One or more tumors‡ (≥1 cm diameter) |
| $T_4$ | Confluence of erythema covering ≥80% body surface area |
| **Lymph nodes** | |
| $N_0$ | No clinically abnormal peripheral lymph nodes§; biopsy not required |
| $N_1$ | Clinically abnormal peripheral lymph nodes; histopathology Dutch grade 1 or NCI LN0-2 |
| | $N_{1a}$ Clone negative or equivocal |
| | $N_{1b}$ Clone positive and identical to skin |
| $N_2$ | Clinically abnormal peripheral lymph nodes; histopathology Dutch grade 2 or NCI LN3 |
| | $N_{2a}$ Clone negative or equivocal |
| | $N_{2b}$ Clone positive and identical to skin |
| $N_3$ | Clinically abnormal peripheral lymph nodes; histopathology Dutch grades 3–4 or NCI LN4 |
| | $N_{3a}$ Clone negative or equivocal |
| | $N_{3b}$ Clone positive and identical to skin |
| $N_x$ | Clinically abnormal peripheral lymph nodes; no histologic confirmation |
| **Visceral** | |
| $M_0$ | No visceral organ involvement |
| $M_{1a}$ | Bone marrow only involvement |
| | Clone negative or equivocal |
| | Clone positive and identical to skin |
| $M_{1b}$ | Nonbone marrow visceral involvement |
| | Clone negative or equivocal |
| | Clone positive and identical to skin |
| $M_x$ | Visceral involvement is neither confirmed nor refuted by available pathologic or imaging assessment |
| **Blood**& | |
| $B_0$ | Absence of significant blood involvement: ≤250/μL of CD4+/CD26- or CD4+/CD7-cells |
| | $B_{0a}$ Clone negative or equivocal |
| | $B_{0b}$ Clone positive and identical to skin |
| $B_1$ | Low blood tumor burden: does not meet the criteria for $B_0$ or $B_2$ |
| | $B_{1a}$ Clone negative or equivocal |
| | $B_{1b}$ Clone positive and identical to skin |
| $B_2$ | High blood tumor burden: ≥1000/μL of CD4+/CD26− or CD4+/CD7-cells or other aberrant population of lymphocytes identified by flow cytometry |
| | $B_{2a}$ Clone negative or equivocal |
| | $B_{2b}$ Clone positive and identical to skin |
| $B_X$ | Unable to quantify blood involvement according to agreed upon guidelines |
| | $B_{Xa}$ Clone negative or equivocal |
| | $B_{Xb}$ Clone positive and identical to skin |

| **Stage**(z) | | | | | |
|---|---|---|---|---|---|
| IA | $T_1N_0M_0B_{0,1}$ | IB | $T_2N_0M_0B_{0,1}$ | | |
| IIA | $T_{1,2}N_{1,2}M_0B_{0,1}$ | IIB | $T_3N_{0-2}M_0B_{0,1}$ | | |
| IIIA | $T_4N_{0-2}M_0B_0$ | IIIB | $T_4N_{0-2}M_0B_1$ | | |
| IVA1 | $T_{1-4}N_{0-2}M_0B_2$ | IVA2 | $T_{1-4}N_3M_0B_{0-2}$ | IVB | $T_{1-4}N_{0-3}M_{1A,B}B_{0-2}$ |

* For skin, a patch indicates any size skin lesion without significant elevation or induration. The presence/absence of hypo- or hyperpigmentation, scale, crusting, and/or poikiloderma should be noted.

† For skin, plaque indicates any size skin lesion that is elevated or indurated. The presence or absence of scale, crusting, and/or poikiloderma should be noted. Histologic features such as folliculotropism or large cell transformation (>25% large cells), CD30+ or CD30−, and clinical features such as ulceration are important to document.

‡ For skin, the tumor indicates at least one ≥1 cm diameter solid or nodular lesion with evidence of depth and/or vertical growth. Note a total number of lesions, total volume of lesions, largest size lesion, and region of body involved. Also note if histologic evidence of large cell transformation has occurred. Phenotyping for CD30 is encouraged.

§ For node, Abnormal lymph nodes are those >1.5 cm longest diameter according to the Lugano classification [10] and confirmed by imaging. The pathological findings of a representative abnormal lymph node may apply to all abnormal lymph nodes.

¶ For viscera, the spleen and liver may be diagnosed by imaging criteria.

& For blood, it is expected that patients with high blood tumor burden ($B_2$) will have a clone in the blood that is identical to that in the skin. Nonidentical T-cell clones are often detected in peripheral blood with increasing age and are of unknown clinical significance. Patients with lymphopenia (defined as <1000 absolute lymphocytes) may potentially have an underestimation of aberrant lymphocyte burden if assessed only by the absolute number and not also by the percentage of immunophenotypically abnormal lymphocytes.

(z) Folliculotropism is a histologic feature that can occur irrespective of stage. Histologic evidence of FMF is associated with a higher risk of disease progression. In selected cases or inadequate response, consider primary treatment for stage IIB (tumor stage disease). Adapted from Olsen *et al.* [11].

**Table 1.3** TNM classification system for cutaneous lymphomas other than mycosis fungoides and Sézary syndrome

| Classification | Description |
|---|---|
| $T_1$ | Solitary skin involvement |
| | $T_{1a}$: Solitary lesion <5 cm in diameter |
| | $T_{1b}$: Solitary lesion ≥5 cm in diameter |
| $T_2$ | Regional involvement of skin: multiple lesions limited to 1 body region or 2 contiguous body regions |
| | $T_{2a}$: All disease encompassing a <15-cm-diameter circular area |
| | $T_{2b}$: All disease encompassing a ≥15 to <30-cm-diameter circular area |
| | $T_{2c}$: All disease encompassing a ≥30-cm-diameter circular area |
| $T_3$ | Generalized skin involvement |
| | $T_{3a}$: Multiple lesions involving 2 noncontiguous body regions |
| | $T_{3b}$: Multiple lesions involving ≥3 body regions |
| $N_0$ | No clinical or pathologic involvement of lymph nodes |
| $N_1$ | Involvement of 1 peripheral lymph node region that drains an area of current or previous skin involvement; biopsy positive for lymphoma |
| $N_2$ | Involvement of ≥2 peripheral lymph node regions or involvement of any lymph node region that does not drain an area of current or previous skin involvement; biopsy positive for lymphoma |
| $N_3$ | Involvement of central lymph nodes; biopsy positive for lymphoma |
| $N_X$ | Clinically abnormal peripheral or central LN but no pathologic determination. |
| $M_0$ | No visceral involvement |
| $M_1$ | Visceral involvement |
| $M_X$ | Visceral involvement is neither confirmed nor refuted by available pathologic or imaging assessment |

Adapted from Olsen *et al.* [11].

broad surface of the biopsy may be more useful than a small punch biopsy – provided, of course, that the shave biopsy is deep enough to include the superficial part of the reticular dermis. Punch biopsies may provide sufficient diagnostic information, particularly in tumors with homogeneous populations of cells, but may be too small for phenotypic and genetic analyses, if needed. Particularly in biopsy of suspect early mycosis fungoides, it is a good rule to perform more biopsies on different lesions, in order to get as much information as possible.

### Surgical artifacts

Surgical specimens should be carefully removed, paying particular attention not to crush the tissue and not to put surgical specimens on a gauze. Unfortunately, many dermatological surgeons are unaware of the deleterious effects of gauzes on surgical specimens, particularly in biopsies of small dimensions, and even more regrettably, many dermatology textbooks describe the use of gauzes for placing surgical specimens as a standard procedure. Upon contact with a gauze, otherwise adequate biopsies show variable alterations of cell morphology, similar to what can be seen in fixation artifacts (Fig. 1.2). Drying artifacts may render a precise diagnosis impossible even in a large, seemingly well-done punch biopsy (Fig. 1.3). Some cell types get these artifacts in a matter of a few moments (e.g., blastoid cells of large cell lymphomas/leukemias), whereas other are more resistant. The same deleterious effect can be observed in other cutaneous tumors (e.g., Merkel cell carcinoma). Immunohistochemical analyses may still offer some information on specimens with drying artifacts, but as a morphologic-phenotypic correlation is no longer possible, the histologic report should mention that the evaluation of immunohistology is seriously hindered by the artifacts. Other surgical and technical artifacts may reduce, sometimes dramatically, the ability of a dermatopathologist to render a precise diagnosis, such as crushing of a specimen, reduced fixation (due often to the insufficient amount of formalin used to send the specimen to the processing laboratory), heat and freezing artifacts (evident in hot summers and cold winters, particularly in specimens that are processed at sites distant from the surgical theatre), and cauterization artifacts (due to the use of cauterizing surgical blades – so-called "harmonic scalpels"). It is imperative that dermatological surgeons submitting specimens with such artifacts are made aware of the problem, in order to avoid in future unnecessary repetition of the biopsies.

## Histopathology, immunophenotype, and molecular genetics

### Histopathology

Sections should be cut with a maximum thickness of 4 μm (we use 3.5 μm) and subsequently stained with hematoxylin and eosin (H&E). Stainings with periodic acid–Schiff (PAS) and Giemsa are not performed routinely on skin specimens but may be helpful in specific settings. High-quality sections are necessary for a correct diagnosis.

Morphologic examination of a biopsy specimen should assess the following criteria:

1. Architecture of the infiltrate (e.g., superficial, superficial and deep, subcutaneous, etc.)
2. Involvement of particular structures (e.g., epidermotropism, pilotropism, etc.)
3. Cell composition (e.g., monomorphous infiltrate, mixed cell infiltrate, etc.)
4. Cell morphology
5. Other specific clues and criteria (e.g., deposition of mucin within the hair follicles, angiocentricity/angiodestruction, etc.).

Much information can be gathered at low power by examination of the pattern of growth, and basic morphologic assessment is also useful for the selection of appropriate panels of antibodies necessary for phenotypic analyses, and of other ancillary techniques useful in the study of the biopsy specimen.

### Immunophenotype

Staining techniques and automated immunostainers have allowed the standardization of phenotypic studies on formalin fixed, paraffin-embedded (FFPE) tissue sections. A list of antibodies

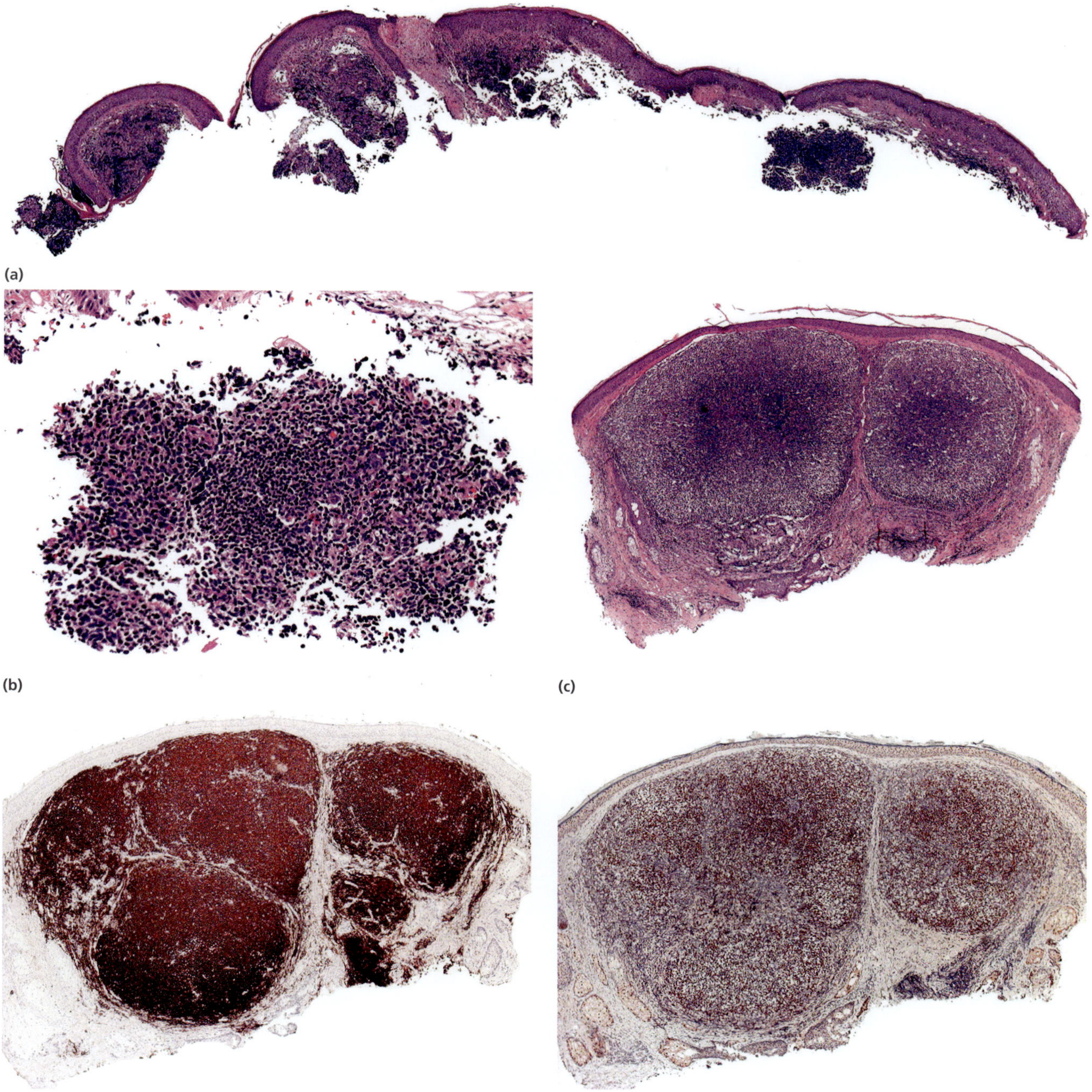

(a) (b) (c) (d) (e)

Figure 1.1 Surgical artifact due to a superficial shave biopsy. (a) Superficial shave biopsy taken from the nose under the clinical diagnosis of "r/o basal cell carcinoma" revealed a flat epidermis and fragments of lymphoid infiltrates. (b) Some of the cells within the infiltrate had large nuclei and a new, deeper biopsy was advised. (c) An adequate, new biopsy showed nodular lymphoid infiltrates with a biphasic pattern characterized by mid-sized and large cells arranged at the periphery of the nodules, suggestive of follicle center lymphoma. (d) Positivity for CD20. (e) Bcl-6 confirmed the diagnosis. A high level of suspicion should be exerted when atypical lymphoid infiltrates are only partially sampled. In this context, a punch biopsy is a better type of partial sampling of a cutaneous lymphoid infiltrate than a shave biopsy.

reactive with lymphocyte subsets and accessory cells in FFPE tissue sections is provided in Table 1.4. It should be emphasized that immunohistochemical stainings are not necessary in each and every case of cutaneous lymphoma/pseudolymphoma. In early lesions of mycosis fungoides, for example, I seldom use immunohistology as a routine investigation: in fact, correlation with the clinical picture is faster, cheaper, and gives better information in order to establish the diagnosis. Sometimes, however, staining for pan-T-cell markers may be useful in better displaying the number and distribution of intraepithelial lymphocytes.

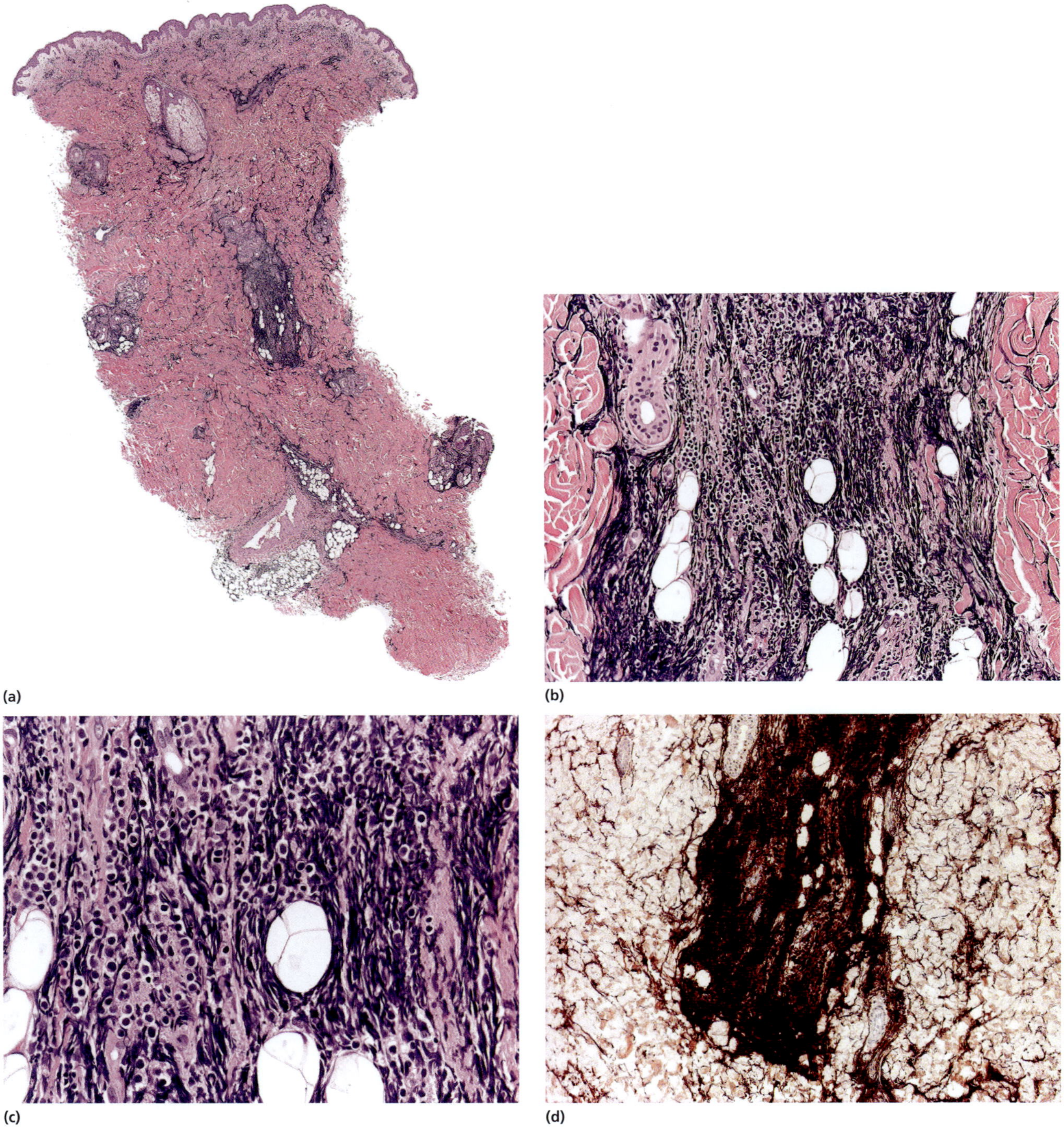

Figure 1.2 Surgical artifact due to placing the biopsy on a gauze (drying artifacts). (a) A 4 mm punch biopsy originally well taken and deep enough (b) shows at high power severe drying artifacts that affect most of the neoplastic cells within the infiltrate; (c) some of the evaluable cells show a mid-sized blastoid appearance. (d) Staining for TdT shows a possible positivity of the cells, but the exact interpretation is hindered by the artifacts. The diagnosis of T lymphoblastic lymphoma was subsequently confirmed by a new biopsy.

Although phenotypic investigations provide crucial information for the diagnosis and classification of cutaneous lymphomas, it should be remembered that malignant cells are characterized by a "plasticity" that may transcend the relatively rigid schemes of our classifications. Besides aberrant expressions of phenotypic markers ("lineage infidelity"), cases with so-called "transdifferentiation," that is, the evolution of a tumor into a clonally related neoplasm of a different cell line has been

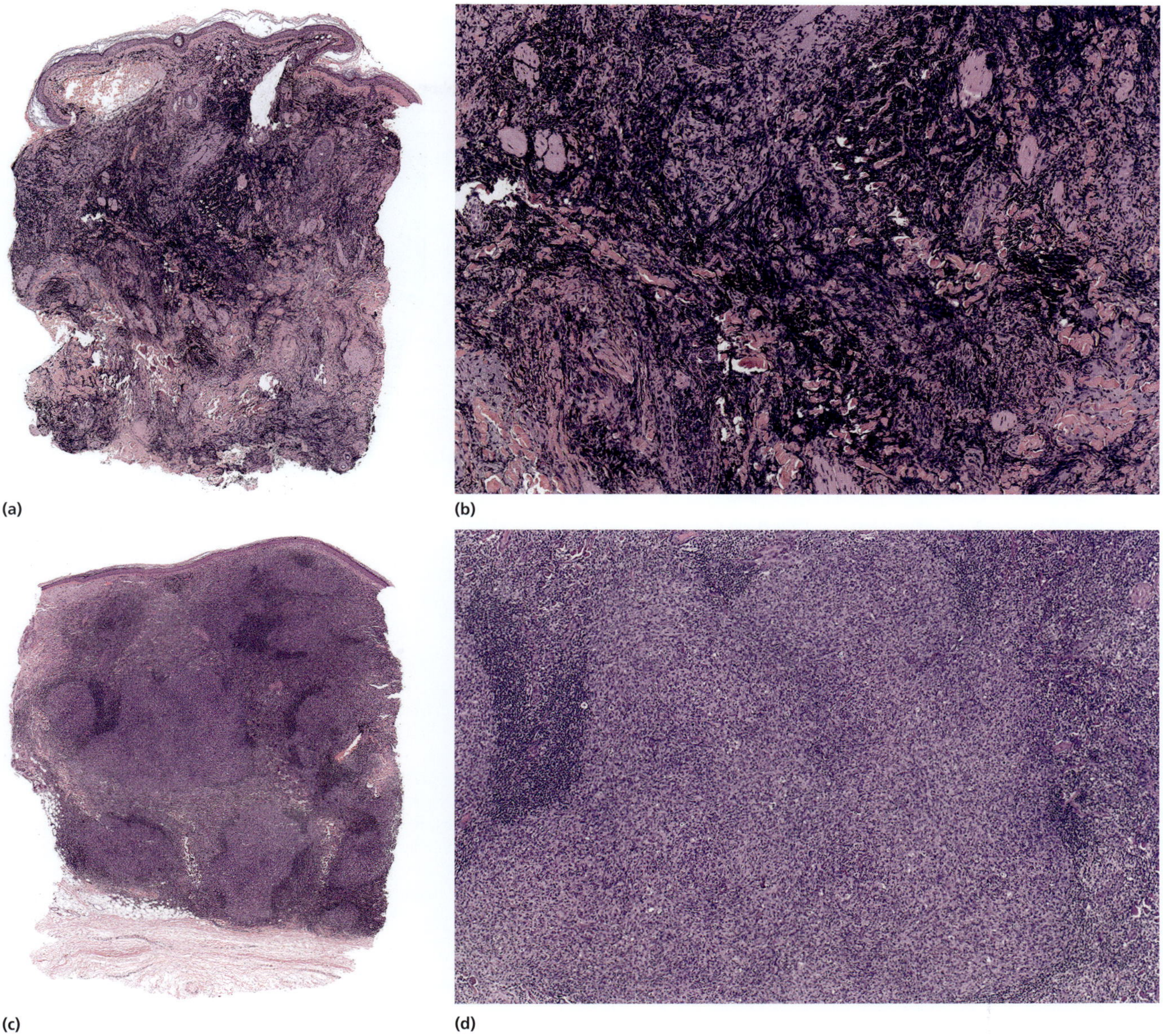


**Figure 1.3** Surgical artifact due to placing the biopsy on a gauze (drying artifacts). (a) A 5 mm punch biopsy originally well taken (b) shows severe drying artifacts that affect most of the neoplastic cells within the infiltrate; (c) a repeat biopsy without artifacts shows the same architectural pattern of the infiltrate, (d) and allows to clearly recognize the histopathological features of cutaneous follicle center lymphoma.

described [13]. Although transdifferentiation was thought to be peculiar to precursor lymphomas/leukemias, it has been observed also in mature B-cell neoplasms that have evolved into clonally related dendritic or histiocytic tumors [14]. Overlapping myeloid and lymphoid features can be observed in chronic myelogenous leukemia, in which blast crisis in 10% of the cases reveals a B- or, more rarely, a T-cell phenotype. In some cases, molecular data have provided a rational explanation for the association of different diseases, such as the presence of *TET2* mutations in both angioimmunoblastic T-cell lymphoma and chronic myelomonocytic leukemia, explaining the observation of patients presenting with both diseases. The concept of transdifferentiation expands the traditional model of hematopoiesis based on the unidirectional maturation of hematopoietic precursors into lineage-committed cells. Even normal lymphocytes, particularly B-cells, under appropriate environmental conditions may transdifferentiate into macrophages or other hematopoietic cell types [15].

## Gene rearrangement studies

Analysis of the T-cell receptor (TCR) and immunoglobulin (Ig) genes provides useful information for the study of

**Table 1.4** Panel of antibodies for immunohistologic analysis of cutaneous lymphomas and pseudolymphomas on routinely fixed, paraffin-embedded sections of tissue

| Antigen/antibody | Main immunostaining in cutaneous lymphomas/pseudolymphomas and/or specificity |
|---|---|
| CD1a | Positive in reactive and neoplastic Langerhans cells. Positivity also in most precursor T-cell lymphomas/leukemias. Useful also in the differential diagnosis of dendritic cell proliferations in patients with chronic myeloid neoplasms. |
| CD2 | Pan T-cell marker. Loss of expression is never found in reactive T-cell infiltrates. Positive also in systemic mastocytosis and in a subset of myeloid neoplasms. |
| CD2AP | Plasmacytoid dendritic cells; Positive in blastic plasmacytoid dendritic cell neoplasm. |
| CD3 | Pan T-cell marker. Loss of expression is never found in reactive T-cell infiltrates. |
| CD3ε | T-cells (epsilon chain of CD3). Positive in T cells and also in some NK-cell neoplasms. |
| CD4 | Positive in T-helper cells and related T-cell lymphomas. Commonly positive also in myeloid neoplasms and in blastic plasmacytoid dendritic cell neoplasm. |
| CD5 | Pan T-cell marker. Loss of expression is never found in reactive T-cell infiltrates. Also positive in B lymphocytes in some B-cell lymphoma/leukemia (e.g., B-CLL, mantle cell lymphoma). |
| CD7 | Pan T-cell marker. Although loss of expression may be observed in some cutaneous T-cell lymphomas, the expression may be downregulated also in cases of inflammatory dermatoses, thus not providing a robust criterion for diagnosis. |
| CD8 | Positive in T-cytotoxic cells. |
| CD10 | CALLA. Positive in neoplastic cells of follicle center lymphomas (follicular > diffuse). Positivity found also in follicular T-helper lymphocytes and derived lymphomas. Positivity in single cells in cutaneous biopsies difficult to evaluate because of background staining of dermal fibers. |
| CD11c | Marker of normal monocytes/macrophages. Also positive in acute myeloid leukemia and in hairy cell leukemia. |
| CD13 | Marker of myeloid cells. Useful in the diagnosis of myeloid leukemias. |
| CD14 | Marker of monocytes/macrophages. Useful in the diagnosis of myeloid leukemias. |
| CD15 | Hodgkin and Reed-Sternberg cells in Hodgkin lymphoma; Also positive in granulocytes and monocytes and in some myeloid neoplasm. |
| CD16 | Expressed by NK lymphocytes and some T cells. |
| CD19 | Positive in B-cells. |
| CD20 | Positive in B-cells. Expression may be lost after therapy with rituximab. |
| CD21 | Follicular dendritic cells in both benign and malignant infiltrates with lymphoid follicles. |
| CD23 | Positive in the majority of cells of B-CLL; stains also follicular dendritic cells. |
| CD25 | IL-2 receptor, expressed on activated lymphocytes. Positive in ATLL and in some cases of mycosis fungoides. Neoplastic mast cells in systemic mastocytosis are positive for CD25 as well as for CD2. |
| CD30 | Activated T- and B-cells; Hodgkin and Reed-Sternberg cells in Hodgkin lymphoma. Positivity defines a group of cutaneous T-cell lymphomas including cutaneous anaplastic large cell lymphoma and lymphomatoid papulosis. Variable numbers of positive cells may be observed in most cutaneous lymphoproliferative disorders, thus the diagnostic value is only in conjunction with other markers. Positivity required for treatment with brentuximab vedotin. |
| CD31 | Positive in endothelial cells (but not specific for them). Does not discriminate between blood and lymphatic vessels. |
| CD33 | Positive in early myeloid cells, and in subsets of myeloid leukemia. |
| CD34 | Positive in precursor T or B cells and in some case of myeloid leukemia. Positive in endothelial cells (does not discriminate between blood and lymphatic vessels). |
| CD35 | Follicular dendritic cells in both benign and malignant infiltrates with lymphoid follicles. |
| CD37 | Expressed in most T and B cells. May be useful in cases treated with anti-CD37 antibodies (e.g., otlertuzumab). |
| CD38 | Plasma cells in benign and malignant conditions, including plasmablastic lymphoma. Positive in a subset of B-CLL. |
| CD43 | Pan T-cell marker; positive also in myeloid cells. B-cell neoplasms is positive in neoplastic cells of B-CLL and mantle cell lymphoma. |
| CD45 | Leukocyte common antigen (utility in confirming the hematolymphoid origin of a given tumor) (negative in some hematological neoplasms, e.g., plasma cell neoplasms, some anaplastic large cell lymphoma) |
| CD45RA | Naive T-cells. Positive in primary cutaneous aggressive epidermotropic $CD8^+$ cytotoxic T-cell lymphoma (but diagnosis cannot be based on this marker only). |
| CD45RO | Memory T-cells. Useful in some cases to confirm T-cell differentiation of neoplastic cells. |
| CD52 | Mature lymphocytes. Positivity is a pre-requisite for treatment with an anti-CD52 antibody (alemtuzumab). |
| CD54 | Intracellular adhesion molecule 1 (ICAM-1). Expressed on endothelial cells. May be implicated in the pathogenesis of intravascular lymphomas. |
| CD56 | Positive in NK-cells and a good marker for the majority of cases of extranodal NK/T-cell lymphoma, nasal-type. Also positive in neoplastic plasma cells. |
| CD57 | Positive in NK-cells (neoplastic cells in extranodal NK/T-cell lymphoma, nasal-type are usually negative) |
| CD68 | Positive in normal and neoplastic histiocytes and macrophages. Positivity in a subset of myeloid leukemias. Two different epitopes marked by the clones KP-1 and PGM-1 may show completely different staining patterns in neoplastic conditions (and sometimes in reactive conditions as well). |
| CD79a | B-cells. Expression in B lymphocytes starts earlier than that of CD20, thus some precursor B-cell neoplasms may be $CD79a^+$ but $CD20^-$. |
| CD99 | Positive in a subset of precursor cells. Expression is found also in several non-lymphoid neoplasms and should be evaluated only in the general context. |
| CD103 | In cutaneous lymphoproliferative disorders positive mostly in ATLL and in some cases of mycosis fungoides. |
| CD117 | c-kit; positive in both reactive and neoplastic mast cells. Positive in a subset of myeloid leukemias. |

**Table 1.4** *(cont'd)*

| Antigen/antibody | Main immunostaining in cutaneous lymphomas/pseudolymphomas and/or specificity |
|---|---|
| CD123 | Plasmacytoid dendritic cells in both benign and malignant conditions (blastic plasmacytoid dendritic cell neoplasm and dendritic cell neoplasms in chronic myeloid leukemia). |
| CD138 | Plasma cells in benign and malignant conditions, including plasmablastic lymphoma. |
| CD163 | Positive in normal and neoplastic histiocytes and macrophages. More sensitive than CD68. Positivity in a subset of myeloid leukemias. |
| CD200 | Positive in B-cell chronic lymphocytic leukemia. |
| CD207 | Marker of Langerin, specific for Langerhans cells (both benign and malignant). |
| CD246 | ALK-1 (anaplastic large cell lymphoma kinase). Only rarely positive in cases of cutaneous anaplastic large cell lymphoma; positivity may be more common in pediatric cases. The pattern may be nuclear and/or cytoplasmatic, with different patterns associated in part with specific genetic aberrations involving *ALK*. |
| CD279 | PD-1. Positive in follicular T-helper lymphocytes as well as in a subset of activated lymphocytes. |
| PD-L1 | PD-1 ligand. Utility mostly in the setting of specific treatment. |
| CD303 | BDCA2. Expressed in reactive and neoplastic plasmacytoid dendritic cells. Reliable marker of blastic plasmacytoid dendritic cell neoplasm. |
| Ig heavy chains (IgA, IgD, IgE, IgG, IgM) | B-cells. IgM is important in two main contexts: non-class-switched cutaneous marginal zone lymphoma, and cutaneous diffuse large B-cell lymphoma, leg-type. |
| IgG4 | IgG4-producing plasma cells. Positive in some cutaneous disorders (e.g., granuloma faciale), but not linked with certainty to cutaneous lymphoproliferative disorders. |
| Ig light-chains (kappa, lambda) | Used to test clonality in infiltrates with prominent B-cell populations; in situ hybridization provides better results but can only be applied in cases with plasma cell differentiation. |
| Ki-67 | Proliferating cells. Useful in two main ways: (i) to determine the proliferation rate (e.g., the proliferation of nearly 100% of neoplastic ells is required for a diagnosis of Burkitt lymphoma), and (ii) to detect the pattern of proliferation and eventual "hot spots" in cases with mixed cell infiltrates. "Aberrant" patterns may be observed in neoplastic lymphoid follicles (decreased proliferation as opposed to the high proliferation typical of reactive follicles), and in band-like T-cell infiltrates related to drugs (very high proliferation as opposed to the low proliferation typical of early mycosis fungoides). |
| Pan-Cytokeratin | Marker of epithelial cells. Useful in the differential diagnosis of undifferentiated tumors (but it may be aberrantly expressed in non-epithelial neoplasms). Useful also in better visualizing the pattern of intraepithelial lymphocytes, particularly in adnexotropic mycosis fungoides. |
| EMA | Epithelial membrane antigen. Positive in epithelial tumors and in a subset of lymphocytes and plasma cells. In lymphoproliferative disorders used mainly in multiple myeloma and cutaneous anaplastic large cell lymphoma, but does not give more information than those provided by more specific markers. |
| S100 protein | Positive in benign and malignant Langerhans cells and in interdigitating reticulum cells. Useful also in the differential diagnosis of dendritic cell proliferations in patients with chronic myeloid neoplasms. |
| TdT | Terminal deoxynucleotidyl transferase. Nuclear staining (cytoplasmic staining is not specific and mostly due to artifacts, and should be ignored). Positive in precursor lymphomas of both B- and T-cell phenotype. Positivity can be observed in a small subset of myeloid leukemias. |
| TCR-$\beta$ ($\beta$F1) | $\alpha/\beta$ T-cells. Positive in some cases of cutaneous $\gamma/\delta$ T-cell lymphoma with expression of both $\alpha/\beta$ and $\gamma/\delta$ markers. The expression may be lost in some $\alpha/\beta$ cutaneous T-cell lymphomas, thus negativity cannot be considered as a surrogate for TCR-$\gamma$ or TCR-$\delta$ positivity. |
| TCR-$\gamma$ | $\gamma/\delta$ T-cells. Positivity for either TCR-$\gamma$ or TCR-$\delta$ pre-requisite for the diagnosis of cutaneous $\gamma/\delta$ T-cell lymphoma. |
| TCR-$\delta$ | $\gamma/\delta$ T-cells. Positivity for either TCR-$\gamma$ or TCR-$\delta$ pre-requisite for the diagnosis of cutaneous $\gamma/\delta$ T-cell lymphoma. |
| TIA-1 | Present in all cytotoxic T-cells (granular cytoplasmic positivity). |
| Granzyme-B | Present in activated cytotoxic T-cells (granular cytoplasmic positivity). |
| Perforin | Present in activated cytotoxic T-cells (granular cytoplasmic positivity). |
| Bcl-2 | Expressed in most mature T- and B-cells. Lack of expression in germinal center B lymphocytes in the lymph nodes is used to confirm benignancy of the germinal centers, but malignant lymphoid follicles in cutaneous follicular lymphoma are mostly Bcl-2-negative. Positivity in neoplastic large B lymphocytes aids in the diagnosis of cutaneous diffuse large B-cell lymphoma, leg-type. |
| Bcl-6 | Nuclear expression in follicular B-cells (both benign and malignant). Positive also in follicular T-helper lymphocytes. |
| Bcl-10 | Nuclear expression in marginal zone lymphoma may be associated with a worse prognosis. |
| HGAL | B-cells in the germinal center; in general does not provide better information than Bcl-6 in that setting. |
| LMO-2 | B-cells in the germinal center; in general does not provide better information than Bcl-6 in that setting. |
| IRTA1 | Immunoglobulin superfamily receptor translocation-associated 1. Membranous expression. Positive in most cutaneous and other extranodal marginal zone lymphomas; lower percentage of cases of nodal marginal zone lymphoma positive as well. |
| Anti-HLA-DR | Expression of HLA-DR, a human MHC class II molecule expressed on antigen-presenting cells (subsets of dendritic cells, B lymphocytes, monocytes, macrophages). |
| CXCL-13 | Positive in follicular T-helper lymphocytes and T-cell lymphomas with TFH phenotype. |
| ICOS | Inducible co-stimulator protein; Positive in follicular T-helper lymphocytes, both benign and malignant. |
| Cyclin-D1 | Uniform positivity in mantle cell lymphoma (a minority of cases is negative); variable numbers of positive cells may be observed in other B-cell neoplasms, particularly plasma cell myeloma. |
| Cyclin D2, D3 | Mantle cell lymphoma (cases negative for cyclin D1). |

*(Continued)*

**Table 1.4** *(cont'd)*

| Antigen/antibody | Main immunostaining in cutaneous lymphomas/pseudolymphomas and/or specificity |
|---|---|
| SOX11 | Mantle cell lymphoma (including cases negative for cyclin D1). Negativity in mantle cell lymphoma linked to a more indolent course. |
| LEF1 | Nuclear expression in B-CLL (negative in mantle cell lymphoma and marginal zone lymphoma) |
| FOX-P1 | Forkhead box protein 1; Nuclear expression in cutaneous diffuse large B-cell lymphoma, leg type (negative in cutaneous follicle center lymphoma, diffuse type). |
| FOX-P3 | Forkhead box protein 3; T-regulatory cells; nuclear expression. Positive in neoplastic cells ATLL and in a subset of cases of mycosis fungoides. |
| IRF8 | Interferon regulatory factor 8. Highly expressed in myeloid cells. Expressed in neoplastic cells of follicle center lymphoma. |
| IRF4/MUM-1 | Multiple myeloma oncogene 1. Positive in plasma cell neoplasms. Useful mostly in the differentiation of cutaneous diffuse large B-cell lymphoma, leg type (positive) from cutaneous follicle center lymphoma, diffuse type (negative or positive in a small minority of cells). |
| TRAF1 | TNF receptor encoded factor 1. Positive in cutaneous $CD30^+$ lymphoproliferative disorders. |
| ZAP-70 | Zeta-associated protein 70. Nuclear positivity in B-CLL is associated with unmutated status and a worse prognosis. Positive also in normal T lymphocytes. |
| MYC | Overexpression of MYC (nuclear staining). Expression of the antibody is not synonymous with the presence of a chromosomal translocation. Useful in the definition of a subset of diffuse large B-cell lymphoma, leg type with "double" or "triple" expression status (Bcl-2, Bcl-6, MYC). The cut-off point to define positivity is 40% of neoplastic cells. |
| OCT2 | Nuclear expression. Usually used in conjunction with BOB1; positive in most B-cell lymphomas. |
| BOB1 | Nuclear expression. Usually used in conjunction with OCT2; positive in most B-cell lymphomas. |
| p16 | Loss of expression if gene silenced. May have a prognostic value in a subset of cases of cutaneous diffuse large B-cell lymphoma, leg type. |
| HHV-8 | Human herpes virus 8. Positive in all cases of Kaposi sarcoma (both HIV and non-HIV-related). In lymphoproliferative disorders positive in primary effusion lymphoma and a subset of cases of Castleman disease. |
| EBER-1† | Small nuclear RNA associated with EBV. Nuclear positivity in all cells infected by EBV. |
| LMP-1 | EBV latent membrane protein. Expressed only in latency types 2 and 3, thus does not stain all EBV infected cells. |
| TP | *Treponema pallidum*, specific for syphilis. The staining pattern reveals the typical morphology of the *Treponema*. The staining should be performed in all cases of lymphoproliferative disorders associated with HIV infection. |
| Myeloperoxidase | Positive in reactive myeloid cells and in a subset of cases of myeloid leukemia. |
| MNDA | Myeloid cell nuclear differentiation antigen. Positive in reactive myeloid cells and in a subset of cases of myeloid leukemia. Positive also in a subset of marginal zone lymphoma but negative in cutaneous follicle center lymphoma. |
| Lysozyme | Positive in reactive myeloid cells and in a subset of cases of myeloid leukemia. Robust marker in cases otherwise negative for most markers. |
| PAX-5 | Paired box gene 5, Immature and mature B-cells. In precursor, B-cell lymphomas may be used as a surrogate marker of CD19 when other B-cell markers are negative. Positive within the nuclei of Hodgkin and Reed-Sternberg cells. A pitfall is represented by positivity for PAX-5 in some cases of Merkel cell carcinoma. |
| TCL-1 | A subset of CD4-/CD8-T-cells. Positive in plasmacytoid dendritic cells. In hematological neoplasms positive in T-cell prolymphocytic leukemia and in blastic plasmacytoid dendritic cell neoplasm. |
| D2-40 | Surrogate marker for podoplanin. Positive in endothelial cells of lymphatic vessels. Crucial for the differential diagnosis of intravascular neoplasms (vessels negative in intravascular B- and NK/T-cell lymphoma, positive in intralymphatic anaplastic large cell lymphoma). |
| TCF4 (E2-2) | Positive in blastic plasmacytoid dendritic cell neoplasm. |
| P24 | HIV p24-gag viral capsid protein, useful for immunohistochemical demonstration of HIV infection. Positivity is found in follicular dendritic cells and in cutaneous Langerhans cells. |
| SPIB | Positive in blastic plasmacytoid dendritic cell neoplasm. |
| Annexin A1 | Encoded by the ANXA1 gene which is upregulated in hairy cell leukemia. Considered as the most sensitive and specific marker for the diagnosis of hairy cell leukemia. Expression is mostly membranous, sometimes cytoplasmatic. |
| NPM1 | Aberrant cytoplasmic expression in acute myeloid leukemia with mutated *NPM1*. |
| FDCSP | Follicular dendritic cell secreted peptide, expressed in follicular dendritic cell sarcoma. |
| SRGN | Serglycin, expressed in follicular dendritic cell sarcoma. |

† In situ hybridization.

cutaneous lymphomas. Early in their differentiation, T and B lymphocytes rearrange their TCR and Ig genes, respectively. Analysis of the gene rearrangement provides clues to the clonality of a given infiltrate. Benign (reactive) lymphoid proliferations are characterized by a polyclonal pattern of TCR and/or Ig gene rearrangement. In contrast, malignant lymphomas reveal a monoclonal population of lymphocytes. A standardized assay (BIOMED-2) has been introduced in order to homogenize the different methods and to allow a better comparison of results of gene rearrangement studies and is still used in most centers [16, 17]. Besides indubitable advantages, analysis of TCR and Ig genes rearrangement also has limitations. In fact, benign inflammatory dermatoses may present with a monoclonal pattern, and a "germline" or polyclonal pattern may be observed in clear-cut lymphomas (e.g., in NK-cell neoplasms or in blastic plasmacytoid dendritic cell neoplasms, among others). In addition, the presence of only a few neoplastic cells may give rise to false negative results in cases of early cutaneous T- or B-cell lymphoma, and the finding of small clones of reactive lymphocytes may be falsely interpreted as a monoclonal population of cells in benign infiltrates ("pseudoclonality"). Next-generation sequencing (NGS), known also as "high-throughput sequencing" has been proposed as a more reliable method for analysis of T-cell clonality [18–20]. This technique provides indubitable advances over standard polymerase chain reaction (PCR) protocols, providing also data on the quantity of neoplastic cells present in a given infiltrate. In a recent overview of published literature, the sensitivity of NGS ranged between 69% and 100% (sensitivity of standard PCR methods was 44–72%), and specificity ranged between 86% and 100% (specificity of standard PCR methods was 77–88%) [21], thus showing an improvement in the diagnostic utility compared to standard methods. On the other hand, data from non-lymphoma patients (i.e., patients with inflammatory conditions) are still scarce, and the method is expensive, and not yet widely accessible.

## Other methods used in the study of cutaneous lymphoid infiltrates

### Fluorescence in situ hybridization (FISH)

The fluorescence in situ hybridization (FISH) technique is based on the annealing of single-stranded DNA to a complementary genomic target sequence in a neoplastic cell. Depending on the probes selected, the FISH method can be used to detect different types of chromosomal abnormalities, including monosomy, trisomy, and other aneuploidies, as well as translocations and deletions. This method can be used routinely and can provide valuable information for precise diagnosis and classification.

There are two main types of probes for the detection of translocations, namely, dual-fusion and break-apart probes [22]. Dual-fusion probes consist of two probes labeled in different colors, each of them binding to a distinct chromosome. They are designed to detect translocations of part of one chromosome to another chromosome. In cells not bearing the translocation that is being investigated, four distinct signals (two for each color) are recognized, corresponding to the two alleles of each separate chromosome. By contrast, cells bearing the translocation will show two distinct signals (one for each color), corresponding to the intact alleles, and two fused signals, corresponding to the translocated chromosomes. Dual-fusion probes are highly specific, the main limitation being that they recognize only the translocation for which they have been designed. They are particularly useful for the detection of translocations that are common in a given lymphoma (e.g., the t(14;18) in nodal follicle center lymphoma). Break-apart probes consist of two distinct probes labeled in different colors, binding to DNA sequences flanking the known region of a chromosome. If the region is split, then two signals appear separated, representing the split chromosome, and two are together, representing the normal allele. If the region is intact, four close signals represent the two alleles of the chromosome without breaks. Break-apart probes are very sensitive for detecting chromosomal splits, but do not provide any information concerning the other gene involved in the translocation. They are particularly useful in lymphomas that show different translocations involving one part of a given chromosome with various partner chromosomes (this is the case, for example, for *MYC* translocations).

### Other molecular investigations

A detailed discussion of molecular techniques used in the study of cutaneous lymphomas is beyond the scope of this book. Besides, methods that seem to be innovative at the time of writing may be obsolete when the book is out in print. In addition, cost and availability are still a limiting factor, as most dermatopathology laboratories are not equipped with molecular techniques, or have only limited possibilities. With the exception of analysis of TCR and Ig genes rearrangement and of FISH techniques, genomic analyses cannot yet be considered routine in the diagnosis of cutaneous lymphomas in most dermatopathological laboratories. On the other hand, new genetic insights into malignant tumors are providing not only diagnostic clues but also allowing the identification of molecules that represent potential therapeutic targets [23]. Genetic and epigenetic alterations relevant to different types of cutaneous T- and B-cell lymphomas will be discussed in the respective chapters. A review of molecular techniques useful in hematopathology (that is, not only for cutaneous lymphomas) has been recently published [24].

## Lymphoma microenvironment and lymphoma-associated microorganisms

Lymphomas are not constituted by pure populations of malignant lymphocytes, and the presence of accessory (non-neoplastic) cells admixed with neoplastic ones is well known. In mycosis fungoides, for example, a population of interdigitating reticulum cells has been observed in specific lesions, and several studies demonstrated that their number varies in different stages of the disease, decreasing in more advanced stages. There is good evidence that non-neoplastic lymphoid and other accessory cells are crucial for the development and maintenance of malignant lymphomas, particularly low-grade ones, and a large number of such cells has been identified and better characterized ("lymphoma microenvironment"). The interaction of neoplastic cells with their microenvironment is a two-way relationship: the microenvironment helps in sustaining the neoplastic cells and at the same time malignant lymphocytes recruit accessory and other reactive cells. A typical example is represented by angioimmunoblastic T-cell lymphoma, a peculiar neoplasm deriving from specific subsets of follicular T-helper (TFH) lymphocytes with a $CD4^{+}/PD\text{-}1^{+}/Bcl\text{-}6^{+}/CXCL\text{-}13^{+}/ICOS^{+}$ phenotype, which is invariably associated with a reactive compartment of B lymphocytes and other accessory cells.

Besides accessory cells, in many lymphomas, a pivotal role is played by microorganisms, particularly viruses. The Epstein–Barr virus (EBV) is involved in several types of lymphomas, and the demonstration of EBV integration in neoplastic cells is an important diagnostic criterion in many lymphoma types. Besides EBV, other viruses are involved in some lymphoproliferative conditions (e.g., human herpes virus (HHV)-8 and human T-lymphotropic virus 1 (HTLV-1)). Bacteria, too, have been implicated in the etiology of some cases of non-Hodgkin lymphoma (e.g., *Borrelia burgdorferi* in cutaneous marginal zone lymphoproliferative disorder, *Helicobacter pylori* in gastric MALT-lymphoma). In short, several microorganisms are linked to different types of lymphoproliferative conditions, and demonstration of infection is important for both diagnosis and (sometimes) treatment.

## Pseudomalignancy, premalignancy, and early malignancy

One of the major conceptual problems in the field of cutaneous lymphomas is the precise classification of "early" manifestations of it, and their distinction from benign infiltrates. The concept of the "parapsoriases," introduced by the French dermatologist Brocq in 1902, is paradigmatic of this problem and shows that, in spite of over 100 years of research, we are still unable to provide a precise conceptual frame for "pseudo" malignancies, "pre" malignancies, and "early" malignancies (see also Chapter 2) [25, 26]. This difficulty is not unique to cutaneous lymphomas (actinic keratosis and melanoma in situ represent two other typical examples), and is not confined to skin neoplasms, but rather is an intrinsic problem of most "cancers."

In my opinion, some of the difficulties that we encounter in daily routine in the diagnosis of early cutaneous lymphomas are, in truth, conceptual rather than practical: the search for criteria that allow diagnosis of the earliest stages of malignant tumors brings us to the grey zone between clearly benign and clearly malignant neoplasms, in a cloudy area where conventional definitions and criteria do not always work. Increased knowledge and improved diagnostic techniques are changing the very concept of cancer, not only in the skin but in other organs as well. Autopsy investigations of men older than 80 years demonstrated that nearly all of them have small prostatic carcinomas that were clinically silent and that did not affect their life span. In fact, it seems likely that in many (if not all) organs there are forms of early cancer that are clinically silent and that do not cause overt disease. This problem is well known to epidemiologists, and is defined as "over diagnosis" of cancer, thereby meaning not a false positive result (i.e., a wrong diagnosis of cancer) but a diagnosis of a tumor that fulfills all pathologic criteria of cancer, but that would not have grown to become clinically evident [27]. In short, the major difficulty lies in defining precisely what is early cancer and in drawing an unambiguous line between what is clearly benign and what is already malignant.

In the realm of lymphoproliferative disorders, a paradigmatic example of the problem of drawing a precise line between "benignancy" and "malignancy" is represented by monoclonal gammopathy of undetermined significance (MGUS). Patients with MGUS are at risk of progression into a lymphoproliferative malignancy (usually a plasma cell myeloma). On the other hand, it has been demonstrated that, although not all patients with MGUS develop malignant lymphoma, almost all patients with multiple myeloma had a preceding MGUS, thus clearly showing that this is more an "early malignancy" than a "non-neoplastic" process. To further complicate the issue, the concept of "monoclonal gammopathy of clinical significance" has been introduced [28], again splitting the "grey area" into small "entities" with different names, all of which reflect different stages of the same pathological process. Similar conceptual problems in hematology are represented by monoclonal B-cell lymphocytosis, follicular lymphoma "in situ," myelodysplastic syndromes, clonal hematopoiesis of indeterminate potential and other "borderline" conditions, and in the skin by "parapsoriasis en plaques" and lymphomatoid papulosis, among others. There is sufficient evidence that not all "early malignant" tumors must invariably progress to metastatic disease and kill the patient, and in my opinion, our main difficulty is probably more of a semantic nature, namely, the exact definition (and nomenclature) of what is "early" cancer.

So where do we draw the line? Where do we set the boundary between benign and malignant diseases? In my opinion, any boundary – like any classification – is clearly arbitrary and artificial. On the other hand, in order to treat patients we need classifications, precise diagnostic criteria, and clear-cut boundaries between diseases. In this context, it should be unambiguously stated that our definitions and criteria work in the vast majority of cases of cutaneous lymphoma (and, of course, of other diseases as well). In patients with "borderline" disorders, a pragmatic approach seems to be the most appropriate, avoiding unnecessary aggressive treatment. What is radically changing, on the other hand, is the concept of "early cancer" and the way we convey this diagnosis to our patients. It is the responsibility of managing physicians to provide accurate information to their patients, clearly explaining to them the problems related to a diagnosis of "parapsoriasis" or early mycosis fungoides, as well as the existence and the meaning of the "grey zone" between benign and malignant conditions.

## References


1. Campo E, Jaffe ES, Cook JR, *et al.* The International Consensus Classification of Mature Lymphoid Neoplasms: a report from the Clinical Advisory Committee. *Blood* 2022;**140**:1229–1253.
2. Arber DA, Borowitz MJ, Cook JR, *et al.*, eds. *The International Consensus Classification of Myeloid and Lymphoid Neoplasms.* Wolters Kluver: Philadelphia (US), 2025.
3. Alaggio R, Amador C, Anagnostopoulos I, *et al.* The 5th edition of the World Health Organization Classification of Haematolymphoid Tumours: Lymphoid Neoplasms. *Leukemia* 2022;**36**:1720–1748.
4. Khoury JD, Solary E, Abla O, *et al.* The 5th edition of the World Health Organization Classification of Haematolymphoid Tumours: Myeloid and Histiocytic/Dendritic Neoplasms. *Leukemia* 2022;**36**: 1703–1719.
5. WHO Classification of Tumours Editorial Board. *Haematolymphoid Tumours.* 5th edition. Lyon (France): IARC, 2024.
6. Willemze R, Kerl H, Sterry W, *et al.* EORTC classification for primary cutaneous lymphomas: a proposal from the Cutaneous Lymphoma Study Group of the European Organization for Research and Treatment of Cancer. *Blood* 1997;**90**:354–371.
7. Kempf W, Mitteldorf C, Cerroni L. Classifications of cutaneous lymphomas and lymphoproliferative disorders: An update from the EORTC cutaneous lymphoma histopathology group. *J Eur Acad Dermatol Venereol* 2024;**38**:1491–1503.
8. Senff NJ, Kluin-Nelemans JC, Willemze R. Results of bone marrow examination in 275 patients with histological features that suggest an indolent type of cutaneous B-cell lymphoma. *Br J Haematol* 2008;**142**:52–56.
9. Olsen E, Vonderheid E, Pimpinelli N, *et al.* Revisions to the staging and classification of mycosis fungoides and Sezary syndrome: a proposal of the International Society for Cutaneous Lymphomas (ISCL) and the cutaneous lymphoma task force of the European Organization of Research and Treatment of Cancer (EORTC). *Blood* 2007;**110**:1713–1722.
10. Cheson BD, Fisher RI, Barrington SF, *et al.* Recommendations for initial evaluation, staging, and response assessment of Hodgkin and non-Hodgkin lymphoma: the Lugano classification. *J Clin Oncol* 2014;**32**:3059–3068.
11. Olsen EA, Whittaker S, Willemze R, *et al.* Primary cutaneous lymphoma: recommendations for clinical trial design and staging update from the ISCL, USCLC, and EORTC. *Blood* 2022;**140**:419–437.
12. National Comprehensive Cancer Network. Primary Cutaneous Lymphomas (Version 3.2025). Accessed September 20, 2025. https://www.nccn.org/professionals/physician_gls/pdf/primary_cutaneous.pdf.
13. Kumar R, Khan SP, Joshi DD, *et al.* Pediatric histiocytic sarcoma clonally related to precursor B-cell acute lymphoblastic leukemia with homozygous deletion of CDKN2A encoding p16INK4A. *Pediatr Blood Cancer* 2011;**56**:307–310.
14. West DS, Dogan A, Quint PS, *et al.* Clonally related folliculari lymphomas and langerhans cell neoplasms – expanding the spectrum of transdifferentiation. *Am J Surg Pathol* 2013;**37**:978–986.
15. Montecino-Rodriguez E, Leathers H, Dorshkind K. Bipotential B-macrophage progenitors are present in adult bone marrow. *Nat Immunol* 2001;**2**:83–88.
16. Van Dongen JJM, Langerak AW, Brüggemann M, *et al.* Design and standardization of PCR primers and protocols for detection of clonal immunoglobulin and T-cell receptor gene recombinations in suspect lymphoproliferations: report of the BIOMED-2 Concerted Action BMH4-CT98-3936. *Leukemia* 2003;**17**:2257–2317.
17. Van Krieken JH, Langerak AW, Macintyre EA, *et al.* Improved reliability of lymphoma diagnostics via PCR-based clonality testing: report of the BIOMED-2 Concerted Action BHM4-CT98-3936. *Leukemia* 2007;**21**:201–206.
18. Scherer F, Kurtz DM, Diehn M, Alizadeh AA. High-throughput sequencing for noninvasive disease detection in hematologic malignancies. *Blood* 2017;**130**:440–452.
19. Kirsch IR, Watanabe R, O'Malley JT, *et al.* TCR sequencing facilitates diagnosis and identifies mature T cells as the cell of origin in CTCL. *Sci Transl Med* 2015;**7**:308ra158.
20. Matos TR, de Rie MA, Teunissen MBM. Research techniques made simple: high-throughput sequencing of the T-cell receptor. *J Invest Dermatol* 2017;**137**:e131–e138.
21. Shinohara MM, Rieger KE, Sundram U, *et al.* Assessing T-cell receptor clonality by next-generation sequencing in atypical cutaneous lymphoid infiltrates and cutaneous T-cell lymphoma: a scoping review. *J Cutan Pathol* 2024;**51**:813–819.
22. Ventura RA, Martin-Subero JI, Jones M, *et al.* FISH analysis for the detection of lymphoma-associated chromosomal abnormalities in routine paraffin-embedded tissue. *J Mol Diagn* 2006;**8**:141–151.
23. Gallardo F, Pujol RM. Genetics abnormalities with clinical impact in primary cutaneous lymphomas. *Cancers* 2022;**14**:4972.
24. Chatterjee G, He R, Patkar N, *et al.* Molecular techniques in haematopathology: what and how? *Histopathology* 2025;**86**:38–57.
25. Cerroni L. Cutaneous lymphoid proliferations: a clinicopathological continuum? *Diagn Histopathol* 2009;**16**:417–424.
26. Ganapathi KA, Pittaluga S, Odejide OO, *et al.* Early lymphoid lesions: conceptual, diagnostic and clinical challenges. *Haematologica* 2014;**99**:1421–1432.
27. Welch HG, Black WC. Overdiagnosis in cancer. *J Natl Cancer Inst* 2010;**102**:605–613.
28. Fermand JP, Bridoux F, Dispenzieri A, *et al.* Monoclonal gammopathy of clinical significance: a novel concept with therapeutic implications. *Blood* 2018;**132**:1478–1485.

## SECTION 1

# Cutaneous NK/T-cell lymphomas and lymphoproliferative disorders

# CHAPTER 2
# The "parapsoriases"

A specific chapter on "parapsoriasis" was introduced for the first time in the fifth edition of this book. As the debate on the use of this terminology is far from being settled, in spite of the controversies and ongoing discussions, for two main reasons I decided to keep the chapter also in this edition of the book: (i) physicians dealing with skin lymphomas will likely be confronted with such cases and with patients diagnosed with "parapsoriasis," and (ii) to explain the historical background behind the "concept" of the parapsoriases, in order to allow readers to form their own opinion on this debated and controversial terminology.

Although it is virtually impossible to *understand* what the parapsoriases really are, in order to be able to at least understand the debate which is going on for more than one century, one has to get some basic information about how the term itself was born. After the first description of mycosis fungoides by Alibert, dermatologists realized that the aggressive tumor stage of the disease was preceded by a long-standing phase characterized by patches and plaques (first described by the French dermatologist Pierre-Antoine Bazin in 1870) [1], and at the same time also recognized that this "flat-stage" of the disease could present with many different clinical features (reflected in terms such as "porokeratosis variegata," "xanthoerythrodermia perstans," and "poikiloderma vasculare atrophicans" among others). The discussion soon began as to whether the patch-, plaque- and tumor-stages represented one and the same disease, or not. In addition, at the beginning of the twentieth century, there was a search for a "general" classification of skin diseases arranged in a kind of tree with different branches according to specific variants. In 1902, and again in 1903 Louis-Anne-Jean Brocq, a brilliant French dermatologist, introduced the concept and scheme of "parapsoriasis" (Fig. 2.1) [2, 3]. The term parapsoriasis was not intended to denote a new disease, but rather to refer to a group of separate diseases, all of which had been described previously, and which had certain features in common. The term represented also part of an ambitious scheme to classify and relate all inflammatory dermatoses. The features that these diseases had in common were unknown etiology, chronicity, failure to respond to therapy, and lack of pruritus. Brocq was aware of the shortcomings of his term, given the variety of eruptions included under it, and spoke of a "dénomination fort discutable, mais courte et non-encore utilisée" (denomination highly questionable, but short and not yet used) [2]. Brocq published the term as singular, but he meant it as plural – a group of related diseases.

When speaking of "unknown etiology, chronicity, and failure to respond to therapy," we should understand that the concept of Brocq was proposed in 1902, a year when the ambulances were pulled by horses, hospital wards had >20 beds each, antibiotics and steroids (to mention only two of hundreds of drugs) had not yet been "discovered," and heroin was a legal pharmaceutical drug developed by Bayer in 1897 (for several complains including bronchitis, pain, and asthma among many others), sold in >20 countries, and in 1902 representing alone 5% of all profits of the drug company. It seems less understandable to think that today, in a new millennium and in what has been called the "era of precision medicine," we are still using a term that was meant to be only provisional (and highly debatable) over 100 years ago. If you would have to hurry to a hospital with an ambulance, or would try to produce or sell heroin as a medicine today, you would immediately appreciate the differences between now and then; the parapsoriases, on the other hand, are still here …

In fact, over a century later the dermatological community is still using this ill-defined term, and the debate over the exact nosology of the parapsoriases seems far from being settled [4]. This is even more surprising if one thinks that already in 1938 Harry Keil, an American dermatologist working in New York City, wrote: "Parapsoriasis en plaques disséminées, parapsoriasis lichenoides of French authors, parakeratosis variegata, and the retiform type of parapsoriasis with their evolution into poikiloderma probably represent different phases of a single disease, which invariably progresses to mycosis fungoides. (…) The nomenclature of parapsoriasis, mycosis fungoides, and poikiloderma vascolare atrophicans should be revised in the light of collected data." [5]. Rather than following the suggestion by Keil, in 1953 parapsoriasis en plaques was further divided by Degos into "small plaque" and "large plaque" types [6]. In 1981, 77 years after Brocq's original publication, Lambert and Everett, wrote: "Whereas the opinion of the average physician regarding dermatologic nomenclature is at least partially based on ignorance of the

*Skin Lymphoma: The Illustrated Guide*, Sixth Edition. Lorenzo Cerroni.

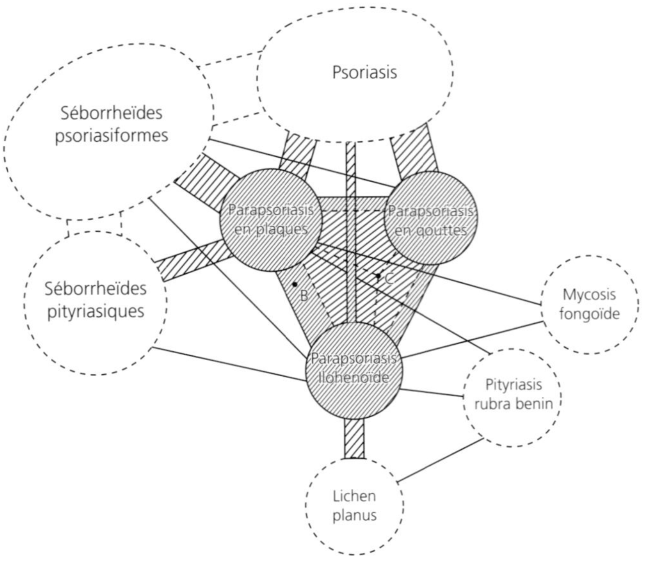


**Figure 2.1** The original scheme of the "parapsoriasis" proposed by Brocq in 1902.

subject, even dermatologists who are keenly versed in the entities that comprise the parapsoriasis group find the nomenclature difficult." [7]. LeBoit and Pincus in 2017 wrote: "In our opinion, the term *parapsoriasis* is invalid scientifically, although it may have some functional utility in that it is a shorthand for 'I suspect that this is an early patch of mycosis fungoides but am not sure'" [8]. Some authors suggested to exclude the term parapsoriasis from the medical vocabulary [9], while others advocated its utility [10]. In short, more than 120 years after Brocq and more than 40 years after Lambert and Everett, the difficulty is still unabated. Both terms "large plaque" and "small plaque" parapsoriasis are in use, and are the source of vivid debate. What is even more confounding, a term that had been devised for a *group of disorders* is now used to define a single "*entity*" [11].

Besides semantic issues (the term parapsoriasis conveys a wrong sense of relationship to psoriasis – but mycosis fungoides, after all, is also a misnomer), the exact nosology of the parapsoriases (small- and large-plaque) is still a matter of discussion. In this context, the term "plaque" is also wrong, as we are referring to lesions that clinically are patches. In my opinion, there is no doubt that large-patch parapsoriasis belongs to the clinical spectrum of mycosis fungoides and cannot (and should not) be distinguished from other early manifestations of the disease. Thus, in what follows I will only concentrate on small-patch parapsoriasis, as this is a much more slippery subject. At the beginning, however, it should be underlined that distinction of "small-patch" from "large-patch" parapsoriasis is a matter of the discussion, too, as (i) it only relies on the size of lesions (the size of either type of parapsoriasis was never defined precisely) and (ii) often both small and large lesions are present in one and the same patient. Besides, it is well known that small patches of disease are common in patients with otherwise "conventional" mycosis fungoides.

Having briefly discussed the historical background and the problems of the definition of the "parapsoriases," I must admit that, as a matter of fact, I use this terminology in the daily routine (exclusively "small patch parapsoriasis"). This is mainly due to two reasons: (i) A diagnosis of early mycosis fungoides is bound with considerable distress for the patients; small patch parapsoriasis represents a term that is not identified as a malignant disorder by them; (ii) in some cases of early mycosis fungoides the histopathological features are not clearly diagnostic, particularly because biopsies are often performed under different types of treatment; in such cases I find the phrasing "spectrum small-patch parapsoriasis/early mycosis fungoides" useful. I admit that my approach to the parapsoriases is neither better nor less problematic than any other, and only wish to explain here what I do in the daily routine. On the other hand, I don't think that the term "small patch parapsoriasis" is better or worse than other terms such as "clonal dermatitis," "T-cell lymphocytic dyscrasia," or "chronic superficial dermatitis" – all of them are similar attempts to avoid to use the term "early mycosis fungoides." Regardless of the academic discussion, it is important to underline that patients with small-patch parapsoriasis should not be treated aggressively, as progression of the disease is rare and, when it happens, takes place usually only after very long periods of time.

I refer to small-patch parapsoriasis as a disease presenting exclusively with small patches (not larger than a few centimeters). Numbers defining exactly the size of the patches would only add a false sense of precision that in my opinion does not exist, and in spite of a similar distribution the size of the lesions may vary markedly in different patients or in the same patient at different times (Fig. 2.2). The lesions are located mostly on the trunk, particularly the flanks, and proximal part of the upper extremities, and correspond clinically for the most part to what has been defined also "digitate dermatosis." Histology shows variable hyperplasia of the epidermis with focal spongiosis, focal parakeratosis, and variably dense superficial lympho-histiocytic infiltrates, which sometimes tend to confluence in an early band in area devoid of prominent spongiosis (Fig. 2.3). Intraepidermal lymphocytes are present as a rule, but they are usually found in area of spongiosis and are never numerous (Fig. 2.3b). In this context, it must be clearly underlined that any given biopsy specimen showing uncontroversial histopathological features of mycosis fungoides should be classified as such. Immunohistology with pan-T-cell markers (CD3, CD5) may be used in order to better visualize the intraepidermal lymphocytes and better quantify their number. In my opinion, staining for CD7 does not have any diagnostic value in distinguishing between "dermatitis" and early mycosis fungoides. Molecular genetic techniques reveal that in some of the lesions of small-patch parapsoriasis a monoclonal population of T lymphocytes can be found.

As already mentioned, the exact relationship between small-patch parapsoriasis and mycosis fungoides is still a matter of debate. Some authors think that they represent one and the same disease [12, 13]. In Graz, we have observed patients with

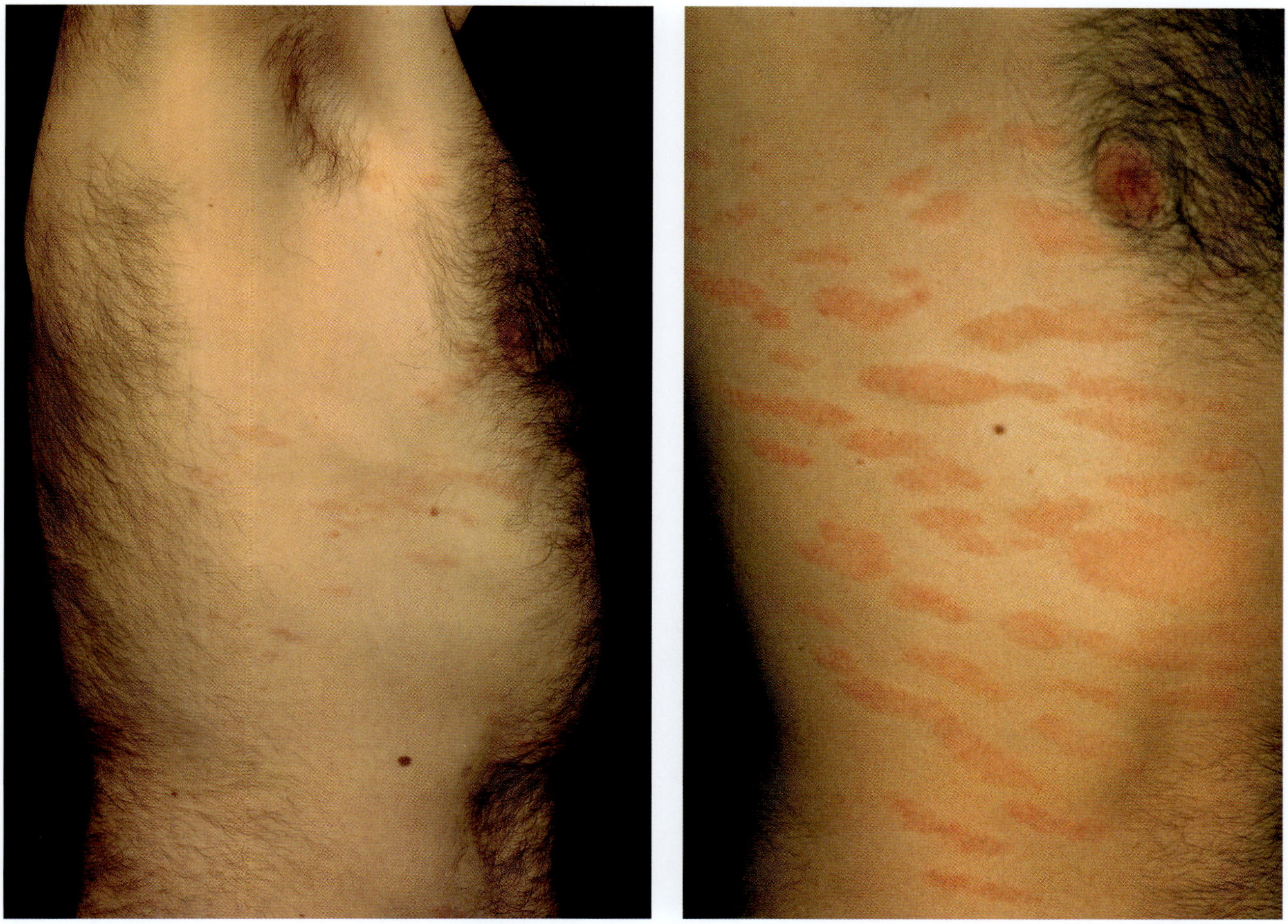

(a) (b)

**Figure 2.2** Small-patch parapsoriasis ("digitate dermatitis," "fingerprint dermatitis"). (a) and (b): similar distribution and shape, but different size of the lesions in two different patients.

small digitate lesions on the trunk who on follow-up developed typical plaques and tumors of mycosis fungoides, or even erythroderma (Fig. 2.4), as well as patients with "digitate" lesions on the flank and other lesions at sites typical for mycosis fungoides (Fig. 2.5), sometimes with the characteristic "parchment-like" surface of patch lesions of the disease (Fig. 2.6). These observations suggested us that small-patch parapsoriasis most likely represents an early manifestation of the disease. A similar observation has been made by Väkevä and co-workers, who reported that 10% of their patients with small-patch parapsoriasis developed mycosis fungoides during the course of the disease [14], and by Belousova and co-workers [15]. A similar spectrum of presentations can be observed between the two diseases, and cases of hypopigmented parapsoriasis have been reported [16]. However, it must be mentioned that divergent opinions exist, and other authors think that the two diseases are unrelated [7, 17]. In addition, in my experience, the percentage of patients who develop clear-cut mycosis fungoides is minimal (probably <1%), and certainly much lower than the 10% reported by Väkevä and co-workers. An exhaustive summary of the published literature with plenty of citations from old sources, useful to better understand this subject, can be found in the monography published by Ackerman and coworkers in 2008 [12], and a review of reported cases of "parapsoriasis" eventuating into mycosis fungoides has been published [18].

Finally, it must be clearly stated once again that "large-patch parapsoriasis" represents one of the most typical early manifestations of conventional mycosis fungoides [19]. The lesions are commonly located on the buttocks, trunk, proximal medial upper extremities, or breast in women, and show typical histopathological features, and behavior, of early mycosis fungoides (Fig 2.7). In this context, it is interesting that a recent study on analysis of clonality by single-cell sequencing revealed a monoclonal T-cell population in 6/8 cases of large-patch and in 1/7 of small-patch parapsoriasis, respectively, confirming that large-patch parapsoriasis belongs to the spectrum of early mycosis fungoides, and suggesting that the majority of cases of small-patch parapsoriasis may represent a non-neoplastic condition [20].

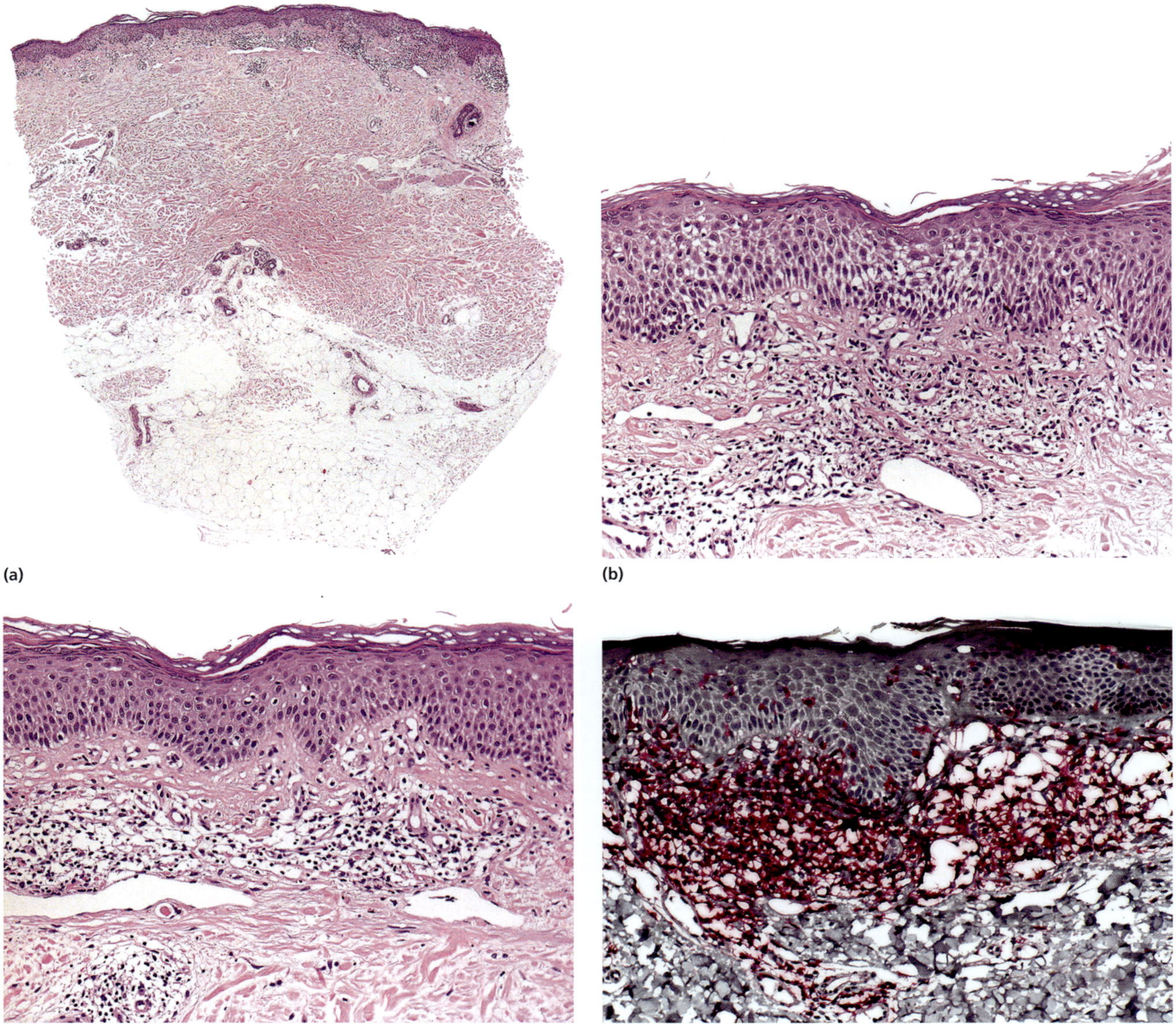


**Figure 2.3** Small-patch parapsoriasis. Histology shows (a) a moderately hyperplastic, focally spongiotic epidermis with a superficial lymphoid infiltrate. (b) Some areas are characterized by prominent spongiosis, whereas other (c) show minimal spongiosis, slight fibrosis of the papillary dermis, and a band-like lymphoid infiltrate, similar to what can be seen in early lesions of mycosis fungoides. (d) Staining for CD3 highlights some intraepidermal lymphocytes.

## Résumé

| | **The "parapsoriases" ("small patch" and "large patch" parapsoriasis)** |
|---|---|
| **Clinical** | Adults.<br>***Small patch parapsoriasis:*** corresponds mostly to so-called "digitate" dermatosis; elongated, patch, scaly erythematous lesions on the trunk and proximal part of upper extremities. Progression to clear-cut mycosis fungoides may be observed, but only in a minimal percentage of cases (<1%).<br>***Large patch parapsoriasis:*** corresponds to conventional, early lesions of mycosis fungoides; commonly located on the buttocks, trunk, and upper extremities, as well as on the breast in women. |
| **Morphology** | ***Small patch parapsoriasis:*** Irregular, sometimes psoriasiform epithelial hyperplasia with scant spongiosis and focal parakeratosis; superficial lympho-histiocytic infiltrate, sometimes with hints of a band-like arrangement. Variable numbers of intraepidermal lymphocytes but lack of "disproportionate" epidermotropism.<br>***Large patch parapsoriasis:*** Identical to patch-stage mycosis fungoides. |
| **Immunohistochemistry** | Not relevant; staining for pan-T-cell markers (CD3, CD5) may better highlight the number and distribution of intraepidermal lymphocytes. |
| **Genetics** | Monoclonal rearrangement of the TCR genes in a proportion of cases. |
| **Treatment guidelines** | ***Small patch parapsoriasis:*** PUVA, UVB 311 nm, topical steroids; watchful waiting.<br>***Large patch parapsoriasis:*** see Chapter 3. |

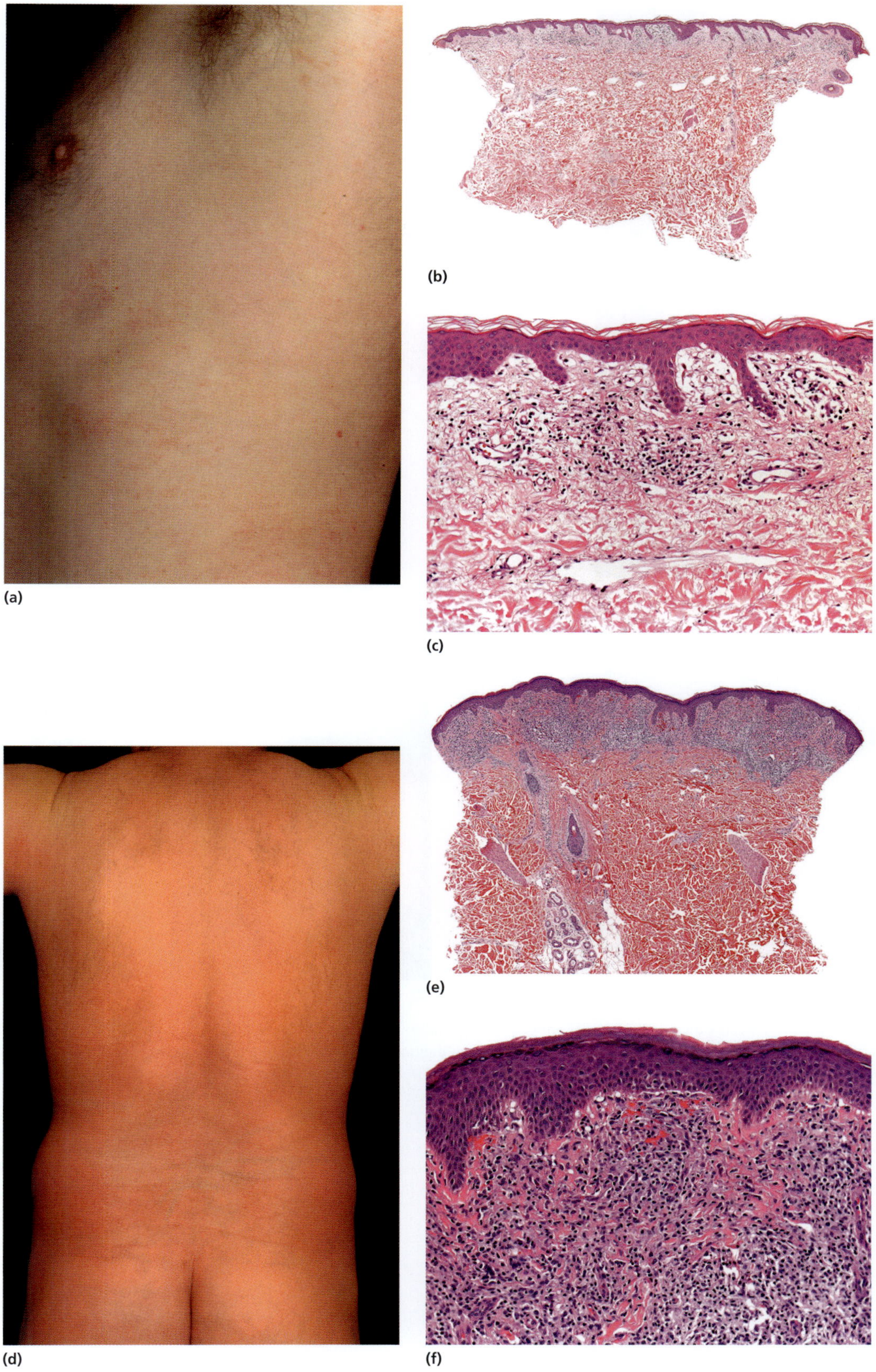

Figure 2.4 Small-patch parapsoriasis ("digitate dermatitis," "fingerprint dermatitis") evolving into erythroderma. (a) Small, partly digitate lesions at the onset of the disease. (b, c) Histology confirmed features of small-patch parapsoriasis. (d) Some years later erythroderma developed, (e, f) with histopathological features of mycosis fungoides.

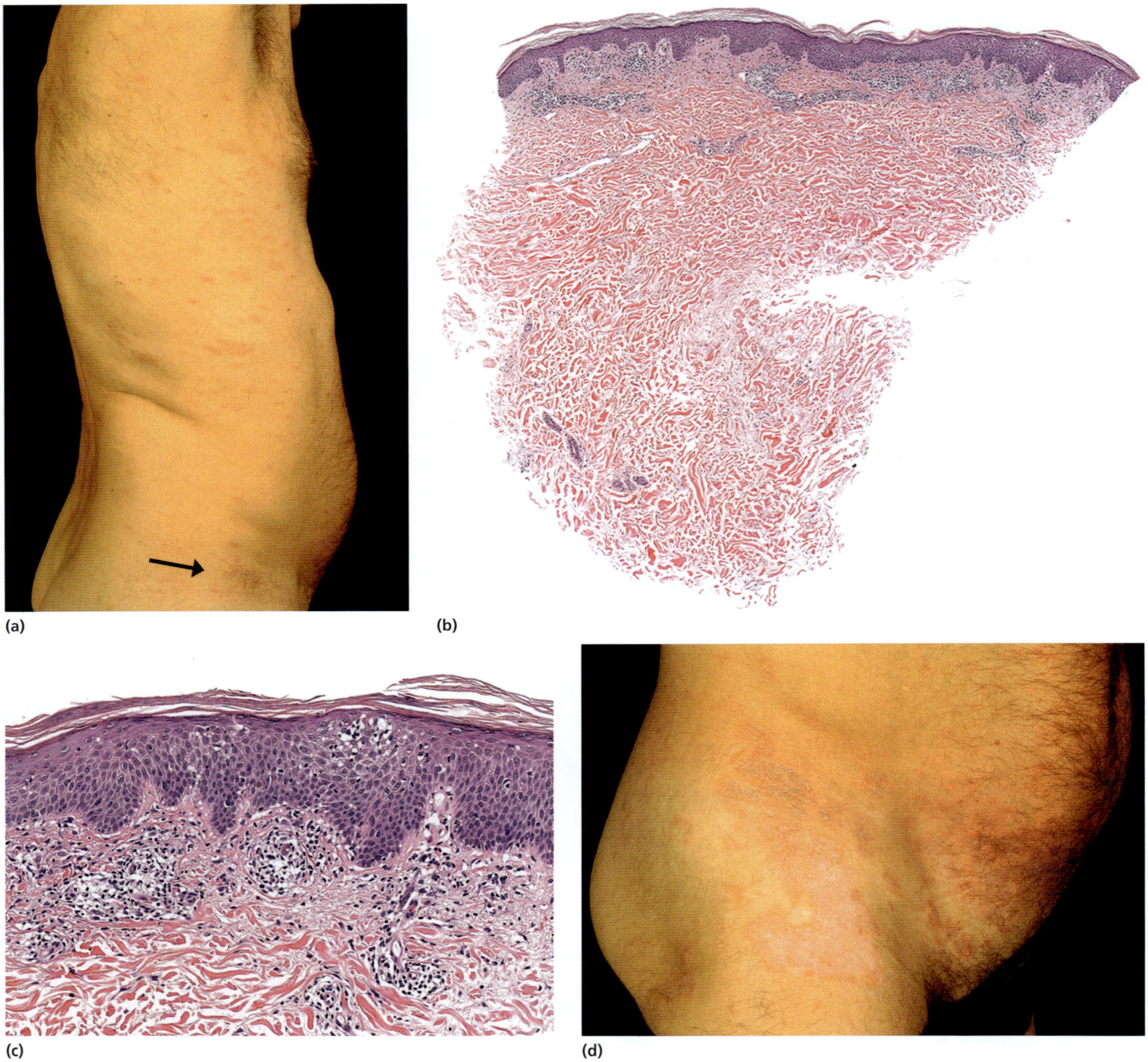


Figure 2.5 Small-patch parapsoriasis ("digitate dermatitis," "fingerprint dermatitis"). (a) This patient had typical lesions on the upper flank, but also a more irregular, infiltrated area on the lower flank (arrow). A biopsy from a "digitate" lesion showed (b) a relatively dense, superficial infiltrate with (c) several intraepidermal lymphocytes in areas of relatively scant spongiosis. (d) Two months later the lesion on the lower flank was growing and becoming partly hypopigmented, and new lesions were appearing on the waistband. Cases like this one are uncommon yet paradigmatic of the difficulties that may arise in clearly separating "digitate dermatitis" from early mycosis fungoides.

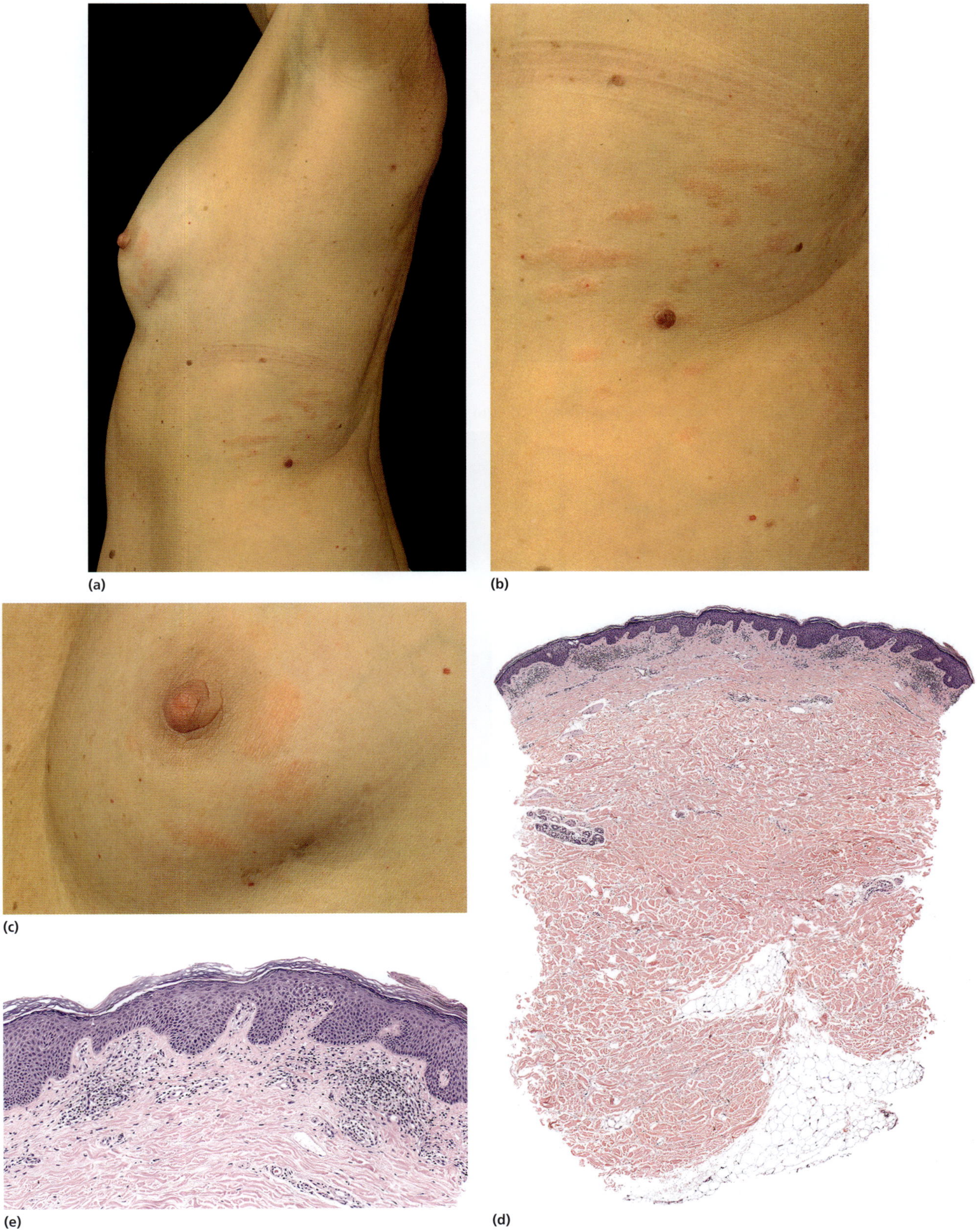


**Figure 2.6** Small-patch parapsoriasis ("digitate dermatitis," "fingerprint dermatitis"). (a, b) "Digitate" lesions coexisting with (c) lesions on the breast showing a "parchment-like" surface. Histological examination from one of the digitate lesions showed (d) a band-like infiltrate with (e) a few epidermotropic lymphocytes.

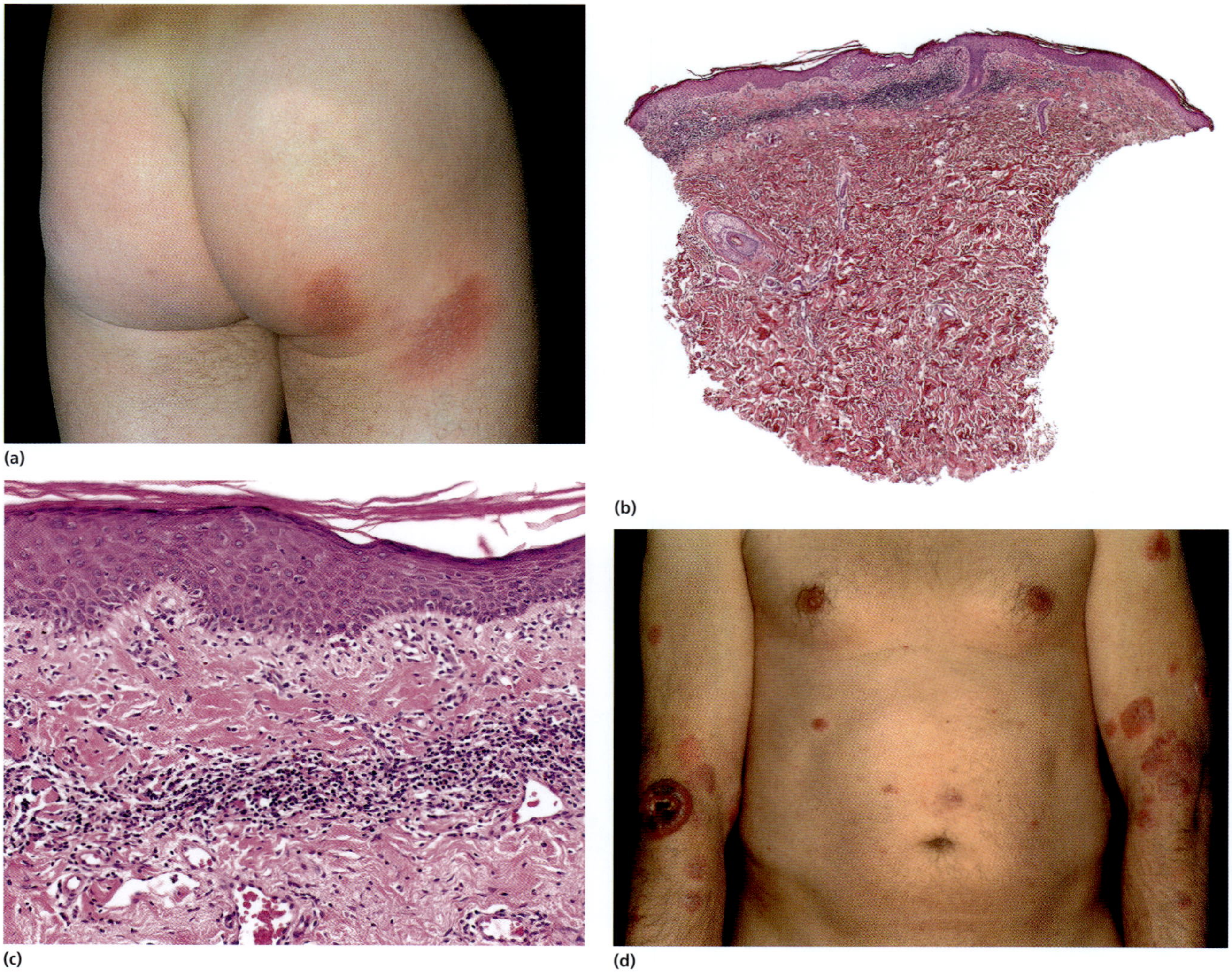


**Figure 2.7** This 28-year-old man presented (a) with two erythematous lesions on the proximal area of the right posterior thigh and buttock (clinical features of so-called "large-patch parapsoriasis"). A biopsy revealed (b) a superficial, band-like infiltrate with (c) only a few intraepidermal lymphocytes. A diagnosis of mycosis fungoides was made. 21 years later he presented with infiltrated plaques on the abdomen, shortly afterwards followed by (d) ulcerated tumors on the trunk and limbs. He received total body electron beam therapy with complete remission but relapsed a few months after the end of the treatment, and eventually succumbed to mycosis fungoides 25 years after the first diagnosis, and 38 years after the first manifestations of the disease.

## References

1. Bazin PAE. *Lecons sur le traitment des maladies chronique en général, affections de la peau en particulier*. Paris: Adrein Delahaye, 1870: 425 and 436–438,.
2. Brocq L. Les parapsoriasis. *Ann Dermatol Syphiligr (Paris)* 1902; **35**:433–468.
3. Brocq L. Parapsoriasis. *J Cutan Dis* 1903;**21**:315–322.
4. Cerroni L. Past, present and future of cutaneous lymphomas. *Semin Diagn Pathol* 2017;**34**:3–14.
5. Keil H. Parapsoriasis en plaques disséminées and incipient mycosis fungoides. Supplementary data on their relationship. *Arch Dermatol Syphil* 1938;**38**:545–554.
6. Degos R. Dermatoses érythémato-squameuses. In: *Traité de Dermatologie*. Paris: Flammarion, 1953: 188–194.
7. Lambert WC, Everett MA. The nosology of parapsoriasis. *J Am Acad Dermatol* 1981;**5**:373–395.
8. LeBoit PE, Pincus LB. Mycosis fungoides and Sèzary syndrome. In: Jaffe ES, Arber DA, Campo E, *et al*., eds. *Hematopathology*. 2nd edition. Elsevier, 2017: 713–729.
9. Caldeira Xavier Jr JC, Polizel Ocanha-Xavier J, Alencar Marques ME. Shall we exclude parapsoriasis from the medical vocabulary? *J Cutan Pathol* 2021;**48**:833–836.
10. de Castro e Souza B, Sanches JA. Reasons we should not exclude the term parapsoriasis from the medical vocabulary. *J Cutan Pathol* 2021;**48**:1436–1437.
11. Holubar K. Psoriasis and parapsoriasis: since 200 and 100 years, respectively. *J Eur Acad Dermatol Venereol* 2003;**17**:126–127.
12. Ackerman AB, Denianke K, Sceppa J, *et al. Mycosis Fungoides: Perspective Historical Allied with Critique Methodical for the Purpose of Illumination Maximal*. New York: Ardor Scribendi, 2008.
13. Ackerman AB, Schiff TA. If small plaque (digitate) parapsoriasis is a cutaneous T-cell lymphoma, even an abortive one, it must be mycosis fungoides. *Arch Dermatol* 1996;**132**:562–566.

14. Väkevä L, Sarna S, Vaalasti A, *et al.* A retrospective study of the probability of the evolution of parapsoriasis en plaques into mycosis fungoides. *Acta Derm Venereol (Stockh)* 2005;**85**:318–323.
15. Belousova IE, Vanecek T, Samtsov AV, *et al.* A patient with clinicopathologic features of small plaque parapsoriasis presenting later with plaque-stage mycosis fungoides: report of a case and comparative retrospective study of 27 cases of "nonprogressive" small plaque parapsoriasis. *J Am Acad Dermatol* 2008;**59**:474–482.
16. El-Darouti MA, Fawzy MM, Hegazy RA, Abdel Hay RM. Hypopigmented parapsoriasis en plaque, a new, overlooked member of the parapsoriasis family: a report of 34 patients and a 7-year experience. *J Am Acad Dermatol* 2012;**67**:1182–1188.
17. Burg G, Dummer R, Nestle FO, *et al.* Cutaneous lymphomas consist of a spectrum of nosologically different entities including mycosis fungoides and small plaque parapsoriasis. *Arch Dermatol* 1996;**132**:567–572.
18. Sibbald C, Pope E. Systematic review of cases of cutaneous T-cell lymphoma transformation in pityriasis lichenoides and small plaque parapsoriasis. *Br J Dermatol* 2016;**175**:807–809.
19. Sanchez JL, Ackerman AB. The patch stage of mycosis fungoides: criteria for histologic diagnosis. *Am J Dermatopathol* 1979;**1**:5–26.
20. Alkon N, Chennareddy S, Cohenour ER, *et al.* Single cell sequencing delineates T-cell clonality and pathogenesis of the parapsoriasis disease group. *J Allergy Clin Immunol* 2024;**155**:461–478.

## CHAPTER 3

# Mycosis fungoides

Mycosis fungoides is the most common type of cutaneous lymphoma, representing almost 50% of all lymphomas arising primarily in the skin [1–5]. It is defined as a tumor composed of small/medium-sized, epidermotropic T-helper lymphocytes (but T-cytotoxic variants are not uncommon, and neoplastic cells may be medium/large in advanced stages).

Mycosis fungoides is the oldest entity in the field of cutaneous lymphomas, having been described more than two centuries ago, in 1806, by the French dermatologist Alibert. Traditionally it is divided into three clinical phases: patch, plaque, and tumor stage. The clinical course can be protracted over years or decades. In the 2024 update of the classification of cutaneous lymphomas and lymphoproliferative disorders by the European Organization for Research and Treatment of Cancer (EORTC) [6], in the International Consensus Classification (ICC) *of Myeloid and Lymphoid Neoplasms* proposed by the Clinical Advisory Committee (CAC) in 2022 [7] and published as a book in 2025 [5], as well as in the 5th edition of the World Health Organization (WHO) *Classification of Haematolymphoid Tumours* [3], the term "mycosis fungoides" is restricted to the classic type of the disease (so-called "Alibert–Bazin"), characterized by the typical slow evolution and protracted course. It is estimated that over 90% of patients with early mycosis fungoides neither progress to tumor stage nor show extracutaneous manifestations of the disease [8, 9]. Phenotypic and genetic studies showed that entities described in the past as "rapidly progressive" mycosis fungoides (e.g., mycosis fungoides *a tumeur d'emblée*, generalized pagetoid reticulosis – Ketron–Goodman) are better classified among the group of aggressive cutaneous cytotoxic natural killer (NK)/T-cell lymphomas (see Chapters 7 and 8).

The incidence of the disease worldwide is probably around 6–7 cases/$10^6$, with many regional variations and with a regular increase in recent decades [10, 11]. A stabilization of the incidence has been noted in the United States in the period 1998–2009 [12]. There is a higher incidence in black patients [13] and the average age of onset seems to be younger for black than for white patients [14a].

Although mycosis fungoides is considered as the prototype of primary cutaneous lymphomas, the origin of the disease from lymphocytes resident within the skin has been questioned, and an alternative model suggesting that mycosis fungoides is a systemic disease, where the spread of malignant cells through the blood to the skin is an essential component of the pathogenesis, has been proposed [14b]. However, in most patients the disease remains confined to the skin for a long time, and the discussion concerning the systemic versus primary cutaneous origin does not bear relevance for the management of patients.

In spite of decades of research, the etiology of mycosis fungoides remains unknown. A genetic predisposition may play a role in some cases. A familial occurrence of the disease has been reported in a few instances including disease onset in identical twins [15–17], but a large study on Danish patients showed that twins of patients affected by mycosis fungoides or Sézary syndrome did not develop the disease after a median period of observation of 20 years (range: 3–40 years) [18]. A study conducted among Israeli Jewish patients showed a significantly greater allele frequency of HLA DQBI*03, suggesting that genetic factors may play a role in the etiology of the disease, at least in selected groups of patients [19]. On the other hand, mycosis fungoides has been rarely observed in unrelated married individuals, pointing to the existence of environmental factors [20]. In this context, a study on Iranian veterans confirmed to have exposure to sulfur mustard during the Iraq–Iran War of the 1980s showed an increased incidence of mycosis fungoides compared to the Iranian general population [21]. Association with long-term exposure to various allergens and association with chronic skin disorders have also been suggested as possible etiologic factors, but no epidemiologic study confirmed these hypotheses beyond doubt. In this context, it has been suggested that bacterial triggers may be involved in disease onset and progression, and staphylococcal enterotoxin A stimulates STAT3 activation and IL-17 expression [22, 23]. STAT3 is involved in neoplastic cell survival in mycosis fungoides [24]. In fact, antibiotic treatment induces a reduction of the tumor burden in advanced stages (see section on therapy below in this chapter). A relationship with *Borrelia burgdorferi* infection, human T lymphotropic virus I (HTLV-I), cytomegalovirus (CMV), human herpes virus (HHV)-6, HHV-8, Merkel cell polyoma virus (MCPyV), and Epstein–Barr virus (EBV) has

*Skin Lymphoma: The Illustrated Guide*, Sixth Edition. Lorenzo Cerroni.

also been investigated, but so far a link to infectious agents could not be demonstrated [25, 26]. Chronic inflammation due to different mechanisms, eventually resulting in the development of lymphoma, has been termed "malignant inflammation," an oxymoron, that to my eyes, does not add clarity to an already unclear field [27]. Interestingly, mycosis fungoides has been observed rarely in patients who received solid organ transplantation, suggesting that immune suppression may contribute to the development of the disease [28, 29]. In one exceptional case, mycosis fungoides has been acquired as a donor-derived malignancy following reduced-intensity hematopoietic stem cell transplantation from a matched unrelated donor [30]. In short, genetic background, environmental factors, chronic antigenic stimulation, and exposure to cancerogenic agents seem to play a role in mycosis fungoides (as in many other human cancers), but the frame keeping all of these factors together is still elusive.

A recent molecular study revealed the high complexity of mycosis fungoides, with a median of 135 different genomic alterations per lesion (including 67 samples of early and late lesions from 48 patients with newly diagnosed disease) [31]. Activation of genes belonging to pathways associated with inflammation, immune activation, and regulation of apoptosis have been identified in the early phases, but also in chronic inflammatory dermatoses [32]. Recent developments in the analysis of clonality using high-throughput sequencing showed that neoplastic T cells in early mycosis fungoides may represent as little as 10% of the infiltrate [33], thus explaining the difficulties in the histopathological diagnosis. The small number of neoplastic cells admixed with a predominant inflammatory infiltrate should also suggest to exert caution in the interpretation of molecular features of early lesions.

Mycosis fungoides has been described in patients with other cutaneous or extracutaneous hematologic disorders, especially lymphomatoid papulosis and Hodgkin lymphoma. In occasional patients, the same clone has been detected in mycosis fungoides and associated lymphomas, raising questions about a common origin of the diseases, while in others the clone was different [33–38]. In addition, patients with mycosis fungoides are at higher risk of developing a second malignancy [39, 40]. In a Dutch study, patients with mycosis fungoides had a statistically significant higher incidence of cutaneous melanoma, cutaneous squamous cell carcinoma, and extracutaneous hematological malignancies, whereas there was no association between mycosis fungoides and other extracutaneous solid organ tumors [41].

A staging classification system for mycosis fungoides was proposed by a joint working group of the International Society of Cutaneous Lymphoma (ISCL) and the EORTC Cutaneous Lymphoma Task Force [42]. This system has been validated by a study on large numbers of cases [43], and has been subsequently only slightly modified in conjunction with the United States Cutaneous Lymphoma Consortium (USCLC) (see Chapter 1, Table 1.2) [44, 45]. In patients presenting only with patches of the disease (early mycosis fungoides), staging investigations are not necessary, and only clinical examination is performed (assessment of the percentage of body involvement and of superficial lymph nodes). A bone marrow biopsy is not necessary in early mycosis fungoides, and results of real-time quantitative polymerase chain reaction (PCR) analyses do not support its routine use at this stage [46]. Patients with infiltrated plaques, tumors, or erythroderma should be screened for extracutaneous involvement (laboratory investigations, sonography of lymph nodes, CT and/or PET scan of chest, abdomen and pelvis, bone marrow biopsy, examination of the peripheral blood). Suspect lymph nodes (lymph nodes that are either >1.5 cm in diameter and/or irregular, clustered, or fixed) should be biopsied. Although the presence of a monoclonal population of T lymphocytes within the peripheral blood has been observed by the PCR technique in some patients with early mycosis fungoides, in many of these cases the clone was different from the one detected in the skin lesions [47]. Evaluation of the peripheral blood is crucial in erythrodermic patients with suspected Sézary syndrome, but of little relevance in those with patches of early mycosis fungoides. Updated criteria for blood staging have been proposed in the setting of the Prospective Cutaneous Lymphoma International Prognostic Index study (PROCLIPI – a large, multicenter, ongoing study) (see also Chapter 4) [48], and have been included with minor modifications in current staging systems [44, 45]. Interestingly, in this context a recent study showed that the same T-cell clone could be demonstrated by high-throughput TCR sequencing in the blood and skin lesions of 5% of patients with early mycosis fungoides, suggesting that subclinical blood involvement may be more common than previously thought (an unrelated T-cell clone was found in the blood of another 23.3% of cases) [49]. On the other hand, these data refer to a small group of patients, and the finding of an identical clone in the blood and skin was not associated with a shorter time to systemic treatment in that study [49].

Although the staging of mycosis fungoides in early phases of the disease is based on the distinction of patches from plaques as defined by Olsen *et al.* [42], a recent survey clearly showed that for staging of mycosis fungoides, there is limited consensus among experts concerning the validity of the identification of plaques, the relevance of histopathological analysis in the classification of the disease as patch- or plaque-stage, and the distinction between thin and thick plaques [50], suggesting that other histopathological features or biomarkers may be necessary to achieve a more precise staging of the early phases of the disease.

Many studies have addressed the identification of clinical markers of the disease, but at present there is no investigation other than conventional physical examination and radiologic imaging that can allow reliable and repeatable monitoring of mycosis fungoides, particularly in the early stages. Several markers have been the subject of investigations, including cancer antigen 27.29 (CA27.29) [51], transthyretin [52], peripheral blood mononuclear cell cytokine expression [53], circulating CD8$^+$ lymphocytes [54], testis-specific protein 10 (TSGA10) [55], and B-cell activating factor (BAFF) [56] among others, but their value, if any, is yet unclear. Flow cytometry immunophenotyping and analysis of T-cell receptor Vβ repertoires are effective in demonstrating and quantifying small numbers of circulating tumor cells in patients with mycosis fungoides [57]. In general, a diagnostic delay between first symptom development and initial diagnosis is frequent [58], highlighting the difficulties due to lack of a singular diagnostic test for mycosis fungoides. The finding of the same T-cell clone from different skin sites has been proposed as highly specific for mycosis fungoides compared to inflammatory dermatoses [59]. However, the duration of symptoms does not correlate with the presence/absence of a T-cell clone at first diagnosis [60], suggesting that at least in some patients the prodromic symptoms may be non-specific and/or unrelated to the disease.

The relationship between mycosis fungoides and Sézary syndrome has been the subject of innumerable studies. In the past, Sézary syndrome was considered to be the leukemic variant of mycosis fungoides, and both entities were lumped in the non-specific group of cutaneous T-cell lymphoma (CTCL). Indeed, this term is still being used in publications on the subject, often hindering a precise analysis of the data reported. Although the term CTCL has helped focus the attention on a group of lymphomas arising primarily in the skin, its use should be discouraged, and cases should be classified according to precise categories. In fact, there are phenotypic and genetic data supporting the distinction of mycosis fungoides from Sézary syndrome [61–63]. Mycosis fungoides is a disease of skin resident, effector memory T-cells, whereas Sézary syndrome is a malignancy of central memory T-cells [64]. These two types of cutaneous T-cell lymphoma have many overlapping but also several distinguishing features, and should be kept separate for purposes of diagnosis, staging, and treatment.

Finally, one of the main controversies in mycosis fungoides is the relationship with the so-called "parapsoriases." A detailed discussion on this subject is provided in Chapter 2.

## Onset of mycosis fungoides or exacerbation of undiagnosed disease under treatment with immunomodulatory agents

Several cases of undiagnosed mycosis fungoides progressing to the tumor stage under treatment with different immunologic agents (in the medical jargon often referred to as "biologicals") have been described [65–70]. In some cases, it may be that a genuine association of two diseases (mycosis fungoides and an antecedent inflammatory disorder) may have occurred. In other cases, however, a wrong diagnosis of inflammatory dermatosis (usually atopic dermatitis or psoriasis) had been made initially, and a treatment with one of the many immunomodulatory agents had been started, resulting in rapid progression of the mycosis fungoides with an aggressive clinical course [71]. These cases underline the need for an accurate and precise diagnosis of inflammatory skin disorders that shall be treated with immunomodulatory agents, as a misdiagnosis can bear catastrophic consequences. In particular, treatment with dupilumab, a modulator of both the interleukin-4 and interleukin-13 pathways, has been suspected to be the reason for progression of undiagnosed mycosis fungoides with an accelerated, aggressive course [72]. In many centers, histologic verification of the diagnosis is required before starting treatment with immunomodulatory drugs, but due to the difficulties in the histopathologic diagnosis of early mycosis fungoides, some cases may still be missed even after biopsy. On the other hand, recent data suggest that, at least for patients under dupilumab treatment for atopic dermatitis, some of the atypical lymphoid proliferations occurring under treatment may be reactive rather than represent true examples of mycosis fungoides [73, 74]. In a report from a single center, no case of progression to mycosis fungoides was observed after treatment of severe atopic dermatitis by Janus kinase inhibitors (JAKi) or tralokinumab, an anti-IL13 antibody, whereas 30 patients were diagnosed with mycosis fungoides after treatment with dupilumab (in one of these cases the histopathological diagnosis of atopic dermatitis was revised to mycosis fungoides after review of the original specimens, yet biopsies from only 5 cases were subjected to review, thus reclassification occurred in 20% of cases) [75a].However, in patients with subclinical mycosis fungoides, the inhibition of interleukin-4 by dupilumab may disrupt the balance between neoplastic and microenvironment cells, leading to the unmasking of mycosis fungoides [75b].

In the onset of mycosis fungoides under immunomodulatory drugs used for inflammatory dermatoses, anti-tumor necrosis factor (TNF)α compounds were those predominantly involved [76, 77]. The "onset" of mycosis fungoides may be explained in three possible ways: (i) pre-existing mycosis fungoides misdiagnosed as inflammatory dermatosis with an aggressive outcome (aggravating role of immunomodulatory drugs); (ii) coexistence of mycosis fungoides and inflammatory dermatosis (the immunomodulatory drugs improve the inflammatory dermatosis and at the same time undercover mycosis fungoides); and (iii) mycosis fungoides arises de novo in association with an inflammatory dermatosis (either fortuitously or triggered by immunomodulatory drugs, eventually on a predisposed background). It should be remembered that besides mycosis fungoides (including pilotropic mycosis fungoides), also other cutaneous T- and B-cell lymphomas have been observed in patients treated with immunomodulatory drugs for inflammatory dermatoses (including lymphomatoid papulosis, Sézary syndrome, subcutaneous panniculitis-like T-cell lymphoma, cutaneous peripheral T-cell lymphoma, NOS, cutaneous extranodal NK/T-cell lymphoma, nasal-type, cutaneous aggressive epidermotropic CD8$^+$ cytotoxic T-cell lymphoma, cutaneous γ/δ T-cell lymphoma, cutaneous follicle center lymphoma, cutaneous marginal zone lymphoma, and cutaneous diffuse large B-cell lymphoma, leg-type) [76, 77].

In this context, however, the true risk of developing a cutaneous lymphoma in patients with genuine inflammatory dermatoses treated with immunomodulatory agents seems to be negligible: in fact, in contrast to the very large numbers of patients who are treated with these compounds worldwide, only a few cases of cutaneous lymphoma have been reported, some of which were later reclassified as cutaneous lymphoma (mycosis fungoides) misdiagnosed initially as an inflammatory dermatosis. In addition, as already mentioned and at least for what concerns dupilumab, some of the lymphoid proliferations arising under treatment may be reactive rather than truly neoplastic and regress upon discontinuation of the drug [73, 74, 78].

## Clinical features

Most patients are adults, but it should be remembered that mycosis fungoides represents the most common cutaneous lymphoma in children and adolescents (see the specific section in this chapter and pictures of various clinical features in children in Chapter 30). Although the same spectrum of clinical presentations can be observed worldwide, some clinical differences exist among patients of different racial backgrounds (see below). In some developing countries, patients may present with more advanced disease due to poor health education, lack of access to appropriate health services, and financial constraints [79].

Lesions of mycosis fungoides can be divided morphologically into patches, plaques, and tumors, and clinical morphology has been used in the past to classify the disease in three clinical stages according to the presence of such lesions. The widely accepted definition of "patch" refers to a lesion of any size without significant elevation or induration, and of "plaque" to a lesion of any size that is elevated or indurated [42]. The three "stages" reflect disease activity and correlate well with prognosis. In fact, although patches and plaques are considered as a single morphologic criterion in the ISCL–EORTC staging system, two studies clearly showed that the presence of plaques is associated with a worse prognosis in terms of survival and progression risk as compared with that of patches only [43, 80a]. However, as already mentioned, there is no consensus among experts on the definition and staging utility of "patches," "thin plaques," and "thick plaques" (not to mention flat tumors - see below in this section) [50].

Although patches are considered a clinical feature of early mycosis fungoides, it should be underlined that patients with advanced mycosis fungoides who are in complete remission after successful treatment may relapse with either patches, plaques, or tumors, and that patches are frequently seen together with tumors in patients with advanced mycosis fungoides. Thus, for staging purposes, the most infiltrated specific lesion should be considered.

Patches of mycosis fungoides are characterized by variably large, erythematous, finely scaling, non-elevated, and/or indurated lesions. They can be generalized (Fig. 3.1) or localized; when localized, there is often a predilection for the buttocks and other sun-protected areas (Figs. 3.2 and 3.3). Generalized patches may present as large, irregular erythematous lesions (Fig. 3.4). Scaling is variable and may also depend on previous local treatment (Fig. 3.5). Partial loss of elastic fibers and atrophy of the epidermis may confer on the lesions a typical wrinkled appearance, and terms such as "parchment-like" or "cigarette paper-like" have been used to describe them (Fig. 3.6). These morphological features are characteristic of a long-standing lesion and represent a clue against an inflammatory dermatosis. Sometimes the single patches have a yellowish hue, conferring a "xanthomatous"-like aspect to the lesions (in the past referred to as "xanthoerythroderma perstans") (Fig. 3.7). As mycosis fungoides is an itchy condition, scratching artifacts, similar to those observed in eczematous dermatoses, may be visible (Fig. 3.8).

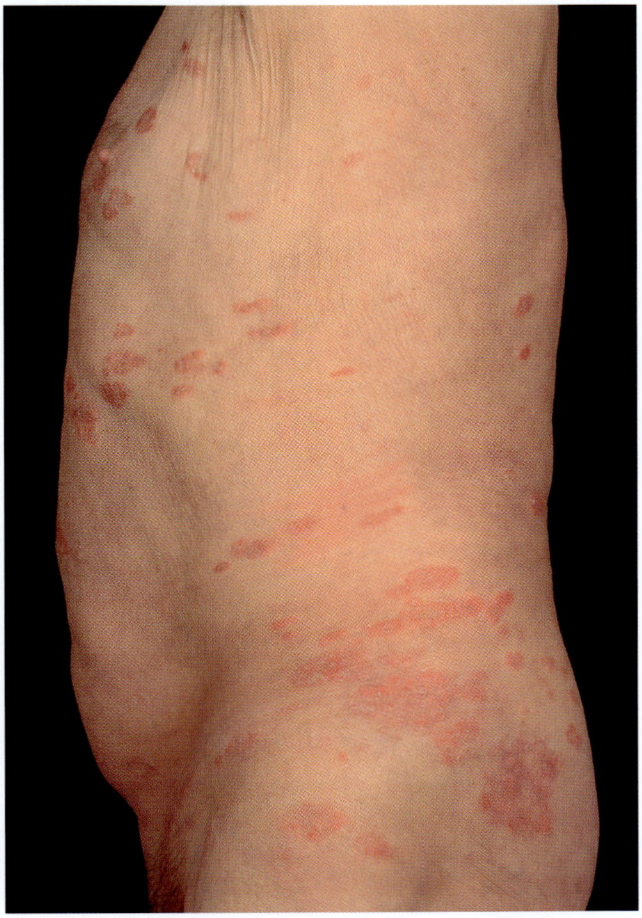

**Figure 3.1** Mycosis fungoides, patch stage. Generalized, scaly patches on the trunk. Note the "digitate dermatitis"-like pattern on the flank.

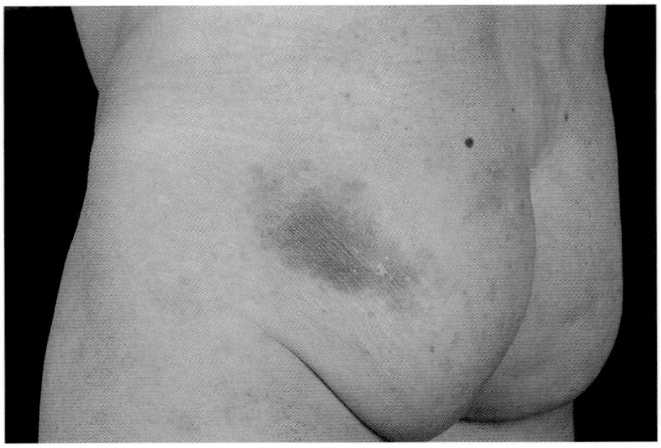

**Figure 3.2** Mycosis fungoides, patch stage. Localized, early patches on the buttocks.

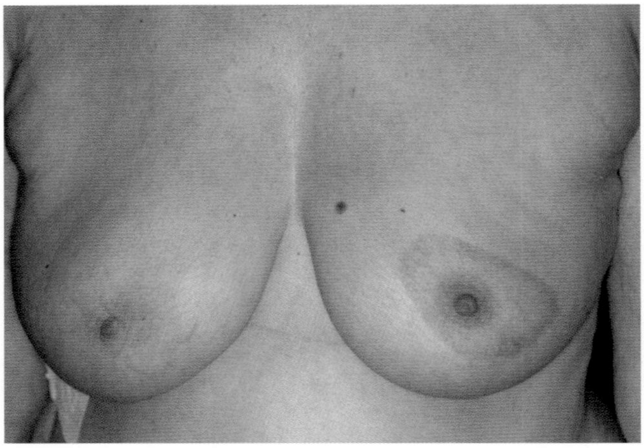

**Figure 3.3** Mycosis fungoides, patch stage. Localized, annular patch on the breast.

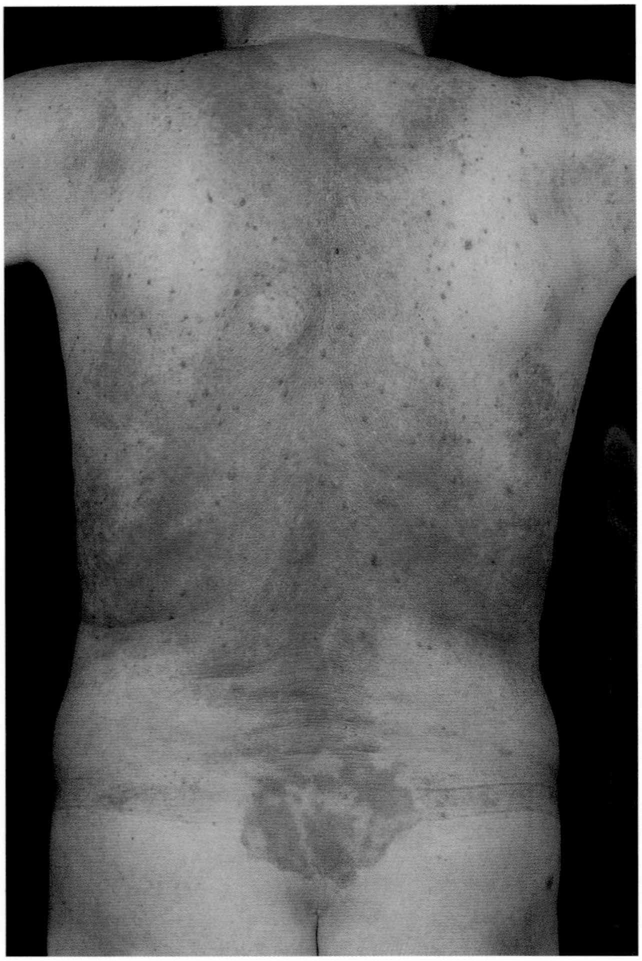

**Figure 3.4** Mycosis fungoides, patch stage. Irregular, large, confluent erythematous patches covering most of the back.

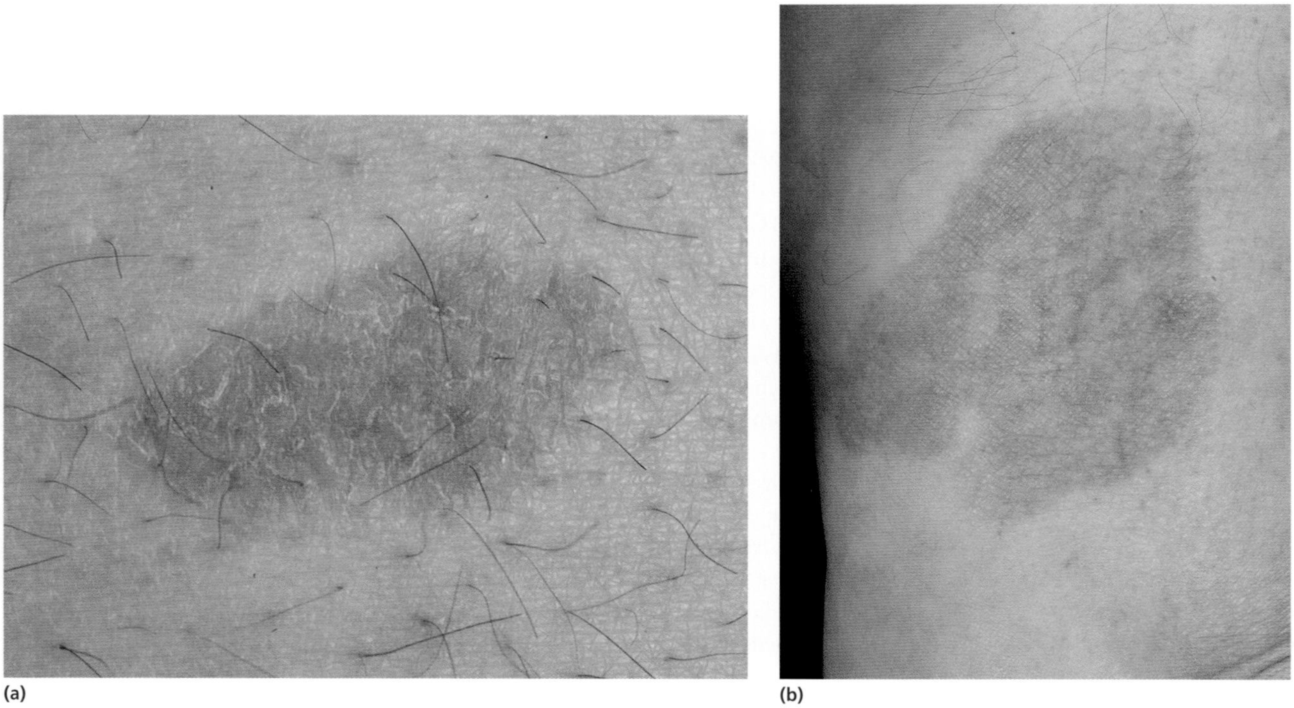

**Figure 3.5** Mycosis fungoides, patch stage. (a) Detail of one patch with focal scaling. (b) Detail of a patch without scaling and with focal atrophy after local steroid treatment.

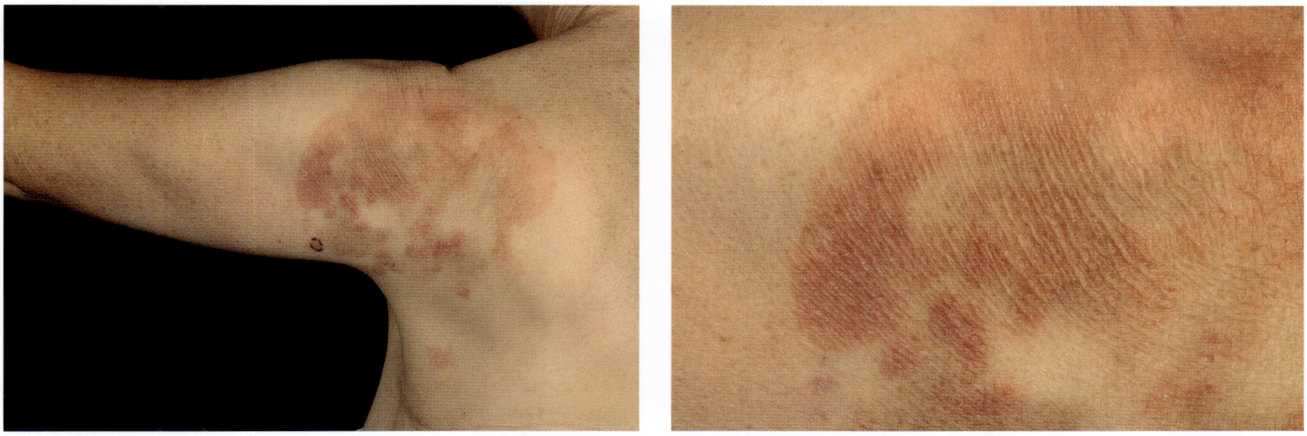

(a) (b)

Figure 3.6 Mycosis fungoides, patch stage. (a, b) Note loss of elasticity in affected skin with "parchment-like" appearance, as compared to unaffected skin in the surrounding.

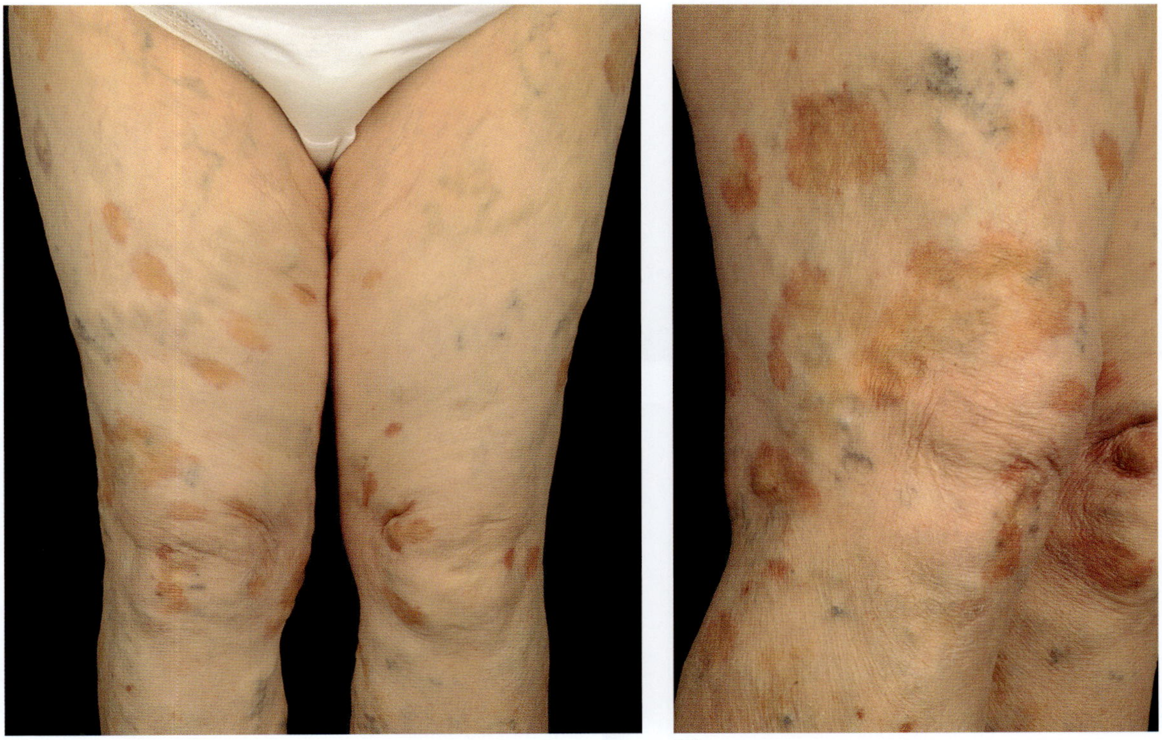

(a) (b)

Figure 3.7 Mycosis fungoides, patch stage. (a) Several patches with a yellowish-orange color ("xanthoerythroderma perstans"). (b) Detail of the lesions.

Plaques of mycosis fungoides are characterized by infiltrated (elevated and/or indurated), variably scaling, reddish-brown lesions (Figs. 3.9 and 3.10). Typical patches are usually observed contiguous to plaques or at other sites of the body. The size and form of the plaques are variable. Ulceration is uncommon; in some cases superficial crusts convey some resemblance to impetiginized lesions (and secondary impetiginization may also occur). Plaques with brownish color may mimic granulomatous lesions, particularly those of sarcoidosis (Fig. 3.11). Plaques of mycosis fungoides should be distinguished from flat tumors of the disease, but the differentiation of plaques from flat tumors may be very subjective clinically, and can be better achieved by correlation with the histopathological features; besides, in some cases the degree of skin infiltration may be difficult to

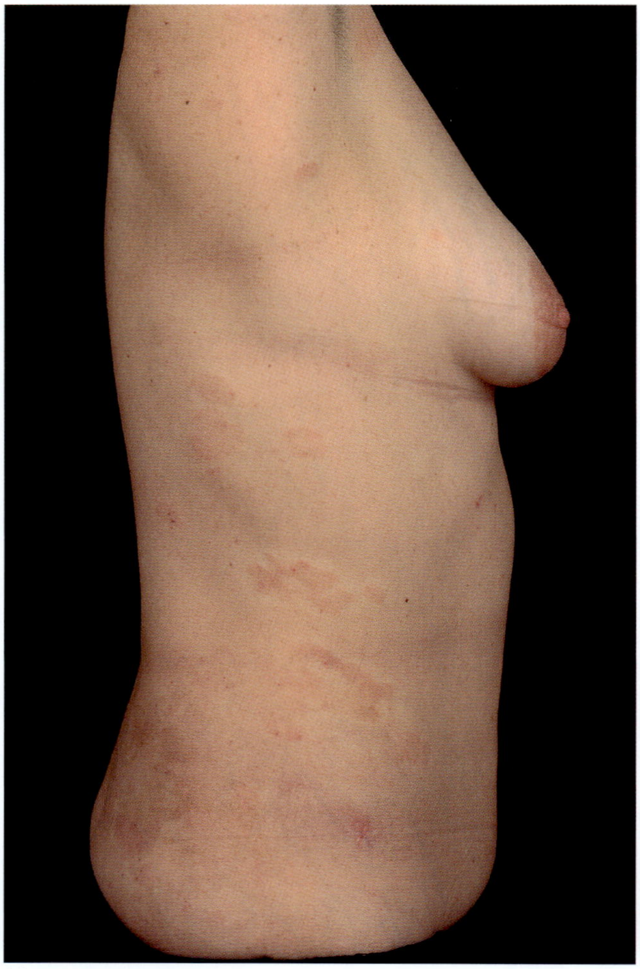

(a)

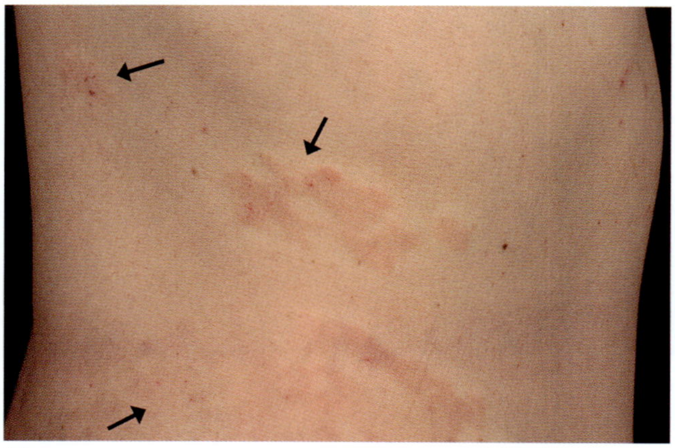

(b)

**Figure 3.8** Mycosis fungoides, patch stage. (a) Generalized lesions with (b) several small scratching artifacts (arrows).

determine, and lesions that are clearly infiltrated (i.e., "plaques") histopathologically may not look so clinically (Fig. 3.12). In fact, distinction of patches from plaques may be difficult even histopathologically [80b].

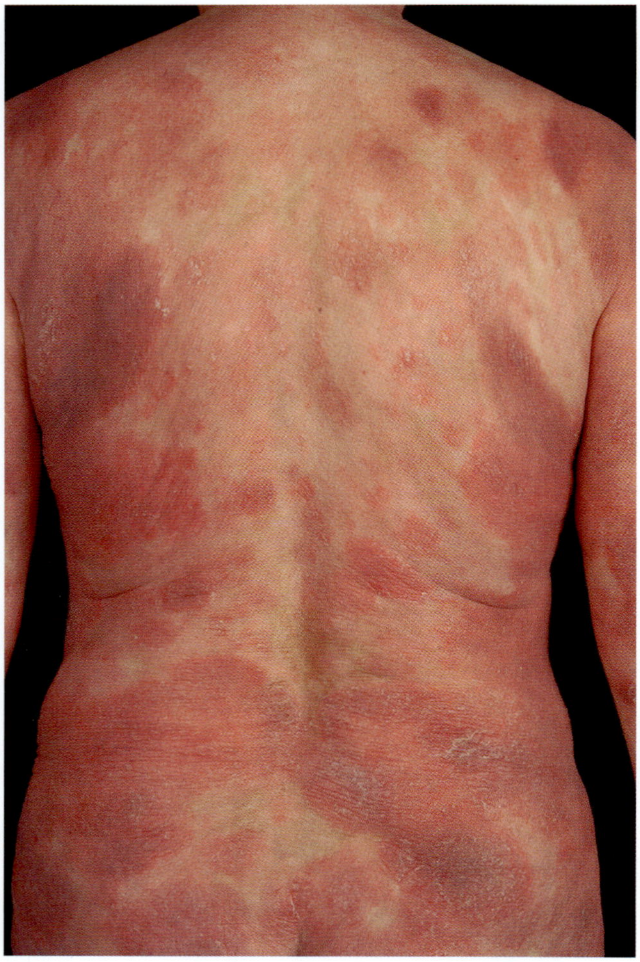

**Figure 3.9** Mycosis fungoides, plaque stage. Generalized, erythematous, partly scaly patches and thin plaques on the trunk.

Patches and plaques of mycosis fungoides may have a different morphology on dark skin ("skin of color"). Besides the hypopigmented variant, which is seen more often in black patients, lesions usually appear less erythematous and have a grayish or silver hue instead (Figs. 3.13a and b). Both hyperpigmentation and hypopigmentation may be present, often at the same time. Asiatic patients often present with hyperpigmentation at the site of active lesions (Fig. 3.13c).

Tumors in mycosis fungoides may be solitary, localized, or generalized, and are often (but not always) observed in combination with patches and plaques (Figs. 3.14 and 3.15). Ulceration is common, and in some cases flat, ulcerated tumors may be misconstrued as patches or plaques (Fig. 3.16). For practical purposes, patches and plaques of mycosis fungoides are almost never ulcerated and bleeding (unless traumatized). Large ulceration of flat tumors may mimic the picture of so-called ulcus rodens (Fig. 3.17), and fungating tumors may destroy underlying structures (Fig. 3.18). Flat tumors and associated plaques may present as large, marginated, sometimes "geographical" lesions

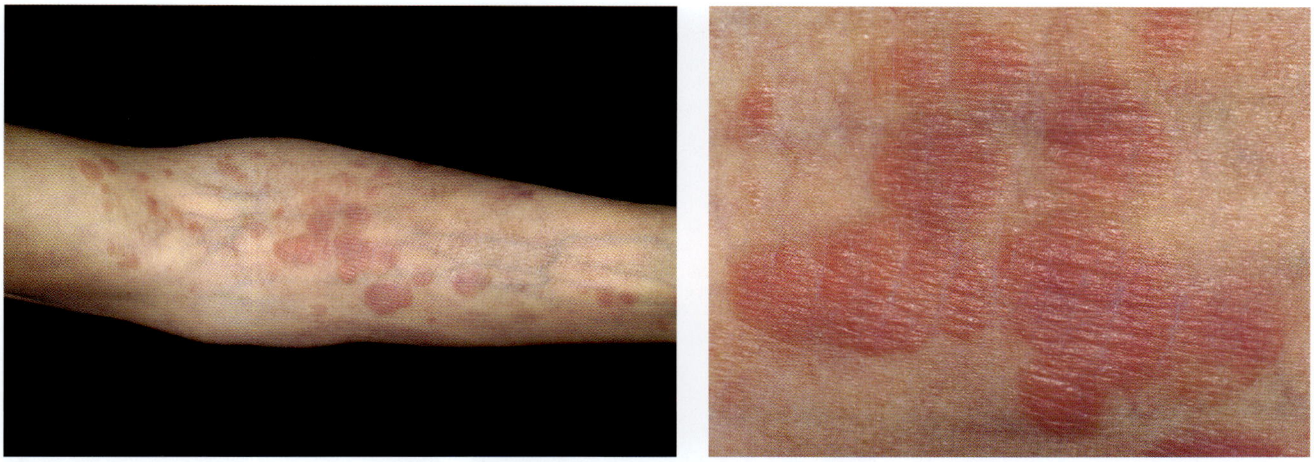

(a) (b)

Figure 3.10 Mycosis fungoides, plaque stage. (a) Several erythematous plaques on the arm. (b) Detail of the plaques.

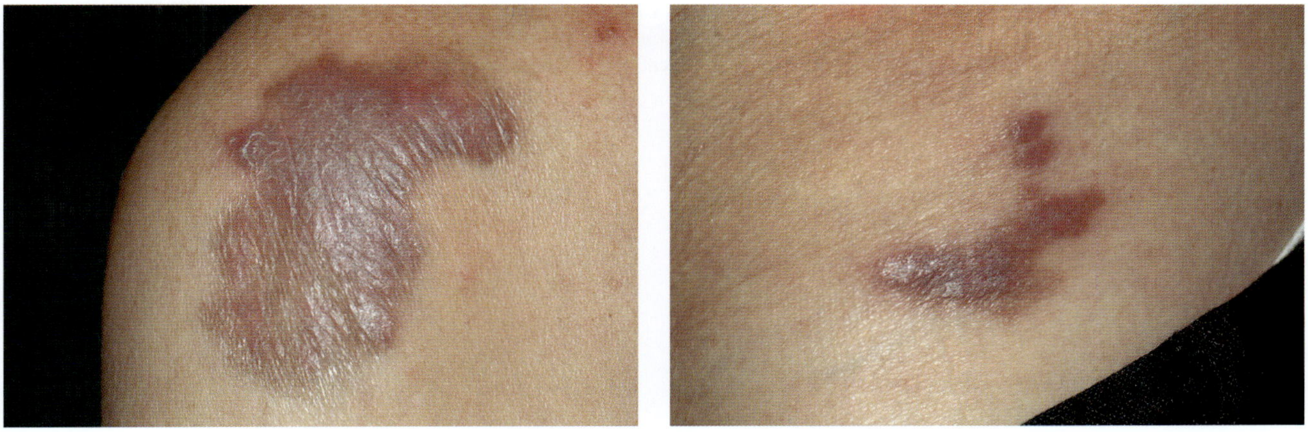

(a) (b)

Figure 3.11 Mycosis fungoides, plaque stage. (a, b). Brownish plaques mimicking the picture of a granulomatous dermatitis, particularly sarcoidosis.

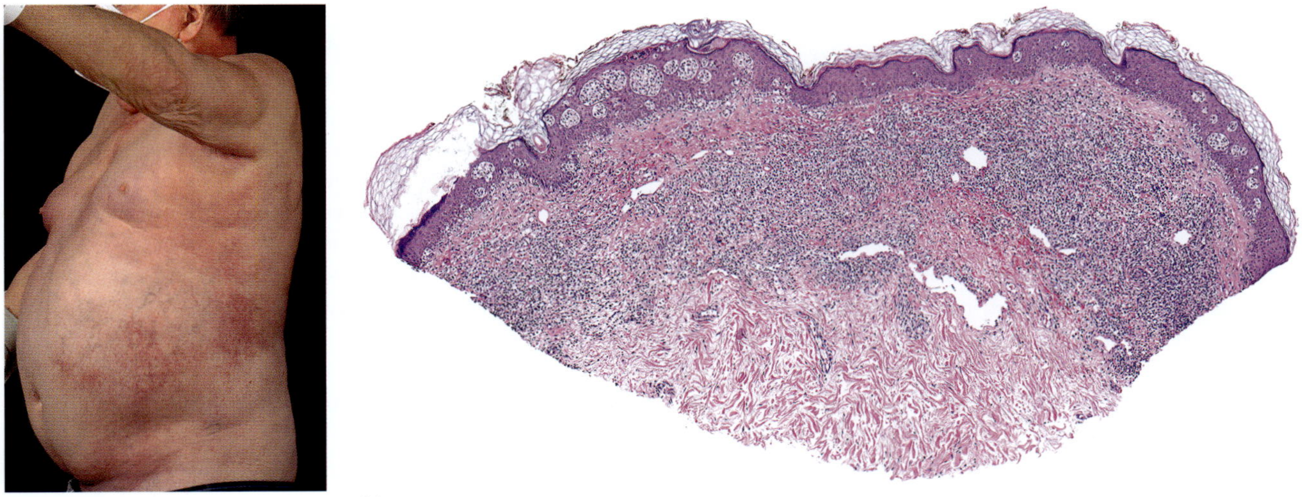

(a) (b)

Figure 3.12 Mycosis fungoides, plaque stage. (a) diffuse infiltrate of the trunk without clear-cut clinical plaques; (b) histological examination reveals a dense, band-like lymphoid infiltrate with many Darier nests within the epidermis, corresponding to a plaque rather than a patch.

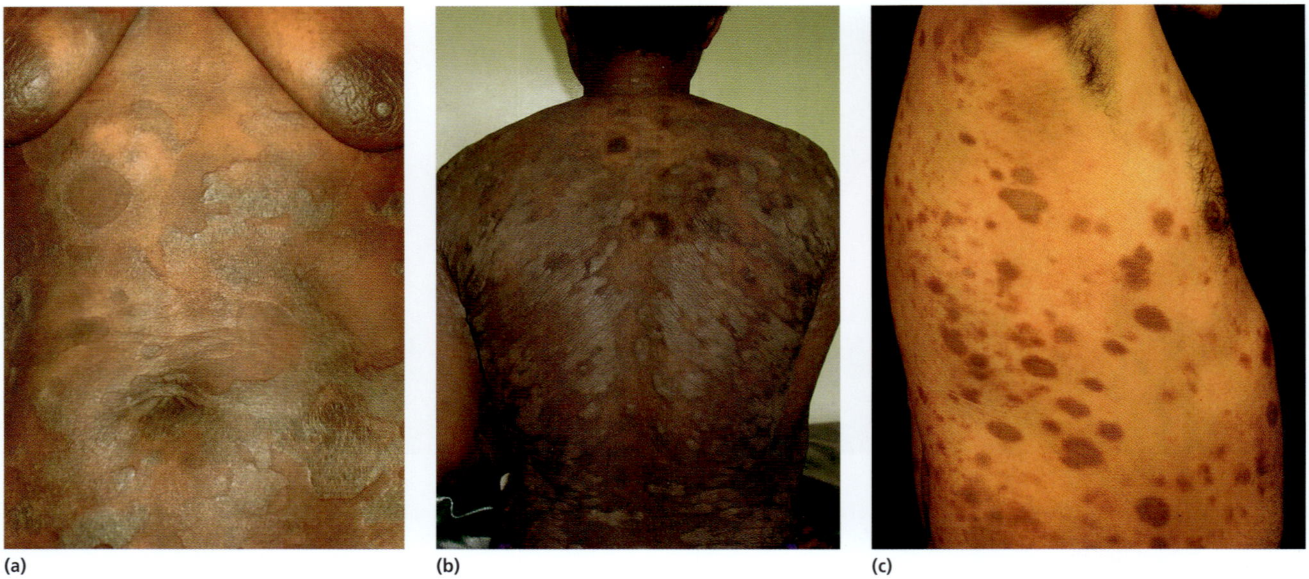


**Figure 3.13** Mycosis fungoides on dark skin ("skin of color") and Asiatic skin. (a) Note the silver hue of patches and plaques, and absence of erythematous features in an African patient; (b) another African patient showing mostly hypopigmented and partly hyperpigmented, generalized patches and plaques (*Courtesy of Dr. Cesare Massone, Genova, Italy*). (c) Asiatic patients and patients from Middle East often present with hyperpigmented rather than erythematous patches and plaques.

(Fig. 3.19a), and a similar figurate arrangement may be observed also in earlier phases of the disease (Fig. 3.19b). The annular or figurate appearance of some lesions of mycosis fungoides is likely due to partial spontaneous regression of part of the lesion (in general, partial regression is not uncommon in mycosis fungoides). On the scalp, confluent, flat tumors may confer on the lesion features similar to those of "cutis verticis gyrata" (Fig. 3.20). The growth rate of tumors in mycosis fungoides is variable: in some cases they grow rapidly in a matter of weeks, and in others they are relatively stable for months.

Besides the skin, tumors of mycosis fungoides may involve the mucosal regions (Fig. 3.21). Involvement of the mucosal surfaces is very unusual in the early phases, but less so in advanced stages. As oral and genital mucosa are frequently involved in cytotoxic NK/T-cell lymphomas, care should be taken to classify these cases correctly. Precise clinical history taking, re-evaluation of previous biopsies, and complete phenotypic and genotypic investigations are mandatory to make the diagnosis of mucosal involvement in mycosis fungoides.

Itch is often a prominent symptom in all stages of the disease and may be very difficult to treat [81]. Onychodystrophy may be prominent in advanced mycosis fungoides (similarly to Sézary syndrome) (Fig. 3.22) [82]. Other nail alterations include nail discoloration, thickening, crumbling, onycholysis, onychomadesis, splinter hemorrhages, subungual hyperkeratosis, and anonychia [83]. Erythroderma can develop in the course of the disease, rendering distinction from Sézary syndrome difficult without a proper clinical history (see also the section on erythrodermic mycosis fungoides in this chapter and Chapter 4). The palms and soles may be affected in some patients, either with diffuse or with patchy, scaly erythema (Fig. 3.23). Involvement of these regions is more common in the syringotropic variant of the disease. It is crucial to understand that lesions of mycosis fungoides *restricted* to the palms and soles (so-called palmoplantar mycosis fungoides) are exceedingly rare, if they exist at all (see below in this chapter and also Chapter 31). Tumors in acral locations are not unusual and sometimes represent the first sign of disease's progression (Fig. 3.24).

Conventional clinical examination is sufficient for evaluation of the clinical features of the disease. The utility of confocal microscopy as first-line investigation in patients with mycosis fungoides has been discussed [84], but in my opinion it does not provide information that goes beyond what can be obtained by the naked eyes examination followed by biopsy. The same holds true for dermatoscopy, which does not offer any information that is not already provided by conventional clinical examination, and, in my opinion, does not play any role in the diagnosis of the disease.

Clinical variants of mycosis fungoides are discussed in specific sections in this chapter.

## Extracutaneous involvement

Lymph nodes, lung, spleen, and liver are the most frequent sites of extracutaneous involvement in mycosis fungoides, but specific lesions can arise in all organs [85]. The bone marrow is

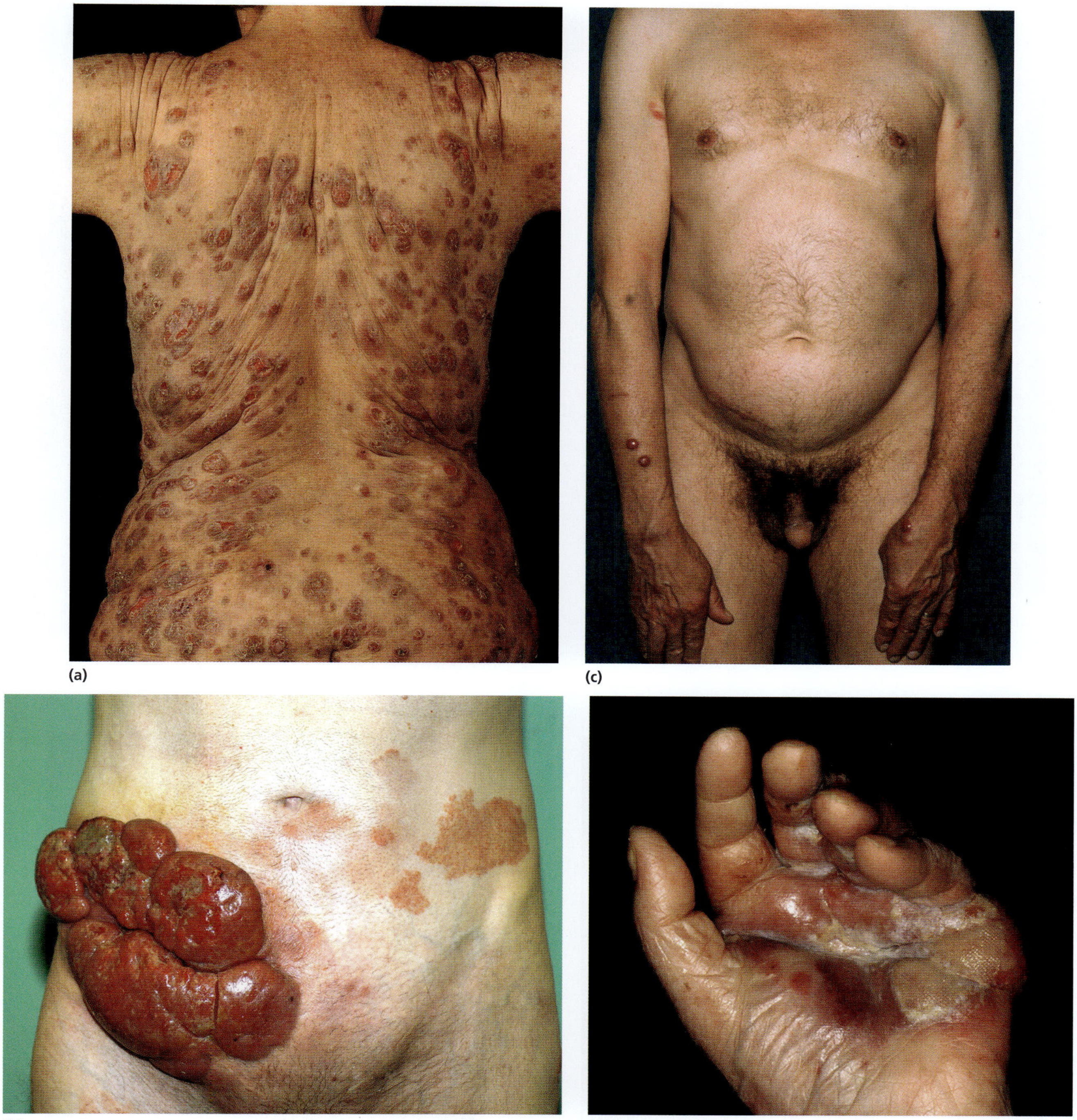

(a) (c) (b) (d)

**Figure 3.14** Mycosis fungoides, tumor stage. (a) Generalized, confluent patches, plaques, and tumors. (b) Large, fungating, ulcerated tumor contiguous to patches and plaques of the disease (*Courtesy of Dr. Cornelia Müller, Homburg/Saar, Germany*). (c) Several small tumors on both arms with only few, noncontiguous patches. (d) Large, infiltrated, partly tumoral lesion on the hand.

usually spared. Lymph node involvement may be difficult to differentiate histopathologically from so-called dermopathic lymphadenopathy, and it has been demonstrated that, irrespective of the histopathologic features, enlarged lymph nodes represent a bad prognostic sign [43].

Because of the presence of ulcerated tumors and immune deficiency (due to both the lymphoma and the many treatments typically administered to these patients during the course of the disease), septicemia and/or pneumonia are the major causes of death.

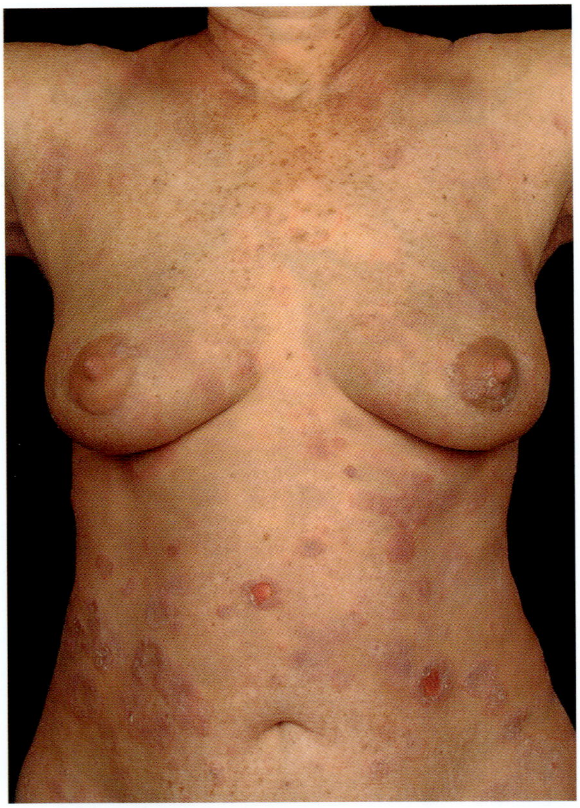

**Figure 3.15** Mycosis fungoides, tumor stage. Generalized plaques and flat tumors, some with superficial erosions.

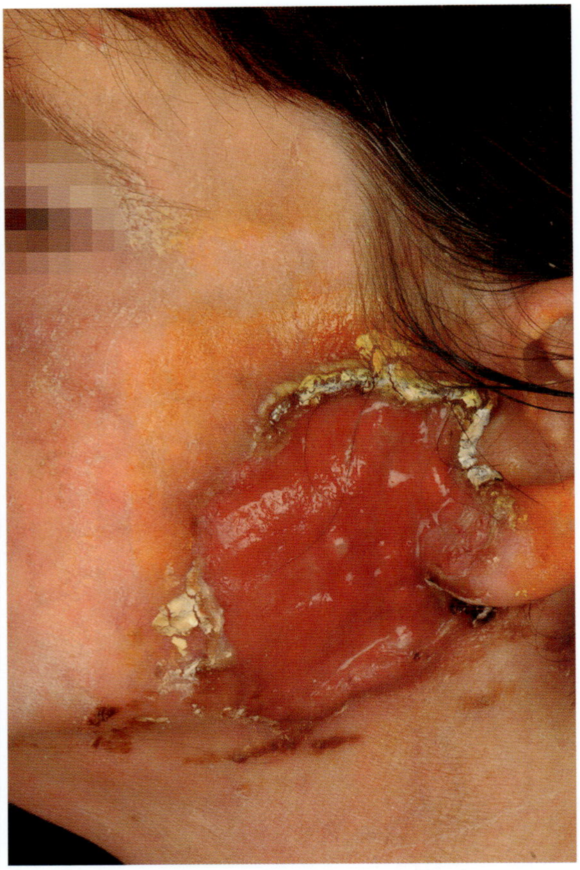

**Figure 3.17** Mycosis fungoides, tumor stage. Large, ulcerated flat tumor on the face mimicking the clinical picture of so-called ulcus rodens.

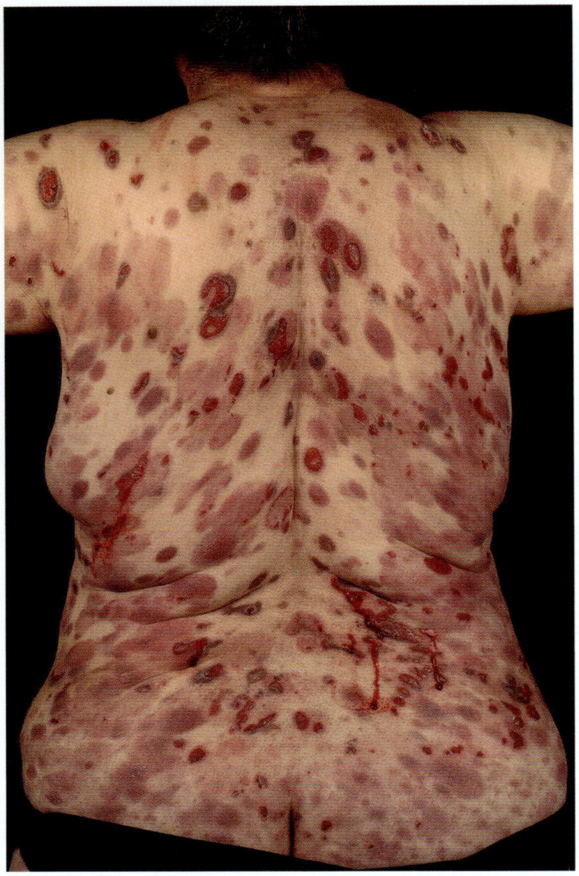

**Figure 3.16** Mycosis fungoides, tumor stage. Generalized, partly ulcerated, bleeding flat tumors in association with patches and plaques.

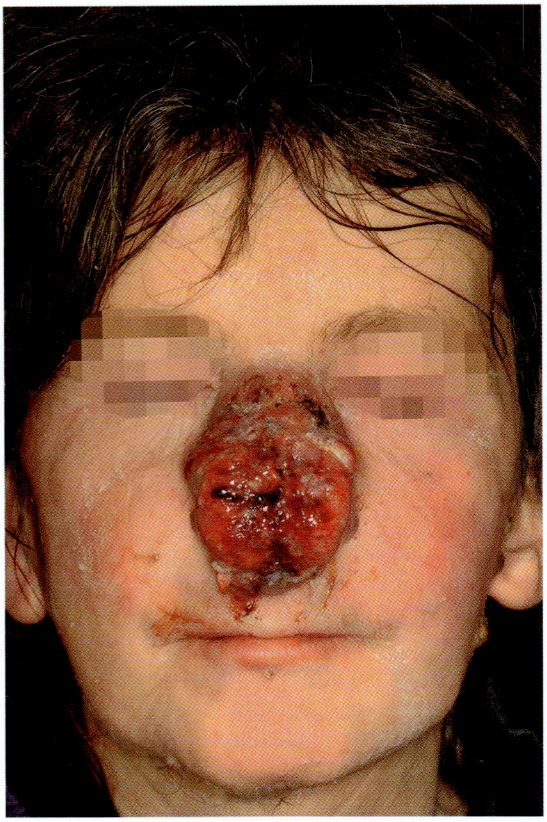

**Figure 3.18** Mycosis fungoides, tumor stage. Large ulcerated tumor destroying the nose and mimicking the picture of "lethal midline granuloma." It is crucial to distinguish such cases from cutaneous extranodal NK/T-cell lymphoma, nasal-type.

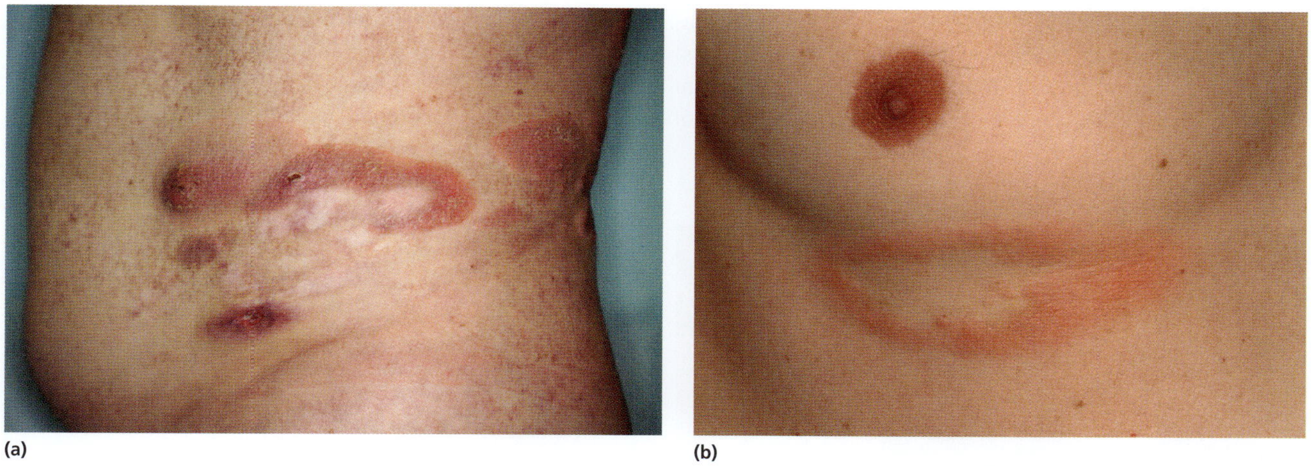

Figure 3.19 Mycosis fungoides. (a) Bizarre, partly annular configuration of confluent plaques and tumors. (b) A similar annular configuration in another patient with early mycosis fungoides mimicking erythema migrans.

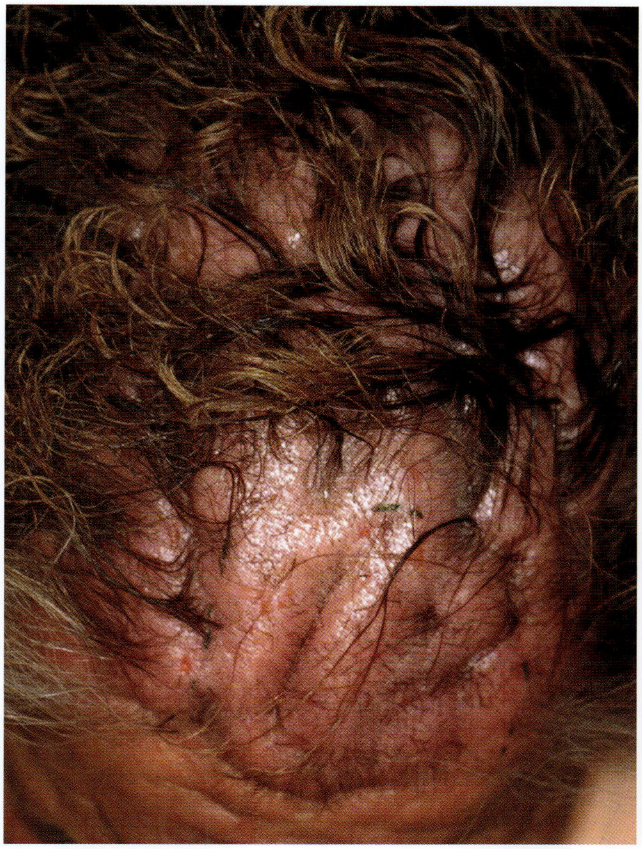

Figure 3.20 Mycosis fungoides, tumor stage. Involvement of the scalp with the clinical picture of "cutis verticis gyrata."

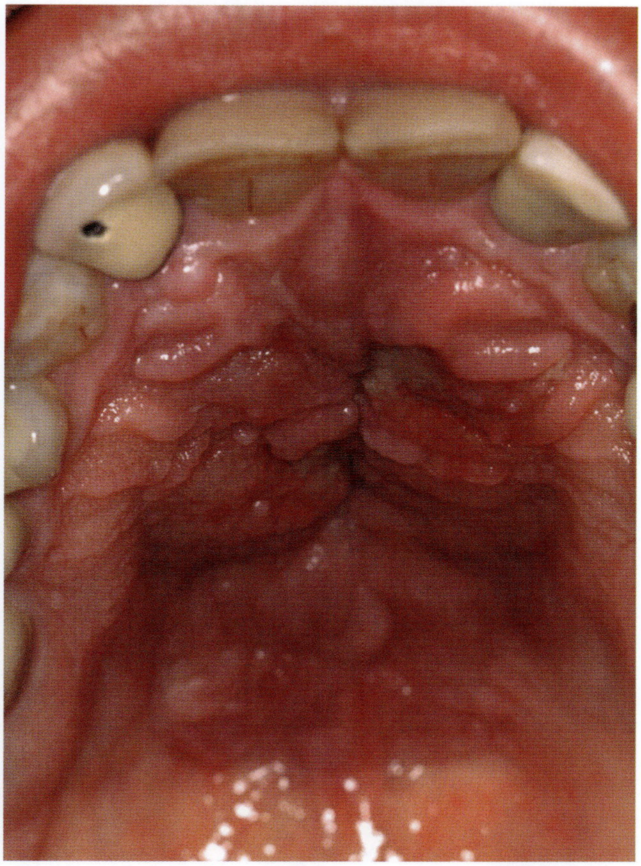

Figure 3.21 Mycosis fungoides, tumor stage. Involvement of the oral mucosa.

## Association with other diseases

As mentioned before, mycosis fungoides can be observed in association with other hematological diseases such as lymphomatoid papulosis, anaplastic large cell lymphoma, and Hodgkin lymphoma. The onset of these disorders may precede, be concomitant with, or occur later than the diagnosis of mycosis fungoides. It may be extremely difficult (if not impossible) to differentiate tumor-stage mycosis fungoides from lesions of lymphomatoid papulosis and anaplastic large cell lymphoma (see also Chapter 5). Some of the cases reported as lymphomatoid papulosis or cutaneous anaplastic large cell lymphoma arising after the onset of mycosis fungoides may in fact represent lesions of tumor-stage mycosis fungoides with expression of CD30. In this context, as already mentioned, it should be underlined that spontaneous regression (usually partial regression) of single tumors of mycosis fungoides is not uncommon, and that in a patient with mycosis fungoides regression of any lesion is not a criterion for diagnosis of lymphomatoid papulosis. Besides these disease entities, mycosis fungoides has been observed also in association with other non-Hodgkin lymphomas of T- or B-cell lineage [86–88]. In rare cases, mycosis fungoides may be

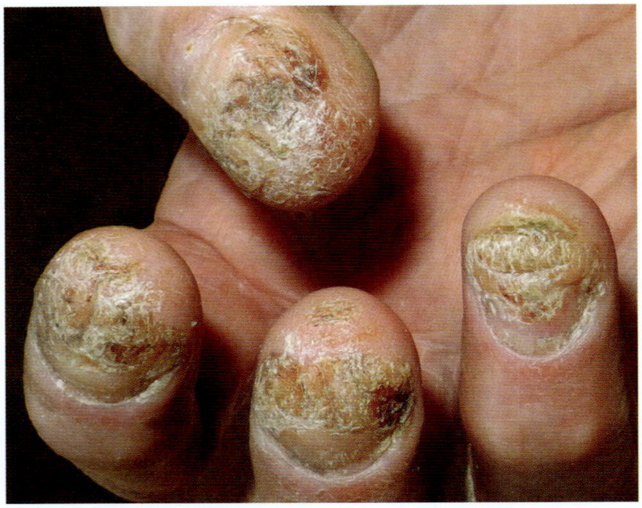

**Figure 3.22** Pronounced onychodystrophy in advanced mycosis fungoides. (*Courtesy of Dr. Carlo Cota, Rome, Italy.*)

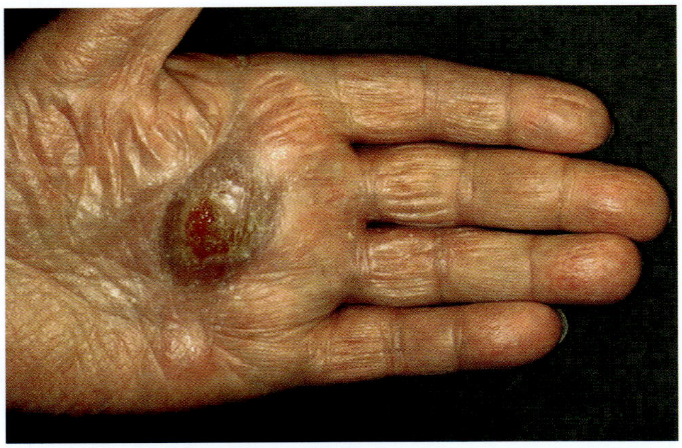

**Figure 3.24** Mycosis fungoides. Large, ulcerated tumor on the palm.

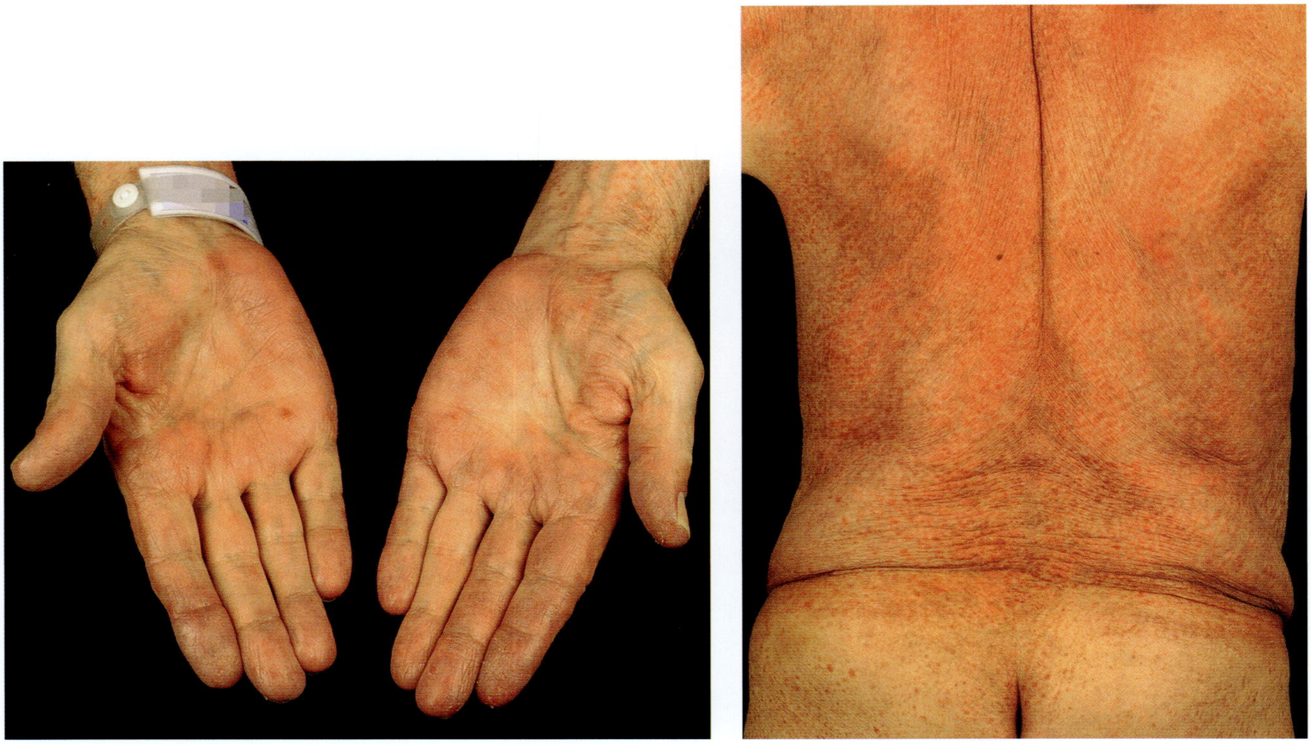

(a) (b)

**Figure 3.23** Mycosis fungoides. (a) Erythematous, partly scaly, partly erosive lesions on both palms. (b) This patient had also infiltrated erythematous lesions on the trunk with a "cobblestone" appearance.

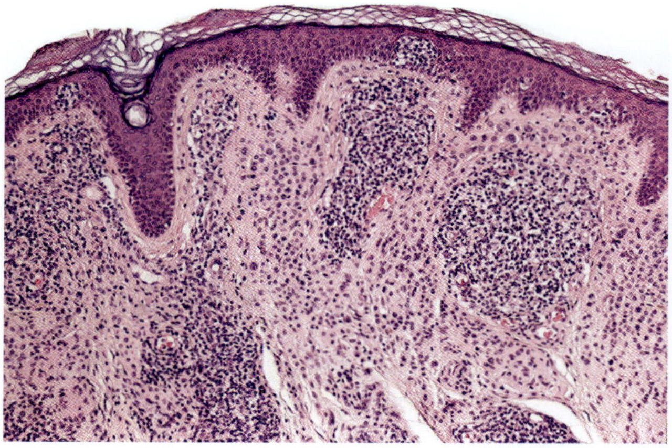

Figure 3.25 Mycosis fungoides. Specific infiltrate of the disease within a pre-existent melanocytic nevus. Note clusters of intraepidermal lymphocytes (Darier nests).

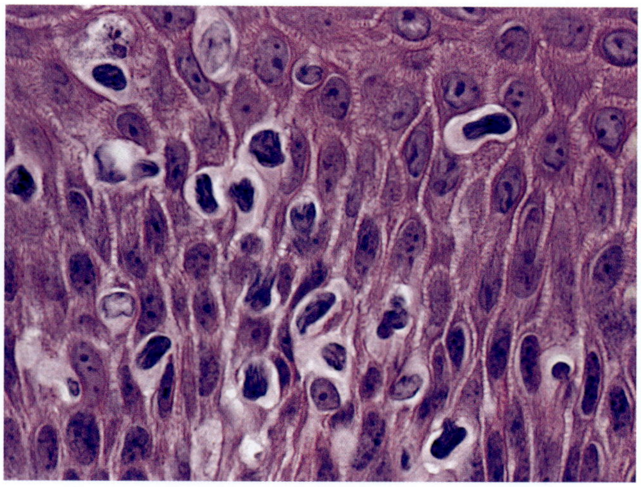

Figure 3.26 Mycosis fungoides. Intraepidermal lymphocytes with predominance of medium-sized pleomorphic ("cerebriform") lymphocytes.

associated with a second, unrelated lymphoma at the same skin site ("composite lymphoma") (see Chapter 28) [89].

An increased incidence of cancers other than lymphomas has been observed in patients with mycosis fungoides [40, 86]. In these patients, mycosis fungoides may represent either the primary or the subsequent malignancy. Besides Hodgkin and non-Hodgkin lymphomas, the most frequent second malignancies are melanoma, lung carcinoma, colon carcinoma, and renal carcinoma, as well as breast carcinoma in females and prostate carcinoma in males [40]. As already mentioned, in a Dutch study, patients with mycosis fungoides had a statistically significant higher incidence of cutaneous melanoma, cutaneous squamous cell carcinoma, and extracutaneous hematological malignancies, whereas there was no association between mycosis fungoides and other extracutaneous solid organ tumors [41]. Infections, too, are more common and sometimes more severe than in the general population [90].

Specific infiltrates of mycosis fungoides can be observed in benign and malignant skin tumors such as melanocytic nevi, malignant melanoma, and seborrheic keratoses, among others (Fig. 3.25). In these cases, the association of the two diseases represents an example of so-called "collision tumors," due to colonization of a second neoplasm by neoplastic cells of mycosis fungoides (composite lymphomas are also conceptually, at least in part, a variant of "collision tumors").

## Histopathology, immunophenotype, and molecular genetics

Mycosis fungoides is a cutaneous T-cell lymphoma characterized cytomorphologically by the proliferation of small- to medium-sized pleomorphic ("cerebriform") lymphocytes (Fig. 3.26). Intraepidermal collections of lymphocytes (so-called "Pautrier microabscesses") (Fig. 3.27), considered the hallmark of the disease, are present only in a minority of early patches of mycosis fungoides and can be absent from more advanced lesions as well. Parenthetically, the first description of the "microabscesses" was not by Pautrier but by Jean Ferdinand Darier several decades before [91]. Pautrier was puzzled by the attribution of this observation to himself and acknowledged that the intraepidermal collections of lymphocytes should have been termed "Darier nests" (a term that was used in the 1920s) instead [91]. Thus, the term "Pautrier microabscess" is twice wrong: first because Pautrier did not describe this histopathological feature of mycosis fungoides, and second because these collections of cells are not "microabscesses." Giessinger and coworkers recently summarized the history of the mistaken attribution of the intraepidermal collections of lymphocytes to Pautrier rather than to Darier, explaining that it was due to American dermatologists and dermatopathologists who were not aware of the original description by Darier [92]. In this book the correct terminology of Darier nests will be used, and I strongly advocate to use in the medical literature this term rather than the wrong "Pautrier microabscesses," in order not to perpetuate a mistake that has been repeated for almost one century.

Another curious semantic issue is the variable use of the terms "epidermotropism" and "exocytosis" to describe intraepidermal lymphocytes [93]. Epidermotropism is used for referring to the presence of neoplastic lymphocytes within the epidermis, whereas exocytosis is used to refer to the presence of non-neoplastic intraepidermal lymphocytes in inflammatory conditions. To my eyes, the use of different terms in order to describe one and the same finding, that is, the presence of intraepidermal lymphocytes, is a typical example of the lack of precision in medical language. Personally, I refer to intraepidermal

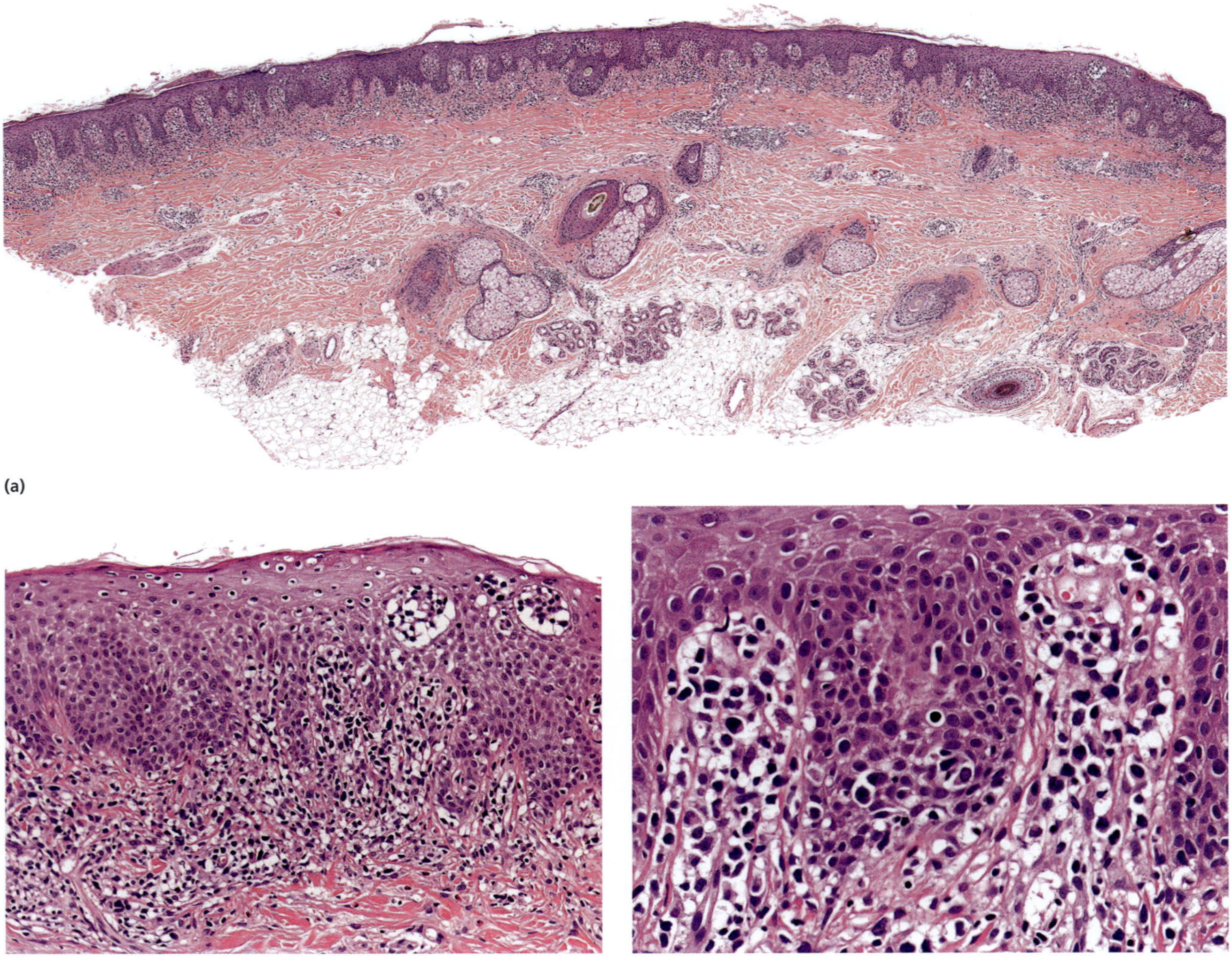

(a)

(b)

(c)

**Figure 3.27** Histopathologic features of a clear-cut patch of mycosis fungoides. (a) Psoriasiform epidermal hyperplasia and band-like infiltrate of lymphocytes within the superficial dermis. (b) Epidermotropism of lymphocytes with Darier nests. (c) Detail of pleomorphic lymphocytes.

lymphocytes as "epidermotropic lymphocytes" regardless of the background condition. Parenthetically, there may be "exocytosis" of reactive lymphocytes in cases of mycosis fungoides, thus presenting with both "epidermotropism" and "exocytosis" of lymphocytes in the same specimen.

It should be emphasized that, although precise histopathologic criteria for the diagnosis of early mycosis fungoides have been identified (Table 3.1), in many cases a definitive diagnosis can be made only after a careful correlation with the clinical features of the disease [94, 95]. Further problems can arise when biopsies are taken after different types of local treatment that alter the histopathologic features of the lesions. As a general rule, it is advisable to take multiple biopsies from morphologically different lesions (Fig. 3.28), if necessary to repeat biopsies after a 2-week period without local treatment, and to perform repeat biopsies on recurrent lesions after successful treatment, in order to check whether the histopathologic features are stable or changing (i.e., occurrence of large cell transformation, which may be observed also in flat lesions) (see Figs. 3.51 and 3.52).

Scoring systems and algorithms for the diagnosis of mycosis fungoides have been proposed, combining the clinical aspect with the immunophenotypic and molecular features of the infiltrate [96]. The algorithm proposed by the ISCL was found useful but limited by low specificity [97]. However, in my view and in that of others [98], the diagnosis of mycosis fungoides can be achieved in most cases by accurate clinicopathologic correlation, without the need of more or less complex algorithms. In this context, our group described several histopathologic patterns of early mycosis fungoides that were previously poorly characterized, showing the protean nature of the disease and the difficulties in histopathologic diagnosis [94]. As already mentioned, high-throughput sequencing showed that neoplastic

**Table 3.1** Histopathologic criteria for the diagnosis of early mycosis fungoides[#]

| Epidermis |
|---|
| Intraepidermal collections of lymphocytes (Darier nests) |
| Lymphocytes aligned along the dermoepidermal junction ("basilar epidermotropism") |
| Intraepidermal lymphocytes larger than lymphocytes in the dermis |
| Intraepidermal lymphocytes with "haloed" nuclei |
| "Disproportionate" epidermotropism (large numbers of epidermotropic lymphocytes in areas of scant spongiosis)* |
| **Dermis** |
| Expanded papillary dermis with slight fibrosis and coarse bundles of collagen |
| Band-like or patchy-lichenoid infiltrate of lymphocytes |

[#] No single criterion (not even the presence of Darier nests) is pathognomonic for mycosis fungoides or other cutaneous T-cell lymphomas (see also Chapter 31).
* This criterion is only valid for sections stained with hematoxylin and eosin, and it is not applicable to sections stained immunohistochemically for pan-T-cell markers.

T cells in mycosis fungoides may represent a very small percentage of the infiltrate [33], explaining the difficulties in the histopathological diagnosis of early lesions of the disease.

Teledermatopathology with the use of computerized (digital) slides may be useful particularly for obtaining a second expert opinion, and it is sufficiently reliable in that setting [99, 100], but it is being increasingly used in routine diagnostics as well. Artificial intelligence (AI) has been tested for the histopathological differentiation of mycosis fungoides from benign inflammatory dermatoses, but the results were slightly worse than the evaluation made by expert dermatopathologists [101], suggesting that AI-based histopathological evaluation is not yet ripe for this differential diagnosis.

## Histopathology

Early lesions of mycosis fungoides reveal in the vast majority of cases a patchy lichenoid or band-like infiltrate in an expanded, partly fibrotic papillary dermis (Fig. 3.29). The epidermis may be hyperplastic, normal, or atrophic, and the pattern may be different in different biopsies taken on the same day (Fig. 3.28). Small lymphocytes predominate and atypical cells can be observed only in a minority of cases (usually confined almost exclusively within the epidermis). Epidermotropism of solitary lymphocytes is usually found (Fig. 3.30a), whereas large, clear-cut Darier nests (Fig. 3.30b) as well as prominent ("pagetoid") epidermotropism (Fig. 3.30c) are uncommon. Pagetoid epidermotropism is present as a rule in pagetoid reticulosis (see below in this chapter) but is infrequent in other lesions of mycosis fungoides, and this pattern should always prompt to consider the differential diagnosis with other entities such as lymphomatoid papulosis, aggressive epidermotropic $CD8^+$ cytotoxic T-cell lymphoma, and cutaneous $\gamma/\delta$ T-cell lymphoma. Pagetoid epidermotropism in mycosis fungoides is often observed in cases with cytotoxic phenotype.

Useful diagnostic clues are the presence of epidermotropic lymphocytes with nuclei slightly larger than those of lymphocytes within the upper dermis (Figs 3.31a), the presence of lymphocytes aligned along the basal layer of the epidermis ("basilar epidermotropism") (Fig. 3.31b), as well as, in areas with spongiosis, the presence of many intraepidermal lymphocytes (Fig. 3.31c) [94, 102–106]. This last feature is referred to as "disproportionate" epidermotropism because a few intraepidermal lymphocytes may be observed in areas of spongiosis in many inflammatory dermatoses (see also Fig. 3.117c). In some cases, the intraepidermal lymphocytes have a clear halo around the cell and are referred to as "haloed" lymphocytes (Fig. 3.31a). Although haloed lymphocytes are considered typical of cutaneous T-cell lymphomas, particularly mycosis fungoides, they are present as a rule in lichen sclerosus as well (see Chapter 31). The papillary dermis shows a moderate to marked fibrosis with coarse bundles of collagen and a band-like or patchy-lichenoid infiltrate of lymphocytes. Dermal edema is usually not found, but exceptions exist (see below). Eosinophils may be present (Fig. 3.27b), but large numbers are not a common finding in patches and plaques of mycosis fungoides [107]. Langerhans cells are usually increased in the epidermis and dermis in early lesions of mycosis fungoides (see the section on immunophenotype in this chapter).

Particularly in biopsies taken under local skin-directed treatment modalities (e.g., local steroids, ultraviolet irradiation) the infiltrate may be scant, but focal epidermotropism may still allow a specific diagnosis (Fig. 3.32). On the other hand, although mycosis fungoides is considered by definition an epidermotropic lymphoma, in a few cases (about 5% of the total) epidermotropism may be minimal or be missing altogether (Fig. 3.33), in some cases likely related to previous treatment (particularly if the diagnosis is not yet known, biopsies are often taken during therapy because of poor response of the lesions, and are submitted as "therapy-resistant dermatitis").

Unusual histopathologic patterns of mycosis fungoides in early phases include the presence of a perivascular (as opposed to patchy-lichenoid or band-like) superficial infiltrate (Fig. 3.34), prominent spongiosis (Fig. 3.31c) [108], sometimes with Darier nests mimicking spongiotic vesicles (Fig. 3.35), interface dermatitis, sometimes with several necrotic keratinocytes similar to the picture of erythema multiforme (Fig. 3.36), marked pigment incontinence with melanophages in the papillary dermis (see the section on hyperpigmented mycosis fungoides in this chapter), prominent epidermal hyperplasia like in lichen simplex chronicus (Fig. 3.37), prominent sclerosis of the papillary dermis mimicking lichen sclerosus (Fig. 3.38) [109], and prominent extravasation of erythrocytes simulating the picture of lichenoid purpura (see the section on pigmented purpura-like mycosis fungoides in this chapter).

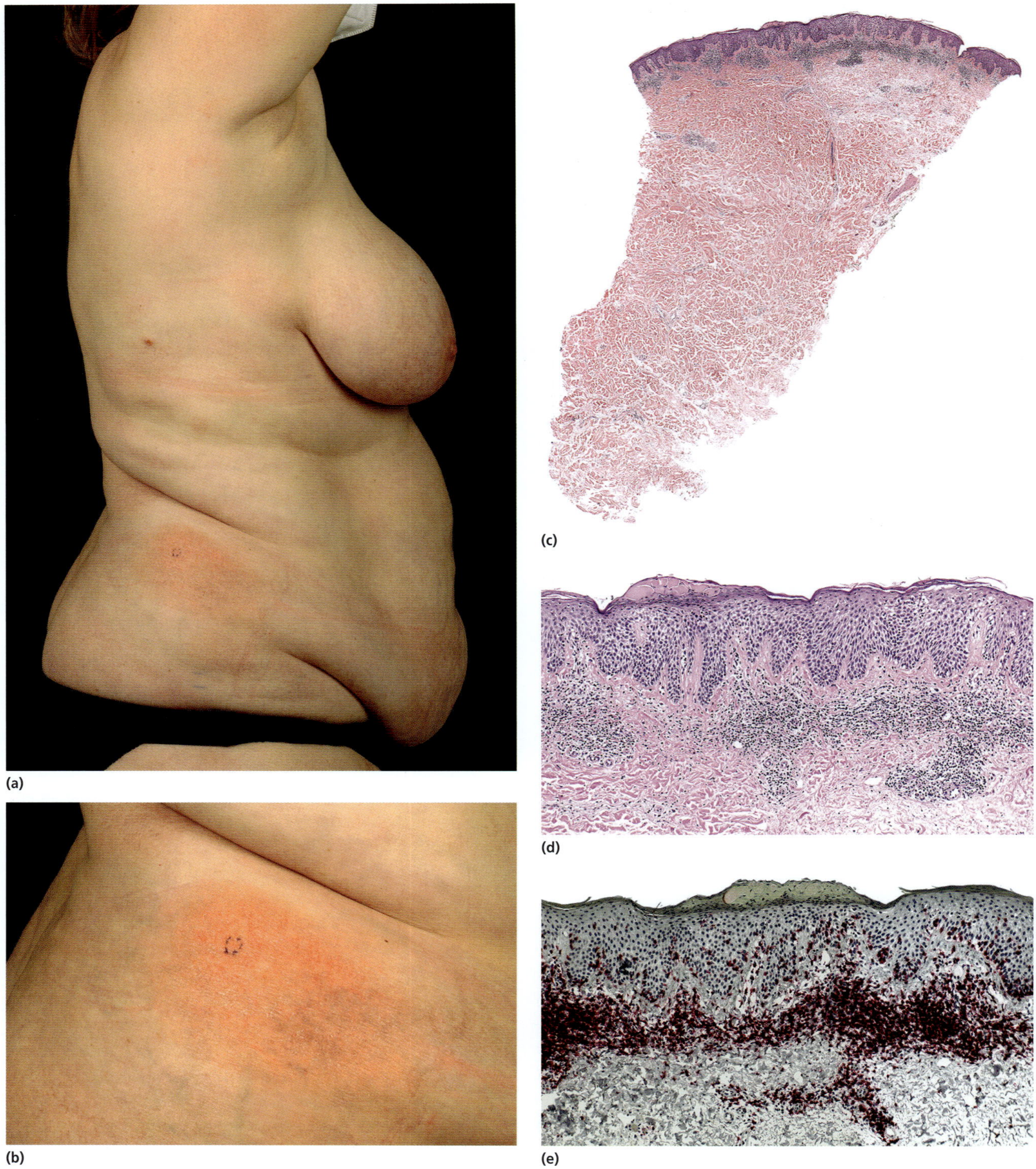


**Figure 3.28** Early mycosis fungoides with different clinical and histopathologic features in different biopsies taken on the same day. (a, b) Erythematous lesions with a scaly surface on the right flank, corresponding histopathologically to (c, d) a psoriasiform-spongiotic pattern with a dense lymphoid infiltrate and many intraepidermal lymphocytes, (e) better highlighted by a staining for CD3. (f, g) Poikilodermatic, atrophic lesions on the left flank, corresponding histopathologically to (h, i) a flat epidermis with a band-like lymphoid infiltrate characterized by (j) numerous intraepidermal lymphocytes positive for CD3.

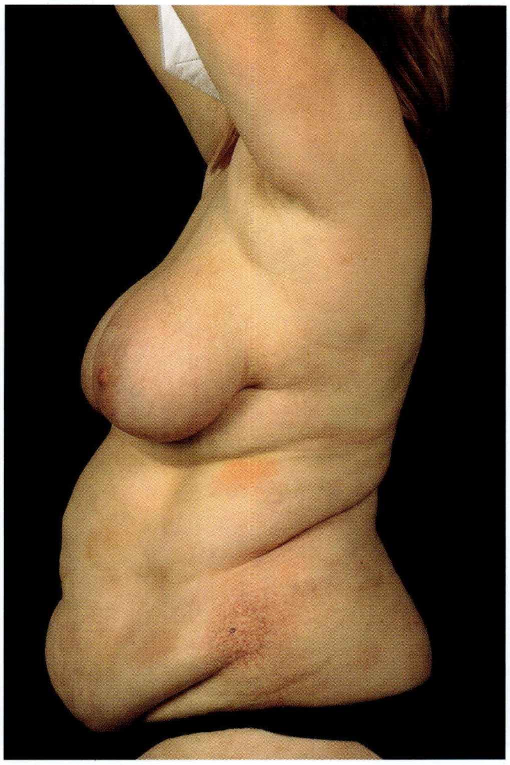

(f)

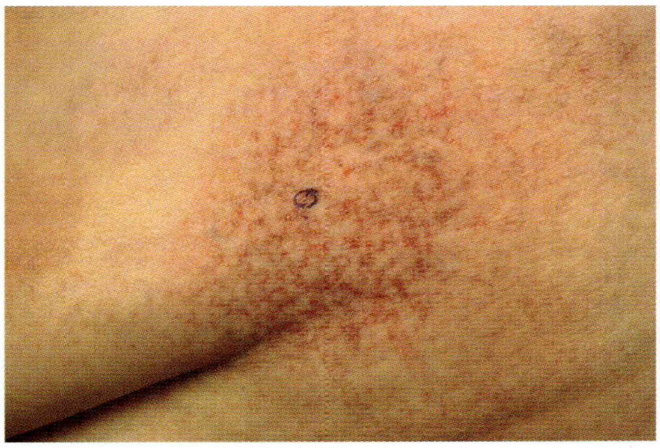

(g)

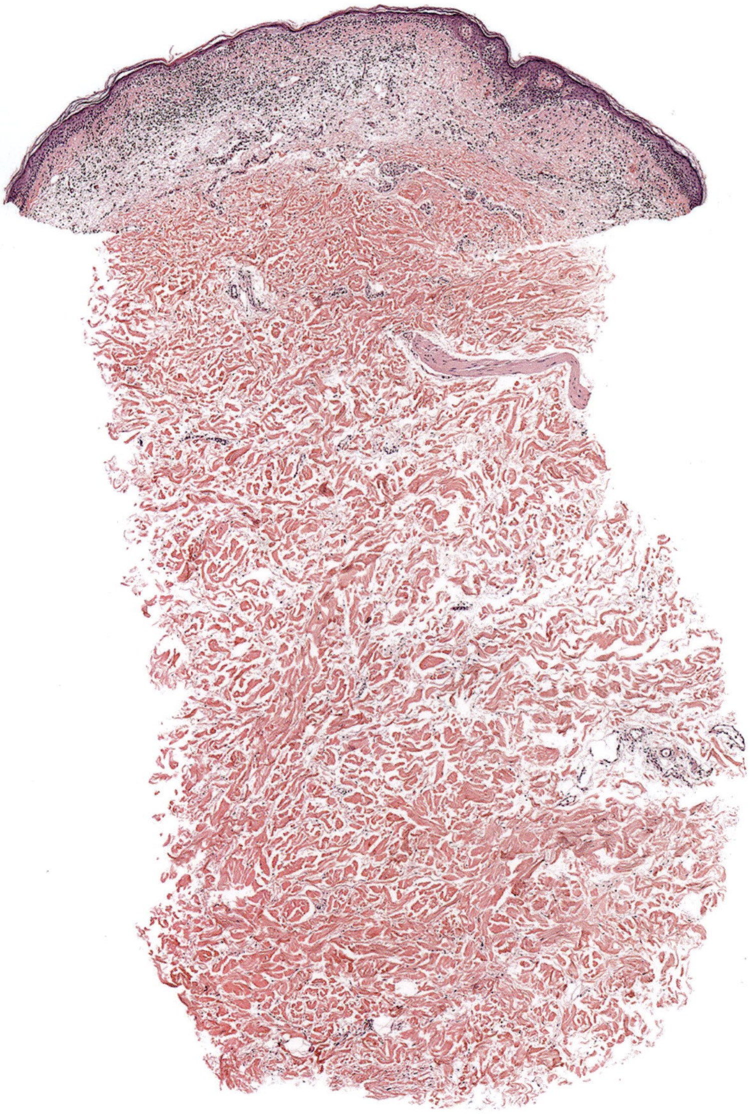

(h)

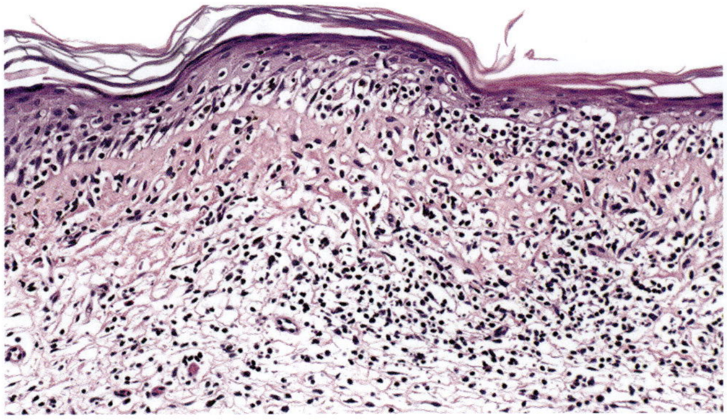

(i)

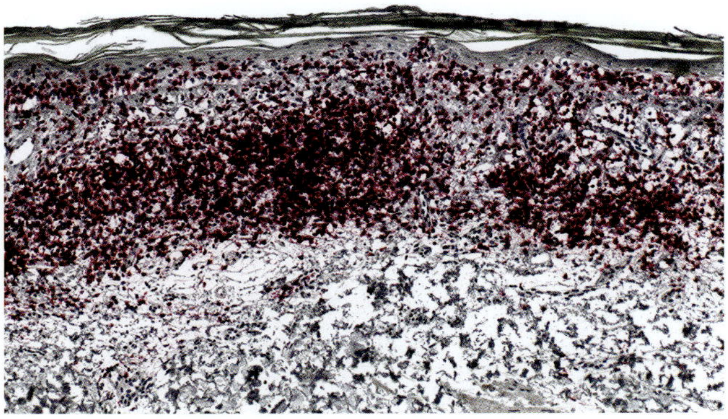

(j)

Figure 3.28 (Continued)

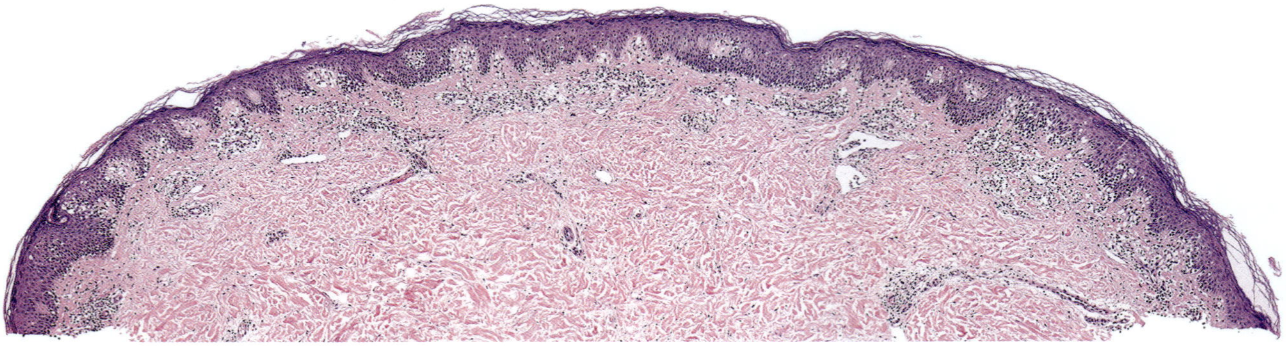

**Figure 3.29** Histopathologic features of early mycosis fungoides. "Patchy-lichenoid" (early band-like) lymphocytic infiltrate with focal fibrosis of the papillary dermis and with many epidermotropic lymphocytes.

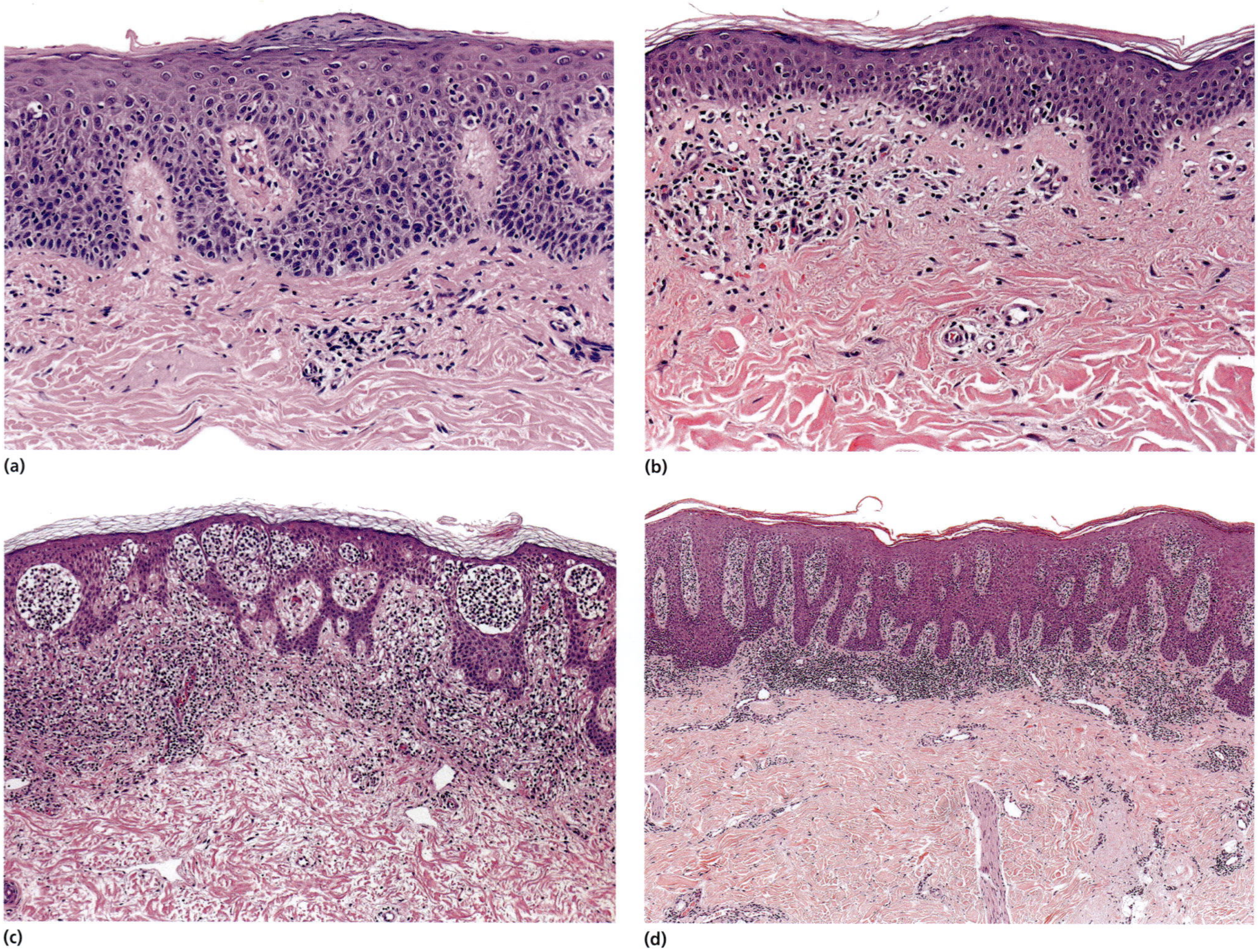

**Figure 3.30** Variable histopathologic features of early mycosis fungoides. (a) Several intraepidermal lymphocytes without Darier nests. (b) Sparse infiltrate with some intraepidermal lymphocytes. (c) Epidermotropism of lymphocytes with several, large Darier nests. (d) Pagetoid epidermotropism characterized by hyperplastic epidermis with innumerous intraepidermal lymphocytes. Presence of many, large Darier nests or of pagetoid epidermotropism is unusual in early mycosis fungoides.

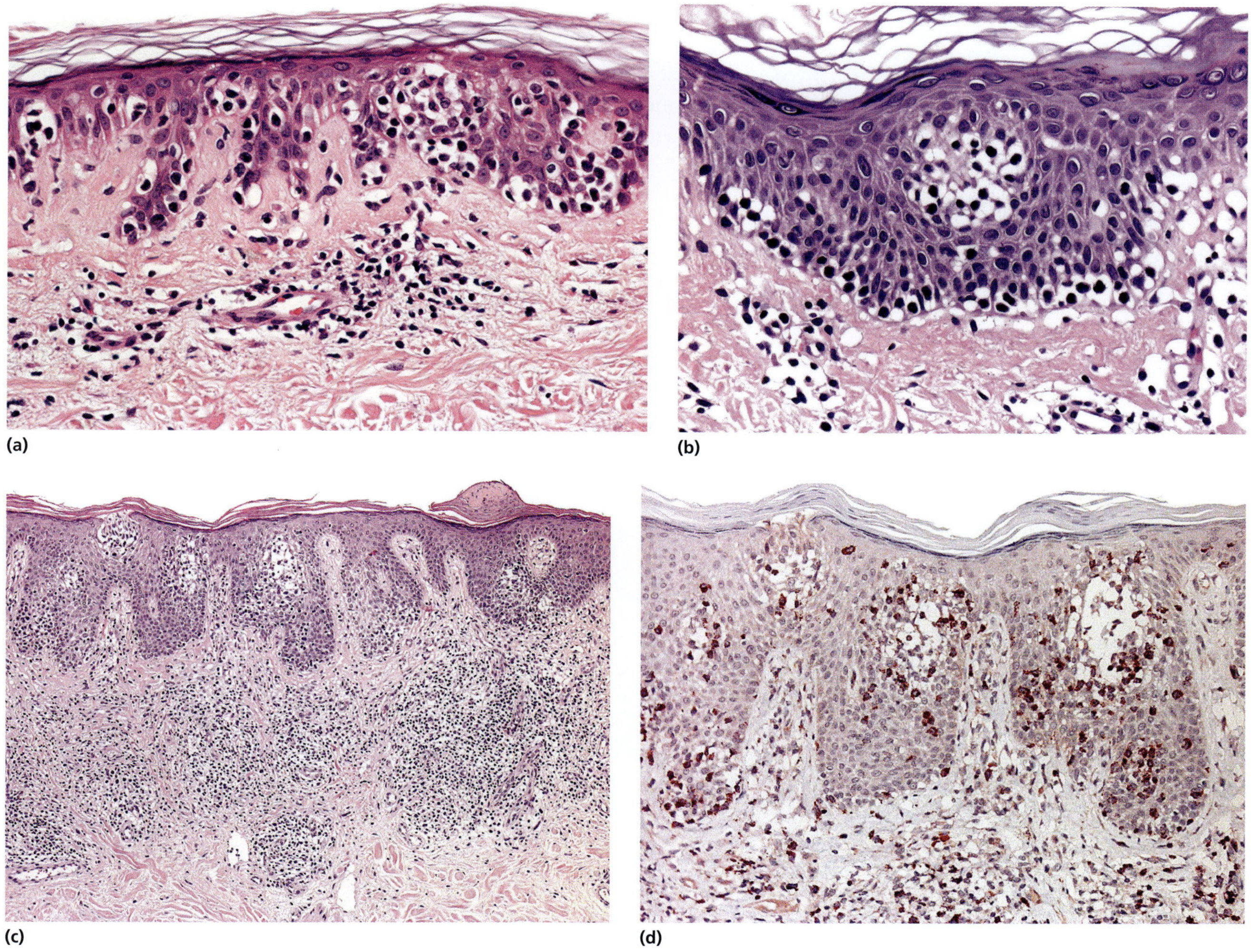

Figure 3.31 Histopathologic features of early mycosis fungoides. (a) Epidermotropic lymphocytes with nuclei larger than those of the lymphocytes within the superficial dermis. Note also lymphocytes with a clear halo around the nuclei ("haloed lymphocytes"). (b) Epidermotropism of lymphocytes aligned along the basal layer of the epidermis ("basilar epidermotropism"). (c) "Disproportionate" epidermotropism (presence of many intraepidermal lymphocytes on the background of epidermal spongiosis). (d) Staining for CD3 (or other pan T-cell markers) allows a better visualization of the intraepidermal lymphocytes in cases with a spongiotic pattern.

A pattern characterized by a markedly flattened epidermis, a lichenoid infiltrate in the dermis, and increased, dilated vessels in the papillary dermis is the histopathologic counterpart of poikilodermatous mycosis fungoides (see the specific section in this chapter). In rare cases subcorneal neutrophils may be prominent (in the absence of a secondary epidermomycosis), and may be related to a pustular appearance clinically (Fig. 3.39). Although edema is considered not typical of mycosis fungoides and, when present, is often used to "rule out" the disease, cases with edema in the superficial dermis can be observed, and presence of prominent edema cannot be considered diagnostic of inflammatory conditions (Fig. 3.40). Finally, in some patients the histopathological features may resemble those observed in pityriasis lichenoides and varioliformis acuta (PLEVA) (see the specific section in this chapter). This last pattern is found more frequently, but not exclusively, in children.

Finally, I have observed in several cases a histopathological pattern characterized by hyperplastic epidermis with many epidermotropic lymphocytes arranged as solitary units and/or along the basal membrane, and by only sparse superficial dermal infiltrates (Fig. 3.41). Minimal or absent spongiosis allows differentiation from an eczematous dermatitis, but correlation with the clinical picture is crucial in order to establish the correct diagnosis. This pattern can be observed irrespective of the size and distribution of the lesions (Fig. 3.42), and in my experience is not related to previous treatment. The epidermotropic lymphocytes in this cases may be better visualized by immunohistochemical staining for pan-T-cell markers.

Some histopathological features of early mycosis fungoides, namely, higher infiltrate density and depth, more large cells, and a higher proliferative index, have been linked to the subsequent development of tumors [110]. However, in my experience higher infiltrate density and depth, large cells, and a high proliferative index are not common features of *early* mycosis fungoides, and there are no histopathological aspects of early lesions that can be used reliably to predict the behavior of the disease in any given patient.

Plaques of mycosis fungoides are characterized by a dense, band-like infiltrate of lymphocytes within the upper dermis (Fig. 3.43). Epidermotropism shows the same pattern described for patches of the disease, but Daier's nests are more common (pagetoid epidermotropism, as for patches of mycosis fungoides, is uncommon and usually related to a cytotoxic phenotype). Cytomorphologically, small/medium pleomorphic (cerebriform) lymphocytes predominate (Fig. 3.44).

In tumors of mycosis fungoides a nodular or diffuse infiltrate is found within the entire dermis, usually involving the subcutaneous fat (Fig. 3.45). Epidermotropism may be lost. Flat tumors are characterized histopathologically by dense

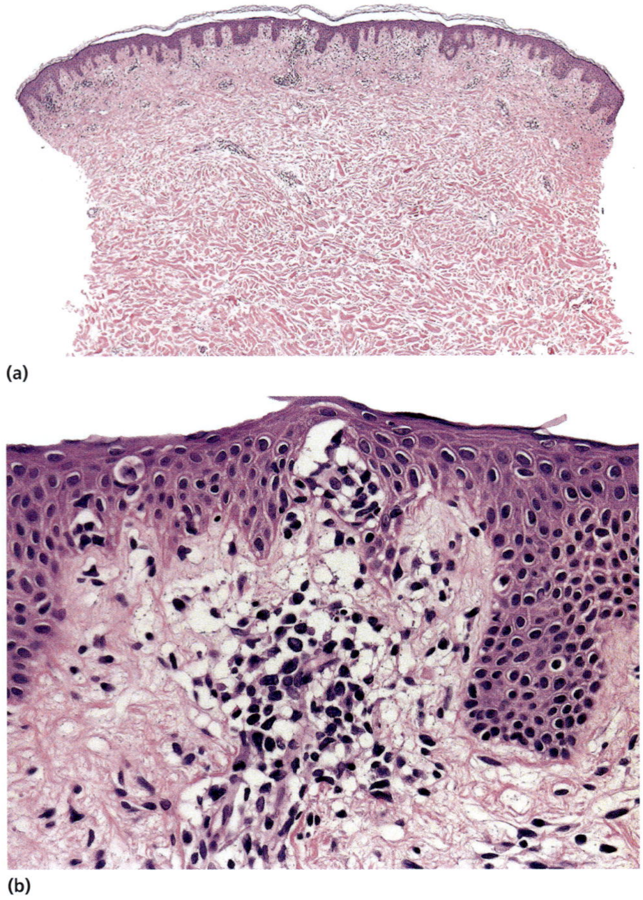

**Figure 3.32** Histopathologic features of early mycosis fungoides. (a) Sparse, superficial infiltrate with (b) only focally small aggregates of intraepidermal lymphocytes.

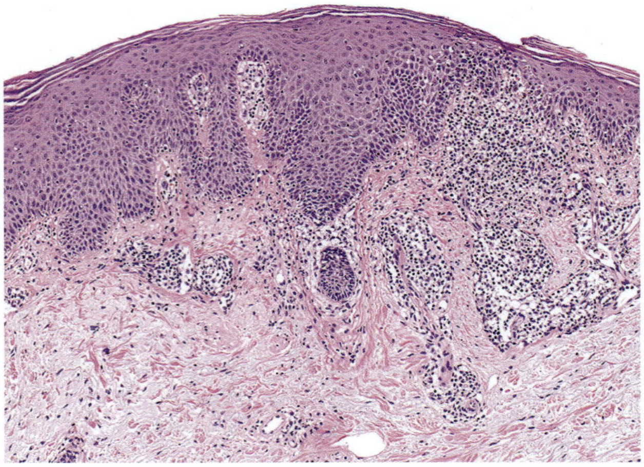

**Figure 3.34** Histopathologic features of early mycosis fungoides. Mostly perivascular, superficial infiltrate of lymphocytes with epidermotropism.

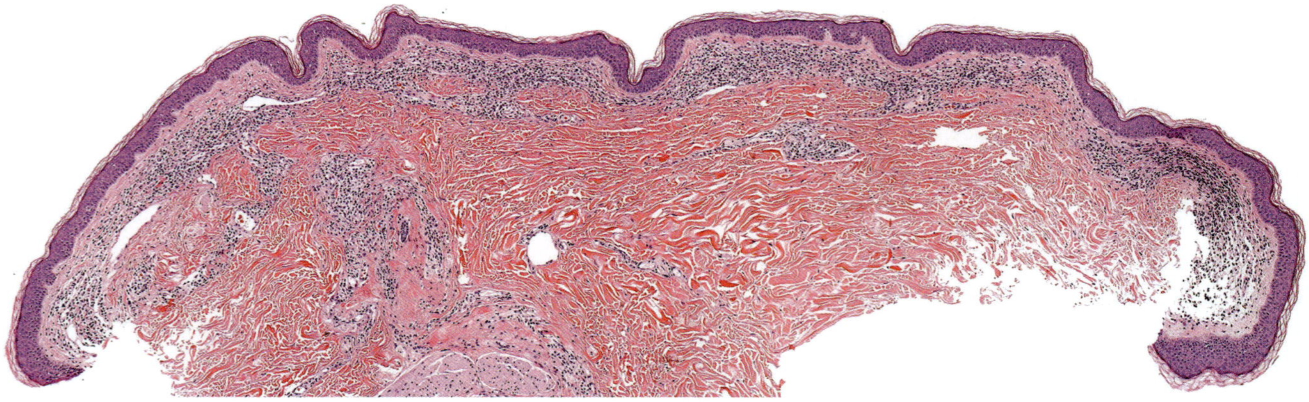

**Figure 3.33** Histopathologic features of early mycosis fungoides. Band-like infiltrate of lymphocytes in the papillary dermis without epidermotropism.

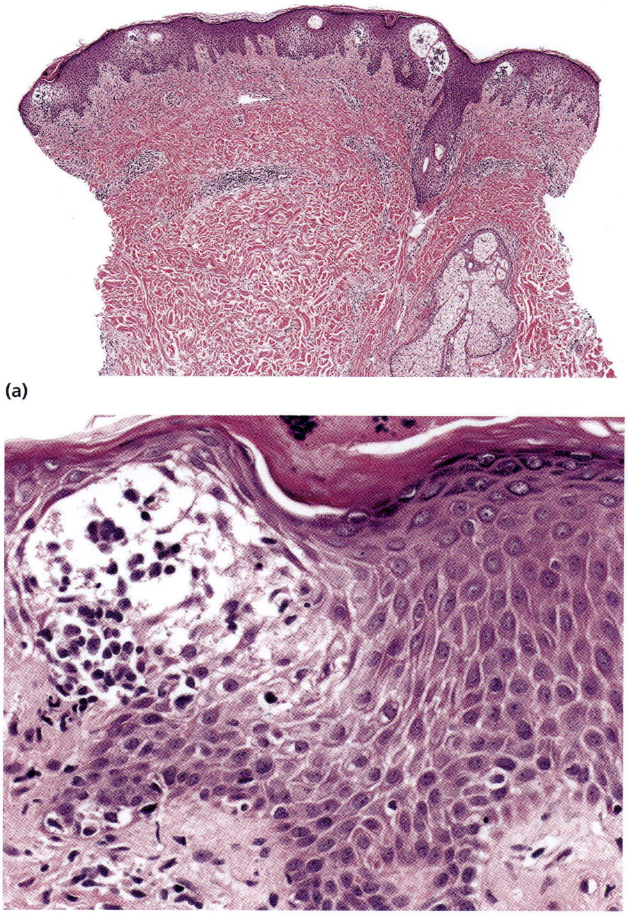

(a)

(b)

**Figure 3.35** Histopathologic features of early mycosis fungoides. (a) Psoriasiform hyperplasia of the epidermis with prominent spongiosis and spongiform vesicles. (b) Detail of a vesicle with several lymphocytes.

infiltrates confined to the superficial and mid parts of the dermis (Fig. 3.46). In some cases flat tumors of mycosis fungoides may present with a predominantly interstitial infiltrate (see the section on interstitial mycosis fungoides in this chapter). Prominent involvement of the subcutaneous fat may be observed in some cases (Fig. 3.47), as well as very rarely angiocentricity/angiodestruction (Fig. 3.48). It should be underlined that tumors of mycosis fungoides are morphologically indistinguishable from those of other types of primary or secondary cutaneous NK/T-cell lymphoma.

Neurotropism can be rarely observed in tumors of mycosis fungoides (Fig. 3.49) [111]; in my experience this is a rare finding, and is not related to a possible involvement of the central nervous system. Xanthomatous infiltrates have been observed in tumor-stage mycosis fungoides after treatment with brentuximab vedotin [112], but the significance of this finding, if any, is unclear.

### Large cell transformation

In advanced stages, patients with mycosis fungoides may develop lesions with many large cells (immunoblasts, large pleomorphic cells, or large anaplastic cells) (Fig. 3.50) [113, 114]. Large cell transformation in mycosis fungoides is defined as the presence of large cells exceeding 25% of the infiltrate or of large cells forming microscopic nodules, and has been detected in more than 50% of patients with tumor-stage mycosis fungoides [113]. Clusters of large cells may sometimes be observed in plaques of mycosis fungoides (usually in patients having tumors at other sites of the body), and rarely even in patches of the disease (these patients, too, usually also have plaques and tumors of mycosis fungoides at other sites of the body) (Fig. 3.51). Large cell transformation may be rarely observed also in long-standing lesions of solitary mycosis fungoides (Fig. 3.52). A high Ki-67 index and positivity for p53 have been reported as useful in confirming large cell transformation in mycosis fungoides [115]. However, large cell transformation should be diagnosed exclusively according to the histopathological-morphological features described above.

Tumors with a large cell morphology may or may not express CD30. Negativity for CD30 has been related to a poor prognosis in transformed mycosis fungoides [116], but this finding is questionable (see section on prognosis). Mycosis fungoides with large cell transformation and CD30 expression should be distinguished from cutaneous anaplastic large cell lymphoma and lymphomatoid papulosis [117, 118]. Spontaneous regression of some lesions and/or CD30 expression by neoplastic cells may suggest the diagnosis of anaplastic large cell lymphoma or lymphomatoid papulosis in these patients, but such a diagnosis should be made only upon compelling evidence in patients with known mycosis fungoides. In this context, most cases of mycosis fungoides with $CD30^+$ large cell transformation are negative for IRF4 translocations, whereas primary cutaneous large cell anaplastic lymphomas are positive [119–121]. In addition, the percentage of $CD30^+$ cells rarely reaches the 75% mark necessary for a diagnosis of anaplastic large cell lymphoma [116, 117]. Multiple myeloma-1/interferon regulatory factor-4 (MUM1/IRF4), a member of the interferon regulatory factor (IRF) family of transcription factors, is positive in cutaneous $CD30^+$ lymphoproliferative disorders and in $CD30^+$ large cell transformation of mycosis fungoides, but it is otherwise negative in mycosis fungoides. Although lymphomatoid papulosis may be associated with mycosis fungoides, the highest degree of caution should be exercised in making this diagnosis when mycosis fungoides precedes the putative lymphomatoid papulosis. In fact, one patient with mycosis fungoides whom we published several years ago as "PUVA-induced lymphomatoid papulosis in mycosis fungoides" [122] turned out to have a $CD30^+$ large cell transformation with bad prognosis, and similar patients have been described as well [123, 124]. Large cell transformation of mycosis fungoides bears a poor prognosis and usually heralds the terminal stage of the disease, but I have observed rare cases with prolonged survival (>10 years).

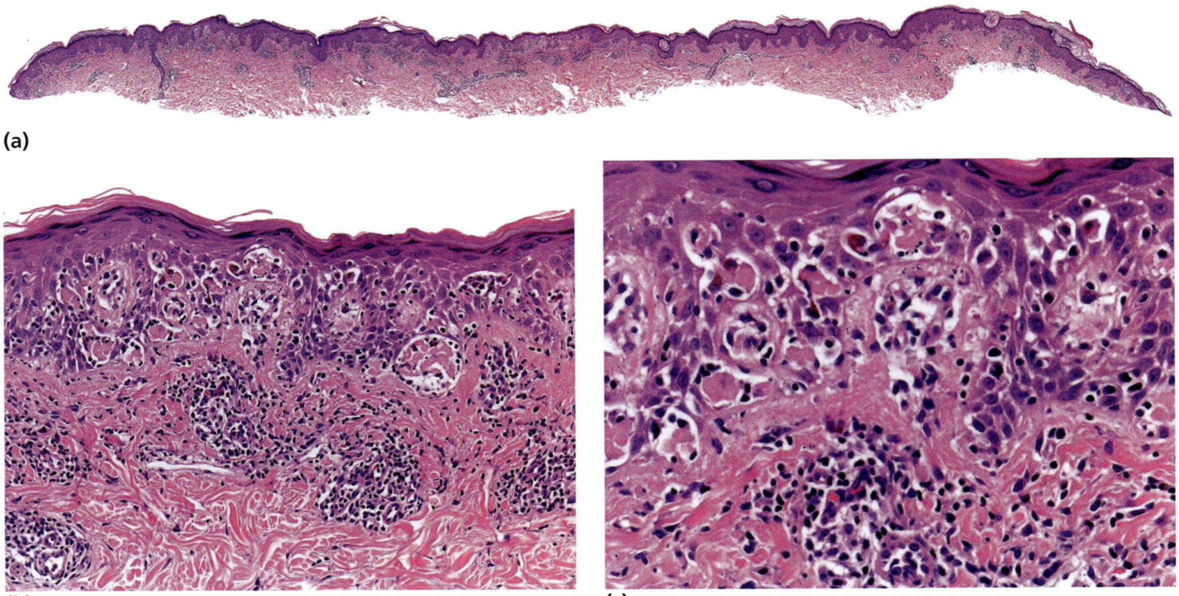

(a) (b) (c)

**Figure 3.36** Mycosis fungoides. (a) Patchy-lichenoid superficial infiltrate with focal epidermotropism of lymphocytes and with (b, c) many necrotic keratinocytes mimicking the pattern of erythema multiforme; note the epidermotropic lymphocytes.

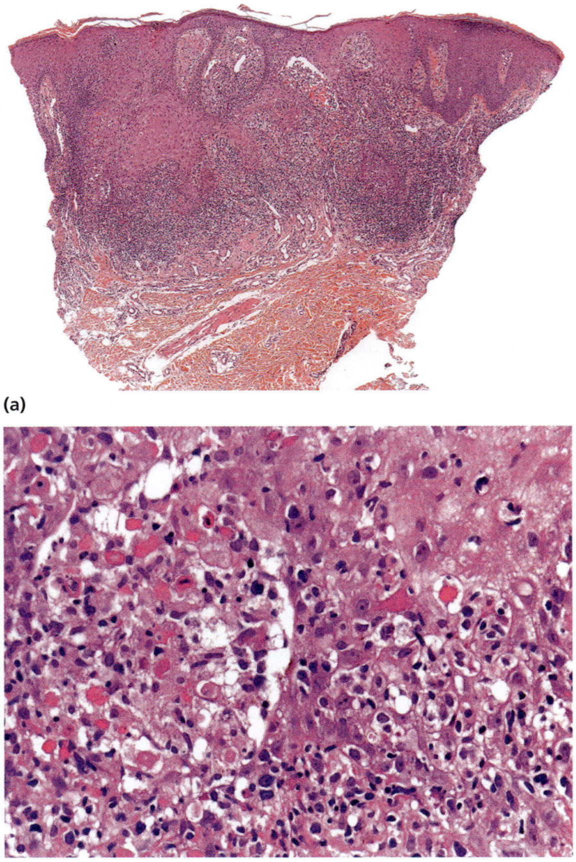

(a) (b)

**Figure 3.37** Mycosis fungoides. (a) Irregular, pseudoepitheliomatous epidermal hyperplasia mimicking lichen simplex chronicus and dense, superficial lymphoid infiltrates. (b) Cluster of necrotic keratinocytes admixed with epidermotropic lymphocytes.

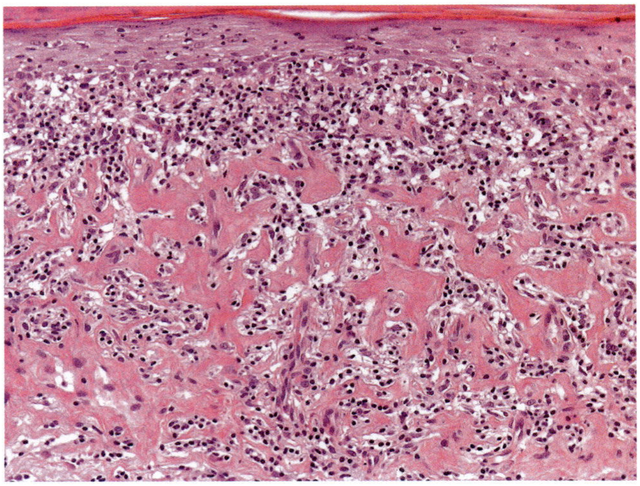

**Figure 3.38** Mycosis fungoides. Prominent sclerosis of the papillary dermis and infiltrate of lymphocytes with epidermotropism mimicking the histopathologic pattern of lichen sclerosus.

## Immunophenotype

Mycosis fungoides is characterized by an infiltrate of $\alpha/\beta$ T-helper memory lymphocytes ($\beta F1^+$, $TCR\gamma^-$, $TCR\delta^-$, $CD3^+$, $CD4^+$, $CD5^+$, $CD8^-$, $CD45Ro^+$, TIA-$1^-$) (Fig. 3.53). Only a minority of cases exhibit a T-cytotoxic ($\beta F1^+$, $TCR\gamma^-$, $TCR\delta^-$, $CD3^+$, $CD4^-$, $CD5^+$, $CD8^+$, TIA-$1^+$) (Fig. 3.54) or $\gamma/\delta$ T-cell phenotype ($\beta F1^-$, $TCR\gamma^+$, $TCR\delta^+$, $CD3^+$, $CD4^-$, $CD5^+$, $CD8^+$, TIA-$1^+$) (Fig. 3.55), which show no clinical and/or prognostic differences [125–127]. In these cases, correlation with the clinical features is crucial, in order to rule out skin involvement by aggressive cytotoxic lymphomas such as cutaneous aggressive

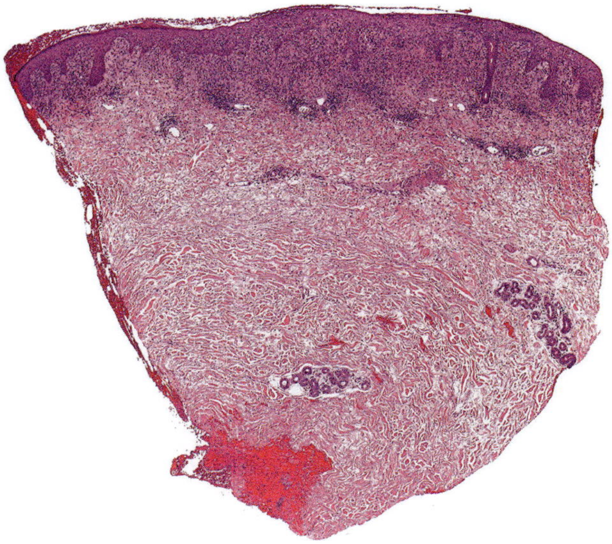

(a)

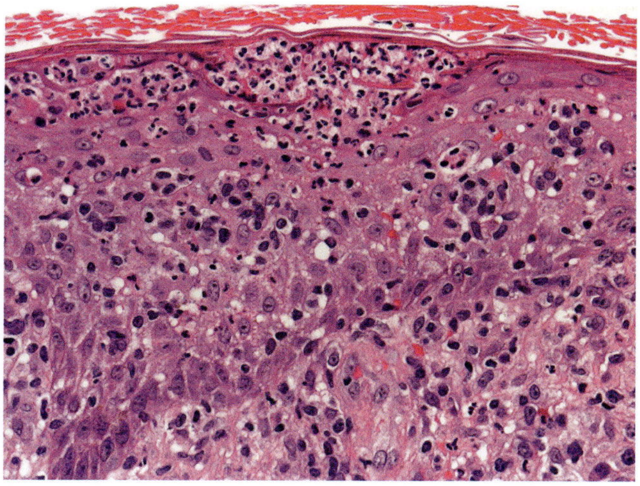

(b)

Figure 3.39 Mycosis fungoides. (a) Band-like infiltrate of lymphocytes with (b) many epidermotropic lymphocytes and prominent subcorneal collections of neutrophils.

epidermotropic CD8$^+$ cytotoxic T-cell lymphoma or cutaneous γ/δ T-cell lymphoma (see also Chapter 7).

Positivity for the C-C chemokine receptor 4 (CCR4) is found in a subset of cases with either helper or cytotoxic phenotype, and may be exploited for specific therapy [128, 129].

In late stages there may be a (partial) loss of pan-T-cell antigens (CD2, CD3, CD5) and/or CD4/CD8 expression (Fig. 3.56). Loss of pan-T-cell markers is a helpful sign for the diagnosis of mycosis fungoides (and of T-cell lymphomas in general), but in my experience it is very rare in early lesions of the disease. Rarely, early mycosis fungoides displays an aberrant CD4$^+$/CD8$^+$ or CD4$^-$/CD8$^-$ phenotype (double positivity or double negativity is less infrequent in advanced lesions) [130, 131]. Double negative cases may be positive for PD-1 [132]. Although this molecule is considered a marker of follicular helper T-cells (TFH), it is not specific for these cells [133]. In mycosis fungoides, the amount of PD-1$^+$ cells is smaller than in Sézary syndrome [134, 135], but staining for PD-1 alone cannot be considered reliable for distinguishing mycosis fungoides from Sèzary syndrome. Some cases show the complete phenotype of TFH cells (PD-1$^+$, Bcl-6$^+$, CXCL13$^+$, CD10$^+$) (Fig. 3.57) [136–139], and a TFH phenotype has been observed also in biopsies showing large cell transformation [140].

Cytotoxic-associated markers such as T-cell intracellular antigen (TIA)-1, granzyme B, and perforin are negative in mycosis fungoides (with the obvious exception of cases with cytotoxic phenotype). In cases that displayed previously a conventional T-helper phenotype, sometimes biopsies of tumor lesions may reveal positivity for cytotoxic proteins [141], even in some biopsies in which the CD4-positivity is retained (Fig. 3.58). These cases should not be classified as cytotoxic lymphoma, but as tumor-stage mycosis fungoides with a cytotoxic phenotype. Cases with a cytotoxic phenotype may also express CD56 [142], but CD56-positivity has been observed rarely also in specimens of otherwise conventional CD4$^+$ mycosis fungoides [143]. Besides expression of cytotoxic granules, sequential biopsies of mycosis fungoides may show a phenotypic switch with expression of different markers, sometimes even in biopsies taken from different lesions at the same time [144–146]. This is particularly important when evaluating phenotypic features of biomarkers relevant for therapy, as a marked variability of expression may be observed in different biopsies [147].

As already mentioned, in plaque and tumor lesions (and rarely focally in patches, too) neoplastic T-cells may express the CD30 antigen (Fig. 3.59). It has been suggested that a higher expression of CD30 in non-transformed mycosis fungoides is associated with a worse prognosis [148]. On the other hand, CD30-negativity has been linked with a worse prognosis in transformed mycosis fungoides [116]. In my opinion, it is conceptually difficult to conceive of a marker that is associated with both good and bad prognoses depending only on the type of lesion where it is detected (transformed versus non-transformed, respectively), and I think that the prognostic value of CD30 expression (or lack of expression) should be critically considered. In addition, variability in expression has been detected in different biopsies taken at the same time [147, 149], thus showing that CD30 expression, or lack of it, may be due at least in part to a sampling problem. In this context, as anti-CD30 treatment with brentuximab vedotin is an option for tumor stage mycosis fungoides, biopsies should be performed from multiple lesions, as a single skin biopsy might lead to misinterpretation of CD30 with risk of inadequate therapeutic decisions [149].

Aberrant expression of the B-cell antigen CD20 by neoplastic T lymphocytes has been observed exceptionally [150, 151] and

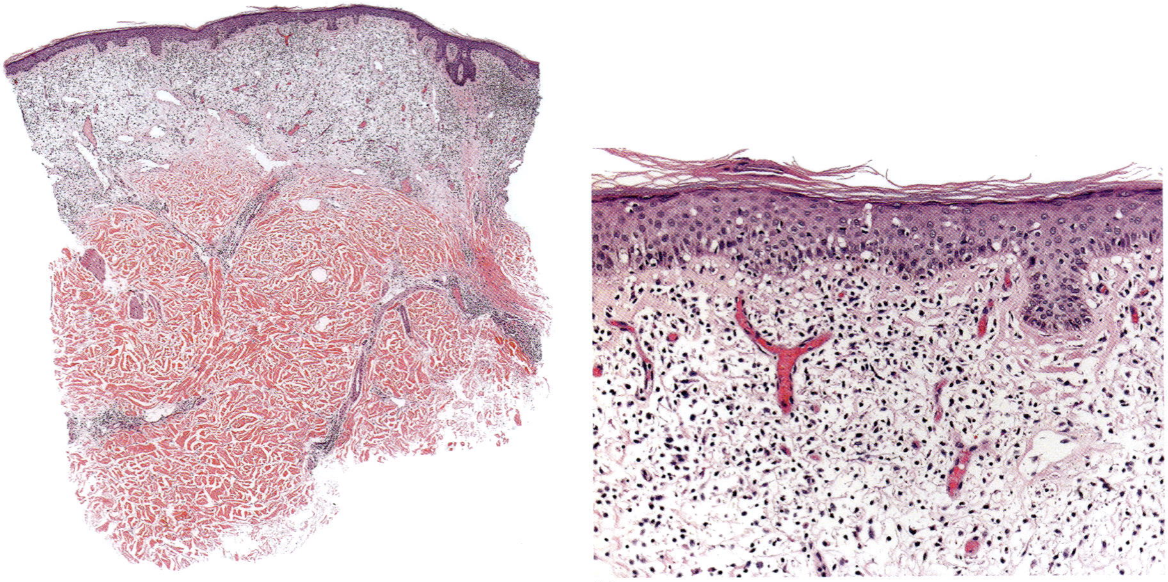

(a) (b)

**Figure 3.40** Mycosis fungoides. (a) Widely expanded, edematous papillary dermis with a band-like lymphoid infiltrate and (b) a few intraepidermal lymphocytes in a patient with a long history of mycosis fungoides and in the absence of specific treatment (refused by the patient).

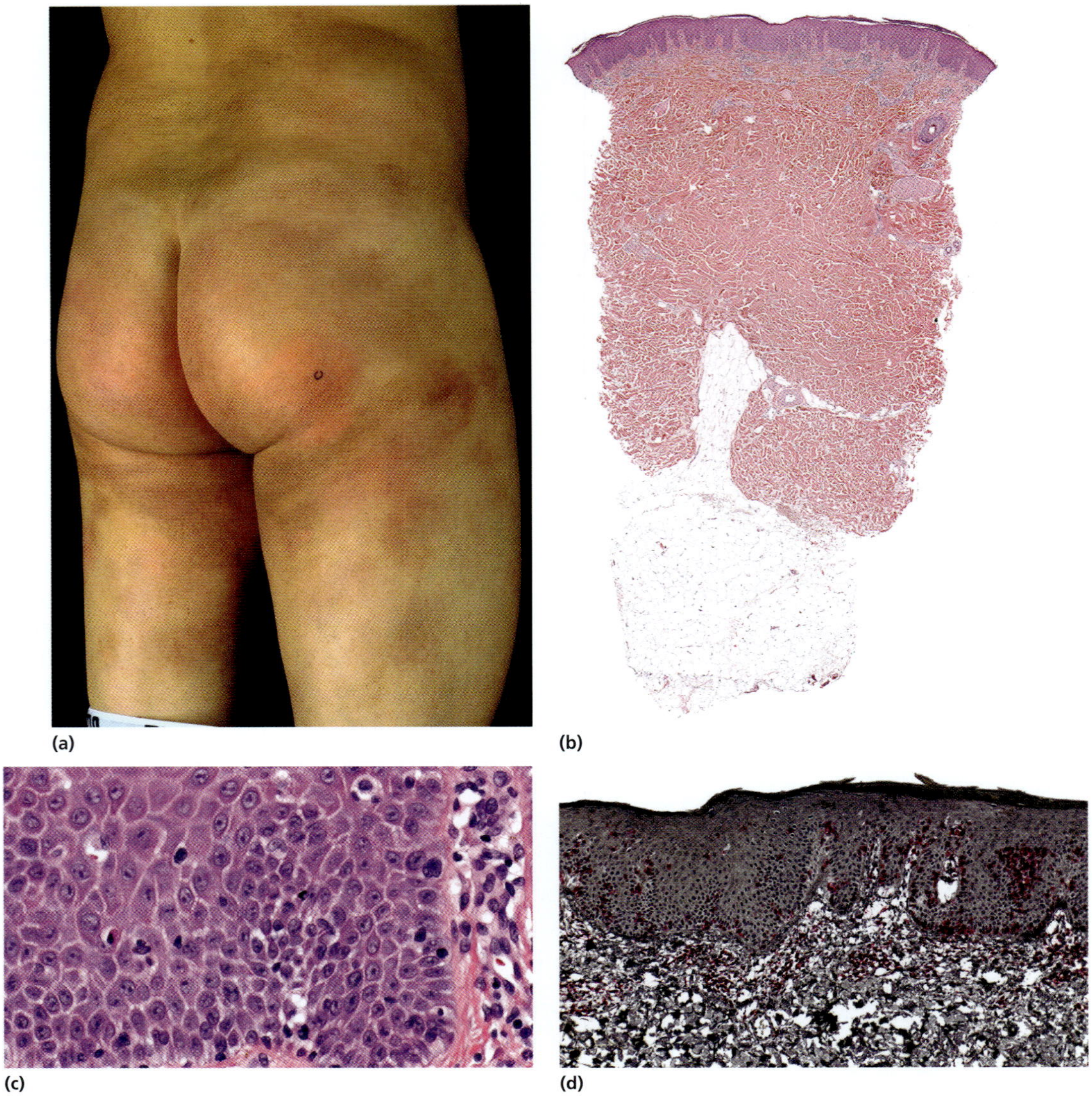

(a) (b) (c) (d)

**Figure 3.41** Mycosis fungoides. (a) Confluent erythematous-livid patches on the buttocks and thighs. (b) Histopathologically, hyperplastic epidermis with (c) several epidermotropic lymphocytes arranged as solitary units. (d) Staining for CD3 allows to better visualize the epidermotropic lymphocytes.

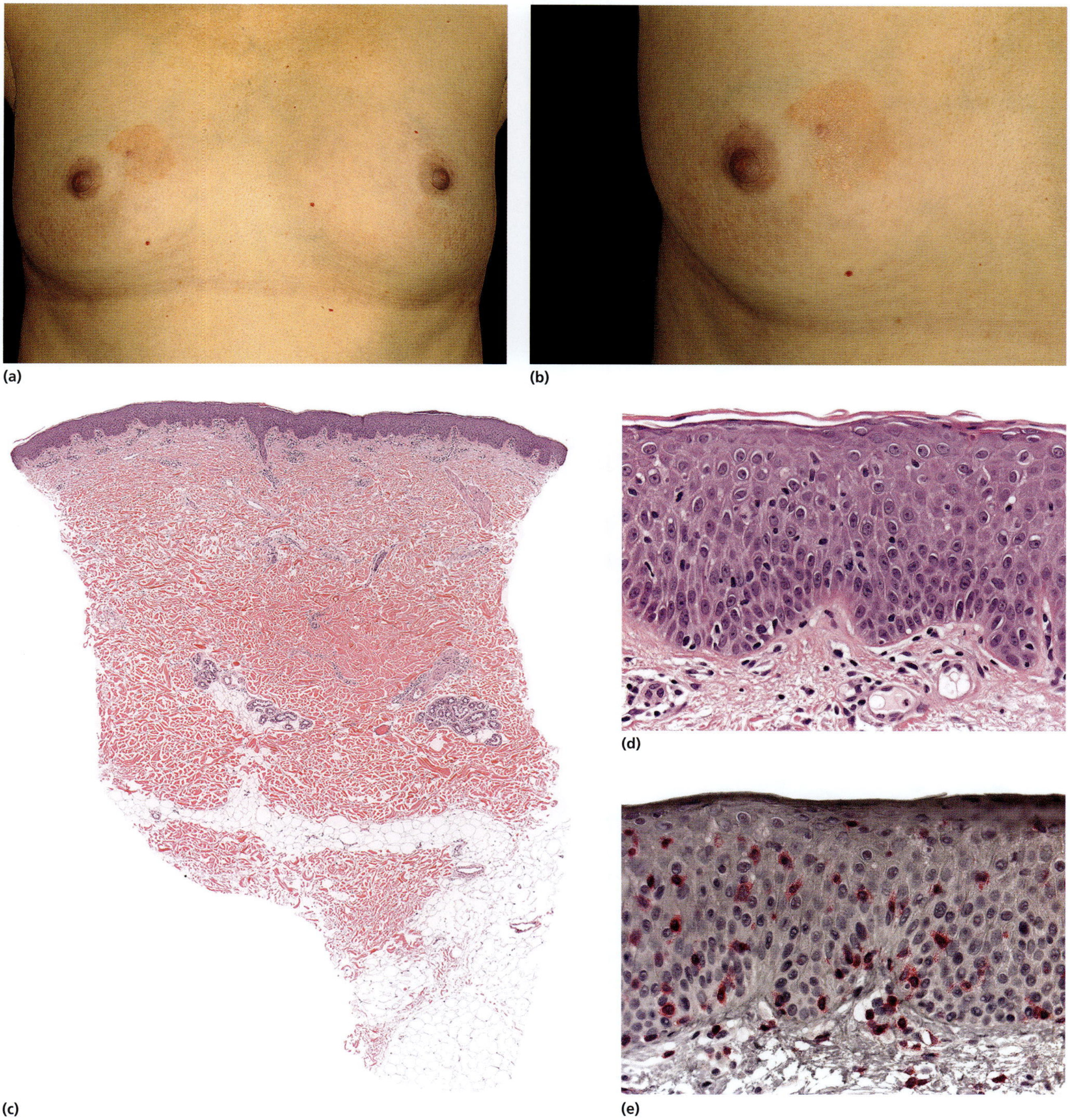


Figure 3.42 Mycosis fungoides. (a, b) Small erythematous patches on the breast. (c) Histopathologically, hyperplastic epidermis with (d) several intraepidermal lymphocytes arranged as solitary units. (e) Staining for CD3 allows to better visualize the epidermotropic lymphocytes.

seems to be more frequent in large cell transformation [152]. In these cases, negativity for other B-cell markers such as CD79a or PAX-5 and positivity for T-cell markers helps in determining the exact lineage of the cells.

T-regulatory (T*reg*) cells comprise a T-cell population that can influence other cell types with suppression of the immune response, and that shows mostly a $CD4^+/CD25^+/FOX\text{-}P3^+$ phenotype. In contrast to previous findings, studying sequential lesions of patients with mycosis fungoides, we could not find a significant difference in the percentage of T*reg* cells between patch/plaque and tumor stage biopsies, nor any association with prognosis [153], and other cases with conventional behavior

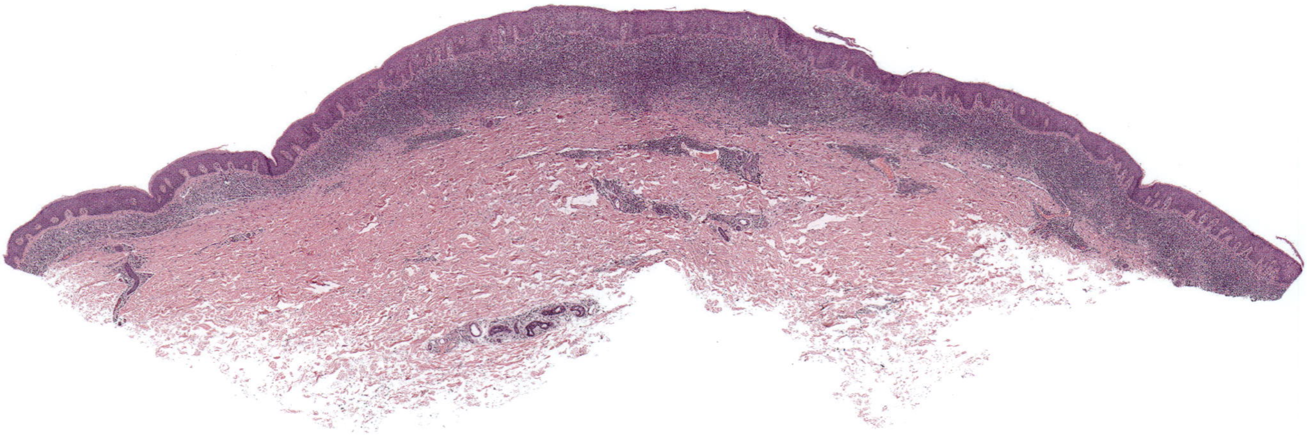

Figure 3.43 Mycosis fungoides, plaque stage. Dense band-like lymphoid infiltrate involving the papillary and superficial part of reticular dermis.

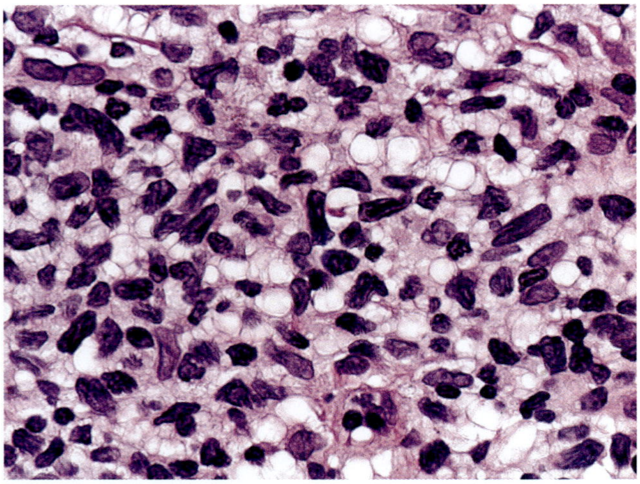

Figure 3.44 Mycosis fungoides, plaque stage. Cytomorphology of a plaque reveals predominance of small- and mid-sized pleomorphic lymphocytes.

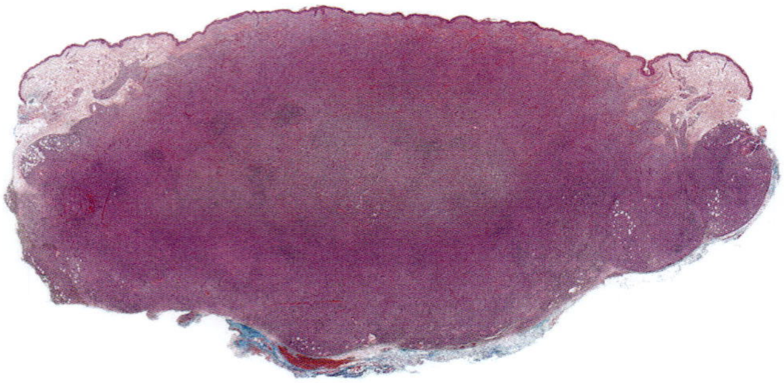

(a)

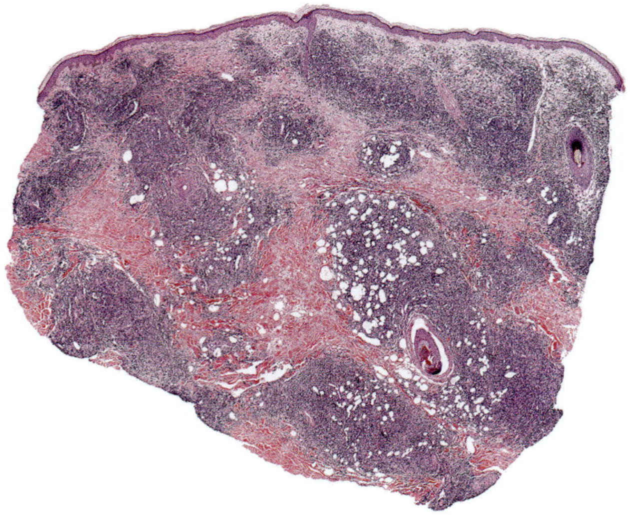

(b)

Figure 3.45 Mycosis fungoides, tumor stage. (a) Dense, diffuse lymphoid infiltrates replacing the entire dermis and subcutaneous fat. (b) Dense nodular infiltrates within the entire dermis.

have been reported as well [154]. Additionally, neoplastic lymphocytes with the phenotype of T*reg* cells can be observed in mycosis fungoides (Fig. 3.60) [153, 155]. It has been suggested that the number of intraepidermal FOX-P3$^+$ cells is higher in inflammatory conditions than in mycosis fungoides [156], but I would exert the greatest caution in using this criterion for the differential diagnosis of early mycosis fungoides.

An increased number of CD1a$^+$ Langerhans cells as well as of other, mostly immature dendritic cells can be observed in mycosis fungoides, particularly in non-tumoral lesions [157, 158a]. An increased number of Langerhans cells may be observed both in the dermal component of the infiltrate (Fig. 3.61) and within the epidermis, sometimes mimicking the histopathologic features of Langerhans cell histiocytosis (Fig. 3.62). These clusters represent most likely a reactive hyperplasia of Langerhans cells. To my eyes, cases reported as "concomitant" mycosis fungoides and Langerhans cell histiocytosis represent marked Langerhans cell hyperplasia rather than genuine Langerhans cell histiocytosis [158b]. In this context, it should be remembered that the occurrence of clonally related dendritic or histiocytic tumors has been observed rarely in

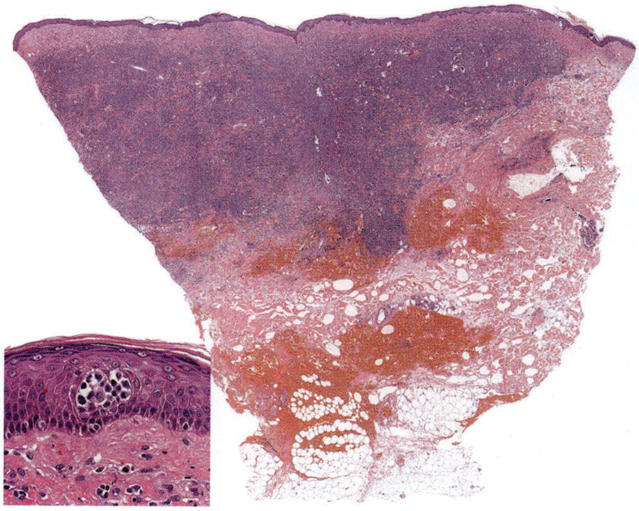

Figure 3.46 Mycosis fungoides, histopathologic features of a flat tumor. "Top-heavy," dense lymphoid infiltrates within the dermis. Note focal epidermotropism (inset).

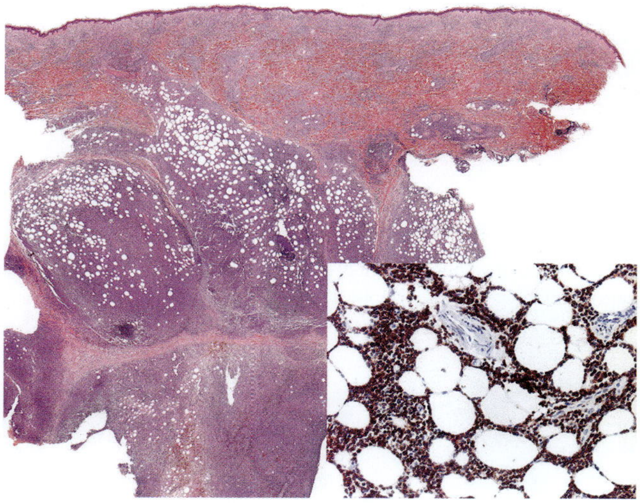

Figure 3.47 Mycosis fungoides with prominent involvement of the subcutaneous fat tissue. Both the density of the infiltrate, replacing the fat rather than mimicking the features of a lobular panniculitis, and the involvement of the dermis represent differential diagnostic clues from subcutaneous panniculitis-like T-cell lymphoma. However, in areas of fat involvement rimming of adipocytes is usually present (inset, staining for TCR-ß), indistinguishable from that observed in subcutaneous panniculitis-like T-cell lymphoma.

mature B-cell neoplasms (so-called "transdifferentiation" – see Chapter 1), but has never been described in mycosis fungoides. Although "Langerhans cell microabscesses" are considered as a differential diagnostic tool for lymphomatoid contact dermatitis (see Chapter 31), they can be rarely observed in mycosis fungoides as well. The number of Langerhans cells and other dendritic cell populations varies according to the stage, suggesting that changes in the microenvironment of mycosis fungoides occur during the course of the disease [159].

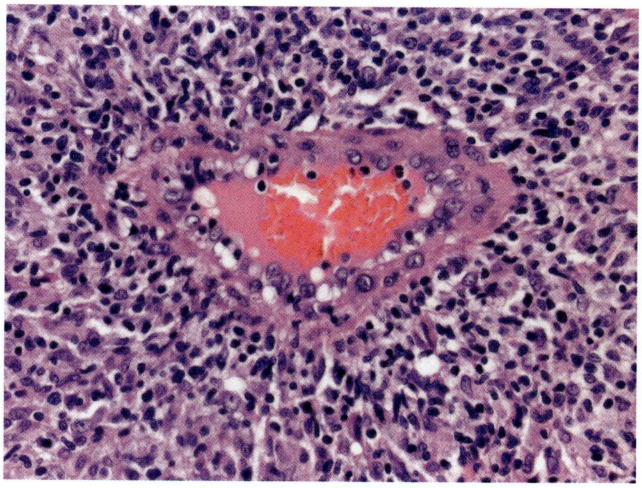

Figure 3.48 Mycosis fungoides with angiocentricity and angiotropic lymphocytes.

Lesions of mycosis fungoides, particularly in advanced stages, may show a prominent amount of reactive $CD20^+$ B lymphocytes, even forming germinal centers (Fig. 3.63) [160–162]. The B lymphocytes may be prominent and mask the true T-cell nature of the neoplastic infiltrate. These cases should not be misinterpreted as B-cell lymphoma. On the other hand, it should be kept in mind that exceptional cases of composite lymphoma (mycosis fungoides and a primary cutaneous B-cell lymphoma within the same lesion) have been observed [89]. B-cell lymphomas composite with mycosis fungoides are mostly cases of B-cell chronic lymphocytic leukemia (B-CLL) colonizing the lesions of mycosis fungoides (see Chapter 28) [163, 164]. As already mentioned, CD20 may also be expressed aberrantly by neoplastic T lymphocytes, thus underlining the need for complete phenotypic analyses of every case.

## Molecular genetics

A monoclonal rearrangement of the T-cell receptor (TCR) genes is commonly found in plaques and tumors of mycosis fungoides. Using a sensitive technique (Biomed-2), the majority (>80%) of patch lesions also show monoclonality of T lymphocytes. Next generation sequencing (NGS), known also as "high-throughput sequencing" has been proposed as a more reliable method for analysis of T-cell clonality [33, 165]. This technique offers indubitable advances over standard PCR protocols, providing also data on the quantity of neoplastic cells present in a given infiltrate. In an overview of published literature, sensitivity of NGS ranged between 69% and 100% (sensitivity of standard PCR methods was 44–72%), and specificity ranged between 86% and 100% (specificity of standard PCR methods was 77–88%) [166], thus showing an improvement in the

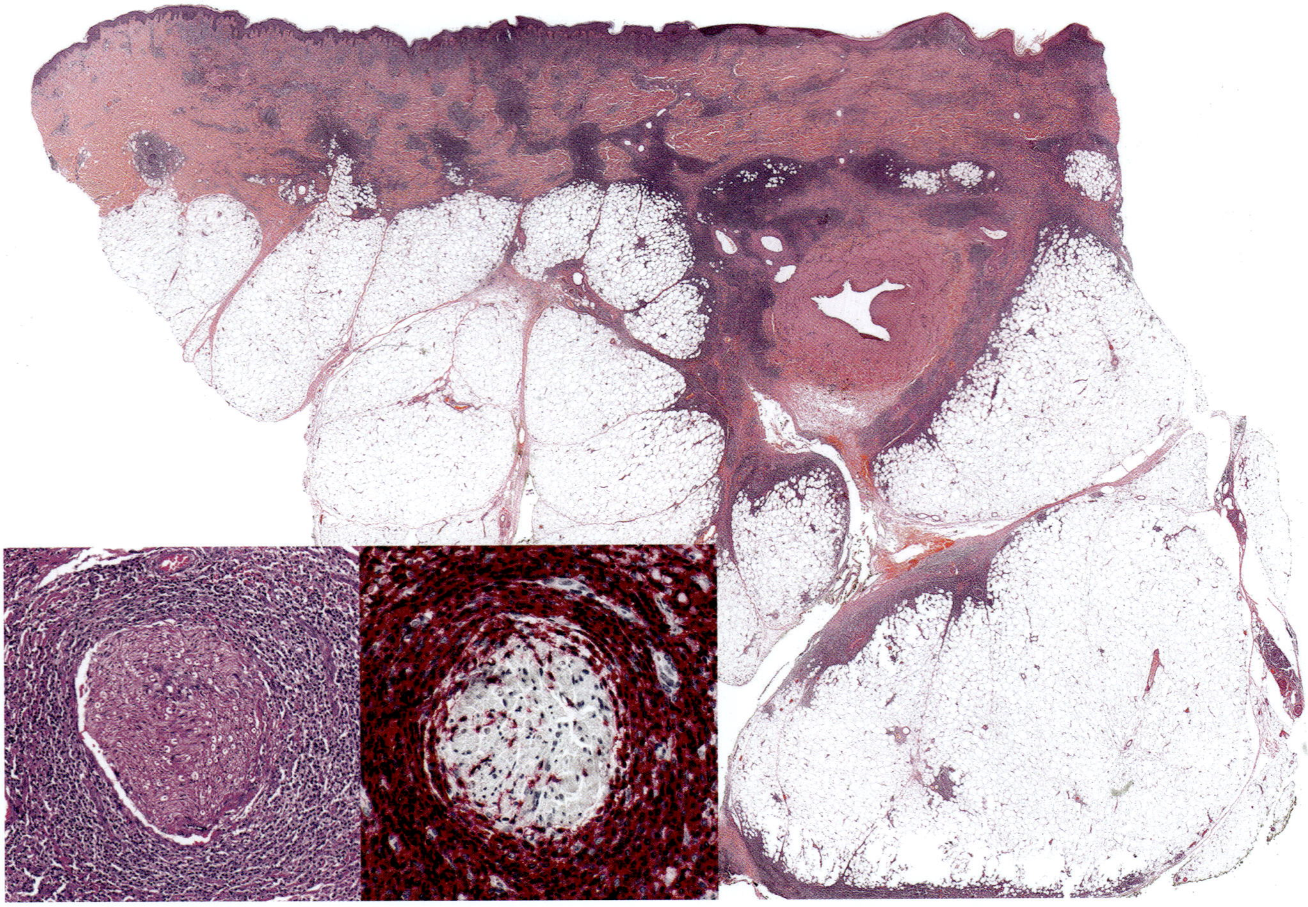

**Figure 3.49** Mycosis fungoides with neurotropism. Tumor stage mycosis fungoides with prominent involvement of the subcutaneous tissue; note the superficial band-like infiltrate. In the deeper part of the specimen several nerves are surrounded by dense lymphoid infiltrates (inset left). Staining for CD5 highlights neurotropic lymphocytes (inset right).

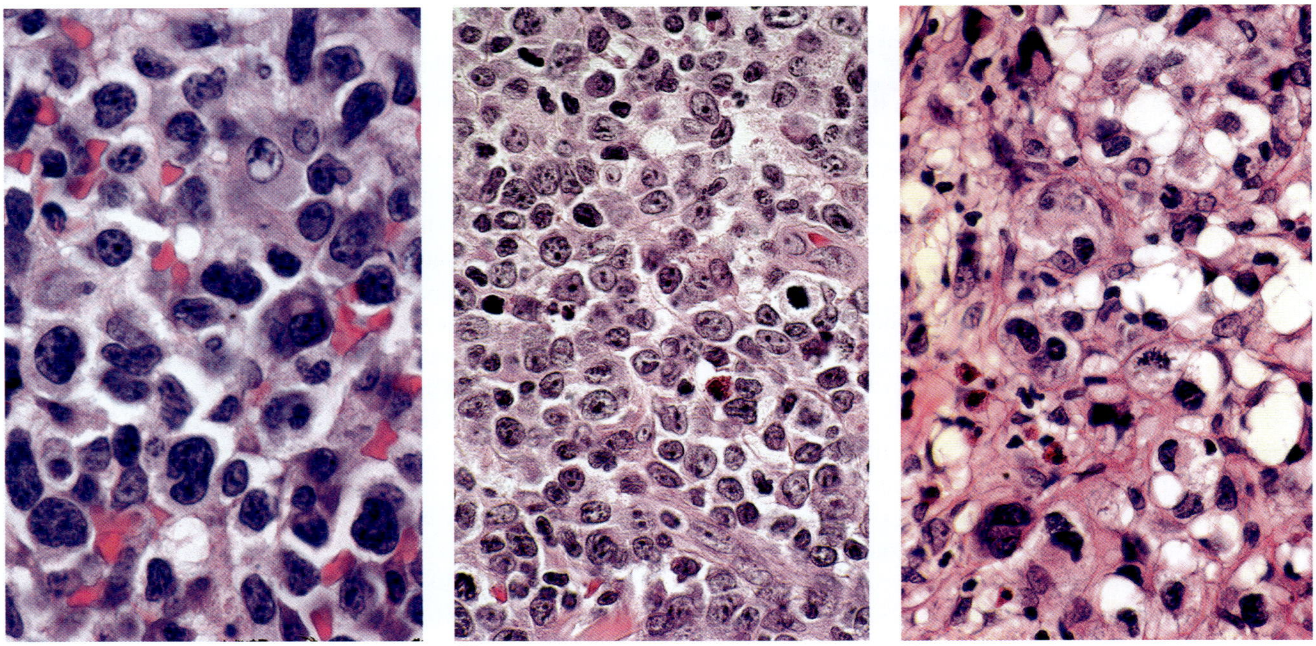

(a) (b) (c)

**Figure 3.50** Mycosis fungoides with large cell transformation. (a) Medium- and large-sized pleomorphic lymphocytes. (b) Immunoblasts admixed with reactive lymphocytes. (c) Large anaplastic cells admixed with pleomorphic cells and reactive lymphocytes.

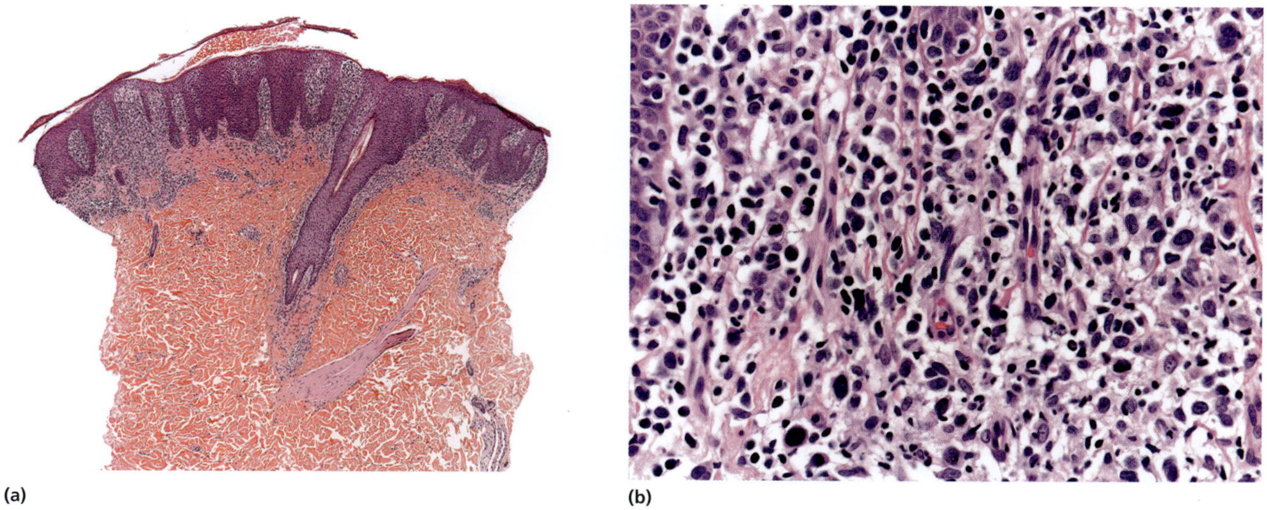

Figure 3.51 Mycosis fungoides with large cell transformation in a flat lesion. (a) Superficial band-like infiltrate of lymphocytes with prominent epidermotropism and Darier nests. (b) Cytomorphology reveals predominance of mid-sized and large, pleomorphic lymphocytes.

diagnostic utility compared to standard methods. On the other hand, data from non-lymphoma patients (i.e., patients with inflammatory conditions) are still scarce [167a, 167b], and the method is expensive and not yet widely accessible. Comprehensive whole-exome sequencing showed that the majority of the samples of mycosis fungoides presented multiple TCRγ, TCRα, and TCRβ clonotypes, suggesting that the initial malignant transformation may not occur in mature memory T cells but rather at the level of T-lymphocyte progenitors before TCRβ or TCRα rearrangements [168]. Single-cell gene expression profiling studies in advanced phases of the disease revealed a large inter- and intra-tumor gene expression heterogeneity, as well as a common gene expression signature in highly proliferating lymphocytes [169].

Demonstration of T-cell clonality with standard methods at the first diagnostic biopsy does not affect the prognosis of patients with early mycosis fungoides [125]. However, the tumor clone frequency in the skin, as detected by high-throughput sequencing, is an independent prognostic parameter (a tumor clone frequency of >25% was a strong predictor of progression) [170]. Development of "patient-specific" DNA probes can identify the neoplastic clone also in lesions that are not specific histopathologically [171], and may be a useful method (though not routinely available) for detection of residual disease.

The presence of a monoclonal population of T lymphocytes has been detected in the peripheral blood in patients with early-stage mycosis fungoides. In many of these patients, the clone was different from that detected within the skin, but in some cases the same clone was present both in the peripheral blood and in the cutaneous lesions of mycosis fungoides, even after successful treatment and complete clinical remission [47]. An older study by the French Group of Cutaneous Lymphomas suggested that the presence of an identical clone in the skin and blood is an independent prognostic factor in early mycosis fungoides [172]. However, as already mentioned, in the study by Joffe *et al.*, the finding of an identical clone in the blood and skin was not associated with a shorter time to systemic treatment [49]. The exact diagnostic and prognostic value of molecular genetic analysis of the TCR genes rearrangement within the peripheral blood in patients with early mycosis fungoides is still unclear. Detection of monoclonality within lymph nodes that are not affected clinically and/or histopathologically has been associated with a worse prognosis [173]. The analysis of the rearrangement of TCR genes in the peripheral blood and/or uninvolved lymph nodes is not part of routine investigations in early mycosis fungoides, but the determination of clonality is paramount in lymph nodes showing histopathologically the picture of dermopathic lymphadenopathy.

Interestingly, recent data demonstrated the monoclonal origin of malignant T cells in different skin lesions from a single patient, suggesting a multistep and parallel transformation model in which a single lymphocyte expands and seeds at different cutaneous sites long before the lesions are clinically detectable [174]. Parallel subclonal evolution occurs independently over time, resulting in the development of new skin lesions. Further onset of new lesions is due to multiple waves of dissemination of subclones, thus providing a possible explanation for the intra- and interlesional heterogeneity of mycosis fungoides, as well as for the difference in the therapeutic response of lesions located at different anatomical sites [174].

Several studies have addressed early genetic events in mycosis fungoides [175, 176], but results have been sometimes contradictory [177, 178]. Some of the differences may be related to the methods used, other to patients' selection and/or patients' number, still other may reflect the molecular heterogeneity of mycosis fungoides and other cutaneous T-cell lymphomas. In this context, it should be underlined that molecular analysis of early lesions of mycosis fungoides is hindered by the intrinsic difficulties in the identification of neoplastic cells, which are a small minority and may look morphologically and phenotypically identical to reactive lymphocytes. As genetic techniques,

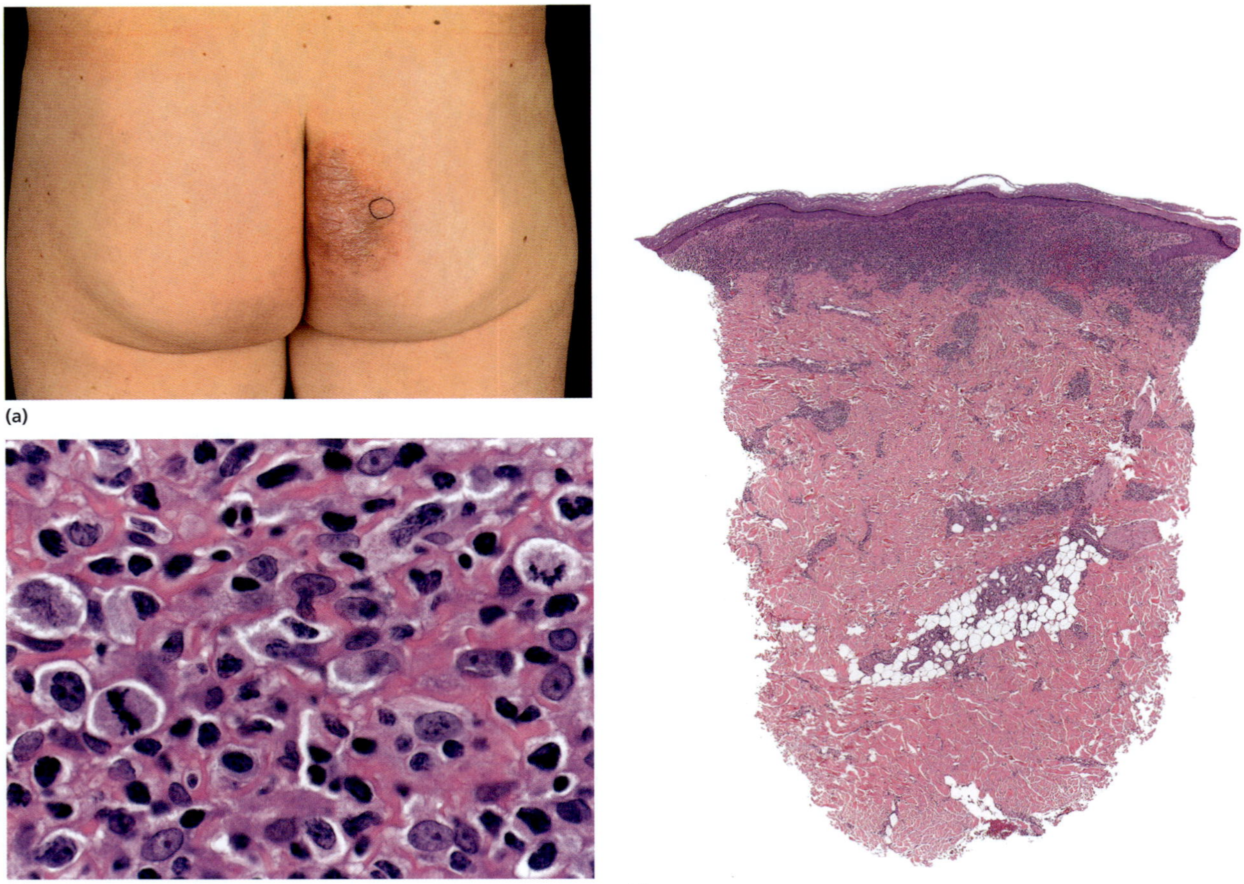
(a) (b) (c)

**Figure 3.52** Solitary mycosis fungoides of >10 years duration in a 46-year-old man. (a) Solitary plaque on the gluteal region. (b) Histology reveals a dense band-like infiltrate with focal hemorrhage and with (c) predominance of large, atypical lymphocytes (large cell transformation in a flat lesion).

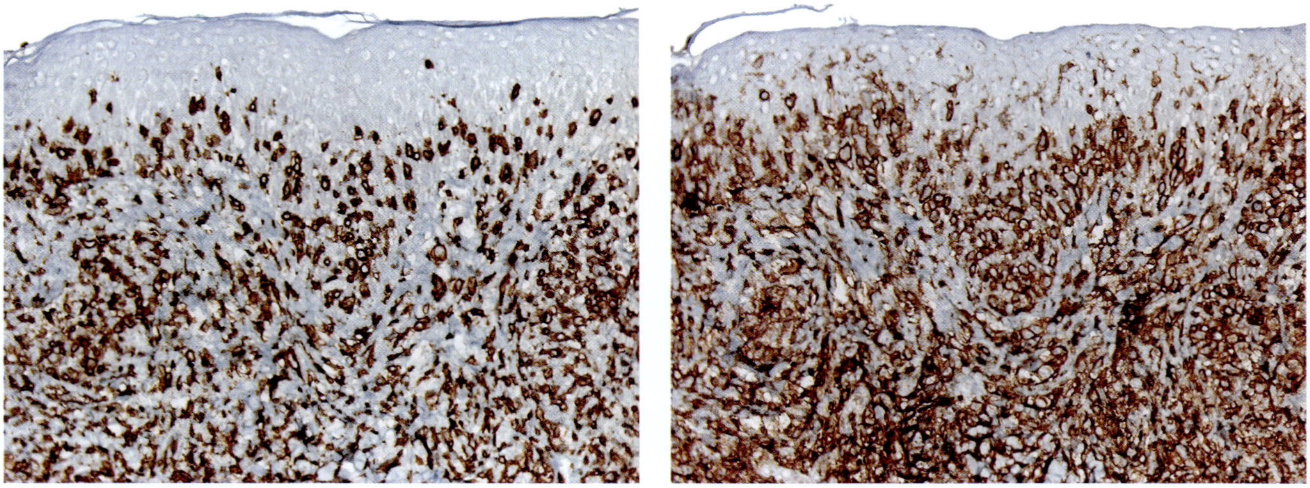
(a) (b)

**Figure 3.53** Mycosis fungoides. Positivity of neoplastic cells for (a) CD3 and (b) CD4. Note that CD4 also decorates some intraepidermal Langerhans cells.

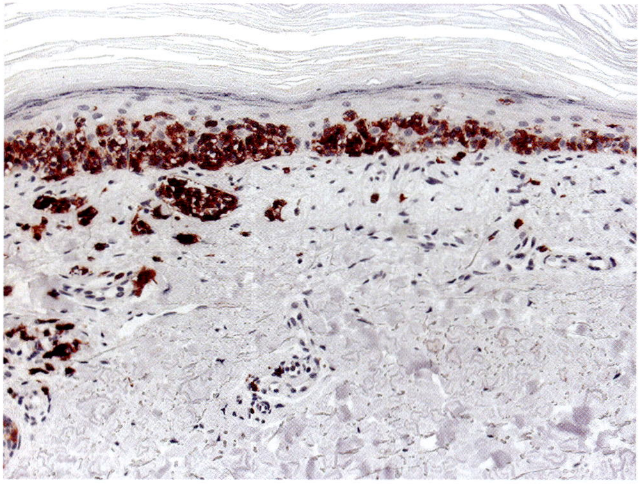

**Figure 3.54** Cytotoxic mycosis fungoides with neoplastic cells positive for CD8.

especially on routinely fixed specimens, require a certain threshold of tumor DNA, it may be difficult to analyze early lesions of mycosis fungoides where only a few neoplastic cells can be observed.

Genes regulating several key functions of the cells are altered in mycosis fungoides, including genes involved in cell cycle and apoptosis regulators, DNA damage repair, histone remodelers, and epigenetic modifiers [179, 180]. In spite of previous suggestions, the role of UV radiation seems to be negligible [181a], and a srecent tudy from Australia confirmed the lack of correlation with UV exposure [181b]. Aberrant activation of the JAK–STAT signaling pathway represents an important molecular feature of the disease [182]. Somatic copy number variants comprise >90% of all driver mutations, a frequency much higher than that observed in other forms of adults' cancer [179]. A significant proportion of these mutations are represented by focal deletions resulting in frequent hemizygous loss of target tumor suppressor gene loci [179]. *MAPK1*, *BRAF*, *CARD11*, and *PRKG1* mutations are driving increased MAPK, NF-κB, and NFAT activity upon T cell receptor stimulation [180]. Dysregulation of the pathway involving the nuclear factor κ-light-chain enhancer of activated B-cells (NF-κB) has been demonstrated in several studies [183, 184]. In a minority of patients, there are recurrent point mutations and genomic gains of *TNFRSF1B*, encoding the tumor necrosis factor receptor TNFR2 involved in NF-κB signaling [185]. Whole-genome sequencing of tumors of mycosis fungoides revealed interleukin-2 signaling pathway mutations, including activating Janus kinase 3 (JAK3) mutations, which may be targeted pharmacologically [186]. Although *RHOA* alterations can be found in a distinct subset of cases of mycosis fungoides, they are different from those commonly found in angioimmunoblastic T-cell lymphoma and related disorders [187]. A study on early lesions showed that many genes belonging to pathways associated with inflammation, regulation of apoptosis, and immune activation are upregulated in both early mycosis fungoides and inflammatory disorders [27]. Only a few genes had a discriminatory diagnostic value, and among these *TOX* (a transcription factor) and *PDCD1* (a pro-apoptosis regulator) were considered to be more helpful for identification of early lesions of the disease [32]. Oncogenes such as *p16* and *p53* do not show alterations in early lesions, but are often mutated in late (tumor) phases of the disease [188–190]. These results are in keeping with the demonstration that Twist, a transcription factor blocking p53 and inhibiting c-myc-induced apoptosis, is overexpressed only in biopsies from advanced stages [191]. Dysregulated expression of *JUNB* and *JUND* has

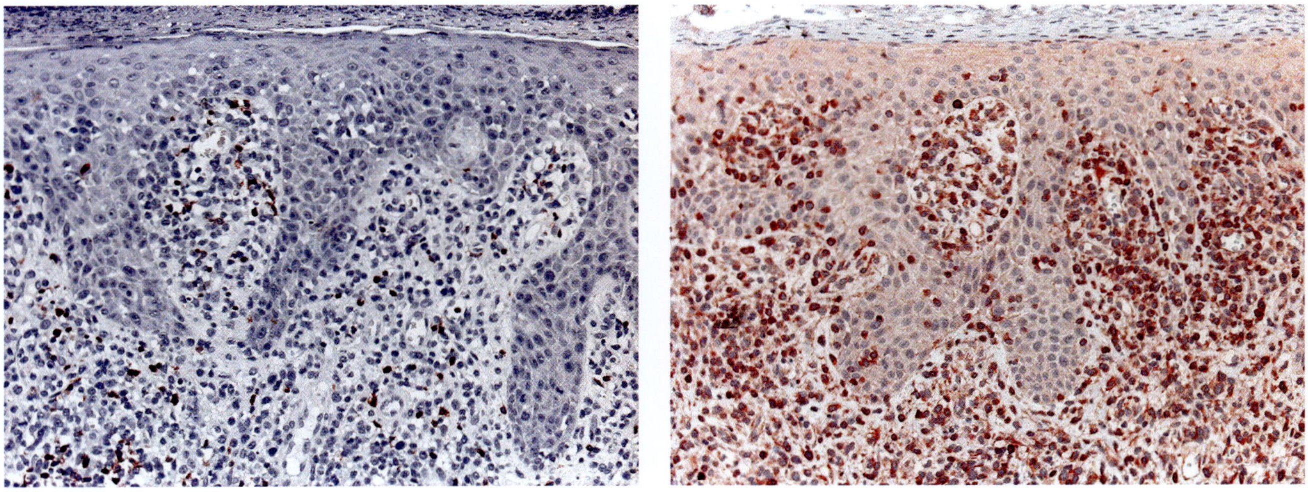

**(a)** **(b)**

**Figure 3.55** Cytotoxic mycosis fungoides with γ/δ phenotype. (a) Negative staining for βF1 and (b) positivity for TCRγ.

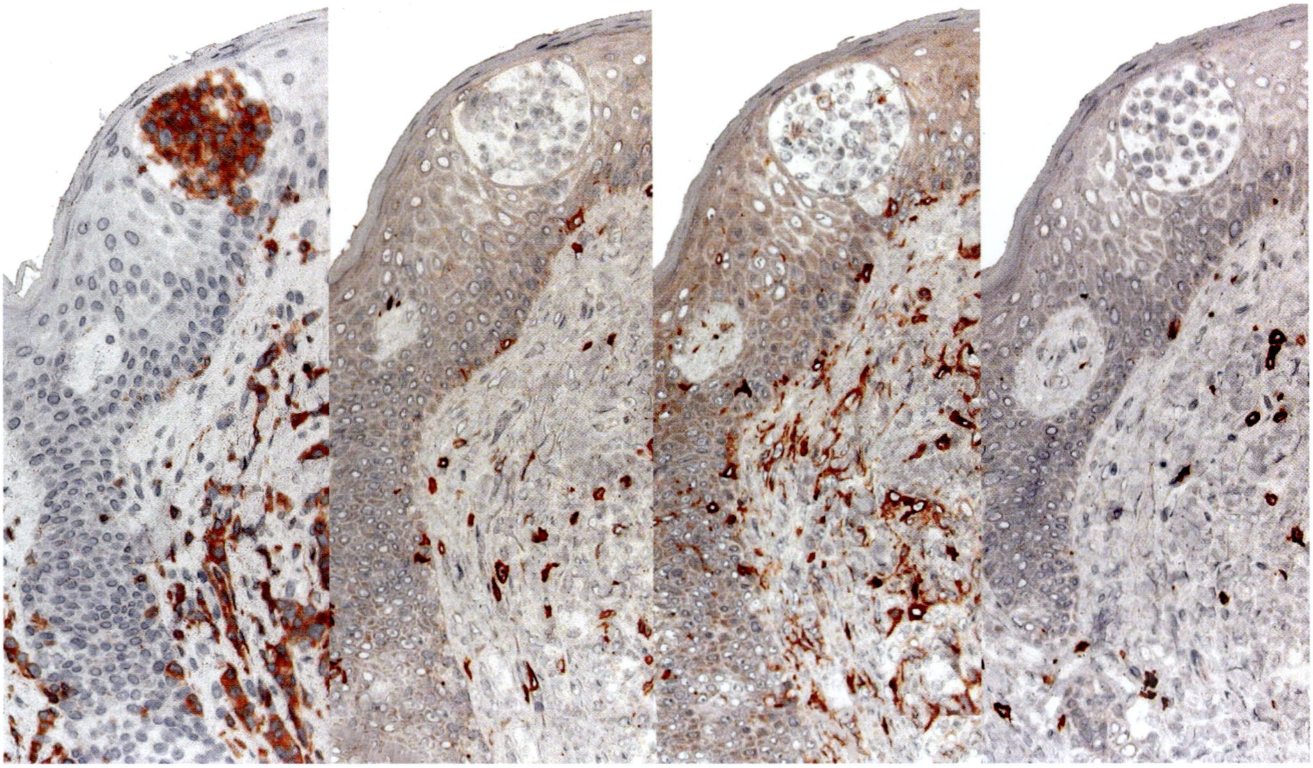

**Figure 3.56** Advanced mycosis fungoides with aberrant phenotype. From the left to the right: positivity of epidermotropic lymphocytes within a Darier nest for CD3, and negativity for CD5, CD4, and CD8.

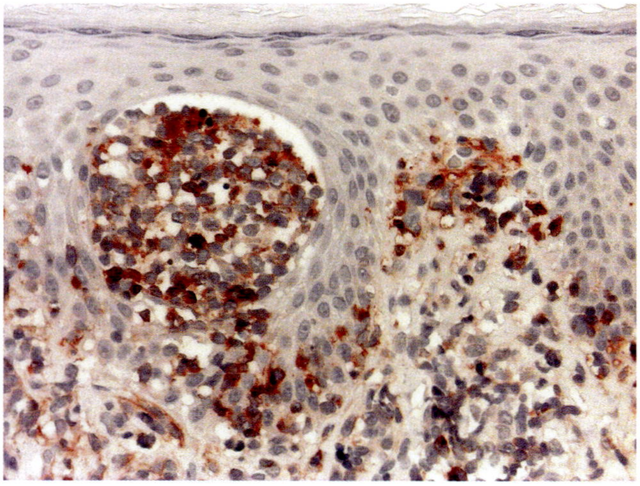

**Figure 3.57** Mycosis fungoides with TFH phenotype. Positivity of epidermotropic neoplastic lymphocytes for CD10.

been found in some cases [192] and *FAS* mutations in others [189]. Recurrent deletions of tumor suppressor genes *BCL7A*, *SMAC/DIABLO*, and *RHOF* have been detected by comparative genome hybridization in cases of early mycosis fungoides [193]. Del6q16.3 (*TNFAIP3*) was recently found to represent a molecular alteration in patients with early-stage mycosis fungoides and higher risk of progression, thus potentially being helpful in the identification of patients who may have a more aggressive disease [31]. Gain7q, gain10p15.1 (*IL2RA* and *IL15RA*), del10p11.22 (*ZEB1*), and mutations in *JUNB* and *TET2* were other molecular alterations associated with high-risk disease stages [31].

Using cDNA microarray analysis, a signature of 27 genes, including oncogenes and other genes involved in the control of apoptosis, has been identified in cases of early- and late-stage mycosis fungoides, and a six-gene prediction model capable of distinguishing mycosis fungoides from inflammatory diseases has been proposed, including *FJX1*, *Hs.127160*, *STAT4*, *SYNE-1B*, *TRAF1*, and *BIRC3* [194]. In a similar study, consensus clustering revealed the presence of two clusters that tended to include mostly patients with mycosis fungoides in the early stages (Ia and Ib), and of a third cluster limited mostly to patients with more advanced disease [195]. However, the number of cases was relatively small and overlapping data were observed. Using reverse transcription-PCR, 593 genes overexpressed in mycosis fungoides were identified, allowing stratification of the disease into three different prognostic groups [196]. Mutations in genes like *APC*, *AK2*, *TYRO3*, and *ITPKB* that regulate tumor proliferation and apoptosis were noted. Using NGS,

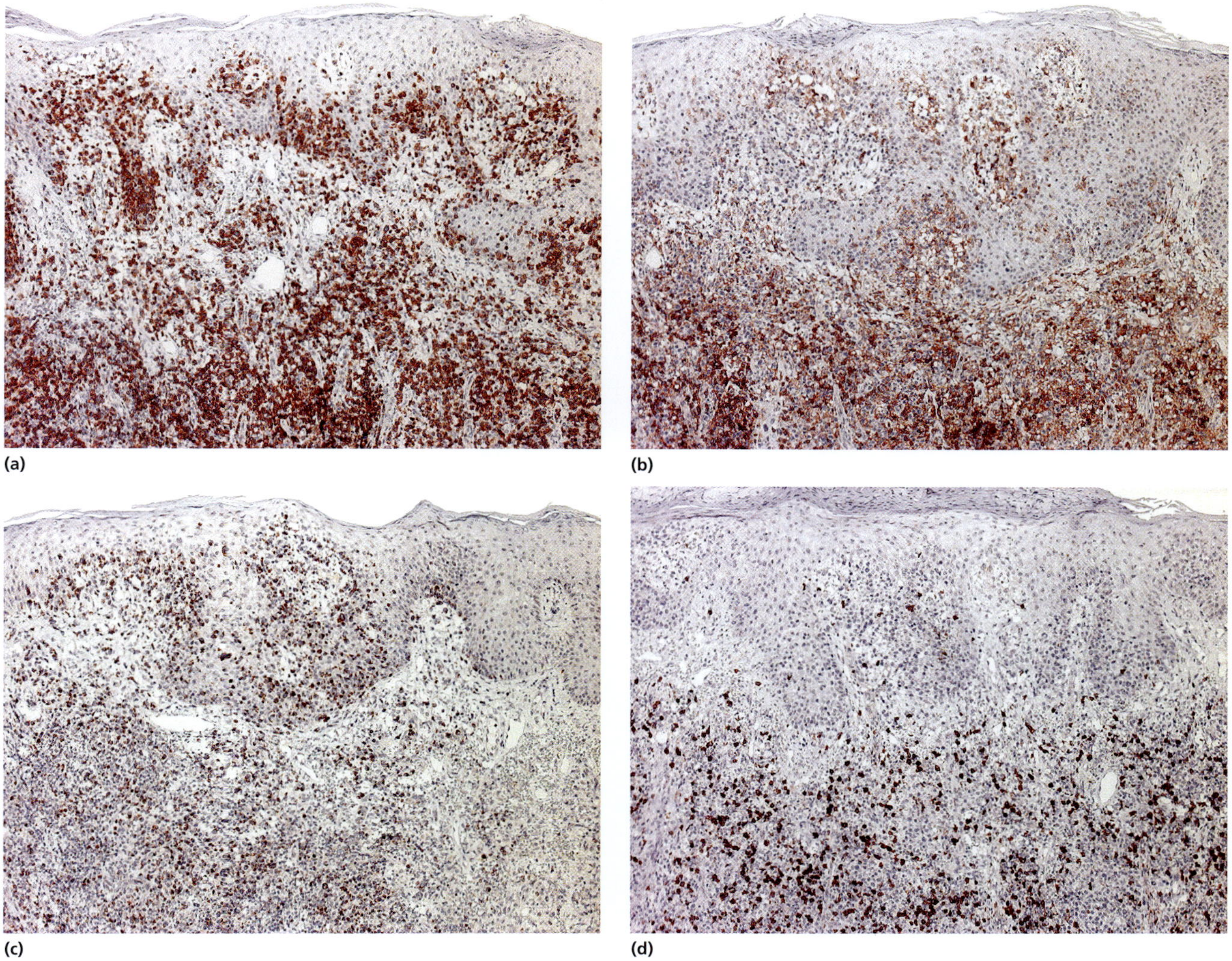


Figure 3.58 Mycosis fungoides, tumor stage with cytotoxic phenotype. Neoplastic cells are positive for (a) CD3, (b) CD4 (dim expression) and (c) granzyme B, and (d) negative for CD8.

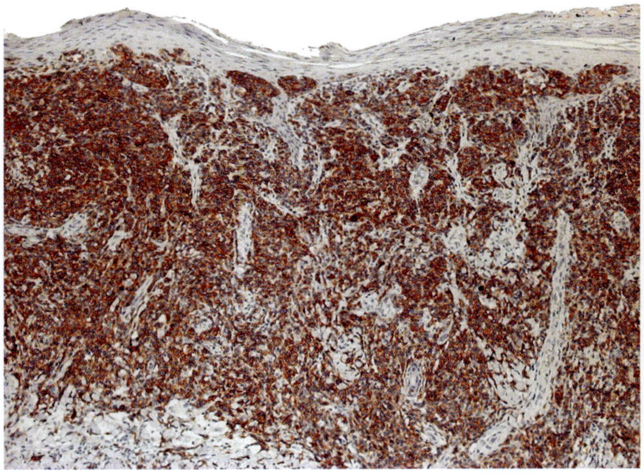

Figure 3.59 Mycosis fungoides, tumor stage. Strong positivity for CD30 in both epidermotropic and dermal neoplastic lymphocytes.

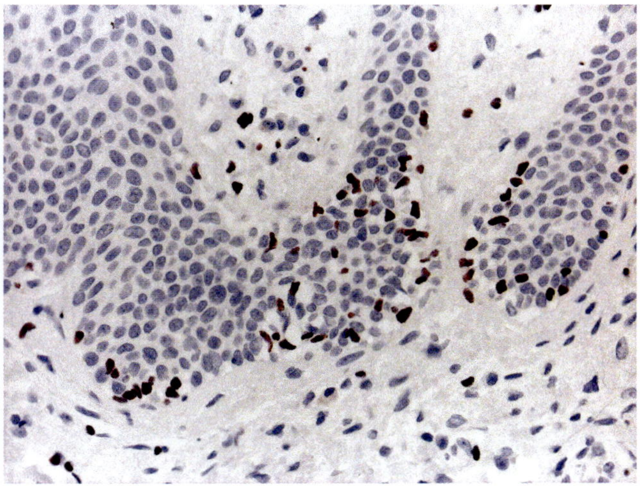

Figure 3.60 Mycosis fungoides with Treg phenotype. Positivity of epidermotropic neoplastic lymphocytes for FOX-P3.

mutations in genes involved in apoptotic, NF-kB, JAK–STAT, and TCR signaling pathways, including *HLA-DRB1*, *AK2*, *ITPKB*, *HLA-B*, *TYRO3*, and *CHD2* were found, as well as previously reported MF-associated mutations such as *DNMT3A* and *STAT5B* [197].

Several studies focused on micro RNA (miRNA) expression profiling; miR-92a and miR-155 are upregulated and miR-203 and miR-205 are downregulated in mycosis fungoides as compared to inflammatory disorders [198–201]. However, as miR-203 and miR-205 are expressed by keratinocytes, their "downregulation" in mycosis fungoides may be due also to the different amount of epidermis in specimens of mycosis fungoides with many epidermotropic lymphocytes (lower amount of epidermal tissue) as opposed to those of inflammatory dermatoses without or with only a few intraepidermal lymphocytes (higher amount of epidermal tissue) [182]. miR-155 may be relevant also for disease progression by contributing to apoptosis resistance and increased tumor growth [202], and miR-155 inhibitors are being tested in clinical trials [203]. In addition, miR-155 and miR-200b were significantly associated with overall survival [204]. Diminished levels of miR-29b that contributed to overexpression of the epigenetic reader bromodomain-containing protein 4 (BRD4) have been observed in one patient [205]. Different miRNA expression profiles have been found in mycosis fungoides when compared with cutaneous anaplastic large cell lymphoma [206], but another study found similar profiles with overexpression of the onco-microRNAs miR-155, miR-21, or miR-142 and low expression of miR-141/200c cluster in both diseases [207]. Different miRNA expression profiles have been detected also in mycosis fungoides and atopic dermatitis, representing a potentially useful diagnostic tool [208].

Recent data showed that genetic alterations of class I human leukocyte antigen (HLA-I), including loss of heterozygosity and allele-specific mutations, occur in about half of the patients with advanced-stage mycosis fungoides, possibly resulting in immune evasion and resistance to immunotherapy [209]. Interestingly, single-cell RNA sequencing showed that the genetic alterations in HLA-I were subclonal and reversible, with some alleles disrupted or restored over time, indicating a dynamic, ongoing immune selection of neoplastic clones.

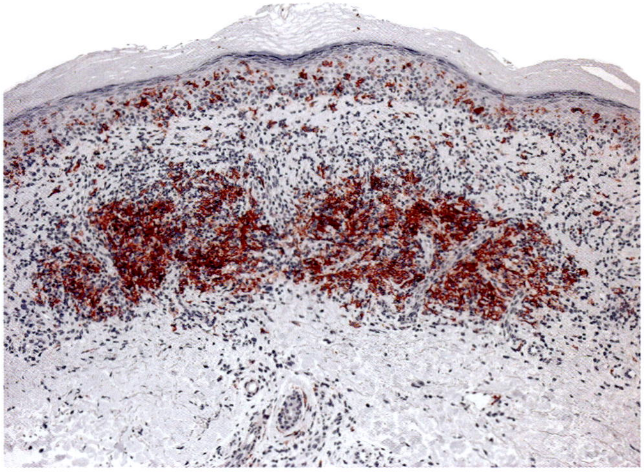

**Figure 3.61** Mycosis fungoides with clusters of dermal Langerhans cells positive for CD1a.

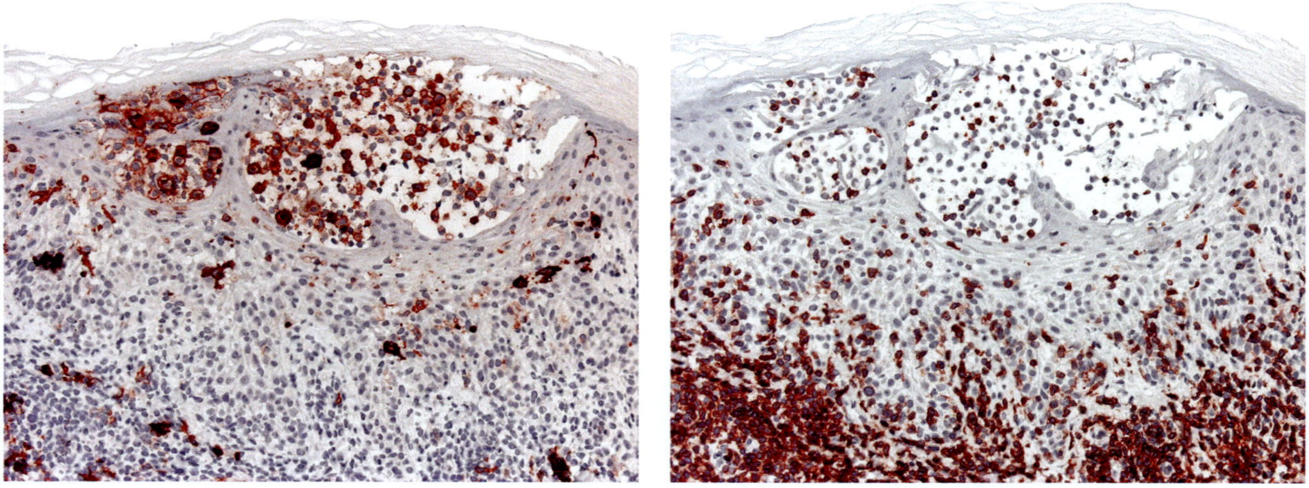

(a) (b)

**Figure 3.62** Mycosis fungoides with clusters of intraepidermal Langerhans cells mimicking the picture of Langerhans cell histiocytosis. (a) Staining for CD1a highlights numerous Langerhans cells. (b) Staining for CD3 shows only a few T lymphocytes within the intraepidermal clusters.

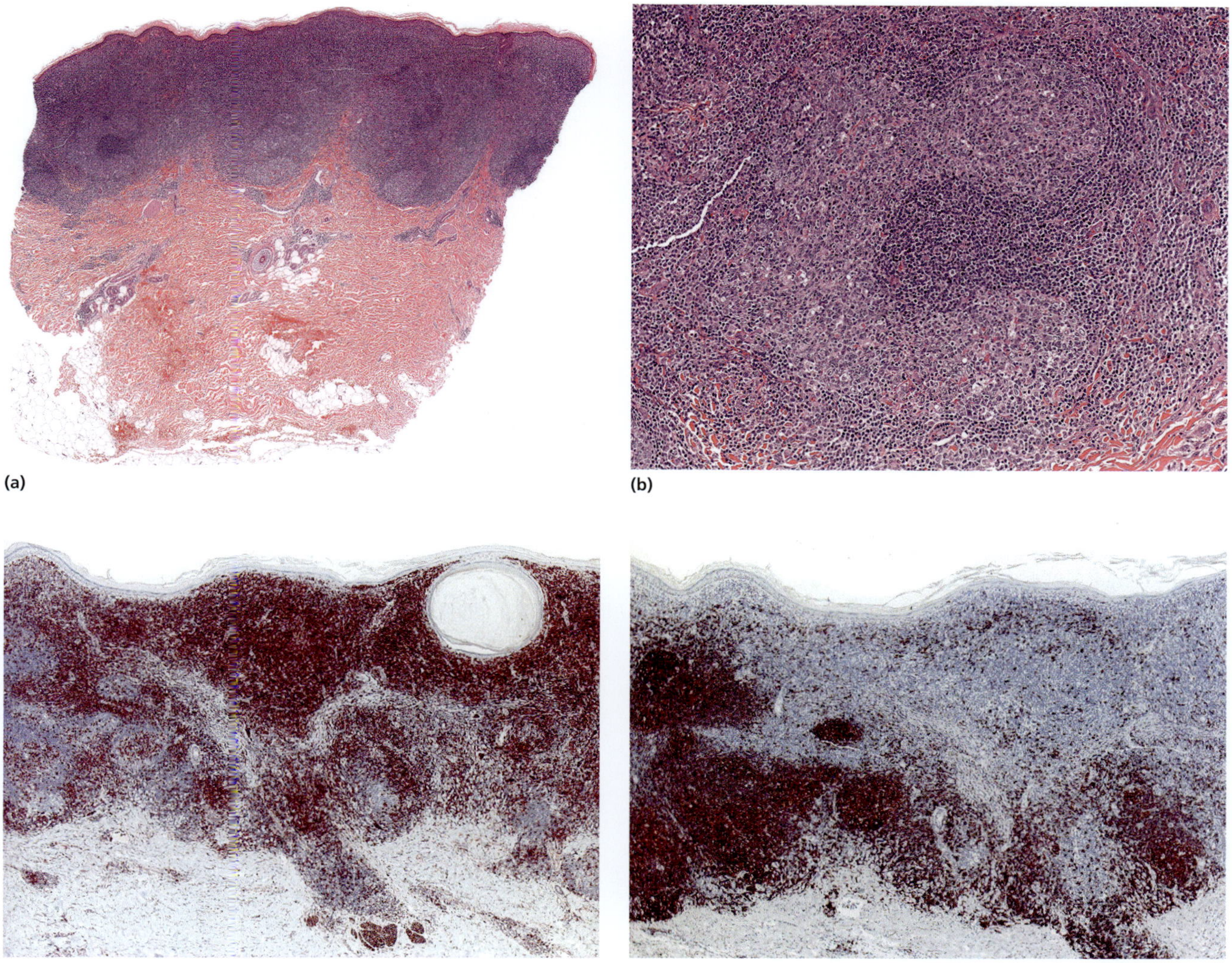

**Figure 3.63** Mycosis fungoides with prominent B-cell reaction. (a) Dense, band-like lymphoid infiltrate in the superficial and mid-dermis. (b) Note reactive germinal centers within the infiltrate. (c) Staining for CD3 shows predominance of T lymphocytes with epidermotropism. (d) Staining for CD20 highlights the numerous B lymphocytes.

## Histopathologic differential diagnosis from inflammatory conditions

The histopathologic diagnosis of early mycosis fungoides may be extremely difficult. In fact, in some instances differentiation from inflammatory skin conditions (e.g., atopic dermatitis, chronic contact dermatitis) may be impossible on histopathologic grounds alone. In these cases clinical correlation is crucial to make a definitive diagnosis. It should be underlined that in many cases the presence of "non-specific" histopathologic features does not allow one to rule out a diagnosis of mycosis fungoides if the clinical presentation is suggestive of the disease. In such cases I describe the histopathologic aspects as "consistent with" the clinical diagnosis, rather than simply issuing a report of "nonspecific chronic dermatitis." If only biopsies with marked epidermotropism and/or the presence of Darier nests were to be reported as diagnostic, then the majority of early lesions of mycosis fungoides would be missed on histopathologic grounds. The ISCL proposed a scoring system for diagnosis of early patches of mycosis fungoides [96], but clinicopathologic correlation, integration of all available data, and especially repeated biopsies are crucial. A detailed discussion of the histopathological features of different types of inflammatory lesions mimicking mycosis fungoides is provided in Chapter 31, and a list of clinicopathological mimickers in Table 31.1.

Immunohistologic features of mycosis fungoides are not distinctive and are similar to those observed in many inflammatory skin conditions. Staining for CD2, CD3, or CD5 may help highlighting epidermotropic T lymphocytes, but presence of intraepidermal lymphocytes cannot be considered pathognomonic of mycosis fungoides. The presence of several intraepidermal lymphocytes in areas with only scant spongiosis is considered suspicious for mycosis fungoides ("disproportionate epidermotropism," i.e., too many lymphocytes for too little spongiosis); on the other hand, using pan-T-cell immunohistochemical markers, several epidermotropic lymphocytes can be observed in many inflammatory dermatoses; in this context, the interpretation of the ratio of epidermotropic lymphocytes/spongiosis should be made with caution, particularly on sections stained by immunohistochemistry. It has been suggested that in early stages of mycosis fungoides, in contrast to benign (inflammatory) cutaneous infiltrates of T lymphocytes, there is a loss of expression of the T-cell-associated antigen CD7, but in my opinion this finding is of limited relevance. In addition, T lymphocytes in some cases of benign inflammatory dermatosis show loss of CD7 as well. Expression of thymocyte selection-associated high-mobility group box (TOX) is usually higher in mycosis fungoides (>50% of cells) than in inflammatory dermatoses (<50% of cells), but to my eyes this marker does not seem to represent a reliable differential diagnostic tool.

Molecular analysis of TCR genes rearrangement is a further method helpful in the differentiation of mycosis fungoides from benign skin conditions. In particular, detection of the same clone in lesions from different skin sites seems to be highly specific for mycosis fungoides as compared to inflammatory disorders [59]. It must be underlined, however, that several benign dermatoses have been shown to harbor a monoclonal population of T lymphocytes (e.g., lichen planus and lichen sclerosus, among others). In short, absence of clonality should not be considered as a criterion to rule out mycosis fungoides, and presence of clonality should not be considered diagnostic for mycosis fungoides. Analysis of clonality with high-throughput sequencing seems to be a more reliable method for analysis of T-cell clonality [33, 165]. This method also provides an explanation for the difficulties found in the histopathological diagnosis of early lesions, as neoplastic T cells may represent as little as 10% of the infiltrate [33].

Besides the differential diagnosis with inflammatory (reactive) conditions, mycosis fungoides should be differentiated from other cutaneous lymphomas, particularly Sézary syndrome and cutaneous cytotoxic NK/T-cell lymphomas (see Chapters 4, 7, 8, and 9).

## Clinical and histopathologic variants

Mycosis fungoides has been defined as a "dermatologic masquerader" [210, 211], and several clinical and/or histopathologic variants have been described (Table 3.2). It must be underlined that some of these "variants" are peculiar clinical or histopathologic presentations observed only in a few patients,

**Table 3.2** Clinicopathologic and phenotypic variants of mycosis fungoides

| |
|---|
| **Clinical variants with "conventional" histopathological features** |
| Atopic dermatitis-like mycosis fungoides[§] |
| Erythrodermic mycosis fungoides |
| Hypopigmented mycosis fungoides |
| Ichthyosiform mycosis fungoides |
| Palmo-plantar mycosis fungoides[$] |
| Papular mycosis fungoides |
| Papuloerythroderma Ofuji |
| Parapsoriasis ("large patch") (for a discussion on small patch parapsoriasis see Chapter 2) |
| Pityriasis lichenoides-like mycosis fungoides (clinical variant) |
| Psoriasiform mycosis fungoides |
| Unilesional (solitary) mycosis fungoides |
| Waistband mycosis fungoides |
| Zosteriform mycosis fungoides |
| **Clinical variants with peculiar histopathological features** |
| Acanthosis nigricans-like mycosis fungoides |
| Adnexotropic mycosis fungoides, including pilotropic (folliculotropic) mycosis fungoides (with or without follicular mucinosis), mycosis fungoides with eruptive infundibular cysts and comedones, acneiform mycosis fungoides, lichen spinulosus-like mycosis fungoides, and syringotropic mycosis fungoides* |
| Anetodermic mycosis fungoides (mycosis fungoides with secondary anetoderma) (secondary anetoderma may be observed also in generalized follicular mucinosis) |
| Bullous (vesiculobullous) mycosis fungoides |
| Dyshidrotic mycosis fungoides |
| Granulomatous slack skin |
| Hyperpigmented mycosis fungoides |
| "Invisible" mycosis fungoides |
| Pagetoid reticulosis (Woringer–Kolopp type) |
| Poikilodermatous mycosis fungoides |
| Purpuric mycosis fungoides |
| Pustular mycosis fungoides |
| Verrucous/hyperkeratotic mycosis fungoides |
| **Histopathological variants** |
| Annular lichenoid dermiatitis of youth-like mycosis fungoides |
| Granulomatous mycosis fungoides |
| Interstitial mycosis fungoides |
| Large cell transformation |
| Mycosis fungoides with epidermal mucinosis |
| Pityriasis lichenoides-like mycosis fungoides (histopathological variant) |
| Sclerosing mycosis fungoides (lichen sclerosus-like) |
| **Phenotypic variants**[#] |
| Cytotoxic mycosis fungoides (CD8+ and/or $\gamma/\delta$+; rarely CD4+ with expression of cytotoxic proteins) |
| Mycosis fungoides with T follicular helper (TFH) phenotype |
| Mycosis fungoides with T-regulatory (T*reg*) phenotype |

§ Histopathologically characterized often by variable spongiotic changes.
[$] Most reported cases may represent in truth a pseudolymphomatous variant of palmoplantar psoriasis (see also Chapter 31).
* Pilotropic mycosis fungoides and syringotropic mycosis fungoides may be observed independently from one another, but in many instances of syringotropic mycosis fungoides the hair follicles are involved as well, thus the term adnexotropic mycosis fungoides better reflects the clinicopathological features of this variant of the disease.
\# A phenotypic switch may occur in sequential biopsies, and sometimes different phenotypic features are present in different biopsies taken on the same day.

but others are more frequent and may represent a true pitfall in the diagnosis of the disease. Patients with these variants often also show aspects of "conventional" mycosis fungoides at other sites of the body or develop more typical lesions during follow-up. Clinical and/or histopathologic features of a variant of mycosis fungoides may be restricted to a body site or to a time frame.

Three variants of mycosis fungoides were considered peculiar enough to be listed separately in the WHO–EORTC classification of cutaneous lymphomas [1, 6], namely, pilotropic (folliculotropic) mycosis fungoides, localized pagetoid reticulosis (Woringer–Kolopp), and granulomatous slack skin.

In addition to the variants listed in Table 3.2, a plethora of terms have been used in the past for mycosis fungoides (such as parakeratosis variegata and poikiloderma vasculare atrophicans among others), and unfortunately some of them are still in use today. The use of these terms has brought much confusion to this field and should be discouraged.

## Adnexotropic mycosis fungoides

Mycosis fungoides may present clinically and histopathologically with prominent involvement of adnexal structures, particularly the hair follicles and eccrine glands. Such cases are classified as pilotropic and syringotropic mycosis fungoides, respectively. Although traditionally considered as two separate variants of mycosis fungoides, pilotropic and syringotropic mycosis fungoides to my eyes represent a spectrum of adnexotropic mycosis fungoides that shows more overlapping than distinguishing features. In fact, many cases of syringotropic mycosis fungoides show concomitant, prominent involvement of the hair follicles (hence the old term of "syringolymphoid hyperplasia with alopecia" for this variant of the disease) (Fig. 3.64). For practical purposes, discussion of pilotropic and syringotropic mycosis fungoides will be summarized herein in two separate sections, but it should be underlined that they represent two overlapping faces of adnexotropic mycosis fungoides.

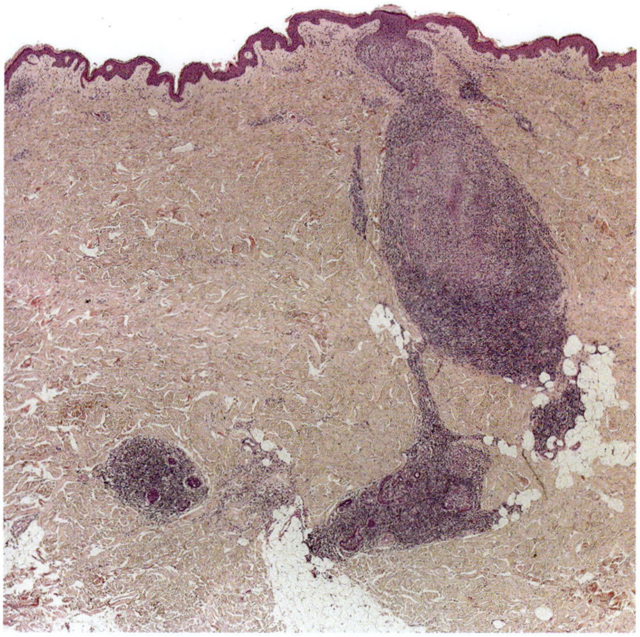

**Figure 3.64** Adnexotropic mycosis fungoides. Prominent involvement of both a hair follicle ("pilotropic" mycosis fungoides) and eccrine glands ("syringotropic" mycosis fungoides) in the same biopsy specimen.

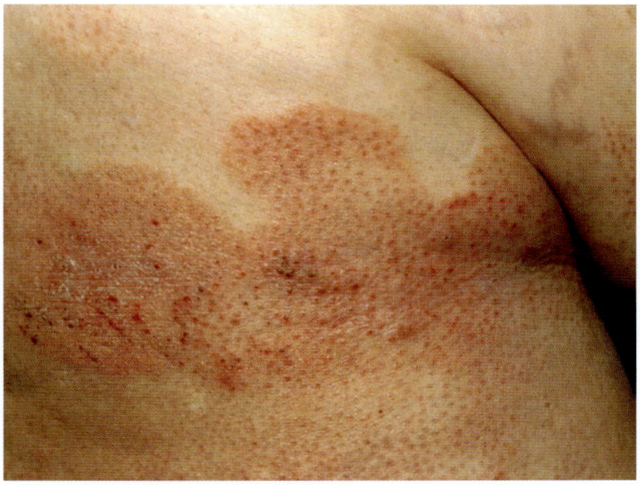

**Figure 3.65** Pilotropic mycosis fungoides. Confluent follicular erythematous papules on the thigh. Note small, superficial erosions representing scratching artifacts.

## Pilotropic (folliculotropic) mycosis fungoides (with or without follicular mucinosis) and relationship with so-called "benign" follicular mucinosis

Some patients with mycosis fungoides present with lesions characterized by prominent involvement of the hair follicles (Figs. 3.65) [212]. Clinically, sometimes only small areas of patchy alopecia on different parts of the body are visible (Fig. 3.66). On the face, due to the large number of hair follicles, lesions often look more infiltrated (Fig. 3.67). The ears can be involved (Fig. 3.68). At body sites with only vellus hairs, lesions may be very subtle, and it may be difficult to appreciate the extent of the disease (Fig. 3.69). Follicular hyperkeratosis may confer on the lesion some resemblance to lichen spinulosus (Fig. 3.70a), and rarely long, tiny keratotic spines may protrude from affected follicles (Fig. 3.70b) [213–215]. In fact, it is debatable whether cases published in the literature as "lichen spinulosos with follicular mucinosis" do not represent in truth an early variant of folliculotropic mycosis fungoides ("idiopathic generalized follicular mucinosis") [216], and cases of lichen spinulosos-like pilotropic mycosis fungoides in children have been reported [200]. In several cases the prominent follicular distribution of the lesions without involvement of the

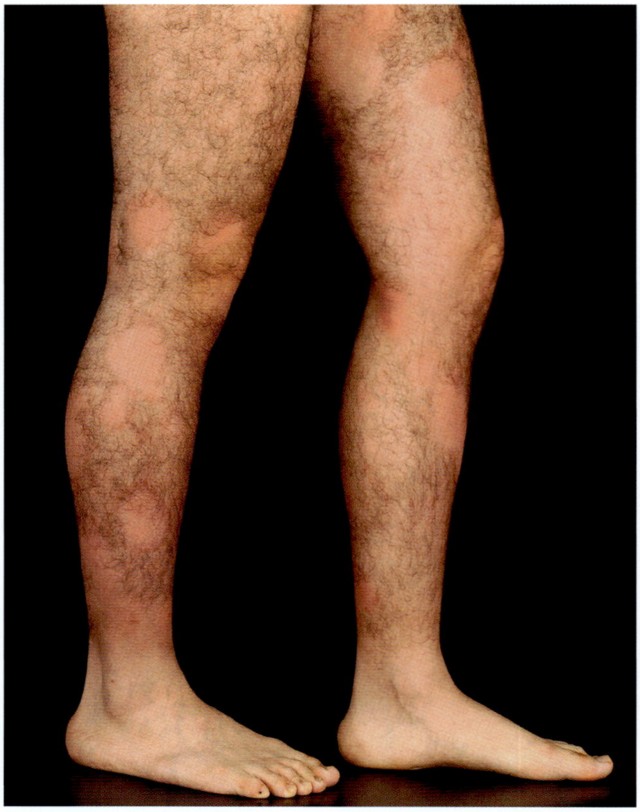

**Figure 3.66** Pilotropic mycosis fungoides. Patchy areas of alopecia on both legs.

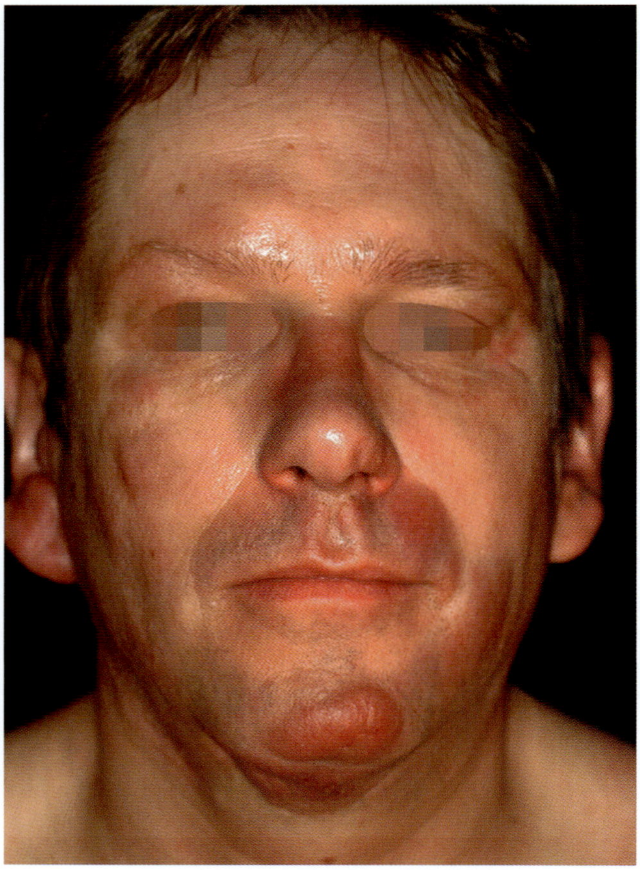

**Figure 3.67** Pilotropic mycosis fungoides. Lesions on the face present with a more infiltrated aspect due to the larger number of hair follicles as well as to the presence of hair follicles reaching deeper within the subcutaneous fat in this region of the body.

interfollicular epidermis produces a characteristic "agminated" appearance of the lesions (Fig. 3.71). Rarely, pilotropic mycosis fungoides presents with solitary lesions [217–220]. Itching is severe and represents a major problem in this variant of mycosis fungoides, and may be nonresponsive to standard treatments. Prurigo-like lesions as well as small, superficial erosions caused by scratching may complicate the clinical picture and lead to the erroneous diagnosis of an eczematous dermatitis (Fig. 3.72). Although pilotropic mycosis fungoides is considered a distinct clinicopathological variant of the disease, it should be underlined that in many cases of otherwise conventional mycosis fungoides some biopsy specimens may show variable involvement of the hair follicles, particularly in infiltrated and/or advanced lesions (Fig. 3.73). I refer to these cases as "mycosis fungoides with focal pilotropism." The term pilotropic mycosis fungoides should be restricted to cases presenting with the characteristic clinicopathological features (focal areas of alopecia clinically; infiltrate involving mostly or only the hair follicles histopathologically).

The histopathological features of pilotropic mycosis fungoides vary according to the number and depth of the hair follicles in the affected body area. In general and in any body area, particularly in early lesions of pilotropic mycosis fungoides the epidermis between affected hair follicles does not show conventional features of mycosis fungoides, and the pathological changes are restricted to the hair follicle(s) (Fig. 3.74). In areas rich in follicles that extend into the subcutaneous fat, like the head and neck region, the histopathological aspect is completely different than in areas with a small number of shorter follicles. Lesions on the head and neck region are characterized by dense infiltrates extending into the subcutaneous tissue and showing variable numbers of pilotropic lymphocytes within many hair follicles (Fig. 3.75). Eosinophils are a common bystander in these lesions (Fig. 3.75b). By contrast, lesions located on the trunk and extremities are characterized by less dense and more superficial infiltrates with frequent cystic dilatation of the hair follicles (Fig. 3.76). In rare cases, the hair follicles are completely wiped off by the lymphocytes, and the vertical arrangement of the infiltrate is the only histopathological feature betraying the nature of the disease (Fig. 3.77). Mucin deposition may be present or absent in pilotropic mycosis fungoides, and in my experience is almost invariably found in the head and neck area (Fig. 3.75) and less frequent and abundant on the trunk and extremities (Fig. 3.78). The deposition of

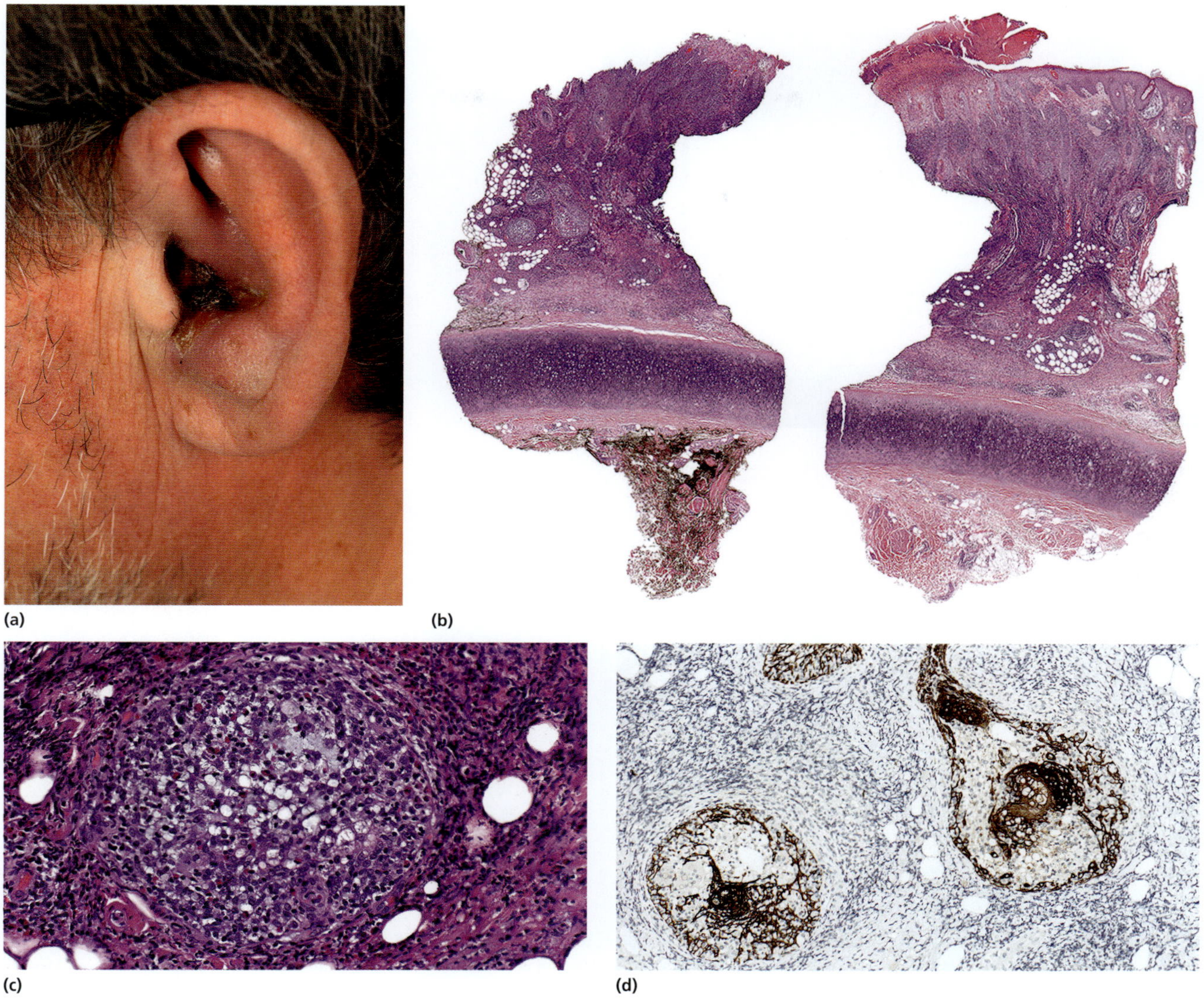

**Figure 3.68** Pilotropic mycosis fungoides. (a) Crusted lesions located in the external ear canal. (b) Histology shows dense lymphoid infiltrates and a serum crust; (c) remnants of a hair follicle with mucin deposition can be appreciated and (d) better visualized with a staining for pan-cytokeratin.

mucin is restricted to the hair follicles (follicular mucinosis), and may be markedly variable within different hair follicles (Fig. 3.74). Deposition of mucin and/or prominent pilotropism of lymphocytes may disrupt the follicle and make it more difficult to appreciate the typical histopathological features; in such cases, staining for pan-cytokeratin helps visualize remnants of hair follicles that are masked by lymphoid infiltrates (Fig. 3.68b–d). In some patients, mucin deposition may be observed in one biopsy but not in other specimens, again showing the variability of clinicopathological findings in mycosis fungoides [221, 222]. In lesions of mycosis fungoides involving the hair follicles, a prominent perifollicular granulomatous reaction may be observed, sometimes replacing the entire follicle (Fig. 3.79) [223, 224]. The onset of pustules and/or of impetiginized lesions is more frequent in pilotropic mycosis fungoides than in other variants of the disease (Fig. 3.80).

The phenotype of pilotropic mycosis fungoides is invariably characterized by predominance of $CD4^+$ T lymphocytes, and only exceptionally $CD8^+$ cases may be observed [225]. In my experience, the rare cases of pilotropic mycosis positive for CD8 do not show exclusive involvement of the hair follicles, and neoplastic lymphocytes are present within the epidermis as well (Fig. 3.81).

As already mentioned, alopecia due to destruction of the follicles is common (so-called alopecia mucinosa), either generalized or localized. The pattern of alopecia in mycosis fungoides is often distinctive and is characterized by irregular areas of hair loss, patchy erythema, and follicular papules and/or comedones (Figs. 3.72 and 3.82c). In some patients, alopecia areata-like lesions or even alopecia universalis may be observed [226]. Sometimes alopecia can be present in patients who do not have other lesions of follicular mycosis fungoides,

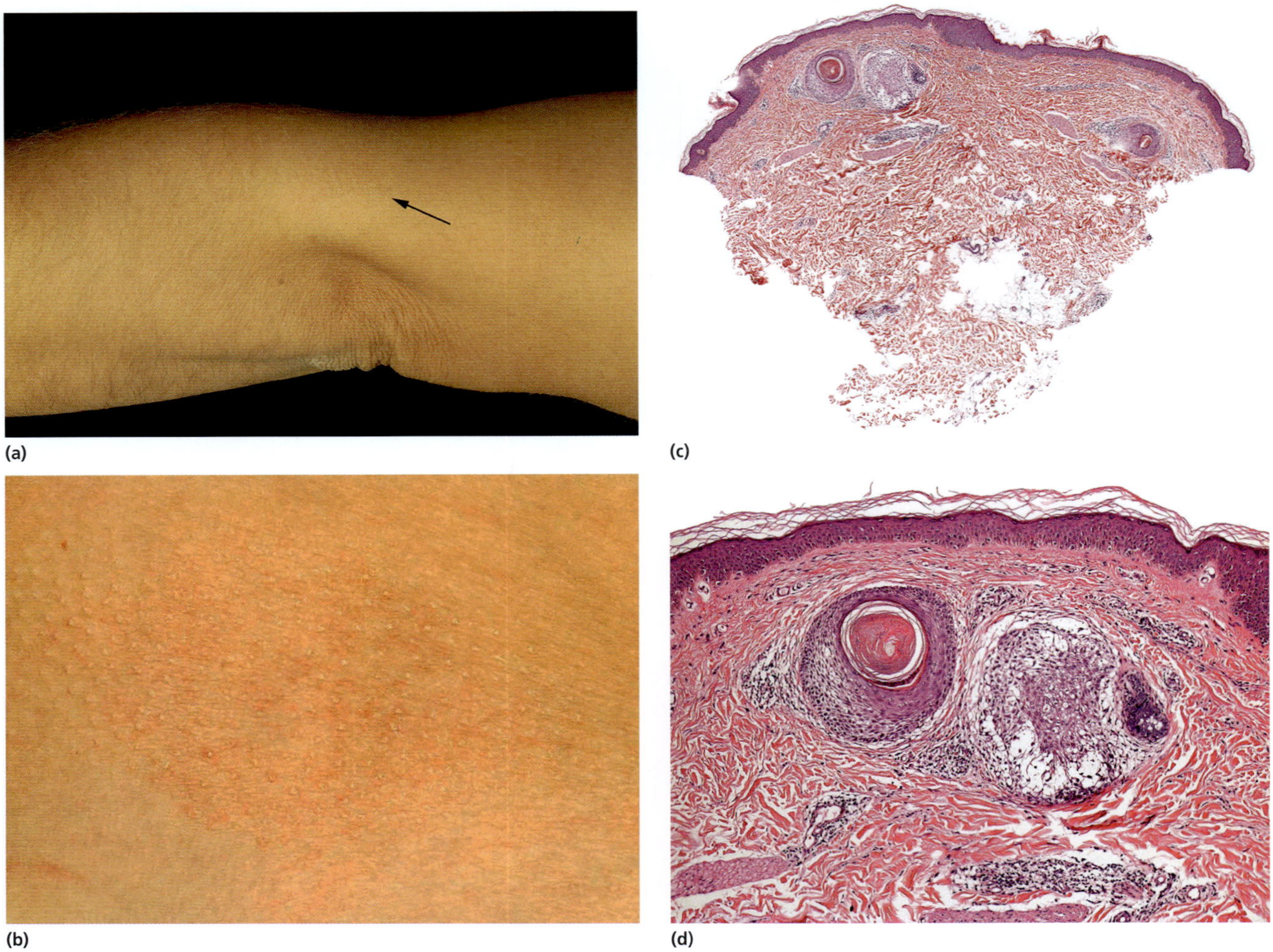


**Figure 3.69** Early lesions of pilotropic mycosis fungoides. (a) Small, inconspicuous area of alopecia with follicular keratoses. (b) Detail of the clinical features. (c, d) Histopathology reveals deposition of mucin within the hair follicle and perifollicular lymphoid infiltrates with intraepithelial lymphocytes.

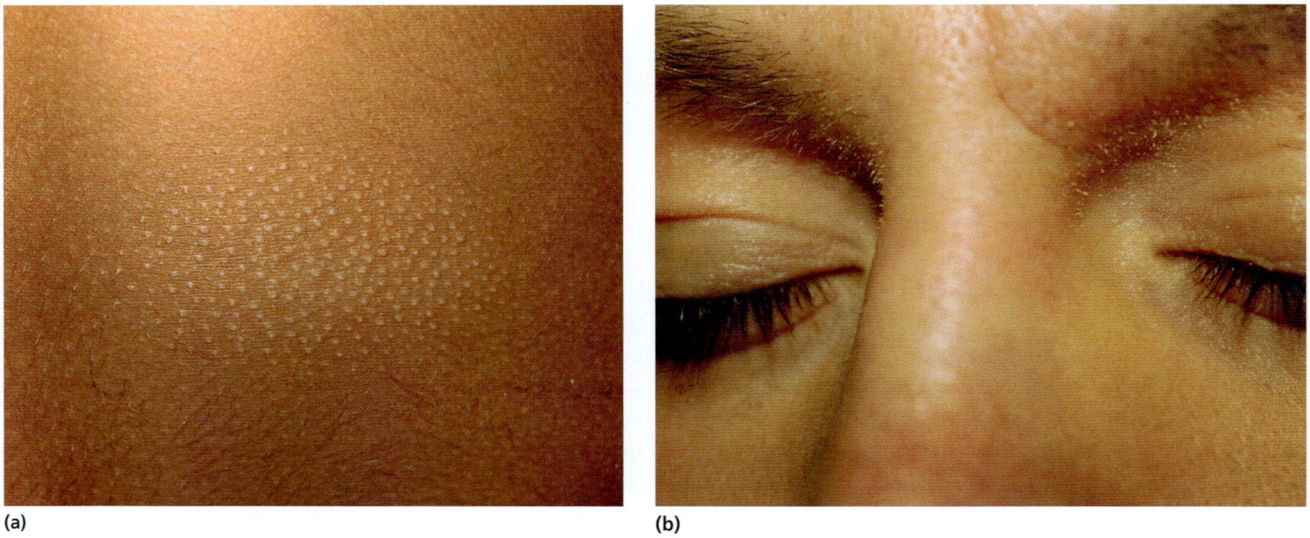


**Figure 3.70** Pilotropic mycosis fungoides. (a) Follicular hyperkeratosis resembling the clinical aspects of lichen spinulosus. (*Courtesy of Prof. Luis Requena, Madrid, Spain.*) (b) Tiny keratotic spikes protruding from the hair follicles ("spiky" pilotropic mycosis fungoides). (*Courtesy of Prof. Ketty Peris, Rome, Italy.*)

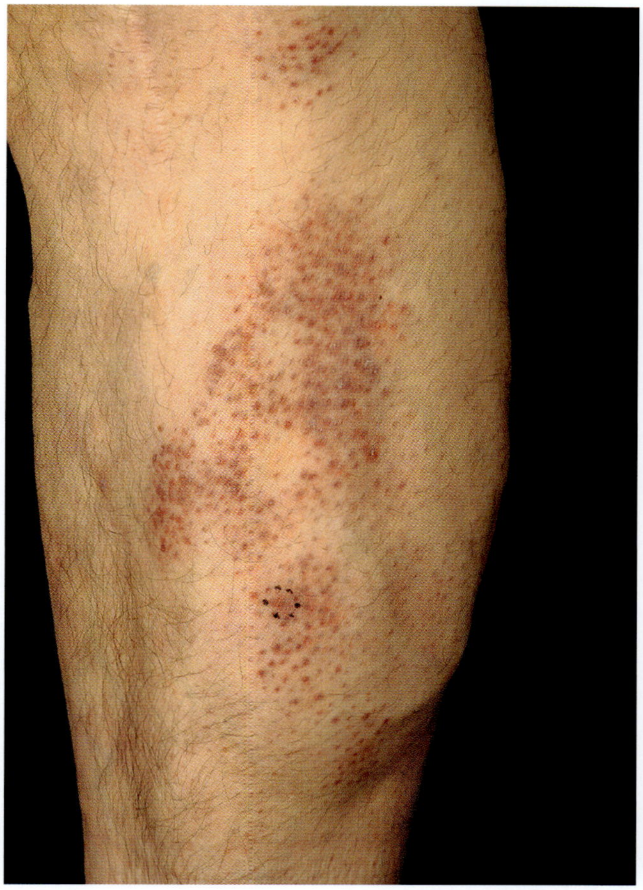

Figure 3.71 Pilotropic mycosis fungoides with agminated, livid follicular papules.

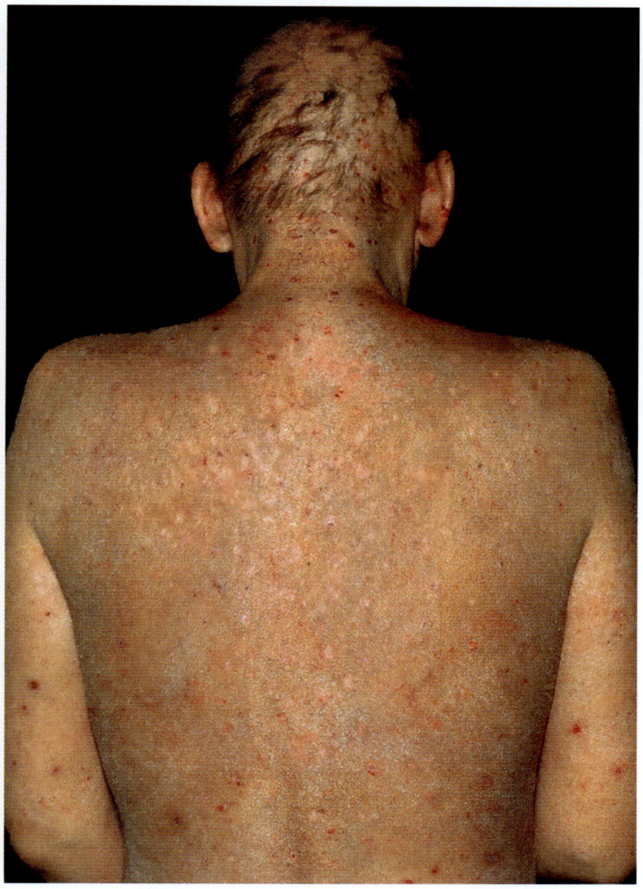

Figure 3.72 Pilotropic mycosis fungoides. Note irregular loss of hairs ("alopecia mucinosa") and superficial erosions representing scratch artifacts resulting from intense itching, mimicking the clinical picture of generalized atopic dermatitis. The pattern of scalp alopecia seen in this patient is typical of mycosis fungoides.

but it is most prominent in the pilotropic variant of the disease [226]. Besides alopecia, in patients with marked involvement of the hair follicles, with or without deposition of mucin, a localized or rarely widespread eruption of small infundibular cysts and/or comedones infiltrated by neoplastic T lymphocytes can be observed ("mycosis fungoides with eruptive cysts and comedones") (Figs. 3.82a and b) [227]. Histology of comedones is characterized by wide cystic openings on the surface of the epidermis, surrounded by mainly pericystic, usually sparse lymphoid infiltrates (Fig. 3.82d). Confluent, small infundibular cysts may result in the clinical picture of so-called "milia en plaques," a condition that besides mycosis fungoides can be associated with several inflammatory disorders (Figs. 3.83 and 3.84). Variable numbers of small epidermal cysts may also be visible as a result of chronic "inflammation" of the hair follicles (Fig. 3.85a). In such cases, the pericystic infiltrate is variably dense and may be sparse. Helpful clues for the differentiation from inflamed epidermal cysts are the presence around the cyst of a mainly lymphoid infiltrate without suppurative aspects or granulomatous formation (Fig. 3.85b). When present, concomitant involvement of the eccrine glands with syringometaplasia represents a helpful diagnostic clue (Fig. 3.86). Prominent involvement of the hair follicles with follicular hyperplasia may lead to the formation of elevated lesions, clinically resembling tumors of the disease, even in the absence of true neoplastic tumors ("pseudotumoral mycosis fungoides") (Fig. 3.87) [228].

Another clinical variant of pilotropic mycosis fungoides, observed almost exclusively in advanced stages of the disease, is characterized by prominent involvement of the eyelids with marked swelling and complete loss of the eyelashes (Fig. 3.88) [229]. In patients with conventional mycosis fungoides with involvement of the hair follicles, I have observed rarely a histopathological pattern characterized by a band-like infiltrate associated to prominent involvement of the subcutaneous fat, in spite of a minimal involvement of the reticular dermis (Fig. 3.89). It is conceivable that in such cases the infiltrate extends to the depth along the hair follicles and other adnexal structures, and then becomes diffuse within the subcutaneous

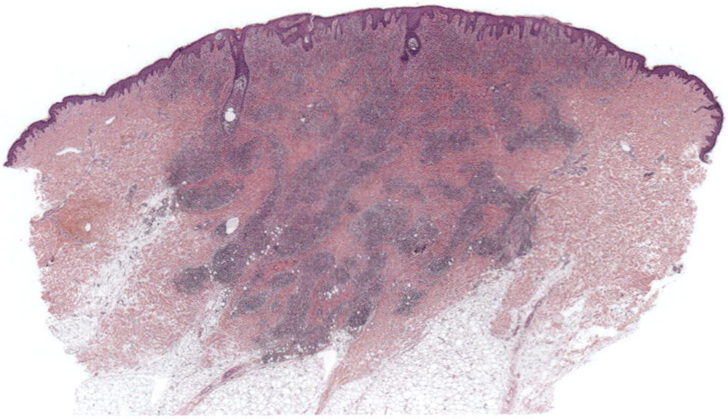

(a)

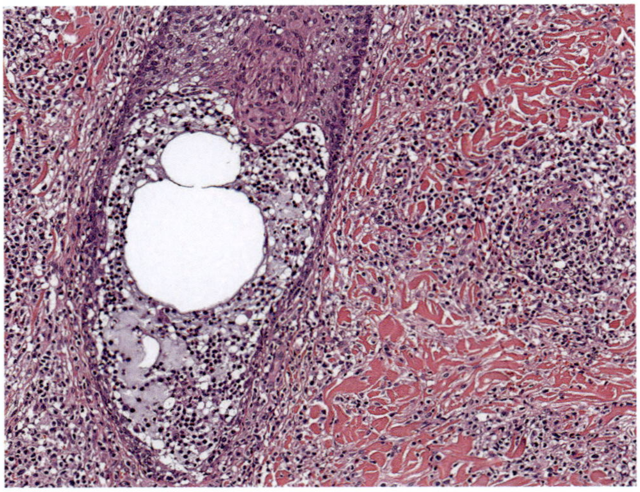

(b)

Figure 3.73 Mycosis fungoides with involvement of a hair follicle. (a) Dermal tumor of mycosis fungoides with involvement of the epidermis and (b) focal pilotropism with mucin deposition within a hair follicle.

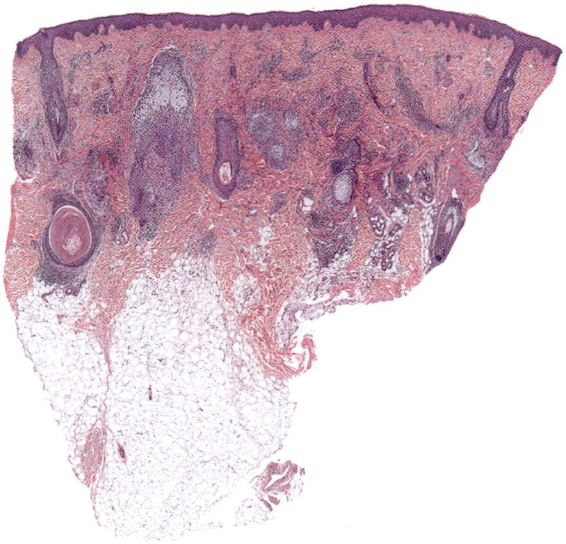

Figure 3.74 Pilotropic mycosis fungoides. Dense lymphoid infiltrates and mucin deposition within several hair follicles but without involvement of the interfollicular epidermis.

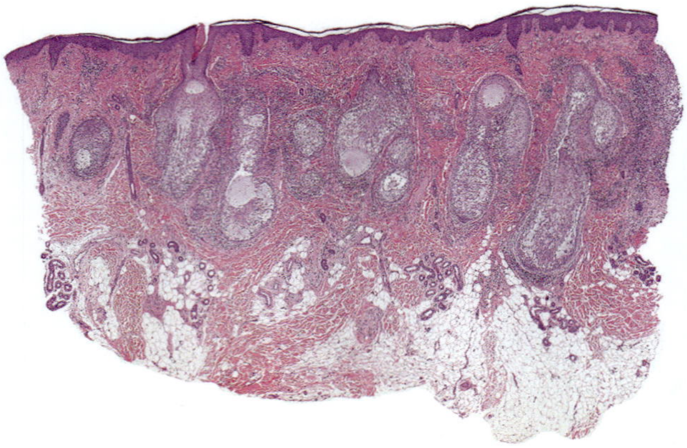

(a)

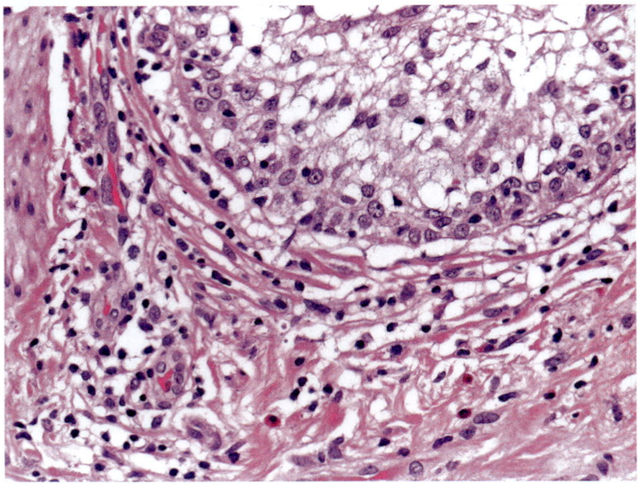

(b)

Figure 3.75 Pilotropic mycosis fungoides on the head and neck region. (a) Dense lymphoid infiltrates and mucin deposits within several hair follicles. (b) Pilotropic infiltrates and mucin deposition; note eosinophils within the dermal infiltrate.

tissue, but the exact reason(s) for this peculiar (and potentially misleading) histopathological feature is unknown.

There is no consensus on the exact nosology of so-called "idiopathic generalized follicular mucinosis" [212], and some authors do not believe that it represents a manifestation of mycosis fungoides. These cases are characterized by non-infiltrated, generalized lesions with hair loss in affected areas (Figs. 3.66, 3.69, and 3.80). The term "pilotropic T-cell dyscrasia" has been proposed for this condition [230]. However, cases of "idiopathic generalized follicular mucinosis" with progression to advanced mycosis fungoides and death have been well documented (Fig. 3.90) [212]. I have observed patients with clear-cut pilotropic mycosis fungoides who entered clinical remission after conventional treatments, and who subsequently relapsed with skin lesions showing clinical and histopathologic features of "idiopathic" follicular mucinosis. Interestingly, generalized follicular mucinosis may rarely present with

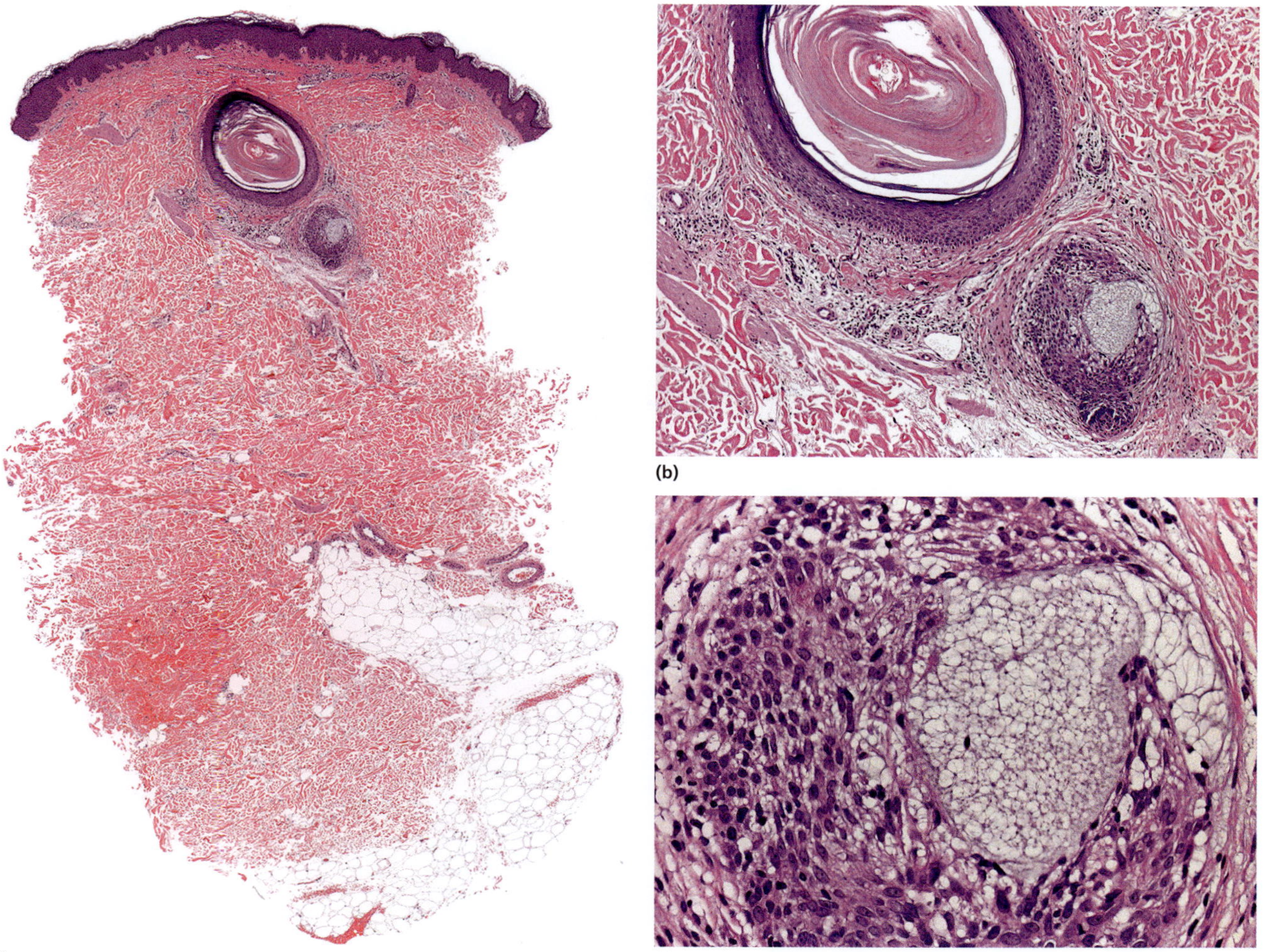

(a) (b) (c)

**Figure 3.76** Pilotropic mycosis fungoides on the trunk. (a) Sparse, superficial, perifollicular lymphoid infiltrates with cystic dilatation of the hair follicle. (b) Besides cystic dilatation, the affected hair follicle shows pilotropic lymphocytes and (c) focal mucin deposition.

hypopigmented lesions, indistinguishable from hypopigmented mycosis fungoides (Fig. 3.91) [231]. In my opinion, "idiopathic generalized follicular mucinosis" represents a variant of mycosis fungoides, and association with the disease has been observed even in children [232, 233]. The discussion is not only academic, however, as some authors reported a worse prognosis in patients with pilotropic mycosis fungoides as compared to those with "conventional" variants of the disease [234–238]. However, patients with "idiopathic" generalized follicular mucinosis were not included in these studies, thus introducing a selection bias. Other reports revealed a prognosis of pilotropic mycosis fungoides similar to that of the conventional variant of the disease [239], and the same group that first reported a worse prognosis subsequently described cases with a more indolent behavior and proposed the distinction of pilotropic mycosis fungoides into two groups ("indolent" and "aggressive" follicular mycosis fungoides) [240]. In this context, even recently it has been stated that predicting the evolution of patients with follicular mucinosis is a "sticky" situation [241]. A study by Van Santen *et al.* suggested that decreased survival is associated with percentage of atypical cells, cell size, percentage of Ki-67⁺ cells, and presence of epidermotropism not restricted to the hair follicles, whereas extensive follicular mucinosis is associated with increased survival, and the extent of perifollicular infiltrates has no prognostic value [242].

The nosology of "benign" solitary follicular mucinosis is unclear. Patients are usually children or young adults presenting with a single infiltrated patch on the face and alopecia in the affected region (Fig. 3.92). Although "benign" follicular mucinosis may be compared conceptually to the "solitary" variant of mycosis fungoides with good prognosis, in children and adolescents presenting with solitary lesions, I have never observed progression to advanced stages of the disease. I have seen, however, rare cases of pilotropic mycosis fungoides in adults

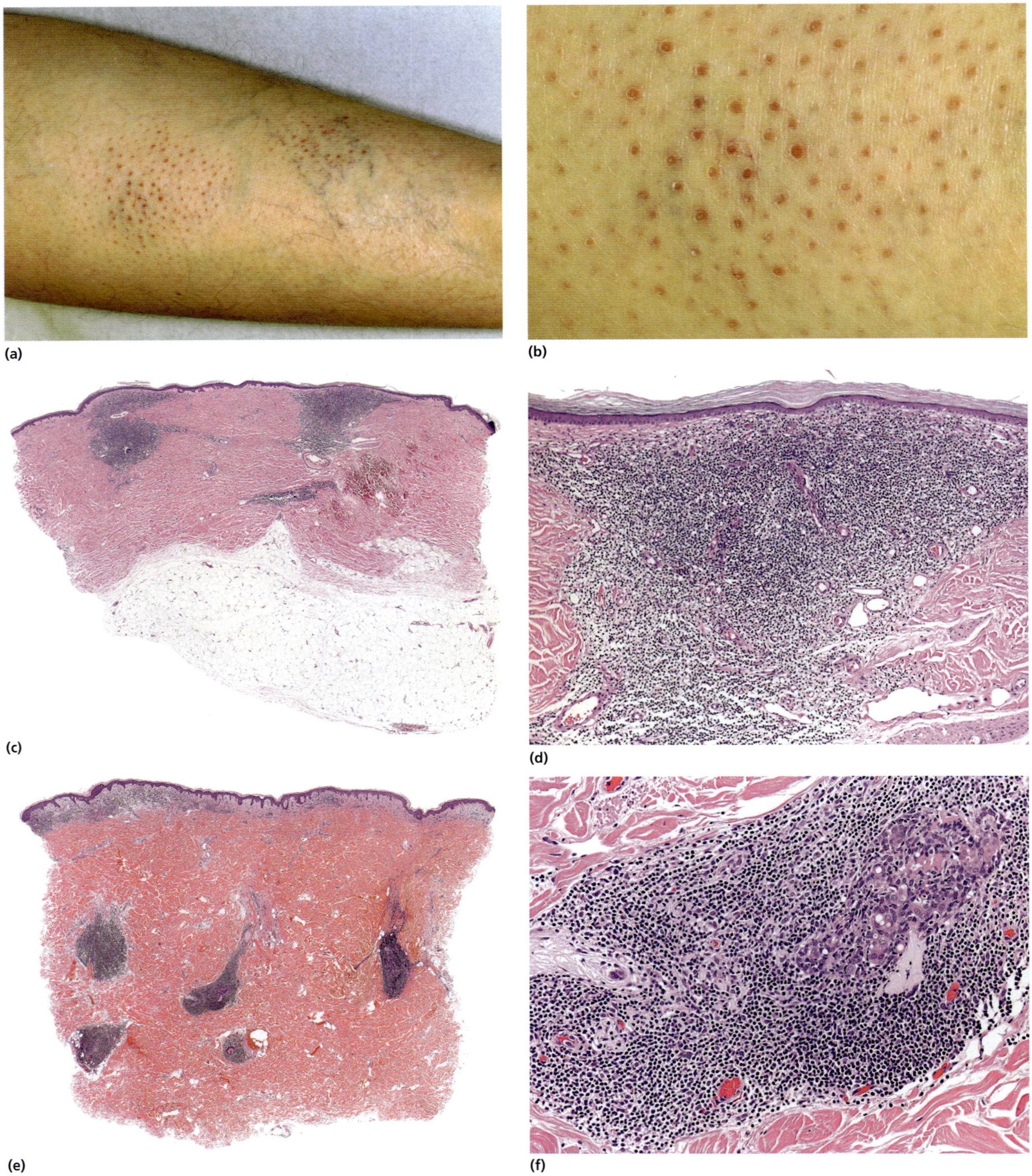

**Figure 3.77** Follicular mycosis fungoides without visible follicles. A 58-year-old man had a previous diagnosis of solitary mycosis fungoides treated by local radiotherapy with complete resolution. (a, b) Short after the end of radiotherapy he relapsed with multiple, follicular lesions on the trunk and extremities (*Courtesy of Dr. Martin Laimer, Salzburg, Austria*). (c) A biopsy showed dense, localized lymphoid infiltrates in the superficial and mid-dermis with an arrangement consistent with a follicular distribution. (d) Although hair follicles could not be observed in several deeper sections of tissue, smooth muscles were visible in the immediate vicinity of the lymphoid infiltrates. (e) A review of the biopsy of the initial solitary lesions showed a band-like infiltrate in the superficial dermis as well as (f) dense aggregates of lymphocytes around and within the eccrine glands with syringometaplasia, confirming the diagnosis of adnexotropic mycosis fungoides.

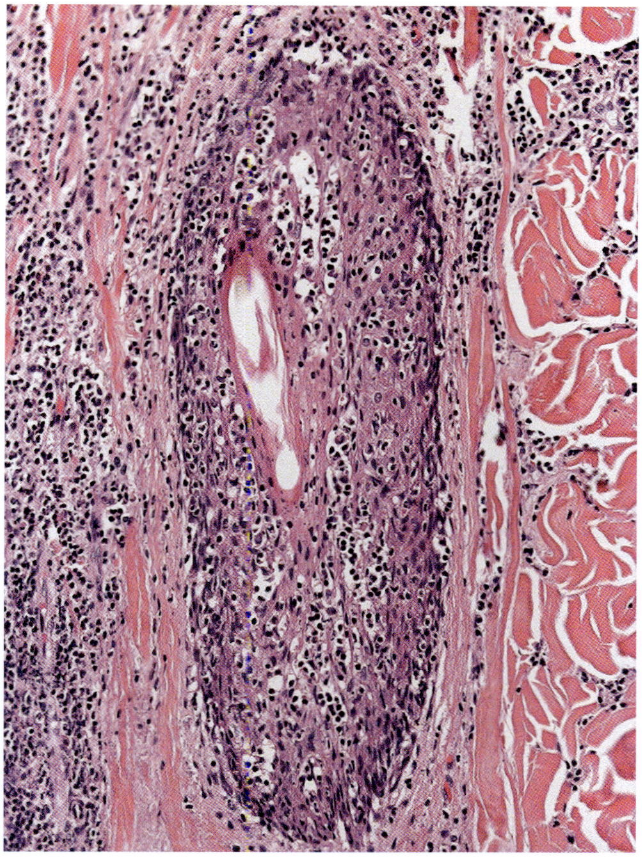

Figure 3.78 Pilotropic mycosis fungoides on the trunk. Note many pilotropic lymphocytes and complete absence of mucin.

beginning with a solitary lesion on the face, and subsequently showing progression to widespread disease (Fig. 3.93). The clinicopathologic features of solitary follicular mucinosis are indistinguishable from those of pilotropic mycosis fungoides, and monoclonality of T lymphocytes can be demonstrated in about half of the cases [212]. In addition, as already mentioned, cases of "unilesional" pilotropic mycosis fungoides have been reported, even in children and also on the face [188]. It has been suggested that current diagnostic criteria for early mycosis

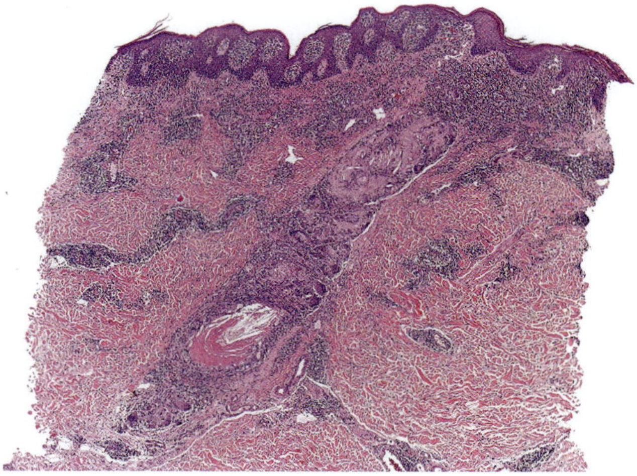

Figure 3.79 Mycosis fungoides with involvement of a hair follicle. The affected hair follicle is replaced by granulomatous inflammation. Note conventional features of mycosis fungoides in the epidermis.

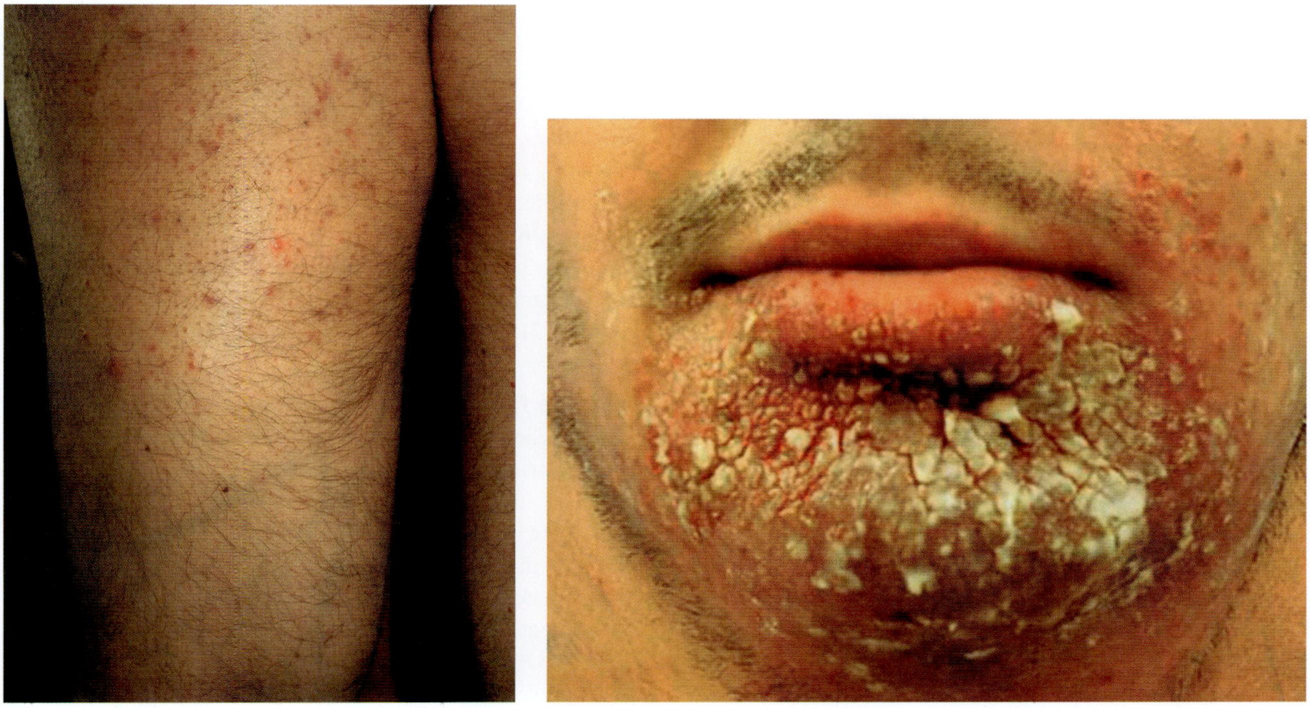

(a) (b)

Figure 3.80 Pilotropic mycosis fungoides. (a) Several, tiny follicular hyperkeratoses and small pustules in an area with loss of hairs in many of the affected follicles. (*Courtesy of Dr. Carlo Cota, Rome, Italy.*) (b) Impetiginization and keratotic scales on confluent lesions of pilotropic mycosis fungoides on the chin.

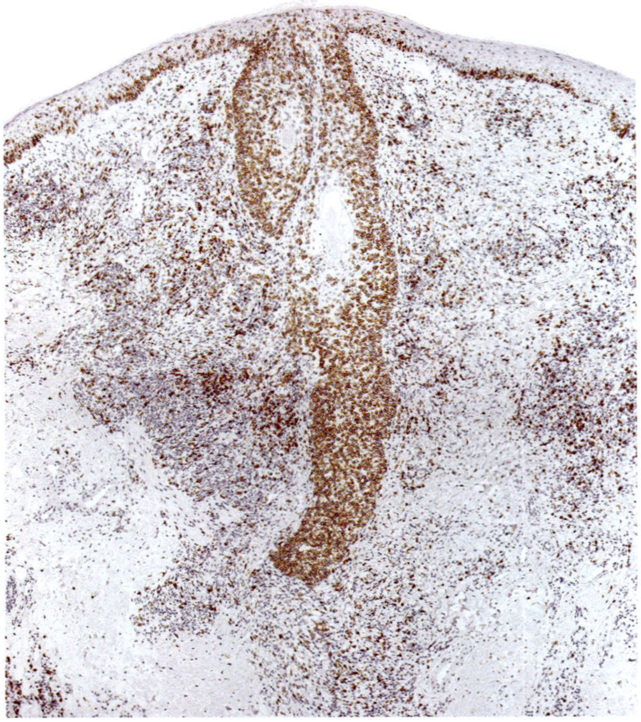

**Figure 3.81** Mycosis fungoides with involvement of a hair follicle. Staining for CD8 shows a pagetoid pilotropism as well as the presence of many positive intraepidermal lymphocytes. Positivity for CD8 is extremely rare in pilotropic mycosis fungoides.

fungoides should not be applied to children with alopecia mucinosa [243], but I would agree only for those presenting with solitary lesions of the disease, as pediatric patients with generalized involvement of the skin in my opinion have mycosis fungoides. For practical purposes, I do not use the term "pilotropic mycosis fungoides" for cases characterized by solitary lesions, particularly in children and adolescents, but mention the need for follow-up. Management should be conservative, and spontaneous resolution may occur.

Another clinical variant of follicular mucinosis, the so-called acneiform type, is very rare. It is characterized by follicular, erythematous papules on the head and neck area and on the upper trunk, and the histopathological findings are indistinguishable from those of conventional follicular mucinosis (Fig. 3.94). In this type, too, a relationship with mycosis fungoides has been proposed [244], yet it is unclear whether these cases are really part of the spectrum of adnexotropic mycosis fungoides, and a follow-up study showed an invariably benign course [245]. I have seen only a few patients, and none of them developed clear-cut mycosis fungoides. However, "acneiform" follicular lesions have been described in patients with mycosis fungoides [239], and a monoclonal T-cell population may be observed in the infiltrate [246].

Besides these variants, I have seen one case of generalized follicular mucinosis with anetoderma in all of the lesions (see below the paragraph on anetodermic mycosis fungoides). Follicular mucinosis with linear distribution of the lesions has also been rarely described, but it may be that these cases represent peculiar nevoid forms of the hair follicles with secondary mucin deposition, rather than genuine follicular mucinosis [247–249].

In advanced stages of the disease, patients with pilotropic mycosis fungoides may sometimes present with tumors contiguous to areas showing clinical features of follicular involvement (Fig. 3.90c). However, in other cases the features of pilotropic mycosis fungoides may be inconspicuous clinically, and histopathologically the hair follicles may be almost completely or entirely wiped off by the infiltrate. In such cases, sometimes the architecture of the infiltrate may still betray the prominent involvement of the adnexal structures, and immunohistology may confirm the presence of numerous lymphocytes within the remnants of the hair follicles (Figs. 3.77, 3.95).

The clinical differential diagnosis of pilotropic mycosis fungoides is broad, including mainly lichen spinulosus, lichen planopilaris, acneiform dermatoses, nevus comedonicus, milia en plaques due to other conditions, atopic dermatitis, and keratosis pilaris. Clinical differentiation from lichen spinulosus may be extremely difficult, but the finding of mucin deposition within the hair follicles in more than one biopsy in my opinion suggests the diagnosis of follicular mucinosis rather than lichen spinulosus (Fig. 3.96) [200]; as already mentioned, cases published in the literature as "lichen spinulosos with follicular mucinosis" may represent examples of folliculotropic mycosis fungoides [216]. The histopathological presentation is very distinctive and allows differentiation from these entities (notwithstanding the problems in distinguishing among the different types of "follicular mucinosis"). Therapeutic options for pilotropic mycosis fungoides are summarized below in the section on treatment of mycosis fungoides.

Finally, it should be mentioned that deposition of mucin within the hair follicle is not synonymous with alopecia mucinosa/follicular mucinosis, and it may be an incidental finding in biopsy specimens of different conditions (including other cutaneous hematological malignancies) (see Chapter 31 and Figs. 31.11 and 31.17) [250, 251].

### Mycosis fungoides with epidermal mucinosis

Although in most cases mucin deposition in mycosis fungoides is restricted to the epithelium of the hair follicles, in some cases the epidermis may be involved as well (Fig. 3.97). Prominent intraepidermal mucin may be misconstructed as spongiform vesicles, and such cases may be misinterpreted as an eczematous dermatitis (Fig. 3.98) [252, 253]. These cases do not present the typical clinical features of pilotropic mycosis fungoides (Fig. 3.97a), and are otherwise indistinguishable from conventional cases of early mycosis fungoides. Unlike follicular mucinosis, epidermal mucinosis is an incidental

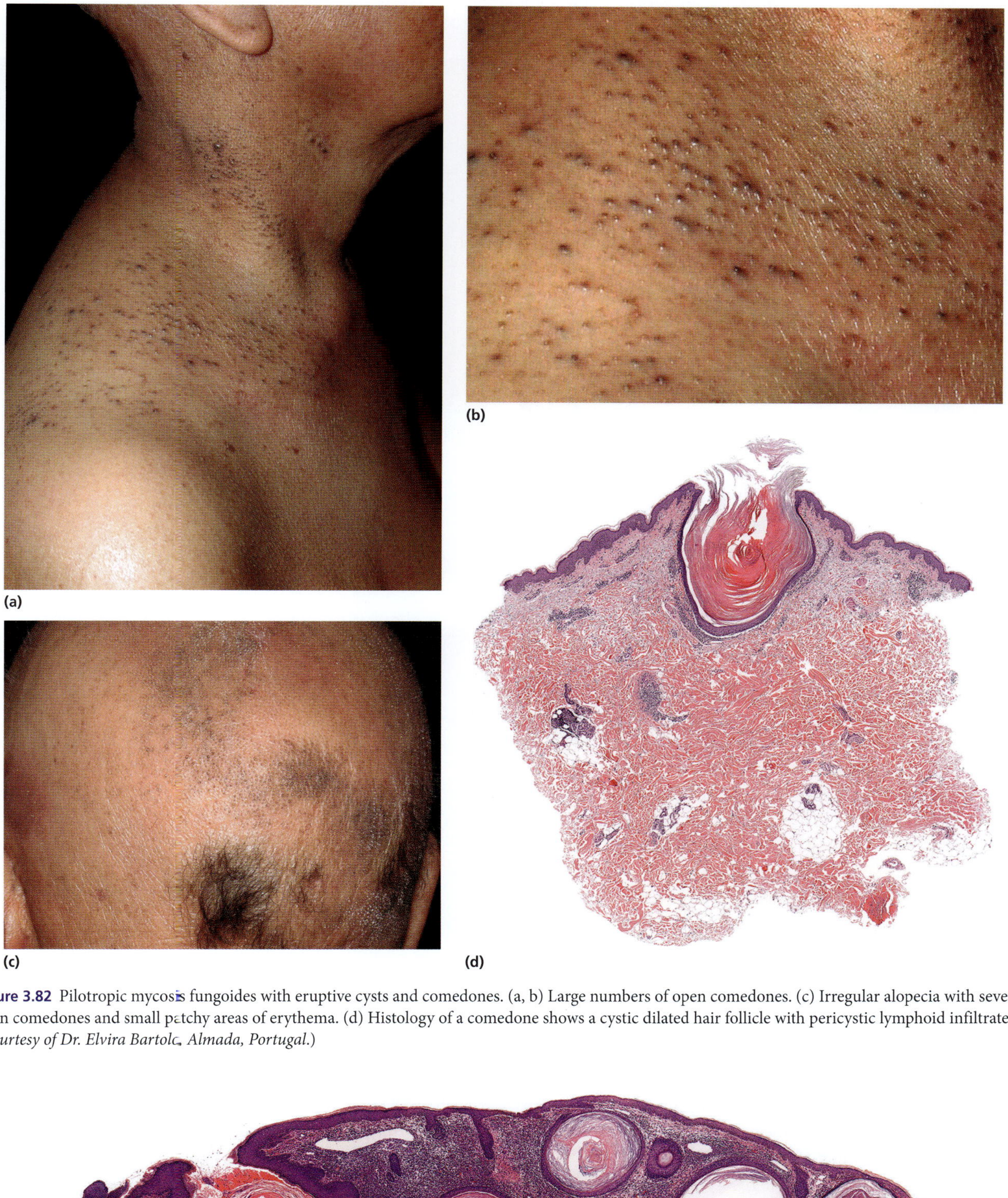

**Figure 3.82** Pilotropic mycosis fungoides with eruptive cysts and comedones. (a, b) Large numbers of open comedones. (c) Irregular alopecia with several open comedones and small patchy areas of erythema. (d) Histology of a comedone shows a cystic dilated hair follicle with pericystic lymphoid infiltrates. (*Courtesy of Dr. Elvira Bartolo, Almada, Portugal.*)

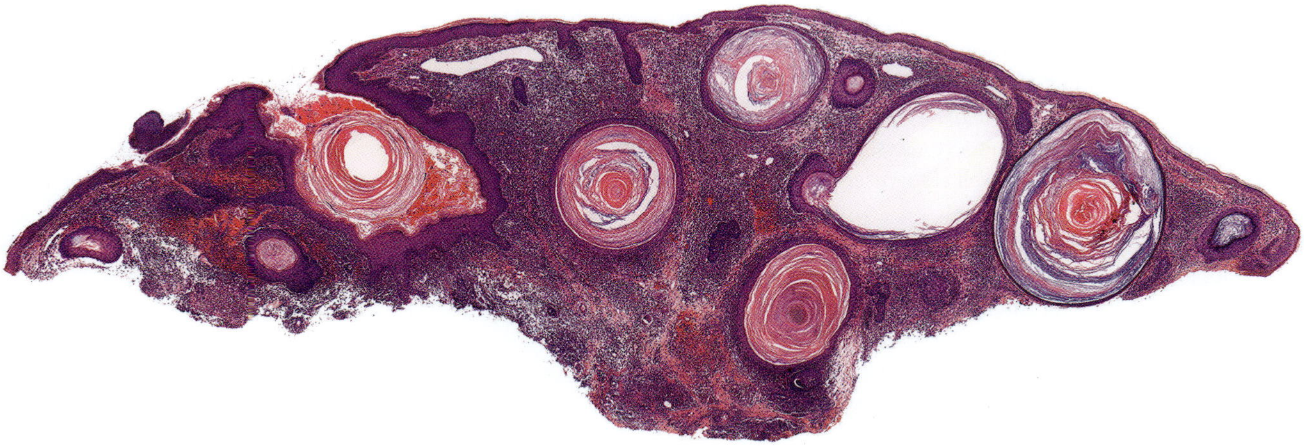

**Figure 3.83** Pilotropic mycosis fungoides with eruptive cysts and comedones. Several small infundibular cysts and dense lymphoid infiltrates in so-called milia en plaque.

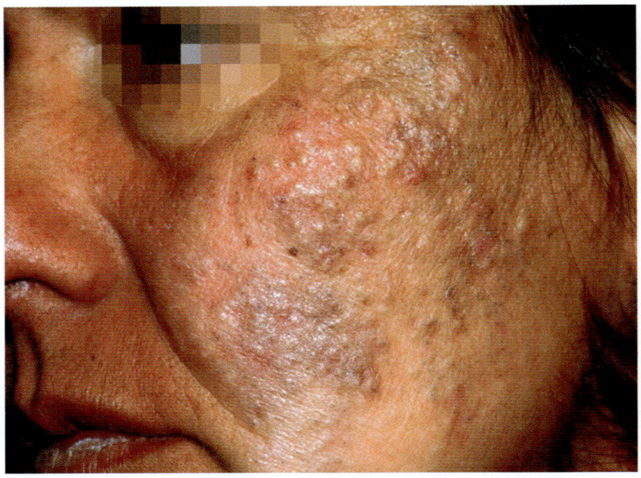

**Figure 3.84** Pilotropic mycosis fungoides with eruptive cysts and comedones. Confluent, small epidermal cysts on the cheek ("milia en plaque").

finding which is usually present only in one biopsy from a given patient. I have never observed epidermal mucinosis in tumor stage mycosis fungoides.

## Syringotropic mycosis fungoides

Syringotropic mycosis fungoides is the other adnexotropic pattern of the disease, and is often combined with more or less prominent involvement of the hair follicles. Clinically, in many cases distinction from pilotropic mycosis fungoides is not possible, and lesions may show a similar follicular plugging with agminated arrangement (Fig. 3.99). Lesions may be generalized or solitary. Palms and soles are involved more commonly than in other variants of the disease (Fig. 3.100). In some cases, conventional patches of mycosis fungoides are present at other body sites. Histopathologically, the lesions are characterized by dense lymphoid infiltrates located mainly around hyperplastic eccrine glands and coils, often with syringometaplasia (Fig. 3.101) [254, 255]. The hair follicles are usually involved as well and are surrounded by dense lymphoid infiltrates with pilotropism. A concomitant band-like infiltrate in the papillary dermis is observed in the majority of the specimens. Particularly in cases without band-like infiltrate, however, the histopathologic diagnosis may be very difficult (Fig. 3.102).

The term "syringolymphoid hyperplasia with alopecia" has been used in the past to refer to these cases, but the relationship to mycosis fungoides has been well recognized [254].

## Pustular mycosis fungoides

A variant of mycosis fungoides characterized by pustular lesions was described for the first time by Ackerman in 1966 [256]. A few other cases have been reported subsequently [257–259]. The pustules are visible histopathologically (mostly as intracorneal aggregates of neutrophils, similar to what can be observed in generalized pustular psoriasis and in acute generalized exanthematous pustulosis – AGEP), but may be not evident clinically; thus, this type of mycosis fungoides represents preeminently a histopathological variant of the disease (Fig. 3.103). Cases with visible pustules resemble clinically generalized pustular psoriasis or AGEP. In some patients the pustules are in continuity with the hair follicles [191], thus representing a variant of pilotropic mycosis fungoides, but in several cases they are unrelated to the follicles [260]. Pustular mycosis fungoides has been associated with progression of the disease [261, 262], and in a large study it was characterized by a worse prognosis compared to conventional mycosis fungoides [260]. However, I think that, at least in a proportion of the cases, the onset of pustules may be a consequence of the advanced disease rather than

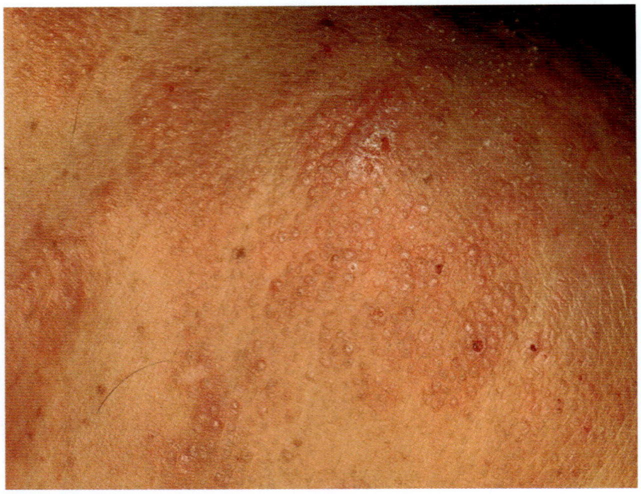

(a)

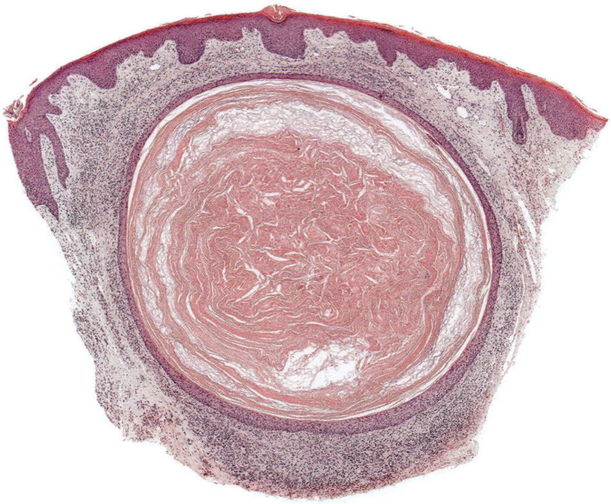

(b)

**Figure 3.85** Pilotropic mycosis fungoides. (a) Several small cysts and infiltrated erythematous lesions in a patient with long-standing pilotropic mycosis fungoides. (b) A small epidermal cyst surrounded by lymphoid infiltrate devoid of neutrophils or granulomatous features.

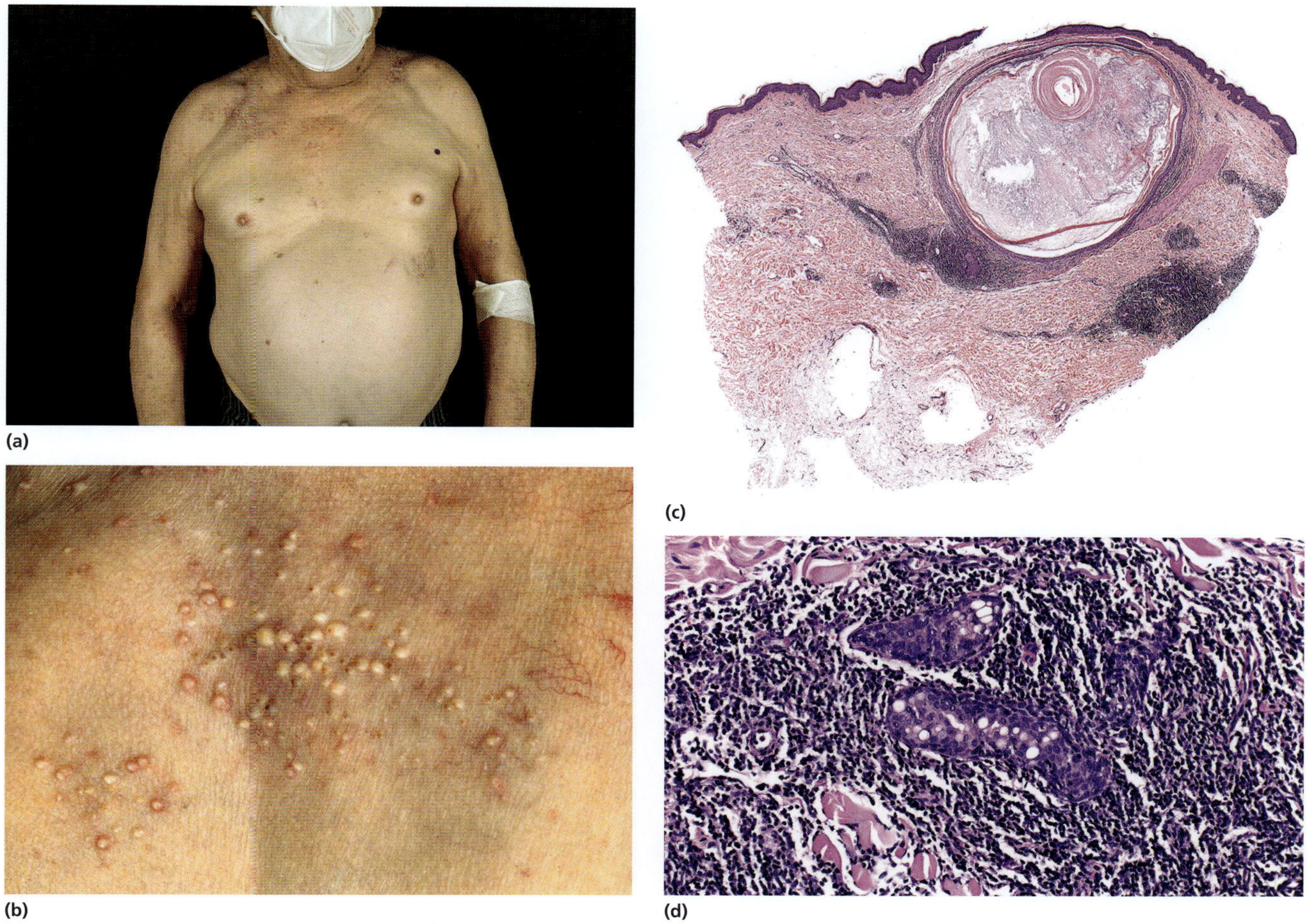

Figure 3.86 Pilotropic mycosis fungoides. (a) Irregular distribution of (b) variably large cysts, most of which are surrounded by a thin inflammatory halo. (c) Histology reveals an infundibular cyst with pericystic lymphoid infiltrate and (d) with involvement of the eccrine glands with syringometaplasia.

the reason for a worse prognosis, possibly representing impetiginization or other microbial superinfections in patients with impaired immune system.

## Localized pagetoid reticulosis (Woringer–Kolopp type)

Localized pagetoid reticulosis is a variant of mycosis fungoides presenting with psoriasiform, scaly erythematous patches or plaques, usually located on the extremities (Fig. 3.104). The lesions are either solitary or localized to one acral site. The clinical presentation can be deceptive, simulating that of benign conditions such as warts or eczematous dermatitis (Fig. 3.105). The histologic picture shows a markedly hyperplastic epidermis with striking ("pagetoid") epidermotropism of medium-sized pleomorphic lymphocytes (Figs. 3.106a and b). The lymphocytes may show a tropism for adnexal structures and grow along the eccrine coils (Figs. 3.106c and d), thus cautioning against superficial treatment modalities. Pagetoid reticulosis is usually characterized by a T-cytotoxic phenotype (Fig. 3.106d), but a helper phenotype or double negativity for both CD4 and CD8 have been reported [263, 264], as well as double expression of TCRαβ and TCRγδ [265].

The term "pagetoid reticulosis" should be restricted to solitary or localized lesions only (Woringer–Kolopp type). Most patients presenting with the "generalized" form of pagetoid reticulosis (Ketron–Goodman type) have one of the cutaneous aggressive cytotoxic NK/T-cell lymphomas (cutaneous aggressive epidermotropic $CD8^+$ cytotoxic T-cell lymphoma, cutaneous γ/δ T-cell lymphoma, extranodal NK/T-cell lymphoma, nasal type) (see Chapters 7, 8, and 9).

It should be emphasized that a histopathologic picture characterized by markedly hyperplastic epidermis with pagetoid epidermotropism of innumerable T lymphocytes is not restricted to pagetoid reticulosis or aggressive cytotoxic NK/T-cell lymphomas: other lymphomas may rarely present with similar features, and a definitive diagnosis should be made only upon compelling clinicopathologic evidence and after complete phenotypic and genotypic studies [266]. Lymphomatoid papulosis, type D, may be indistinguishable from pagetoid reticulosis histopathologically, but shows the typical waxing and waning course clinically, and usually does not arise on acral sites (see Chapter 5). The presence of intraepidermal CD30$^+$ neoplastic cells in "pagetoid reticulosis" should raise suspicion of such a variant of lymphomatoid papulosis; a precise classification of these cases can be achieved only upon clinicopathologic correlation.

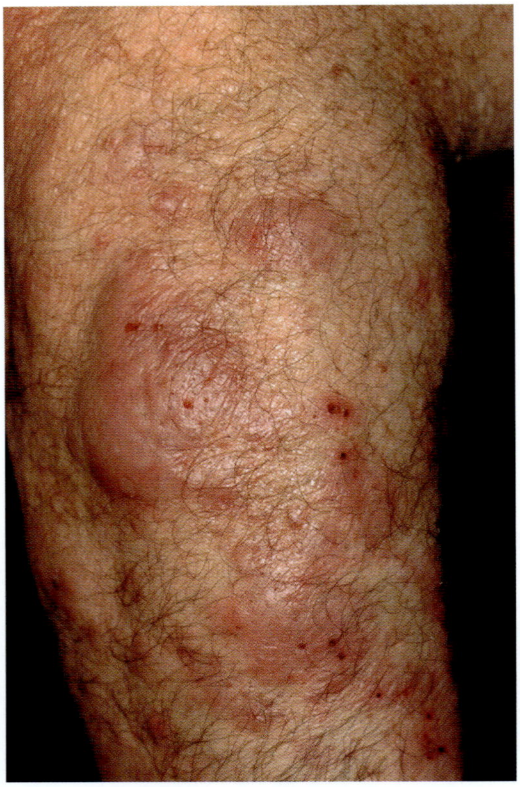

**Figure 3.87** Pilotropic mycosis fungoides with several involved follicles and a tumoral infiltrate ("pseudotumor") on the upper arm, resulting from confluence of several affected follicles.

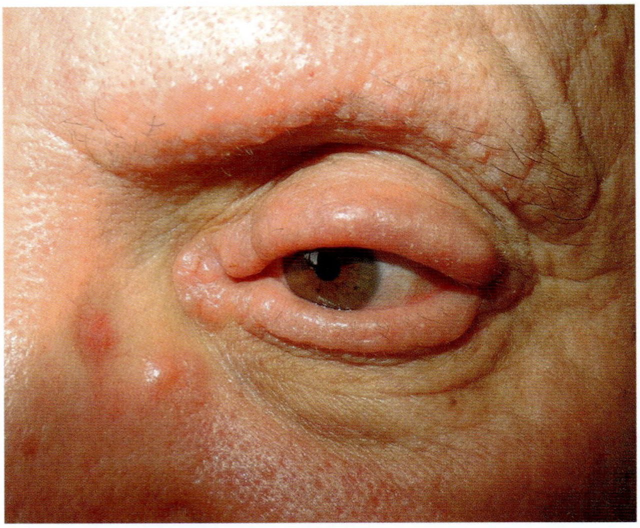

**Figure 3.88** Pilotropic mycosis fungoides. Almost complete loss of eyelashes with swelling of the eyelids in advanced stage of the disease. Note also almost complete loss of the eyebrow. (*Courtesy of Dr. Carlo Cota, Rome, Italy.*)

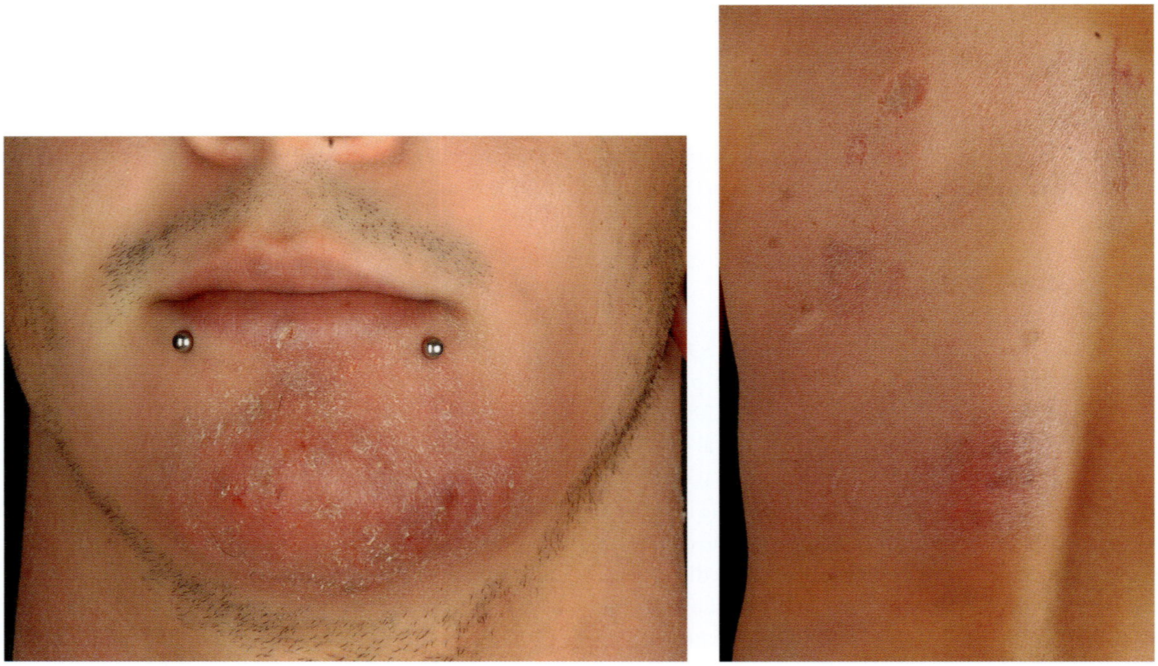

(a) (b)

**Figure 3.89** Mycosis fungoides with involvement of the subcutaneous tissue. (a) This patient had typical lesions of follicular mucinosis on the chin, and (b) conventional lesions of mycosis fungoides on the trunk and extremities. (c) A biopsy from the trunk showed a band-like infiltrate with minimal involvement of the reticular dermis, but (d) prominent involvement of the subcutaneous tissues as well as (e) a band-like infiltrate in the superficial dermis. Note that the infiltrate extends to the depth along the adnexal structures.

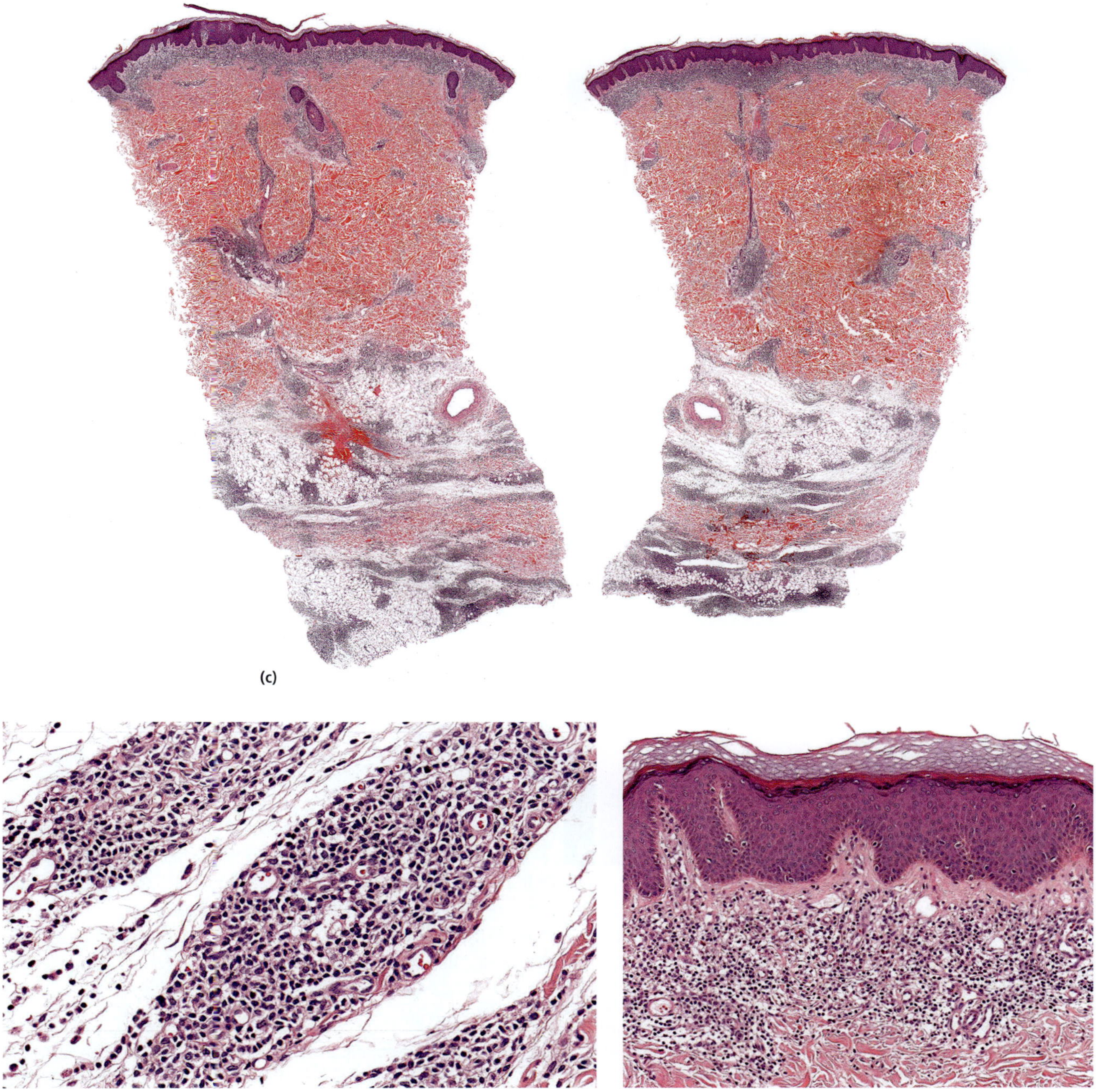

(c)

(d) (e)

Figure 3.89 (Continued)

The prognosis of patients with solitary pagetoid reticulosis is excellent, and involvement of internal organs has never been observed. Development of conventional mycosis fungoides has been documented in a few patients. The treatment of choice is surgical excision or local radiotherapy. Other skin-directed therapies may be used for more extensive lesions, including topical or intralesional steroids, topical nitrogen mustard, photodynamic therapy, laser ablation, PUVA, and narrow-band UV-B irradiation [267, 268], but superficial treatment modalities may be ineffective in cases showing deeper extension along the adnexal structures (see Fig. 3.106d).

## Unilesional ("solitary") mycosis fungoides

Besides localized pagetoid reticulosis, a solitary variant of mycosis fungoides with clinicopathologic features similar to "common" mycosis fungoides has been described [269–271].

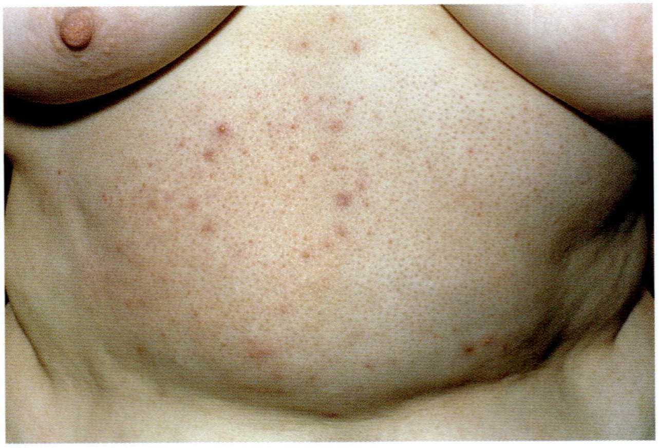

(a)

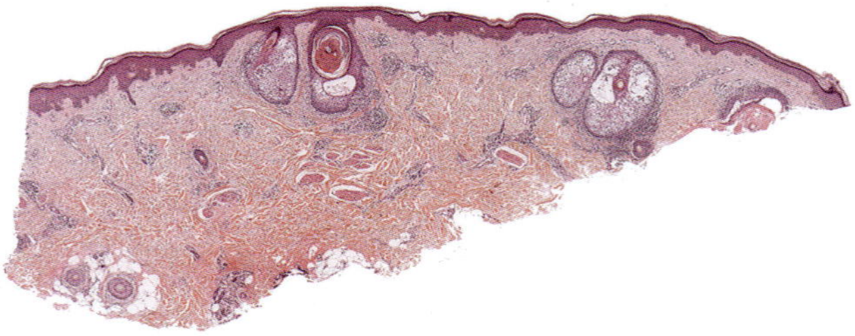

(b)

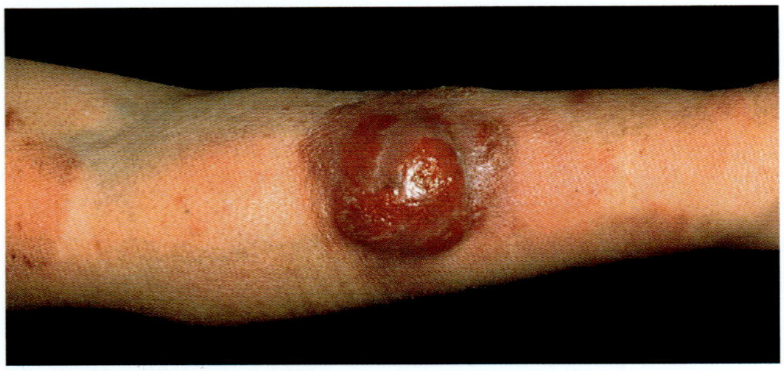

(c)

Figure 3.90 Pilotropic mycosis fungoides ("idiopathic generalized follicular mucinosis"). (a) Generalized follicular papules, pustules, and small patches in a 38-year-old woman in a picture taken in 1981. According to the patient, the first manifestations of the diseases dated back to 1976. (b) A biopsy revealed follicular mucinosis with scant lymphoid infiltrates ("idiopathic follicular mucinosis"). (c) The same patient with tumor stage mycosis fungoides in 1985. The patient died of progressive disease 4 years later at the age of 46, 8 years after first presentation and 13 years after onset of the disease.

The literature about this subject is confusing, as in the past disparate cases were lumped together in this category, including pagetoid reticulosis and "mycosis fungoides en tumeur d'emblée" among others. In addition, many of the cases reported in the literature probably represent in truth examples of lichenoid keratosis or other pseudolymphomas (including some of the cases published by our group – see the section on lichenoid [lymphomatoid] keratosis in Chapter 31) [269]. On the other hand, I have rarely observed patients with solitary lesions of genuine mycosis fungoides (Figs. 3.52a and 3.107), and some cases have been reported (reviewed in [272]). Solitary mycosis fungoides is localized mostly on sun-protected areas. The clinical presentation and histopathological features are identical to those of conventional mycosis fungoides, but rare cases may present with peculiar clinical (and histopathological) aspects [273]. In some patients with long-standing solitary lesions, large cell transformation may occur even in the absence of a more widespread skin involvement (see Figs. 3.52b and c). Increased expression of microRNA-17 ~ 92 has been observed in one case [274].

It is yet unclear whether solitary mycosis fungoides has a better prognosis [275], but in some instances development of generalized lesions of the disease has been observed over time [276]. As in other variants of the disease, the presence of large cell transformation should be regarded as a bad prognostic sign.

## Granulomatous mycosis fungoides

Granulomatous mycosis fungoides is an unusual histologic variant of the disease described first by Ackerman and Flaxman in 1970, who reported a patient with tumor-stage mycosis fungoides with histiocytic giant cells scattered within the dermal infiltrate [277].

Granulomatous lesions may either precede, be concomitant with, or follow "classic" mycosis fungoides; they can be observed in patches, plaques, and tumors of the disease, and in some cases even within affected lymph nodes [278]. Clinically there may be irregular areas of induration (Fig. 3.108), but in most cases the clinical aspect does not betray the presence of granulomas histopathologically. In my experience, a granulomatous reaction is observed mostly in tumors of mycosis fungoides, and sometimes may be secondary to treatment. Granulomas can also be observed in the context of pilotropic mycosis fungoides, due to destruction of hair follicles (see the section on pilotropic mycosis fungoides in this chapter and Fig. 3.79). Especially at first biopsy, the disease shows prominent granulomatous features, the diagnosis of mycosis fungoides may be missed, and the histopathologic picture may be misinterpreted as that of a "granulomatous dermatitis." Epidermotropism is a helpful clue (Fig. 3.109), but it is often minimal or missing in granulomatous tumors (Fig. 3.110).

Histopathologically, granulomatous mycosis fungoides may also be difficult or even impossible to distinguish from other cutaneous T-cell lymphoproliferative diseases with granulomatous features (e.g., $CD4^+$ small/medium T-cell lymphoproliferative disorders) [279], and clinicopathologic correlation is crucial for the diagnosis. Although the infiltrate in granulomatous mycosis fungoides usually involves the entire dermis, in rare cases the granulomatous features may be observed in the context of superficial infiltrates [280]. Small clusters of $CD123^+$ plasmacytoid dendritic may be observed in lesions of granulomatous mycosis fungoides [281]. However, in my experience they do not represent a helpful diagnostic clue, as plasmacytoid dendritic cells may be observed in a variety of cutaneous inflammatory and neoplastic conditions.

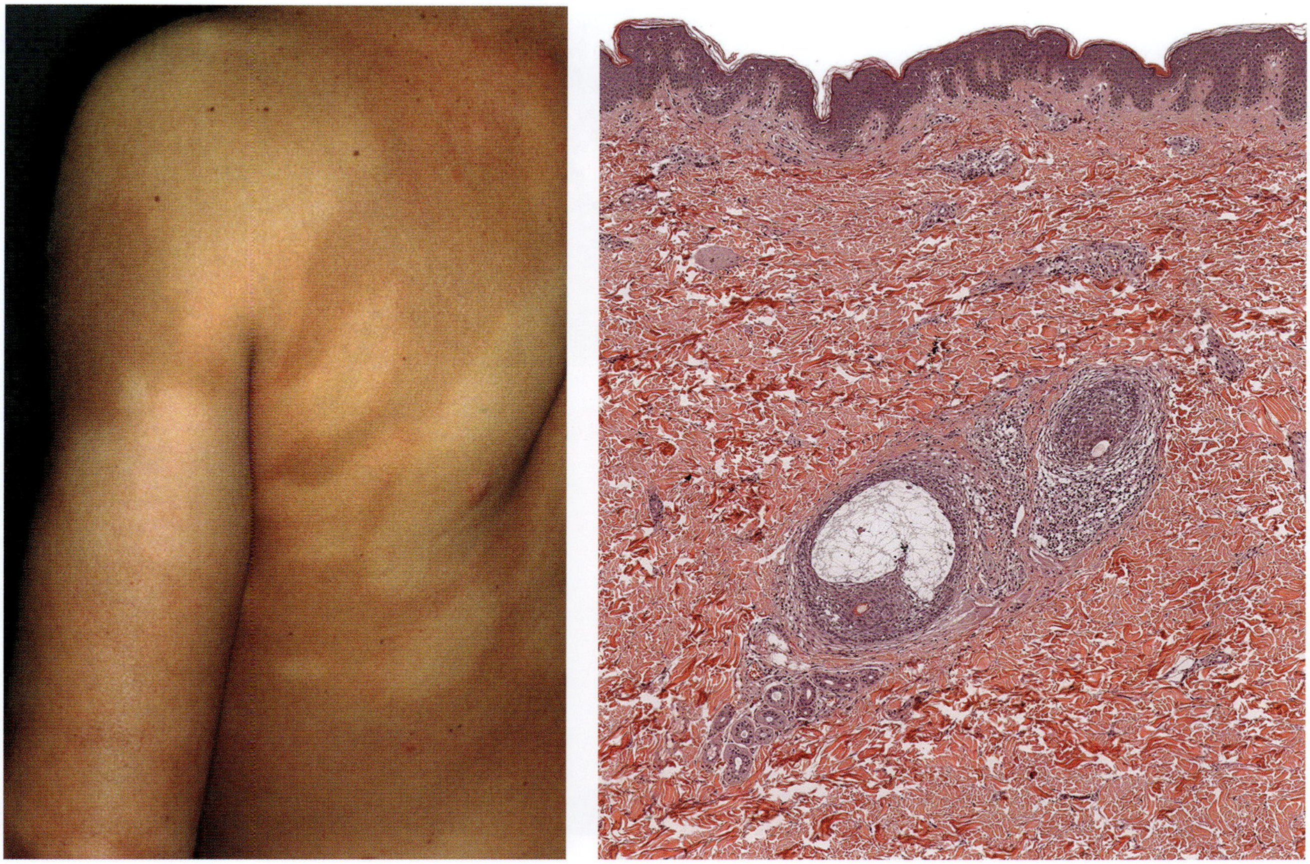

(a) (b)

**Figure 3.91** Pilotropic mycosis fungoides. (a) Hypopigmented patches on the trunk and upper extremities, indistinguishable from hypopigmented mycosis fungoides (*Courtesy of Dr Luca Muscardin, Rome, Italy*). (b) Histology reveals typical features of follicular mucinosis.

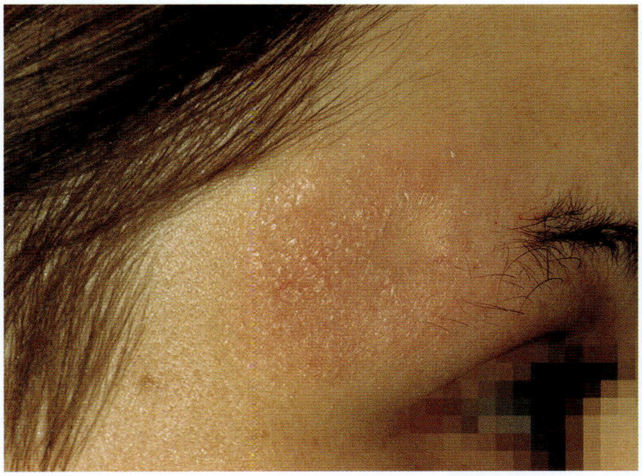

**Figure 3.92** Solitary "benign" follicular mucinosis. Solitary erythematous patch with follicular accentuation and alopecia on the eyebrow of an 18-year-old girl.

Granulomatous mycosis fungoides seems to have a worse prognosis than that of conventional variants of the disease, and patients have a higher risk of developing a second lymphoma [282]. On the other hand, the amount of the granulomatous reaction is often variable in different biopsies from a single patient, suggesting that the term "granulomatous mycosis fungoides" should be used as a description of histopathologic specimens, and not for classifying the disease in a given patient. It is also important to realize that differentiation of "conventional" granulomatous mycosis fungoides from granulomatous slack skin cannot be achieved on histopathologic grounds only, and that correlation with the clinical picture is crucial for a precise classification [283].

## Granulomatous slack skin

A rare variant of granulomatous mycosis fungoides is represented by granulomatous slack skin, which is characterized clinically by the occurrence of bulky, pendulous skinfolds, usually located in flexural areas (Fig. 3.111) [284–286]. It is a variant observed almost exclusively in adults and elderly patients, but rare cases in children have been reported [287]. Granulomatous slack skin is considered in most cases as a specific manifestation of mycosis fungoides, and is included as a variant of mycosis fungoides in the ICC and WHO classifications [1, 3]. Association

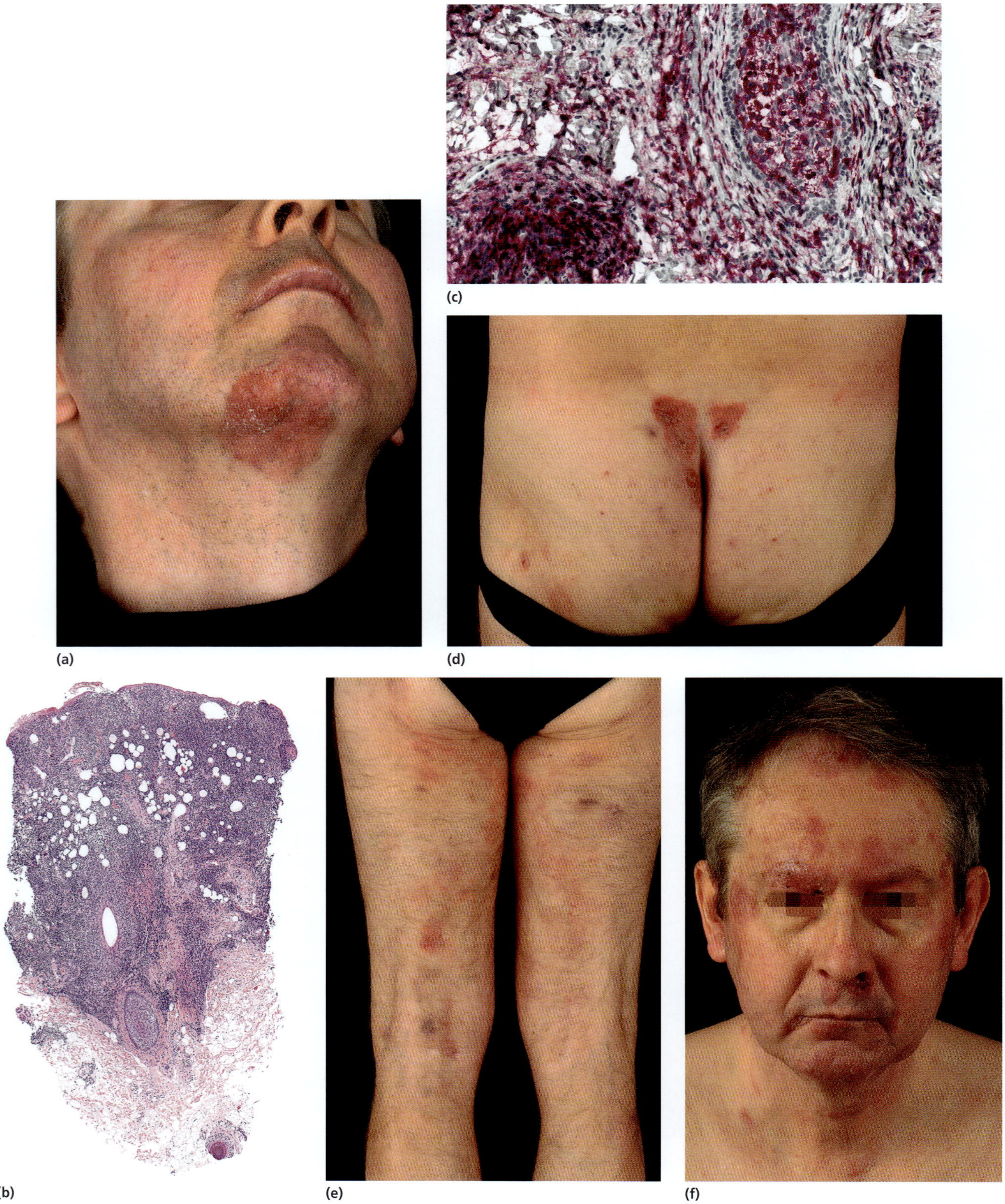


**Figure 3.93** Follicular mycosis fungoides. (a) The disease in this patient started with a long-standing, solitary plaque on the chin, revealing histopathologically (b) a dense lymphoid infiltrate with only remnants of affected hair follicles with some mucin deposition, and (c) several intraepithelial lymphocytes. Three years later, several partly "acneiform" lesions were visible on the buttocks (d) and thighs (e), and (f) two more years later a diffuse infiltration of the face was present.

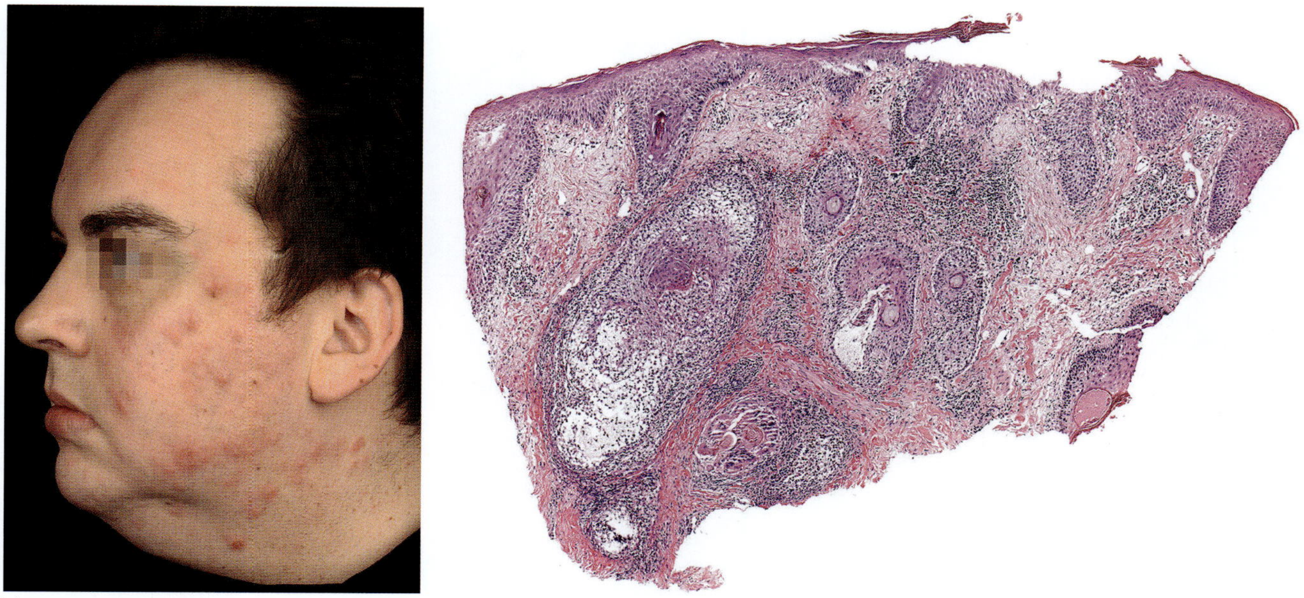


Figure 3.94 Acneiform follicular mucinosis. (a) Acneiform papules on the face. Note the lack of involvement of the eyebrows. (b) Histology reveals typical features of follicular mucinosis.

with other lymphomas, including Hodgkin lymphoma, has been reported in the past. In most of these cases, on the other hand, granulomatous slack skin probably represented a manifestation of mycosis fungoides associated with a second lymphoma, rather than a clinicopathologic variant of the second lymphoma. Interestingly, a recent series showed extracutaneous involvement in 38% of patients [288]; on the other hand, my experience and that acquired through published cases is that the prognosis of granulomatous slack skin is excellent. Treatment with methotrexate seems to represent a valid alternative to surgery of the bulky skin in these patients [288].

The granulomatous infiltrate in granulomatous slack skin is usually diffuse and involves the subcutaneous tissues, in contrast to the patchy, dermal granulomas observed in "conventional" granulomatous mycosis fungoides (Fig. 3.112), but differentiation between the two variants may not be possible on histopathological grounds alone. Histiocytic giant cells with many nuclei and with intracytoplasmic phagocyted leukocytes are a common finding (Fig. 3.113). Elastophagocytosis is typically present. Interestingly, elastolysis has been observed also in cases of conventional mycosis fungoides [289]. The same rearrangement of T-cells has been observed in skin and nodal lesions in one patient [290], and a t(3,9)(q12;p24) has been detected in another case [291].

As already mentioned, a diagnosis of granulomatous slack skin can only be made when the typical clinical presentation is observed, as histopathological differentiation from "conventional" granulomatous mycosis fungoides is not possible [283]. On the other hand, in some patients, lesions located at typical sites of granulomatous slack skin (axillae, groins), but that do not show bulky, pendulous skin folds, may be considered as early manifestations of the disease if the characteristic histopathologic features described above are present (Fig. 3.114). Whether these patients, if untreated, progress to overt granulomatous slack skin is unclear.

## Erythrodermic mycosis fungoides

Patients with mycosis fungoides may develop erythroderma during the course of their disease (Fig. 3.115). Rarely, swelling of the lymph nodes and the presence of circulating neoplastic cells ("Sézary cells") are observed as well, thus showing overlapping clinical features with Sézary syndrome. The histopathologic and phenotypic features are identical to those of conventional mycosis fungoides. However, patients with erythrodermic mycosis fungoides show more commonly a B0 or B1 blood involvement, whereas a B2 involvement is needed for the diagnosis of Sézary syndrome (see also Chapter 1, Table 1.2) [292]. On the other hand, B1 is considered a "pre-Sézary syndrome" stage; thus, patients with erythrodermic mycosis fungoides and positive blood biomarkers are at higher risk of developing aggressive disease [292]. After successful treatment, patients may relapse with conventional patches, plaques, or tumors of mycosis fungoides or with new flares of erythroderma. In this context, in my experience erythroderma alone without blood involvement does not put patients in a high-risk category, which should be considered only for patients with erythroderma and positive blood biomarkers.

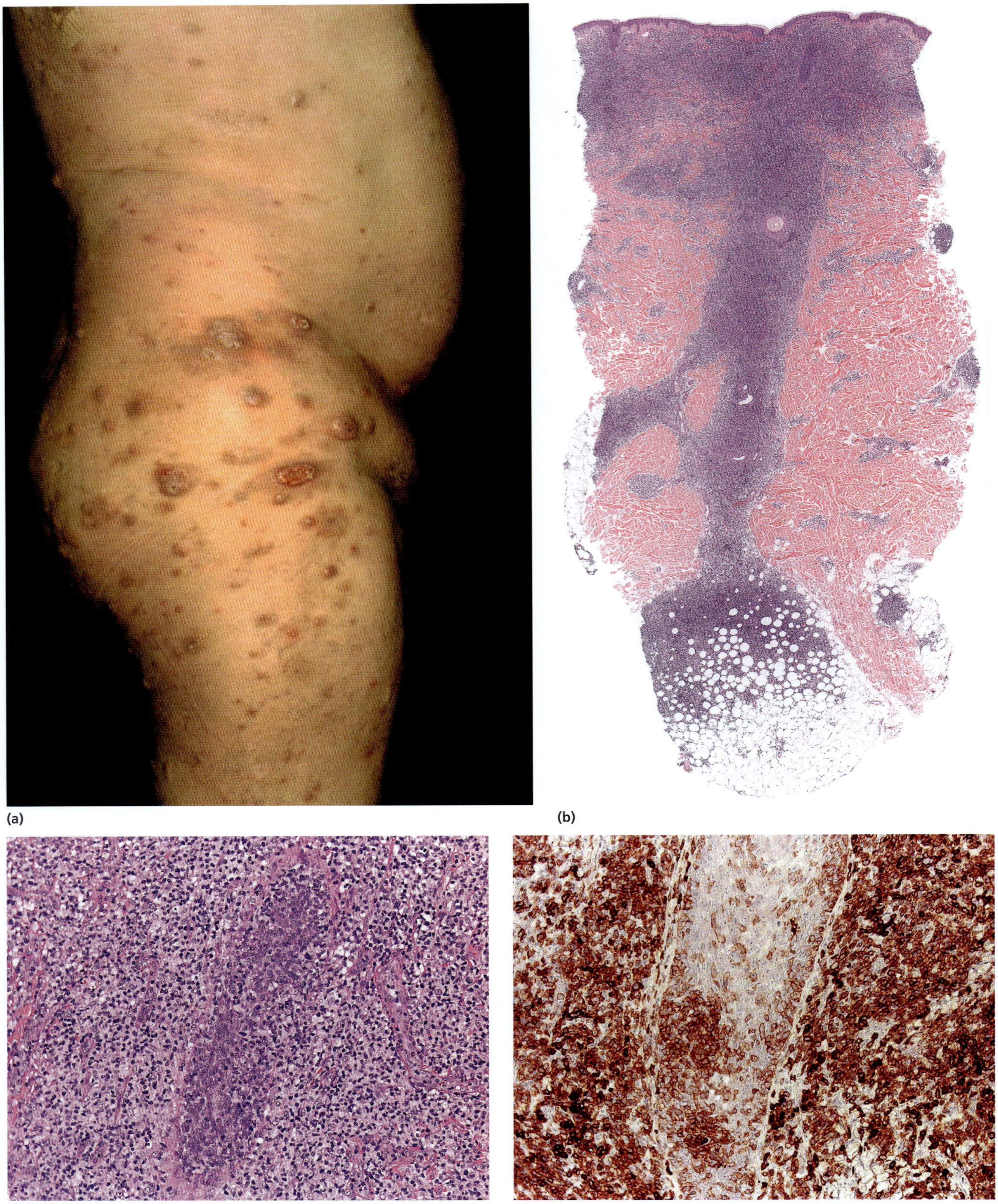

(a) (b) (c) (d)

Figure 3.95 Pilotropic mycosis fungoides in tumor stage. This 50-year-old patient had a 17-year history of pilotropic mycosis fungoides. (a) The clinical presentation is characterized by multiple, partly ulcerated plaques and tumors and many papules, some with follicular openings. Histology of one lesion shows (b) dense lymphoid infiltrates involving the subcutaneous fat and growing along the dermal adnexal structures. (c) Only remnants of hair follicles with several pilotropic lymphocytes are visible. (d) Immunohistology highlights numerous pilotropic lymphocytes positive for CD5.

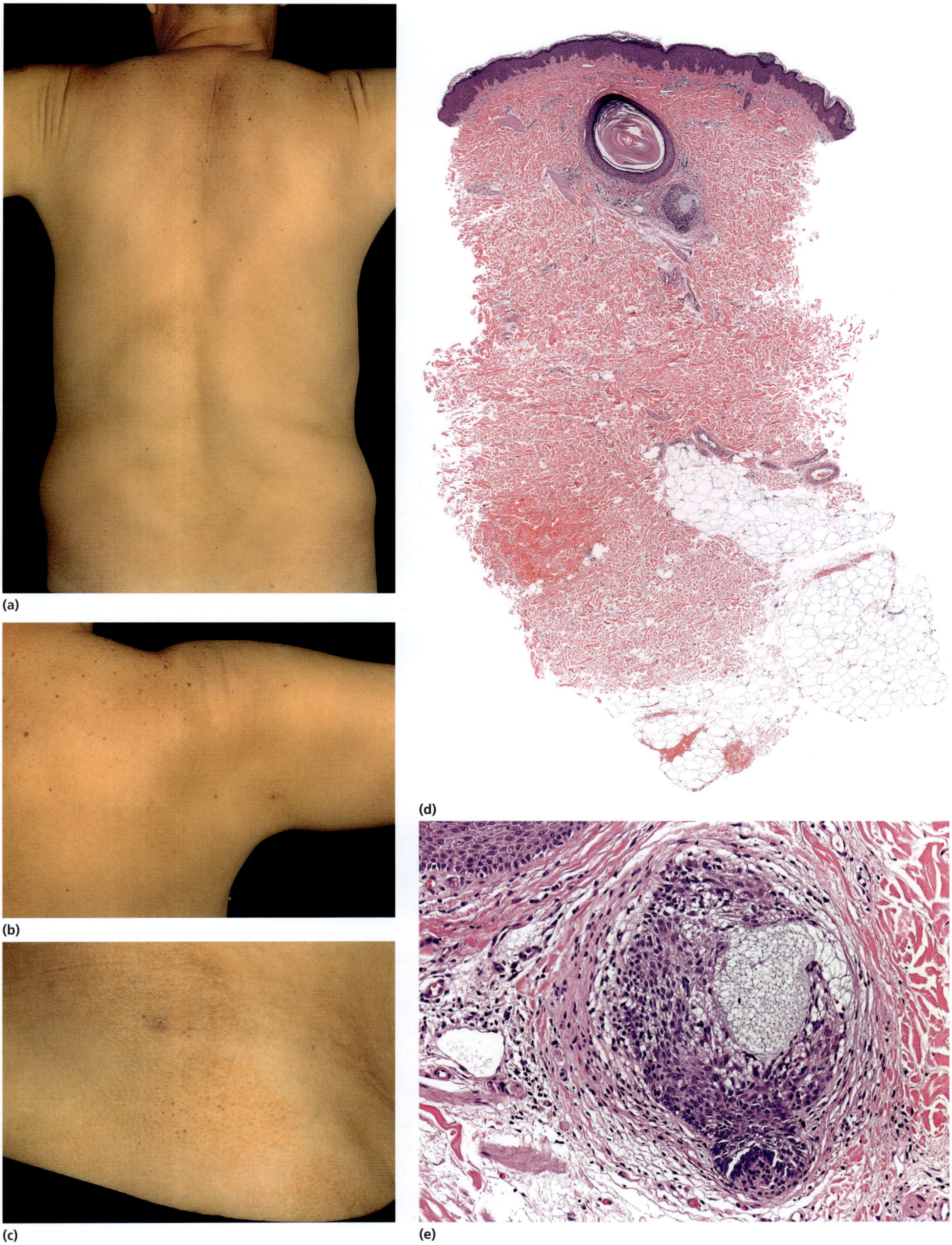

(a) (b) (c) (d) (e)

Figure 3.96 Pilotropic mycosis fungoides mimicking clinically lichen spinulosus. (a), (b) and (c) Irregular distribution of tiny follicular hyperkeratoses, some with small open comedones. (d) Histology shows a dilated hair follicle with (e) prominent mucin deposition.

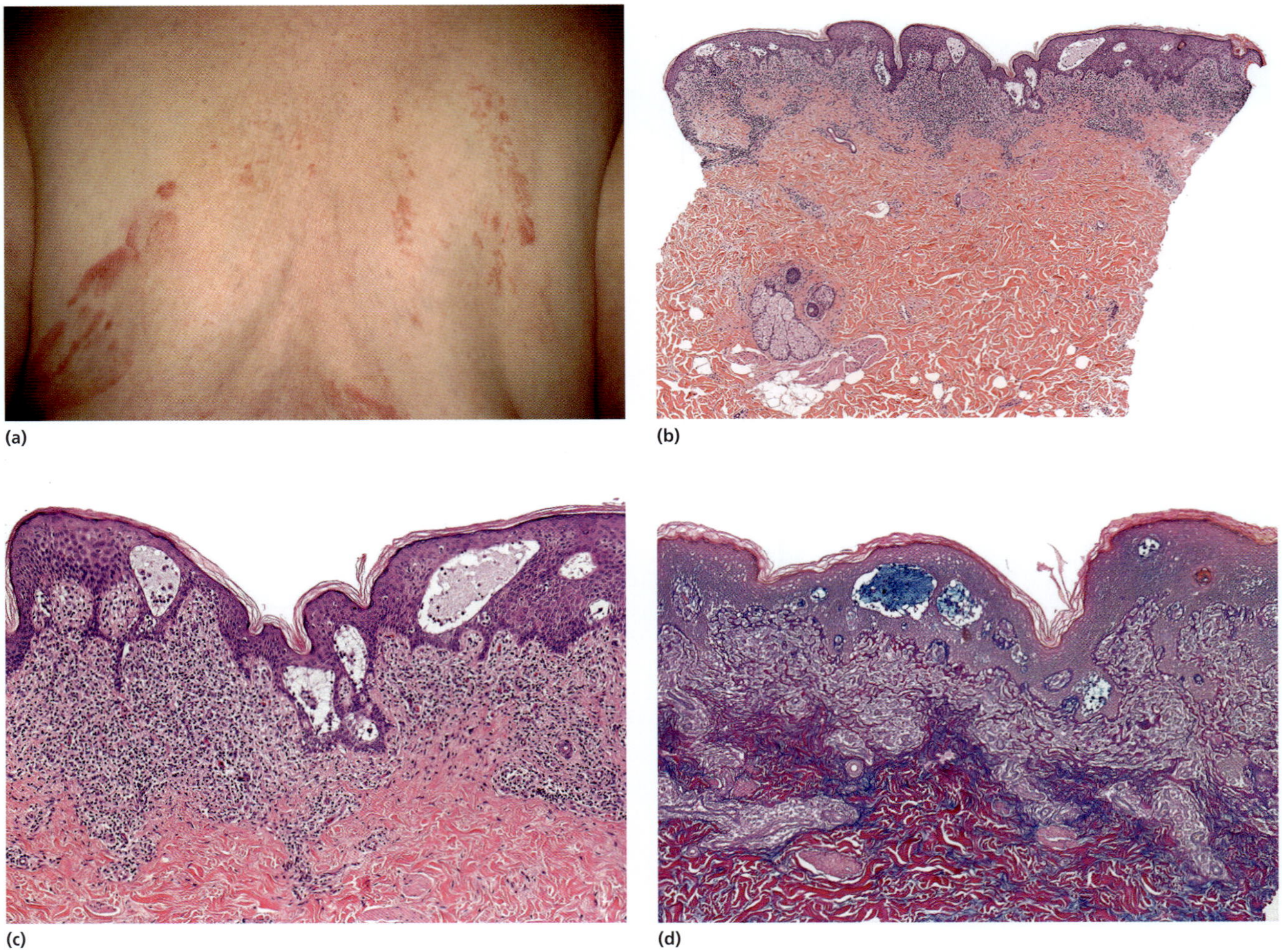

Figure 3.97 Mycosis fungoides with intraepidermal mucinosis. (a) The clinical presentation is similar to conventional mycosis fugoides and does not show follicular accentuation. Histology shows (b) a band-like lymphoid infiltrate with epidermotropic lymphocytes and (c) large deposits of mucin within the epidermis. (d) Staining for colloidal iron highlights the intraepidermal mucin.

The relationship between erythrodermic mycosis fungoides and Sézary syndrome is still unclear. The CAC and WHO classifications suggest that these cases should not be classified as Sézary syndrome but as erythrodermic mycosis fungoides, and the diagnosis of Sézary syndrome should be reserved for those patients presenting with the typical features of the disease from the outset [1, 3]. In fact, a strong support to the distinction of mycosis fungoides from Sézary syndrome has been provided by phenotypic and genetic analyses that showed major differences between the two diseases [61–64]. On the other hand, similarities in blood biomarkers may suggest the existence of a spectrum between the two diseases [292], or it may suggest that once blood involvement takes place in mycosis fungoides, it shares a common clinical and prognostic pathway with Sézary syndrome. At the present state of knowledge, in patients presenting with erythroderma, precise history taking and complete blood analyses are crucial for proper diagnosis, in order to distinguish erythrodermic mycosis fungoides from genuine Sézary syndrome.

Differentiation of erythrodermic mycosis fungoides from Sézary syndrome on histopathological grounds is usually not possible. A perivascular infiltrative pattern, predominance of small/mixed lymphoid cells and of eosinophils have been observed more often in erythrodermic mycosis fungoides, whereas lower numbers of $CD8^+$ cells were more common in Sézary syndrome in one study [293]. A high number of PD-$1^+$ lymphocytes, too, seems to be more common in Sèzary syndrome than in mycosis fungoides [134, 135]. However, I would caution against attempting to distinguish erythrodermic mycosis fungoides from Sézary syndrome based on histopathological features alone.

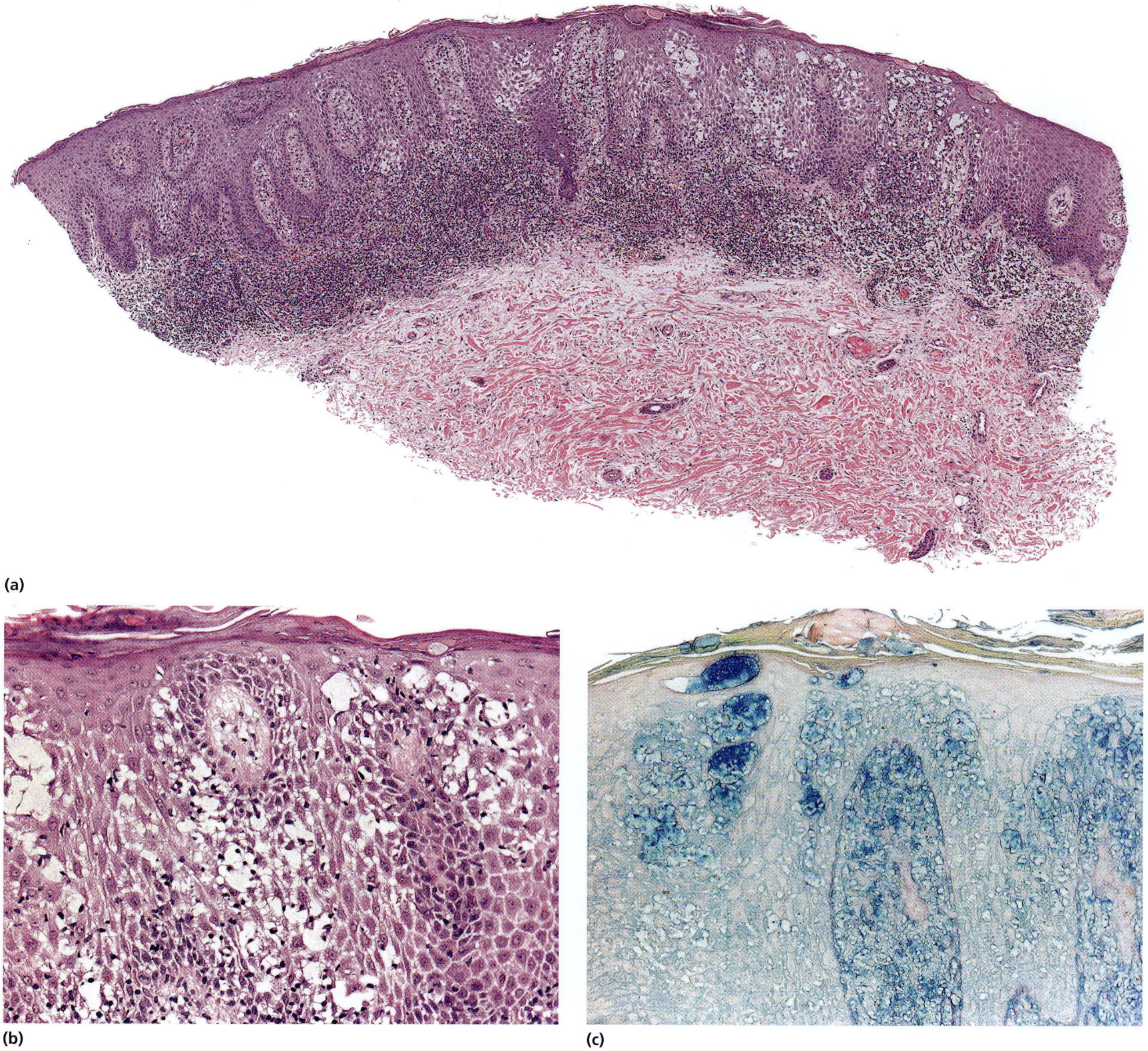


Figure 3.98 Mycosis fungoides with intraepidermal mucinosis. (a) Psoriasiform hyperplasia of the epidermis and band-like dermal lymphoid infiltrate; (b) intraepidermal mucin may be misinterpreted as spongiosis and the biopsy misdiagnosed as "pseudolymphomatous" eczematous dermatitis; (c) staining for colloidal iron highlights abundant intraepidermal deposits of mucin.

## Mycosis fungoides mimicking eczematous dermatoses

Mycosis fungoides is an itchy condition (particularly pilotropic mycosis fungoides), and in some patients artifacts induced by rubbing and scratching may confer an "eczematous" aspect to the clinical picture, mimicking particularly late-onset atopic dermatitis. This is more common in generalized, suberythrodermic or erythrodermic forms of the disease, but may be occasionally observed also in localized patches and plaques (Figs. 3.116 and 3.117a). Histopathological features in these cases show variable amount of spongiosis, and differentiation from atopic dermatitis or other eczematous dermatoses may be difficult, particularly in biopsies taken under treatment (which unfortunately are the vast majority of biopsies in this setting). Presence of "disproportionate epidermotropism" (see above in this chapter and Fig. 3.31c) is a helpful clue, but it may be difficult to appreciate or even missing under treatment (Fig. 3.117b). Staining for pan-T cell markers helps highlighting the epidermotropic lymphocytes (Fig. 3.104c), and it is helpful particularly in cases with a scant infiltrate.

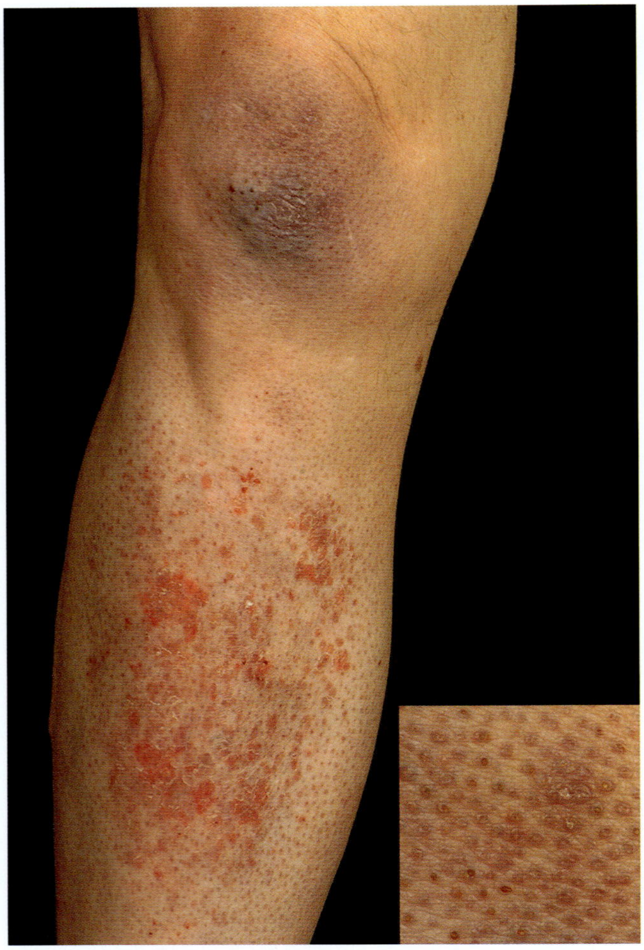

Figure 3.99 Syringotropic mycosis fungoides. Erythematous patches with focal erosions on the knee and leg. Note follicular plugging (inset).

## Interstitial mycosis fungoides

Interstitial mycosis fungoides is a variant of the disease that does not have a characteristic clinical presentation, but shows histopathologically a pattern that may be misinterpreted as that of an inflammatory dermatosis (particularly interstitial granuloma annulare and inflammatory stage of localized scleroderma) [294–296]. Clinically it is usually found in flat tumors of mycosis fungoides or in ill-defined, large infiltrated lesions that clinically don't betray their neoplastic nature (Fig. 3.118). Interstitial mycosis fungoides usually is a histopathological pattern found occasionally in patients with otherwise conventional mycosis fungoides, but some patients may repeatedly show this pattern in different biopsies taken over several years. It is a rare pattern documented mostly in short case reports, with only two larger studies published [295, 297].

Epidermotropism and a band-like pattern are usually missing, and histology shows dermal infiltrates of lymphocytes dissecting the collagen bundles (Figs. 3.119a and b). Immunohistology confirms that most interstitial cells are T lymphocytes, which is a helpful clue for the differential diagnosis with interstitial inflammatory dermatoses (Fig. 3.119c). A cytotoxic phenotype may be observed [295]. "Free floating" collagen fibers surrounded by neoplastic lymphocytes have been observed in interstitial mycosis fungoides but not in granuloma annulare or morphea [298]. In this context, it should be remembered that granuloma annulare may rarely present with pseudolymphomatous infiltrates, thus complicating the differential diagnosis between the two diseases [299], and that a rare case of genuine granuloma annulare in a patient with mycosis fungoides has been reported [300]. Necrobiotic features have been observed in one case involving the lymph nodes [301]. One study reported frequent granulomatous features and subtle follicular involvement [297], but this is not my experience. In fact, the pictures published in this study in my opinion don't allow to verify whether these cases represent genuine examples of "interstitial" mycosis fungoides, or of conventional mycosis fungoides with small, focal areas of interstitial lymphocytes (a finding that is not infrequent in conventional mycosis fungoides).

Interstitial mycosis fungoides mimics histopathologically the pattern of interstitial granulomatous dermatitis, from which it can be distinguished by the presence of interstitial lymphocytes rather than histiocytes. Other causes of interstitial granulomatous dermatitis should be ruled out (this histopathological pattern may be observed mainly in rheumatoid arthritis, autoimmune diseases, morphea, *Borrelia* infection, drug eruptions, and interstitial granuloma annulare).

## Poikilodermatous mycosis fungoides ("poikiloderma vasculare atrophicans")

Poikilodermatous mycosis fungoides is characterized clinically by atrophic, red-brown macules and patches with prominent telangiectasia (Fig. 3.120). Sites of predilection are the breast and buttocks (where this morphological variant of the disease is not uncommon), but lesions may be generalized. Rarely a widespread "retiform" pattern can be observed, particularly in lesions of long-standing (formerly referred to as "parakeratosis variegata") (Fig. 3.121). Clinically it may mimic a peculiar drug eruption (symmetrical drug-related intertriginous and flexural exanthema – SDRIFE) (Fig. 3.122), but slow onset, persistence of lesions for several months or years and lack of association with any drug allow a differential diagnosis to be made. Histology reveals an atrophic epidermis with loss of rete ridges, an interface dermatitis with a superficial, band-like infiltrate of lymphocytes with epidermotropism, and a thickened papillary dermis (Fig. 3.123). Necrotic keratinocytes and pigment incontinence may be a prominent finding. Dilated capillaries are present within the superficial dermis. This variant has also been referred to as the "lichenoid" type of mycosis fungoides, and in some cases distinction from pigmented atrophic lichen planus may be impossible without correlation with the clinical picture. A case reported as the "teleangiectatic" variant of mycosis fungoides in my opinion represents a presentation of poikilodermatous mycosis fungoides [302].

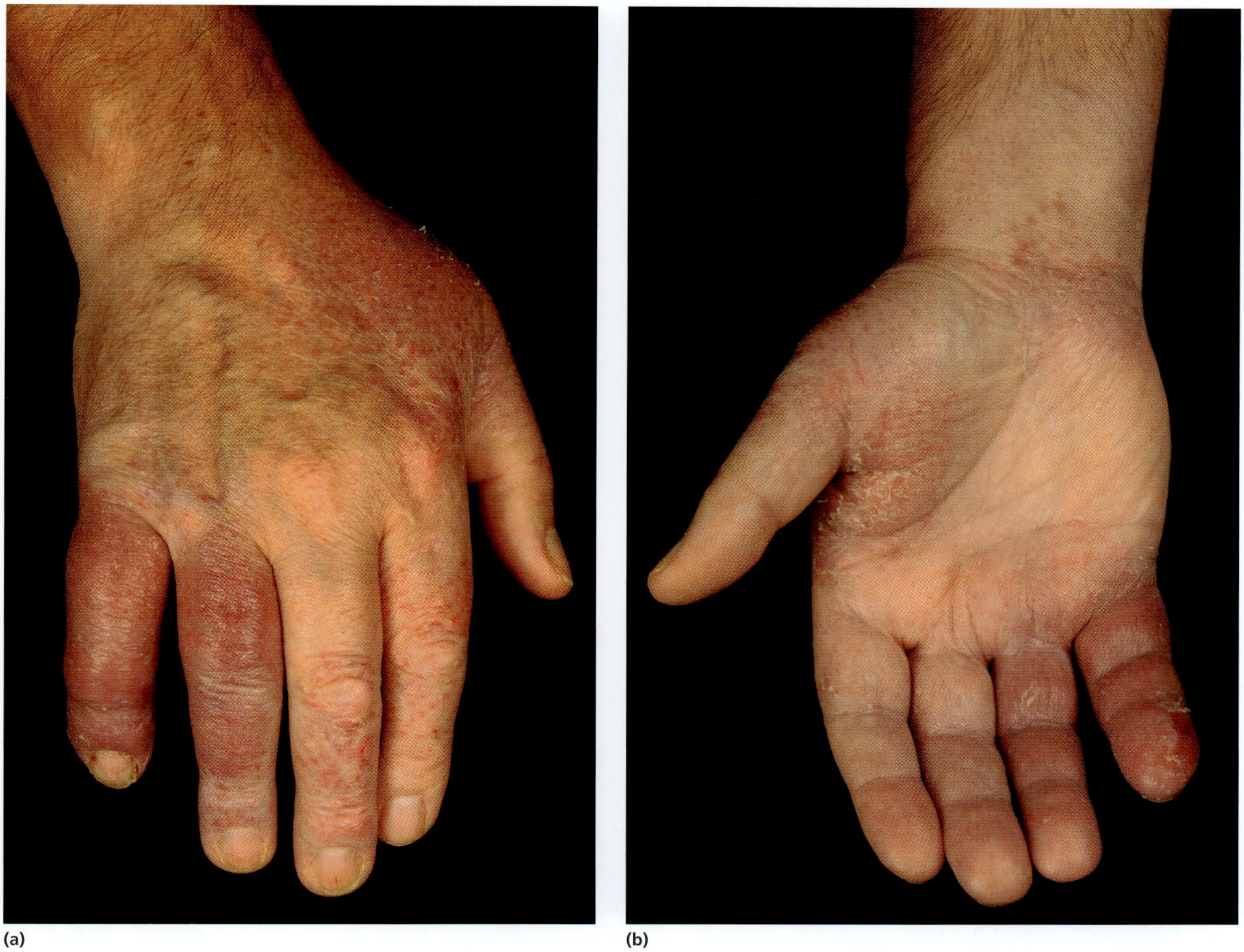

Figure 3.100 Syringotropic mycosis fungoides. (a) Infiltrated, partly erosive, reddish lesions on the dorsal part of the fingers. Note follicular accentuation. (b) The palmar side is also involved.

Clinically, lesions of poikilodermatous mycosis fungoides may persist virtually unchanged for many years irrespective of the amount of lymphoid infiltrate found in sequential biopsies (Fig. 3.124), suggesting that structural changes may take place in the affected skin (variable atrophy of the epidermis, increased vascularity in the superficial dermis, and pigmentation).

A cytotoxic phenotype can be observed in poikilodermatous mycosis fungoides [303]. Prognosis of poikilodermatous mycosis fungoides seems to be better as compared to other variants of the disease [43], and I have observed several patients with stable disease over a period of many years (Fig. 3.124).

## Hypopigmented mycosis fungoides

Patients with mycosis fungoides may develop hypopigmented patches and plaques (Fig. 3.125). These lesions may be misinterpreted clinically as those of pityriasis versicolor, pityriasis alba, or vitiligo. Histology reveals typical features of mycosis fungoides. Hypopigmented mycosis fungoides is observed more frequently in dark-skinned individuals and is one of the most frequent variants seen in children (see Chapter 30, Figs. 30.1j and k) [231, 304, 305]. It is also a common variant of mycosis fungoides observed in Middle-Eastern countries [306]. Repigmentation usually takes place after successful treatment of the lesions, and repigmentation may be used as a marker of treatment's efficacy [305]. Prognosis of hypopigmented mycosis fungoides may be better than that of the conventional variant of the disease [305]; however, this may be due, at least in part, to the inclusion in studies of some patients with hypopigmented inflammatory conditions.

Although hypopigmented lesions may be the sole manifestation of mycosis fungoides, in many cases, especially in Caucasians, careful examination of the patients will show the presence of erythematous lesions to be detected as well (Fig. 3.126). Interestingly, patients with hypopigmented mycosis

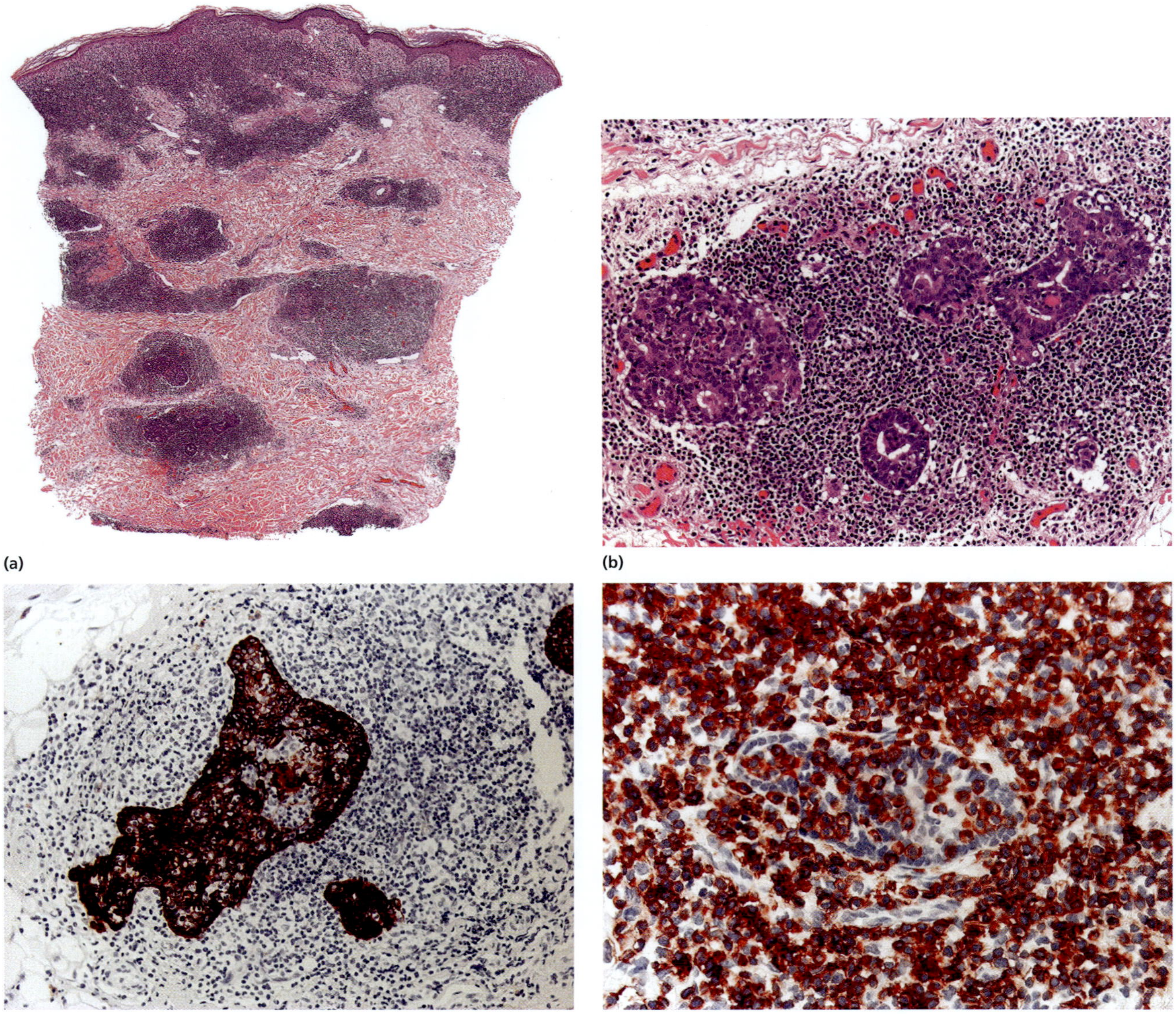


**Figure 3.101** Syringotropic mycosis fungoides. (a) At low power dense, band-like and diffuse lymphoid infiltrates with prominent involvement of the eccrine glands are recognizable. (b) Detail of the eccrine glands with dense lymphoid infiltrates and syringometaplasia. (c) Staining for pan-cytokeratin shows the eccrine gland infiltrated by lymphocytes. (d) Staining for CD5 highlights the intraglandular lymphocytes.

fungoides tend to develop more hypopigmented lesions during the course of the disease, suggesting that this is indeed an unusual variant of mycosis fungoides. In rare cases, a linear distribution has been described in cases of hypopigmented mycosis fungoides [307, 308].

A predominant $CD8^+$ phenotype has been described in patients with hypopigmented mycosis fungoides, possibly underlying some pathogenetic similarities to vitiligo [304]. However, a $CD4^+$ phenotype can be observed as well [231], and most cases of mycosis fungoides that are positive for CD8 are not hypopigmented clinically, suggesting that a cytotoxic phenotype *per se* is not sufficient to induce hypopigmentation clinically. It should be underlined that differential diagnosis of hypopigmented mycosis fungoides from its simulators, including particularly atopic dermatitis and the inflammatory stages of vitiligo, may be extremely difficult, and that at least some of the cases published in the literature may not represent genuine examples of hypopigmented mycosis fungoides. In my experience, this problem is particularly evident in children, and sometimes only follow-up data allow a precise diagnosis (see also Chapter 31). The number of melanocytes is diminished in mycosis fungoides, but melanocytes are not completely absent,

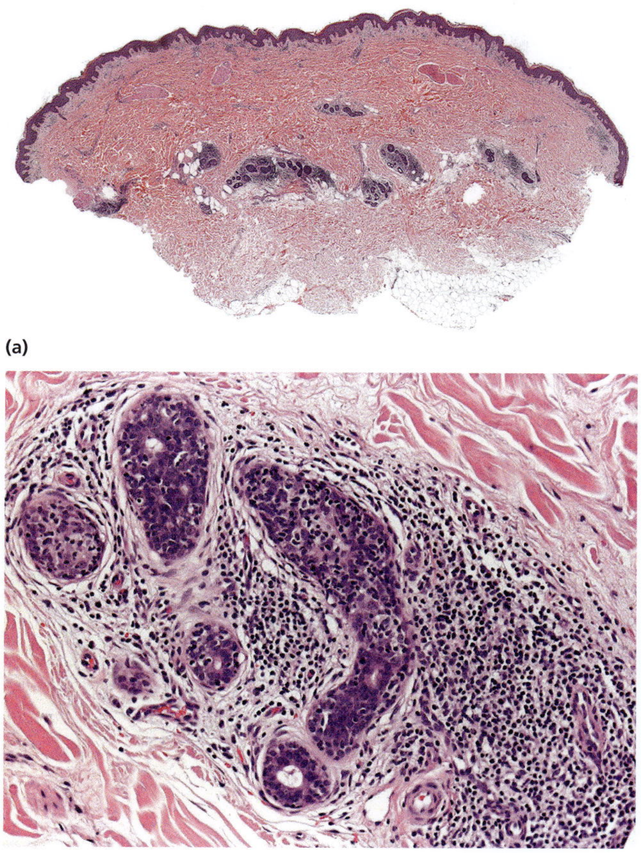

(a)

(b)

Figure 3.102 Syringotropic mycosis fungoides. (a) Neoplastic lymphocytes arranged predominantly around and within sweat glands with only a minimal infiltrate in the papillary dermis. (b) Note syringometaplasia and dense lymphoid infiltrates around the eccrine glands and coils.

unlike the situation in vitiligo, representing a potential diagnostic clue [309, 310].

It is interesting to note that hypopigmented lesions have been described in so-called parapsoriasis en plaques [311] and that an identical clinical presentation may be observed also in "idiopathic generalized follicular mucinosis" (see Fig. 3.91a), again suggesting that these may be variants of mycosis fungoides as well.

## Hyperpigmented mycosis fungoides

Rarely, the clinical picture of mycosis fungoides may be characterized by markedly hyperpigmented lesions, corresponding histopathologically to the presence of pigment incontinence and abundant melanophages in the papillary dermis (Figs. 3.127 and 3.128). The phenotype of these lesions is more often cytotoxic than helper [312], possibly explaining the damage at the dermo-epidermal junction and subsequent pigment incontinence. On the other hand, it should be underlined that most cases of mycosis fungoides with cytotoxic phenotype do not present with hyperpigmented lesions. Hyperpigmented mycosis fungoides may show some overlapping features with poikilodermatous mycosis fungoides, but in hyperpigmented mycosis fungoides the prominent telangiectasia and retiform pattern are missing clinically, and histopathologically there is no increase in superficial, telangiectatic vessels.

Generalized hyperpigmented lesions covering the entire body have been described as "melanoerythroderma," and are seen more frequently in patients with Sézary syndrome (see Chapter 4 and Fig. 4.11).

## Purpuric mycosis fungoides

In some patients, lesions of mycosis fungoides are characterized clinically by a purpuric hue (Fig. 3.129) and histopathologically by the presence of many extravasated erythrocytes and siderophages (Fig. 3.130). This variant of mycosis fungoides mimics the pigmented purpuric dermatoses both clinically and histopathologically [313].

The differential diagnosis of purpuric mycosis fungoides from lichenoid purpura and lichen aureus can be difficult on histopathologic grounds, and correlation with the clinical features is crucial (see also Chapter 31). The distinction has been rendered even more difficult by the introduction of the term "atypical pigmented purpura" and by the suggestion of a possible relationship between some purpuric dermatoses and mycosis fungoides [314, 315]. Rare patients reported as having "pigmented purpura" progressing to mycosis fungoides probably had purpuric mycosis fungoides from the outset [316, 317]. In this context, it should be emphasized that lichen aureus and lichenoid purpura are wholly benign disorders that should be clearly differentiated from mycosis fungoides. In my experience, patients with genuine lichen aureus or lichenoid purpura never progress to mycosis fungoides (see also Chapter 31).

## Papular mycosis fungoides

In some patients with mycosis fungoides, variably large papules represent the predominant morphologic expression of the disease, and small and/or large patches are absent (Figs. 3.131–3.133) [318, 319]. The papules are not centered on the hair follicles, and these last are not involved histopathologically. Besides the original report of 6 cases by our group [318], only a few case reports have been published [320–324], as well as a larger follow-up study by our group including several new cases [319]. Sometimes the lesions may resemble clinically those of pityriasis lichenoides (see next section).

Histopathologic examination reveals conventional features of mycosis fungoides, but in tiny papules the infiltrate is restricted to a part only of the biopsy specimen (Fig. 3.134). The absence of typical manifestations of the disease renders the clinical diagnosis very difficult. Moreover, differentiation from lymphomatoid papulosis can only be achieved by short-term follow-up of the patients, as the histopathologic features may be indistinguishable (CD30, however, is usually negative in papular

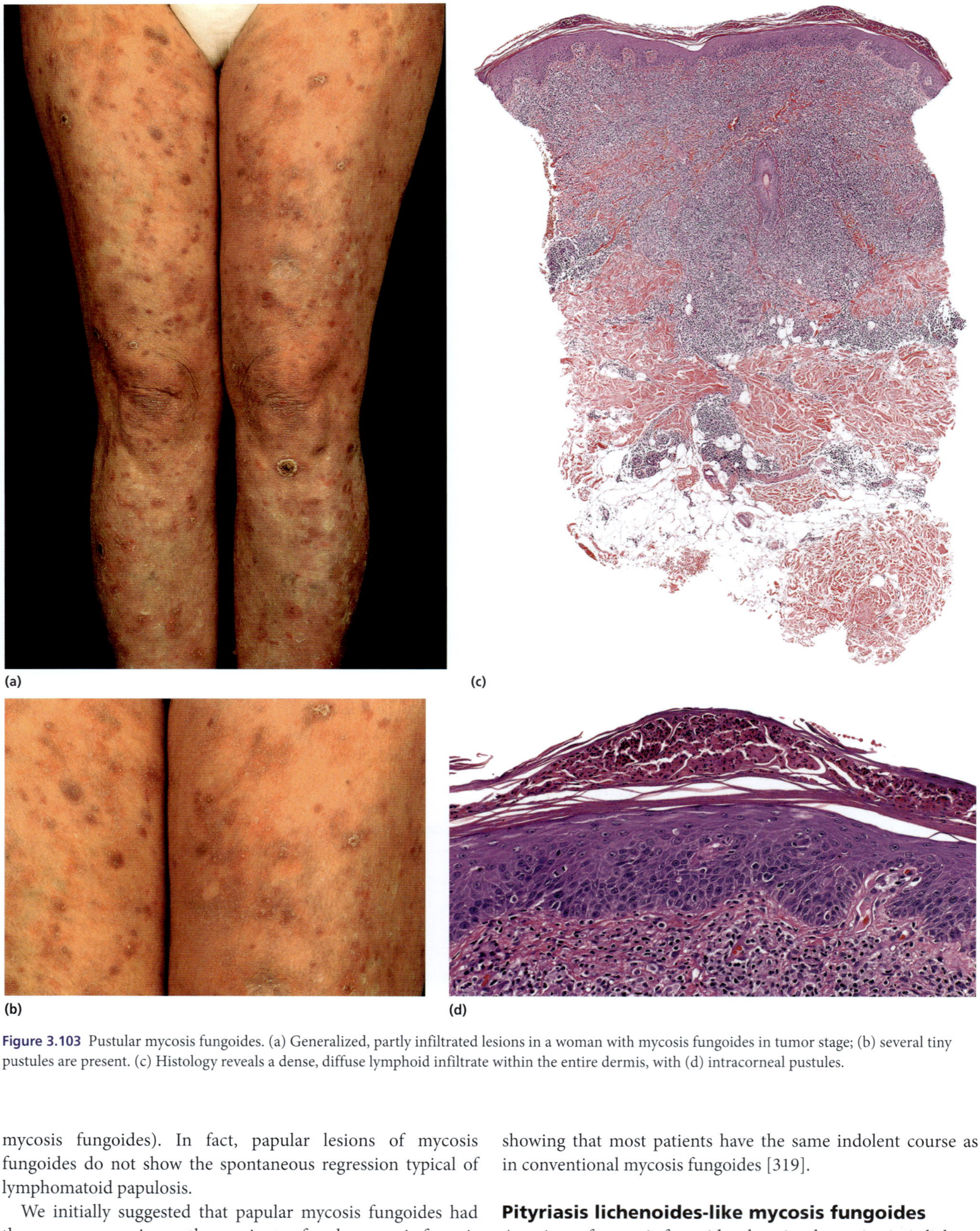


Figure 3.103 Pustular mycosis fungoides. (a) Generalized, partly infiltrated lesions in a woman with mycosis fungoides in tumor stage; (b) several tiny pustules are present. (c) Histology reveals a dense, diffuse lymphoid infiltrate within the entire dermis, with (d) intracorneal pustules.

mycosis fungoides). In fact, papular lesions of mycosis fungoides do not show the spontaneous regression typical of lymphomatoid papulosis.

We initially suggested that papular mycosis fungoides had the same prognosis as other variants of early mycosis fungoides [318]. A follow-up study confirmed that observation, showing that most patients have the same indolent course as in conventional mycosis fungoides [319].

## Pityriasis lichenoides-like mycosis fungoides

A variant of mycosis fungoides that simulates pityriasis lichenoides has been originally described in children [325–327].

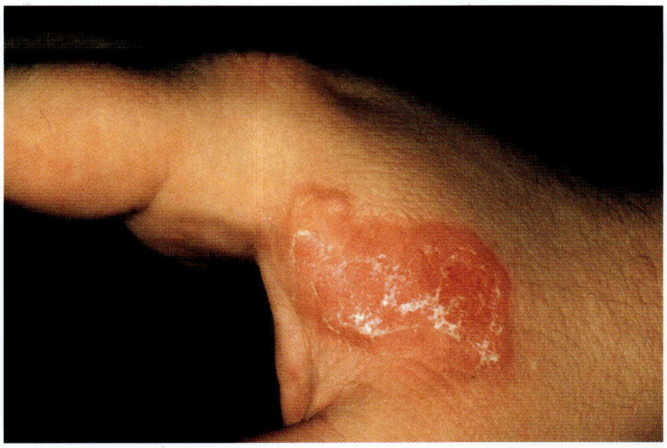

**Figure 3.104** Localized pagetoid reticulosis. Erythematous, scaly plaque on the right hand. (*Courtesy of Prof. Wolfram Sterry, Berlin, Germany.*)

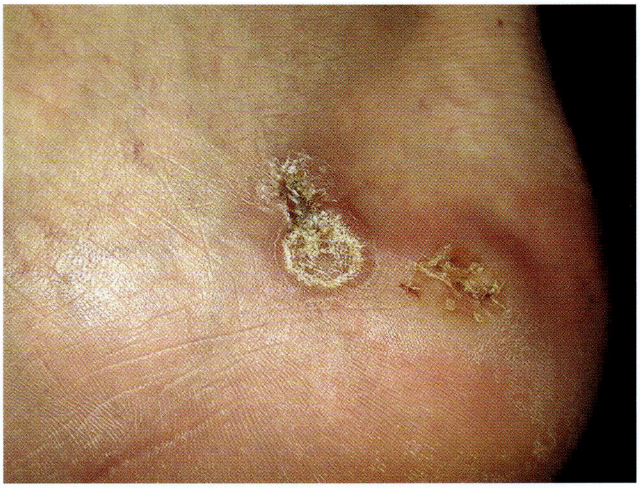

**Figure 3.105** Localized pagetoid reticulosis. Small, warty plaques on the foot. (*Courtesy of Dr. Antonio Perasole, Castelfranco Veneto, Italy.*)

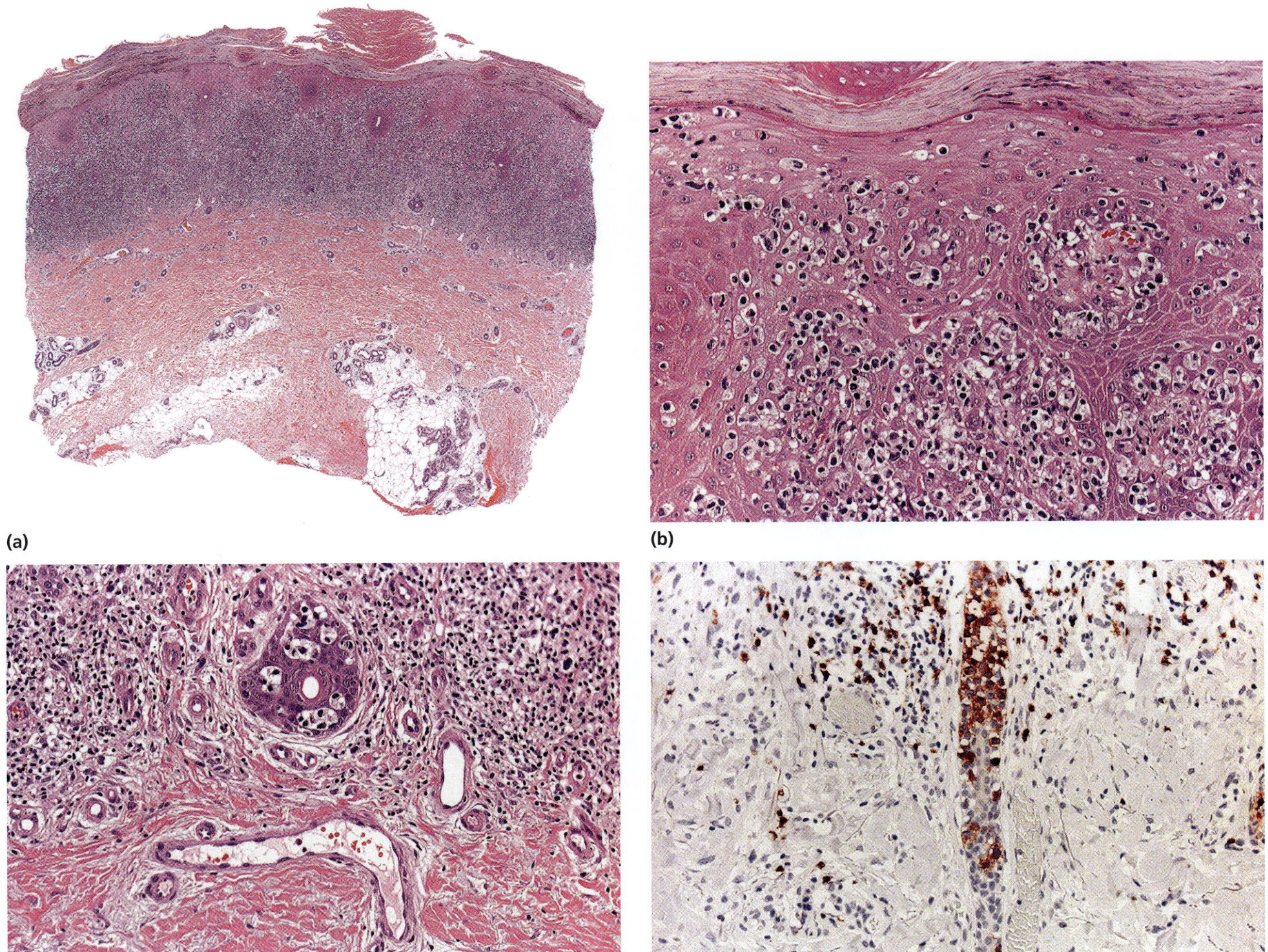

**Figure 3.106** Localized pagetoid reticulosis. (a) Epidermal hyperplasia and dense, band-like lymphoid infiltrate. (b) Prominent ("pagetoid") epidermotropism of small and mid-sized pleomorphic lymphocytes. (c) Neoplastic lymphocytes grow along the eccrine coil. (d) Positivity for CD8 of neoplastic cells within the eccrine coil.

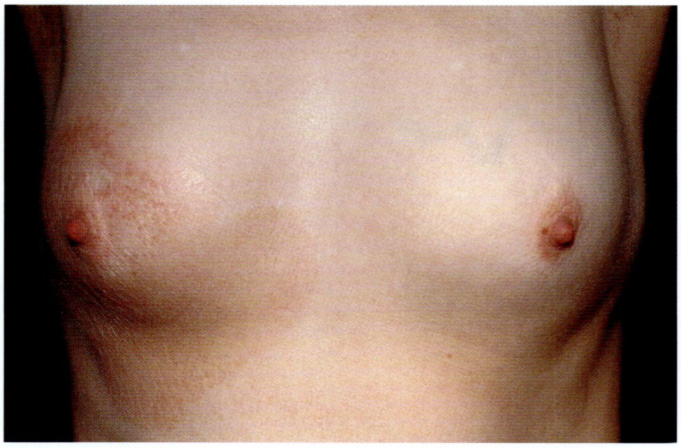

**Figure 3.107** Large, solitary patch of mycosis fungoides on the breast. Note focal atrophy as a sign of a long-standing lesion.

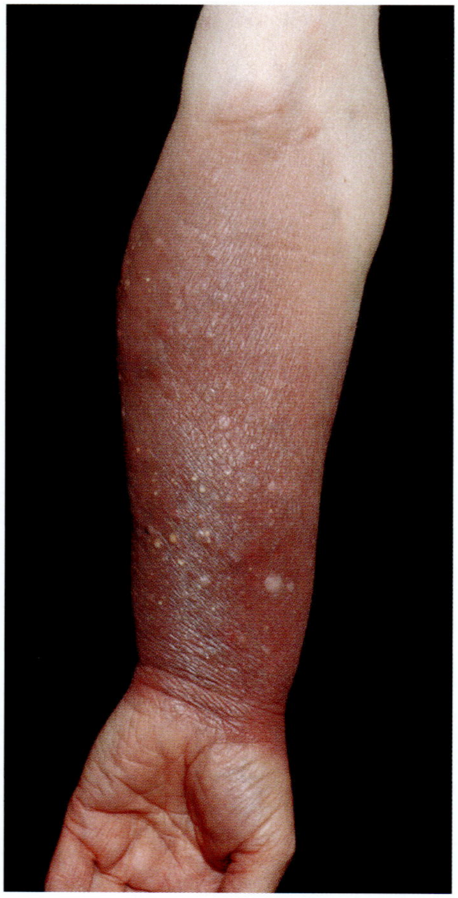

**Figure 3.108** Granulomatous mycosis fungoides. Note reddish-brown plaque with several papules and small nodules on the arm.

Similar cases can be observed also in adults [328–330]. Although the original descriptions were restricted to Caucasian patients, Asian patients with pityriasis lichenoides-like mycosis fungoides (including both children and adults) have been described as well [331].

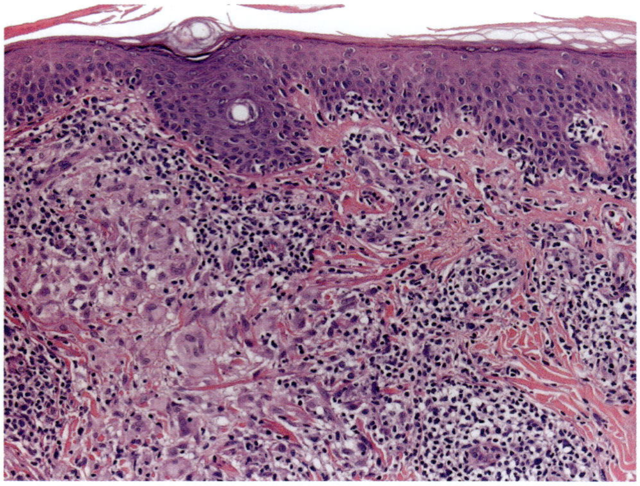

**Figure 3.109** Granulomatous mycosis fungoides. Dense lymphoid infiltrates admixed with large epithelioid granulomas in the dermis. Note focal epidermotropism of lymphocytes.

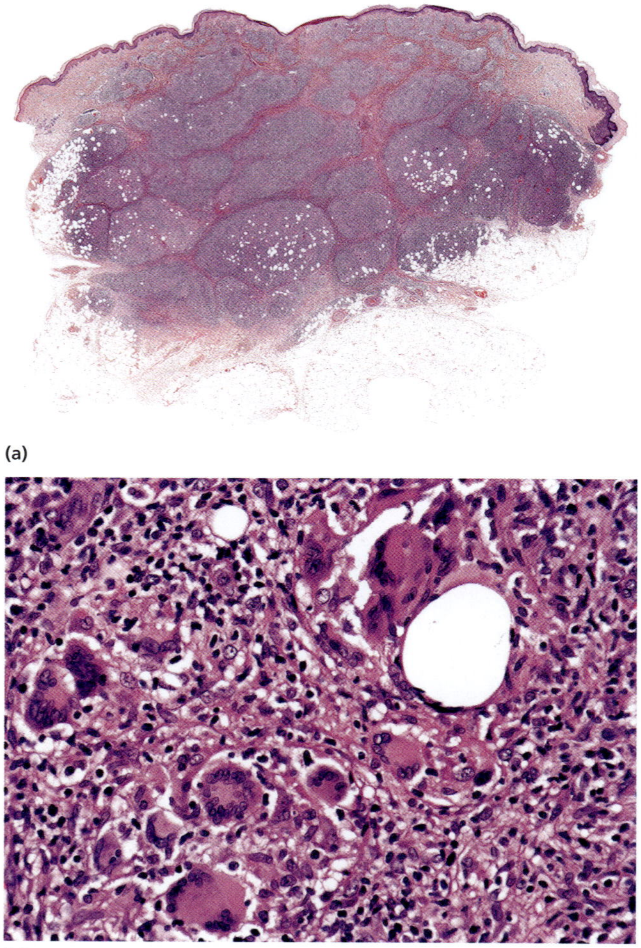

(a)

(b)

**Figure 3.110** Granulomatous mycosis fungoides. (a) Dense, diffuse lymphoid infiltrates within the entire dermis. (b) Several multinucleated histiocytic giant cells.

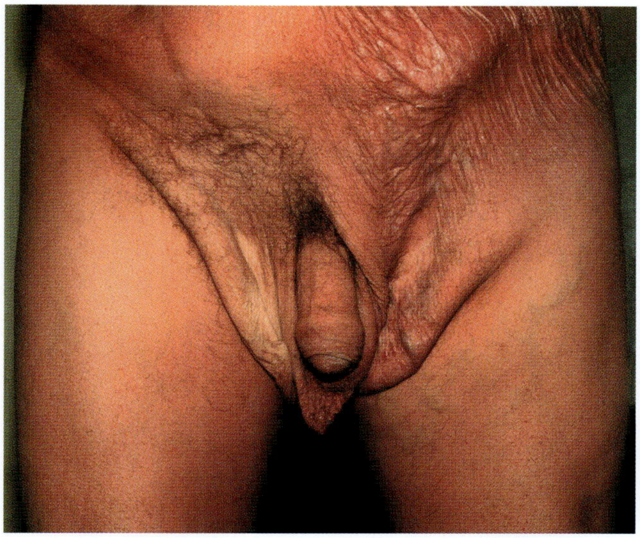

Figure 3.111 Granulomatous slack skin. Prominent atrophy of the skin with bulky pendulous skin folds in the lower abdomen and inguinal region. (*Courtesy of Prof. Giovanni Borroni, Pavia, Italy.*)

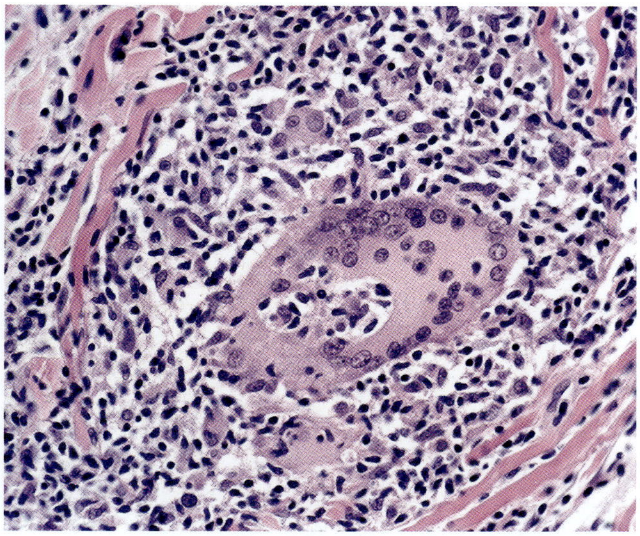

Figure 3.113 Granulomatous slack skin. Histiocytic giant cell with many nuclei and with several intracytoplasmic leukocytes, surrounded by a dense infiltrate of lymphocytes.

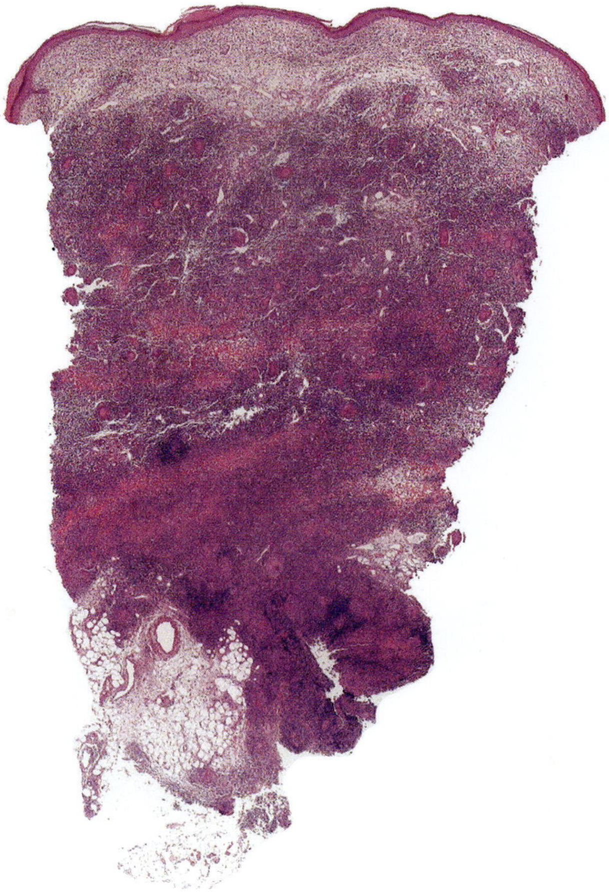

Figure 3.112 Granulomatous slack skin. Dense, diffuse lymphoid infiltrates involving the dermis and subcutaneous fat tissues.

This is a variant of mycosis fungoides with two different and separated aspects: on the one hand, patients may present with lesions reminiscent clinically of pityriasis lichenoides, but with histopathological features of conventional mycosis fungoides. On the other hand, patients with clinically conventional mycosis fungoides may present with histopathological features similar to those of pityriasis lichenoides [330]. These two variants are distinct; that is, a clinical and a histopathological variant of pityriasis lichenoides-like mycosis fungoides exist.

The clinical variant belongs to the group of papular mycosis fungoides (see previous section). In addition to the papules seen in papular mycosis fungoides, some lesions show scales similar to what is observed in pityriasis lichenoides (Fig. 3.135).

The histopathological variant of pityriasis lichenoides-like mycosis fungoides is characterized by superficial lymphoid infiltrates with vacuolar alterations of the basal keratinocytes, necrotic keratinocytes, epidermotropic lymphocytes and so-called "busy" horny layer (parakeratosis and intracorneal neutrophils), similar to what is observed in pityriasis lichenoides (Figs. 3.136a and b). Most of these cases have a $CD8^+$ cytotoxic phenotype (Fig. 3.136c), thus enhancing the similarities to pityriasis lichenoides. In some cases, loss of pan-T-cell markers is very helpful clue to confirm the diagnosis of mycosis fungoides (Fig. 3.136d).

In the literature there are some reports of "atypical pityriasis lichenoides et varioliformis acuta – PLEVA," sometimes with progression to mycosis fungoides [332, 333]. It is unclear whether these patients had mycosis fungoides from the beginning or if an association between the two diseases exists. In addition, we could identify a group of pityriasis lichenoides with aberrant phenotype, showing in a proportion of cases progression to conventional mycosis fungoides [330]. The

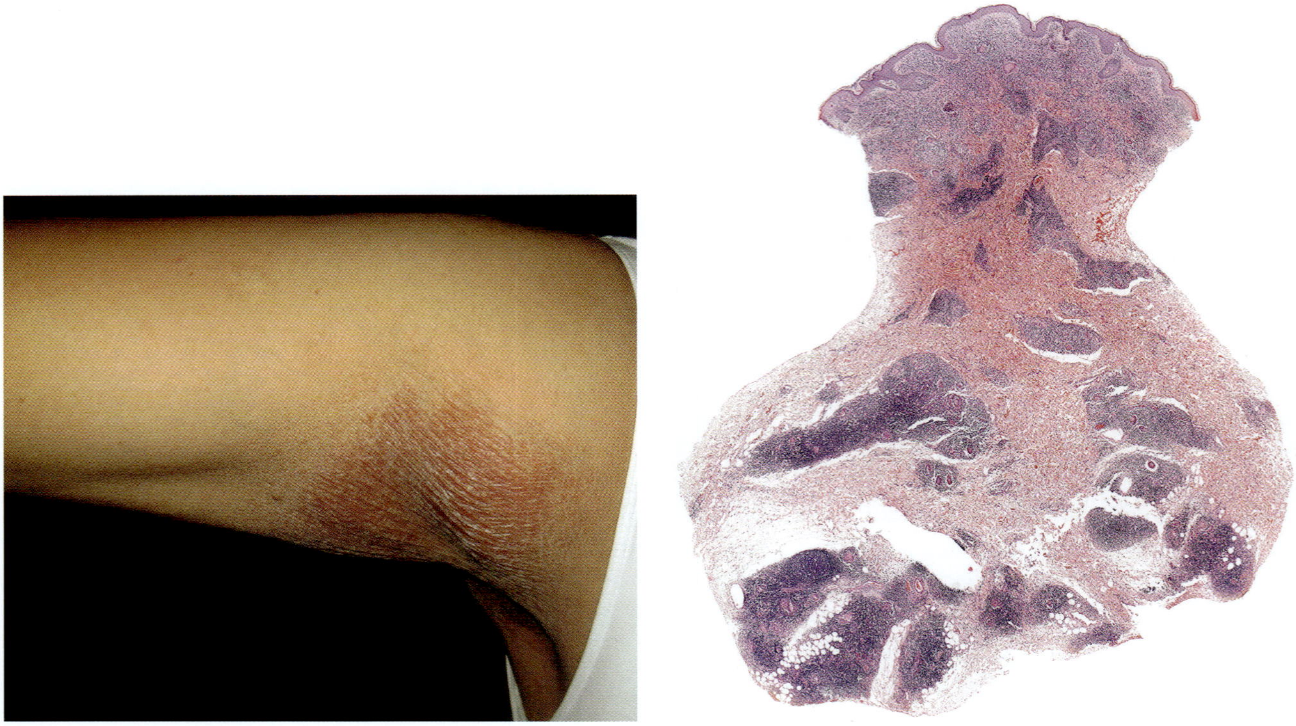

(a) (b)

Figure 3.114 Granulomatous slack skin. (a) Early lesion showing superficial wrinkling and beginning folds. (b) Histology reveals dense lymphoid infiltrates with focal granulomatous features within the dermis and subcutaneous fat tissues. (*Courtesy of Dr. Gerardo Ferrara, Benevento, Italy.*)

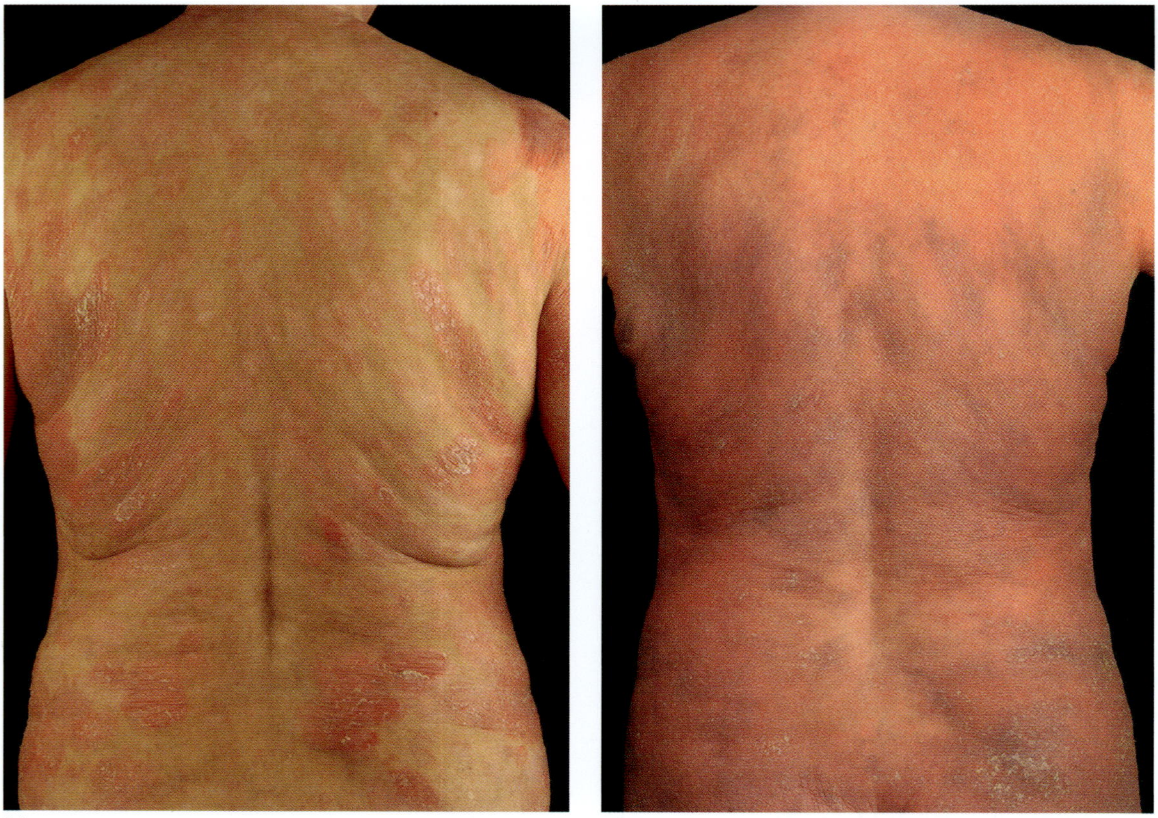

(a) (b)

Figure 3.115 Erythrodermic mycosis fungoides. (a) Clinical picture of a patient with typical plaque-stage mycosis fungoides. (b) The same patient 7 months later showing erythroderma.

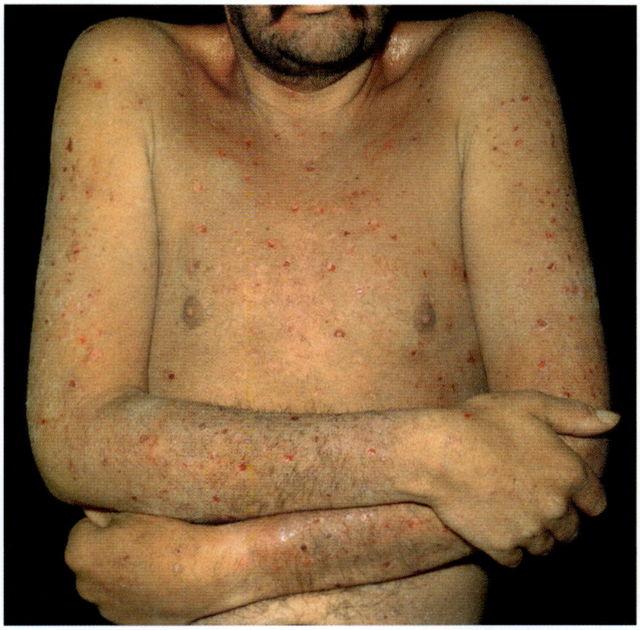

(a)

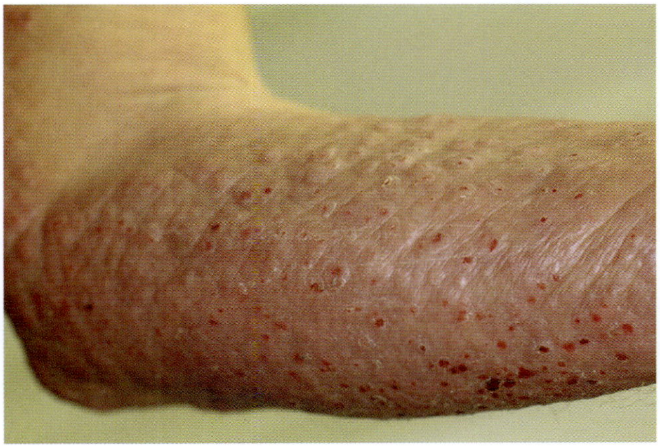

(b)

Figure 3.116 Mycosis fungoides with scratching artifacts. (a) Clinical picture of a patient with generalized pilotropic mycosis fungoides showing an "eczematous" clinical aspect with many superficial erosions due to scratching. (b) Another patient with scratching artifacts on a long-standing plaque of mycosis fungoides on the arm. (*Courtesy of Dr. Martin Laimer, Salzburg, Austria.*)

relationship between pityriasis lichenoides and mycosis fungoides is discussed also in the section on pityriasis lichenoides in Chapter 31.

## Bullous (vesiculobullous) and dyshidrotic mycosis fungoides

Some patients with mycosis fungoides present with vesicular or bullous lesions; these last are sometimes associated with large, superficial erosions. Histologic examination reveals bullous lesions characterized either by cleavage at the dermoepidermal junction or by confluence of large intraepidermal vesicles (Figs. 3.137 and 3.138). Sometimes only superficial erosions are visible clinically, and both the epithelium and the bulla are not visible on the histopathologic specimen (Fig. 3.139a). In these cases, epitheliotropism within remnants of adnexal structures, if present, may be a helpful clue (Fig. 3.139b).

A "dyshidrotic" variant of the disease located on the palms and soles may also present with vesicular lesions (Figs. 3.140 and 3.141). Typical features of mycosis fungoides are commonly present near to the vesicular and bullous ones or at other sites of the body.

The reason(s) for the formation of vesicular and bullous lesions is unclear. Some cases may be due to pre-existent dyshidrotic or vesicular dermatitis and subsequent colonization by neoplastic cells. In other patients a direct cytotoxic effect may be responsible for the detachment of the epidermis from the dermis or pronounced spongiosis may lead to vesiculation, and eventually larger blisters may develop due to confluence of vesicles. Neoplastic cells may also induce directly and/or indirectly degeneration of collagen bundles and the blistering [334]. In some patients, onset of bullous lesions has been related to the use of interferon-α. Rarely, coexistence of mycosis fungoides and an autoimmune bullous disorder may be the reason for this peculiar clinical presentation.

Eczema herpeticatum developing on the background of bullous mycosis fungoides has been described [335].

## Anetodermic mycosis fungoides

Two patients with secondary anetoderma developing on pre-existing lesions of mycosis fungoides have been described [336]. Some of the lesions depicted in this study resembled small tumors clinically, but represented probably just secondary anetodermic changes in flat lesions of mycosis fungoides, thus being a potential pitfall in clinical evaluation of the patients. Although loss of elastic fibers is observed also in granulomatous slack skin, anetoderma secondary to mycosis fungoides has completely different clinical and histopathologic features, and there is no relationship between these two variants of the disease.

I have observed anetoderma also in the context of generalized follicular mucinosis (Fig. 3.142), again underlining the fact that different variants of mycosis fungoides may show overlapping clinicopathologic features. Interestingly, in this patient anetodermic lesions with the same clinical and histopathological features could be observed with a time interval of 12 years between two visits, showing a remarkable stability of the clinicopathological features.

## "Invisible" mycosis fungoides

Normal-looking skin in patients with mycosis fungoides may show histopathologic, electron microscopic, immunophenotypic, and/or molecular genetic evidence for the presence of neoplastic lymphocytes [337]. These cases have been termed "invisible" mycosis fungoides in the literature because the

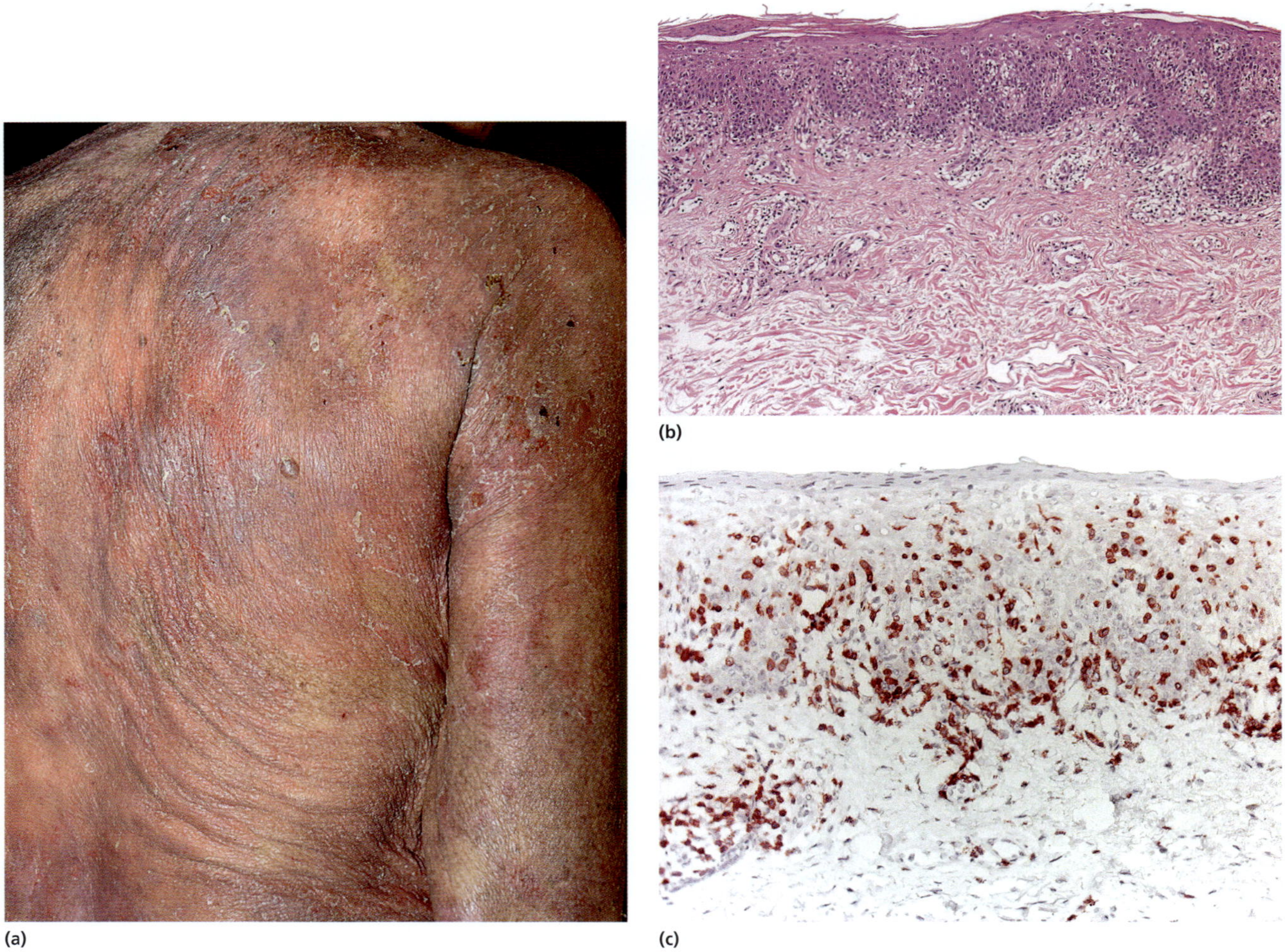


**Figure 3.117** Mycosis fungoides mimicking late-onset atopic dermatitis. (a) Clinical picture characterized by generalized, partly scaly, partly hyperpigmented lesions. (b) Histology shows a hyperplastic epidermis with spongiosis, parakeratosis, and some intraepidermal lymphocytes. Note absence of a band-like infiltrate. (c) Staining for CD3 highlights many intraepidermal lymphocytes ("disproportionate epidermotropism").

lesions are clinically unapparent. The presence of such histologic features in normal-looking skin has been documented at the first diagnosis of mycosis fungoides, in patients with mycosis fungoides at sites distant from erythematous lesions, and in patients in complete clinical remission after treatment. Usually the intraepidermal lymphocytes are only a few (Fig. 3.143).

The finding of neoplastic cells of mycosis fungoides in skin that looks clinically normal poses two main questions: the first relates to the extent of the area that should be treated by skin-targeted therapies, and the second concerns the proper monitoring of patients after treatment. At present, it is difficult to answer either question, as the clinical implications (if any) of "invisible" persistent disease are not clear. In my experience, however, biopsies of normal-looking skin do not add information relevant for further management of patients with mycosis fungoides.

## Psoriasiform mycosis fungoides

Mycosis fungoides may mimic the clinical picture of psoriasis: particularly, in patients with follicular involvement, presence of variably large, confluent psoriasiform scales may be a confounding factor in the clinical differential diagnosis (Figs. 3.144–3.146). Such lesions are observed mainly in patients with long-standing, previously untreated disease. In a recent study, the presence of well-demarcated scaly keratotic patches/plaques resembling psoriasis at the time of initial diagnosis was used as a criterion to classify cases as psoriasiform mycosis fungoides [338], and in this study a more aggressive course for this variant of the disease was observed. However, the percentage of cases of mycosis fungoides classified as psoriasiform in this report was 17.5% (38 out of a total of 217 cases) [338], which is much higher than the occasional, very rare cases that I have observed in the last 4 decades, in my opinion suggesting that

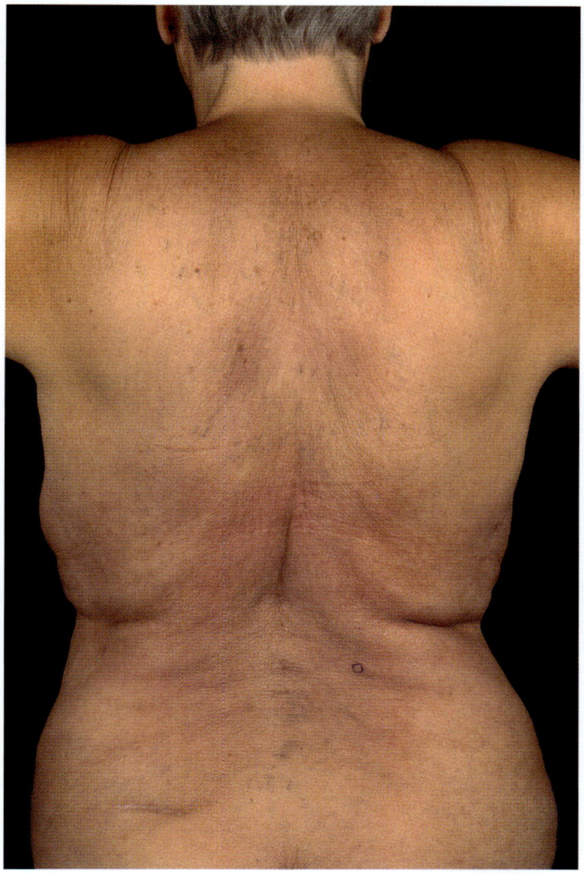

Figure 3.118 Interstitial mycosis fungoides characterized by large, ill-defined, infiltrated, brownish lesions on the back (similar lesions were present also on the abdomen).

inclusion of patients within this group was not very strict (in this context, it should be reminded that "psoriasiform" lesions are not uncommon in patients with mycosis fungoides).

In the context of "psoriasiform mycosis fungoides" it is important to mention cases presenting with lesions restricted to palms and soles, that have been reported in the literature as "mycosis fungoides palmaris et plantaris" (Fig. 3.23) [339–341]. In my opinion, this variant of mycosis fungoides probably does not exist, and these cases represent psoriasis palmo-plantaris with "pseudolymphomatous infiltrates." Some of the published patients had lesions of mycosis fungoides also at other sites of the body, and others had a typical clinical presentation of psoriasis; in this context, it cannot be considered surprising that in one published case the lesions were associated with psoriasis of the nails [342]. A detailed discussion of these subjects is provided in the section on pseudolymphomatous psoriasis in Chapter 31.

## Nevoid hyperkeratosis of the nipple and mycosis fungoides

Several reports pointed at the association of mycosis fungoides and nevoid hyperkeratosis of the nipple. There seems to be a twofold association: on the one hand, some patients with mycosis fungoides may have concomitantly nevoid hyperkeratosis of the nipple (Fig. 3.147) [343–345]; on the other hand, some patients without other clinical manifestations of mycosis fungoides present with nevoid hyperkeratosis of the nipple characterized histopathologically by presence of intraepidermal collections of lymphocytes resembling Darier nests [346, 347]. Conventional lesions of mycosis fungoides did not develop on follow-up [346]. I have observed rarely similar cases (Fig. 3.148). Although the occurrence of nevoid hyperkeratosis of the nipple in patients with mycosis fungoides may be coincidental, and the presence of specific infiltrates histopathologically may be comparable to what can be observed in other cutaneous lesions unrelated to mycosis fungoides (e.g., seborrheic keratosis), lesions of nevoid hyperkeratosis of the nipple showing histopathological features of mycosis fungoides in patients who do not have other manifestations of the disease represent a conceptual and practical problem. In my opinion these cases should be regarded as histopathological simulators of mycosis fungoides rather than as specific manifestations of the disease, akin to lichenoid (lymphomatoid) keratoses, that occasionally can reveal intraepidermal collections of lymphocytes as well (see Chapter 31). However, in contrast to other histopathological simulators of mycosis fungoides, a lymphocytic infiltrate is usually not found in nevoid hyperkeratosis of the nipple. At the present state of knowledge a prudent approach seems to be advisable for these cases: aggressive treatment modalities should be avoided ("watchful waiting" strategy), and patients should be managed with regular follow-up controls.

## Acanthosis nigricans-like mycosis fungoides

In some patients, lesions of mycosis fungoides may resemble clinically acanthosis nigricans (Fig. 3.149) [348]. In the only such case that I have observed, the lesions reminded clinically of a widespread, irregular organoid nevus, and were not restricted to typical areas of acanthosis nigricans but rather generalized. Several biopsy specimens showed an irregular hyperplasia of the epidermis, most likely representing the histopathological counterpart of the clinical presentation, and a surprisingly sparse dermal infiltrate in spite of the presence of several intraepidermal Darier nests (Fig. 3.149d). In some reports, the clinicopathological features were very similar to those observed in my patient [349, 350], whereas in other cases conventional lesions of mycosis fungoides coexisted with the acanthosis nigricans-like presentation [351, 352]. In the context of the rare presence of Darier nests in lesions of clear-cut nevoid hyperkeratosis of the nipple (see paragraph above), one may consider whether these patients, or at least some of them, do really have mycosis fungoides, or a peculiar variant of organoid epidermal hyperplasia with "pseudolymphomatous" infiltrates. At present, given the presence of widespread lesions, this possibility seems unlikely, yet a prudent approach should be considered when managing these patients.

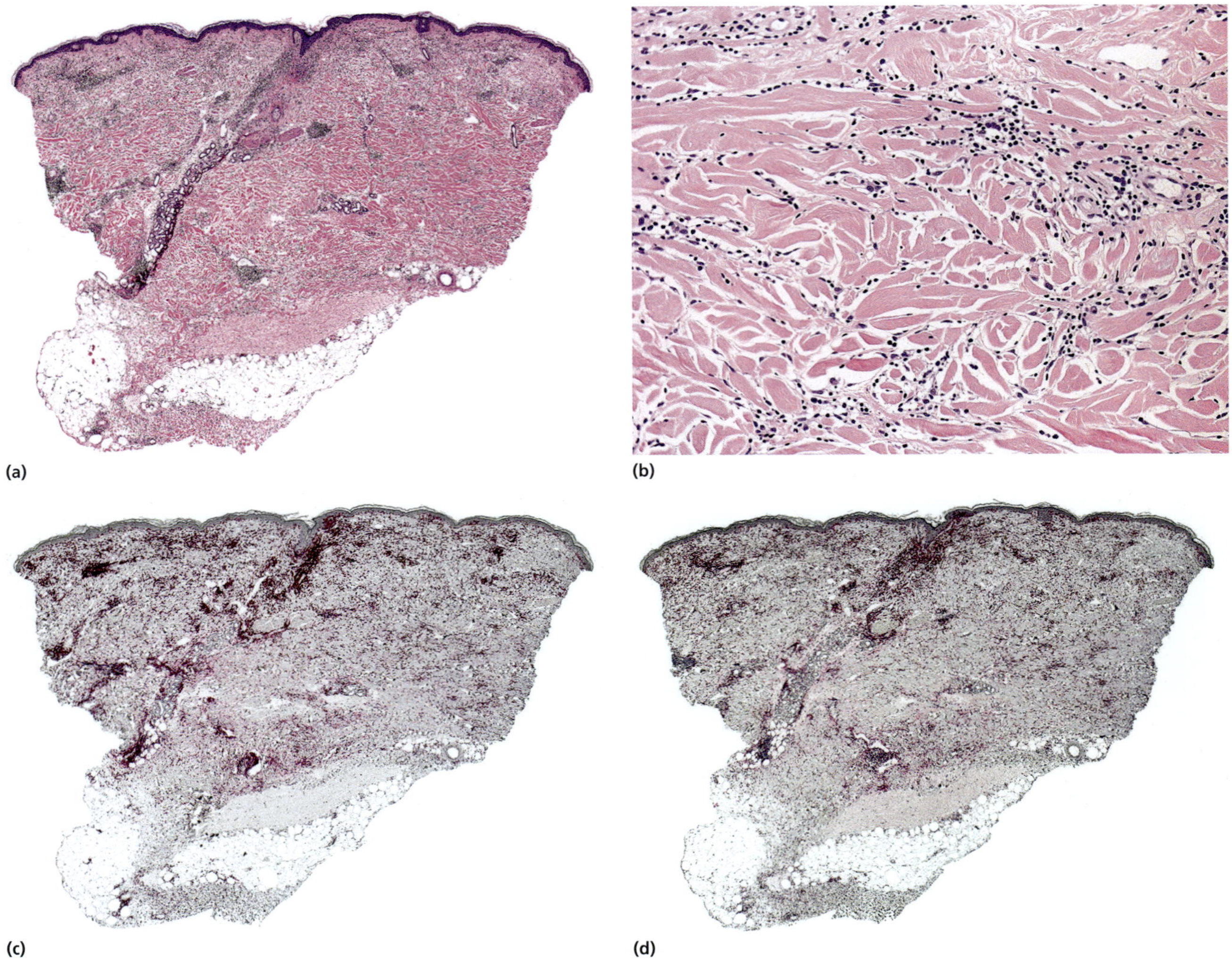

**Figure 3.119** Interstitial mycosis fungoides. (a) Patchy-lichenoid superficial lymphoid infiltrate and interstitial infiltrate within the reticular dermis. (b) Note neoplastic cells arranged in "Indian" files between the collagen fibers. (c) Staining for CD5 and (d) CD8 reveals that most interstitial cells are cytotoxic T lymphocytes and highlights the presence of epidermotropic lymphocytes as well.

## Other unusual clinical presentations of mycosis fungoides

Other clinicopathological variants of mycosis fungoides have been described besides those discussed above in more detail (Table 3.2). ***Ichtyosiform mycosis fungoides*** is characterized by a cobblestone pattern of flat, geometric plaques that remind clinically of ichthyosis vulgaris (Fig. 3.150a). The histopathologic features are identical to those of more conventional variants of the disease. Perioral and nasolabial papules may mimic perioral dermatitis (Fig. 3.150b) [353].

A condition reported in Japan as ***"papuloerythroderma Ofuji"*** [354] in many cases most likely represents a variant of mycosis fungoides characterized by a similar clinical presentation and protracted course. A similar picture can be observed in Caucasian patients as well, in my experience as a feature of advanced disease (Fig. 3.150c). Lesions of mycosis fungoides arising at sites of previous herpes zoster have been classified as ***"zosteriform mycosis fungoides"*** [355].

The presence of lesions arranged predominantly on the waist has been described as ***"waistband mycosis fungoides"*** [356]. I have seen some patients with this clinical presentation (Fig. 3.151), but do not think that it represents a "variant" of the disease, as other lesions are usually present on other parts of the body. Mycosis fungoides accentuated on the waist should be differentiated clinically from other conditions that may show a similar distribution of the lesions, including mostly scleroderma, granuloma annulare, and pigmented atrophic lichen planus.

In one patient with rapidly progressive disease, we have observed innumerable lesions of molluscum contagiosum, similar to the picture of so-called ***"eczema molluscatum,"*** with a peculiar (and unexplained) clearing of the skin

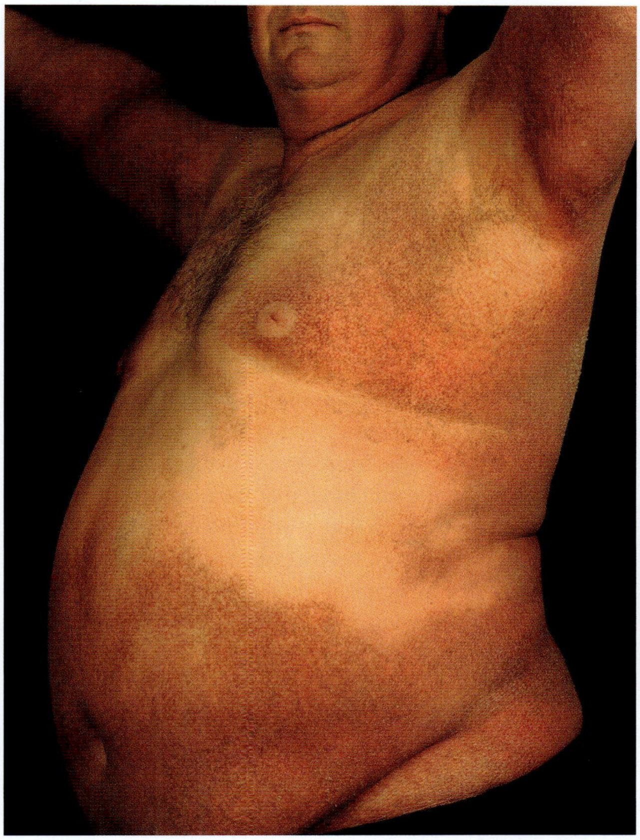

Figure 3.120 Poikilodermatous mycosis fungoides characterized by the presence of confluent, atrophic patches on the trunk and upper extremities.

around most of the viral lesions (Fig. 3.152). Interestingly, eczema molluscatum has been reported rarely in patients with mycosis fungoides [357–360], yet sparing of the areas affected by molluscum contagiosum had not been described. Finally, although ***"squaring" of the rete ridges*** is considered a typical sign of annular lichenoid dermatitis of youth, a histopathological mimicker of mycosis fungoides (see Chapter 31), in rare cases of mycosis fungoides I have observed the same histopathological feature, characterized by clusters of lymphocytes that "cut through" the tip of the rete ridges conferring the typical appearance of "squared" rete ridges (Fig. 3.153).

***Urticarial lesions*** have been described in two patients with blood involvement and positivity of neoplastic cells for CD25 and FOX-P3 [361].

Many of the variants discussed in this and the previous sections have been observed in anecdotal cases only. On the other hand, they underline once again the protean clinicopathologic features of mycosis fungoides and the need for a high level of suspicion when diagnosing cutaneous eruptions that do not fit well into a precise category of inflammatory skin disease.

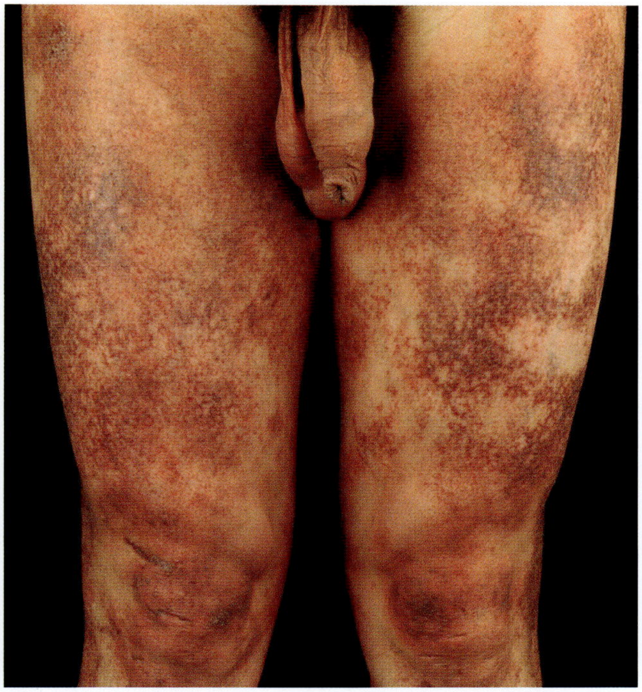

Figure 3.121 Poikilodermatous mycosis fungoides with reticulated, atrophic patches on the thighs ("parakeratosis variegata").

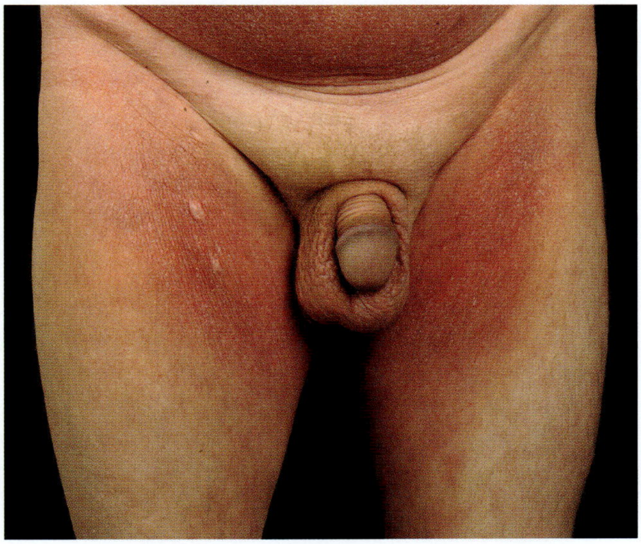

Figure 3.122 Poikilodermatous mycosis fungoides with a clinical distribution and morphology of the lesions resembling those of symmetrical drug-related intertriginous and flexural exanthema (SDRIFE).

## Mycosis fungoides in children and adolescents

Mycosis fungoides is the most common form of cutaneous lymphoma in childhood and adolescence (see also Chapter 30) [362]. In general, in pediatric patients, mycosis fungoides is rare, but

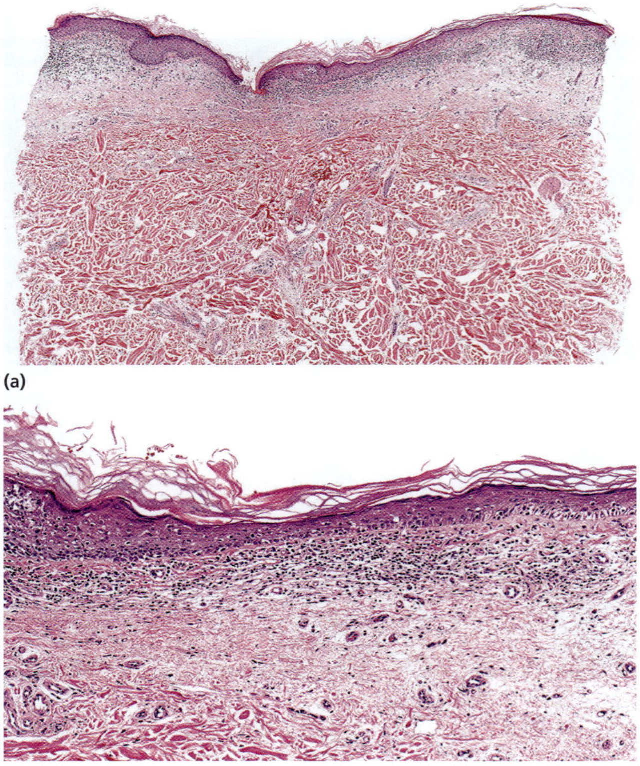

(a)

(b)

**Figure 3.123** Poikilodermatous mycosis fungoides. (a) Band-like infiltrate of lymphocytes. (b) Note epidermotropic lymphocytes, fibrosis of the papillary dermis and increased numbers of telangiectatic vessels.

the true incidence may be higher than assumed because there is often a reluctance to perform biopsies in children, and the diagnosis can be delayed for several years. A national population-based study of the Surveillance, Epidemiology, and End Results (SEER) database and Texas Cancer Registry showed an increase in the incidence of the disease among children and adolescents (until 19 years of age) between 2000 and 2017 [363]. The incidence seems to be higher in Arabic patients compared to United States and European ones [364].

Although all variants of mycosis fungoides may be encountered in young patients, some seem to be more common in this age group. Some typical clinical presentations are pictured in Chapter 30. Hypopigmented mycosis fungoides is more frequent in children than in adults, especially in patients with dark skin [298, 365–368]. A similar prevalence of hypopigmented lesions has been observed in children of Asian and Arab ethnicity [369–371]. Localized pagetoid reticulosis (Woringer–Kolopp type) also occurs more frequently in childhood. The clinical presentation in these cases can be deceiving, and often lesions will be biopsied only after prolonged local treatment for "eczema" or "wart." Purpuric mycosis fungoides was relatively frequent in young patients in one study from Turkey [366]. Pilotropic mycosis fungoides is also a common presentation in young patients [212, 368, 372]. As already mentioned, the exact nosology of cases of follicular mucinosis in children and adolescents presenting with solitary lesions on the head and neck area is still unclear (see the section on pilotropic mycosis fungoides in this chapter). A cytotoxic phenotype of tumor cells seems to be more common in children and adolescents than in adults [365, 368, 373, 374].

A peculiar type of mycosis fungoides in children may simulate either clinically or histopathologically the picture of pityriasis lichenoides, and may be particularly difficult to diagnose (see the section on pityriasis lichenoides-like mycosis fungoides in this chapter, and also the one on pityriasis lichenoides in Chapter 31) [327, 328, 330, 332, 375].

The overall outlook for children or adolescents with mycosis fungoides is difficult to predict, and it has been maintained that mycosis fungoides is more aggressive in pediatric patients [372]. However, most reports suggested that the natural history of the disease is comparable with that of adult patients [366, 368, 369, 376–381]. Indeed, it may be that at least some of the cases reported in the past as "atypical" or "aggressive" mycosis fungoides in children represented examples of cytotoxic NK/T-cell lymphomas, which usually show a more aggressive course and poor prognosis. On the other hand, the onset of lesions of mycosis fungoides in childhood increases the probability of disease progression during the lifetime of the patients. Recommendations for the management of pediatric mycosis fungoides have been recently published, suggesting that addressing clinical severity aspects such as pruritus, functional, or esthetic impairment (e.g., palms, soles, genitalia), quality of life impact, psychological aspects, and parental anxiety is more relevant than TNMB staging [382a]. Recommendations for the diagnosis, staging and treatment of early-stage pediatric mycosis fungoides have been published recently [382a, 382c],

## Treatment

Treatment of mycosis fungoides differs according to the stage of the disease, the extent of the cutaneous and/or extracutaneous manifestations, and the previous therapy (if any). Several guidelines are available for both early and advanced stages of the disease [383–389].

One problem in evaluating treatment strategies is that the level of evidence for any given therapy is usually low, as large, double-blinded studies have been performed only rarely. Another major problem is the lack of standardized end points and response criteria for studies on the efficacy of therapy, an issue that has recently been the subject of a consensus statement of the EORTC, ISCL, and USCLC [390]. Complete response in the skin is defined as 100% clearance of skin lesions, partial response as 50–99% clearance without new tumors, stable disease as <25% increase to <50% clearance in skin disease without new tumors, and progressive disease as ≥25% increase in skin disease or new tumors [390]. Several end points have been identified and

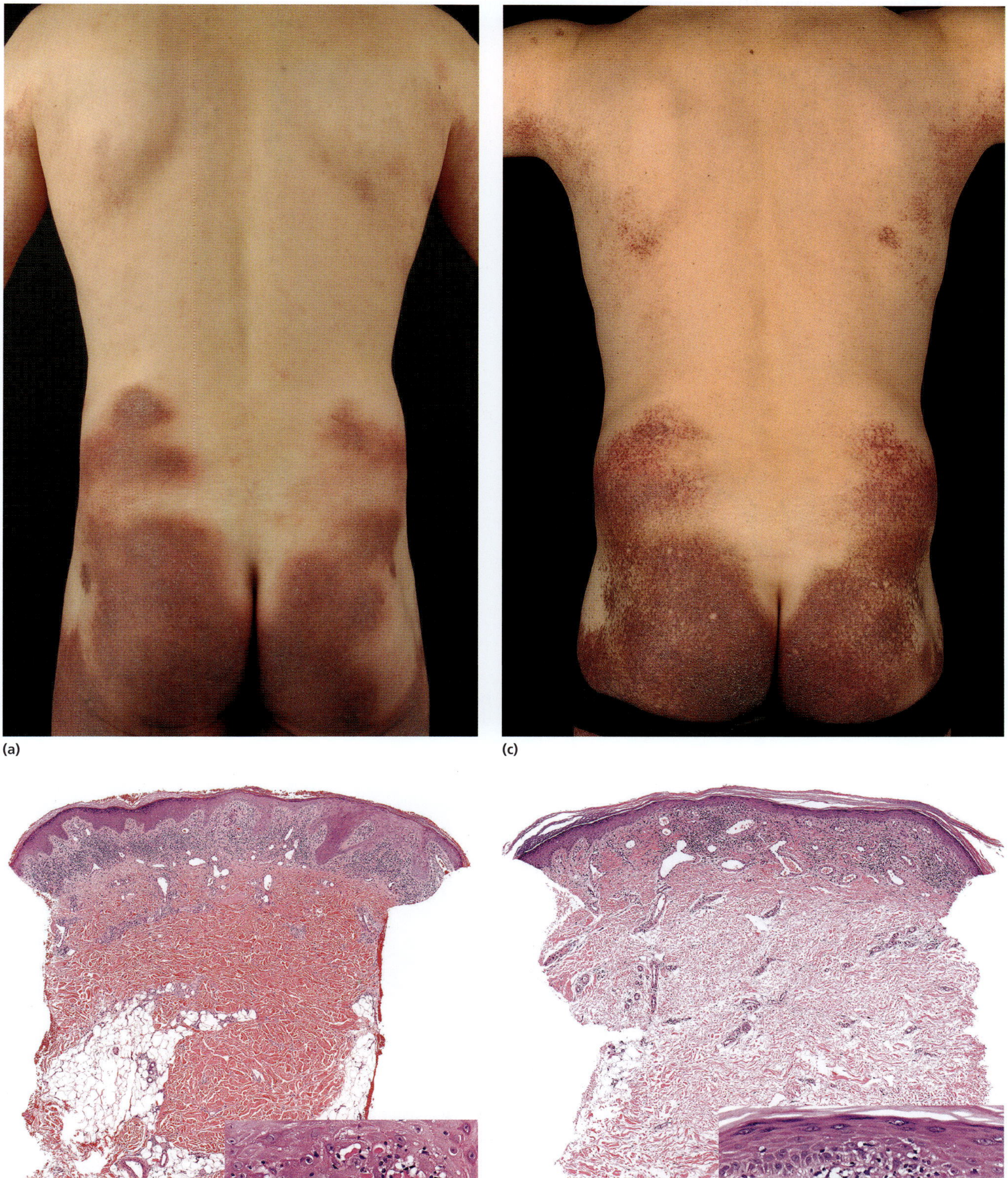

Figure 3.124 Poikilodermatous mycosis fungoides. (a) A 30-year-old man at first presentation with poikilodermatic lesions covering most of the buttocks and only minimal involvement of the back and upper extremities. (b) A biopsy specimen showed a band-like infiltrate of lymphocytes within an expanded papillary dermis with teleangiectatic vessels; note epidermotropic lymphocytes with necrotic keratinocytes (inset). (c) More than 10 years later, the patient still had similar lesions with a more pronounced reticulated pattern and with more accentuated involvement of the back and upper extremities. (d) A new biopsy showed a decrease in the density of the infiltrate with more pronounced telangiectasia; note a few epidermotropic lymphocytes (inset).

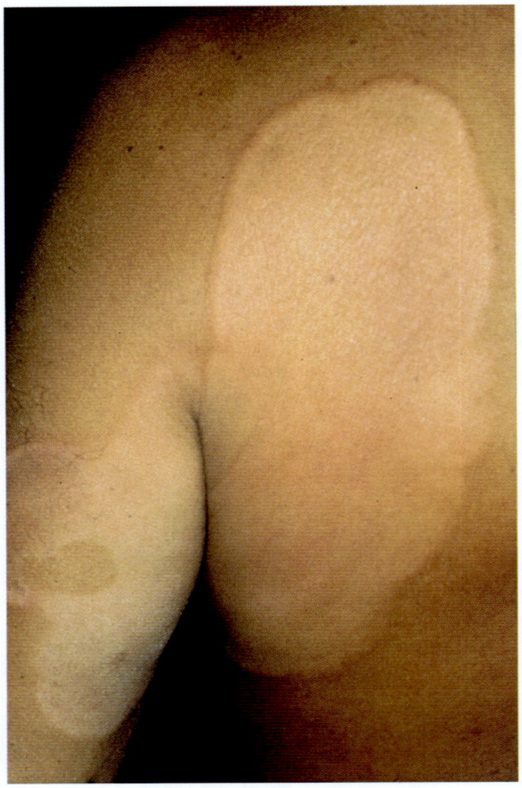

**Figure 3.125** Hypopigmented patches of mycosis fungoides on the left shoulder and arm. Note elevated, slightly erythematous margins.

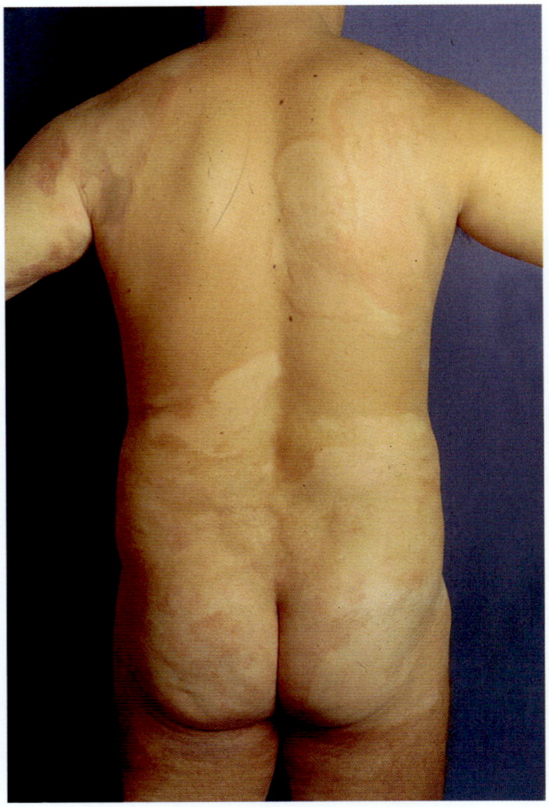

**Figure 3.126** Hypopigmented mycosis fungoides covering large parts of the body. Note erythematous areas as well.

defined precisely, including objective response rate, time to response, response duration, time to relapse/freedom from relapse, time to treatment failure/freedom from treatment failure, time to progression, progression-free survival, disease-free survival, and relapse-free survival [390]. Applying the same end points and response criteria is a crucial step in order to compare different studies and/or different treatment modalities.

The first-line treatment of early lesions of mycosis fungoides includes different skin-directed modalities. Topical application of steroids (e.g., clobetasole propionate) or of chemotherapeutic agents (chlormethine gel, carmustine, methotrexate) is usually efficacious [391, 392], and it has been suggested that chlormethine gel should be considered as a first-line treatment in selected patients [393, 394]. Topical retinoids (bexarotene 1% gel) may also be considered; tazarotene and alitretinoin are other retinoids available for topical treatment in cream or gel formulas. An inflammatory reaction on treated skin is the main side effect of topical retinoids, being a limiting factor for their application to large areas of the body. Topical toll-like receptor antagonists (imiquimod, resiquimod) have also some efficacy in early-stage mycosis fungoides [395]. All topical treatments have some degree of efficacy, but recurrences are the rule. It should be also noted that the administration of placebo as a topical vehicle devoid of active principle was found to produce an objective response in 24% of patients with early mycosis

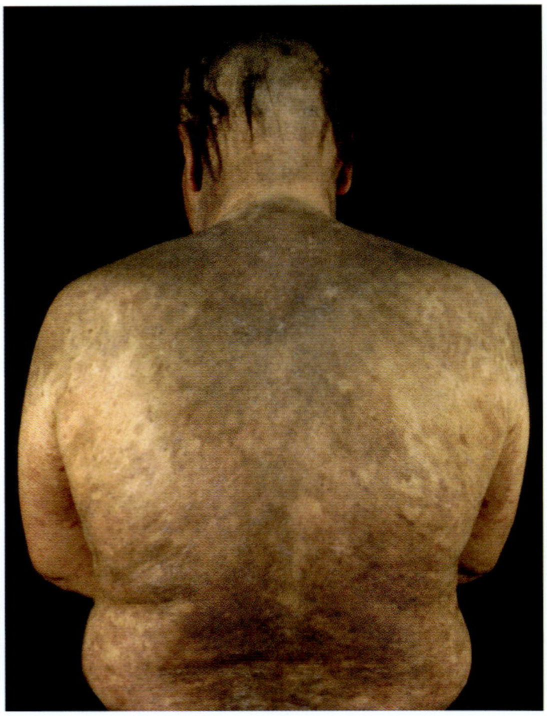

**Figure 3.127** Hyperpigmented mycosis fungoides. Note diffuse brown color and irregular alopecia. (*Courtesy of Dr. Maria Cristina Coccia, Genova, Italy.*)

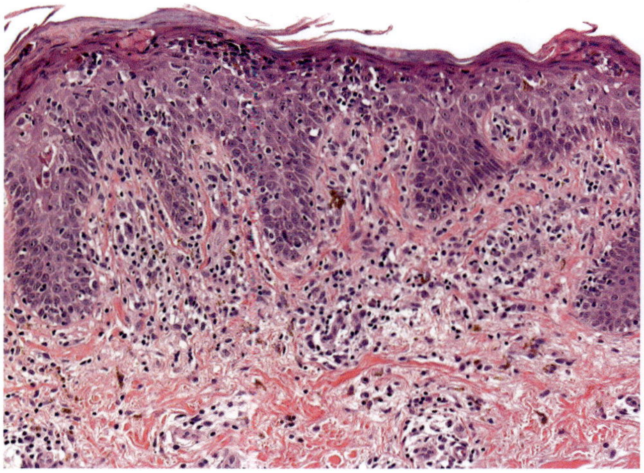

Figure 3.128 Hyperpigmented mycosis fungoides. Lymphoid infiltrates with epidermotropic lymphocytes, necrotic keratinocytes, and several melanophages in the papillary dermis.

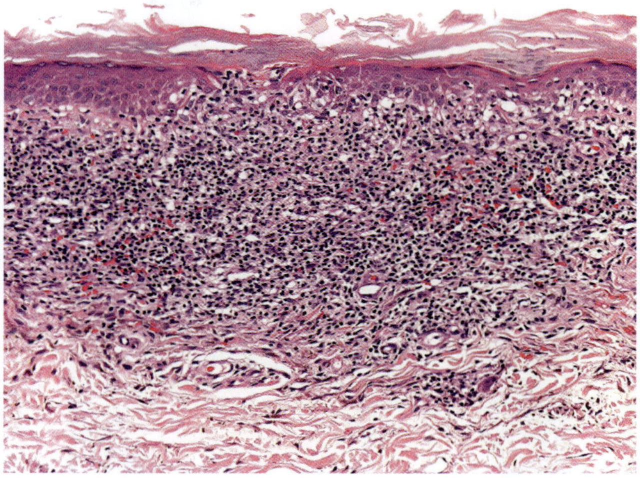

Figure 3.130 Purpuric mycosis fungoides. Dense, band-like lymphoid infiltrate with epidermotropic lymphocytes, extravasated erythrocytes, and siderophages.

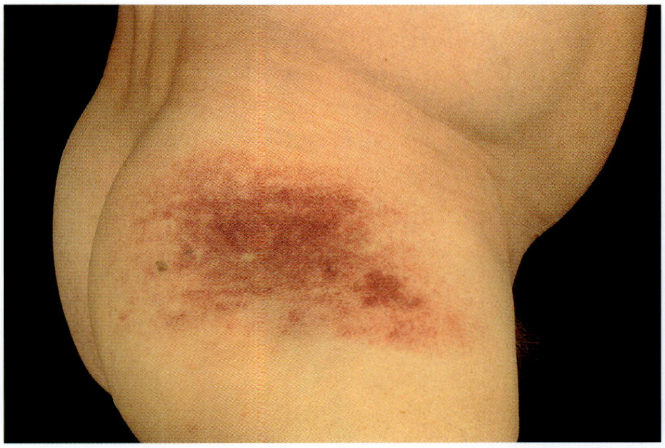

Figure 3.129 Purpuric mycosis fungoides. Purpuric, irregular, infiltrated patch on sun-covered skin of the flank.

fungoides in a double-blind, randomized study [396]. The notion that a considerable proportion of patients with patch-stage mycosis fungoides shows a complete clinical response upon local application of placebo suggests that in early phases the disease may be controlled also with a watchful waiting strategy.

The use of psoralens in association with UV-A irradiation (PUVA), interferon-α, retinoids, or a combination of these three modalities is one of the first-line treatments of early mycosis fungoides [397–400]. Interferon α-2a has shown an overall response rate of 53.3% in a recent large study by the EORTC-Cutaneous Lymphoma Tumour Group, with better results obtained when combination regimens were used [401]. PUVA treatment has also been administered in the form of so-called bath-PUVA. In many cases, patients with localized patches of the disease can also be managed with local steroid ointments.

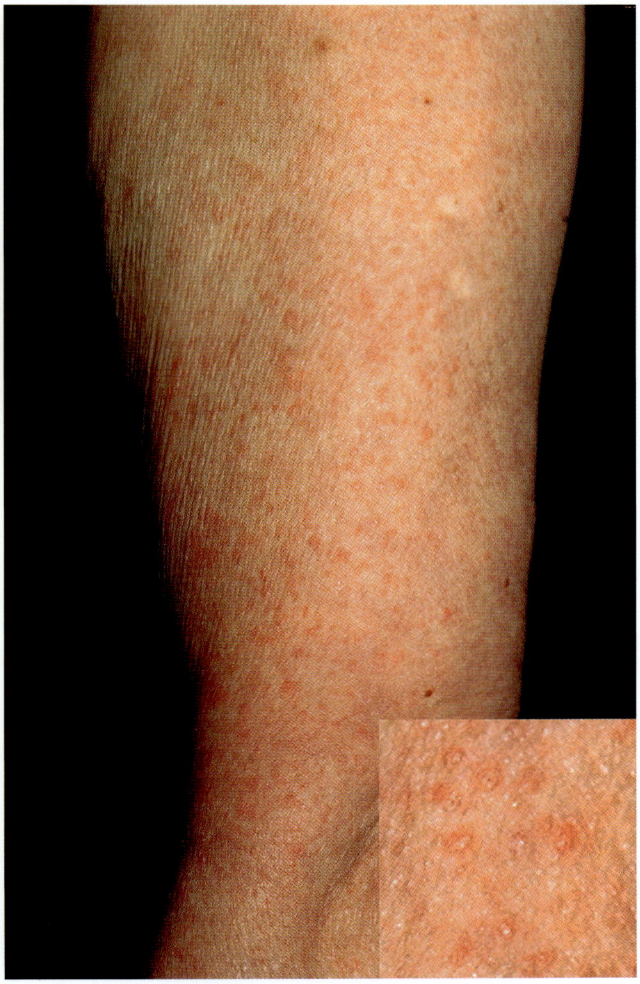

Figure 3.131 Papular mycosis fungoides. Tiny erythematous papules on the arm. Inset: detail of the papules.

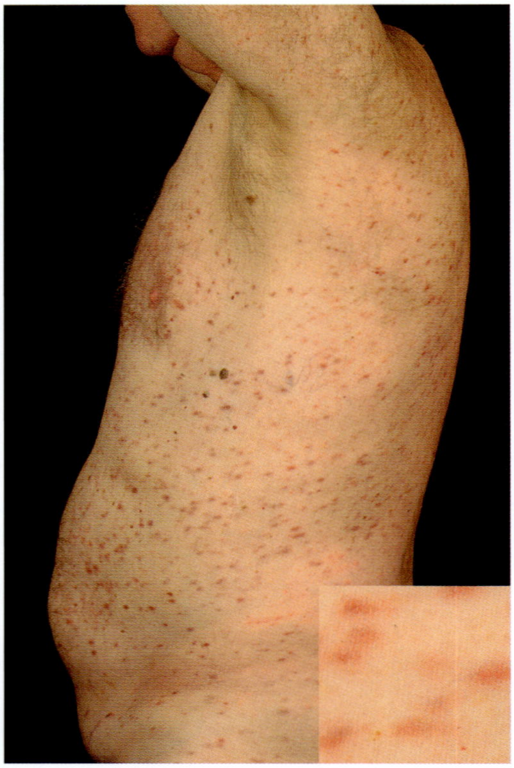

Figure 3.132 Papular mycosis fungoides. Generalized erythematous, partly brownish papules. Inset: detail of the papules.

UV-B irradiation (or narrow-band UV-B – 311 nm) may be used alternative to PUVA [402, 403]. Among the retinoids, bexarotene has been used frequently for the treatment of mycosis fungoides (in both early and late stages), either alone or, more often, in combination with other agents [399, 404, 405]. No differences in outcome could be found in a large multicenter study comparing PUVA alone versus PUVA + bexarotene in early mycosis fungoides [406]. Phototherapy may be administered also as photodynamic therapy with 5-aminolaevulinic acid [407], with good response of superficial lesions of mycosis fungoides (the size of the area that can be treated is a limiting factor for photodynamic therapy, which on the other hand is a good alternative for small, solitary lesions).

The administration of total body irradiation [408–410], proposed by some authors as a first-line treatment, should probably be restricted to patients with mycosis fungoides in advanced stages. The EORTC guidelines include this therapy as a second-line option for the disease presenting with plaques +/− patches covering ≥10% of the body surface (T2b) [388]. Radiation therapy is a good option for solitary lesions of pilotropic/syringotropic mycosis fungoides, and is efficacious also in cases of localized pagetoid reticulosis. Recommendations from the EORTC cutaneous lymphoma tumor group for radiation therapy have been published recently [411]. Brentuximab vedotin, an anti-CD30 monoclonal antibody, represents one of the most promising treatment modalities in cases expressing

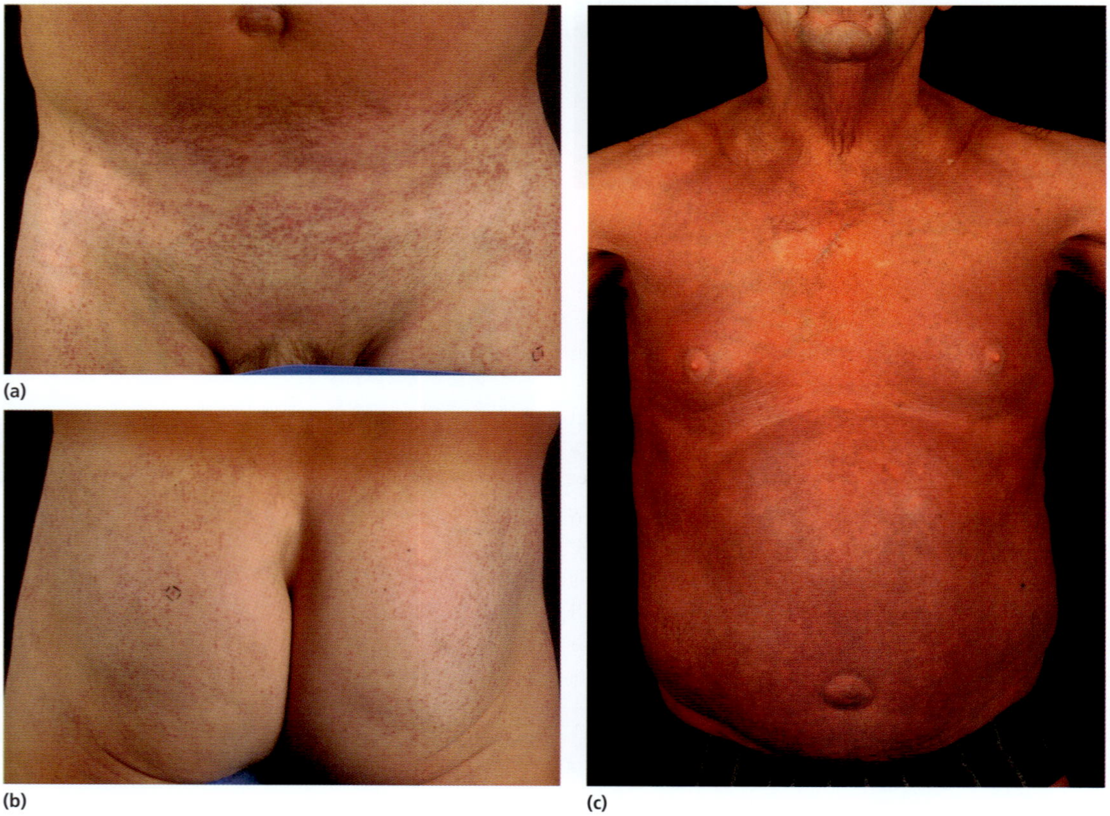


Figure 3.133 Papular mycosis fungoides. (a), (b) Tiny papules arranged mostly on sun-protected skin of the inguinal area and buttocks. (c) Ten years later the patient developed erythroderma.

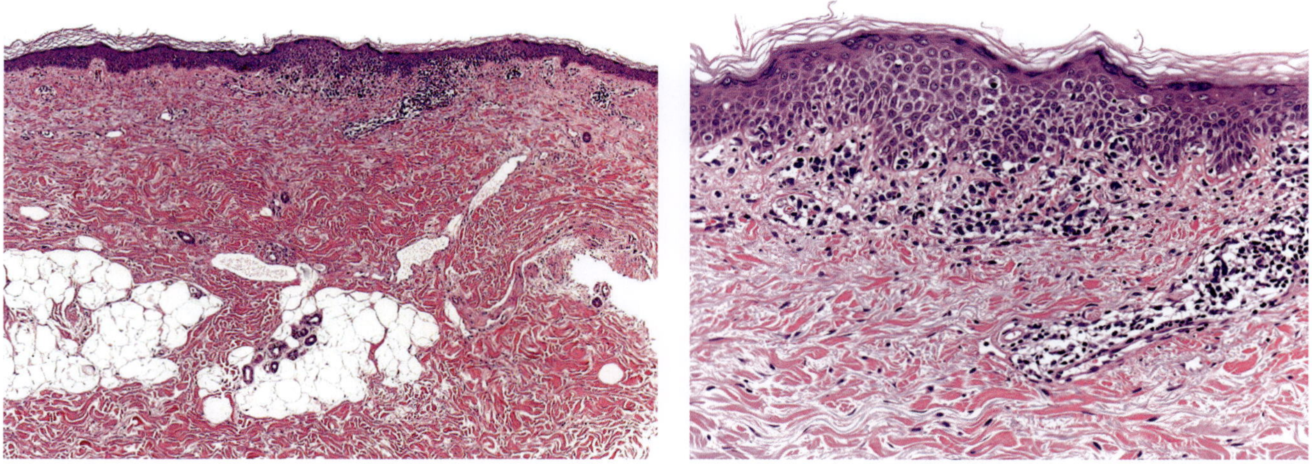

(a) (b)

Figure 3.134 Papular mycosis fungoides. (a) Histology of a tiny papule reveals an infiltrate confined to a small portion of the specimen. (b) Detail shows typical changes of mycosis fungoides (same patient as Fig. 3.131).

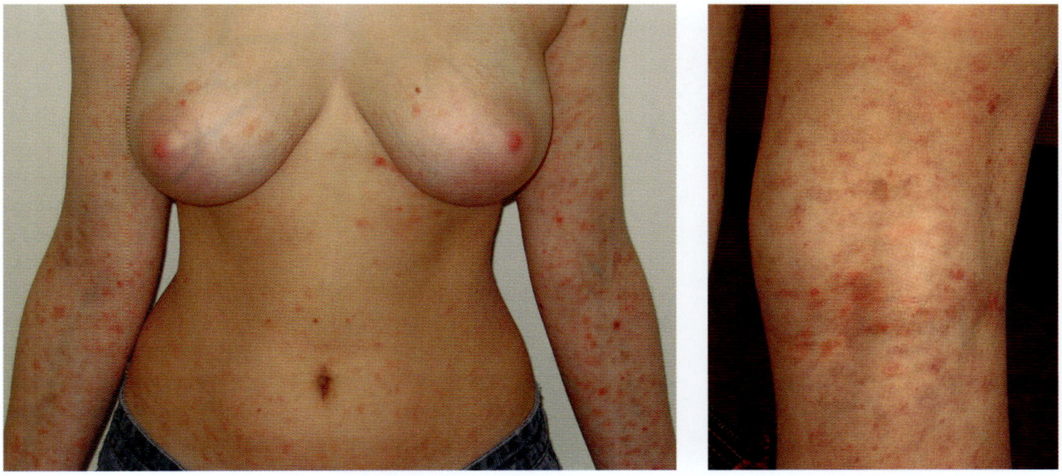

(a) (a)

Figure 3.135 Pityriasis lichenoides-like mycosis fungoides (clinical variant). (a, b) Papular, partly scaly eruption clinically similar to pityriasis lichenoides. *(Courtesy of Dr. Annika Volke, Tartu, Estonia.)*

CD30 [412–414]. Brentuximab vedotin has been included as a second-line treatment option for mycosis fungoides in stages IA, IB, and IIA [388], but in our center we never use it for stage IA. The ALCANZA study showed that a significant improvement in objective response lasting at least 4 months was seen with brentuximab vedotin versus physician's choice of methotrexate or bexarotene in CD30+ pre-treated mycosis fungoides [415]. Although brentuximab vedotin should be used in cases that are positive for CD30, several reports pointed at the efficacy of the treatment also in CD30-negative cases [416, 417]. Finally, mogamulizumab represents a further treatment alternative [418, 419], and it has been recently added to the second-line therapeutical options for mycosis fungoides in stages IA, IB, and IIA [388]. However, it is more commonly used for management of advanced disease or of Sézary syndrome [418]. It may be that the development of a granulomatous cutaneous reaction after drug administration represents a marker of good response to mogamolizumab [420].

Even in advanced stages of the disease, when evaluating the efficacy of any given therapy, it should be remembered that in some patients a progression-free survival time of some months may be observed with the use of placebo [421]. Many different treatment modalities have been proposed over the years for advanced mycosis fungoides. Conventional systemic

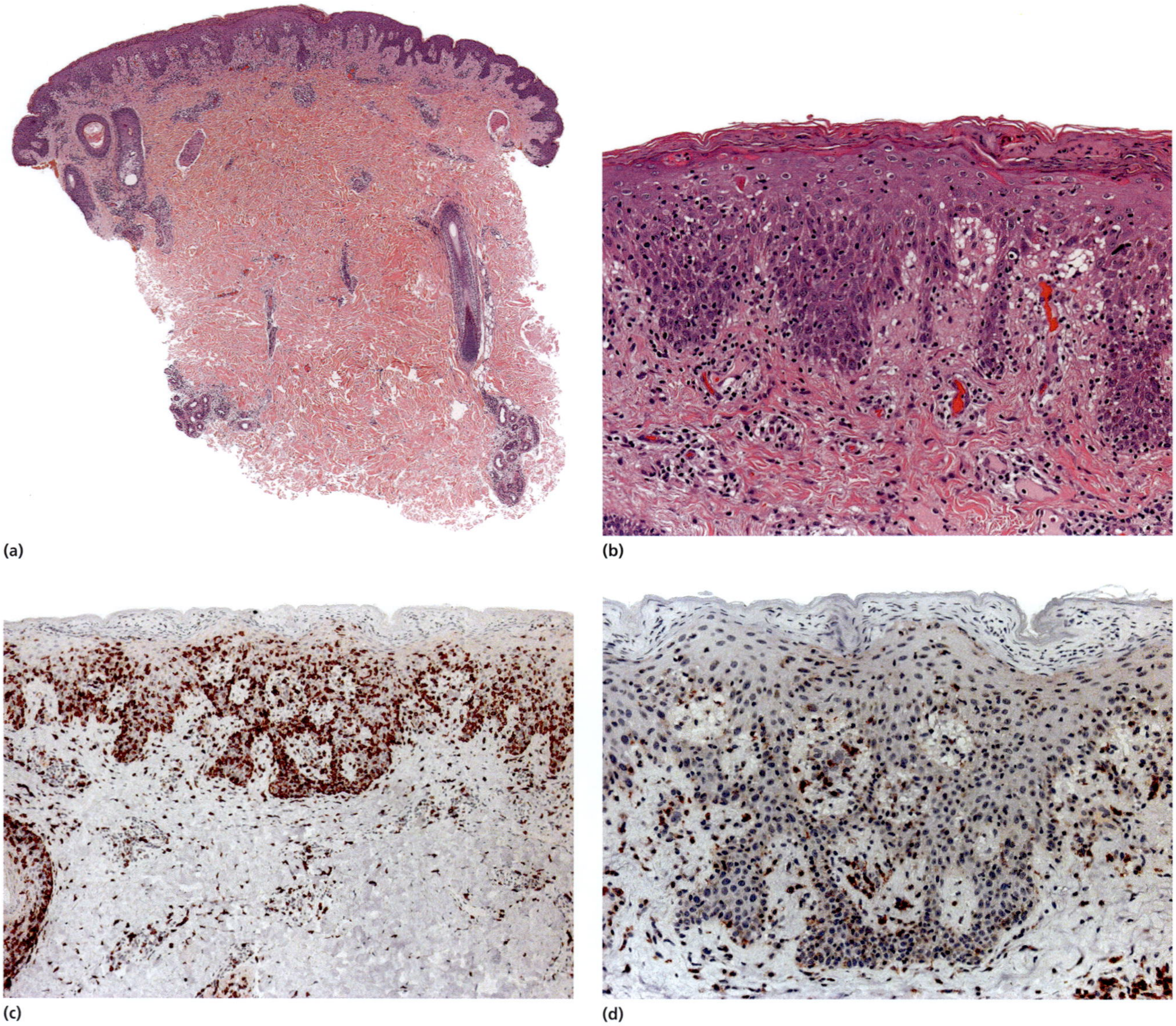

Figure 3.136 Pityriasis lichenoides-like mycosis fungoides (histological variant). (a) Superficial infiltrate with (b) epidermal hyperplasia, parakeratosis, necrotic keratinocytes, and lymphoid infiltrates with intraepidermal lymphocytes mimicking the histopathologic features of pityriasis lichenoides. Immunohistology shows (c) positivity for CD8 and (d) loss of CD5 expression.

chemotherapy (CHOP), single-agent chemotherapy, and other immunomodulatory treatments usually give good results in tumor-stage mycosis fungoides, but recurrences are the rule. Many compounds have been tested, including, among others, the histone deacetylase inhibitors romidepsin [422–424] vorinostat [425] and quisinostat [426], bortezomib (a proteasome inhibitor used in the treatment of myeloma), ixazomib (another proteasome inhibitor used in the treatment of myeloma, which may have utility in appropriately selected patients and/or in combination with other agents) [427], gemcitabine [428], fludarabine, panobinostat (a pan-deacetylase inhibitor), pegylated liposomal doxorubicin (Caelyx) [429], lenalidomide (a derivative of thalidomide) [430], interleukin-12, interferon gamma [431], and $DAB_{389}$-IL-2 fusion protein (Ontak, denileukin diftitox) [432]. Romidepsin gave good results also in controlling pruritus [422], and patients with prior chemotherapy were able to achieve durable responses similar to those observed in patients who were chemotherapy naïve [423]. Methotrexate has been used alone or in combination with other agents and may function through upregulation of Fas and enhancement of sensitivity to apoptosis [433].

New insights into the pathogenesis of mycosis fungoides provided a rationale for innovative treatment strategies.

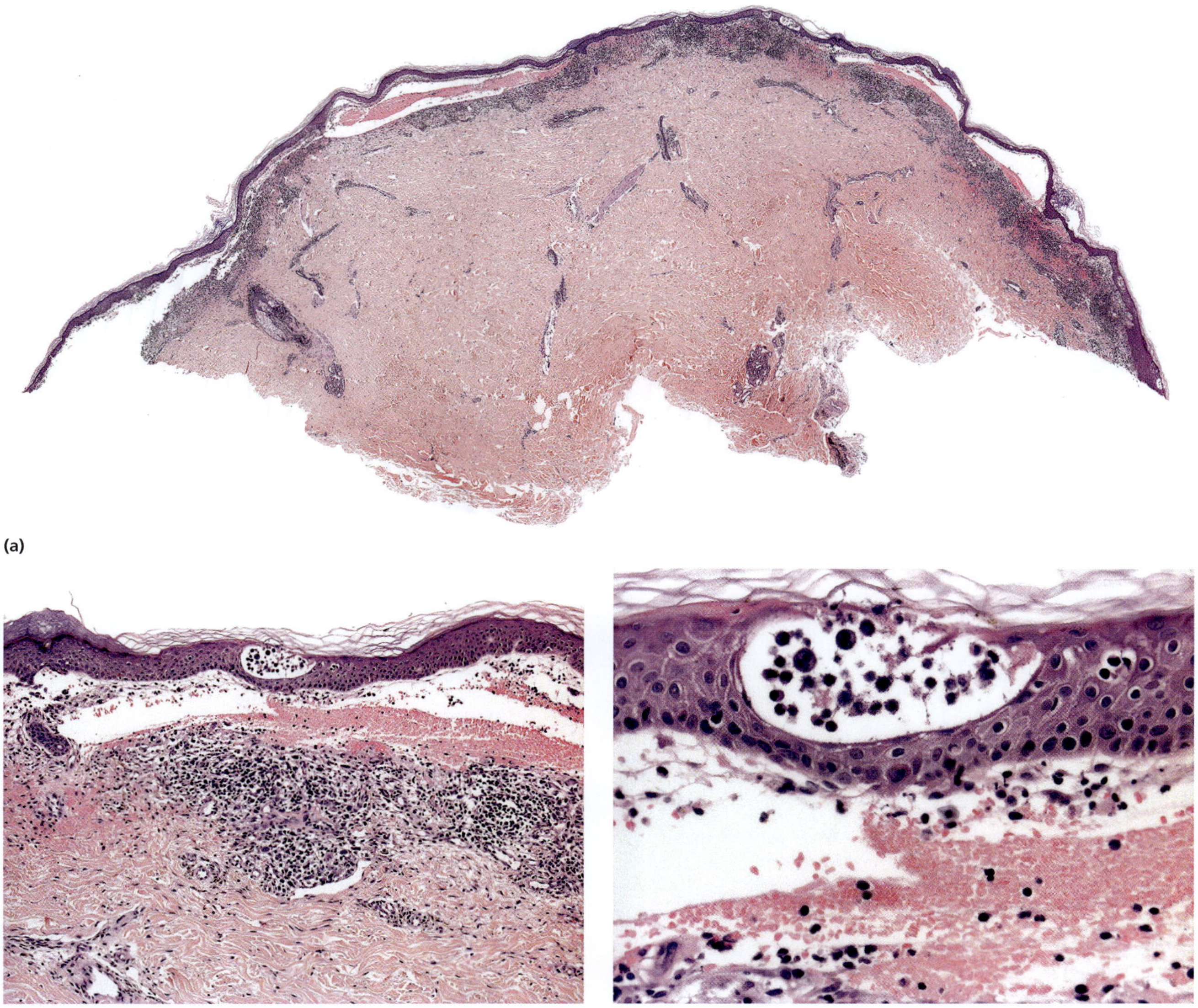

(a)

(b)

(c)

**Figure 3.137** Bullous mycosis fungoides. (a) Subepidermal bulla with dense band-like infiltrates of lymphocytes in the papillary dermis. (b, c) Detail of the bulla with epidermotropic lymphocytes.

Alemtuzumab, an anti-CD52 monoclonal antibody, induces remissions in some patients [434, 435]; it seems that toxicity (particularly potentially serious infections) is best controlled by administering low subcutaneous doses in short courses. The anti-CD4 antibody zanolimumab has been used in a few patients [435]. Therapeutic targeting of the immune checkpoint pathway using monoclonal antibodies (e.g., ipilimumab, pembrolizumab, nivolumab) represents a further possibility for treatment of mycosis fungoides [436]. The combination of dimethyl fumarate (an inhibitor of NF-κB acting as a survival factor in mycosis fungoides) and an inhibitor of the antiapoptotic protein Bcl-2 may also be another treatment modality [437]. Antiangiogenetic drugs have been tested in experimental settings [438].

Extracorporeal photopheresis and total skin electron beam irradiation have been applied in advanced mycosis fungoides [408, 439, 440a]. Radiotherapy of large tumors is a good palliative modality to improve quality of life. A retrospective study showed that a single 6Gy dose has the same efficacy as 2x4Gy doses in managing localized lesions of the disease [440b]. Some patients have also been treated with different types of tumor vaccines [441–443], but results are disappointing.

Several reports showed that allogeneic stem cell transplantation is a potentially curative option, even in advanced stages of the disease [444–460]. Encouraging results have been confirmed by a recent large series, suggesting that allogeneic stem cell transplantation should be considered for patients with high-risk,

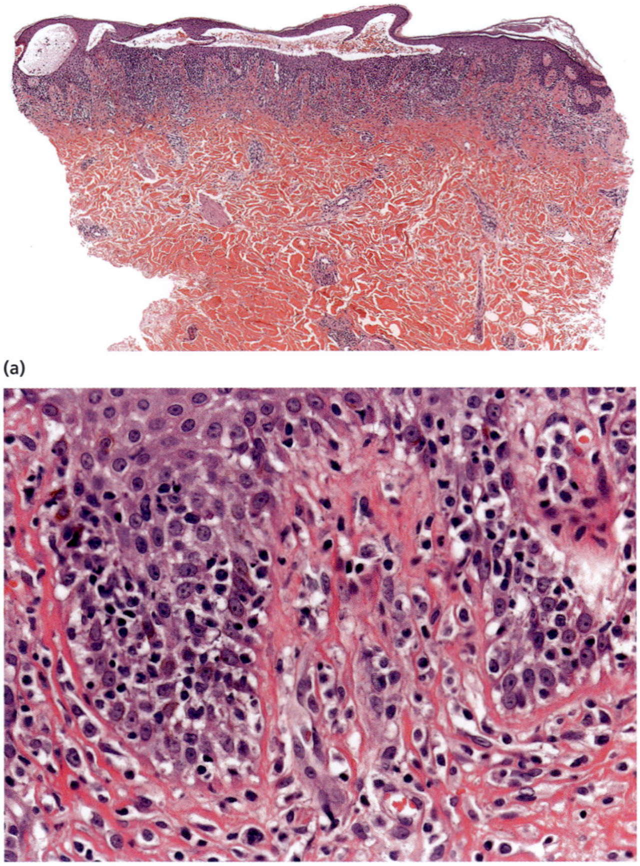

(a) (b)

**Figure 3.138** (a) Vesicular mycosis fungoides. Large, partly confluent intraepidermal vesicles with only a few lymphocytes. (b) Note several epidermotropic lymphocytes.

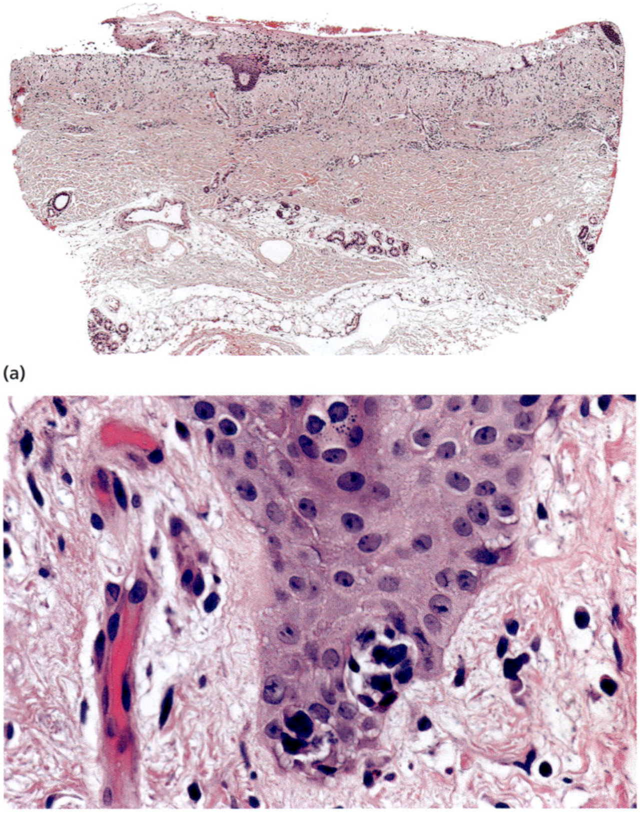

(a) (b)

**Figure 3.139** Bullous mycosis fungoides. (a) The epithelium is almost completely absent, and only a superficial erosion with small remnants of the acrosyringium is visible, together with a superficial, sparse lymphoid infiltrate. (b) Note two small clusters of intraepithelial lymphocytes within the acrosyringium.

advanced-stage mycosis fungoides who achieve pre-transplant disease remission [461]. Although toxicity is high, this option is one of the most promising for advanced-stage disease in selected patients. Allogeneic stem cell transplantation is usually preceded by reduced-intensity conditioning regimens, and patients with complete response or very good partial response before transplantation have a lower cumulative incidence of relapse than those with a higher disease burden [458]. Caution should be advised if previous treatments included alemtuzumab (interference with post-transplant cyclophosphamide effect and reactivation of cytomegalovirus) or mogamulizumab (increased risk of acute graft-versus-host disease) [462]. Check point inhibitors may also be associated with increased risk of acute graft-versus-host disease. A graft-versus-lymphoma mechanism may contribute to the beneficial effect of this treatment modality, as more than 50% of relapsing patients respond to donor lymphocyte infusions. Autologous bone marrow transplantation showed good results with complete clinical responses, but recurrence within short periods of time is the rule, and this modality is no longer suggested. In a recent survey among hematologists, criteria have been proposed for consideration of allogeneic stem

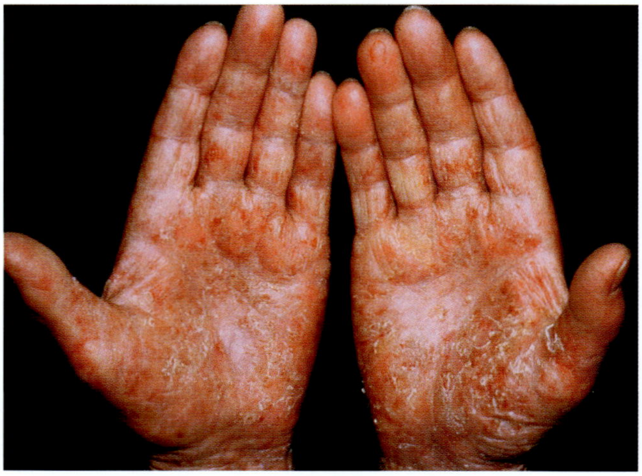

**Figure 3.140** Dyshidrotic mycosis fungoides. Dyshidrotic vesicles and small erosions on the palms.

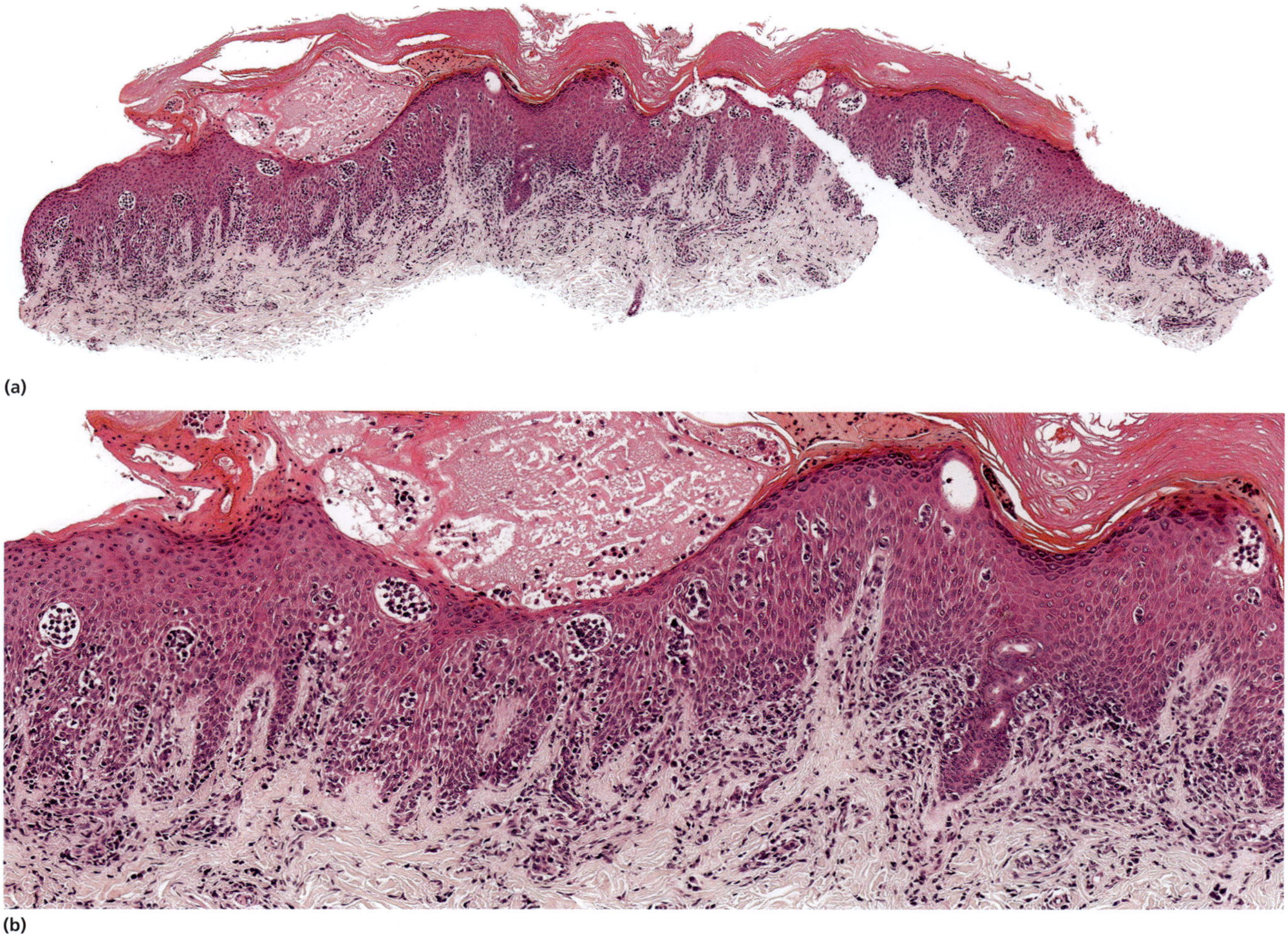

Figure 3.141 Dyshidrotic mycosis fungoides. (a) Histology reveals a band-like infiltrates of lymphocytes with epidermotropism. (b) Detail of epidermotropic lymphocytes (same patient as Fig. 3.140.)

cell transplantation, preparative regimens and procedures, evaluation of disease status at the time of allogeneic stem cell transplantation, and multidisciplinary management in the pre- and post-transplant settings [463a]. Clinical practice recommendations for allogeneic stem cell transplantation in mycosis fungoides have been issued recently [463b].

Recently, chimeric antigen receptor (CAR) T-cell therapy has shown promising results for systemic B-cell lymphomas, and it has been tested in peripheral T-cell lymphomas as well. However, in T-cell lymphomas, the treatment-related cytotoxicity on normal T cells, which share target antigens with tumor T lymphocytes, still represents a problem. On the other hand, CAR T-cells targeting CD5, a pan-T-cell marker, have been used to treat relapsed and refractory mature T-cell lymphomas [464, 465]. In addition, the CC chemokine receptor 4 (CCR4) is highly expressed in mycosis fungoides, and optimized anti-CCR4 CAR T cells have been recently identified, which could be beneficial for the treatment of patients with mycosis fungoides while limiting toxicity on normal T lymphocytes [466]. At present CAR T-cell therapy for T-cell lymphomas has yet to be optimized, but it may represent a further option for advanced and/or relapsed disease.

A particular problem is represented by treatment of pilotropic or syringotropic mycosis fungoides, as skin-directed therapies may fail to reach a depth sufficient to achieve good results. Treatment should be tailored on the clinical picture ("indolent" vs. "aggressive," see above in this chapter). Topical treatments are usually less efficacious, as neoplastic cells reside within the hair follicles and reach deep in the dermis or even in the subcutaneous fat. Phototherapy with narrowband UVB (311 nm) or PUVA is usually associated with other systemic treatments (interferon alpha, bexarotene). An excellent response has been reported with the use of hydroxychloroquine in so-called "idiopathic generalized follicular mucinosis." Methotrexate, gemcitabine, liposomal doxorubicin, brentuximab vedotin, polychemotherapy, pralatrexate, and alemtuzumab represent some options for aggressive cases [467]. Extracorporeal photopheresis has been anecdotally used with success in generalized

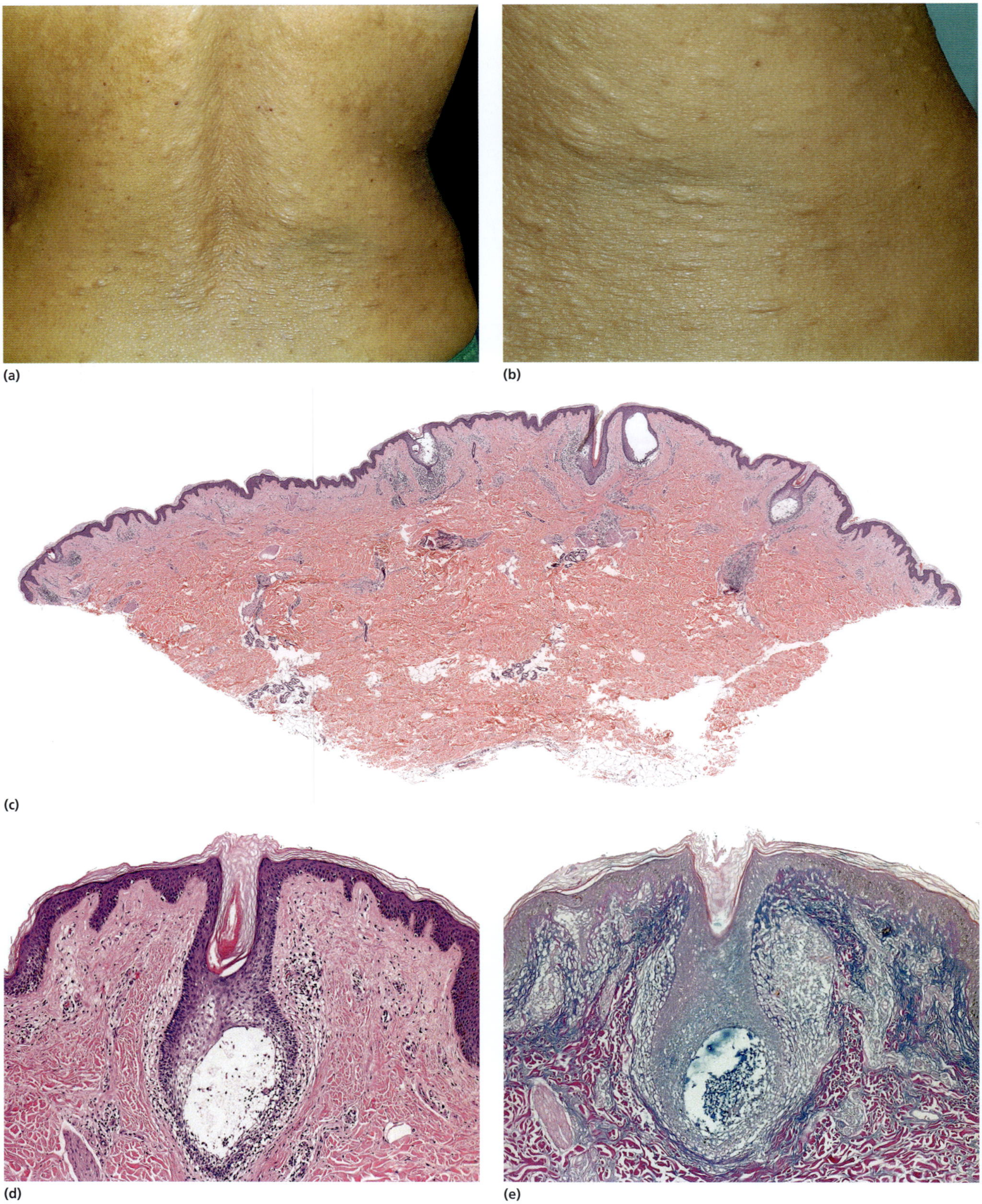


**Figure 3.142** Anetodermic follicular mucinosis. (a, b) Generalized anetodermic papules on the back. (c) Histology reveals prominent follicular mucinosis within all visible hair follicles; (d) detail of a follicle. (e) A colloidal iron stain confirms the presence of mucin within the hair follicles. (f) Orcein staining shows focal loss of elastic fibers (area delimited by arrows). The patient presented again 12 years later with similar anetodermic lesions on the trunk, and also with patchy alopecia of the scalp. (*Courtesy of Prof. Sergio Chimenti, Rome, Italy.*)

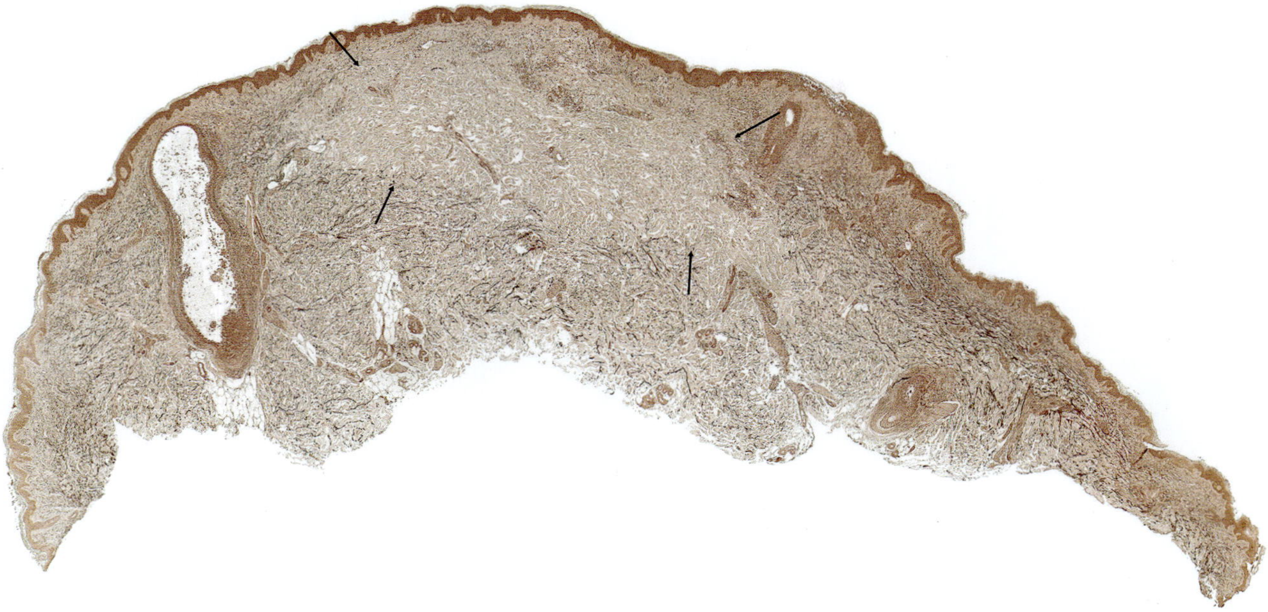

(f)

Figure 3.142 (Continued)

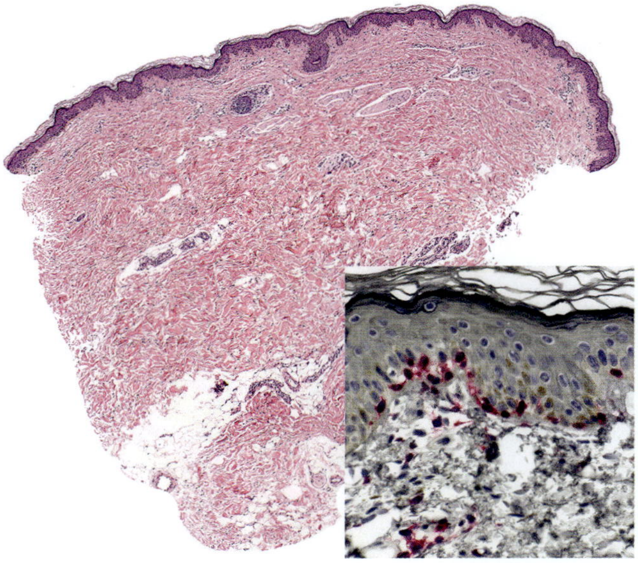

Figure 3.143 "Invisible" mycosis fungoides. Biopsy of seemingly unaffected skin of a patient in remission after PUVA treatment shows only a few intraepidermal lymphocytes ("basilar epidermotropism") highlighted by a staining for CD5 (inset). The clinical relevance of this finding is unclear.

syringotropic mycosis fungoides [468]. Radiation therapy may be administered locally or with total body irradiation. As for conventional mycosis fungoides, stem cell transplantation may represent an option in highly selected patients.

Another particular problem is represented by management of the disease in the pediatric population. Consensus-based recommendations for the approach to mycosis fungoides in children have been recently issued [382].

The knowledge that infection with *Staphylococcus aureus* may enhance neoplastic progression in patients with mycosis fungoides has prompted the investigation of transient antibiotic treatment in patients with advanced stages of the disease, showing that a significant decrease in the percentage of neoplastic cells could be observed following antibiotic treatment (without other changes in the treatment regimen), and suggesting that aggressive antibiotic treatment may inhibit the growth of malignant T lymphocytes in lesional skin [469].

An issue that only rarely has been properly addressed in controlled studies, but that should be carefully evaluated, concerns the quality of life in patients with late-stage mycosis fungoides [470, 471]. In fact, patients may have tumor-stage disease for several years, underlying the need for proper palliation and alleviation of symptoms. In some patients, particularly those with pilotropic mycosis fungoides, pruritus may be intractable and so severe as to induce suicide, underlining the need for a proper, aggressive treatment of this symptom. Recently, aprepitant, a substance P antagonists which blocks the neurokinin 1 receptor, was shown to be efficacious in reducing refractory pruritus in patients with mycosis fungoides [472].

## Prognosis

Mycosis fungoides is a lymphoma of low-grade malignancy with prolonged survival, and progression from cutaneous disease to extracutaneous spread usually takes place over many

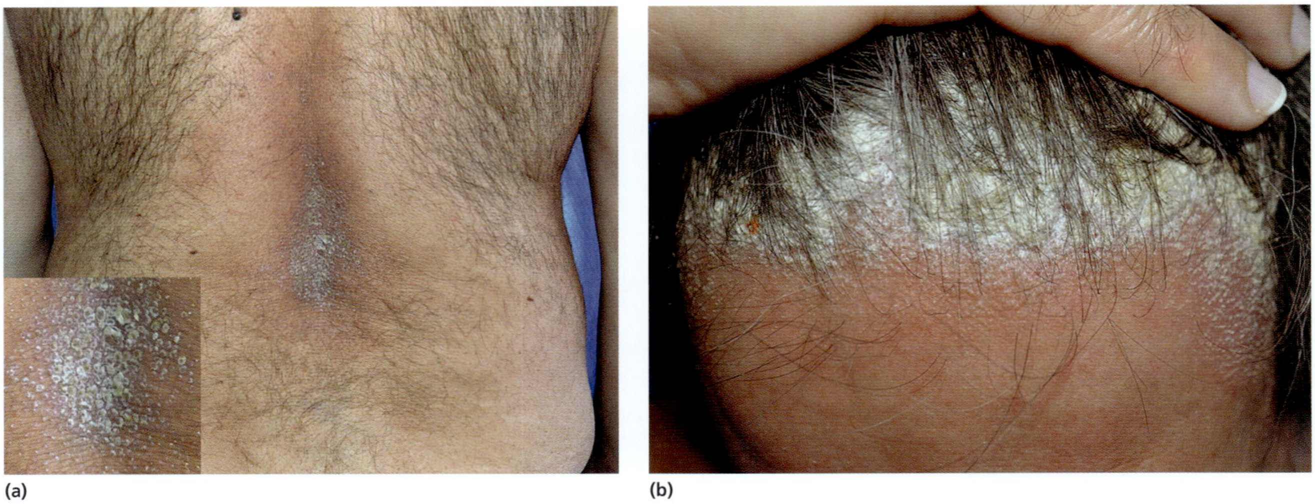

**Figure 3.144** Psoriasiform mycosis fungoides in a patient with prominent involvement of the hair follicles. (a) Psoriasiform scales on the trunk with detail of the scales (inset). (b) Psoriasiform plaque on the scalp, clinically similar to severe scalp psoriasis; note the follicular papules and spiky keratosis that allow a correct diagnosis to be made. (*Courtesy of Dr. Paolo Bauer, Trento, Italy.*)

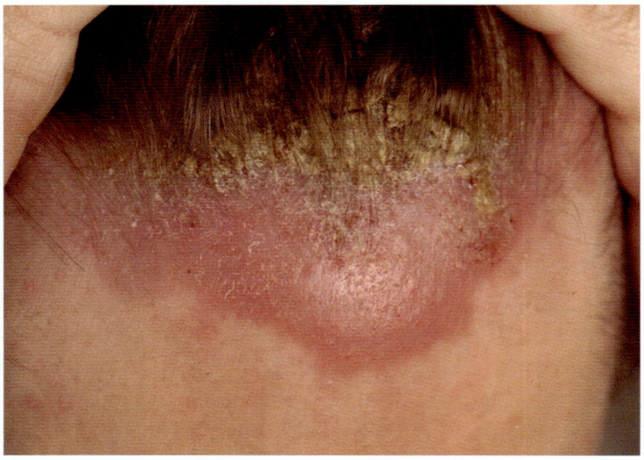

**Figure 3.145** Psoriasiform mycosis fungoides. The scales on the scalp are similar to those of Fig. 3.144b, but there is a larger infiltrated area on the forehead.

years to decades [1–6, 473]. As the disease arises more commonly in the elderly, most patients never progress to advanced stages and die of unrelated causes [474]. In fact, it has been estimated that only 15–20% of patients die of their disease [8]. In patients with stage IA/IB, the annual incidence of disease progression to the tumor stage is around 1–2% [475].

Development of tumors or of large cell transformation usually heralds the terminal stages of the disease (in my experience and that of others, however, patients may survive several years with tumor-stage mycosis fungoides [116]). In this context, it should be underlined that many patients in tumor stage, even those with huge, ulcerated tumor masses, but for the skin lesions are in excellent general conditions (Fig. 3.154). These patients usually succumb to infective complications, particularly sepsis, caused by the presence of large ulcerative lesions on the background of an impaired immune system (due to both the lymphoma and the many treatments that they have received over the years). The challenge in treating such patients would be to target the skin lesions without impairing the immune system, which is paramount for control of both the neoplastic progression and the infective complications. Unfortunately, this medical need has not been met yet.

The most important prognostic parameters are stage at diagnosis, absence of complete remission after first treatment, age, serum LDH level, and race (black patients have a worse prognosis, but this may be related to difficulties in gaining access to proper therapy) [8, 9, 43, 474, 476, 477]. Another study, however, suggested that demographic and socioeconomic factors do not have a clear prognostic role [478]. In a large study on >1.200 patients with advanced mycosis fungoides/Sézary syndrome, four variables were identified as carrying a poor prognosis: stage IV, age >60 years, large-cell transformation, and increased levels of serum LDH [479]; in another one advanced stage, high serum levels of LDH, and loss of CD26 and CD7 expression in the peripheral blood were identified as poor prognostic factors in tumor-stage mycosis fungoides [480]. Gender had an impact on prognosis in a large study (women had a better prognosis) [43], but not so in another large one [475]. Large cell transformation, plaques of the disease as opposed to patches, follicular involvement, and dermopathic nodes as opposed to no enlarged lymph nodes are associated with a worse prognosis [43, 481, 482a]. The presence of numerous $CD20^+$ cells in cases with large cell transformation may be associated with a worse prognosis [152]. In transformed mycosis fungoides, CD30-negativity and follicular involvement were associated with a worse prognosis in one

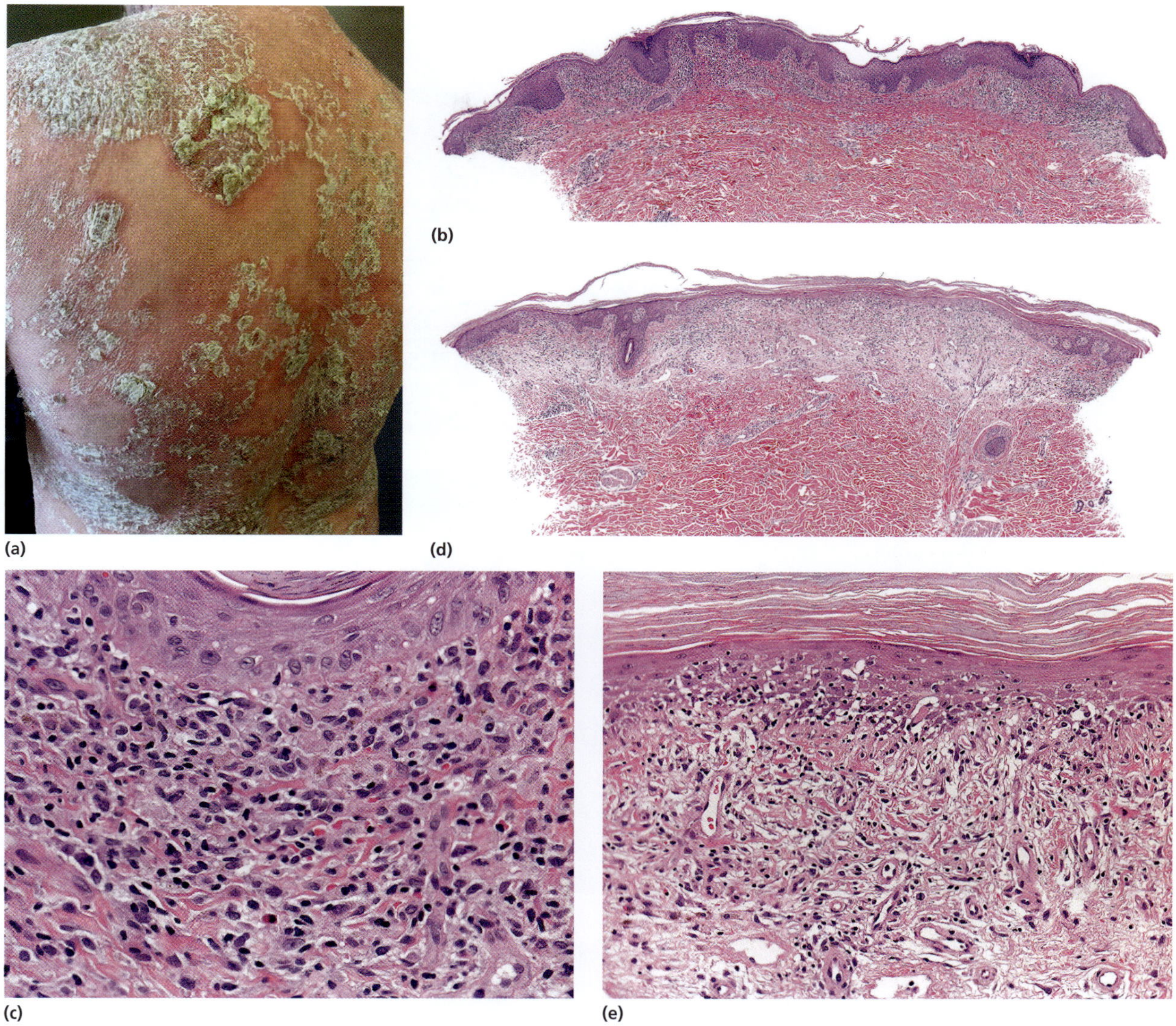

**Figure 3.146** Psoriasiform mycosis fungoides. (a) Generalized lesions with large, thick scales similar to those observed in untreated lesions of psoriasis. (*Courtesy of Dr. Carlo Cota, Rome, Italy.*) Two biopsies taken on the same day show different patterns allowing a clear-cut distinction from psoriasis; the first biopsy is characterized by (b) a psoriasiform epidermal hyperplasia with (c) atypical small and mid-sized lymphocytes within the infiltrate; the second one by (d) a poikilodermatic pattern with flat epidermis and (e) numerous apoptotic keratinocytes and epidermotropic lymphocytes.

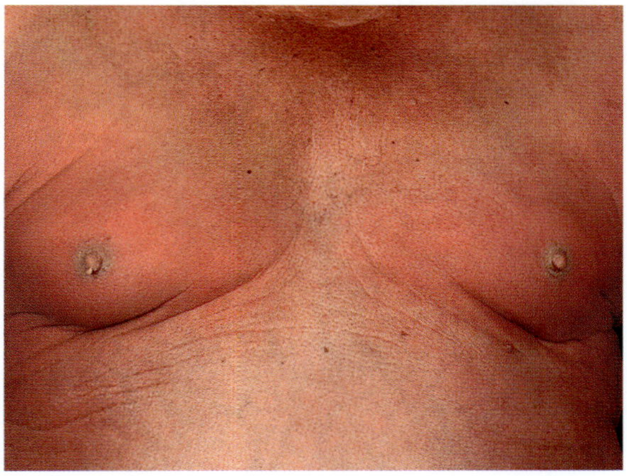

**Figure 3.147** Nevoid hyperkeratosis of the nipple in a patient with erythrodermic mycosis fungoides.

study [116]. However, as already mentioned, CD30-positivity in non-transformed cases was associated with a worse prognosis in another study [148], and the exact prognostic role of CD30, if any, is unclear. The prognostic role of CD30 alone seems to be even more questionable, as remarkable inter- and intra-lesional variability in CD30 expression was found in biopsies taken from two different lesions or within one and the same lesion from a single patient [147]. This variability should be kept in mind also when selecting patients for brentuximab vedotin treatment. Finally, another study suggested that increased body surface area involvement is associated with decreased survival, and proposed a second cut-off point at 40% surface body area in addition to the 10% currently used for separating stage IA from stage IB [482b].

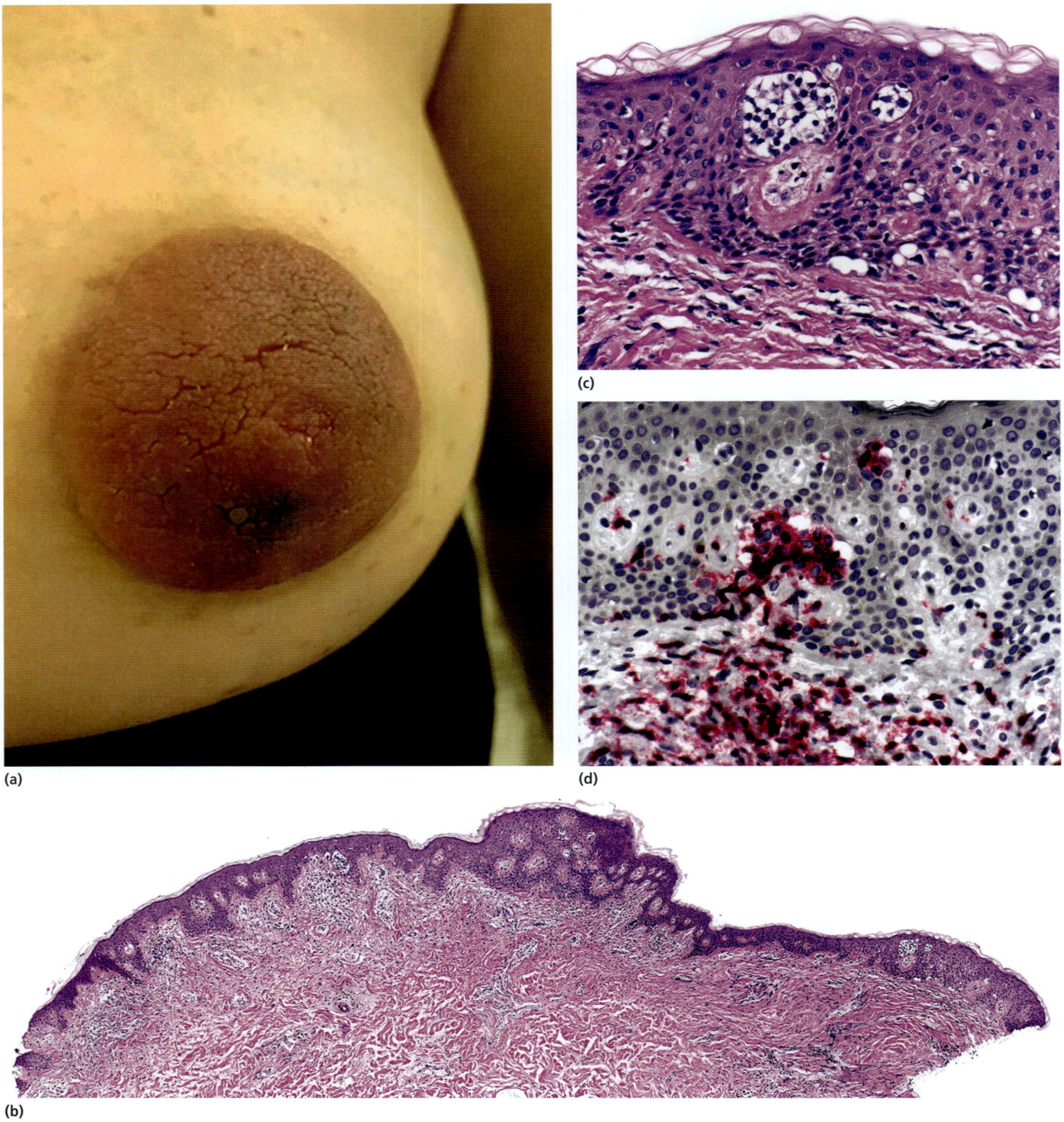

Figure 3.148 Nevoid hyperkeratosis of the nipple in a patient without mycosis fungoides. (a) This 34-year-old woman presented with clinical lesions of nevoid hyperkeratosis of the nipple without other clinical manifestations of mycosis fungoides. (b) A biopsy shows only a superficial lymphoid infiltrate with (c) intraepidermal collections of lymphocytes (Darier nests) which are (d) positive for CD3.

A better prognosis has been reported for poikilodermatous mycosis fungoides [42], and the hypopigmented variant seems to show a better prognosis, too [483]. A worse prognosis, on the other hand, has been observed in patients with pustular mycosis fungoides [260]. There seem to be no relevant prognostic differences between tumors as compared to erythroderma [475]. Although at present the definition of early mycosis fungoides does not include differentiation between patches and plaques, patients with plaques are more likely to progress to advanced stages of disease [43, 80a]. Once extracutaneous spread takes place, initial prognostic parameters have no influence on survival and the prognosis is bad [85].

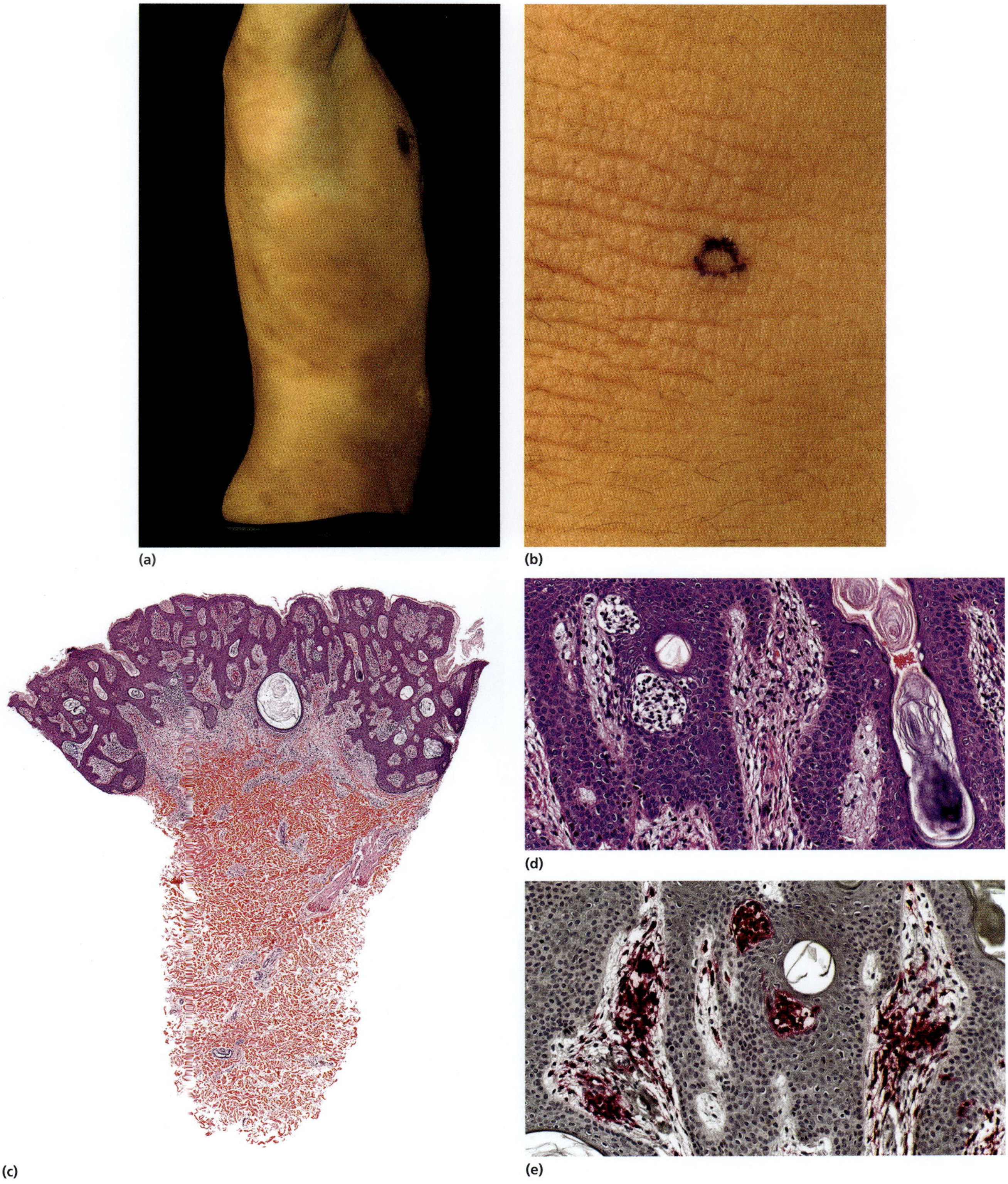

**Figure 3.149** Acanthosis nigricans-like mycosis fungoides. (a) Generalized lesions with (b) a verrucous surface reminiscent of epidermal nevi. Histopathology shows (c) prominent hyperplasia of the epidermis with (d) Darier nests of lymphocytes; (e) staining for CD3 highlights the epidermotropic nests.

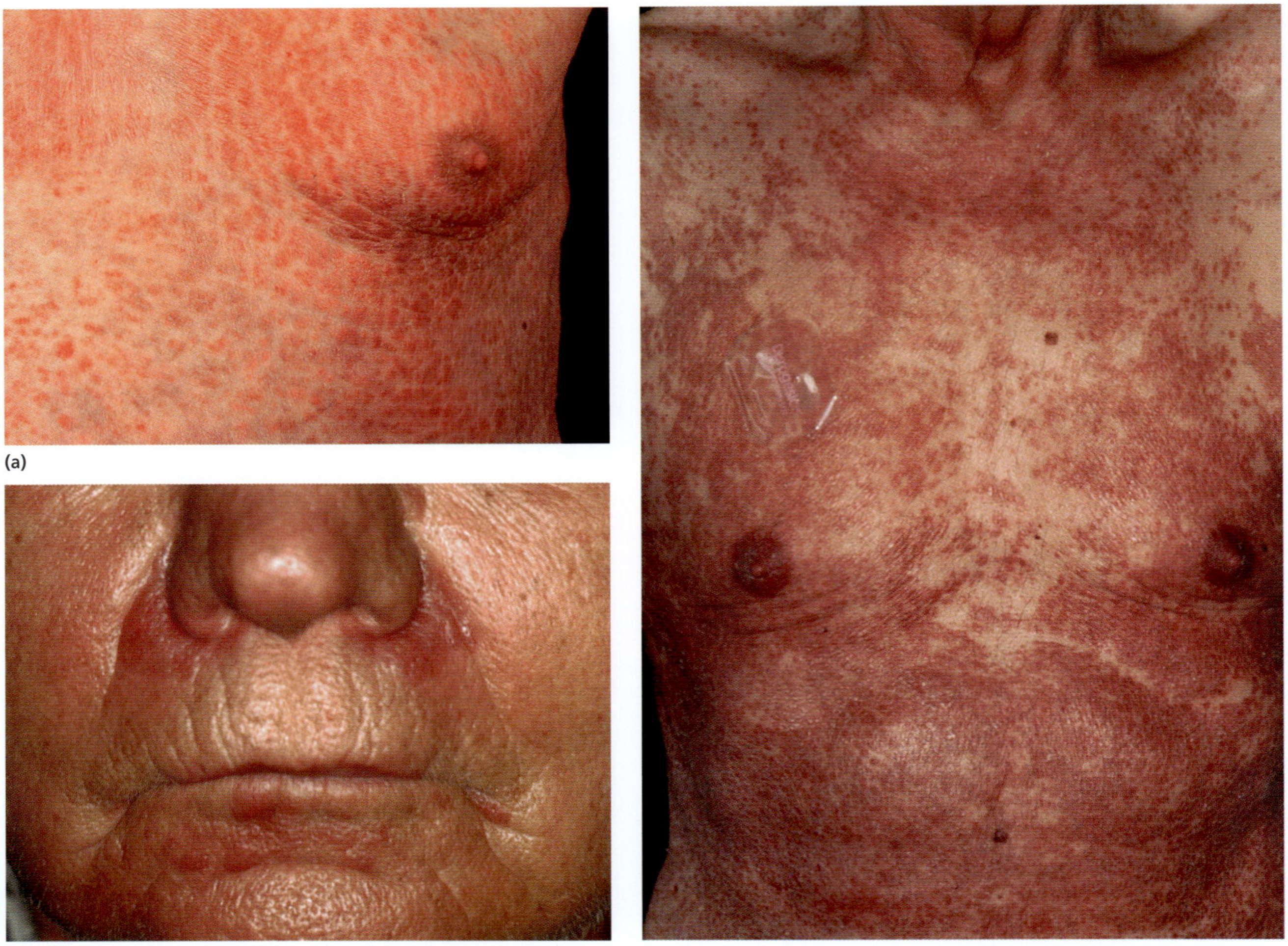

(a)

(b)

(c)

Figure 3.150 Unusual clinical presentations of mycosis fungoides. (a) Mycosis fungoides with ichthyosiform clinical features. (b) Mycosis fungoides with lesions on the nasolabial folds and in perioral location mimicking the clinical picture of perioral dermatitis. (c) Mycosis fungoides with clinical features similar to those of "papuloerythroderma Ofuji" in a Caucasian patient.

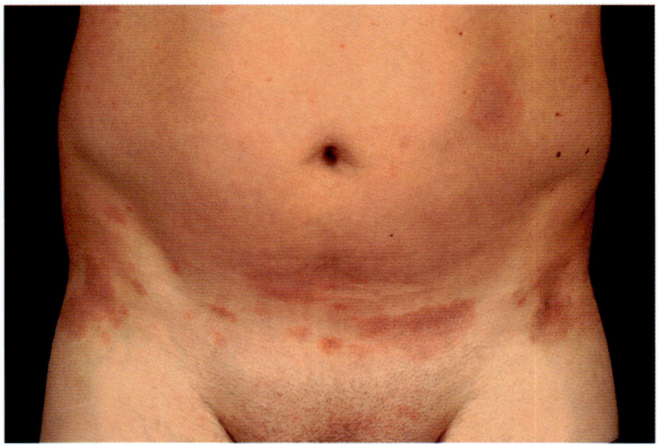

Figure 3.151 Waistband mycosis fungoides. Infiltrated patches and thin plaques mostly located along the waistline.

A Cutaneous Lymphoma International Prognostic index (CLIPi) was proposed for assessing the prognosis of patients with mycosis fungoides and Sézary syndrome [484], but it failed to identify prognostic groups in a cohort of Spanish patients [485a]. In a new version tailored for advanced disease, nodal N3 status, age>60yrs, raised serum lactate dehydrogenase, and large-cell transformation in the skin were associated with worse prognosis [485b]. In the CLIPi study, male gender, age >60, presence of plaques, involvement of the hair follicles (folliculotropic disease), and stage N1/Nx were associated with a worse prognosis in early-stage mycosis fungoides, and male gender, age >60, stages B1/B2 and N2/3, and visceral involvement were associated with worse prognosis in patients with advanced disease [484]. Two models were developed for early and late stages using these prognostic variables, stratified

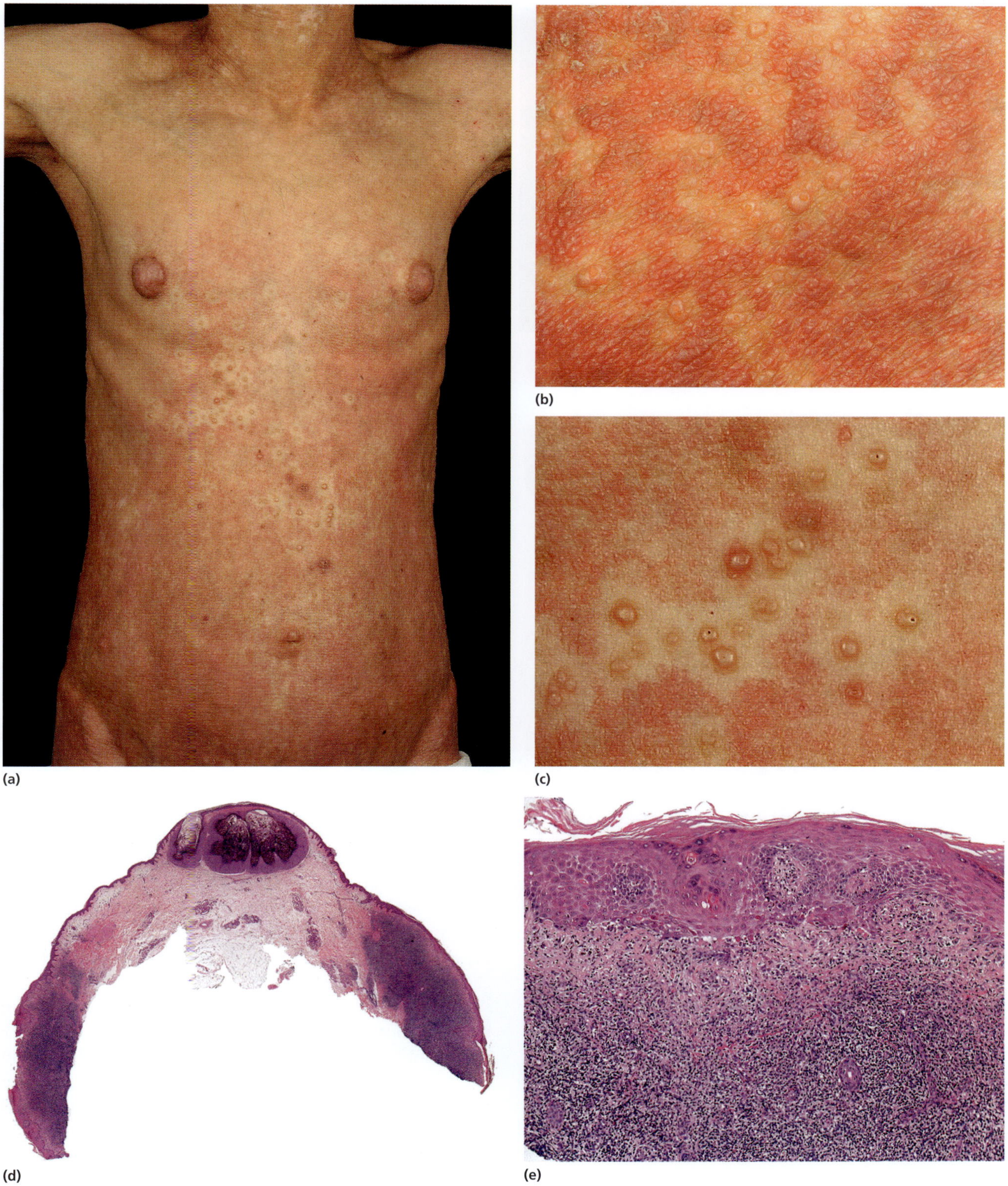


**Figure 3.152** Eczema molluscatum in mycosis fungoides in a 45-year-old man. (a) Generalized plaques and flat tumors of mycosis fungoides with also nevoid hyperkeratosis of the nipples and with (b, c) innumerable mollusca contagiosa, mostly with a perilesional area of spared epidermis. Biopsy of one molluscum contagiosum showed (d) typical features of the viral disease and spared skin in the vicinity of it, (e) whereas the skin distant from the molluscum contagiosum shows dense lymphoid infiltrates with epidermotropism. The conditions of the patient rapidly deteriorated, and he died of mycosis fungoides 5 months after the first observation.

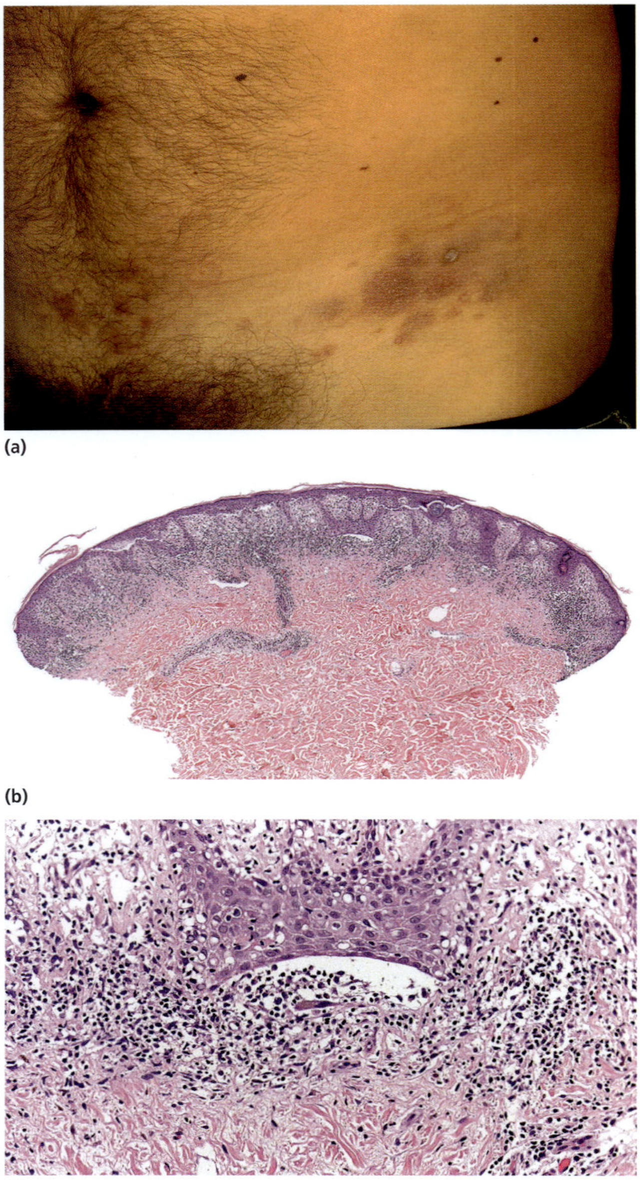

(a)

(b)

(c)

Figure 3.153 Mycosis fungoides on the waistline mimicking histopathologically annular lichenoid dermatitis of youth. (a) Irregular, infiltrated lesions on the abdomen along the waistline. Histology shows (b) a dense band-like lymphoid infiltrate with (c) "squaring" of the rete ridges.

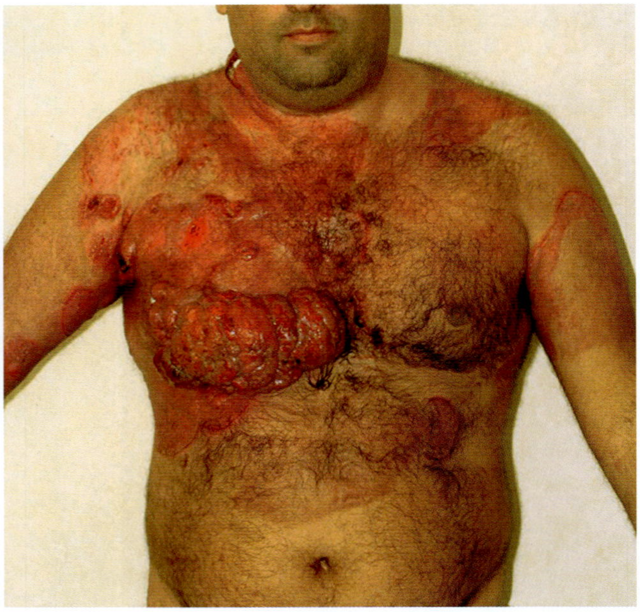

Figure 3.154 Mycosis fungoides, tumor stage. This patient presented with huge, ulcerated tumor masses as well as disseminated patches and plaques, but was otherwise in excellent general conditions. Prognosis in such cases is usually not related to the mycosis fungoides per se, rather to the complications that occur as a consequence of large ulcerations on the background of an impaired immune system due to both the mycosis fungoides and the many treatments typically received by such patients. Over 2 years after this picture was taken, the patient was still alive and in good general conditions, but for persisting skin patches, plaques, and tumors of the disease. (*Courtesy of Dr. Carlo Cota, Rome, Italy.*)

according to the risk as follows: 0–1 factor (low risk), 2 factors (intermediate risk), and 3–5 factors (high risk) [484].

A severity index of mycosis fungoides that assigns different scores to various categories (body surface area, number of tumors, lymph node status, atypical cells in the peripheral blood, and visceral involvement) has been proposed as a valuable tool for measuring disease activity [486]. In my opinion, like many other "numerical" values in assessing tumor prognosis, it conveys a sense of precision that in some cases may be an oversimplification.

The finding of an identical clone in the blood and skin is associated with a worse prognosis [43, 487, 488]. The finding of a cutaneous clone alone at first diagnosis does not have prognostic implications [489], but the presence of a T-cell clone frequency of >25%, identified by high-throughput sequencing, may predict a more aggressive course in early mycosis fungoides [170]. The detection in the peripheral blood of a clone unrelated to the cutaneous one does not have prognostic implications. Finally, the finding of molecular residual disease at follow-up in patients in complete remission is not a prognostic factor of clinical outcome at 4 years [489].

In one study, the presence of large Darier nests with 10 or more lymphocytes, the presence of atypical lymphocytes in the dermal infiltrate, and the presence of small numbers of $CD8^+$ cells in the dermal infiltrate have been related to a worse prognosis [490], but in my experience and in that of others [491] histopathologic features in early stages of mycosis fungoides do not provide useful information in order to predict the course of the disease. In stage IIb, the number of tumors and time interval between tumor formation seem to correlate with survival [492].

Molecular investigations provided new genetic criteria for stratification of patients with mycosis fungoides [196, 493], but these methods are not used routinely, and results should be validated in larger cohorts. A shorter survival has been observed in patients with *CDKN2A-CDKN2B* inactivation [494, 495]. Promoter methylation of specific biomarkers was associated with disease progression in early stage mycosis fungoides, with *PPARG* methylation being a significant predictor of disease progression within 6 years [496]. Aberrant CD137 ligand expression induced by GATA6 overexpression seems to contribute to tumor progression [497a]. One study suggested that tumor microenvironment, particularly M2 macrophages and cancer-associated fibroblasts, could contribute to progression in early-stage mycosis fungoides, and that significant transcriptomic changes can be observed during progression of the disease [497b].

Finally, the microenvironment of mycosis fungoides may also be linked to prognosis. Using TCR β chain variable region-specific staining to discriminate between tumor-infiltrating lymphocytes and neoplastic cells, disease progression was found to be associated with increasing divergence of the tumor-phenotype away from that of tumor-infiltrating lymphocytes, and with reduced functional activity of tumor infiltrating lymphocytes [498].

| **Résumé** | |
|---|---|
| **Clinical** | Adults. Rarely observed in children (but the most common cutaneous lymphoma in this age group!). Patches, plaques, and tumors can be found. Preferential location: buttocks, other sun-protected areas (early phases). Several clinical variants have been described, some very distinctive on clinical grounds (e.g., adnexotropic mycosis fungoides). |
| **Morphology** | Small/medium pleomorphic (cerebriform) cells. During the course of the disease, large cell transformation may occur and is associated with a worse prognosis. Epidermotropism is common but may be rarely missing; Darier nests (Pautrier microabscesses) are infrequent in early lesions. Some variants have peculiar histopathological features (e.g., adnexotropic mycosis fungoides). |
| **Immunohistochemistry** | CD2, CD3, CD4, CD5, βF1 + <br> CD8, TCR-γ, TCR-δ, CD56, TIA-1 −(+) <br><br> CD30 may be positive in variable proportions of cells in plaque and tumors, particularly in those with large cell morphology; rare cells may be positive in early patches. <br><br> Phenotypic variations and phenotypic switch may occur, particularly in advanced disease! |
| **Genetics** | Monoclonal rearrangement of the TCR genes may be undetectable in early phases using conventional PCR methods (higher sensitivity has been demonstrated with NGS). Aberrant activation of the JAK-STAT signaling pathway. Genes regulating several key functions of the cells are altered in mycosis fungoides, including genes involved in cell cycle and apoptosis regulators, DNA damage repair, histone remodelers, and epigenetic modifiers. |
| **Treatment guidelines** | *Early phases*: PUVA, UVB 311 nm, interferon-α2a, bexarotene (alone or in combination); topical chemotherapy (chlormethine); topical steroids; watchful waiting if treatment can be postponed. Solitary lesions (e.g., pagetoid reticulosis) can be managed by local radiotherapy. <br><br> *Advanced disease*: allogeneic stem cell transplantation may represent a curative option in selected patients. Monochemotherapy (gemcitabine, pegylated liposomal doxorubicin); total body electron beam irradiation; low-dose methotrexate; Brentuximab vedotin (also in cases negative for CD30); Mogamulizumab; Palliative radiation therapy of large tumors. Polychemotherapy (CHOP or CHOP-like) in stage IV. <br><br> Other immune modulators can be considered in advanced stages of mycosis fungoides. Alemtuzumab (in patients with blood involvement), zanolimumab, ipilimumab, pembrolizumab, and nivolumab have been tested in single cases or in small series. |

## References


1. Willemze R, Cerroni L, Kempf W, *et al.* The 2018 update of the WHO-EORTC classification for primary cutaneous lymphomas. *Blood* 2019;**133**:1703–1714.
2. Fink-Puches R, Zenahlik P, Bäck B, *et al.* Primary cutaneous lymphomas: applicability of current classification schemes (European Organization for Research and Treatment of Cancer, World Health Organization) based on clinicopathologic features observed in a large group of patients. *Blood* 2002;**99**:800–805.
3. Pulitzer M, Pimpinelli N, Berti E, *et al.* Mycosis fungoides. In: *WHO Classification of Tumours Editorial Board.* Haematolymphoid Tumours. 5th edition. Lyon (France): IARC, 2024: 688–693.
4. Cerroni L. Mycosis fungoides – clinical and histopathologic features, differential diagnosis, and treatment. *Semin Cut Med Surg* 2018; **37**:2–10.
5. Comfere NI, Calonje E, Cerroni L. Mycosis fungoides. In: Arber DA, Borowitz MJ, Cook JR, *et al.*, eds. *The International Consensus Classification of Myeloid and Lymphoid neoplasms.* Philadelphia (US): Wolters Kluver, 2025: 672–679.

6. Kempf W, Mitteldorf C, Cerroni L, *et al.* Classifications of cutaneous lymphomas and lymphoproliferative disorders: an update from the EORTC cutaneous lymphoma histopathology group. *J Eur Acad Dermatol Venereol* 2024;**38**:1491–1503.
7. Campo E, Jaffe ES, Cook JR, *et al.* The International Consensus Classification of mature lymphoid neoplasms: a report from the Clinical Advisory Committee. *Blood* 2022;**140**:1229–1253.
8. Zackheim HS, Amin S, Kashani-Sabet M, McMillan A. Prognosis in cutaneous T-cell lymphoma by skin stage: long-term survival in 489 patients. *J Am Acad Dermatol* 1999;**40**:418–425.
9. Kim YH, Liu HL, Mraz-Gernhard S, *et al.* Long-term outcome of 525 patients with mycosis fungoides and Sézary syndrome. *Arch Dermatol* 2003;**139**:857–866.
10. Criscione VD, Weinstock MA. Incidence of cutaneous T-cell lymphoma in the United States, 1973–2002. *Arch Dermatol* 2007;**143**:854–859.
11. Saunes M, Lund Nilsen TI, Johannesen TB. Incidence of primary cutaneous T-cell lymphoma in Norway. *Br J Dermatol* 2009;**160**:376–379.
12. Korgavkar K, Xiong M, Weinstock M. Changing incidence trends of cutaneous T-cell lymphoma. *JAMA Dermatol* 2013;**149**:1295–1299.
13. Hinds GA, Heald P. Cutaneous T-cell lymphoma in skin of color. *J Am Acad Dermatol* 2009;**60**:359–375.
14. (a)Zampella JG, Hinds GA. Racial differences in mycosis fungoides: a retrospective study with a focus on eosinophilia. *J Am Acad Dermatol* 2013;**68**:967–971.(b) Gniadecki R, Guenova E, Querfeld C, *et al.* Hematogenous seeding in mycosis fungoides and Sézary syndrome: current evidence and clinical implications. *Br J Dermatol* 2025;**192**:381–389.
15. Hodak E, Friedman E. Familial mycosis fungoides: model of genetic susceptibility. *Clin Lymphoma Myeloma* 2010;**10**(suppl. 2): s67–s69.
16. Naji AA, Waiz MM, Sharquie KE. Mycosis fungoides in identical twins. *J Am Acad Dermatol* 2001;**44**:532–533.
17. Schneider BF, Christian M, Hess CE, Williams ME. Familial occurrence of cutaneous T cell lymphoma: a case report of monozygotic twin sisters. *Leukemia* 1995;**9**:1979–1981.
18. Odum N, Lindahl LM, Wod M, *et al.* Investigating heredity in cutaneous T-cell lymphoma in a unique cohort of Danish twins. *Blood Cancer J* 2017;**7**:e517.
19. Hodak E, Klein T, Gabay B, *et al.* Familial mycosis fungoides: report of 6 kindreds and a study of the HLA system. *J Am Acad Dermatol* 2005;**52**:393–402.
20. Schmidt AN, Robbins JB, Greer JP, Zic JA. Conjugal transformed mycosis fungoides: the unknown role of viral infection and environmental exposures in the development of cutaneous T-cell lymphoma. *J Am Acad Dermatol* 2006;**54**:s202–s205.
21. Emadi SN, Shiri M, Shiri Z, *et al.* Mycosis fungoides two decades after exposure to sulphur mustard: a follow-up of 1100 victims. *J Eur Acad Dermatol Venereol* 2017;**31**:432–437.
22. Fanok MH, Sun A, Fogli LK, *et al.* Role of dysregulated cytokine signaling and bacterial triggers in the pathogenesis of cutaneous T-cell lymphoma. *J Invest Dermatol* 2018;**138**:1116–1125.
23. Willerslev-Olsen A, Krejsgaard T, Lindahl LM, *et al.* Staphylococcal enterotoxin A (SEA) stimulates STAT3 activation and IL-17 expression in cutaneous T-cell lymphoma. *Blood* 2016;**127**:1287–1296.
24. Vieyra-Garcia PA, Wei T, Naym DG, *et al.* STAT3/5-dependent IL9 overexpression contributes to neoplastic cell survival in mycosis fungoides. *Clin Cancer Res* 2016;**22**:3328–3339.
25. Mirvish ED, Pomerantz RG, Geskin LJ. Infectious agents in cutaneous T-cell lymphoma. *J Am Acad Dermatol* 2011;**64**:423–431.
26. Du-Thanha A, Dereurea O, Guillota B, Foulongne V. Merkel cell polyomavirus: its putative involvement in a particular subset of cutaneous lymphoma with possibly unfavorable outcome. *J Clin Virol* 2014;**61**:161–165.
27. Gordon ER, Fahmy LM, Trager MH, *et al.* From molecules to microbes: tracing cutaneous T-cell lymphoma pathogenesis through malignant inflammation. *J Invest Dermatol* 2024;**144**: 1954–1962.
28. Rodriguez-Gil Y, Palencia SI, Lopez-Rios F, *et al.* Mycosis fungoides after solid organ transplantation: report of 2 new cases. *Am J Dermatopathol* 2008;**30**:150–155.
29. Amin A, Burkhart C, Groben P, *et al.* Primary cutaneous T-cell lymphoma following organ transplantation in a 16-year-old boy. *Ped Dermatol* 2009;**26**:112–113.
30. Kinsella FA, Amel Kashipaz MR, Scarisbrick J, Malladi R. Donor-derived mycosis fungoides following reduced intensity haematopoietic stem cell transplantation from a matched unrelated donor. *BMJ Case Rep* 2017 January 10:pii: bcr2016216331. doi: 10.1136/bcr-2016-216331.
31. Flechon L, Arib I, Dutta AK, *et al.* Genomic profiling of mycosis fungoides identifies patients at high risk of disease progression. *Blood Adv* 2024;**8**:3109–3119.
32. Zhang Y, Wang Y, Yu R, *et al.* Molecular markers of early-stage mycosis fungoides. *J Invest Dermatol* 2012;**132**:1698–1706.
33. Kirsch IR, Watanabe R, O'Malley JT, *et al.* TCR sequencing facilitates diagnosis and identifies mature T cells as the cell of origin in CTCL. *Sci Transl Med* 2015;**7**:308ra158.
34. Davis TH, Morton CC, Miller-Cassman R, *et al.* Hodgkin's disease, lymphomatoid papulosis, and cutaneous T-cell lymphoma derived from a common T-cell clone. *N Engl J Med* 1992;**326**:1115–1122.
35. Wood GS, Crooks CF, Uluer AZ. Lymphomatoid papulosis and associated cutaneous lymphoproliferative disorders exhibit a common clonal origin. *J Invest Dermatol* 1995;**105**:51–55.
36. Kremer M, Sandherr M, Geist B, *et al.* Epstein–Barr virus-negative Hodgkin's lymphoma after mycosis fungoides: molecular evidence for distinct clonal origin. *Mod Pathol* 2001;**14**:91–97.
37. Zackheim HS, Jones C, PE LB, *et al.* Lymphomatoid papulosis associated with mycosis fungoides: a study of 21 patients including analyses for clonality. *J Am Acad Dermatol* 2003;**49**:620–623.
38. de la Garza Bravo MM, Patel KP, Loghavi S, *et al.* Shared clonality in distinctive lesions of lymphomatoid papulosis and mycosis fungoides occurring in the same patients suggests a common origin. *Hum Pathol* 2015;**46**:558–569.
39. Väkevä L, Pukkala E, Ranki A. Increased risk of secondary cancers in patients with primary cutaneous T cell lymphoma. *J Invest Dermatol* 2000;**115**:62–65.
40. Goyal A, O'Leary D, Goyal K, *et al.* Increased risk of second primary hematologic and solid malignancies in patients with mycosis fungoides: a Surveillance, Epidemiology, and End Results analysis. *J Am Acad Dermatol* 2020;**83**:404–411.
41. Ottevanger R, Vermaas E, Willemze R, *et al.* Mycosis fungoides and associated malignancies in a Dutch nationwide retrospective cohort study. *Acta Derm Venereol* 2024 Sep 15;**104**:adv40065.
42. Olsen E, Vonderheid E, Pimpinelli N, *et al.* Revisions to the staging and classification of mycosis fungoides and Sezary syndrome: a proposal of the International Society for Cutaneous Lymphomas

(ISCL) and the cutaneous lymphoma task force of the European Organization of Research and Treatment of Cancer (EORTC). *Blood* 2007;**110**:1713–1722.
43. Agar NS, Wedgeworth E, Crichton S, *et al.* Survival outcomes and prognostic factors in mycosis fungoides/sezary syndrome: validation of the Revised International Society for Cutaneous Lymphomas/European Organisation for Research and Treatment of Cancer staging proposal. *J Clin Oncol* 2010;**28**:4730–4739.
44. Olsen EA, Whittaker S, Willemze R, *et al.* Primary cutaneous lymphoma: recommendations for clinical trial design and staging update from the ISCL, USCLC, and EORTC. *Blood* 2022;**140**: 419–437.
45. National Comprehensive Cancer Network. Primary Cutaneous Lymphomas (Version 3.2025). Accessed September 20, 2025. https://www.nccn.org/professionals/physician_gls/pdf/primary_cutaneous.pdf.
46. Kamstrup MR, Madsen HO, Skovgaard GL, *et al.* Analysis of extracutaneous spread in mycosis fungoides. *J Invest Dermatol* 2009;**129**:2905–2907.
47. Delfau-Larue MH, Laroche L, Wechsler J, *et al.* Diagnostic value of dominant T-cell clones in peripheral blood in 363 patients presenting consecutively with a suspicion of cutaneous lymphoma. *Blood* 2000;**96**:2987–2992.
48. Scarisbrick JJ, Hodak E, Bagot M, *et al.* Blood classification and blood response criteria in mycosis fungoides and Sezary syndrome using flow cytometry: recommendations from the EORTC cutaneous lymphoma task force. *Eur J Cancer* 2018;**93**:47–56.
49. Joffe D, Bhatti S, Banner L, *et al.* The overlap of skin and blood T-cell clones in early-stage mycosis fungoides. *Blood Adv* 2023;**7**:6206–6210.
50. Quaglino P, Scarisbrick J, Roccuzzo G, *et al.* Identifying unmet needs and challenges in the definition of a plaque in mycosis fungoides: an EORTC-CLTG/ISCL survey. *J Eur Acad Dermatol Venereol* 2023;**37**:680–688.
51. Cen P, Duvic M, Cohen PR, Kurzrock R. Increased cancer antigen 27.29 (CA27.29) level in patients with mycosis fungoides. *J Am Acad Dermatol* 2008;**58**:382–386.
52. Escher N, Kaatz M, Melle C, *et al.* Posttranslational modifications of transthyretin are serum markers in patients with mycosis fungoides. *Neoplasia* 2007;**9**:254–259.
53. Chong BF, Wilson AJ, Gibson HM, *et al.* Immune function abnormalities in peripheral blood mononuclear cell cytokine expression differentiates stages of cutaneous T-cell lymphoma/mycosis fungoides. *Clin Cancer Res* 2008;**14**:646–653.
54. Abeni D, Frontani M, Sampogna F, *et al.* Circulating CD8+ lymphocytes, white blood cells, and survival in patients with mycosis fungoides. *Br J Dermatol* 2005;**153**:324–330.
55. Theinert SM, Pronest MM, Peris K, *et al.* Identification of the testis-specific protein 10 (TSGA10) as serologically defined tumor-associated antigen in primary cutaneous T-cell lymphoma. *Br J Dermatol* 2005;**153**:639–641.
56. Ohmatsu H, Sugaya M, Miyagaki T, *et al.* BAFF levels are increased in lesional skin and sera in patients with cutaneous T-cell lymphoma. *Br J Dermatol* 2012;**167**:359–367.
57. Feng B, Jorgensen JL, Jones D, *et al.* Flow cytometric detection of peripheral blood involvement by mycosis fungoides and Sézary syndrome using T-cell receptor Vb chain antibodies and its application in blood staging. *Mod Pathol* 2010;**23**:284–295.
58. Scarisbrick JJ, Quaglino P, Prince HM, *et al.* The PROCLIPI international registry of early-stage mycosis fungoides identifies substantial diagnostic delay in most patients. *Br J Dermatol* 2019; **181**:350–357.
59. Thurber SE, Zhang B, Kim YH, *et al.* T-cell clonality analysis in biopsy specimens from two different skin sites shows high specificity in the diagnosis of patients with suggested mycosis fungoides. *J Am Acad Dermatol* 2007;**57**:782–790.
60. Larson AR, Rodig S, Granter SR. Duration of symptoms does not correlate with results of T-cell gene rearrangement studies in patients evaluated for cutaneous T-cell lymphoma. *J Cutan Pathol* 2015;**42**:618–621.
61. Laharanne E, Oumouhou N, Bonnet F, *et al.* Genome-wide analysis of cutaneous T-cell lymphomas identifies three clinically relevant classes. *J Invest Dermatol* 2010;**130**:1707–1718.
62. van Doorn R, van Kester MS, Dijkman R, *et al.* Oncogenomic analysis of mycosis fungoides reveals major differences with Sézary syndrome. *Blood* 2009;**113**:127–136.
63. Dobos G, De Cevins C, So SLK, *et al.* The value of five blood markers in differentiating mycosis fungoides and Sèzary syndrome: a validation cohort. *Br J Dermatol* 2021;**185**:405–411.
64. Campbell JJ, Clark RA, Watanabe R, *et al.* Sézary syndrome and mycosis fungoides arise from distinct T-cell subsets: a biologic rationale for their distinct clinical behaviors. *Blood* 2010;**116**:761–777.
65. Hernandez C, Worobec SM, Gaitonde S, *et al.* Progression of undiagnosed cutaneous T-cell lymphoma during efalizumab therapy. *Arch Dermatol* 2009;**145**:92–94.
66. Lafaille P, Bouffard D, Provost N. Exacerbation of undiagnosed mycosis fungoides during treatment with etanercept. *Arch Dermatol* 2009;**145**:94–95.
67. Chuang GS, Wasserman DI, Byers HR, Demierre MF. Hypopigmented T-cell dyscrasia evolving to hypopigmented mycosis fungoides during etanercept therapy. *J Am Acad Dermatol* 2008;**59**:s121–s122.
68. Lourari S, Prey S, Livideanu C, *et al.* Cutaneous T-cell lymphoma following treatment of rheumatoid arthritis with tumour necrosis factor-a blocking agents: two cases. *J Eur Acad Dermatol Venereol* 2009;**23**:967–968.
69. Geller S, Pulitzer M, Horwitz SM, *et al.* Mycosis fungoides, psoriasis and anti-PD-1 – a new aspect of known associations. *J Dtsch Dermatol Ges* 2019;**17**:186–188.
70. Biondo G, Cerroni L, AMG B, *et al.* Risk of mycosis fungoides in psoriatic patients: a critical review. *J Eur Acad Dermatol Venereol* 2020;**34**:1186–1195.
71. Foo SH, Shah F, Chaganti S, *et al.* Unmasking mycosis fungoides/Sézary syndrome from preceding or co-existing benign inflammatory dermatoses requiring systemic therapies: patients frequently present with advanced disease and have an aggressive clinical course. *Br J Dermatol* 2016;**174**:901–904.
72. Chiba T, Nagai T, Osada SI, Manabe M. Diagnosis of mycosis fungoides following administration of dupilumab for misdiagnosed atopic dermatitis. *Acta Derm Venereol* 2019;**99**:818–819.
73. Boesjes CM, van der Gang LF, Bakker DS, *et al.* Dupilumab-associated lymphoid reactions in patients with atopic dermatitis. *JAMA Dermatol* 2023;**159**:1240–1247.
74. Guitart J. Dupilumab, atopic dermatitis, and mycosis fungoides – new insights on an evolving story. *JAMA Dermatol* 2023; **159**:1177–1178.

75. (a) Liao V, Lavin L, Pulitzer MP, *et al.* Diagnosis of cutaneous T-cell lymphoma following exposure to biologic agents for atopic dermatitis: a retrospective cohort study from a single tertiary cancer center. *J Am Acad Dermatol* 2025;**92**:1394–1395. (b) Guglielmo A, Borghi A, Schettini N, *et al.* Mycosis fungoides and IL-4/13 inhibitors: what is known and unmet needs. *Expert Rev Clin Immunol* 2025;**21**:723–729.
76. Dequidt L, Franck N, Sanchez-Pena P, *et al.* Cutaneous lymphomas appearing under biologics: 44 cases from the French study group on cutaneous lymphomas and French pharmacovigilance database. *Br J Dermatol* 2019;**181**:616–618.
77. Martinez-Escala ME, Posligua AL, Wickless H, *et al.* Progression of undiagnosed cutaneous lymphoma after anti-tumor necrosis factor-alpha therapy. *J Am Acad Dermatol* 2018;**78**:1068–1076.
78. Buffon S, Alberti Violetti S, Avallone G, *et al.* Mycosis fungoides and Sézary syndrome following dupilumab treatment: experience of two Italian tertiary care centres. *Clin Exp Dermatol* 2023;**48**: 1376–1378.
79. Grijsen ML, Mtayangulwa RG, Naafs B, *et al.* The clinical spectrum of mycosis fungoides in Tanzania, East Africa. *Br J Dermatol* 2017;**176**:1653–1656.
80. (a) Wernham AG, Shah F, Amel-Kashipaz R, *et al.* Stage I mycosis fungoides: frequent association with a favourable prognosis but disease progression and disease-specific mortality may occur. *Br J Dermatol* 2015;**173**:1295–1297.(b) Kersten JM, Ottevanger R, Doeleman T, *et al.* Histopathologic evaluation of density and depth of the lymphoid infiltrate in clinically defined patches and plaques in early stage mycosis fungoides. *J Cutan Pathol* 2025;**52**:406–409.
81. Meyer N, Paul C, Misery L. Pruritus in cutaneous T-cell lymphomas: frequent, often severe and difficult to treat. *Acta Derm Venereol (Stockh)* 2010;**90**:12–17.
82. Grande-Sarpa H, Callis Duffin KP, Florell SR. Onychodystrophy and tumor-stage mycosis fungoides confined to a single digit: report of a case and review of nail findings in cutaneous T-cell lymphoma. *J Am Acad Dermatol* 2008;**59**:154–157.
83. Bishop BE, Wulkan A, Kerdel F, *et al.* Nail alterations in cutaneous T-cell lymphoma: a case series and review of nail manifestations. *Skin Appendage Disord* 2015;**1**:82–86.
84. Mancebo SE, Cordova M, Myskowski PL, *et al.* Reflectance confocal microscopy features of mycosis fungoides and Sézary syndrome: correlation with histopathologic and T-cell receptor rearrangement studies. *J Cutan Pathol* 2016;**43**:505–515.
85. de Coninck EC, Kim YH, Varghese A, Hoppe RT. Clinical characteristics and outcome of patients with extracutaneous mycosis fungoides. *J Clin Oncol* 2001;**19**:779–784.
86. Huang KP, Weinstock MA, Clarke CA, *et al.* Second lymphomas and other malignant neoplasms in patients with mycosis fungoides and Sézary syndrome. Evidence from population-based and clinical cohorts. *Arch Dermatol* 2007;**143**:45–50.
87. Hallermann C, Kaune MK, Tiemann M, *et al.* High frequency of primary cutaneous lymphomas associated with lymphoproliferative disorders of different lineage. *Ann Hematol* 2007;**86**:509–515.
88. Herzo E, DiCaudo DJ, Davis MDP, *et al.* Review of contemporaneous mycosis fungoides and B-cell malignancy at Mayo Clinic. *J Am Acad Dermatol* 2009;**61**:271–275.
89. Whitling NA, Shanesmith R, Jacob L, *et al.* Composite lymphoma of mycosis fungoides and cutaneous small B-cell lymphoma in a 73-year-old male patient. *Hum Pathol* 2013;**44**:670–675.
90. Blaizot R, Ouattara E, Fauconneau A, *et al.* Infectious events and associated risk factors in mycosis fungoides/Sézary syndrome: a retrospective cohort study. *Br J Dermatol* 2018;**179**:1322–1328.
91. Cribier BJ. The myth of Pautrier's microabscesses. *J Am Acad Dermatol* 2003;**48**:796–797.
92. Giessinger J, LeBoit PE, Cribier B. Pautrier microabscess: a topic of great controversy. *Am J Dermatopathol* 2021;**43**:848–849.
93. Fung MA. 'Epidermotropism' vs. 'exocytosis' of lymphocytes 101: definition of terms. *J Cutan Pathol* 2010;**37**:525–529.
94. Massone C, Kodama K, Kerl H, Cerroni L. Histopathologic features of early (patch) lesions of mycosis fungoides. A morphologic study on 745 biopsy specimens from 427 patients. *Am J Surg Pathol* 2005;**29**:550–560.
95. Hadi R, Miller TI, May C, *et al.* Impact of clinical photographs on the accuracy and confidence in the histopathological diagnosis of mycosis fungoides. *J Cutan Pathol* 2021;**48**:842–846.
96. Pimpinelli N, Olsen EA, Santucci M, *et al.* Defining early mycosis fungoides. *J Am Acad Dermatol* 2005;**53**:1053–1063.
97. Vandergriff T, Nezafati KA, Susa J, *et al.* Defining early mycosis fungoides: validation of a diagnostic algorithm proposed by the International Society for Cutaneous Lymphomas. *J Cutan Pathol* 2015;**42**:318–328.
98. Furmanczyk PS, Wolgamot GM, Kussick SJ, *et al.* Diagnosis of mycosis fungoides with different algorithmic approaches. *J Cutan Pathol* 2010;**37**:8–14.
99. Gru AA, Kim J, Pulitzer M, *et al.* The use of central pathology review with digital slide scanning in advanced-stage mycosis fungoides and Sézary syndrome: a multi-institutional and international pathology study. *Am J Surg Pathol* 2018;**42**:726–734.
100. Fertig RM, Gaudi S, Cervantes J, *et al.* Feasibility study in teledermatopathology: an examination of the histopathologic features of mycosis fungoides and spongiotic dermatitis. *J Cutan Pathol* 2017;**44**:919–924.
101. Doeleman T, Brussee S, Hondelink LM, *et al.* Deep learning-based classification of early-stage mycosis fungoides and benign inflammatory dermatoses on hematoxylin and eosin-stained whole-slide images: a retrospective, proof-of-concept study. *J Invest Dermatol* 2025;**145**:1127–1134.
102. Shapiro PE, Pinto FJ. The histologic spectrum of mycosis fungoides/Sezary syndrome (cutaneous T-cell lymphoma): a review of 222 biopsies, including newly described patterns and the earliest pathologic changes. *Am J Surg Pathol* 1994;**18**:645–667.
103. Santucci M, Biggeri A, Feller AC, *et al.* Efficacy of histologic criteria for diagnosing early mycosis fungoides: an EORTC Cutaneous Lymphoma Study Group investigation. *Am J Surg Pathol* 2000;**24**:40–50.
104. Sanchez JL, Ackerman AB. The patch stage of mycosis fungoides: criteria for histologic diagnosis. *Am J Dermatopathol* 1979;**1**:5–26.
105. Smoller BR, Bishop K, Glusac E, *et al.* Reassessment of histologic parameters in the diagnosis of mycosis fungoides. *Am J Surg Pathol* 1995;**19**:1423–1430.
106. Guitart J, Kennedy J, Ronan S, *et al.* Histologic criteria for the diagnosis of mycosis fungoides: proposal for a grading system to standardize pathology reporting. *J Cutan Pathol* 2001;**28**: 174–183.
107. Dalton SR, Chandler WM, Abuzeid M, *et al.* Eosinophils in mycosis fungoides: an uncommon finding in the patch and plaque stages. *Am J Dermatopathol* 2012;**34**:586–591.

108. Shamim H, Johnson EF, Gibson LE, Comfere N. Mycosis fungoides with spongiosis: a potential diagnostic pitfall. *J Cutan Pathol* 2019;**46**:645–652.
109. Tekin B, Kempf W, Seckin D, *et al.* Interstitial mycosis fungoides with lichen sclerosus – like clinical and histopathological features. *Am J Dermatopathol* 2016;**38**:138–143.
110. Wehkamp U, Weichenthal M, Egberts F, *et al.* Clinically defined subgroups of mycosis fungoides display differing histopathological features at initial biopsy. *Leuk Lymphoma* 2018;**59**:2871–2879.
111. Rodriguez G, Tellez A. Perineural and intraneural cutaneous granulomas in granulomatous mycosis fungoides mimicking tuberculoid leprosy. *Int J Dermatol* 2016;**55**:1336–1340.
112. Buchely N, Al-Rohil RN, Aung PP, *et al.* Dermal xanthomatous infiltrates after brentuximab vedotin therapy in mycosis fungoides with large-cell transformation: a novel histologic finding. *J Cutan Pathol* 2018;**45**:711–715.
113. Cerroni L, Rieger E, Rödl S, Kerl H. Clinicopathologic and immunologic features associated with transformation of mycosis fungoides to large-cell lymphoma. *Am J Surg Pathol* 1992;**16**:543–552.
114. Vergier B, De Muret A, Beylot-Barry M, *et al.* Transformation of mycosis fungoides: clinicopathologic and prognostic features of 45 cases. *Blood* 2000;**95**:2212–2218.
115. Raghavan SS, Hong EK, Kim YH, Kim J. Utility of CD30, Ki-67, and p53 in assisting with the diagnosis of mycosis fungoides with large cell transformation. *J Cutan Pathol* 2019;**46**:33–43.
116. Benner MA, Jansen PM, Vermeer MH, *et al.* Prognostic factors in transformed mycosis fungoides: a retrospective analysis of 100 cases. *Blood* 2012;**119**:1643–1649.
117. Kadin ME, Hughey LC, Wood GS. Large-cell transformation of mycosis fungoides-differential diagnosis with implications for clinical management: a consensus statement of the US Cutaneous Lymphoma Consortium. *J Am Acad Dermatol* 2014;**70**:374–376.
118. Fauconneau A, Pham-Ledard A, Cappellen D, *et al.* Assessment of diagnostic criteria between primary cutaneous anaplastic large-cell lymphoma and CD30-rich transformed mycosis fungoides; a study of 66 cases. *Br J Dermatol* 2015;**172**:1547–1554.
119. Pham-Ledard A, Prochazkova-Carlotti M, Laharanne E, *et al.* IRF4 gene rearrangements define a subgroup of CD30-positive cutaneous T-cell lymphoma: a study of 54 cases. *J Invest Dermatol* 2010;**130**:816–825.
120. Karai LJ, Kadin ME, Hsi ED, *et al.* Chromosomal rearrangements of 6p25.3 define a new subtype of lymphomatoid papulosis. *Am J Surg Pathol* 2013;**37**:1173–1181.
121. Wada DA, Law ME, Hsi ED, *et al.* Specificity of IRF4 translocations for primary cutaneous anaplastic large cell lymphoma: a multicenter study of 204 skin biopsies. *Mod Pathol* 2011;**24**:596–605.
122. Wolf P, Cerroni L, Smolle J, Kerl H. PUVA-induced lymphomatoid papulosis in a patient with mycosis fungoides. *J Am Acad Dermatol* 1991;**25**:422–426.
123. Ogino J, Saga K, Kagaya M, *et al.* CD30+ large cell transformation of mycosis fungoides after psoralen plus ultraviolet A photochemotherapy. *Br J Dermatol* 2006;**156**:148–151.
124. Nakahigashi K, Ishida Y, Matsumura Y, *et al.* Large cell transformation mimicking regional lymphomatoid papulosis in a patient with mycosis fungoides. *J Dermatol* 2008;**35**:283–288.
125. Massone C, Crisman G, Kerl H, Cerroni L. The prognosis of early mycosis fungoides is not influenced by phenotype and T-cell clonality. *Br J Dermatol* 2008;**159**:881–886.
126. Rodríguez-Pinilla SM, Ortiz-Romero PL, Monsalvez V, *et al.* TCR-γ expression in primary cutaneous T-cell lymphomas. *Am J Surg Pathol* 2013;**37**:375–384.
127. Martinez-Escala ME, Kantor RW, Cices A, *et al.* CD8+ mycosis fungoides: a low-grade lymphoproliferative disorder. *J Am Acad Dermatol* 2017;**77**:489–496.
128. Geller S, Hollmann TJ, Horwitz SM, *et al.* CCR4 expression in CD8+ cutaneous T-cell lymphomas and lymphoproliferative disorders and its implications for diagnosis and treatment. *Histopathology* 2020;**76**:222–232.
129. Jour G, Aung PP, Merrill ED, *et al.* Differential expression of CCR4 in primary cutaneous gamma/delta (γ/δ) T cell lymphomas and mycosis fungoides: significance for diagnosis and therapy. *J Dermatol Sci* 2018;**89**:88–91.
130. Tournier E, Laurent C, Thomas M, *et al.* Double-positive CD4/CD8 mycosis fungoides: a rarely reported immunohistochemical profile. *J Cutan Pathol* 2014;**41**:58–62.
131. Bekel L, Chaby G, Lok C, *et al.* Primary cutaneous T-cell lymphoma presenting as mycosis fungoides with a T-/null-cell phenotype: report of two cases. *Br J Dermatol* 2015;**172**:1637–1641.
132. Kempf W, Kazakov DV, Cipolat C, *et al.* CD4/CD8 double negative mycosis fungoides with PD-1 (CD279) expression – A disease of follicular helper T cells? *Am J Dermatopathol* 2012;**34**:757–761.
133. Guitart J, Gammon B. The difficulties in defining follicular T helper phenotype in cutaneous lymphomas. *Am J Dermatopathol* 2013;**35**:691.
134. Cetinözman F, Jansen PM, Vermeer MH, *et al.* Differential expression of programmed death-1 (PD-1) in Sezary syndrome and mycosis fungoides. *Arch Dermatol* 2012;**148**:1379–1385.
135. Di Raimondo C, Rubio-Gonzalez B, Palmer J, *et al.* Expression of immune checkpoint molecules programmed death protein 1, programmed death-ligand 1 and inducible T-cell co-stimulator in mycosis fungoides and Sèzary syndrome: association with disease stage and clinical outcome. *Br J Dermatol* 2022;**187**:234–243.
136. Gammon B, Guitart J. Intertriginous mycosis fungoides. A distinct presentation of cutaneous T-cell lymphoma that may be caused by malignant follicular helper T cells. *Arch Dermatol* 2012;**148**:1040–1044.
137. Meyerson HJ, Awadallah A, Pavlidakey P, *et al.* Follicular center helper T-cell (TFH) marker positive mycosis fungoides/Sezary syndrome. *Mod Pathol* 2013;**26**:32–43.
138. Park JH, Han JH, Kang HY, *et al.* Expression of follicular helper T-cell markers in primary cutaneous T-cell lymphoma. *Am J Dermatopathol* 2014;**36**:465–470.
139. Bosisio FM, Cerroni L. Expression of T-follicular helper markers in sequential biopsies of progressive mycosis fungoides and other primary cutaneous T-cell lymphomas. *Am J Dermatopathol* 2015;**37**:115–121.
140. Bosisio FM, Cerroni L. Mycosis fungoides with large cell transformation and T follicular helper phenotype. *Pathol Case Rev* 2014;**19**:208–211.
141. Vermeer MH, Geelen FAMJ, Kummer JA, *et al.* Expression of cytotoxic proteins by neoplastic T cells in mycosis fungoides increases with progression from plaque stage to tumor stage disease. *Am J Pathol* 1999;**154**:1203–1210.

142. Kim M, Park M, Lim M, Kim J. Cytotoxic variant of mycosis fungoides with CD8+ CD56+ phenotype: a case report and review of literature. *Korean J Pathol* 2014;**48**:390–393.
143. Horst BA, Kasper R, LeBoit P. CD4+, CD56+ mycosis fungoides: case report and review of the literature. *Am J Dermatopathol* 2009;**31**:74–76.
144. Aung PP, Climent F, Muzzafar T, *et al.* Immunophenotypic shift of CD4 and CD8 antigen expression in primary cutaneous T-cell lymphomas: a clinicopathologic study of three cases. *J Cutan Pathol* 2014;**41**:51–57.
145. Endo C, Naka Y, Miyagaki T, *et al.* Immunophenotypic shift from CD4(+) to CD8(+) in mycosis fungoides. *Br J Dermatol* 2016;**175**:830–833.
146. Kash N, Massone C, Fink-Puches R, Cerroni L. Phenotypic variation in different lesions of mycosis fungoides biopsied within a short period of time from the same patient. *Am J Dermatopathol* 2016;**38**:541–545.
147. Rahbar Z, Li S, Tavallaee M, *et al.* Variability in the expression of immunohistochemical markers: implications for biomarker interpretation in cutaneous T-cell lymphoma. *J Invest Dermatol* 2018;**138**:1204–1206.
148. Edinger JT, Clark BZ, Pucevich BE, *et al.* CD30 expression and proliferative fraction in nontransformed mycosis fungoides. *Am J Surg Pathol* 2009;**33**:1860–1868.
149. Mitteldorf C, Kampa F, Ströbel P, *et al.* Intraindividual variability of CD30 expression in mycosis fungoides –implications for diagnostic evaluation and therapy. *Histopathology* 2022;**81**:55–64.
150. Sen F, Kang S, Cangiarella J, *et al.* CD20 positive mycosis fungoides: a case report. *J Cutan Pathol* 2008;**35**:398–403.
151. Harms KL, Harms PW, Anderson T, *et al.* Mycosis fungoides with CD20 expression: report of two cases and review of the literature. *J Cutan Pathol* 2014;**41**:494–503.
152. Jullié ML, Carlotti M, Vivot A Jr, *et al.* CD20 antigen may be expressed by reactive or lymphomatous cells of transformed mycosis fungoides: diagnostic and prognostic impact. *Am J Surg Patho* 2013;**37**:1845–1854.
153. Fried I, Cerroni L. FOXP3 in sequential biopsies of progressive mycosis fungoides. *Am J Dermatopathol* 2012;**34**:263–265.
154. Satou A, Asano N, Kato S, *et al.* FoxP3-positive T cell lymphoma arising in non-HTLV1 carrier: clinicopathological analysis of 11 cases of PTCL-NOS and 2 cases of mycosis fungoides. *Histopathology* 2016;**68**:1099–1108.
155. Marzano AV, Vezzoli P, Fanoni D, *et al.* Primary cutaneous T-cell lymphoma expressing FOXP3: a case report supporting the existence of malignancies of regulatory T cells. *J Am Acad Dermatol* 2009;**61**:348–355.
156. Wada DA, Wilcox RA, Weenig RH, *et al.* Paucity of intraepidermal FoxP3-positive T cells in cutaneous T-cell lymphoma in contrast with spongiotic and lichenoid dermatitis. *J Cutan Pathol* 2010;**37**:535–541.
157. Christie LJ, Evans AT, Bray SE, *et al.* Lesions resembling Langerhans cell histiocytosis in association with other lymphoproliferative disorders: a reactive or neoplastic phenomenon? *Hum Pathol* 2006;**37**:32–39.
158. (a)Schlapbach C, Ochsenbein A, Kaelin U, *et al.* High numbers of DC-SIGN+ dendritic cells in lesional skin of cutaneous T-cell lymphoma. *J Am Acad Dermatol* 2010;**62**:995–1004.(b) Carrasco Mendoza CA, Arana I, Cassarino DS. Rare concomitant langerhans cell histiocytosis in a patient with folliculotropic mycosis fungoides. *J Cut Pathol* 2025;**52**:474–477.
159. Pileri A, Agostinelli C, Sessa M, *et al.* Langerhans, plasmacytoid dendritic and myeloid-derived suppressor cell levels in mycosis fungoides vary according to the stage of the disease. *Virchows Arch* 2017;**470**:575–582.
160. Ishida M, Okabe H. Reactive lymphoid follicles with germinal centers in granulomatous mycosis fungoides: a case report with review of the literature. *J Cutan Pathol* 2013;**40**:284–285.
161. Ferrara G, Chiarelli C, Simonetti S. B-cell lymphofollicular infiltrates in mycosis fungoides. *Tumori* 2010;**96**:487–491.
162. Ferrara G, Stefanato CM. Mycosis fungoides with reactive lymphoid follicles may represent an early histopathologic picture of granulomatous slack skin. *J Cutan Pathol* 2013;**40**:611–613.
163. Barzilai A, Trau H, David M, *et al.* Mycosis fungoides associated with B-cell malignancies. *Br J Dermatol* 2006;**155**:179–186.
164. Grange F, Avril MF, Esteve E, *et al.* Coexistent cutaneous T-cell lymphoma and B-cell malignancy. *J Am Acad Dermatol* 1994;**31**:724–731.
165. Scherer F, Kurtz DM, Diehn M, Alizadeh AA. High-throughput sequencing for noninvasive disease detection in hematologic malignancies. *Blood* 2017;**130**:440–452.
166. Shinohara MM, Rieger KE, Sundram U, *et al.* Assessing T-cell receptor clonality by next-generation sequencing in atypical cutaneous lymphoid infiltrates and cutaneous T-cell lymphoma: a scoping review. *J Cutan Pathol* 2024;**51**:813–819.
167. (a) Wehkamp U, Pietzka S, Kotrová M, *et al.* Mycosis fungoides: differentiation from inflammation and detection of circulating tumour cells with the EuroClonality next-generation sequencing assay. *Br J Dermatol* 2025;**192**:492–500.(b) Wehkamp U, Pietzka S, Kotrová M, *et al.* Mycosis fungoides: differentiation from inflammation and detection of circulating tumour cells with the EuroClonality next-generation sequencing assay. *Br J Dermatol* 2025;**192**:492–500.
168. Iyer A, Hennessey D, O'Keefe S, *et al.* Clonotypic heterogeneity in cutaneous T-cell lymphoma (mycosis fungoides) revealed by comprehensive whole-exome sequencing. *Blood Adv* 2019;**3**:1175–1184.
169. Gaydosik AM, Tabib T, Geskin LJ, *et al.* Single-cell lymphocyte heterogeneity in advanced cutaneous T-cell lymphoma skin tumors. *Clin Cancer Res* 2019;**25**:4443–4454.
170. de Masson A, O'Malley JT, Elco CP, *et al.* High-throughput sequencing of the T cell receptor β gene identifies aggressive early-stage mycosis fungoides. *Sci Transl Med* 2018 May 9;**10**(440):pii: eaar5894. doi: 10.1126/scitranslmed.aar5894.
171. Volkenandt M, Soyer HP, Cerroni L, *et al.* Molecular detection of clone-specific DNA in histopathologically unclassified lesions of a patient with mycosis fungoides. *Arch Dermatol Res* 1992;**284**:22–23.
172. Beylot-Barry M, Sibaud V, Thiebaut R, *et al.* Evidence that an identical T cell clone in skin and peripheral blood lymphocytes is an independent prognostic factor in primary cutaneous T cell lymphomas. *J Invest Dermatol* 2001;**117**:920–926.
173. Assaf C, Hummel M, Steinhoff M, *et al.* Early TCR- and TCR-PCR detection of T-cell clonality indicates minimal tumor disease in lymph nodes of cutaneous T-cell lymphoma: diagnostic and prognostic implications. *Blood* 2005;**105**:503–510.
174. Liu X, Jin S, Hu S, *et al.* Single-cell transcriptomics links malignant T cells to the tumor immune landscape in cutaneous T cell lymphoma. *Nature Comm* 2022;**13**:1158.

175. Barba G, Matteucci C, Girolomoni G, *et al.* Comparative genomic hybridization identifies 17q11.2 approximately q12 duplication as an early event in cutaneous T-cell lymphomas. *Cancer Genetics Cytogen* 2008;**184**:48–51.
176. Wain EM, Mitchell TJ, Russell-Jones R, Whittaker SJ. Fine mapping of chromosome 10q deletions in mycosis fungoides and Sezary syndrome: identification of two discrete regions of deletion at 10q23.33–24.1 and 10q24.33–25.1. *Genes Chromos Cancer* 2005;**42**:184–192.
177. Karenko L, Hahtola S, Paivinen S, *et al.* Primary cutaneous T-cell lymphomas show a deletion or translocation affecting NAV3, the human UNC-53 homologue. *Cancer Res* 2005;**65**:8101–8110.
178. Marty M, Prochazkova M, Laharanne E, *et al.* Primary cutaneous T-cell lymphomas do not show specific NAV3 gene deletion or translocation. *J Invest Dermatol* 2008;**128**:2458–2466.
179. Choi J, Goh G, Walradt T, *et al.* Genomic landscape of cutaneous T cell lymphoma. *Nat Genet* 2015;**47**:1011–1019.
180. da Silva Almeida AC, Abate F, Khiabanian H, *et al.* The mutational landscape of cutaneous T cell lymphoma and Sezary syndrome. *Nat Genet* 2015;**47**:1465–1470.
181. (a) Gniadecki R, O'Keefe S, Hennessey D, Iyer A. Is cutaneous T-cell lymphoma caused by ultraviolet radiation? A comparison of UV mutational signatures in malignant melanoma and mycosis fungoides. *Cells* 2023;**12**:1616.(b) Campbell BA, Baade PD, Dasgupta P, *et al.* Geospatial analyses demonstrate variation of cutaneous T-cell lymphomas across Australia, providing insights into possible causes. *Br J Dermatol* 2025;**92**:1018–1028.
182. Tensen CP, Quint KD, Vermeer MH. Genetic and epigenetic insights into cutaneous T-cell lymphoma. *Blood* 2022;**139**:15–33.
183. Krejsgaard T, Vetter-Kauczok CS, Woetmann A, *et al.* Ectopic expression of B-lymphoid kinase in cutaneous T-cell lymphoma. *Blood* 2009;**113**:5896–5904.
184. van Kester MS, Borg MK, Zoutman WH, *et al.* A meta-analysis of gene expression data identifies a molecular signature characteristic for tumor-stage mycosis fungoides. *J Invest Dermatol* 2012;**132**:2050–2059.
185. Ungewickell A, Bhaduri A, Rios E, *et al.* Genomic analysis of mycosis fungoides and Sézary syndrome identifies recurrent alterations in TNFR2. *Nat Genet* 2015;**47**:1056–1060.
186. McGirt LY, Jia P, Baerenwald DA, *et al.* Whole-genome sequencing reveals oncogenic mutations in mycosis fungoides. *Blood* 2015;**126**:508–519.
187. Park J, Yang J, Wenzel AT, *et al.* Genomic analysis of 220 CTCLs identifies a novel recurrent gain-of-function alteration in RLTPR (p.Q575E). *Blood* 2017;**130**:1430–1440.
188. Navas IC, Ortiz-Romero PL, Villuendas R, *et al.* p16(INK4a) gene alterations are frequent in lesions of mycosis fungoides. *Am J Pathol* 2000;**156**:1565–1572.
189. Dereure O, Levi E, Vonderheid EC, Kadin ME. Infrequent Fas mutations but no bax or p53 mutations in early mycosis fungoides: a possible mechanism for the accumulation of malignant T lymphocytes in the skin. *J Invest Dermatol* 2002;**118**:949–956.
190. Scarisbrick JJ, Woolford AJ, Calonje E, *et al.* Frequent abnormalities of the p15 and p16 genes in mycosis fungoides and Sezary syndrome. *J Invest Dermatol* 2002;**118**:493–499.
191. Goswami M, Duvic M, Dougherty A, *et al.* Increased twist expression in advanced stage of mycosis fungoides and Sezary syndrome. *J Cutan Pathol* 2012;**39**:500–507.
192. Mao X, Orchard G, Lillington DM, *et al.* Amplification and overexpression of JUNB is associated with primary cutaneous T-cell lymphomas. *Blood* 2003;**101**:1513–1519.
193. Carbone A, Bernardini L, Valenzano F, *et al.* Array-based comparative genomic hybridization in early-stage mycosis fungoides: recurrent deletion of tumor suppressor genes BCL7A, SMAC/DIABLO, and RHOF. *Genes Chromos Cancer* 2008;**47**:1067–1075.
194. Tracey L, Villuendas R, Dotor AM, *et al.* Mycosis fungoides shows concurrent deregulation of multiple genes involved in the TNF signaling pathway: an expression profile study. *Blood* 2003;**102**:1042–1050.
195. Shin J, Monti S, Aires DJ, *et al.* Lesional gene expression profiling in cutaneous T-cell lymphoma reveals natural clusters associated with disease outcome. *Blood* 2007;**110**:3015–3027.
196. Litvinov IV, Jones DA, Sasseville D, *et al.* Transcriptional profiles predict disease outcome in patients with cutaneous T-cell lymphoma. *Clin Cancer Res* 2010;**16**:2106–2114.
197. Shrestha S, Newsom K, Chaffin JM, Seifert RP. Pathogenic variants of mycosis fungoides identified using next-generation sequencing. *J Hematop* 2024;**17**:209–214.
198. Maj J, Jankowska-Konsur A, Sadakierska-Chudy A, *et al.* Altered microRNA expression in mycosis fungoides. *Br J Dermatol* 2012;**166**:331–336.
199. Ralfkiaer U, Hagedorn PH, Bangsgaard N, *et al.* Diagnostic microRNA profiling in cutaneous T-cell lymphoma (CTCL). *Blood* 2011;**118**:5891–5900.
200. van Kester MS, Ballabio E, Benner MF, *et al.* miRNA expression profiling of mycosis fungoides. *Mol Oncol* 2011;**5**:273–280.
201. Moyal L, Yehezkel S, Gorovitz B, *et al.* Oncogenic role of microRNA-155 in mycosis fungoides: an in vitro and xenograft mouse model study. *Br J Dermatol* 2017;**177**:791–800.
202. Tensen CP, Vermeer MH. MicroRNA-155 potentiates tumour development in mycosis fungoides. *Br J Dermatol* 2017;**177**:618–620.
203. Seto AG, Beatty X, Lynch JM, *et al.* Cobomarsen, an oligonucleotide inhibitor of miR-155, coordinately regulates multiple survival pathways to reduce cellular proliferation and survival in cutaneous T-cell lymphoma. *Br J Haematol* 2018;**183**:428–444.
204. Shen X, Wang B, Li K, *et al.* MicroRNA signatures in diagnosis and prognosis of cutaneous T-cell lymphoma. *J Invest Dermatol* 2018;**138**:2024–2032.
205. Kohnken R, Wen J, Mundy-Bosse B, *et al.* Diminished microRNA-29b level is associated with BRD4-mediated activation of oncogenes in cutaneous T-cell lymphoma. *Blood* 2018;**131**:771–781.
206. Benner MF, Ballabio E, van Kester MS, *et al.* Primary cutaneous anaplastic large cell lymphoma shows a distinct miRNA expression profile and reveals differences from tumor-stage mycosis fungoides. *Exp Dermatol* 2012;**21**:630–642.
207. Sandoval J, Dıaz-Lagares A, Salgado R, *et al.* MicroRNA expression profiling and DNA methylation signature for deregulated microRNA in cutaneous T-cell lymphoma. *J Invest Dermatol* 2015;**135**:1128–1137.
208. Ralfkiaer U, Lindal L, Litman T, *et al.* MicroRNA expression in early mycosis fungoides is distinctly different from atopic dermatitis and advanced cutaneous T-cell lymphoma. *Anticancer Res* 2014;**34**:7207–7218.
209. Kwang AC, Duran GE, Fernandez-Pol S, *et al.* Genetic alteration of class I HLA in cutaneous T-cell lymphoma. *Blood* 2025;**145**:311–324.

210. Nashan D, Faulhaber D, Ständer S, *et al.* Mycosis fungoides: a dermatological masquerader. *Br J Dermatol* 2007;**156**:1–10.
211. Zackheim HS, McCalmont TH. Mycosis fungoides: the great imitator. *J Am Acad Dermatol* 2002;**47**:914–918.
212. Cerroni L, Fink-Puches R, Bäck B, Kerl H. Follicular mucinosis: a critical reappraisal of clinicopathologic features and association with mycosis fungoides and Sézary syndrome. *Arch Dermatol* 2002;**138**:182–189.
213. Tomasini C, Kempf W, Novelli M, *et al.* Spiky follicular mycosis fungoides: a clinicopathologic study of eight cases. *J Cutan Pathol* 2015;**42**:164–172.
214. Baykal C, Atci T, Ozturk SS, *et al.* Underrecognized clinical features of folliculotropic mycosis fungoides: a large clinical series. *J Dtsch Dermatol Ges* 2017;**15**:289–299.
215. Wakosa A, Binois R, Kerdraon R, *et al.* Mycosis fungoides associated with follicular mucinosis manifested by lichen spinulosus in skin folds. *Ann Dermatol Venereol* 2014;**141**:482–484.
216. Gallo JC, de Wet J, Visser WI, *et al.* Generalized lichen spinulosus and secondary follicular mucinosis. *J Am Acad Dermatol Case Reports* 2023;**33**:101–104.
217. Kempf W, Kazakov D, Schermesser M, *et al.* Unilesional follicular mycosis fungoides: report of two cases with progression to tumor stage and review of the literature. *J Cutan Pathol* 2012;**39**:853–860.
218. Amitay-Laish I, Feinmesser M, Ben-Amitai D, *et al.* Unilesional folliculotropic mycosis fungoides: a unique variant of cutaneous lymphoma. *J Eur Acad Dermatol* 2016;**30**:25–29.
219. Magro CM, Telang GH, Momtahen S. Unilesional follicular mycosis fungoides: report of 6 cases and review of the literature. *Am J Dermatopathol* 2018;**40**:329–336.
220. van Santen S, Jansen PM, Vermeer MH, Willemze R. Folliculotropic mycosis fungoides presenting with a solitary lesion: Clinicopathological features and long-term follow-up data in a series of 9 cases. *J Cutan Pathol* 2018;**45**:122–128.
221. Flaig MJ, Cerroni L, Schuhmann K, *et al.* Follicular mycosis fungoides: a histopathologic analysis of nine cases. *J Cutan Pathol* 2001;**28**:525–530.
222. Gerami P, Guitart J. The spectrum of histopathologic and immunohistochemical findings in folliculotropic mycosis fungoides. *Am J Surg Pathol* 2007;**31**:1430–1438.
223. Wang L, Wang G, Gao T. Granulomatous syringotropic mycosis fungoides with two lesions having reactive B-cell proliferation. *J Cutan Pathol* 2014;**41**:400–406.
224. Demirkesen C, Esirgen G, Engin B, *et al.* The clinical features and histopathologic patterns of folliculotropic mycosis fungoides in a series of 38 cases. *J Cutan Pathol* 2015;**42**:22–31.
225. Marschalko M, Erös N, Kontar O, *et al.* Folliculotropic mycosis fungoides: clinicopathological analysis of 17 patients. *J Eur Acad Dermatol Venereol* 2015;**29**:964–972.
226. Bi MY, Curry JL, Christiano AM, *et al.* The spectrum of hair loss in patients with mycosis fungoides and Sézary syndrome. *J Am Acad Dermatol* 2011;**64**:53–63.
227. Torres T, Velho G, Alves R, *et al.* Widespread comedones as the sole clinical manifestation of follicular mycosis fungoides. *Eur J Dermatol* 2010;**20**:534–535.
228. Kossard S, Weller P. Pseudotumorous folliculotropic mycosis fungoides. *Am J Dermatopathol* 2005;**27**:224–227.
229. Gül Ü, Soylu S, Aslan E, *et al.* Uncommon presentation of mycosis fungoides: eyelid margin involvement. *J Dermatology* 2008;**35**:581–584.
230. Magro CM, Crowson AN. Folliculotropic T-cell lymphocytosis as a distinct form of pilotropic T-cell dyscrasia. *Am J Clin Pathol* 2011;**135**:221–229.
231. Ardigó M, Borroni G, Muscardin L, *et al.* Hypopigmented mycosis fungoides in Caucasian patients: a clinicopathologic study of 7 cases. *J Am Acad Dermatol* 2003;**49**:264–270.
232. Alikhan A, Griffin J, Nguyen N, *et al.* Pediatric follicular mucinosis: presentation, histopathology, molecular genetics, treatment, and outcomes over an 11-year period at the Mayo Clinic. *Pediatr Dermatol* 2013;**30**:192–198.
233. Santos-Briz A, Cañueto J, García-Dorado J, *et al.* Pediatric primary follicular mucinosis: further evidence of its relationship with mycosis fungoides. *Pediatr Dermatol* 2013;**30**:e218–e220.
234. van Doorn R, Scheffer E, Willemze R. Follicular mycosis fungoides, a distinct disease entity with or without associated follicular mucinosis. *Arch Dermatol* 2002;**138**:191–198.
235. Gerami P, Rosen S, Kuzel T, *et al.* Folliculotropic mycosis fungoides. An aggressive variant of cutaneous T-cell lymphoma. *Archiv Dermatol* 2008;**144**:738–746.
236. Mantaka P, Helsing P, Gjersvik P, *et al.* Clinical and histopathological features of folliculotropic mycosis fungoides: a Norwegian patient series. *Acta Derm Venereol* 2013;**93**:325–329.
237. Lehman JS, Cook-Norris RH, Weed BR, *et al.* Folliculotropic mycosis fungoides. Single-center study and systematic review. *Arch Dermatol* 2010;**146**:607–613.
238. Wieser I, Wang C, Alberti-Violetti S, *et al.* Clinical characteristics, risk factors and long-term outcome of 114 patients with folliculotropic mycosis fungoides. *Arch Dermatol Res* 2017;**309**:453–459.
239. Muniesa C, Estrach T, Pujol RM, *et al.* Folliculotropic mycosis fungoides: clinicopathologic features and outcome in a series of 20 patients. *J Am Acad Dermatol* 2010;**62**:418–426.
240. van Santen S, Roach REJ, van Doorn R, *et al.* Clinical staging and prognostic factors in folliculotropic mycosis fungoides. *JAMA Dermatol* 2016;**152**:992–1000.
241. Heymann WR. Predicting the nature of follicular mucinosis: still a sticky situation. *J Am Acad Dermatol* 2019;**80**:1524–1525.
242. Van Santen S, Jansen PM, Quint KD, *et al.* Plaque stage folliculotropic mycosis fungoides: histopathologic features and prognostic factors in a series of 40 patients. *J Cutan Pathol* 2020;**47**:241–250.
243. Zvulunov A, Shkalim V, Ben-Amitai D, *et al.* Clinical and histopathologic spectrum of alopecia mucinosa/follicular mucinosis and its natural history in children. *J Am Acad Dermatol* 2012;**67**:1174–1181.
244. Shamim H, Riemer C, Weenig R, *et al.* Acneiform presentations of folliculotropic mycosis fungoides. *Am J Dermatopathol* 2021;**43**:85–92.
245. Brau-Javier CN, Santos-Arroyo AE, De Sanctis-González IM, Sánchez JL. Follicular mucinosis presenting as an acneiform eruption: a follow-up study. *Am J Dermatopathol* 2013;**35**:792–796.
246. Wittenberg GP, Gibson LE, Pittelkow MR, el Azhary RA. Follicular mucinosis presenting as an acneiform eruption: report of four cases. *J Am Acad Dermatol* 1998;**38**:849–851.
247. Fahrner LJ, Solomon AR. Persistent papular plaques on the face. *Pediatr Dermatol* 1989;**6**:254–245.
248. Tosti A, Fanti PA, Peserico A, Varotti C. Linear alopecia mucinosa along Blaschko lines. *Acta Derm Venereol (Stockh)* 1992;**72**:155–156.
249. Tadini G, Boldrini MP, Brena M, *et al.* Nevoid follicular mucinosis: a new type of hair follicle nevus. *J Cutan Pathol* 2013;**40**:844–847.

250. Mir-Bonafé JM, Cañueto J, Fernández-López E, Santos-Briz A. Follicular mucinosis associated with nonlymphoid skin conditions. *Am J Dermatopathol* 2014;**36**:705–709.
251. Geller S, Gomez CJ, Myskowski PL, Pulitzer M. Follicular mucinosis in patients with hematologic malignancies other than mycosis fungoides: a clinicopathologic study. *J Am Acad Dermatol* 2019;**80**:1704–1711.
252. Hu SW, Ratech H, Naeem R, *et al.* Mycosis fungoides with epidermal mucinosis: a variant of mycosis fungoides with a spongiosis-like pattern. *J Cutan Pathol* 2015;**42**:730–738.
253. Riveiro-Falkenbach E, Ruano Y, Garrido M, *et al.* Acral mycosis fungoides with epidermal microvesiculation mucinosis. *Am J Dermatopathol* 2015;**37**:632–634.
254. Pileri A, Facchetti F, Rütten A, *et al.* Syringotropic mycosis fungoides: a rare variant of the disease with peculiar clinicopathologic features. *Am J Surg Pathol* 2011;**35**:100–109.
255. Yost JM, Do TT, Kovalszki K, *et al.* Two cases of syringotropic cutaneous T-cell lymphoma and review of the literature. *J Am Acad Dermatol* 2009;**61**:133–138.
256. Ackerman AB, Miller RC, Shapiro L. Pustular mycosis fungoides. *Arch Dermatol* 1966;**93**:221–225.
257. Camisa C, Aulisio A. Pustular mycosis fungoides. *Cutis* 1994;**54**:202–204.
258. Franck N, Carlotti A, Gorin I, *et al.* Mycosis fungoides-type cutaneous T-cell lymphoma and neutrophilic dermatosis. *Arch Dermatol* 2005;**141**:353–356.
259. Pabsch H, Kunze J, Schaller J. Mycosis fungoides presenting as a pustular eruption. *J Am Acad Dermatol* 2009;**61**:908–909.
260. Bontoux C, Badrignans M, Afach S, *et al.* Pustular mycosis fungoides has a poor outcome: a multicentric clinicopathological and molecular case series. *Br J Dermatol* 2024;**192**:125–134.
261. Guillet S, Stokkermans J, Vergier B, *et al.* Acute neutrophilic dermatosis (pustular dermatitis) associated with aggressive transformed mycosis fungoides. *Ann Dermatol Venereol* 2013;**140**: 635–640.
262. Merlet S, Dandurand M, Elmajaoui S, *et al.* Tumoral and pilotropic mycosis fongoides without mucin: evolution towards a pustulous erythroderma. *Ann Dermatol Venereol* 2006;**133**:149–152.
263. Mourtzinos N, Puri PK, Wang G, *et al.* CD4/CD8 double negative pagetoid reticulosis: a case report and literature review. *J Cutan Pathol* 2010;**37**:491–496.
264. Torre-Castro J, Carrasco Santos L, Rodriguez-Pinilla SM, Requena L. Pagetoid reticulosis in a 13-year old female. A unique immunohistochemical profile. *J Cutan Pathol* 2020;**47**:466–469.
265. Tomasini D, Niccoli A, Crivelli F. Pagetoid reticulosis tumor cells with double expression of TCRγδ and TCRαβ: an off-target phenomenon or genuine expression? *J Cutan Pathol* 2015;**42**:427–434.
266. Leinweber B, Chott A, Kerl H, Cerroni L. Epidermotropic precursor T-cell lymphoma with highly aggressive clinical behavior simulating localized pagetoid reticulosis. *Am J Dermatopathol* 2007;**29**:392–394.
267. Lee JL, Viakhireva N, Cesca C, *et al.* Clinicopathologic features and treatment outcomes in Woringer–Kolopp disease. *J Am Acad Dermatol* 2008;**59**:706–712.
268. Osto M, Atify O, Musa A, *et al.* Woringer–Kolopp disease (localized pagetoid reticulosis): a systematic review. *Int J Dermatol* 2023;**62**:312–321.
269. Cerroni L, Fink-Puches R, El-Shabrawi-Caelen L, *et al.* Solitary skin lesions with histopathologic features of early mycosis fungoides. *Am J Dermatopathol* 1999;**21**:518–524.
270. Oliver GF, Winkelmann RK. Unilesional mycosis fungoides: a distinct entity. *J Am Acad Dermatol* 1989;**20**:63–70.
271. Heald PW, Glusac EJ. Unilesional cutaneous T-cell lymphoma: clinical features, therapy, and follow-up of 10 patients with a treatment-responsive mycosis fungoides variant. *J Am Acad Dermatol* 2000;**42**:283–285.
272. Ally MS, Robson A. A review of the solitary cutaneous T-cell lymphomas. *J Cutan Pathol* 2014;**41**:703–714.
273. Belousova IE, Samtsov AV, Kazakov DV. A rare case of solitary hemorrhagic mycosis fungoides with angiocentric features. *Am J Dermatopathol* 2017;**39**:313–315.
274. Moyal L, Gorovitz-Haris B, Yehezkel S, *et al.* Unilesional mycosis fungoides is associated with increased expression of microRNA-17~92 and T helper 1 skewing. *Br J Dermatol* 2019;**180**: 1123–1134.
275. Ally MS, Pawade J, Tanaka M, *et al.* Solitary mycosis fungoides: a distinct clinicopathologic entity with a good prognosis. *J Am Acad Dermatol* 2012;**67**:736–744.
276. Ohtani T, Kikuchi K, Koizumi H, *et al.* A case of CD30+ large-cell transformation in a patient with unilesional patch-stage mycosis fungoides. *Int J Dermatol* 2009;**48**:623–626.
277. Ackerman AB, Flaxman BA. Granulomatous mycosis fungoides. *Br J Dermatol* 1970;**82**:397–401.
278. Scarabello A, Leinweber B, Ardigó M, *et al.* Cutaneous lymphomas with prominent granulomatous reaction: a potential pitfall in the histopathologic diagnosis of cutaneous T- and B-cell lymphomas. *Am J Surg Pathol* 2002;**26**:1259–1268.
279. LeBoit PE, Zackheim HS, White CR Jr. Granulomatous variants of cutaneous T-cell lymphoma: the histopathology of granulomatous mycosis fungoides and granulomatous slack skin. *Am J Surg Pathol* 1988;**12**:83–95.
280. Garrido MC, Maronas-Jimenez L, Ortiz PL, *et al.* Lichenoid granulomatous mycosis fungoides. *Am J Dermatopathol* 2017;**39**: 614–617.
281. Fernandez-Flores A, Cassarino DS. Plasmacytoid dendritic cells in granulomatous variant of mycosis fungoides. *J Cutan Pathol* 2019;**46**:335–342.
282. Li JY, Pulitzer MP, Myskowski PL, *et al.* A case-control study of clinicopathologic features, prognosis, and therapeutic responses in patients with granulomatous mycosis fungoides. *J Am Acad Dermatol* 2013;**69**:366–374.
283. Kempf W, Ostheeren-Michaelis S, Paulli M, *et al.* Granulomatous mycosis fungoides and granulomatous slack skin: a multicenter study of the Cutaneous Lymphoma Histopathology Task Force Group of the European Organization for Research and Treatment of Cancer (EORTC). *Arch Dermatol* 2008;**144**:1609–1617.
284. Ackerman AB. Granulomatous slack skin. In: Ackerman AB, ed. *Histologic Diagnosis of Inflammatory Skin Diseases*. Philadelphia: Lea and Febiger, 1978: 483–485.
285. LeBoit PE. Granulomatous slack skin. *Dermatol Clin* 1994;**12**: 375–389.
286. Clarijs M, Poot F, Laka A, *et al.* Granulomatous slack skin: treatment with extensive surgery and review of the literature. *Dermatology* 2003;**206**:393–397.

287. Rambhia KD, Haldar S, Dongre AM, Khopkar US. Granulomatous slack skin with systemic involvement and a fatal outcome in an adolescent. *Clin Exper Dermatol* 2014;**39**:653–654.
288. Battesti G, Ram-Wolff C, Dobos G, *et al.* Granulomatous slack skin: clinical characteristics, prognosis and response to therapy. A study from the Cutaneous Lymphoma French Study Group. *Br J Dermatol* 2022;**187**:790–793.
289. Bakr F, Ziaj S, Cardoso J, *et al.* Mycosis fungoides and granulomatous slack skin: a single entity with distinct clinical phenotypes. *Am J Dermatopathol* 2024;**46**:14–20.
290. Belousova IE, Nikonova SM, Sima R, Kazakov DV. Granulomatous slack skin with clonal T-cell receptor-γ gene rearrangement in skin and lymph node. *Br J Dermatol* 2007;**157**:405–407.
291. Ikonomou IM, Aamot HV, Heim S, *et al.* Granulomatous slack skin with a translocation t(3;9)(q12;p24). *Am J Surg Pathol* 2007;**31**:803–806.
292. Hurabielle C, Michel L, Ram-Wolff C, *et al.* Expression of Sézary biomarkers in the blood of patients with erythrodermic mycosis fungoides. *J Invest Dermatol* 2016;**136**:317–320.
293. Vonderheid EC, Kantor GR, Telang GH, *et al.* A histo-immunopathologic and prognostic study of erythrodermic cutaneous T cell lymphoma. *J Cutan Pathol* 2019;**46**:913–924.
294. Su LD, Kim YH, LeBoit PE, *et al.* Interstitial mycosis fungoides, a variant of mycosis fungoides resembling granuloma annulare and inflammatory morphea. *J Cutan Pathol* 2002;**29**:135–141.
295. Reggiani C, Massone C, Fink-Puches R, *et al.* Interstitial mycosis fungoides. A clinicopathologic study of 21 patients. *Am J Surg Pathol* 2016;**40**:1360–1367.
296. Shapiro PE, LeBoit PE. Interstitial mycosis fungoides: setting the record straight. *Am J Surg Pathol* 2017;**41**:282–283.
297. Chung C, Wu B, LeWitt T, *et al.* Interstitial mycosis fungoides: a rare presentation of mycosis fungoides with overlapping granulomatous and folliculotropic features. *J Cutan Pathol* 2024;**51**:459–467.
298. Ferrara G, Crisman G, Zalaudek I, *et al.* Free-floating collagen fibers in interstitial mycosis fungoides. *Am J Dermatopathol* 2010;**32**:352–356.
299. Cota C, Ferrara G, Cerroni L. Granuloma annulare with prominent lymphoid infiltrates ("pseudolymphomatous" granuloma annulare). *Am J Dermatopathol* 2012;**34**:259–262.
300. Koochek A, Fink-Puches R, Cerroni L. Coexistence of patch stage mycosis fungoides and interstitial granuloma annulare in the same patient: a pitfall in the clinicopathologic diagnosis of mycosis fungoides. *Am J Dermatopathol* 2012;**34**:198–202.
301. Hamada T, Tada K, Aoyama Y, Iwatsuki K. Necrobiotic features in both cutaneous and lymph node lesions in a patient with interstitial mycosis fungoides. *Intern J Dermatol* 2015;**54**:e122–e125.
302. Garcia-Colmenero L, Curto-Barredo L, Gomez-Martin I, *et al.* Telangiectatic mycosis fungoides: a new clinicopathological presentation mimicking acquired naevoid telangiectasia. *Acta Derm Venereol* 2017;**97**:651–652.
303. Abbott RA, Sahni D, Robson A, *et al.* Poikilodermatous mycosis fungoides: a study of its clinicopathological, immunophenotypic, and prognostic features. *J Am Acad Dermatol* 2011;**65**:313–319.
304. El Shabrawi-Caelen L, Cerroni L, Medeiros LJ, McCalmont TH. Hypopigmented mycosis fungoides: frequent expression of a CD8 T-cell phenotype. *Am J Surg Pathol* 2002;**26**:450–457.
305. Rodney IJ, Kindred C, Angra K, *et al.* Hypopigmented mycosis fungoides: a retrospective clinicohistopathologic study. *J Eur Acad Dermatol Venereol* 2017;**31**:808–814.
306. Abdel-Halim M, El-Nabarawy E, El Nemr R, Hassan AM. Frequency of hypopigmented mycosis fungoides in Egyptian patients presenting with hypopigmented lesions of the trunk. *Am J Dermatopathol* 2015;**37**:834–840.
307. Caytemel C, Gürbüz BÇ. Linear, blaschkoid, hypopigmented and childhood mycosis fungoides. *Indian J Dermatol* 2023;**68**:727.
308. Goldberg DJ, Schinella RS, Kechijian P. Hypopigmented mycosis fungoides: speculations about the mechanism of hypopigmentation. *Am J Dermatopathol* 1986;**8**:326–330.
309. El Darouti MA, Marzouk SA, Azzam O, *et al.* Vitiligo vs. hypopigmented mycosis fungoides (histopathological and immunohistochemical study, univariate analysis). *Eur J Dermatol* 2006;**16**:17–22.
310. Furlan FC, Pereira BAP, da Silva LF, Sanches JA. Loss of melanocytes in hypopigmented mycosis fungoides: a study of 18 patients. *J Cutan Pathol* 2014;**41**:101–107.
311. El-Darouti MA, Fawzy MM, Hegazy RA, *et al.* Hypopigmented parapsoriasis en plaque, a new, overlooked member of the parapsoriasis family: a report of 34 patients and a 7-year experience. *J Am Acad Dermatol* 2012;**67**:1182–1188.
312. Pavlosvky L, Mimouni D, Amitay-Laish I, *et al.* Hyperpigmented mycosis fungoides: an unusual variant of cutaneous T-cell lymphoma with a frequent CD8+ phenotype. *J Am Acad Dermatol* 2012;**67**:69–75.
313. Sacchelli L, Patrizi A, Neri I, *et al.* Brownish asymptomatic lesions on the arms and legs. *J Dtsch Dermatol Ges* 2019;**17**:659–662.
314. Toro JR, Sander CA, LeBoit PE. Persistent pigmented purpuric dermatitis and mycosis fungoides: simulant, precursor, or both? A study by light microscopy and molecular methods. *Am J Dermatopathol* 1997;**19**:108–118.
315. Crowson AN, Magro CM, Zahorchak R. Atypical pigmentary purpura: a clinical, histopathologic, and genotypic study. *Hum Pathol* 1999;**30**:1004–1012.
316. Barnhill RL, Braverman IM. Progression of pigmented purpura-like eruptions to mycosis fungoides: report of three cases. *J Am Acad Dermatol* 1988;**19**:25–31.
317. Viseux V, Schoenlaub P, Cnudde F, *et al.* Pigmented purpuric dermatitis preceding the diagnosis of mycosis fungoides by 24 years. *Dermatology* 2003;**207**:331–332.
318. Kodama K, Fink-Puches R, Massone C, *et al.* Papular mycosis fungoides: a new clinical variant of early mycosis fungoides. *J Am Acad Dermatol* 2005;**52**:694–698.
319. Saggini A, Fink-Puches R, Cota C, *et al.* Papular mycosis fungoides is a distinctive variant of early-stage mycosis fungoides: extended retrospective study with long-term follow-up. *Am J Surg Pathol* 2019;**43**:1129–1134.
320. Martorell-Calatayud A, Botella-Estrada R, Sanmartin-Jimenez O, *et al.* Papular mycosis fungoides: two new cases of a recently described clinicopathological variant of early mycosis fungoides. *J Cutan Pathol* 2010;**37**:330–335.
321. Kim SJ, Schaffer A, Lee HY, *et al.* A case of papular mycosis fungoides: a new clinical variant of early mycosis fungoides. *Ann Dermatol* 2016;**28**:383–384.
322. Santamarina-Albertos A, Munoz-Martinez R, Alvarez-Gago T, *et al.* Papular mycosis fungoides on the legs: a case report. *Actas Dermosifiliogr* 2014;**105**:87–89.

323. Brajon D, Bonnet N, Dales JP, *et al*. Papular mycosis fungoides. *Ann Dermatol Venereol* 2013;**140**:455–458.
324. Liu ZH, Wang YL, Chen SY, *et al*. Papular mycosis fungoides: a new clinic variant of early and benign mycosis fungoides? *J Clin Oncol* 2011;**29**:e381–e383.
325. Fraitag S, Boccara O, Brousse N, *et al*. Mycosis fungoides following pityriasis lichenoides: an exceptional event or a potential evolution? *Pediatr Blood Cancer* 2012;**58**:307.
326. Byul E, Hwan S, Joo E, *et al*. CD8-positive pityriasis lichenoides-like mycosis fungoides. *Eur J Dermatol* 2012;**22**:415–416.
327. Pileri A, Neri I, Raone B, *et al*. Mycosis fungoides following pityriasis lichenoides: an exceptional event or a potential evolution? *Pediatr Blood Cancer* 2012;**58**:306.
328. Wang SH, Hsiao CH, Hsiao PH, Chu CY. Adult pityriasis lichenoides-like mycosis fungoides with high density of CD8-positive T-lymphocytic infiltration. *J Eur Acad Dermatol Venereol* 2007;**21**:401–402.
329. de Unamuno BB, Ferriols AP, Sánchez RB, *et al*. Adult pityriasis lichenoides-like mycosis fungoides: a clinical variant of mycosis fungoides. *Int J Dermatol* 2014;**53**:1331–1338.
330. Borra T, Custrin A, Saggini A, *et al*. Pityriasis lichenoides, atypical pityriasis lichenoides and related conditions: a study of 66 cases. *Am J Surg Pathol* 2018;**42**:1101–1112.
331. Jang MS, Kang DY, Park JB, *et al*. Pityriasis lichenoides-like mycosis fungoides: clinical and histologic features and response to phototherapy. *Ann Dermatol* 2016;**28**:540–547.
332. Magro C, Crowson AN, Kovatich A, Burns F. Pityriasis lichenoides: a clonal T-cell lymphoproliferative disorder. *Hum Pathol* 2002;**33**:788–795.
333. Sibbald C, Pope E. Systematic review of cases of cutaneous T-cell lymphoma transformation in pityriasis lichenoides and small plaque parapsoriasis. *Br J Dermatol* 2016;**175**:807–809.
334. Ueda C, Makino T, Asano Y, *et al*. An ultrastructural examination of a blistering lesion of mycosis fungoides bullosa. *Br J Dermatol* 2011;**165**:213–214.
335. Xu XL, Huang YX, Lin L, *et al*. Bullous mycosis fungoides: report of a case complicated by Kaposi's varicelliform eruption. *J Dermatol* 2013;**40**:841–847.
336. Requena L, Gonzalez-Guerra E, Angulo J, *et al*. Anetodermic mycosis fungoides: a new clinicopathological variant of mycosis fungoides. *Br J Dermatol* 2008;**158**:157–162.
337. Pujol RM, Gallardo F, Llistosella E, *et al*. Invisible mycosis fungoides: a diagnostic challenge. *J Am Acad Dermatol* 2000;**42**:324–328.
338. Jung YM, Cho HS, Kim GH, *et al*. Psoriasiform mycosis fungoides: a clinical and prognostic retrospective cohort study. *Br J Dermatol* 2024;**190**:4[illegible]–434.
339. Stasko T, Van der Ploeg DE, De Villez RL. Hyperkeratotic mycosis fungoides restricted to the palms. *J Am Acad Dermatol* 1982;**7**:792–796.
340. Resnik KS, Kantor GR, Lessin SR, *et al*. Mycosis fungoides palmaris et plantaris. *Arch Dermatol* 1995;**131**:1052–1056.
341. Kim ST, Jeon YS, Sim HJ, *et al*. Clinicopathologic features and T-cell receptor gene rearrangement findings of mycosis fungoides palmaris et plantaris. *J Am Acad Dermatol* 2006;**54**:466–471.
342. Shimomura N, Sugimoto H, Nakayama A, *et al*. Case of mycosis fungoides palmaris et plantaris possibly associated with nail psoriasis. *J Dermatol* 2024;**51**:e13–e15.
343. Allegue F, Soria C, Rocamora A, *et al*. Hyperkeratosis of the nipple and areola in a patient with cutaneous T-cell lymphoma. *Int J Dermatol* 1990;**29**:519–520.
344. Ekinci AP, Sari SO, Buyukbabani N, Baykal C. The dilemma of coexisting nevoid hyperkeratosis of the nipple and areola in mycosis fungoides: a report of three cases. *Dermatopathology* 2015;**2**:61–66.
345. Ahn SK, Chung J, Soo Lee W, *et al*. Hyperkeratosis of the nipple and areola simultaneously developing with cutaneous T-cell lymphoma. *J Am Acad Dermatol* 1995;**32**:124–125.
346. Roustan G, Yus ES, Simón A. Nevoid hyperkeratosis of the areola with histopathological features mimicking mycosis fungoides. *Eur J Dermatol* 2002;**12**:79–81.
347. Rosman IS, Hepper DM, Lind AC, Anadkat MJ. Nevoid hyperkeratosis of the areola misinterpreted as mycosis fungoides. *J Cutan Pathol* 2012;**39**:545–548.
348. Kanitakis C, Tsoitis G. Mycosis fungoides and follicular mucinosis with very prominent papillomatous and verrucous lesions. *Dermatologica* 1977;**155**:268–274.
349. Kim DJ, Van Truong S, Kraus C, *et al*. A case of acanthosis nigricans-like mycosis fungoides. *J Am Acad Dermatol Case Reports* 2021;**16**:144–148.
350. Puig L, Musulèn E, Fernandez-Figueras MT, *et al*. Mycosis fungoides associated with unusual epidermal hyperplasia. *Clin Experim Dermatol* 1996;**21**:61–64.
351. Neill SM, Monk BE, du Vivier A. Mycosis fungoides associated with acanthosis nigricans. *J Royal Soc Med* 1985;**78**:79–81.
352. Willemze R, Scheffer E, Van Vloten WA. Mycosis fungoides simulating acanthosis nigricans. *Am J Dermatopathol* 1985;**7**:365–371.
353. Wolf P, Cerroni L, Kerl H. Mycosis fungoides mimicking perioral dermatitis. *Clin Exp Dermatol* 1992;**17**:132–134.
354. Torchia D, Miteva M, Hu S, *et al*. Papuloerythroderma 2009: two new cases and systematic review of the worldwide literature 25 years after its identification by Ofuji *et al*. *Dermatology* 2010; **220**:311–320.
355. Huang S, Kim EJ, Lewis DJ, *et al*. Mycosis fungoides occurring at the site of previous herpes zoster eruption. *Australas J Dermatol* 2018;**59**:217–219.
356. Oh CW, Thorne A, Duke T, *et al*. Waistband mycosis fungoides: a new clinical variant of early-stage disease. *Skinmed* 2019;**17**:329–332.
357. Melchers RC, Willemze R, Jansen PM, *et al*. Generalized molluscum contagiosum successfully treated with interferon-alpha in a patient with folliculotropic mycosis fungoides. *Case Rep Dermatol* 2019;**11**:52–56.
358. Modschiedler K, Altenhoff J, Von den Driesch P. Lymphoma molluscatum. *Br J Dermatol* 2002;**146**:529–531.
359. Goerz G, Ilgner M. Disseminated molluscum contagiosum in mycosis fungoides during combined glucocorticoid-antineoplastic therapy. *Hautarzt* 1972;**23**:37–40.
360. Ohata C, Fukuda S, Hashikawa K, *et al*. Molluscum contagiosum with CD30+ cell infiltration in a patient with mycosis fungoides. *Am J Dermatopathol* 2014;**36**:685–687.
361. Torre-Castro J, Postigo C, Machan S, *et al*. Urticarial mycosis fungoides: a distinctive presentation with blood involvement and a peculiar immunophenotype. *J Cutan Pathol* 2024;**51**:649–653.
362. Fink-Puches R, Chott A, Ardigò M, *et al*. The spectrum of cutaneous lymphomas in patients under 20 years of age. *Pediatr Dermatol* 2004;**21**:525–533.

363. Jacob JS, Hunt RD. Increasing incidence of pediatric mycosis fungoides from 2000 to 2017: a national population-based study of the Surveillance, Epidemiology, and End Results database and Texas Cancer Registry. *J Am Acad Dermatol* 2023;**88**:185–187.
364. Wohlmut-Wieser I. Primary cutaneous T-cell lymphomas in childhood and adolescence. *J Deutsch Dermatol Ges* 2021; **19**:563–581.
365. Pope E, Weitzman S, Ngan B, *et al.* Mycosis fungoides in the pediatric population: report from an international childhood registry of cutaneous lymphoma. *J Cut Med Surg* 2010;**14**:1–6.
366. Yazganoglu KD, Topkarci Z, Buyukbabani N, *et al.* Childhood mycosis fungoides: a report of 20 cases from Turkey. *J Eur Acad Dermatol Venereol* 2013;**27**:295–300.
367. Jung JM, Lim DJ, Won CH, *et al.* Mycosis fungoides in children and adolescents. a systematic review. *JAMA Dermatol* 2021;**157**:431–438.
368. Welfringer-Morin A, Barroil M, Fraitag S, *et al.* Clinical features, histological characteristics, and disease outcomes of mycosis fungoides in children and adolescents: a nationwide multicentre cohort of 46 patients. *Dermatology* 2023;**239**:132–139.
369. Kim ST, Sim HJ, Jeon YS, *et al.* Clinicopathological features and T-cell receptor gene rearrangement findings of mycosis fungoides in patients younger than age 20 years. *J Dermatol* 2009;**36**:392–402.
370. Nanda A, AlSaleh QA, Al-Ajmi H, *et al.* Mycosis fungoides in Arab children and adolescents: a report of 36 patients from Kuwait. *Ped Dermatol* 2010;**27**:607–613.
371. Heng YK, Koh AMJ, Giam YC, *et al.* Pediatric mycosis fungoides in Singapore: a series of 46 children. *Ped Dermatol* 2014;**31**:477–482.
372. Peters MS, Thibodeau SN, White JW Jr, Winkelmann RK. Mycosis fungoides in children and adolescents. *J Am Acad Dermatol* 1990;**22**:1011–1018.
373. Poppe H, Kerstan A, Böckers M, *et al.* Childhood mycosis fungoides with a CD8+ CD56+ cytotoxic immunophenotype. *J Cutan Pathol* 2015;**42**:258–264.
374. Rovaris M, Colato C, Girolomoni G. Pediatric CD8+/CD56+ mycosis fungoides with cytotoxic marker expression: a variant with indolent course. *J Cutan Pathol* 2018;**45**:782–785.
375. Boccara O, Blanche S, de Prost Y, *et al.* Cutaneous hematologic disorders in children. *Pediatr Blood Cancer* 2012;**58**:226–232.
376. Quaglino P, Zaccagna A, Verrone A, *et al.* Mycosis fungoides in patients under 20 years of age: report of 7 cases, review of the literature and study of the clinical course. *Dermatology* 1999; **199**:8–14.
377. Zackheim HS, McCalmont TH, Deanovic FW, Odom RB. Mycosis fungoides with onset before 20 years of age. *J Am Acad Dermatol* 1997;**36**:557–562.
378. Crowley JJ, Nikko A, Varghese A, *et al.* Mycosis fungoides in young patients: clinical characteristics and outcome. *J Am Acad Dermatol* 1998;**38**:696–701.
379. Wain EM, Orchard GE, Whittaker SJ, *et al.* Outcome in 34 patients with juvenile-onset mycosis fungoides. A clinical, immunophenotypic, and molecular study. *Cancer* 2003;**98**:2282–2290.
380. Boulos S, Vaid R, Aladily TN, *et al.* Clinical presentation, immunopathology, and treatment of juvenile-onset mycosis fungoides: a case series of 34 patients. *J Am Acad Dermatol* 2014;**71**:1117–1126.
381. Virmani P, Levin L, Myskowski PL, *et al.* Clinical outcome and prognosis of young patients with mycosis fungoides. *Pediatr Dermatol* 2017;**34**:547–553.
382. (a) Zvulunov A, Neale H, Stern J, *et al.* Approach to mycosis fungoides in children (ARMFUL study): consensus-based recommendations. *J Am Acad Dermatol* 2024;**91**:1078–1085.(b) Hodak E, Amitay-Laish I, Bagot M, *et al.* ISCL/EORTC-CLTG/USCLC recommendations for the diagnosis, staging and treatment of early-stage paediatric mycosis fungoides - a modified Delphi consensus. Part 1: diagnosis and staging. *Br J Dermatol* 2025;**193**:405–414. (c) Hodak E, Amitay-Laish I, Bagot M, *et al.* ISCL/EORTC-CLTG/USCLC recommendations for the diagnosis, staging and treatment of early-stage paediatric mycosis fungoides - a modified Delphi consensus. Part 2: treatment. *Br J Dermatol* 2025;**193**:653–661.
383. Willemze R, Hodak E, Zinzani PL, *et al.* Primary cutaneous lymphomas: ESMO Clinical Practice Guidelines for diagnosis, treatment and follow-up. *Ann Oncol* 2018 October 1;**29**(Suppl. 4): iv30–iv40.on behalf of the ESMO Guidelines Committee
384. van Santen S, van Doorn R, Neelis KJ, *et al.* Recommendations for treatment in folliculotropic mycosis fungoides: report of the Dutch Cutaneous Lymphoma Group. *Br J Dermatol* 2017;**177**:223–228.
385. Quaglino P, Maule M, Prince HM, *et al.* Global patterns of care in advanced stage mycosis fungoides/Sezary syndrome: a multicenter retrospective follow-up study from the Cutaneous Lymphoma International Consortium. *Ann Oncol* 2017;**28**:2517–2525.
386. Gilson D, Whittaker SJ, Child FJ, *et al.* British Association of Dermatologists and U.K. Cutaneous Lymphoma Group guidelines for the management of primary cutaneous lymphomas 2018. *Br J Dermatol* 2019;**180**:496–526.
387. Olsen EA, Hodak E, Anderson T, *et al.* Guidelines for phototherapy of mycosis fungoides and Sézary syndrome: a consensus statement of the United States Cutaneous Lymphoma Consortium. *J Am Acad Dermatol* 2016;**74**:27–25.
388. Latzka J, Assaf C, Bagot M, *et al.* EORTC consensus recommendations for the treatment of mycosis fungoides/Sèzary syndrome – update 2023. *Eur J Cancer* 2023;**195**:11343.
389. Dippel E, Assaf C, Becker JC, *et al.* S2k-guidelines – cutaneous lymphomas (ICD10 C82-C86): update 2021. *J Dtsch Dermatol Ges* 2022;**20**:537–555.
390. Olsen EA, Whittaker S, Kim YH, *et al.* Clinical end points and response criteria in mycosis fungoides and Sézary syndrome: a consensus statement of the International Society for Cutaneous Lymphomas, the United States Cutaneous Lymphoma Consortium, and the Cutaneous Lymphoma Task Force of the European Organisation for Research and Treatment of Cancer. *J Clin Oncol* 2011;**29**:2598–2607.
391. Lessin SR, Duvic M, Guitart J, *et al.* Topical chemotherapy in cutaneous T-cell lymphoma. *Arch Dermatol* 2013;**149**:25–32.
392. Tacastacas JD, Chan DV, Carlson S, *et al.* Evaluation of O6-benzylguanine-potentiated topical carmustine for mycosis fungoides: a phase 1–2 clinical trial. *JAMA Dermatol* 2017;**153**:413–420.
393. Alberti-Violetti S, Ardigò M, Fava P, *et al.* Multidisciplinary and personalized approach to the management of mycosis fungoides with chlormethine gel: a collection of clinical experiences. *Drugs Context* 2024;**13**.

394. Assaf C, Booken N, Dippel E, *et al.* The optimal use of chlormethine gel for mycosis fungoides: an expert consensus from Germany, Austria and Switzerland (DACH region). *J Dtsch Dermatol Ges* 2022;**20**:579–586.
395. Rook AH, Gelfand JM, Wysocka M, *et al.* Topical resiquimod can induce disease regression and enhance T-cell effector functions in cutaneous T-cell lymphoma. *Blood* 2015;**126**:1452–1461.
396. Duvic M, Olsen EA, Omura GA, *et al.* A phase III, randomized, double-blind, placebo-controlled study of peldesine (BCX-34) cream as topical therapy for cutaneous T-cell lymphoma. *J Am Acad Dermatol* 2001;**44**:940–947.
397. Trautinger F, Knobler R, Willemze R, *et al.* EORTC consensus recommendations for the treatment of mycosis fungoides/Sézary syndrome. *Eur J Cancer* 2006;**42**:1014–1030.
398. Stadler R, Otte HG, Luger T, *et al.* Prospective randomized multicenter clinical trial on the use of interferon a-2a plus acitretin versus interferon a-2a plus PUVA in patients with cutaneous T-cell lymphoma stages I and II. *Blood* 1998;**92**:3578–3581.
399. Straus DJ, Duvic M, Kuzel T, *et al.* Results of a phase II trial of oral bexarotene (Targretin) combined with interferon alfa-2b (Intron-A) for patients with cutaneous T-cell lymphoma. *Cancer* 2007;**109**:1799–1803.
400. Hansen-Abeck I, Geidel G, Abeck F, *et al.* Pegylated interferon-a2a in cutaneous T-cell lymphoma – a multicenter retrospective data analysis with 70 patients. *J Deutsch Dermatol Ges* 2024;**22**:1489–1498.
401. Mitsunaga K, Bagot M, Ram-Wolff C, *et al.* Real-world study of pegylated interferon α-2a to treat mycosis fungoides/Sézary syndrome using time to next treatment as a measure of clinical benefit: an EORTC CLTG study. *Br J Dermatol* 2024;**191**:419–427.
402. Phan K, Ramachandran V, Fassihi H, Sebaratnam DF. Comparison of narrowband UV-B with psoralen-UV-A phototherapy for patients with early-stage mycosis fungoides: a systematic review and meta-analysis. *JAMA Dermatol* 2019;**155**:335–341.
403. Pavlotsky F, Dawood M, Barzilai A. Potential of narrow-band ultraviolet B to induce sustained durable complete remission off-therapy in patients with stage I mycosis fungoides. *J Am Acad Dermatol* 2019;**80**:1550–1555.
404. Gniadecki R, Assaf C, Bagot M, *et al.* The optimal use of bexarotene in cutaneous T-cell lymphoma. *Br J Dermatol* 2007;**157**:433–440.
405. Duvic M, Hymes K, Heald P, *et al.* Bexarotene is effective and safe for treatment of refractory advanced-stage cutaneous T-cell lymphoma: multinational phase II–III trial results. *J Clin Oncol* 2001;**19**:2456–2471.
406. Whittaker S, Ortiz P, Dummer R, *et al.* Efficacy and safety of bexarotene combined with psoralen-ultraviolet A (PUVA) compared with PUVA treatment alone in stage IB-IIA mycosis fungoides: final results from the EORTC Cutaneous Lymphoma Task Force phase III randomized clinical trial (NCT00056056). *Br J Dermatol* 2012;**167**:678–687.
407. Pileri A, Sgubbi P, Agostinelli C, *et al.* Photodynamic therapy: an option in mycosis fungoides. *Photodiagn Photodyn Ther* 2017;**20**:107–110.
408. Jones GW, Kacinski BM, Wilson LD, *et al.* Total skin electron radiation in the management of mycosis fungoides: consensus of the European Organization for Research and Treatment of Cancer (EORTC) Cutaneous Lymphoma Project Group. *J Am Acad Dermatol* 2002;**47**:364–370.
409. Navi D, Riaz N, Levin YS, *et al.* The Stanford University experience with conventional-dose, total skin electron-beam therapy in the treatment of generalized patch or plaque (T2) and tumor (T3) mycosis fungoides. *Arch Dermatol* 2011;**147**:561–567.
410. Morris S, Scarisbrick J, Frew J, *et al.* The results of low-dose total skin electron beam radiation therapy (TSEB) in patients with mycosis fungoides from the UK cutaneous lymphoma group. *Int J Radiat Oncol Biol Phys* 2017;**99**:627–633.
411. Elsayad K, Guenova E, Assaf C, *et al.* Radiotherapy in cutaneous lymphomas: recommendations from the EORTC cutaneous lymphoma tumour group. *Eur J Cancer* 2024;**212**:115064.
412. Schneeweiss M, Porpaczy E, Koch M, *et al.* Transformed mycosis fungoides: bridging to allogeneic stem cell transplantation with brentuximab vedotin. *Leuk Lymphoma* 2016;**57**:206–208.
413. Scarisbrick JJ. Brentuximab vedotin is an effective therapy for CD30(+) mycosis fungoides and cutaneous anaplastic large-cell lymphoma: what is the cost? *Br J Dermatol* 2017;**177**:1474–1475.
414. Stranzenbach R, Dippel E, Schlaak M, *et al.* Brentuximab vedotin in CD30(+) cutaneous lymphoma: how do we treat, how shall we treat? A review of the literature. *Br J Dermatol* 2017;**177**:1503–1509.
415. Prince HM, Kim YH, Horwitz SM, *et al.* Brentuximab vedotin or physician's choice in CD30-positive cutaneous T-cell lymphoma (ALCANZA): an international, open-label, randomised, phase 3, multicentre trial. *Lancet* 2017;**390**:555–566.
416. Mahévas T, Ram-Wolff C, Battistella M, *et al.* Dramatic response to brentuximab vedotin in refractory nontransformed CD30- mycosis fungoides allowing allogeneic stem cell transplant and long-term complete remission. *Br J Dermatol* 2019;**180**:1517–1520.
417. Zhang C, Chairatchaneeboon M, Haun P, *et al.* Treatment of CD30-negative refractory mycosis fungoides with brentuximab vedotin. *JAMA Dermatol* 2018;**154**:109–110.
418. Whittaker S, Hoppe R, Prince HM. How I treat mycosis fungoides and Sezary syndrome. *Blood* 2016;**127**:3142–3153.
419. Khodadoust MS, Mou E, Kim YH. Integrating novel agents into the treatment of advanced mycosis fungoides and Sézary syndrome. *Blood* 2023;**141**:695–703.
420. Chen L, Carson KR, Staser KW, *et al.* Mogamulizumab-associated cutaneous granulomatous drug eruption mimicking mycosis fungoides but possibly indicating durable clinical response. *JAMA Dermatol* 2019;**155**:968–971.
421. Prince HM, Duvic M, Martin A, *et al.* Incidence of spontaneous remission in patients with CD25-positive mycosis fungoides/Sezary syndrome receiving placebo. *J Am Acad Dermatol* 2012;**67**:867–875.
422. Whittaker SJ, Demierre MF, Kim EJ, *et al.* Final results from a multicenter, international, pivotal study of Romidepsin in refractory cutaneous T-cell lymphoma. *J Clin Oncol* 2010;**28**:4485–4491.
423. Duvic M, Bates SE, Piekarz R, *et al.* Responses to romidepsin in patients with cutaneous T-cell lymphoma and prior treatment with systemic chemotherapy. *Leuk Lymphoma* 2018;**59**:880–887.
424. Deschamps O, Ram-Wolff C, Beylot-Barry M, *et al.* Treatment of mycosis fungoides and Sézary syndrome with romidepsin: a series of 32 cases from the French Study Group for Cutaneous Lymphoma. *Br J Dermatol* 2019;**180**:423–424.
425. Duvic M, Talpur R, Ni X, *et al.* Phase 2 trial of oral vorinostat (suberoylanilide hydroxamic acid, SAHA) for refractory cutaneous T-cell lymphoma (CTCL). *Blood* 2007;**109**:31–39.

426. Child F, Ortiz-Romero PL, Alvarez R, *et al.* Phase II multicentre trial of oral quisinostat, a histone deacetylase inhibitor, in patients with previously treated stage IB-IVA mycosis fungoides/Sezary syndrome. *Br J Dermatol* 2016;**175**:80–88.
427. Boonstra PS, Polk A, Brown N, *et al.* A single center phase II study of ixazomib in patients with relapsed or refractory cutaneous or peripheral T-cell lymphomas. *Am J Hematol* 2017;**92**:1287–1294.
428. Zinzani PL, Venturini F, Stefoni V, *et al.* Gemcitabine as single agent in pretreated T-cell lymphoma patients: evaluation of the long-term outcome. *Ann Oncol* 2010;**21**:860–863.
429. Quereux G, Marques S, Nguyen JM, *et al.* Prospective multicenter study of pegylated liposomal doxorubicin treatment in patients with advanced or refractory mycosis fungoides or Sezary syndrome. *Arch Dermatol* 2008;**144**:727–733.
430. Querfeld C, Rosen ST, Guitart J, *et al.* Results of an open-label multicenter phase 2 trial of lenalidomide monotherapy in refractory mycosis fungoides and Sézary syndrome. *Blood* 2014;**123**:1159–1166.
431. Sugaya M, Tokura Y, Hamada T, *et al.* Phase II study of i.v. interferon-gamma in Japanese patients with mycosis fungoides. *J Dermatol* 2014;**41**:50–56.
432. Foss F, Demierre MF, DiVenuti G. A phase-1 trial of bexarotene and denileukin diftitox in patients with relapsed or refractory cutaneous T-cell lymphoma. *Blood* 2005;**106**:454–457.
433. Wu J, Wood GS. Reduction of Fas/CD95 promoter methylation, upregulation of Fas protein, and enhancement of sensitivity to apoptosis in cutaneous T-cell lymphoma. *Arch Dermatol* 2011;**147**:443–449.
434. Lundin J, Hagberg H, Repp R, *et al.* Phase 2 study of alemtuzumab (anti-CD52 monoclonal antibody) in patients with advanced mycosis fungoides/Sézary syndrome. *Blood* 2003;**101**:4267–4272.
435. Kim YH, Duvic M, Obitz E, *et al.* Clinical efficacy of zanolimumab (HuMax-CD4): two phase 2 studies in refractory cutaneous T-cell lymphoma. *Blood* 2007;**109**:4655–4662.
436. Khodadoust MS, Rook AH, Porcu P, *et al.* Pembrolizumab in relapsed and refractory mycosis fungoides and Sézary syndrome: a multicenter phase II study. *J Clin Oncol* 2020;**38**:20–28.
437. Froehlich TC, Müller-Decker K, Braun JD, *et al.* Combined inhibition of Bcl-2 and NFκB synergistically induces cell death in cutaneous T-cell lymphoma. *Blood* 2019;**134**:445–455.
438. Karagianni F, Piperi C, Valero-Diaz S, *et al.* Combination of JAKi and HDACi exerts antiangiogenic potential in cutaneous T-cell lymphoma. *Cancers (Basel)* 2024;**16**:3176.
439. Scarisbrick JJ, Taylor P, Holtick U, *et al.* U.K. consensus statement on the use of extracorporeal photopheresis for treatment of cutaneous T-cell lymphoma and chronic graft-versus-host disease. *Br J Dermatol* 2008;**158**:659–678.
440. (a) King BJ, Lester SC, Tolkachjov SN, *et al.* Skin-directed radiation therapy for cutaneous lymphoma: the mayo clinic experience. *J Am Acad Dermatol* 2020;**82**:634–641.(b) Kersten JM, Ottevanger R, Rademakers SE, *et al.* Modified recommendations for the radiation dose in patients with mycosis fungoides and localised lesional disease based on a retrospective analysis of treatment outcomes. Pract. *Radiat Oncol* 2025;**S1879-8500**(25):00167–00165. doi: 10.1016/j.prro.2025.06.006. Online ahead of print.
441. Kim YH, Gratzinger D, Harrison C, *et al.* In situ vaccination against mycosis fungoides by intratumoral injection of a TLR9 agonist combined with radiation: a phase 1/2 study. *Blood* 2012;**119**:355–363.
442. Maier T, Tun-Kyi A, Tassis A, *et al.* Vaccination of patients with cutaneous T-cell lymphoma using intranodal injection of autologous tumor-lysate-pulsed dendritic cells. *Blood* 2003;**102**: 2338–2344.
443. Heinzerling L, Künzi V, Oberholzer PA, *et al.* Oncolytic measles virus in cutaneous T-cell lymphomas mounts antitumor immune responses in vivo and targets interferon-resistant tumor cells. *Blood* 2005;**106**:2287–2294.
444. Soligo D, Ibatici A, Berti E, *et al.* Treatment of advanced mycosis fungoides by allogeneic stem-cell transplantation with a nonmyeloablative regimen. *Bone Marrow Trans* 2003;**31**:663–666.
445. Guitart J, Wickless SC, Oyama Y, *et al.* Long-term remission after allogeneic hematopoietic stem cell transplantation for refractory cutaneous T-cell lymphoma. *Arch Dermatol* 2002;**138**:1359–1365.
446. Introcaso CE, Leber B, Greene K, *et al.* Stem cell transplantation in advanced cutaneous T-cell lymphoma. *J Am Acad Dermatol* 2008;**58**:645–649.
447. Molina A, Zain J, Arber DA, *et al.* Durable clinical, cytogenetic, and molecular remissions after allogeneic hematopoietic cell transplantation for refractory Sezary syndrome and mycosis fungoides. *J Clin Oncol* 2005;**23**:6163–6171.
448. Duarte RF, Canals C, Onida F, *et al.* Allogeneic hematopoietic cell transplantation for patients with mycosis fungoides and Sezary syndrome: a retrospective analysis of the Lymphoma Working Party of the European Group for Blood and Marrow Transplantation. *J Clin Oncol* 2010;**28**:4492–4499.
449. Jacobsen ED, Kim HT, Ho VT, *et al.* A large single-center experience with allogeneic stem-cell transplantation for peripheral T-cell non-Hodgkin lymphoma and advanced mycosis fungoides/ Sezary syndrome. *Ann Oncol* 2011;**22**:1608–1613.
450. Wu PA, Kim YH, Lavori PW, *et al.* A meta-analysis of patients receiving allogeneic or autologous hematopoietic stem cell transplant in mycosis fungoides and Sézary syndrome. *Biol Blood Marrow Transplant* 2009;**15**:982–990.
451. Shiratori S, Fujimoto K, Nishimura M, *et al.* Allogeneic hematopoietic stem cell transplantation following reduced-intensity conditioning for mycosis fungoides and Sezary syndrome. *Hematol Oncol* 2016;**34**:9–16.
452. Hosing C, Bassett R, Dabaja B, *et al.* Allogeneic stem-cell transplantation in patients with cutaneous lymphoma: updated results from a single institution. *Ann Oncol* 2015;**26**:2490–2495.
453. Virmani P, Zain J, Rosen ST, *et al.* Hematopoietic stem cell transplant for mycosis fungoides and Sézary syndrome. *Dermatol Clin* 2015;**33**:807–818.
454. Oka T, Sugaya M, Cury-Martins J, *et al.* Hematopoietic stem cell transplantation for cutaneous T-cell lymphoma: summary of 11 cases from two facilities in Japan and Brazil. *J Dermatol* 2016;**43**:638–642.
455. Saruta H, Ohata C, Muto I, *et al.* Hematopoietic stem cell transplantation in advanced cutaneous T-cell lymphoma. *J Dermatol* 2017;**44**:1038–1042.
456. Atilla E, Atilla PA, Bozdag SC, *et al.* Allogeneic hematopoietic stem cell transplantation for refractory mycosis fungoides (MF) and Sezary syndrome (SS). *Int J Hematol* 2017;**106**:426–430.
457. Kharfan-Dabaja MA, Kumar A, Ayala E, *et al.* Clinical practice recommendations on indication and timing of hematopoietic

cell transplantation in mature T cell and NK/T cell lymphomas: an international collaborative effort on behalf of the Guidelines Committee of the American Society for Blood and Marrow Transplantation. *Biol Blood Marrow Transplant* 2017;**23**: 1826–1838.
458. Duarte RF, Boumendil A, Onida F, *et al.* Long-term outcome of allogeneic hematopoietic cell transplantation for patients with mycosis fungoides and Sézary syndrome: a European society for blood and marrow transplantation lymphoma working party extended analysis. *J Clin Oncol* 2014;**32**:3347–3348.
459. de Masson A, Beylot-Barry M, Bouaziz JD, *et al.* Allogeneic stem cell transplantation for advanced cutaneous T-cell lymphomas: a study from the French Society of Bone Marrow Transplantation and French Study Group on Cutaneous Lymphomas. *Haematologica* 2014;**99**:527–534.
460. Lechowicz MJ, Lazarus HM, Carreras J, *et al.* Allogeneic hematopoietic cell transplantation for mycosis fungoides and Sezary syndrome. *Bone Marrow Transplant* 2014;**49**:1360–1365.
461. de Masson A, Beylot-Barry M, Ram-Wolff C, *et al.* Allogeneic transplantation in advanced cutaneous T-cell lymphomas (CUTALLO): a propensity score matched controlled prospective study. *Lancet* 2023;**401**:1941–1950.
462. Novelli S, Monter A, Pilar García-Muret M, *et al.* Discussion on the indication of allogeneic stem cell transplantation for advanced cutaneous T cell lymphomas. *Int J Hematol* 2019;**110**:406–410.
463. (a) Goyal A, O'Leary D, Dabaja B, *et al.* ASTCT and USCLC clinical practice recommendations for allogeneic stem cell transplant in mycosis fungoides and Sézary syndrome. *Transplant Cell Ther* 2024;**30**:1047–1050.(b) Goyal A, O'Leary D, Dabaja B, *et al.* ASTCT and USCLC clinical practice recommendations for allogeneic stem cell transplant in mycosis fungoides and Sézary syndrome. *J Am Acad Dermatol* 2025;**93**:387–397.
464. Hill LC, Rouce RH, Wu MJ, *et al.* Antitumor efficacy and safety of unedited autologous CD5.CAR T cells in relapsed/refractory mature T-cell lymphomas. *Blood* 2024;**143**:1231–1241.
465. Grover NS, Beaven AW. T-cell lymphoma: the CAR-T revolution is coming. *Blood* 2024;**143**:1201–1202.
466. Watanabe K, Gomez AM, Kuramitsu S, *et al.* Identifying highly active anti-CCR4 CAR T cells for the treatment of T-cell lymphoma. *Blood Adv* 2023;**7**:3416–3430.
467. Mitteldorf C, Stadler R, Sander CA, *et al.* Folliculotropic mycosis fungoides. *J Dtsch Dermatol Ges* 2018;**16**:543–557.
468. Jennings L, Campbell SM, Yaar R, *et al.* Generalized syringotropic mycosis fungoides responsive to extracorporeal photopheresis. *Br J Dermatol* 2014;**170**:200–202.
469. Lindahl LM, Willerslev-Olsen A, Gjerdrum LMR, *et al.* Antibiotics inhibit tumor and disease activity in cutaneous T cell lymphoma. *Blood* 2019;**134**:1072–1083.
470. LeBon B, Beynon TA, Whittaker SJ. Palliative care in patients with primary cutaneous lymphoma: symptom burden and characteristics of hospital palliative care team input. *Arch Dermatol* 2007;**143**:423–424.
471. Demierre MF, Tien A, Miller D. Health-related quality-of-life assessment in patients with cutaneous T-cell lymphoma. *Arch Dermatol* 2005;**141**:325–330.
472. Maronas-Jimenez L, Estrach T, Gallardo F, *et al.* Aprepitant improves refractory pruritus in primary cutaneous T-cell lymphomas: experience of the Spanish Working Group on Cutaneous Lymphomas. *Br J Dermatol* 2018;**178**:e273–e274.
473. Mourad A, Gniadecki R. Overall survival in mycosis fungoides: a systematic review and meta-analysis. *J Invest Dermatol* 2020;**140**:495–497.
474. van Doorn R, van Haselen CW, van Voorst Vader PC, *et al.* Mycosis fungoides. Disease evaluation and prognosis of 309 Dutch patients. *Arch Dermatol* 2000;**136**:504–510.
475. Quaglino P, Pimpinelli N, Berti E, *et al.* Time course, clinical pathways, and long-term hazards risk trends of disease progression in patients with classic mycosis fungoides. *Cancer* 2012;**118**: 5830–5839.
476. Sun G, Berthelot C, Li Y, *et al.* Poor prognosis in non-Caucasian patients with early-onset mycosis fungoides. *J Am Acad Dermatol* 2009;**60**:231–235.
477. Su C, Nguyen KA, Bai HX, *et al.* Racial disparity in mycosis fungoides: an analysis of 4495 cases from the US National Cancer Database. *J Am Acad Dermatol* 2017;**77**:497–502.
478. Geller S, Lebowitz E, Pulitzer MP, *et al.* Outcomes and prognostic factors in African American/black patients with mycosis fungoides and sezary syndrome: retrospective analysis of 157 patients from a referral cancer center. *J Am Acad Dermatol* 2020;**83**:430–439.
479. Scarisbrick JJ, Prince HM, Vermeer MH, *et al.* Cutaneous Lymphoma International Consortium study of outcome in advanced stages of mycosis fungoides and Sézary syndrome: effect of specific prognostic markers on survival and development of a prognostic model. *J Clin Oncol* 2015;**33**: 3766–3773.
480. Vural S, Akay BN, Botsali A, *et al.* Transformation of mycosis fungoides/Sezary syndrome: clinical characteristics and prognosis. *Turk J Haematol* 2018;**35**:35–41.
481. Diamandidou E, Colome-Grimmer MI, Fayad L, *et al.* Transformation of mycosis fungoides/Sézary syndrome: clinical characteristics and prognosis. *Blood* 1998;**92**:1150–1159.
482. (a)Arulogun SO, Prince HM, Ng J, *et al.* Long-term outcomes of patients with advanced-stage cutaneous T-cell lymphoma and large cell transformation. *Blood* 2008;**112**:3082–3087.(b) Kersten JM, Ottevanger R, Quint KD, *et al.* Prognosis of increasing percentages of lesional body surface area in early stage mycosis fungoides. *J Eur Acad Dermatol Venereol* 2025. doi: 10.1111/jdv.20773. Online ahead of print.
483. Villarreal AM, Gantchev J, Lagacé F, *et al.* Hypopigmented mycosis fungoides: Loss of pigmentation reflects antitumor immune response in young patients. *Cancers (Basel)* 2020;**12**:2007.
484. Benton EC, Crichton S, Talpur R, *et al.* A cutaneous lymphoma international prognostic index (CLIPi) for mycosis fungoides and Sézary syndrome. *Eur J Cancer* 2013;**49**:2859–2868.
485. (a) Sanz-Bueno J, Lora D, Monsalvez V, *et al.* The new Cutaneous Lymphoma International Prognostic index (CLIPi) for early mycosis fungoides failed to identify prognostic groups in a cohort of Spanish patients. *Br J Dermatol* 2016;**175**:794–796.(b) Scarisbrick JJ, Quaglino P, Whittaker SJ, *et al.* A new prognostic index (CLIPI) for advanced cutaneous lymphoma enables precise patient risk stratification. *Blood* 2025. doi: 10.1182/blood.2025029628. Online ahead of print.
486. Evans KG, Troxel AB, DeNardo BJ, *et al.* Validity assessment of the cutaneous T-cell lymphoma severity index to predict prognosis in

advanced mycosis fungoides/Sézary syndrome. *J Am Acad Dermatol* 2011;**64**:682–689.

487. Fraser-Andrews E, Woolford AJ, Russell-Jones R, *et al.* Detection of a peripheral blood T cell clone is an independent prognostic marker in mycosis fungoides. *J Invest Dermatol* 2000;**114**:117–121.
488. Hutchinson CB, Stoecker M, Wang FF, *et al.* Molecular detection of circulating Sezary cells in patients with mycosis fungoides. Could it predict future development of secondary Sezary syndrome? A single institution experience. *Leuk Lymphoma* 2012;**53**:868–877.
489. Hurabielle C, Ingen-Housz-Oro S, Ortonne N, *et al.* Frequency and prognostic value of cutaneous molecular residual disease in mycosis fungoides: a prospective multicentre trial of the Cutaneous Lymphoma French Study Group. *Br J Dermatol* 2015;**173**:1015–1023.
490. Vonderheid EC, Pavlov I, Delgado JC, *et al.* Prognostic factors and risk stratification in early mycosis fungoides. *Leuk Lymphoma* 2014;**55**:44–50.
491. Smoller BR, Detwiler SP, Kohler S, *et al.* Role of histology in providing prognostic informations in mycosis fungoides. *J Cutan Pathol* 1998;**25**:311–315.
492. Boonk SE, Putter H, Koolhof L, *et al.* Quantitation of tumour development correlates with prognosis in tumour stage (stage IIB) mycosis fungoides. *Br J Dermatol* 2014;**170**:1080–1086.
493. Salgado R, Servitje O, Gallardo F, *et al.* Oligonucleotide array – CGH identifies genomic subgroups and prognostic markers for tumor stage mycosis fungoides. *J Invest Dermatol* 2010;**130**:1126–1135.
494. Laharanne E, Chevret E, Idrissi Y, *et al.* CDKN2A–CDKN2B deletion defines an aggressive subset of cutaneous T-cell lymphoma. *Mod Pathol* 2010;**23**:547–558.
495. Nicolae-Cristea AR, Benner MF, Zoutman WH, *et al.* Diagnostic and prognostic significance of CDKN2A/CDKN2B deletions in patients with transformed mycosis fungoides and primary cutaneous CD30-positive lymphoproliferative disease. *Br J Dermatol* 2015;**172**:784–788.
496. Ferrara G, Pancione M, Votino C, *et al.* A specific DNA methylation profile correlates with a high risk of disease progression in stage I classical (Alibert-Bazin type) mycosis fungoides. *Br J Dermatol* 2014;**170**:1266–1275.
497. (a) Kamijo H, Miyagaki T, Shishido-Takahashi N, *et al.* Aberrant CD137 ligand expression induced by GATA6 overexpression promotes tumor progression in cutaneous T-cell lymphoma. *Blood* 2018;**132**(18):1922–1935.(b) Choi ME, Kim G, Shin HJ, *et al.* Spatial transcriptomics of progression gene signature and tumor microenvironment leading to progression in mycosis fungoides. *Blood Adv* 2025;**9**:2871–2885.
498. Murray D, McMurray JL, Eldershaw S, *et al.* Progression of mycosis fungoides occurs through divergence of tumor immunophenotype by differential expression of HLA-DR. *Blood Adv* 2019;**3**:519–530.

## CHAPTER 4

# Sézary syndrome

Sézary syndrome is characterized clinically by pruritic erythroderma, generalized lymphadenopathy, and the presence of circulating malignant T lymphocytes (Sézary cells). Other typical cutaneous changes include palmoplantar hyperkeratosis, alopecia, and onychodystrophy. The syndrome is named after the French dermatologist Albert Sézary, who reported the first patient together with Dr. Yves Bouvrain in 1938 describing a 58-year-old man with "erythroderma with the presence of monstrous cells in dermis and circulation" [1–3]. Sézary subsequently reported further patients and expanded his original description in a series of publications between 1938 and 1949, including the disease among the "reticulosis" (the term used at that time for lymphoproliferative disorders), and stating that it differed from mycosis fungoides [4].

In the International Consensus Classification (ICC) *of Myeloid and Lymphoid Neoplasms*, the 2019 and 2024 updates of classification of cutaneous lymphomas by the European Organization of Research and Treatment of Cancer (EORTC) – Cutaneous Lymphoma Histopathology Group, and the World Health Organization (WHO) *Classification of Haematolymphoid Tumours*, Sézary syndrome is considered as a specific type of T-cell lymphoma, clearly separated from mycosis fungoides [5–8]. In fact, there is a sufficient body of evidence showing that the two diseases represent distinct entities [9, 10]. However, in the WHO *Classification of Haematolymphoid Tumours*, Sézary syndrome is not included in the specific section on cutaneous T-cell lymphomas, a decision that to my eyes is debatable. In the context of the knowledge accumulated over the last decades, it is very unfortunate that many studies, including recent ones, refer to "cutaneous T-cell lymphomas" lumping together cases of mycosis fungoides and Sézary syndrome, and sometimes of other unrelated entities.

The differential diagnosis of erythroderma is considered one of the most vexing problems in dermatology and dermatopathology, and differentiation of Sézary syndrome from non-neoplastic erythroderma may be sometimes impossible [11]. The main causes of erythroderma, besides Sézary syndrome and mycosis fungoides, are atopic dermatitis, psoriasis, and drug reactions, but less frequently other cutaneous inflammatory disorders (and other T-cell lymphomas/leukemias) may present with erythrodermic features as well [12]. In some cases, the precise cause cannot be determined and only a descriptive diagnosis is used ("idiopathic erythroderma," "homme rouge," and "red man syndrome"). For a thorough discussion on differential diagnosis of erythroderma, see the section on non-neoplastic erythroderma in adult patients in Chapter 31. Erythrodermic mycosis fungoides (i.e., erythroderma developing in patients with a previous history of mycosis fungoides) should be distinguished from true Sézary syndrome (see Chapter 3) [5–8]. Several blood markers have been studied in order to distinguish cases of erythrodermic mycosis fungoides or inflammatory erythroderma from those of Sézary syndrome, showing that T-plastin, Twist, and killer cell immunoglobulin-like receptor, three Ig domains and long cytoplasmic tail 2 (KIR3DL2) were associated with Sézary syndrome [13]. Another study on the development of tumor cells showed that Sézary cells are T-helper lymphocytes distinct from those observed in patches, plaques, and tumors of mycosis fungoides [14].

In the past, different diagnostic criteria have been used in studies on Sézary syndrome, hindering comparison of published data. The demonstration of the same monoclonal population of T lymphocytes within the peripheral blood and the skin is considered a crucial criterion for the diagnosis of Sézary syndrome [5–8, 15], combined with an expanded $CD4^+$ population in the peripheral blood resulting in a markedly increased ratio of CD4:CD8 ($\geq$10), and with an increased population in the peripheral blood of $\geq$1000/µL $CD4^+/CD7^-$ or $CD4^+/CD26^-$ cells (or cells with other aberrant phenotype) [5–8, 15, 16]. Blood criteria for the diagnosis of Sézary syndrome and for defining blood involvement in mycosis fungoides have been published by the EORTC [16]. Manual counts of Sézary cells are highly subjective and are being largely replaced by flow cytometry, which provides more objective data [16]. Recent data showed the remarkable plasticity of neoplastic cells in Sézary syndrome, showing that immunophenotypically distinct populations of neoplastic cells are clonally related [17], and explaining some of the difficulties that may be encountered in establishing a precise diagnosis. These new insights may support a revision of criteria for the diagnosis of blood involvement in Sézary syndrome, and provide a better understanding

*Skin Lymphoma: The Illustrated Guide*, Sixth Edition. Lorenzo Cerroni.

for informed treatment decisions [18]. New data suggest also that the study of CD158k and PD-1 expression by leukemic cells may also be helpful in the subclassification of the disease and the selection of proper treatment according to the presence of a $CD158k^+$, $CD158k^-/PD\text{-}1^+$, or $CD158k^-/PD\text{-}1^-$ phenotype [19]. As erythroderma may develop in different inflammatory conditions, and as neoplastic erythroderma may be observed in other cutaneous lymphomas such as mycosis fungoides and T-cell prolymphocytic leukemia, it is important that strict criteria for the diagnosis of Sézary syndrome are used. The presence of clonal T-cells within the peripheral blood alone should not prompt a diagnosis of Sézary syndrome. In fact, detection in the peripheral blood of a T-cell clone without clinical significance is not infrequent in elderly patients, and only the finding of identical clones in the blood and skin together with typical aberrations demonstrated by flow cytometry is considered diagnostic.

The use of standardized end points and response criteria is necessary, too, in order to compare the efficacy of various therapeutic agents on data collected at multiple sites and/or at different time points. The International Society for Cutaneous Lymphomas (ISCL), the United States Cutaneous Lymphoma Consortium (USCLC), and the EORTC–Cutaneous Lymphoma Task Force have published a consensus statement on standardized end point and response criteria [20]. Complete response in the skin is defined as 100% clearance of skin lesions, partial response as 50–99% clearance without new tumors, stable disease as <25% increase to <50% clearance in skin disease without new tumors, and progressive disease as ≥25% increase in skin disease or new tumors [20]. Several end points have been defined, including the objective response rate, time to response, response duration, time to relapse/freedom from relapse, time to treatment failure/freedom from treatment failure, time to progression, progression-free survival, disease-free survival, and relapse-free survival [20].

A staging classification system for mycosis fungoides and Sézary syndrome was proposed by a joint working group of the ISCL and the EORTC–Cutaneous Lymphoma Task Force (see Chapter 1, Table 1.2) [21]. This system has been validated by a study on large numbers of patients [22]. A slightly modified system has been subsequently developed together with the USLCL [23, 24]. Erythroderma (defined as confluence of erythema covering ≥80% of the body surface area) is classified as T4 (corresponding to stages III and IV), and further stage determination is achieved according to the lymph nodes and blood status. The criteria used for quantifying blood involvement are summarized in Table 4.1 (see also Chapter 1, Table 1.2):

**Table 4.1** Values used for quantifying blood burden in patients with Sézary syndrome (see also Chapter 1, Table 1.2) [16, 23, 24].

| | |
|---|---|
| $B_0$ | Absence of significant blood involvement: ≤250/μL of $CD4^+/CD26^-$ or $CD4^+/CD7^-$ cells |
| | $B_{0a}$ Clone negative or equivocal |
| | $B_{0b}$ Clone positive and identical to skin |
| $B_1$ | Low blood tumor burden: does not meet the criteria for $B_0$ or $B_2$ |
| | $B_{1a}$ Clone negative or equivocal |
| | $B_{1b}$ Clone positive and identical to skin |
| $B_2$ | High blood tumor burden: ≥1000/mL of $CD4^+/CD26^-$ or $CD4^+/CD7^-$ cells or other aberrant population of lymphocytes identified by flow cytometry |
| | $B_{2a}$ Clone negative or equivocal |
| | $B_{2b}$ Clone positive and identical to skin |
| $B_X$ | Unable to quantify blood involvement according to agreed-upon guidelines |
| | $B_{Xa}$ Clone negative or equivocal |
| | $B_{Xb}$ Clone positive and identical to skin |

Although the ISCL/EORTC blood staging classification system is generally used for Sézary syndrome, a recent study conducted at a single institution showed that it failed to identify patients with low blood burden, suggesting that inclusion of percentages of $CD4^+/CD7^-$ and $CD4^+/CD26^-$ populations rather than absolute count, as well as of CD4:CD8 ratio of ≥10 in addition to absolute value thresholds may improve sensitivity and specificity [25].

A severity index that assigns different scores to various categories (body surface area, number of tumors, lymph node status, atypical cells in the peripheral blood, and visceral involvement) has been proposed as a tool for measuring disease activity [26]. Although numbers may be useful in assessing disease extent and activity, at the same time, they convey a sense of precision that in some cases may be an oversimplification.

One of the main aspects of Sézary syndrome is the profound alteration of the immune system typical of the disease [27]. An increase in the tumor burden correlates with a decline in multiple arms of the cellular immune response, including natural killer (NK) and cytotoxic T lymphocytes implicated in the antitumoral activity. NK cells and cytotoxic T lymphocytes may also be impaired by the production of interleukin (IL)-10 and transforming growth factor-β (TGFβ) by the tumor cells. The number of myeloid dendritic cells and plasmacytoid dendritic cells is reduced in the peripheral blood, and lack of CD40 ligand expression by neoplastic cells may further contribute to the reduced antitumoral activity and impaired function of the immune system. The immune alterations are reversible upon successful treatment, and normalization occurs if patients achieve complete remission. Due to the severe alterations of the immune system just mentioned, patients with Sézary syndrome have an increased risk of both serious infections and development of further malignancies [28, 29].

The etiology of Sézary syndrome is unknown, and its pathogenesis is only partly understood. An association with viral infections has been postulated in the past, but ruled out in several studies. Although the disease may rarely develop in patients with long-standing inflammatory skin conditions, this association should be considered fortuitous and does not represent a link between Sézary syndrome and other cutaneous diseases. Sézary cells have a mature, memory phenotype with a type 2 helper T-cell (Th2) cytokine profile (characterized by the expression of IL-4, IL-5, and IL-10). The IL-13 and its signaling mediators IL-13Rα1 and IL-13Rα2 are highly expressed in the involved skin of patients with Sézary syndrome, representing potential therapeutic targets for intervention [30]. The vast majority of cases show a high expression of the skin-homing T-cell chemokine receptor 4 (CCR4) [31]. As Sézary cells proliferate poorly, their accumulation in affected tissues may be due to defective T-cell homeostasis involving resistance to apoptosis rather than to increased cell division. Nonfunctional p53 has been detected in several cases [32], and one case with a complex p53 gene mutation has been observed in a Chernobyl survivor, suggesting a possible relationship with environmental factors [33]. Downregulation of the *FAS* gene expression has been demonstrated in several studies, again pointing to a disturbance in the T-cell homeostasis [34–36]. T-plastin, associated with resistance to apoptosis, is expressed in blood lymphocytes of Sézary syndrome but not in those of mycosis fungoides or in healthy individuals, suggesting a role of this molecule in the pathogenesis of the disease [37, 38]. Bacteria may play a direct role in the progression of the disease, and bacterial isolates from the affected skin contain staphylococcal enterotoxin A (SEA) and recombinant SEA, stimulating the activation of signal transducer and activator of transcription 3 (STAT3), and upregulating IL-17 in T cells, thus activating an oncogenic pathway in Sézary syndrome [39]. Recently, it has been suggested that a GATA6/CD137L axis plays a role in tumorigenesis in Sézary syndrome and mycosis fungoides; the overexpression of GATA6 induces aberrant CD137L expression on neoplastic cells, resulting in a CD137-CD137L interaction that promotes cell proliferation and migration [40].

Recent data suggest that neoplastic cells in Sézary syndrome may derive from mutated lymphocyte progenitors that acquire the T-cell receptors (TCRs) in the thymus, and subsequently complete the malignant transformation in the periphery [41]. On the other hand, another study demonstrated the presence of UV signature in cases of Sézary syndrome, suggesting that the disease originates from skin-resident T lymphocytes [42]. Interestingly, in this study, a possible connection between mycosis fungoides, leukemic mycosis fungoides, and Sézary syndrome has been demonstrated, suggesting that the diseases may lie on a continuum, with positive selection of structural variants during leukemogenesis [42].

## Onset/progression under systemic therapies for benign inflammatory dermatoses

As already discussed for mycosis fungoides, Sézary syndrome, too, may arise under systemic therapies for inflammatory dermatoses (either as progression of an undiagnosed dermatosis, or as a lymphoma developing within an immunological altered milieu). Progression occurs especially after antitumor necrosis factor-α therapy. Although mycosis fungoides is more frequent in this setting, a few cases of Sézary syndrome have been described as well [43, 44]. For a detailed discussion on the relationship between systemic biological therapies and onset or unmasking of cutaneous lymphomas, see Chapter 3.

## Clinical features

Sézary syndrome is a rare malignant T-cell lymphoma affecting elderly adults of both genders, with a predilection for males. Patients usually present with an abrupt onset of erythroderma and lymph node enlargement (Fig. 4.1), but itchy eczematous patches indistinguishable from those of an inflammatory condition may be present for some time before erythroderma develops ("prodromic phase"); in some patients, erythroderma may never develop (Fig. 4.2). Large skin folds (groins, axillae) may be spared (Fig. 4.3). In long-standing lesions, lichenification may be observed focally, similar to what is seen in chronic eczematous dermatoses (Fig. 4.4). Even in advanced disease, the clinical presentation may be similar to that of a chronic eczematous dermatitis, due to the presence of scratching artifacts and erosive lesions as the result of the combination of skin fragility and vigorous scratching (Fig. 4.5); focal impetiginization

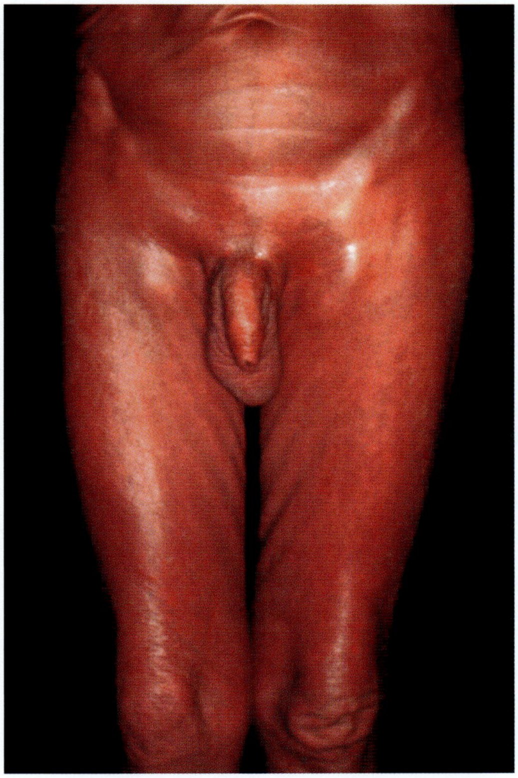

**Figure 4.1** Sézary syndrome. Erythroderma with enlarged inguinal lymph nodes.

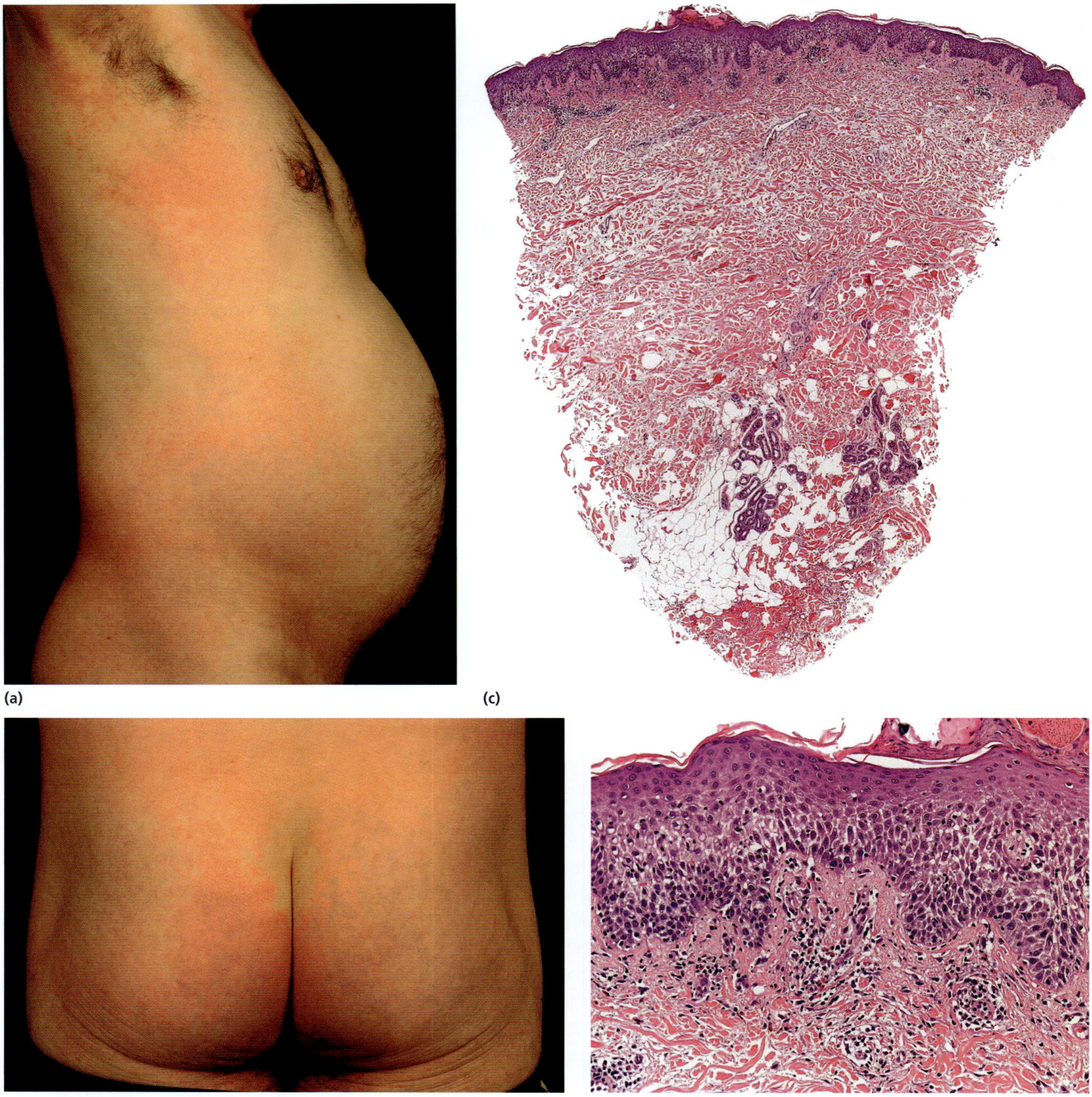

(a) (c) (b) (d)

**Figure 4.2** Sézary syndrome presenting as an "eczematous" dermatitis. (a, b) Itchy eczematous lesions of a few weeks' duration in a 52-year-old man. Histology (c, d) showed irregular epidermal hyperplasia with prominent spongiosis and parakeratosis, and a sparse superficial lymphohistiocytic infiltrate admixed with several eosinophils. The patient subsequently developed palmar hyperkeratosis (e) and onychodystrophy, but (f) was still not erythrodermic. New biopsies over a time of 3 years showed spongiotic features similar to the first one, while other ones (g, h, i) were characterized by a band-like infiltrate with some intraepidermal lymphocytes. Blood examination revealed features consistent with Sézary syndrome ($B_2$ involvement). The patient was treated with extracorporeal photopheresis with only partial response, and eventually succumbed to complications of Sézary syndrome 7 years after the first presentation, without having ever developed erythroderma.

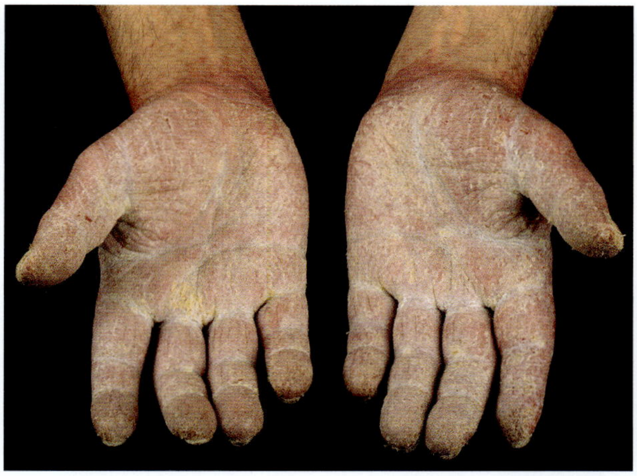

(e)

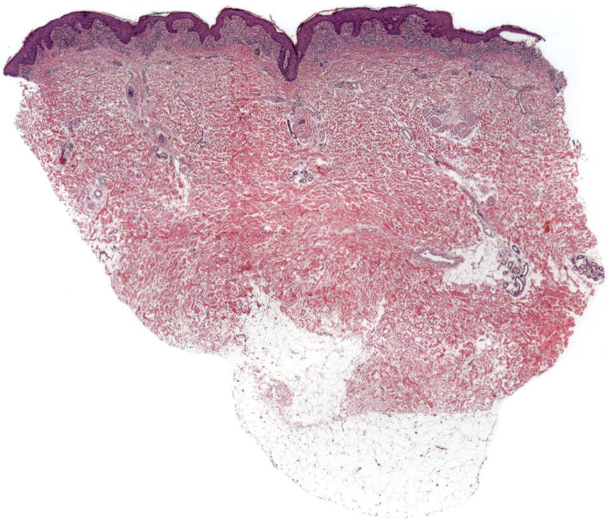

(g)

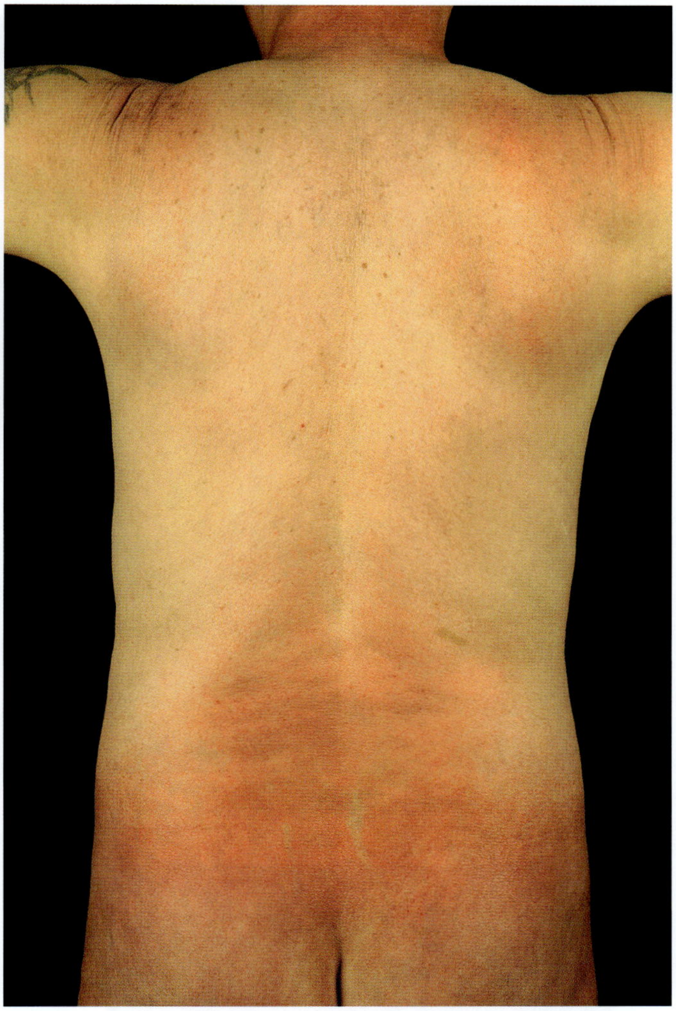

(f)

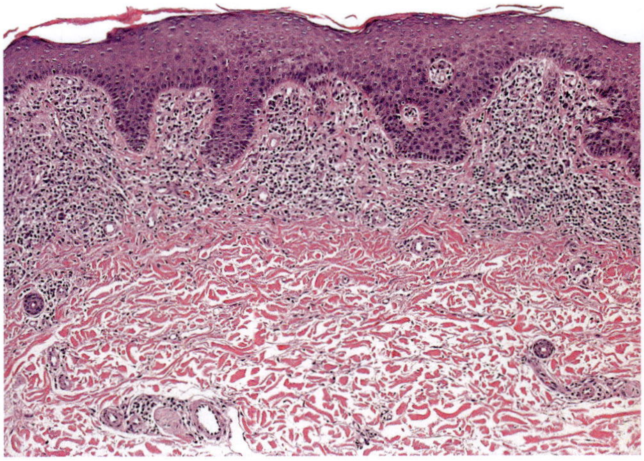

(h)

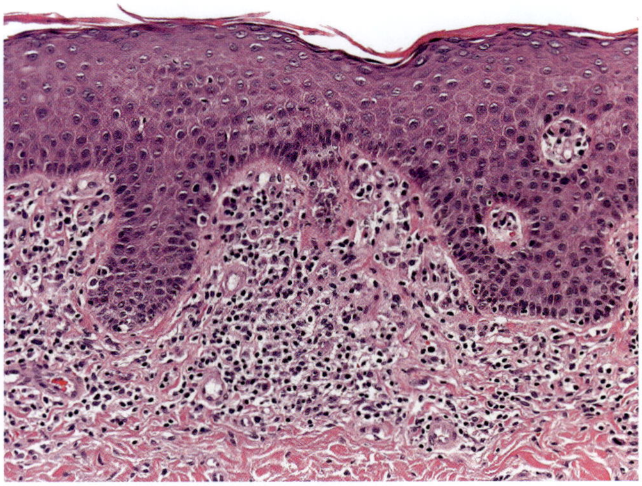

(i)

**Figure 4.2** (Continued)

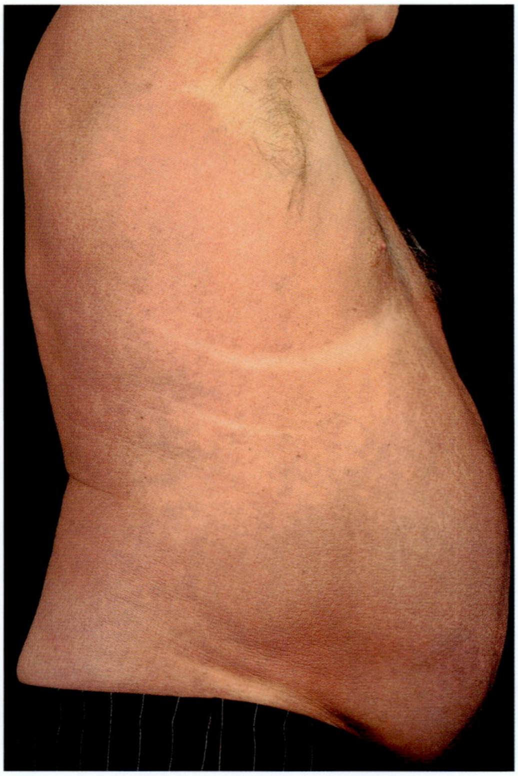

**Figure 4.3** Sézary syndrome. Erythroderma with partial sparing of the skin folds.

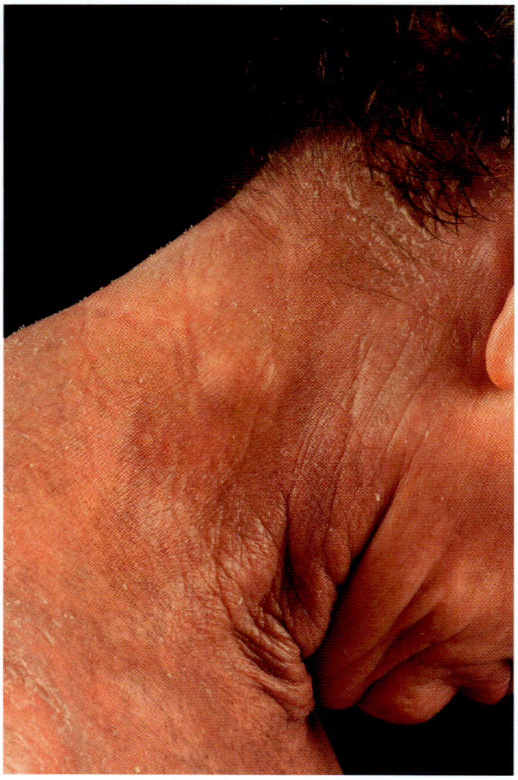

**Figure 4.4** Sézary syndrome. Focal lichenification of the skin on the neck, similar to what is observed in chronic eczematous dermatitis.

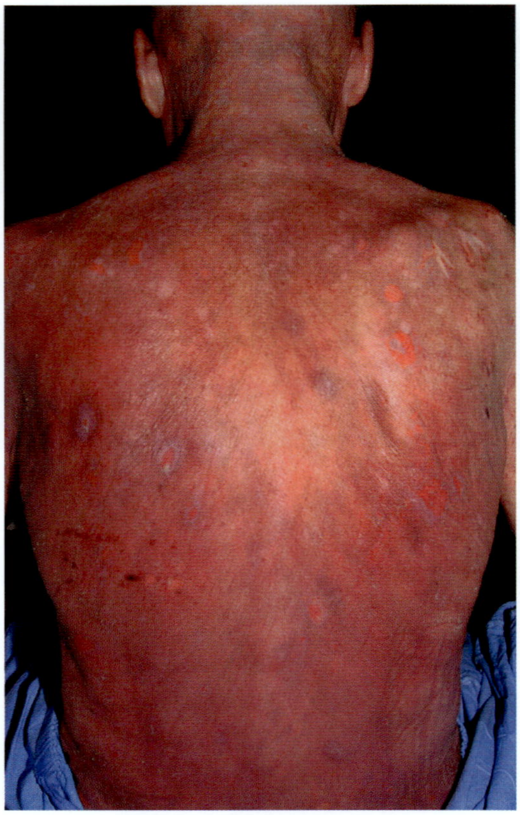

**Figure 4.5** Sézary syndrome. Erythroderma with numerous erosions and scratch artifacts, similar to what can be observed in erythrodermatous eczematous dermatitis in elderly patients.

is common in such cases (Fig. 4.6). The erythroderma is characterized by intense pruritus and scaling, and the pruritus may be intractable. Pruritus may be linked to the production of IL-31 by neoplastic cells, and decreases when IL-31 levels are lower [45]. Common clinical signs are the marked hyperkeratosis of the palms and soles, alopecia, and onychodystrophy (Figs. 4.7–4.9) [46]. Ectropion is a common complication (Fig. 4.10). Sézary syndrome, as well as mycosis fungoides, may also be associated with follicular mucinosis [47, 48]. Other clinical variants include the presence of diffuse hyperpigmentation as a consequence of melanosis or hemosiderosis (melanoerythroderma) (Fig. 4.11) and of vesiculobullous lesions. In fact, melanoerythroderma was already noted in the publication by the Italian dermatologist Baccaredda in 1939, at the same time of the first report by Sézary and Bouvrain, although Baccaredda mistakenly interpreted the features as those of a benign dermatosis [49]. In advanced stages, tumors develop, either on the background of erythroderma or on the suberythroderma (Fig. 4.12a) or in the absence of it (Fig. 4.12b). Palmar purpura characterized by specific infiltrates surmounted by intracorneal haemorrhage can be rarely observed (Fig. 4.13), in some cases in the setting of hyperkeratotic lesions mimicking palmoplantar psoriasis (Fig. 4.14).

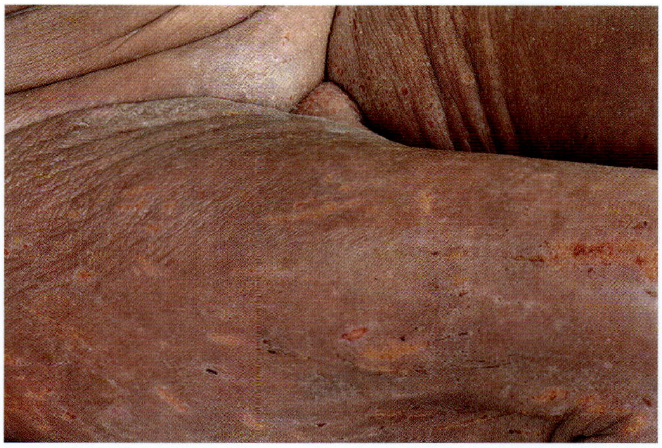

Figure 4.6 Sézary syndrome. Erosions and crusts due to vigorous scratching; note focal impetiginization.

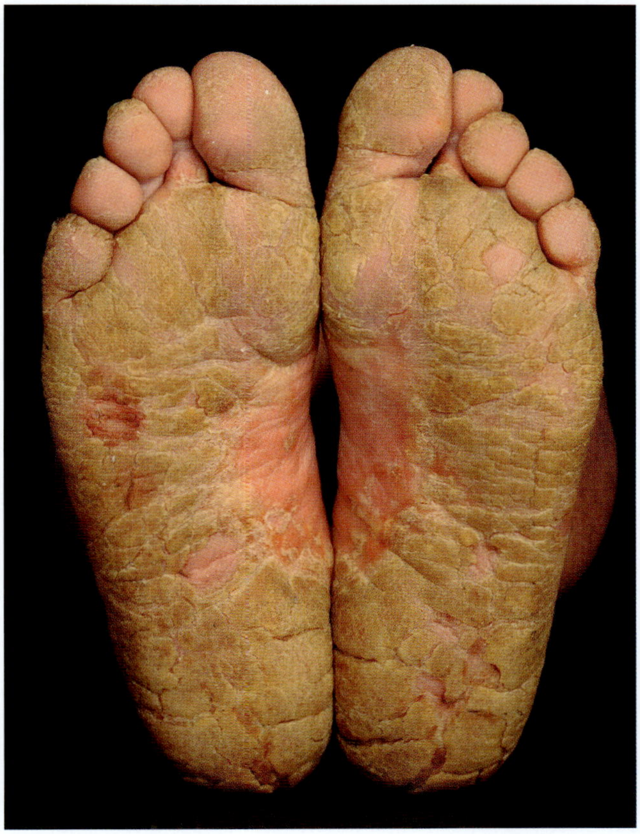

Figure 4.7 Sézary syndrome. Prominent hyperkeratosis of the soles.

It should be noted that several patients with Sézary syndrome present without erythroderma (Fig 4.2) [50, 51]. In a retrospective study, erythroderma was the earliest cutaneous sign of Sézary syndrome only in 25.5% of patients, and only 86.3% developed erythroderma during the disease course [52]. A "non-specific dermatitis" was commonly observed in half of the patients at the first visit [52]. In some patients, prominent photosensitivity may mimic the clinical picture of chronic actinic

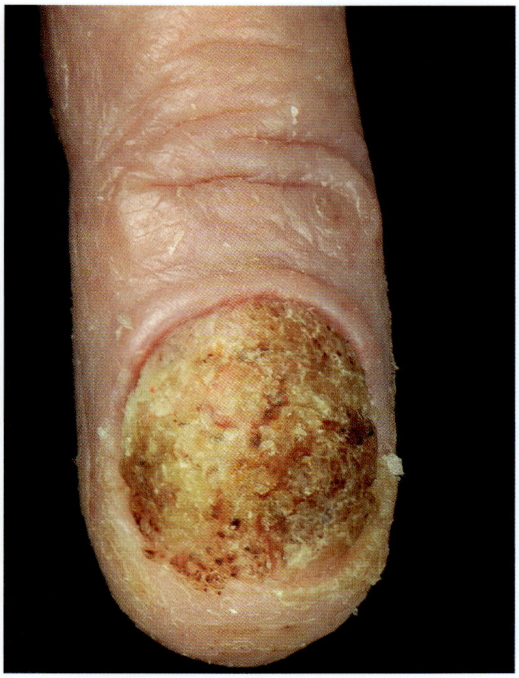

Figure 4.8 Sézary syndrome. Nail dystrophy.

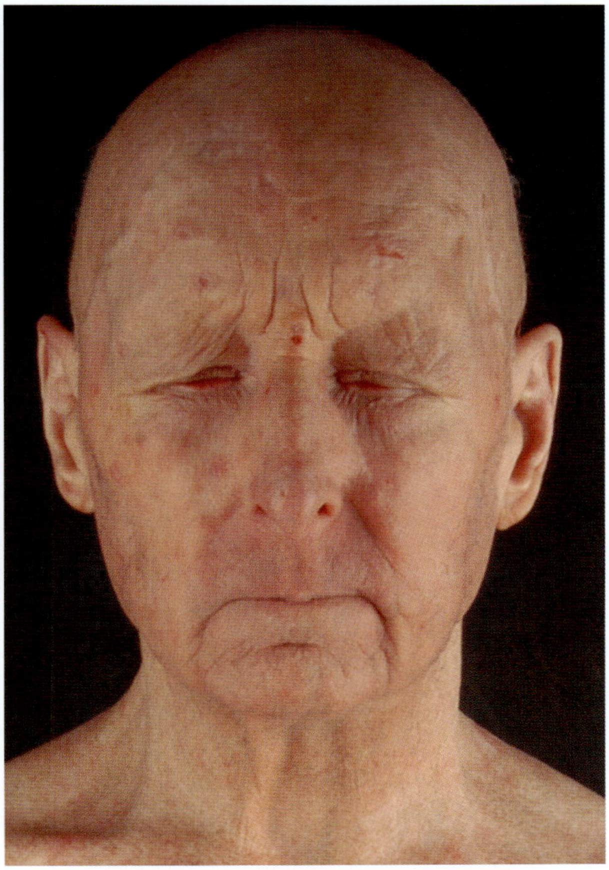

Figure 4.9 Sézary syndrome. Alopecia. Note focally small erosions due to vigorous scratching.

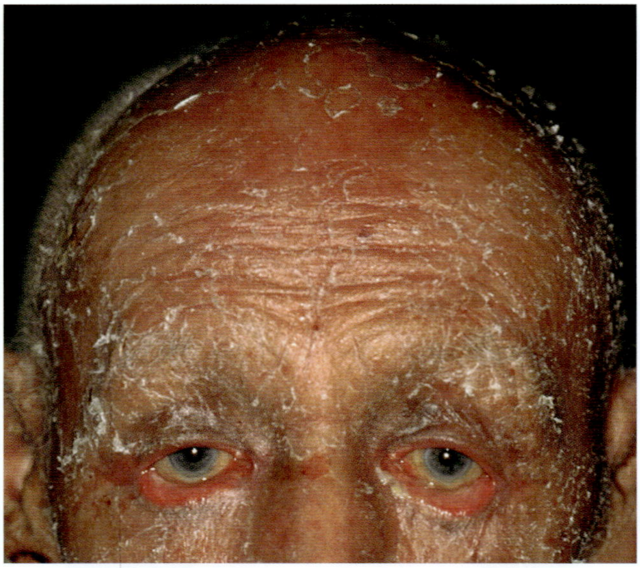

Figure 4.10 Sézary syndrome. Pronounced ectropion. Not also alopecia with complete loss of eyelashes and almost complete loss of eyebrows.

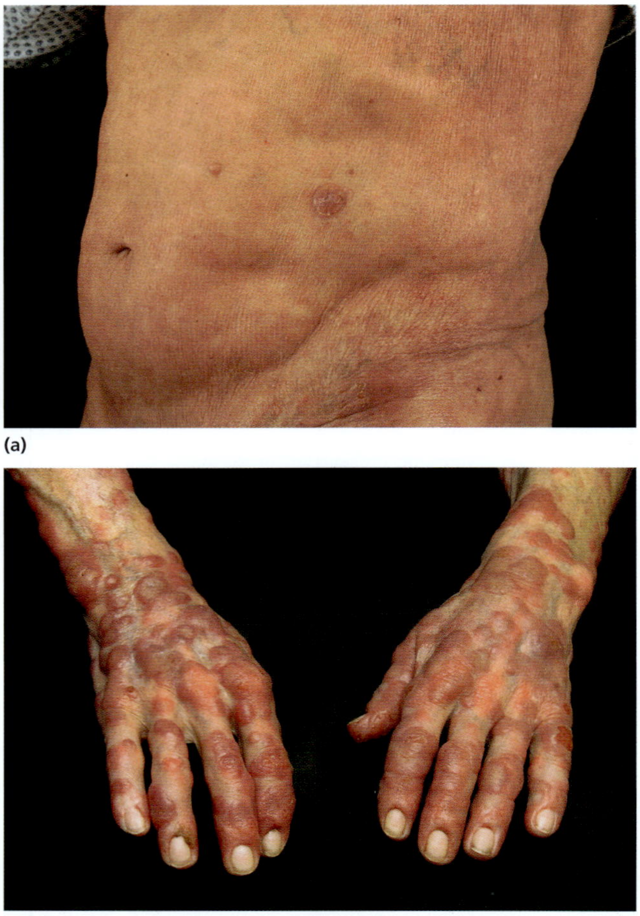

(a)

(b)

Figure 4.12 Sézary syndrome. (a) Tumors on the trunk on the background of erythroderma. (b) Several tumors on both distal arms and hands without erythroderma.

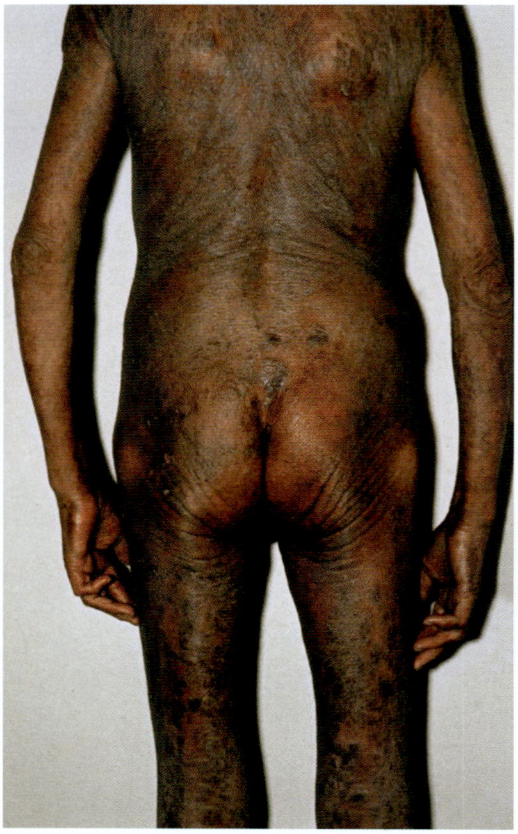

Figure 4.11 Sézary syndrome. Diffuse hyperpigmentation on the background of erythroderma ("melanoerythroderma"). Note also hyperpigmented patches and plaques.

dermatitis/actinic reticuloid, and be the source of a diagnostic pitfall. In fact, patients reported in the past as having actinic reticuloid with transformation into Sézary syndrome probably had Sézary syndrome from the outset (see also Chapter 31).

In rare cases, I have observed in advanced stages of Sézary syndrome generalized, partly confluent papular lesions rather than "conventional" erythroderma (Fig. 4.15). This clinical presentation reminds of papular mycosis fungoides (see Chapter 3), but there is a fundamental difference: papular mycosis fungoides represents an early manifestation of the disease with prognosis similar to conventional mycosis fungoides, whereas in my experience, generalized papular lesions in Sézary syndrome represent progression of the disease, and may be observed in association with tumors (Fig. 4.16).

Peripheral lymph nodes are often (but not always) enlarged. The histopathologic analysis usually shows evidence of nodal involvement, but differentiation from so-called "dermopathic lymphadenopathy" may be very difficult. On the other hand, the presence of dermopathic lymphadenopathy is a bad

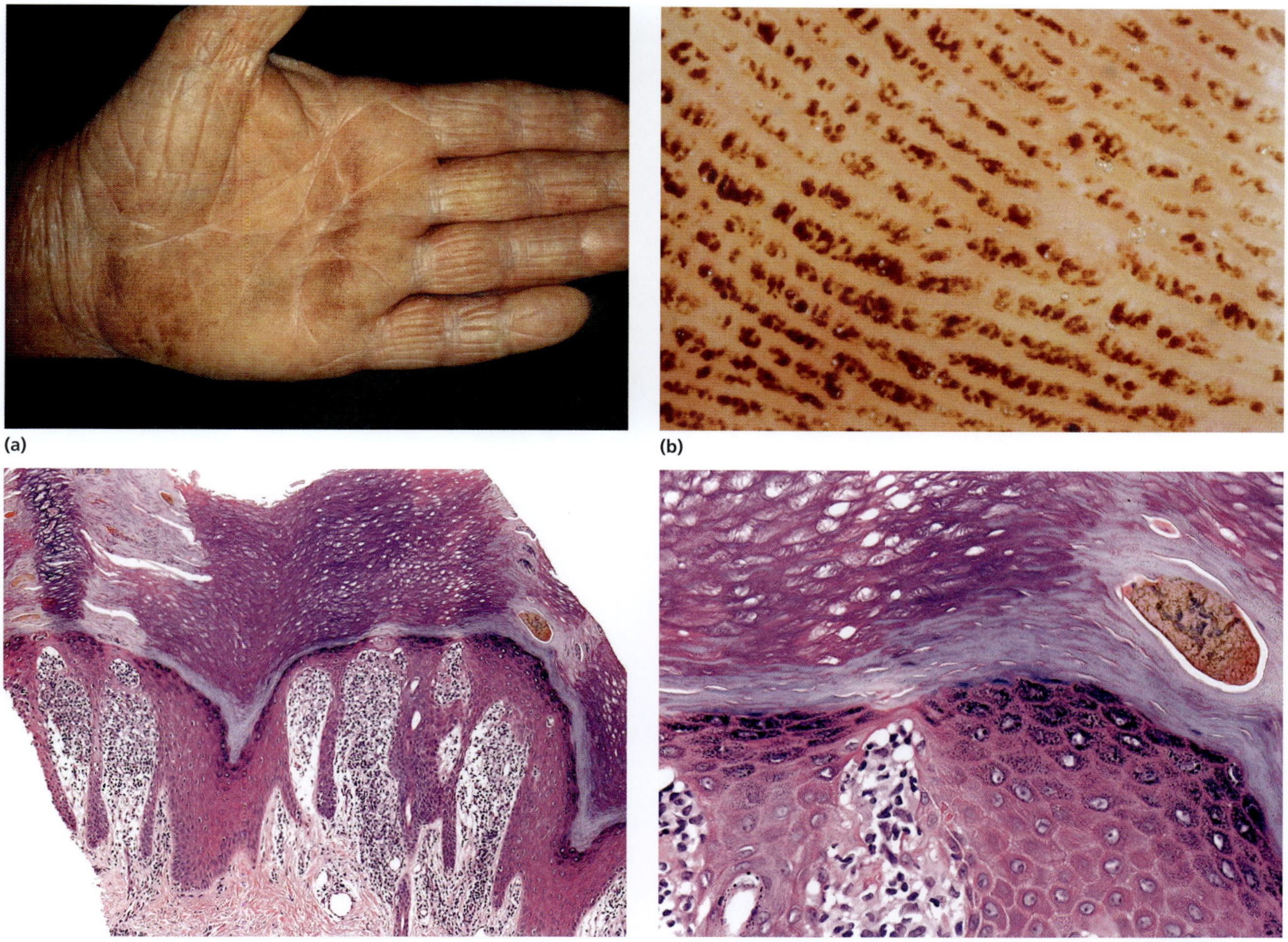

**Figure 4.13** Sézary syndrome. (a) Purpuric lesions on the palms with (b) detail by dermatoscopy. (c) Histology shows irregular epidermal hyperplasia with band-like, epidermotropic lymphoid infiltrate; (d) note epidermotropic lymphocytes and intracorneal hemorrhages responsible for the purpuric appearance of the lesions.

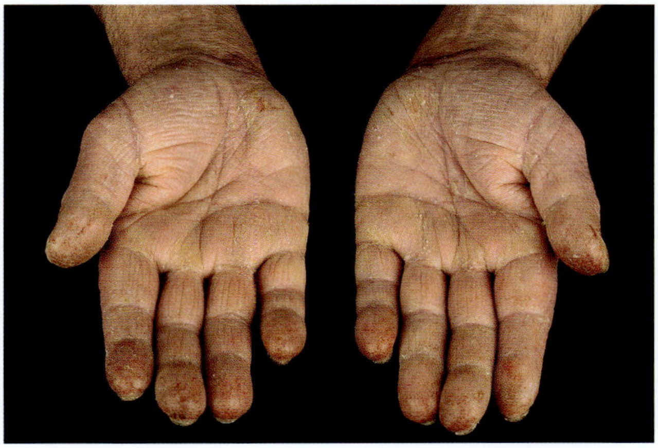

**Figure 4.14** Sézary syndrome. Purpuric lesions on the tips of the fingers and hyperkeratotic lesions on the palms, mimicking the picture of palmoplantar psoriasis.

prognostic sign even if a specific infiltrate cannot be demonstrated beyond doubt [22]. Although Sézary syndrome is regarded as a leukemic variant of cutaneous T-cell lymphoma, involvement of the bone marrow is rare in the early phases (but it may be found in later stages).

The analysis of peripheral blood is necessary for the diagnosis of Sézary syndrome: diagnostic criteria include those mentioned above for $B_2$ involvement (CD4:CD18 $\geq$ 10:1, $\geq$1000/µL $CD4^+/CD7^-$ or $CD4^+/CD26^-$ cells/µL (or other aberrant phenotype). The demonstration of the same monoclonal population of T lymphocytes within the peripheral blood and the skin is a crucial diagnostic criterion. Other useful criteria include Sézary cells (cerebriform lymphocytes) representing more than 20% of circulating lymphocytes, positivity for CD27 in the $CD4^+/CD26^-$ T-cell population, presence of a $CD158k^+$ clonal T-cell population, paucity of forkhead box protein P3 $(FOX\text{-}P3)^+$ circulating cells, and presence of high-scatter T-cells [53, 54].

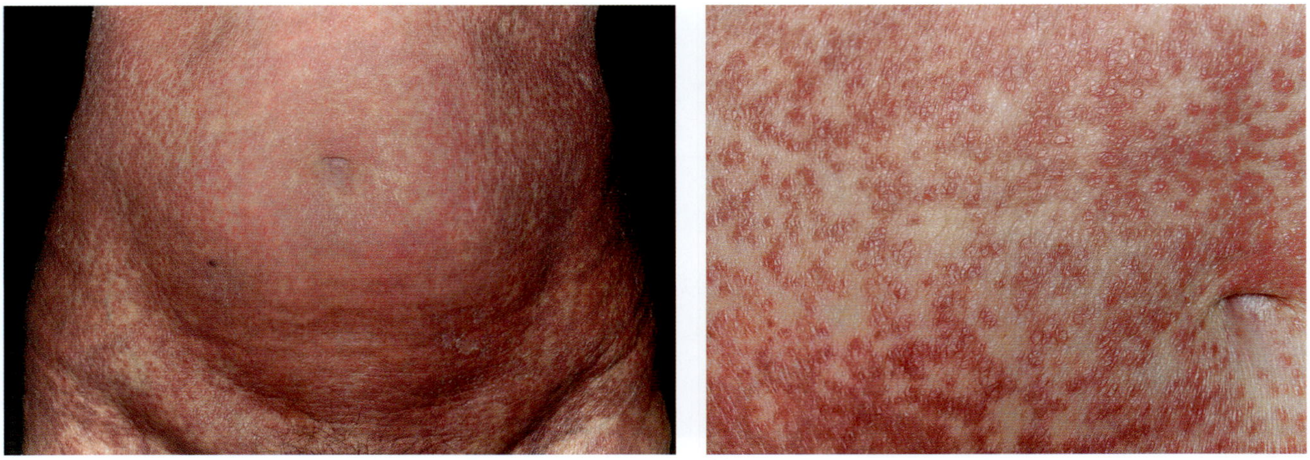

(a) (b)

**Figure 4.15** Sézary syndrome. (a) Generalized papular eruption in a patient with advanced disease. (b) Detail of confluent, flat papules.

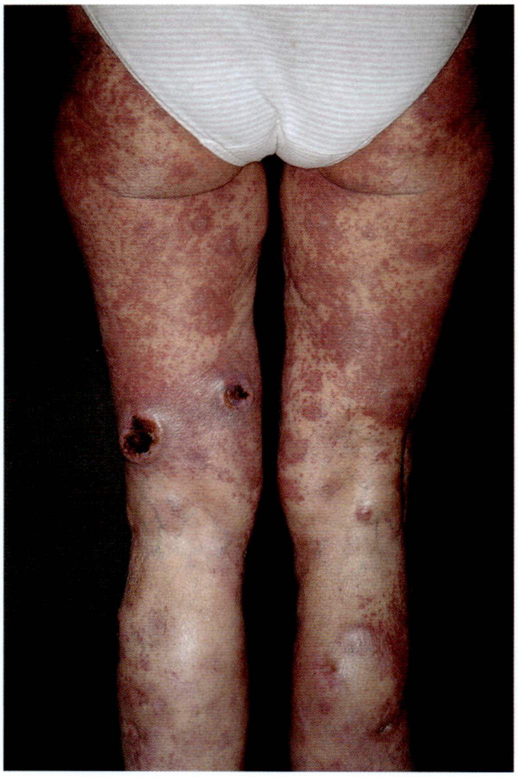

**Figure 4.16** Sézary syndrome. Ulcerated tumors in a patient with advanced disease. On the background, note confluent papular lesions and plaques rather than erythroderma.

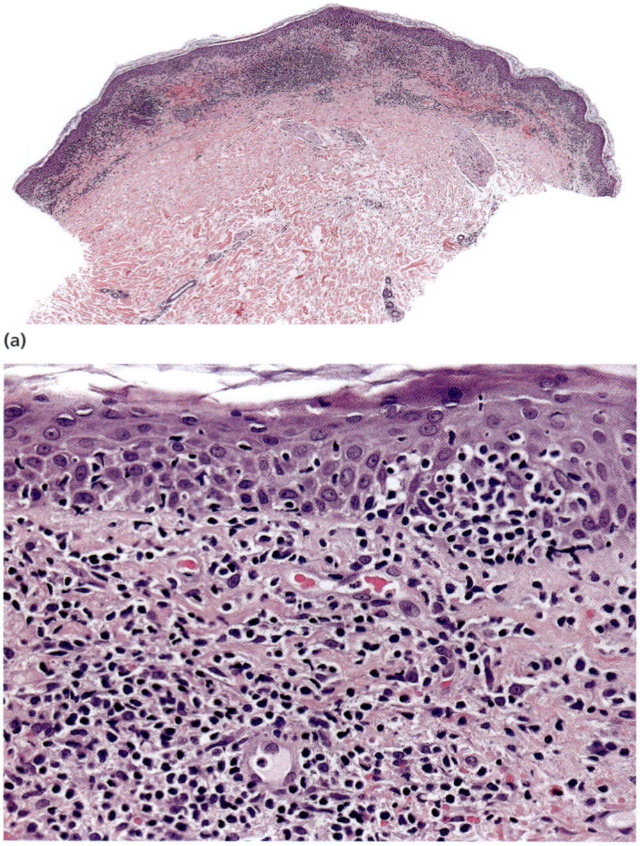

(a)

(b)

**Figure 4.17** Sézary syndrome. (a) Band-like lymphocytic infiltrate in the superficial dermis with (b) epidermotropic lymphocytes.

Inclusion of other markers has been suggested to detect cases with low blood burden (see above in this Chapter) [25]. The flow cytometry analysis and analysis of TCR Vβ repertoires are effective in demonstrating and quantifying small numbers of circulating tumor cells [55]. The analysis of the TCR genes rearrangement by high-throughput sequencing allows to compare the clones in cases suspect for recurrent disease, even with a very low tumor burden [56, 57].

Reflectance confocal microscopy has been reported as an useful adjunct for the clinical diagnosis of Sézary syndrome [58], but in my opinion, it does not add any meaningful information over what is provided by clinical and blood examination.

## Histopathology, immunophenotype, and molecular genetics

### Histopathology

In general, the histopathologic aspects of skin lesions in Sézary syndrome are similar to those of mycosis fungoides [59–61], but epidermotropism is usually less prominent [62]. Because of the lack of or of minimal epidermotropism, the histopathologic features are often difficult to interpret, and differentiation from benign erythroderma due to other diseases may be impossible in some cases [61]. When epidermotropism is present, typical Darier nests may be observed in a minority of cases, indistinguishable from those seen in mycosis fungoides.

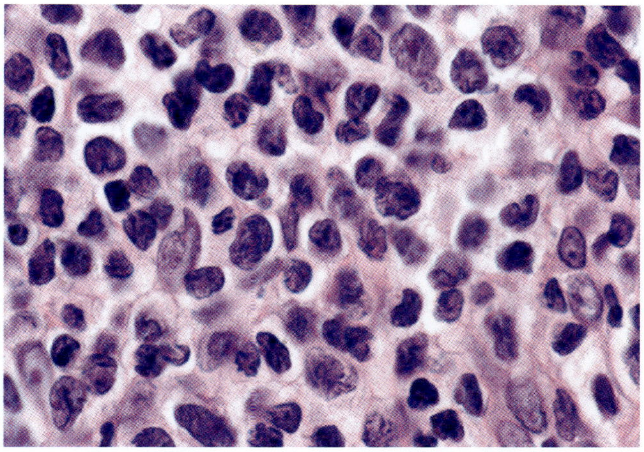

**Figure 4.18** Sézary syndrome. Neoplastic cells are small- to medium-sized pleomorphic ("cerebriform") lymphocytes ("Sézary cells"). Aggregates of such cells are found in infiltrated lesions or in tumors, and are usually not readily identifiable in biopsies of early lesions.

In diagnostic biopsies, a band-like infiltrate of lymphocytes in the superficial dermis combined with epidermotropism allows a proper classification (Fig. 4.17). Cytomorphology reveals predominance of small- to medium-sized pleomorphic (cerebriform) lymphocytes, often referred to as "Sézary cells" (Fig. 4.18). It must be underlined that large numbers of cerebriform cells are observed only in dense infiltrates and only rarely in biopsies of early lesions; thus, for practical purposes, they cannot be considered to be a useful clue for early diagnosis. Because of the overlapping histopathological features, differential diagnosis from mycosis fungoides can be achieved only by correlation with the clinical picture.

In many cases of early Sézary syndrome, the infiltrate is only sparse and not clearly diagnostic of a cutaneous lymphoma (Fig. 4.19). In these nonspecific, "prodromic" lesions, features of a pruritic ("eczematous") dermatosis usually predominate (Figs. 4.20a and b and 4.21a). In fact, I have observed deceptively "inflammatory-like" features in several cases, and refer to this presentation as "pseudodermatitis." In some cases, prurigo-like or eczematous lesions show unusually large, atypical lymphocytes that should always be considered as a worrying sign in this setting (Figs. 4.20c and 4.21b). These cells may be positive for CD30 (Fig. 4.21c), an additional unusual feature

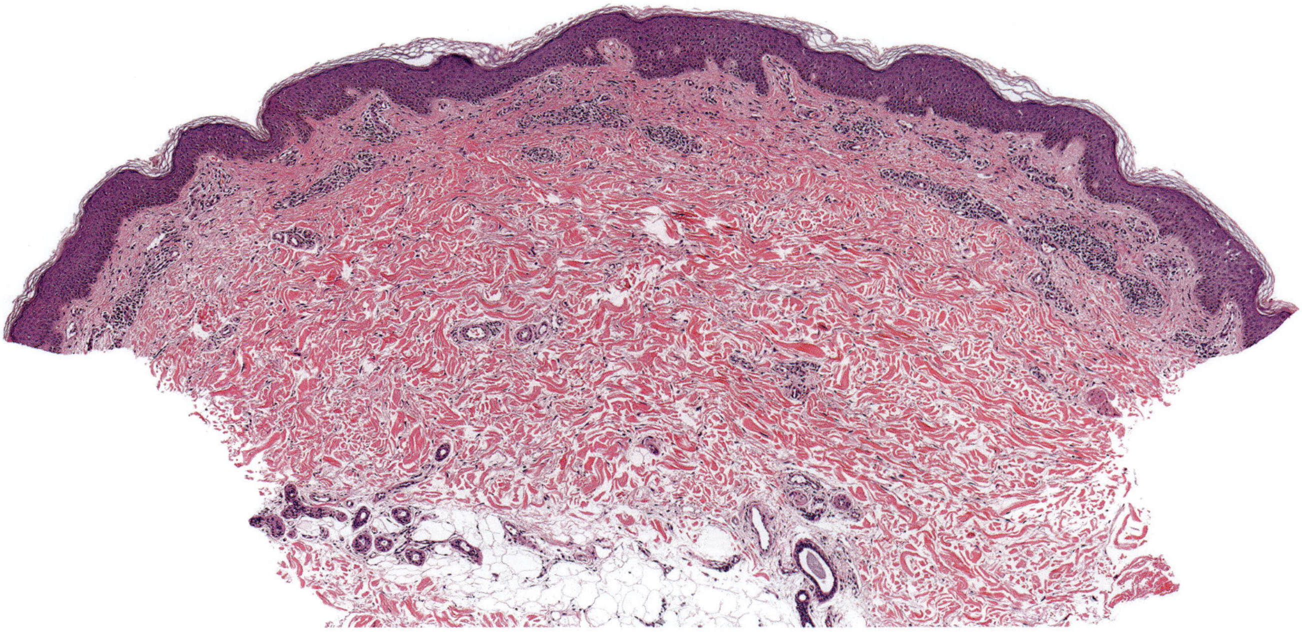

**Figure 4.19** Sézary syndrome. Moderate, irregular epidermal hyperplasia with sparse superficial infiltrate of lymphocytes. These nondiagnostic histopathologic features are commonly found, particularly in biopsies of early lesions ("pseudodermatitis").

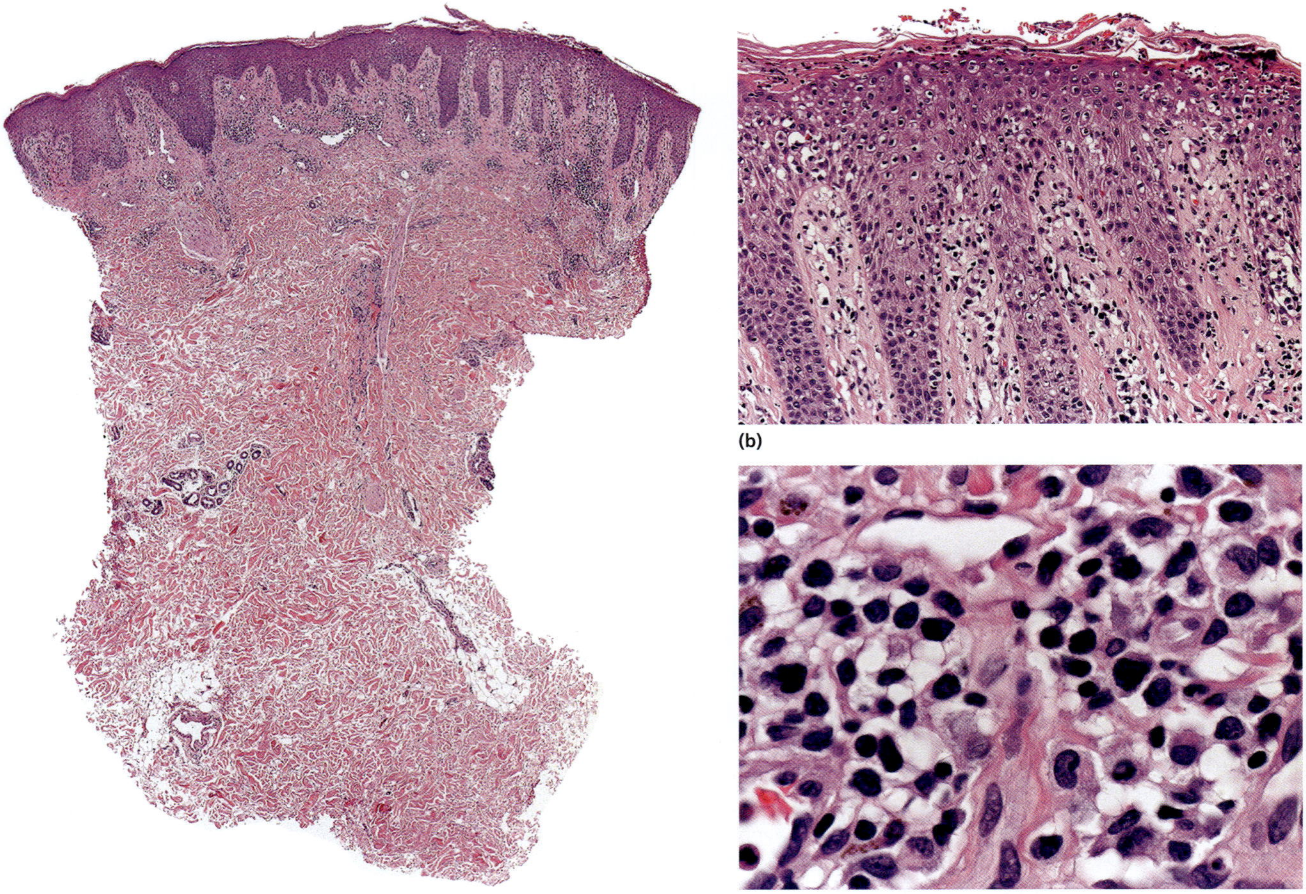

(a) (b) (c)

**Figure 4.20** Sézary syndrome. (a) Psoriasiform hyperplasia of the epidermis with scant spongiosis, parakeratosis and superficial lymphoid infiltrates. (b) Detail of epidermal hyperplasia with intraepidermal lymphocytes and parakeratosis. (c) Some hyperchromatic, atypical cells are present within the infiltrate.

which should prompt to include Sézary syndrome in the differential diagnosis.

Histopathologic variants of Sézary syndrome include the presence of a prominent granulomatous reaction, deposition of mucin within hair follicles (follicular mucinosis), or large cell transformation [47, 48, 63]. Large cell transformation may be detected in skin lesions, lymph nodes, or both, and is indistinguishable from that occurring in advanced mycosis fungoides (see Chapter 3).

Digital slide scanning has been demonstrated a reliable and practical approach to perform central pathology review in cases of mycosis fungoides or Sézary syndrome stage IIb or above, allowing to share difficult cases without the need to send the original glass slide(s) [64]. In my experience, digital histopathological slides with sufficient resolution are equivalent to conventional glass slides also in the early phases of the disease – yet do not overcome the problems intrinsic to the histopathological differential diagnosis of inflammatory versus neoplastic erythroderma.

## Immunophenotype

Immunohistology reveals a predominance of T-helper lymphocytes ($CD3^+$, $CD4^+$, $CD7^-$, and $CD8^-$) (Fig. 4.22a). The findings are indistinguishable from those observed in the majority of cases of mycosis fungoides. CD30 may be expressed in biopsies showing large cell transformation, or on some cells in biopsies of early lesions (see above). The thymocyte selection-associated high-mobility group box (TOX) is associated with the development of $CD4^+/CD8^-$ T cells in the thymus, but is suppressed in mature $CD4^+$ T cells. Aberrant overexpression is observed in Sézary syndrome (as well as in other cutaneous T-cell lymphomas) [65].

Although Sézary syndrome is, by definition, a lymphoma of $CD4^+$ T lymphocytes, exceptional cases may show a double expression of CD4 and CD8 [66]. The presence of double positivity for CD4 and CD8 can be demonstrated also in the circulating lymphocytes in these patients [66, 67].

A different expression of programmed death-1 protein (PD-1, CD279) had been originally described in neoplastic cells of

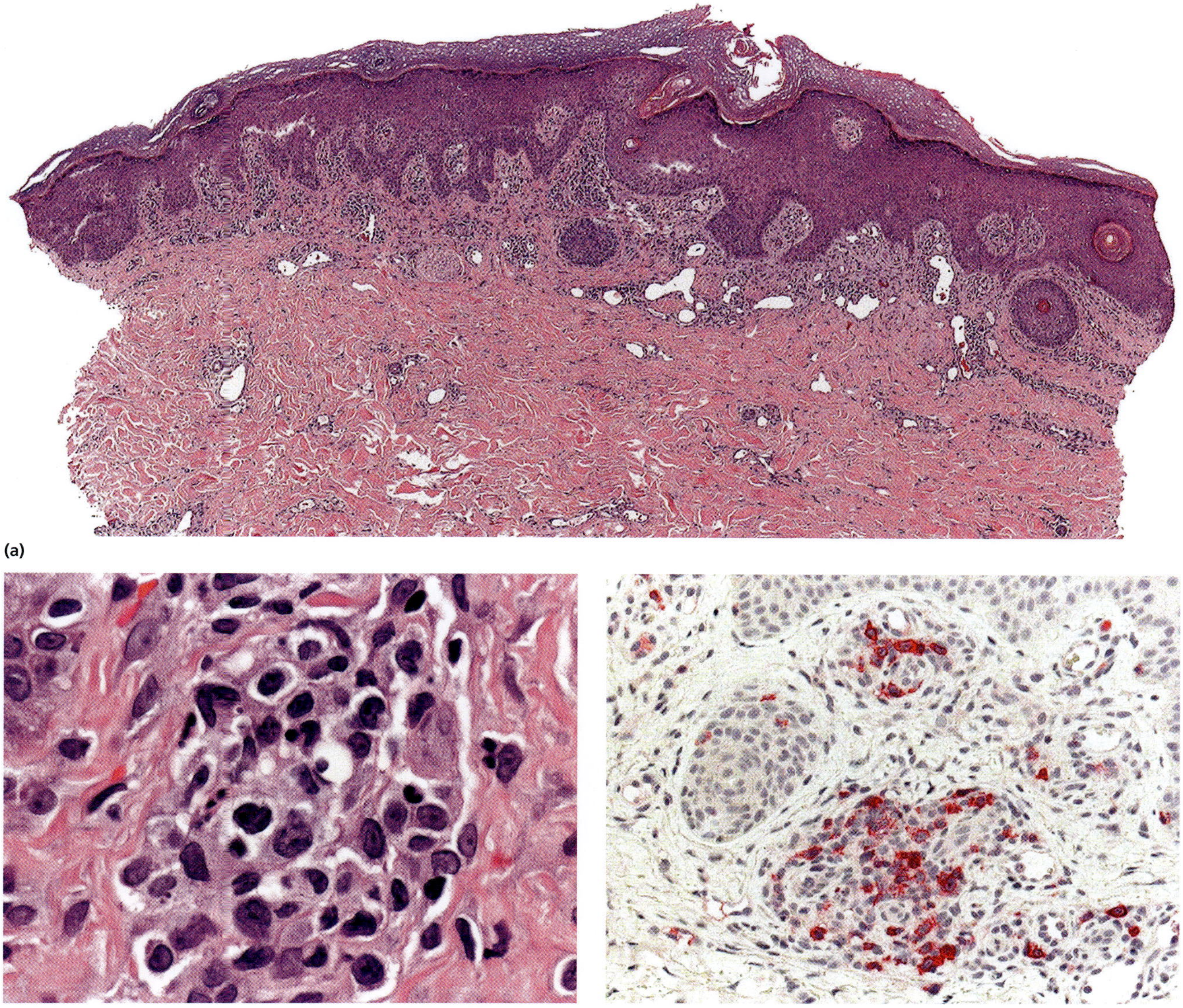

(a) (b) (c)

**Figure 4.21** Sézary syndrome. (a) At scanning magnification features of chronic prurigo predominate. (b) Some large, atypical cells are present within the infiltrate. (c) The large cells are positive for CD30.

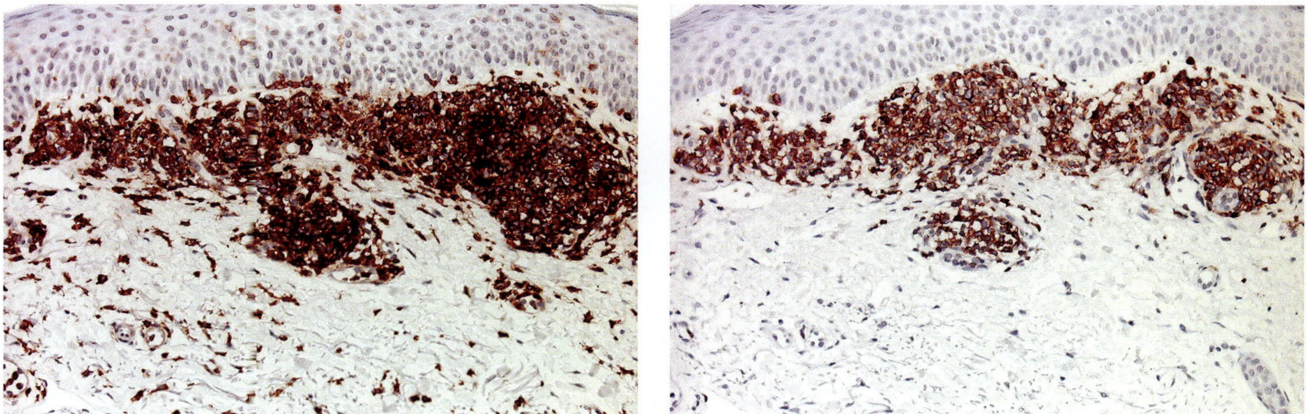

(a) (b)

**Figure 4.22** Sézary syndrome. (a) All cells are positive for CD4. (b) Most of the cells also express PD-1.

Sézary syndrome (positive) as compared to those of mycosis fungoides (negative) [68, 69], but subsequent studies revealed that PD-1$^+$ cells are present in mycosis fungoides as well [70, 71]. However, in a band-like infiltrate with intraepithelial cells, strong positivity of the vast majority of cells for PD-1 is suspicious for Sézary syndrome (Fig. 4.22b). Some of the PD-1$^+$ cases express also CD10, Bcl-6, and CXCL-13, thus showing a true T follicular helper (TFH) phenotype [70, 72]. Interestingly, it seems that in patients with a PD-1$^+$/CD158k$^-$ phenotype, a high number of B-lymphocytes can be observed within the cutaneous infiltrate [19].

A subset of patients with Sézary syndrome shows a FOXP3$^+$/CD25$^-$ phenotype of tumor cells, characterized in some cases by functional features of T-regulatory (Treg) cells [73–75]. The Treg phenotype has been associated with a worse prognosis in one study [73].

Some immunohistochemical markers are important in order to evaluate the feasibility of specific treatments, particularly CD30 (targeted by brentuximab vedotin) and CD52 (targeted by alemtuzumab). In this context, variability in the expression of immunohistochemical markers has been detected in sequential biopsies of mycosis fungoides and Sézary syndrome [76], thus specific treatments may be considered even in cases with negative staining.

## Molecular genetics

Although a large number of investigations is being carried out in Sézary syndrome and other cutaneous T-cell lymphomas, one should always remember that many of the aberrations that have been described are found only in a percentage of patients, and that sometimes results are contradictory. For example, somatic mutations of the Phospholipase C Gamma 1 (*PLCG1*) were described as common in one study (with a frequency of about 20%) [77], and uncommon in another one (5% of cases of Sézary syndrome) [78], with other studies reporting it again as "common" (approximately 10% of cases) [79–81]. Besides the semantic discussion as to whether the presence of a given aberration in 10–20% of cases should be considered as "common" for any disease, some of the differences may be due to the methods used, other to patients' selection and/or patients' number, still others may reflect the molecular heterogeneity of Sézary syndrome (possibly even in different lesions or sequential biopsies from one and the same patient) and other cutaneous T-cell lymphomas, yet they serve as a reminder that results of molecular studies, like all other investigations, should always be confirmed on large numbers of patients.

In the majority of cases of Sézary syndrome, molecular genetic studies of skin lesions show a clonal rearrangement of the TCR genes, but clonality may not be detected in biopsies of early stages. Once again, detection of the same clone within the peripheral blood and the skin is a crucial diagnostic criterion.

Sézary syndrome is characterized by extensive genetic instability with complex karyotypes. Genes regulating several key functions of the cells are altered in, including genes involved in cell cycle and apoptosis regulators, deoxyribonucleic acid (DNA) damage repair, histone remodelers, and epigenetic modifiers [82, 83]. Somatic copy number variants comprise >90% of all driver mutations, a frequency much higher than that observed in other forms of adults' cancer [82]. A significant proportion of these mutations are represented by focal deletions resulting in a frequent hemizygous loss of target tumor suppressor gene loci [82]. *MAPK1, BRAF, CARD11,* and *PRKG1* mutations are driving increased MAPK, nuclear factor κ-light-chain-enhancer of activated B cells (NF-κB) and NFAT activity upon TCR stimulation [83]. In a minority of patients, recurrent point mutations and genomic gains of *TNFRSF1B*, encoding the tumor necrosis factor receptor TNFR2 involved in the NF-κB signaling, have been reported [84]. Interestingly, short telomeres were observed restricted to neoplastic cells [85], suggesting that in Sézary syndrome, telomerase exerts additional functions besides maintenance of telomere length, and that several, disparate mechanisms contribute to disease onset and progression. Using RNA-Seq, an approach to transcriptome profiling that applies deep-sequencing technologies and can be used to obtain global cell transcriptomes, dysregulation of several key cancer pathways, including those involving phosphatidylinositol 3-kinase (PI3K), NF-κB, and TGFβ, have been observed in Sézary syndrome [86]. Interestingly, although *RHOA* alterations can be found in a distinct subset of cases of Sézary syndrome and mycosis fungoides, they are different from those commonly found in angioimmunoblastic T-cell lymphoma and related disorders [81]. In the same study, five novel genes implicated in Sézary syndrome have been detected: *CSNK1A1* (casein kinase 1 alpha 1; involved in the NF-κB signaling), *PTPRN2* (protein tyrosine phosphatase, receptor type N2; involved in the quantities of phosphatidylinositol phospholipids), *RARA* (retinoic acid receptor alpha; encoding a transcription factor important for T-cell differentiation), *ARHGEF3* (Rho guanine nucleotide exchange factor 3; a putative tumor suppressor gene implicated in *RHOA*/cytoskeleton remodeling), and *RLTPR* (RGD, leucine rich repeat, tropomodulin domain containing protein; a putative oncogene encoding a scaffolding protein that has been implicated in CD28 signaling) [81].

Whole-exome and single-nucleotide polymorphism array-based copy number analyses of CD4$^+$ tumor cells in Sézary syndrome showed considerable heterogeneity of candidate driver genes and affected pathways, showing overlaps with other mature T-cell lymphomas, as well as frequent aberrations in genome maintenance and DNA repair genes including protection of telomeres 1 *(POT1)* [87]. Single-cell gene expression profiling studies in advanced phases of the disease revealed a large inter and intratumor gene expression heterogeneity, as well as a common gene expression signature in highly proliferating lymphocytes [88]. Single-cell heterogeneity and presence of drug-resistant clones may be the reason for therapy resistance and treatment failure [89]. Marked heterogeneity has been detected also by analyzing the CD158k$^+$ circulating T lymphocytes, even at the initial diagnosis [90]. All in all, results on single cell analysis in patients with Sézary syndrome revealed a marked heterogeneity of neoplastic cells, suggesting that combination of different drugs targeting different pathways will be needed in order to improve the prognosis of these patients.

No specific karyotype is associated with Sézary syndrome, although genetic instability with recurrent chromosomal abnormalities are observed commonly. A panel of eight genes that can distinguish Sézary syndrome in patients with low numbers of circulating cells has been detected by the cDNA microarray technique [91]. Genome-wide analyses showed gains of 8q23–24.3 and 17q23–24, and losses of 9p21, 10p12–11.2, 10q22–24, 10q25–26, and 17p13–q11.1 [92]. Gains of 8q and 17q and losses of 10q and 17p have been observed also in other studies [42, 93, 94] and could be detected even in cases with limited blood involvement and normal CD4$^+$ cell count, confirming that these are common aberrations in Sézary syndrome. Losses on 10q23 affect the function of *PTEN*, a tumor suppressor gene involved in the regulation of the cell cycle, which is deleted or downregulated in most cases of Sézary syndrome [95]. In another study, copy number losses at 1p36p22, 6q24, and 15q11.2, as well as gains at 22q11.2q13.3, were capable of separating cases of Sézary syndrome from controls [96].

Downregulation of *FAS* and inactivation of p53 and p16 have been observed in several cases [34–36, 97, 98]. In particular, deletion of *TP53* has been reported in 87% of cases of Sézary syndrome, but only in 7% of cases of mycosis fungoides [42]. *BCL2* downregulation and *JUNB* upregulation may also contribute to the resistance to apoptosis [99]. Using quantitative polymerase chain reaction (PCR) analyses, gain of *cMYC* and loss of *cMYC* antagonists (*MXI1* and *MNT*) were observed in the majority of patients with Sézary syndrome, as well as alterations of the IL-2 pathway characterized by gains of *STAT3/STAT5* and IL-2 receptor genes [100]. Derepression of *MYC* may be due also to loss of the transcription factor E2A encoded by the *E2A* gene, resulting in enhanced proliferation and cell cycle progression via activation of *MYC* and of the cell cycle regulator *CDK6* [101].

Studies focused on the microribonucleic acid (miRNA) expression profiling showed that the miR-21 expression is upregulated and miR-342 is downregulated in Sézary syndrome, possibly playing a role in the regulation of apoptosis [102–105], while miR-214 and miR-199a are upregulated in Sézary syndrome but not in patients with erythrodermic atopic dermatitis, providing a possible differential diagnostic criterion [106]. Diminished levels of miR-29b can be observed in neoplastic cells leading to the overexpression of the epigenetic reader bromodomain-containing protein 4 (BRD4), and defining a novel oncogenic pathway featuring IL-15, miR-29b, and BRD4 [107].

## Differential diagnosis

Clinicopathological differentiation of inflammatory erythroderma from Sézary syndrome is one of the most vexing problems in dermatology and dermatopathology. A detailed discussion of differential diagnostic criteria is provided in Chapter 31 and Tables 31.2 and 31.3. A correct histopathological diagnosis (without clinical or laboratory data) could be made only in 51% of cases of Sézary syndrome, and in 80% of cases of inflammatory erythroderma [11], and morphologic criteria do not allow a precise differentiation [108]. Loss of CD7, low numbers of CD8$^+$ lymphocytes, and increased proliferation (as detected by Ki-67) were the strongest indicators predicting the correct diagnosis of Sézary syndrome in one study [11]. The diminished expression of CD7 represented a useful criterion also in another study [109].

The presence of the same T-cell clone in the skin and in the blood is considered one of the main diagnostic criteria of Sézary syndrome, and rules out all inflammatory erythrodermas. Analyzing molecular markers to distinguish Sézary syndrome from inflammatory dermatoses, two combinations of genes were identified: (1) *STAT4, TWIST1*, and *DNM3* or (2) *STAT4, TWIST1*, and *PLS3*, that showed high sensitivity and specificity for the diagnosis of Sézary syndrome [110]. Another study showed some differences between chronic idiopathic erythroderma and Sèzary syndrome, with an expansion of CD8A+KLRK1+ T-cell clones both in blood and skin in the former, and strong expansion of CD4$^+$ clones with a CCR7+SELL+ central memory phenotype in the latter [111]. However, only five patients were included in the group of chronic idiopathic erythroderma and only eight in that of Sèzary syndrome; thus, in my opinion, these results have a very limited value. Epigenomic analyses showed that promoter hypermethylation of *CMTM2, C2orf40, G0S2, HSPB6, PROM1*, and *PAM* was present in 94–100% of cases of Sézary syndrome samples, but not in non-neoplastic erythroderma, and that promoter hypermethylation of the chemokine-like factor *CMTM2* alone was sufficient to accurately distinguish Sézary syndrome from inflammatory erythroderma [112]. Although conventional immunohistochemical staining for CD158k did not allow separation of neoplastic from reactive cases, the mRNA expression of CD158k/KIR3DR2 detected by real-time reverse transcription PCR was significantly higher in lesional skin of Sézary syndrome than in reactive erythrodermic conditions, suggesting that detection of CD158k/KIR3DR2 transcripts may represent a molecular tool for the diagnosis of Sézary syndrome [113].

## Treatment

In spite of many advances, the therapy of Sézary syndrome still represents an unmet medical need with limited efficacy and short duration of responses. The first-line treatment modalities include extracorporeal photopheresis, eventually associated with bexarotene or interferon-α, or low-dose methotrexate. In the past, many patients were managed with chlorambucil combined with prednisone (Winkelmann scheme); although some guidelines include this scheme only as a second-line option, in the last EORTC recommendations, it is mentioned as a first-line modality [114]. Comprehensive reviews of therapeutic options and guidelines are available [27, 115–118]. Guidelines for the use of extracorporeal photopheresis are available as well [119]. Two retrospective studies suggested that extracorporeal photopheresis has a superior time-to-next-treatment in Sézary syndrome, particularly if commenced at an early stage [120, 121]. Treatment modalities may be combined together or with psoralen + UV-A (PUVA), and guidelines for the use of PUVA treatment are available [122].

As for mycosis fungoides, several other treatments have been applied in a limited number of patients with Sézary syndrome, particularly in therapy-refractory cases. The use of total skin electron beam is associated with improvement of the tumor burden in the peripheral blood [123–125]. Other modalities include multiagent and single-agent chemotherapy, particularly gemcitabine, pentostatin [126, 127], histone deacetylase inhibitors like vorinostat, quisinostat, or romidepsin [128–131], and new retinoids such as trimetrexate [132], lenalidomide [133], or liposomal doxorubicin [134]. Although all of these treatments show some degree of efficacy, at least in a proportion of patients, they do not change the natural history of the disease and recurrences are the rule. In addition, rapid progression and/or large cell transformation has been observed, sometimes in patients treated with new therapeutic agents, particularly immunomodulatory drugs [135, 136].

An increasing body of evidence showed that allogeneic stem cell transplantation preceded by reduced-intensity conditioning regimens has emerged as a potentially curative option, even in advanced stages of the disease [137–153]. Allogeneic stem cell transplantation performed in patients with complete response or very good partial response before transplantation has a lower cumulative incidence of relapse compared with those with a higher disease burden [150]. Nonrelapse mortality is lower in patients with good performance status treated with reduced-intensity conditioning regimens and with matched related donor [139]. A graft-versus-lymphoma mechanism may contribute to the beneficial effect of this treatment modality, as more than 50% of relapsing patients respond to donor lymphocytes infusions. The majority of patients are candidates to a reduced intensity conditioning regimen before allogeneic stem cell transplantation in Sézary syndrome [154a]. Caution should be advised if previous treatments included alemtuzumab (interference with post-transplant cyclophosphamide effect) or mogamulizumab (increased risk of acute graft-versus-host disease) [154b]. Treatment with check point inhibitors may also be associated with increased risk of acute graft-versus-host disease. Clinical practice recommendations for allogeneic stem cell transplant in Sézary syndrome have been recently published [154b].

New insights into the pathogenesis of Sézary syndrome is resulting in innovative treatment strategies. Mogamulizumab is currently being used for patients with CCR4-positive disease [155, 156], and it has been included as second-line modality in the EORTC recommendations [114]. A recent study suggested that progressive discontinuation of mogamulizumab may be considered in responsive patients, in order to avoid drug-related complications and/or loss of efficacy due to loss of CCR4 expression, as well as to minimize costs [157]. One problem related to the use of mogamulizumab is represented by the possible onset of a skin rash mimicking a cutaneous T-cell lymphoma clinically and histopathologically (for a detailed discussion of mogamulizumab-associated rash see Chapter 31). Alemtuzumab, an anti-CD52 monoclonal antibody administered in low subcutaneous doses in short courses, induces long-term remissions in some patients with Sézary syndrome [155, 158]. Anti-IL-2 receptor antibody (daclizumab) has been used in Sézary syndrome [159], and brentuximab vedotin, an anti-CD30 monoclonal antibody, represents a treatment possibility in cases expressing CD30 [160]. Therapeutic targeting of the immune checkpoint pathway using targeted monoclonal antibodies (e.g., ipilimumab, pembrolizumab, and nivolumab) represents also a further possibility for treatment of Sézary syndrome [161]. As Notch 1 is overexpressed in tumor cells in a stage-dependent manner, Notch inhibition may represent a possible treatment as well [162, 163]. Notch 1 downregulation induced apoptosis in cutaneous T-cell lymphoma cell lines [162]. Activation of peripheral blood dendritic cells by providing soluble recombinant CD40 ligand may also represent another strategy [164, 165]. Inhibition of the NF-κB/GATA-3 axis by ixazomib may have utility in appropriately selected patients or in combination with other agents [166]. IPH4102, a monoclonal antibody targeting the cell surface protein KIR3DL2 expressed in patents with Sézary syndrome, showed encouraging clinical activity in patients with relapsed or refractory Sézary syndrome [167]. However, p38 has also been identified as a potential therapeutic target that is overexpressed in patients with Sézary syndrome and that can be decreased by synergistic-inhibitor treatment [168]. Ongoing studies are exploring the value of the inhibition of TGF-β, a cytokine with immunosuppressive properties that promote tumor escape by reshaping the tumor microenvironment and inhibiting immune responses, in the treatment of Sézary syndrome [169]. Finally, as disease progression is associated with epigenetic dysregulation and with aberrant miRNAs levels, targeting miRNAs in advanced Sézary syndrome may provide further treatment strategies in the future [170].

One of the major symptoms of Sézary syndrome is pruritus, which may be unbearable and exceedingly difficult to treat. Recently, aprepitant, a substance P antagonists which blocks the neurokinin 1 receptor, was shown to be efficacious in reducing refractory pruritus in patients with Sézary syndrome [171]. Targeting IL-31 production may represent a further promising way of treating pruritus in patients with Sézary syndrome [45].

Recently, chimeric antigen receptor (CAR) T-cell therapy has been tested in peripheral T-cell lymphomas (see also Chapter 3). The CCR4 is expressed in Sézary syndrome, and recently optimized anti-CCR4 CAR T cells have been identified which could be beneficial for the treatment of the disease [172]. At present, however, CAR T-cell therapy for T-cell lymphomas has yet to be optimized, but it may represent a further option for advanced and/or relapsed disease.

## Prognosis

Overall survival of patients with Sézary syndrome depends on the diagnostic criteria used. The five-year survival varies between 11% and almost 50% in published series, thus clearly showing that different criteria for diagnosis and classification were used in different centers. In fact, if strict criteria are adopted, the five-year survival of Sézary syndrome is poor [5, 6], and the disease-specific five-year survival mentioned in the 2019 EORTC/WHO classification of cutaneous lymphomas is 36% [5]. Even with improved therapeutic possibilities, the survival is still very poor [173]. In this context, it should be underlined that patients with erythroderma, even if the cause is not Sézary syndrome or mycosis fungoides (non-neoplastic erythroderma), have a decreased survival compared to healthy individuals [12].

The extent of peripheral blood involvement is a consistently poor prognostic factor. The prognostic value of the $B_1$ and $B_2$ categories of peripheral blood involvement according to the ISCL staging system was supported by one report [174], but a large study found a similar median survival for these two staging categories (3.2 years and 3.1 years, respectively) [22]. Patients with $B_{0a}$ category (<5% of Sézary cells in the peripheral blood and no T-cell clone) have a significantly better median survival than those with $B_{0b}$ (clone detected) (24.5 years and 6.9 years, respectively) [22]. The presence of lymph nodes with dermopathic lymphadenitis ($N_1$) is associated with a worse prognosis in comparison to $N_0$ nodal status, confirming that, in spite of the lack of specific histopathologic criteria, dermopathic changes within the lymph nodes are a bad prognostic feature [22]. Patients with a nodal stage Nx have a greater relative risk for death, underlining the need for excisional biopsies of palpable or radiologically enlarged lymph nodes [22]. The choice of which lymph node to biopsy may also influence the results of the nodal histopathological examination, and the size of the lymph nodes (≥15 mm) was shown to have low specificity for $N_2$ or $N_3$ lymph nodes [175]. The presence of an identical clone in the skin and peripheral blood is an independent prognostic criterion pointing to a worse prognosis [22, 176]. Other factors associated with reduced survival include the stage at diagnosis, failure to undergo remission after the first treatment, advanced age, male gender, race, elevated LDH and $\beta_2$-microglobulin serum levels, presence of a high tumor burden in the peripheral blood, and prior exposure to multiple systemic drugs [177–181]. The expression of FOX-P3 by circulating Sézary cells has also been related to a worse prognosis [73]. The number of circulating Sézary cells may predict the response to treatment, with higher counts showing better responses. The NK-cell activity is significantly enhanced in Sézary syndrome, and higher NK-cell numbers are associated with increased mortality [182]. In one study, high expression of either ICOS or PD-L1 was associated with advanced-stage disease and with the appearance of large-cell transformation [183].

A cutaneous lymphoma international prognostic index (CLIPi) has been proposed for assessing prognosis of patients with mycosis fungoides and Sézary syndrome [184a]. Male gender, age >60, stages B1/B2 and N2/3, and visceral involvement were associated with worse prognosis. Three groups were stratified according to the number of prognostic factors: 0–1 factor (low risk), 2 factors (intermediate risk), and 3–5 factors (high risk). In a new version tailored for advanced disease, nodal N3 status, age>60yrs, raised serum lactate dehydrogenase, and large-cell transformation in the skin were associated with worse prognosis [184b].

Genetic data have also been used to predict prognosis in patients with Sézary syndrome. A panel of 10 genes that can identify a group of patients with survival shorter than 6 months has been identified by the cDNA microarray technique [91]. However, these results have not been verified by larger studies. A shorter survival has been observed in patients with *CDKN2A–CDKN2B* inactivation [185]. Using reverse transcription-PCR, a group of 593 genes overexpressed in mycosis fungoides and Sézary syndrome were identified, allowing stratification of the disease in three different prognostic groups [186]. Genes involved in the Th17 pathway (e.g., *IL-17F*) were expressed in patients with a worse prognosis [186]. However, this study lumped together cases of advanced mycosis fungoides and Sézary syndrome under the term "cutaneous T-cell lymphoma," thus hindering a precise interpretation of the data.

### Résumé

**Sézary syndrome**

| | |
|---|---|
| **Clinical** | Elderly adults. Pruritic erythroderma, generalized lymphadenopathy and circulating Sézary cells. Strict diagnostic criteria include presence of the same neoplastic clone in the blood and skin, a $CD4^+$:$CD8^+$ ratio ≥10 in the peripheral blood, and $B_2$ stage (≥1000/μL $CD4^+$/$CD7^-$ or $CD4^+$/$CD26^-$ cells/μL, or other aberrant phenotype). Aggressive course. |
| **Morphology** | Band-like infiltrates with epidermotropic lymphocytes. Small/medium pleomorphic (cerebriform) cells. In early phases a dermatitis-like pattern is common ("pseudodermatitis"). During the course of the disease, tumors with large cell morphology may arise. |
| **Immunohistochemistry (skin)** | CD2, CD3, CD4, CD5 + <br> CD7, CD8, CD26 – <br> CD52 +/– <br> CD30 –/+ <br> PD-1 + |
| **Genetics** | Same monoclonal rearrangement of the TCR genes in the blood and skin. Alterations of genes regulating several key functions of the cells, including genes involved in cell cycle and apoptosis regulators, DNA damage repair, histone remodelers, and epigenetic modifiers. |
| **Treatment guidelines** | Extracorporeal photopheresis, interferon-α, retinoids (alone or in combination), low-dose methotrexate, alemtuzumab, brentuximab vedotin, mogamulizumab, combination treatments. Several other options, including PUVA associated with other modalities, and single-agent or multiagent chemotherapy (gemcitabine, pegylated liposomal doxorubicin, CHOP, CHOP-like). Chlorambucil with prednisone (Winkelmann scheme) is still included in some guidelines. Allogeneic stem cell transplantation may provide a chance for cure in selected patients. |

## References


1. Sézary A, Bouvrain Y. Erytrodermie avec présence de cellules monstrueuses dans le derme et dans le sang circulant. *Bull Soc Fr Derm Syph* 1938;**45**:254–260.
2. Shakeri A. Albert Sezary-the man, the cell, and the syndrome. *JAMA Dermatol* 2018;**154**:496–497.
3. Steffen C. The man behind the eponym dermatology in historical perspective: Albert Sézary and the Sézary syndrome. *Am J Dermatopathol* 2006;**28**:357–367.
4. Sézary A, Bolgert M. Réticulose érythrodermique avec réticulémie. *Bull Soc Fr Dermatol Syphiligr* 1942;**49**:355–356.
5. Willemze R, Cerroni L, Kempf W, *et al.* The 2018 update of the WHO-EORTC classification for primary cutaneous lymphomas. *Blood* 2019;**133**:1703–1714.
6. Kempf W, Mitteldorf C, Cerroni L, *et al.* Classifications of cutaneous lymphomas and lymphoproliferative disorders: An update from the EORTC cutaneous lymphoma histopathology group. *J Eur Acad Dermatol Venereol* 2024;**38**:1491–1503.
7. Comfere NI, Calonje E, Cerroni L. Sézary syndrome. In: Arber DA, Borowitz MJ, Cook JR, *et al.*, eds. *The International Consensus Classification of Myeloid and Lymphoid Neoplasms*. Philadelphia (US): Wolters Kluwer, 2025: 680–683.
8. Elenitoba-Johnson KSJ, Geddie WR, Ortonne N, *et al.* Sèzary syndrome. In: *WHO Classification of Tumours Editorial Board. Haematolymphoid Tumours*. 5th edition. Lyon (France): IARC, 2024: 674–676.
9. Campbell JJ, Clark RA, Watanabe R, Kupper TS. Sézary syndrome and mycosis fungoides arise from distinct T-cell subsets: a biologic rationale for their distinct clinical behaviors. *Blood* 2010;**116**:767–771.
10. van Doorn R, van Kester MS, Dijkman R, *et al.* Oncogenomic analysis of mycosis fungoides reveals major differences with Sézary syndrome. *Blood* 2009;**113**:127–136.
11. Klemke CD, Booken N, Weiss C, *et al.* Histopathological and immunophenotypical criteria for the diagnosis of Sézary syndrome in differentiation from other erythrodermic skin diseases: a European Organisation for Research and Treatment of Cancer (EORTC) Cutaneous Lymphoma Task Force Study of 97 cases. *Br J Dermatol* 2015;**173**:93–105.
12. Sigurdsson V, Toonstra J, Hezemans-Boer M, van Vloten WA. Erythroderma: a clinical and follow-up study of 102 patients, with special emphasis on survival. *J Am Acad Dermatol* 1996;**35**:53–57.
13. Dobos G, De Cevins C, So SLK, *et al.* The value of five blood markers in differentiating mycosis fungoides and Sèzary syndrome: a validation cohort. *Br J Dermatol* 2021;**185**:405–411.
14. Jiang TT, Kruglov O, Virmani A, *et al.* Deciphering tumor cell evolution in cutaneous T-cell lymphomas: distinct differentiation trajectories in mycosis fungoides and Sézary syndrome. *J Invest Dermatol* 2024;**144**:1088–1098.
15. Vonderheid EC, Bernengo MG, Burg G, *et al.* Update on erythrodermic cutaneous T-cell lymphoma: report of the International Society for Cutaneous Lymphomas. *J Am Acad Dermatol* 2002;**46**:95–106.
16. Scarisbrick JJ, Hodak E, Bagot M, *et al.* Blood classification and blood response criteria in mycosis fungoides and Sezary syndrome using flow cytometry: recommendations from the EORTC cutaneous lymphoma task force. *Eur J Cancer* 2018;**93**:47–56.
17. Najidh S, Tensen CP, van der Sluijs-Gelling AJ, *et al.* Improved Sézary cell detection and novel insights into immunophenotypic and molecular heterogeneity in Sézary syndrome. *Blood* 2021;**138**:2571–2583.
18. Jonak C, Brunner PM. Blood will tell: profiling Sézary syndrome. *Blood* 2021;**138**:2450–2451.
19. Vergnolle I, Dout-Beyries C, Boulinguez S, *et al.* CD158k and PD-1 expressions define heterogeneous subtypes of Sezary syndrome. *Blood Adv* 2022;**6**:1813–1825.

20. Olsen EA, Whittaker S, Kim YH, *et al.* Clinical end points and response criteria in mycosis fungoides and Sézary syndrome: a consensus statement of the International Society for Cutaneous Lymphomas, the United States Cutaneous Lymphoma Consortium, and the Cutaneous Lymphoma Task Force of the European Organisation for Research and Treatment of Cancer. *J Clin Oncol* 2011;**29**:2598–2607.
21. Olsen E, Vonderheid E, Pimpinelli N, *et al.* Revisions to the staging and classification of mycosis fungoides and Sézary syndrome: a proposal of the International Society for Cutaneous Lymphomas (ISCL) and the Cutaneous Lymphoma Task Force of the European Organization of Research and Treatment of Cancer (EORTC). *Blood* 2007;**110**:1713–1722.
22. Agar NS, Wedgeworth E, Crichton S, *et al.* Survival outcomes and prognostic factors in mycosis fungoides/Sézary syndrome: validation of the revised International Society for Cutaneous Lymphomas/European Organisation for Research and Treatment of Cancer staging proposal. *J Clin Oncol* 2010;**28**:4730–4739.
23. Olsen EA, Whittaker S, Willemze R, *et al.* Primary cutaneous lymphoma: recommendations for clinical trial design and staging update from the ISCL, USCLC, and EORTC. *Blood* 2022;**140**:419–437.
24. National Comprehensive Cancer Network. Primary Cutaneous Lymphomas (Version 3.2025). https://www.nccn.org/professionals/physician_gls/pdf/primary_cutaneous.pdf
25. Chrisman LP, Trimark PF, Pang Y, *et al.* Updated cutaneous T-cell lymphoma TNMB staging criteria fail to identify patients with Sézary syndrome with low blood burden. *Blood* 2024;**144**:914–917.
26. Evans KG, Troxel AB, DeNardo BJ, *et al.* Validity assessment of the cutaneous T-cell lymphoma severity index to predict prognosis in advanced mycosis fungoides/Sézary syndrome. *J Am Acad Dermatol* 2011;**64**:682–689.
27. Olsen EA, Rook AH, Zic J, *et al.* Sezary syndrome: immunopathogenesis, literature review of therapeutic options, and recommendations for therapy by the United States Cutaneous Lymphoma Consortium (USCLC). *J Am Acad Dermatol* 2011;**64**:352–404.
28. Scarisbrick JJ, Child FJ, Evans AV, *et al.* Secondary malignant neoplasms in 71 patients with Sézary syndrome. *Arch Dermatol* 1999;**135**:1381–1385.
29. Blaizot R, Ouattara E, Fauconneau A, *et al.* Infectious events and associated risk factors in mycosis fungoides/Sézary syndrome: a retrospective cohort study. *Br J Dermatol* 2018;**179**:1322–1328.
30. Geskin LJ, Viragova S, Stolz DB, Fuschiotti P. Interleukin-13 is overexpressed in cutaneous T-cell lymphoma cells and regulates their proliferation. *Blood* 2015;**125**:2798–2805.
31. Ferenczi K, Fuhlbrigge RC, Pinkus JL, *et al.* Increased CCR4 expression in cutaneous T cell lymphoma. *J Invest Dermatol* 2002;**119**:1405–1410.
32. Lamprecht B, Kreher S, Möbs M, *et al.* The tumour suppressor p53 is frequently nonfunctional in Sézary syndrome. *Br J Dermatol* 2012;**167**:240–246.
33. Fraser-Andrews E, McGregor JM, Crook T, *et al.* Sézary syndrome with a complex, frameshift p53 gene mutation in a Chernobyl survivor. *Clin Dermatol* 2001;**26**:683–685.
34. Jones CL, Wain EM, Chu CC, *et al.* Downregulation of Fas gene expression in Sézary syndrome is associated with promoter hypermethylation. *J Invest Dermatol* 2010;**130**:1116–1125.
35. Wain E, Mitchell T, Russell-Jones R, Whittaker S. Fine mapping of chromosome 10q deletions in mycosis fungoides and Sézary syndrome: identification of two discrete regions of deletion at 10q23.33–24.1 and 10q24.33–25.1. *Genes Chromosomes Cancer* 2005;**42**:184–192.
36. Vermeer MH, van Doorn R, Dijkman R, *et al.* Novel and highly recurrent chromosomal alterations in Sezary Syndrome. *Cancer Res* 2008;**68**:2689–2698.
37. Begue E, Jean-Louis F, Bagot M, *et al.* Inducible expression and pathophysiologic functions of T-plastin in cutaneous T-cell lymphoma. *Blood* 2012;**120**:143–154.
38. Jones CL, Ferreira S, McKenzie RCT, *et al.* Regulation of T-plastin expression by promoter hypomethylation in primary cutaneous T-cell lymphoma. *J Invest Dermatol* 2012;**132**:2042–2049.
39. Willerslev-Olsen A, Krejsgaard T, Lindahl LM, *et al.* Staphylococcal enterotoxin A (SEA) stimulates STAT3 activation and IL-17 expression in cutaneous T-cell lymphoma. *Blood* 2016;**127**:1287–1296.
40. Kamijo H, Miyagaki T, Shishido-Takahashi N, *et al.* Aberrant CD137 ligand expression induced by GATA6 overexpression promotes tumor progression in cutaneous T-cell lymphoma. *Blood* 2018;**132**:1922–1935.
41. Harro CM, Sprenger KB, Chaurio RA, *et al.* Sézary syndrome originates from heavily mutated hematopoietic progenitors. *Blood Adv* 2023;**18**:5586–5602.
42. Park J, Daniels J, Wartewig T, *et al.* Integrated genomic analyses of cutaneous T-cell lymphomas reveal the molecular bases for disease heterogeneity. *Blood* 2021;**138**:1225–1236.
43. Martinez-Escala ME, Posligua AL, Wickless H, *et al.* Progression of undiagnosed cutaneous lymphoma after anti-tumor necrosis factor-alpha therapy. *J Am Acad Dermatol* 2018;**78**:1068–1076.
44. Foo SH, Shah F, Chaganti S, *et al.* Unmasking mycosis fungoides/Sézary syndrome from preceding or co-existing benign inflammatory dermatoses requiring systemic therapies: patients frequently present with advanced disease and have an aggressive clinical course. *Br J Dermatol* 2016;**174**:901–904.
45. Singer EM, Shin DB, Nattkemper LA, *et al.* IL-31 is produced by the malignant T-cell population in cutaneous T-Cell lymphoma and correlates with CTCL pruritus. *J Invest Dermatol* 2013;**133**:2783–2785.
46. Bishop BE, Wulkan A, Kerdel F, *et al.* Nail alterations in cutaneous T-cell lymphoma: a case series and review of nail manifestations. *Skin Appendage Disord* 2015;**1**:82–86.
47. Cerroni L, Fink-Puches R, Bäck B, *et al.* A critical reappraisal of clinicopathologic features and association with mycosis fungoides and Sézary syndrome. *Arch Dermatol* 2002;**138**:182–189.
48. Gerami P, Guitart J. Folliculotropic Sézary syndrome: a new variant of cutaneous T-cell lymphoma. *Br J Dermatol* 2007;**156**:781–783.
49. Baccaredda A. Reticulohistiocytosis cutanea hyperplastica benigna cum melanodermia. *Archiv Dermatol Sifil* 1939;**179**:210.
50. Thompson AK, Killian JM, Weaver AL, *et al.* Sézary syndrome without erythroderma: a review of 16 cases at Mayo Clinic. *J Am Acad Dermatol* 2017;**76**:683–688.
51. Kamijo H, Miyagaki T, Norimatsu Y, *et al.* Sézary syndrome without erythroderma: a case report and review of published work. *J Dermatol* 2019;**46**:61–64.
52. Mangold AR, Thompson AK, Davis MD, *et al.* Early clinical manifestations of Sezary syndrome: a multicenter retrospective cohort study. *J Am Acad Dermatol* 2017;**77**:719–727.
53. Bouaziz JD, Remtoula N, Bensussan A, *et al.* Absolute $CD3^+$ $CD158k^+$ lymphocyte count is reliable and more sensitive than cytomorphology to evaluate blood tumour burden in Sézary syndrome. *Br J Dermatol* 2010;**162**:123–128.
54. Clark RA, Shackelton JB, Watanabe R, *et al.* High-scatter T cells: a reliable biomarker for malignant T cells in cutaneous T-cell lymphoma. *Blood* 2011;**117**:1966–1976.
55. Feng B, Jorgensen JL, Jones D, *et al.* Flow cytometric detection of peripheral blood involvement by mycosis fungoides and Sézary

syndrome using T-cell receptor Vb chain antibodies and its application in blood staging. *Mod Pathol* 2010;**23**:284–295.
56. Scherer F, Kurtz DM, Diehn M, Alizadeh AA. High-throughput sequencing for noninvasive disease detection in hematologic malignancies. *Blood* 2017;**130**:440–452.
57. Kirsch IR, Watanabe R, O'Malley JT, *et al.* TCR sequencing facilitates diagnosis and identifies mature T cells as the cell of origin in CTCL. *Sci Transl Med* 2015;7:308ra158.
58. Mancebo SE, Cordova M, Myskowski PL, *et al.* Reflectance confocal microscopy features of mycosis fungoides and Sézary syndrome: correlation with histopathologic and T-cell receptor rearrangement studies. *J Cutan Pathol* 2016;**43**:505–515.
59. Kohler S, Kim YH, Smoller BR. Histologic criteria for the diagnosis of erythrodermic mycosis fungoides and Sézary syndrome: a critical reappraisal. *J Cutan Pathol* 1997;**24**:292–297.
60. Trotter MJ, Whittaker SJ, Orchard GE, Smith NP. Cutaneous histopathology of Sézary syndrome: a study of 41 cases with a proven circulating T-cell clone. *J Cutan Pathol* 1997;**24**:286–291.
61. Walsh NMG, Prokopetz R, Tron VA, *et al.* Histopathology in erythroderma: review of a series of cases by multiple observers. *J Cutan Pathol* 1994;**21**:419–423.
62. Diwan AH, Prieto VG, Herling M, *et al.* Primary Sézary syndrome commonly shows low-grade cytologic atypia and an absence of epidermotropism. *Am J Clin Pathol* 2005;**123**:510–515.
63. Scarabello A, Leinweber B, Ardigó M, *et al.* Cutaneous lymphomas with prominent granulomatous reaction. A potential pitfall in the histopathologic diagnosis of cutaneous T- and B-cell lymphomas. *Am J Surg Pathol* 2002;**26**:1259–1268.
64. Gru AA, Kim J, Pulitzer M, *et al.* The use of central pathology review with digital slide scanning in advanced-stage mycosis fungoides and Sézary syndrome: a multi-institutional and international pathology study. *Am J Surg Pathol* 2018;**42**:726–734.
65. Schrader AMR, Jansen PM, Willemze R. TOX expression in cutaneous T-cell lymphomas: an adjunctive diagnostic marker that is not tumour specific and not restricted to the $CD4^+/CD8^-$ phenotype. *Br J Dermatology* 2016;**175**:382–386.
66. Miyashiro D, Torrealba MP, Manfrere KC, *et al.* Double-positive CD4 and CD8 Sézary syndrome. *JAAD Case Rep* 2017;**3**:485–488.
67. Uchi H, Hayashida S, Takahara M, *et al.* Serum levels of CC chemokine receptor 4 and CXC chemokine receptor 3 ligands in $CD8^+$ Sézary syndrome. *Acta Derm Venereol* 2012;**92**:280–281.
68. Cetinözman F, Jansen PM, Vermeer MH, *et al.* Differential expression of programmed death-1 (PD-1) in Sézary syndrome and mycosis fungoides. *Arch Dermatol* 2012;**148**:1379–1385.
69. Samimi S, Benoit B, Evans K, *et al.* Increased programmed death-1 expression on $CD4^+$ T cells in cutaneous T-cell lymphoma. *Arch Dermatol* 2010;**146**:1382–1388.
70. Bosisio FM, Cerroni L. Expression of T-follicular helper markers in sequential biopsies of progressive mycosis fungoides and other primary cutaneous T-cell lymphomas. *Am J Dermatopathol* 2015;**37**:115–121.
71. Park JH, Han JH, Kang HY, *et al.* Expression of follicular helper T-cell markers in primary cutaneous T-cell lymphoma. *Am J Dermatopathol* 2014;**36**:465–470.
72. Meyerson HJ, Awadallah A, Pavlidakey P, *et al.* Follicular center helper T-cell (TFH) marker positive mycosis fungoides/Sézary syndrome. *Mod Pathol* 2013;**26**:32–43.
73. Capriotti E, Vonderheid EC, Thoburn CJ, *et al.* Expression of T-plastin, FoxP3 and other tumor-associated markers by leukemic T-cells of cutaneous T-cell lymphoma. *Leuk Lymph* 2008;**49**: 1190–1201.
74. Heid JB, Schmidt A, Oberle N, *et al.* $FOXP3^+$ $CD25^-$ tumor cells with regulatory function in Sézary syndrome. *J Invest Dermatol* 2009;**129**:2875–2885.
75. Wada DA, Pittelkow MR, Comfere NI, *et al.* $CD4^+CD25^+FOXP3^+$ malignant T cells in Sézary syndrome are not necessarily functional regulatory T cells. *J Am Acad Dermatol* 2013;**69**:485–489.
76. Rahbar Z, Li S, Tavallaee M, *et al.* Variability in the expression of immunohistochemical markers: implications for biomarker interpretation in cutaneous T-cell lymphoma. *J Invest Dermatol* 2018;**138**:1204–1206.
77. Vaque JP, Gomez-Lopez G, Monsalvez V, *et al.* PLCG1 mutations in cutaneous T-cell lymphomas. *Blood* 2014;**123**:2034–2043.
78. Caumont C, Gros A, Boucher C, *et al.* PLCG1 gene mutations are uncommon in cutaneous T-cell lymphomas. *J Invest Dermatol* 2015;**135**:2334–2337.
79. Chang LW, Patrone CC, Yang W, *et al.* An integrated data resource for genomic analysis of cutaneous T-cell lymphoma. *J Invest Dermatol* 2018;**138**:2681–2683.
80. Patel VM, Flanagan CE, Martins M, *et al.* Frequent and persistent PLCG1 mutations in Sézary cells directly enhance PLCγ1 activity and stimulate NFκB, AP-1 and NFAT signaling. *J Invest Dermatol* 2020;**140**:380–389.
81. Park J, Yang J, Wenzel AT, *et al.* Genomic analysis of 220 CTCLs identifies a novel recurrent gain-of-function alteration in RLTPR (p.Q575E). *Blood* 2017;**130**:1430–1440.
82. Choi J, Goh G, Walradt T, *et al.* Genomic landscape of cutaneous T cell lymphoma. *Nat Genet* 2015;**47**:1011–1019.
83. da Silva Almeida AC, Abate F, Khiabanian H, *et al.* The mutational landscape of cutaneous T cell lymphoma and Sezary syndrome. *Nat Genet* 2015;**47**:1465–1470.
84. Ungewickell A, Bhaduri A, Rios E, *et al.* Genomic analysis of mycosis fungoides and Sézary syndrome identifies recurrent alterations in TNFR2. *Nat Genet* 2015;**47**:1056–1060.
85. Chevret E, Andrique L, Prochazkova-Carlotti M, *et al.* Telomerase functions beyond telomere maintenance in primary cutaneous T-cell lymphoma. *Blood* 2014;**123**:1850–1859.
86. Lee CS, Ungewickell A, Bhaduri A, *et al.* Transcriptome sequencing in Sézary syndrome identifies Sézary cell and mycosis fungoides-associated lncRNAs and novel transcripts. *Blood* 2012;**120**:3288–3297.
87. Woollard WJ, Pullabhatla V, Lorenc A, *et al.* Candidate driver genes involved in genome maintenance and DNA repair in Sézary syndrome. *Blood* 2016;**127**:3387–3397.
88. Gaydosik AM, Tabib T, Geskin LJ, *et al.* Single-cell lymphocyte heterogeneity in advanced cutaneous T-cell lymphoma skin tumors. *Clin Cancer Res* 2019;**25**:4443–4454.
89. Buus TB, Willerslev-Olsen A, Fredholm S, *et al.* Single-cell heterogeneity in Sézary syndrome. *Blood Adv* 2018;**2**:2115–2126.
90. Moins-Teisserenc H, Daubord M, Clave E, *et al.* CD158k is a reliable marker for diagnosis of Sézary syndrome and reveals an unprecedented heterogeneity of circulating malignant cells. *J Invest Dermatol* 2015;**135**:247–257.
91. Kari L, Loboda A, Nebozhyn M, *et al.* Classification and prediction of survival in patients with the leukemic phase of cutaneous T cell lymphoma. *J Exp Med* 2003;**197**:1477–1488.
92. Laharanne E, Oumouhou N, Bonnet F, *et al.* Genome-wide analysis of cutaneous T-cell lymphomas identifies three clinically relevant classes. *J Invest Dermatol* 2010;**130**:1707–1718.
93. Lin WM, Lewis JM, Filler RB, *et al.* Characterization of the DNA copy-number genome in the blood of cutaneous T-cell lymphoma patients. *J Invest Dermatol* 2012;**132**:188–197.

94. Caprini E, Crsitofoletti C, Arcelli D, *et al.* Identification of key regions and genes important in the pathogenesis of Sézary syndrome by combining genomic and expression microarrays. *Cancer Res* 2009;**69**:8438–8446.
95. Cristofoletti C, Picchio MC, Lazzeri C, *et al.* Comprehensive analysis of PTEN status in Sezary syndrome. *Blood* 2013;**122**: 3511–3520.
96. Mao X, McElwaine S. Functional copy number changes in Sézary syndrome: toward an integrated molecular cytogenetic map III. *Cancer Genet Cytogenet* 2008;**185**:86–94.
97. Scarisbrick JJ, Woolford AJ, Calonje E, *et al.* Frequent abnormalities of the p15 and p16 genes in mycosis fungoides and Sézary syndrome. *J Invest Dermatol* 2002;**118**:493–499.
98. Prasad A, Rabionet R, Espinet B, *et al.* Identification of gene mutations and fusion genes in patients with Sézary syndrome. *J Invest Dermatol* 2016;**136**:1490–1499.
99. Mao X, Orchard G, Lillington DM, *et al.* Amplification and overexpression of JUNB is associated with primary cutaneous T-cell lymphomas. *Blood* 2003;**101**:1513–1519.
100. Vermeer MH, van Doorn R, Dijkman R, *et al.* Novel and highly recurrent chromosomal alterations in Sézary syndrome. *Cancer Res* 2008;**68**:2689–2698.
101. Steininger A, Möbs M, Ullmann R, *et al.* Genomic loss of the putative tumor suppressor gene E2A in human lymphoma. *J Exp Med* 2011;**208**:1585–1593.
102. Ralfkiaer U, Hagedorn PH, Bangsgaard N, *et al.* Diagnostic microRNA profiling in cutaneous T-cell lymphoma (CTCL). *Blood* 2011;**118**:5891–5900.
103. Ballabio E, Mitchell T, van Kester MS, *et al.* MicroRNA expression in Sézary syndrome: identification, function, and diagnostic potential. *Blood* 2010;**116**:1105–1113.
104. van der Fits L, van Kester MS, Qin Y, *et al.* MicroRNA-21 expression in $CD4^+$ T cells is regulated by STAT3 and is pathologically involved in Sézary syndrome. *J Invest Dermatol* 2011;**131**:762–768.
105. van Kester MS, Ballabio E, Benner MF, *et al.* miRNA expression profiling of mycosis fungoides. *Molecular Oncology* 2011;**5**:273–280.
106. Qin Y, Buermans HPJ, van Kester MS, *et al.* Deep-sequencing analysis reveals that the miR-199a2/214 cluster within DNM3os represents the vast majority of aberrantly expressed microRNAs in Sézary syndrome. *J Invest Dermatol* 2012;**132**:1520–1522.
107. Kohnken R, Wen J, Mundy-Bosse B, *et al.* Diminished microRNA-29b level is associated with BRD4-mediated activation of oncogenes in cutaneous T-cell lymphoma. *Blood* 2018;**131**:771–781.
108. Wolff C, Martin-Garcia N, Bensussan A, *et al.* Histopathologic diagnosis of lymphomatous versus inflammatory erythroderma: a morphologic and phenotypic study on 47 skin biopsies. *Am J Dermatopathol* 2010;**32**:755–763.
109. Cetinözman F, Jansen PM, Willemze R. Expression of programmed death-1 in skin biopsies of benign inflammatory vs. lymphomatous erythroderma. *Br J Dermatol* 2014;**171**:499–504.
110. Boonk SE, Zoutman WH, Marie-Cardine A, *et al.* Evaluation of immunophenotypic and molecular biomarkers for Sézary syndrome using standard operating procedures: a multicentre study of 59 patients. *J Invest Dermatol* 2016;**136**:1364e1372.
111. Chennareddy S, Rindler K, Meledathu S, *et al.* Single-cell RNA sequencing of chronic idiopathic erythroderma defines disease-specific markers. *J Allergy Clin Immunol* 2025;**155**: 892–908.
112. van Doorn R, Slieker RC, Boonk SE, *et al.* Epigenomic analysis of Sézary syndrome defines patterns of aberrant DNA methylation and identifies diagnostic markers. *J Invest Dermatol* 2016;**136**:1876–1884.
113. Ortonne N, Le Gouvello S, Mansour H, *et al.* CD158K/KIR3DL2 transcript detection in lesional skin of patients with erythroderma is a tool for the diagnosis of Sézary syndrome. *J Invest Dermatol* 2008;**128**:465–472.
114. Latzka J, Assaf C, Bagot M, *et al.* EORTC consensus recommendations for the treatment of mycosis fungoides/Sèzary syndrome – update 2023. *Eur J Cancer* 2023;**195**:11343.
115. Gilson D, Whittaker SJ, Child FJ, *et al.* British Association of Dermatologists and U.K. Cutaneous Lymphoma Group guidelines for the management of primary cutaneous lymphomas 2018. *Br J Dermatol* 2019;**180**:496–526.
116. Willemze R, Hodak E, Zinzani PL, *et al.* Primary cutaneous lymphomas: ESMO Clinical Practice Guidelines for diagnosis, treatment and follow-up. *Ann Oncol.* 2018;**29**(Supplement_4): iv30–iv40.
117. Quaglino P, Maule M, Prince HM, *et al.* Global patterns of care in advanced stage mycosis fungoides/Sezary syndrome: a multicenter retrospective follow-up study from the Cutaneous Lymphoma International Consortium. *Ann Oncol* 2017;**28**:2517–2525.
118. Dippel E, Assaf C, Becker JC, *et al.* S2k-guidelines – cutaneous lymphomas (ICD10 C82-C86): update 2021. *J Dtsch Dermatol Ges* 2022;**20**:537–555.
119. Scarisbrick JJ, Taylor P, Holtick U, *et al.* U.K. consensus statement on the use of extracorporeal photopheresis for treatment of cutaneous T-cell lymphoma and chronic graft-versus-host disease. *Br J Dermatol* 2008;**158**:659–678.
120. Hanel W, Briski R, Ross CW, *et al.* A retrospective comparative outcome analysis following systemic therapy in Mycosis fungoides and Sezary syndrome. *Am J Hematol* 2016;**91**:E491–E495.
121. Gao C, McCormack C, van der Weyden C, *et al.* Prolonged survival with the early use of a novel extracorporeal photopheresis regimen in patients with Sézary syndrome. *Blood* 2019;**134**:1346–1350.
122. Olsen EA, Hodak E, Anderson T, *et al.* Guidelines for phototherapy of mycosis fungoides and Sézary syndrome: a consensus statement of the United States Cutaneous Lymphoma Consortium. *J Am Acad Dermatol* 2016;**74**:27–58.
123. Jones GW, Rosenthal D, Wilson LD. Total skin electron radiation for patients with erythrodermic cutaneous T-cell lymphoma (mycosis fungoides and the Sézary syndrome). *Cancer* 1999;**85**:1985–1995.
124. Introcaso CE, Micaily B, Richardson SK, *et al.* Total skin electron beam therapy may be associated with improvement of peripheral blood disease in Sézary syndrome. *J Am Acad Dermatol* 2008;**58**:592–595.
125. Klein RS, Dunlop JD, Samimi SS, *et al.* Improvement in peripheral blood disease burden in patients with Sézary syndrome and leukemic mycosis fungoides after total skin electron beam therapy. *J Am Acad Dermatol* 2013;**68**:972–977.
126. Dearden C, Matutes E, Catovsky D. Pentostatin treatment of cutaneous T-cell lymphoma. *Oncology* 2000;**14**(suppl. 2):37–40.
127. Foss FM. Activity of pentostatin (Nipent) in cutaneous T-cell lymphoma: single-agent and combination studies. *Sem Oncol* 2000;**27**(suppl. 5):58–63.
128. Whittaker SJ, Demierre MF, Kim EJ, *et al.* Final results from a multicenter, international, pivotal study of Romidepsin in

refractory cutaneous T-cell lymphoma. *J Clin Oncol* 2010;**28**:4485–4491.
129. Child F, Ortiz-Romero PL, Alvarez R, *et al.* Phase II multicentre trial of oral quisinostat, a histone deacetylase inhibitor, in patients with previously treated stage IB-IVA mycosis fungoides/Sezary syndrome. *Br J Dermatol* 2016;**175**:80–88.
130. Duvic M, Bates SE, Piekarz R, *et al.* Responses to romidepsin in patients with cutaneous T-cell lymphoma and prior treatment with systemic chemotherapy. *Leuk Lymphoma* 2018;**59**:880–887.
131. Deschamps O, Ram-Wolff C, Beylot-Barry M, *et al.* Treatment of mycosis fungoides and Sézary syndrome with romidepsin: a series of 32 cases from the French Study Group for Cutaneous Lymphoma. *Br J Dermatol* 2019;**180**:423–424.
132. Sarris AH, Phan A, Duvic M, *et al.* Trimetrexate in relapsed T-cell lymphoma with skin involvement. *J Clin Oncol* 2002;**20**: 2876–2880.
133. Querfeld C, Rosen ST, Guitart J, *et al.* Results of an open-label multicenter phase 2 trial of lenalidomide monotherapy in refractory mycosis fungoides and Sézary syndrome. *Blood* 2014;**123**:1159–1166.
134. Rupoli S, Goteri G, Pimpinelli N, *et al.* Pegylated liposomal doxorubicin in the treatment of primary cutaneous T-cell lymphomas. *Haematologica* 2007;**92**:686–689.
135. Bouwhuis SA, Davis MDP, el-Azhary RA, *et al.* Bexarotene treatment of late-stage mycosis fungoides and Sézary syndrome: development of extracutaneous lymphoma in 6 patients. *J Am Acad Dermatol* 2005;**52**:991–996.
136. Faguer S, Launay F, Ysebaert L, *et al.* Acute cutaneous T-cell lymphoma transformation during treatment with alemtuzumab. *Br J Dermatol* 2007;**157**:841–842.
137. Molina A, Nademanee A, Arber DA, Forman SJ. Remission of refractory Sézary syndrome after bone marrow transplantation from a matched unrelated donor. *Biol Blood Marrow Transplant* 1999;**5**:400–404.
138. Kahata K, Hashino S, Takahata M, *et al.* Durable remission of Sézary syndrome after unrelated bone marrow transplantation by reduced-intensity conditioning. *Acta Haematol* 2008;**120**:14–18.
139. Duarte RF, Canals C, Onida F, *et al.* Allogeneic hematopoietic cell transplantation for patients with mycosis fungoides and Sézary syndrome: a retrospective analysis of the Lymphoma Working Party of the European Group for Blood and Marrow Transplantation. *J Clin Oncol* 2010;**28**:4492–4499.
140. Schlaak M, Theurich S, Pickenhain J, *et al.* Allogeneic stem cell transplantation for advanced primary cutaneous T-cell lymphoma: a systematic review. *Crit Rev Oncol Hematol* 2013;**85**:21–31.
141. Jacobsen ED, Kim HT, Ho VT, *et al.* A large single-center experience with allogeneic stem-cell transplantation for peripheral T-cell non-Hodgkin lymphoma and advanced mycosis fungoides/Sézary syndrome. *Ann Oncol* 2011;**22**:1608–1613.
142. Wu PA, Kim YH, Lavori PW, *et al.* A meta-analysis of patients receiving allogeneic or autologous hematopoietic stem cell transplant in mycosis fungoides and Sézary syndrome. *Biol Blood Marrow Transplant* 2009;**15**:982–990.
143. Shiratori S, Fujimoto K, Nishimura M, *et al.* Allogeneic hematopoietic stem cell transplantation following reduced-intensity conditioning for mycosis fungoides and Sezary syndrome. *Hematol Oncol* 2016;**34**:9–16.
144. Hosing C, Bassett R, Dabaja B, *et al.* Allogeneic stem-cell transplantation in patients with cutaneous lymphoma: updated results from a single institution. *Ann Oncol* 2015;**26**:2490–2495.
145. Virmani P, Zain J, Rosen ST, *et al.* Hematopoietic stem cell transplant for mycosis fungoides and Sézary syndrome. *Dermatol Clin* 2015;**33**:807–818.
146. Oka T, Sugaya M, Cury-Martins J, *et al.* Hematopoietic stem cell transplantation for cutaneous T-cell lymphoma: Summary of 11 cases from two facilities in Japan and Brazil. *J Dermatol* 2016;**43**:638–642.
147. Saruta H, Ohata C, Muto I, *et al.* Hematopoietic stem cell transplantation in advanced cutaneous T-cell lymphoma. *J Dermatol* 2017;**44**:1038–1042.
148. Atilla E, Atilla PA, Bozdag SC, *et al.* Allogeneic hematopoietic stem cell transplantation for refractory mycosis fungoides (MF) and Sezary syndrome (SS). *Int J Hematol* 2017;**106**:426–430.
149. Kharfan-Dabaja MA, Kumar A, Ayala E, *et al.* Clinical practice recommendations on indication and timing of hematopoietic cell transplantation in mature T cell and NK/T cell lymphomas: an international collaborative effort on behalf of the Guidelines Committee of the American Society for Blood and Marrow Transplantation. *Biol Blood Marrow Transplant* 2017;**23**:1826–1838.
150. Duarte RF, Boumendil A, Onida F, *et al.* Long-term outcome of allogeneic hematopoietic cell transplantation for patients with mycosis fungoides and Sézary syndrome: a European society for blood and marrow transplantation lymphoma working party extended analysis. *J Clin Oncol* 2014;**32**:3347–3348.
151. de Masson A, Beylot-Barry M, Bouaziz JD, *et al.* Allogeneic stem cell transplantation for advanced cutaneous T-cell lymphomas: a study from the French Society of Bone Marrow Transplantation and French Study Group on Cutaneous Lymphomas. *Haematologica* 2014;**99**:527–534.
152. Mori T, Shiratori S, Suzumiya J, *et al.* Outcome of allogeneic hematopoietic stem cell transplantation for mycosis fungoides and Sezary syndrome. *Hematol Oncol* 2020;**38**:266–271.
153. Lechowicz MJ, Lazarus HM, Carreras J, *et al.* Allogeneic hematopoietic cell transplantation for mycosis fungoides and Sezary syndrome. *Bone Marrow Transplant* 2014;**49**:1360–1365.
154. (a) Novelli S, Monter A, Pilar García-Muret M, *et al.* Discussion on the indication of allogeneic stem cell transplantation for advanced cutaneous T cell lymphomas. *Int J Hematol* 2019;**110**:406–410. (b) Goyal A, O'Leary D, Dabaja B, *et al.* ASTCT and USCLC clinical practice recommendations for allogeneic stem cell transplant in mycosis fungoides and Sézary syndrome. *J Am Acad Dermatol* 2025;**93**:387–397.
155. Whittaker S, Hoppe R, Prince HM. How I treat mycosis fungoides and Sezary syndrome. *Blood* 2016;**127**:3142–3153.
156. Khodadoust MS, Mou E, Kim YH. Integrating novel agents into the treatment of advanced mycosis fungoides and Sézary syndrome. *Blood* 2023;**141**:695–703.
157. Tzompa S, Ingen-Housz-Oro S, de Masson A, *et al.* Evolution of patients with Sézary syndrome after mogamulizumab discontinuation for any cause except progression: a multicentre retrospective study (Moga-stop Study). *Br J Dermatol* 2024;**191**:143–144.

158. Bernengo MG, Quaglino P, Comessatti A, *et al.* Low-dose intermittent alemtuzumab in the treatment of Sézary syndrome: clinical and immunologic findings in 14 patients. *Haematologica* 2007;**92**:784–794.
159. Osborne GEN, Pagliuca A, Ho A, du Vivier AWP. Novel treatment of Sézary-like syndrome due to adult T-cell leukaemia/lymphoma with daclizumab (humanized anti-interleukin-2 receptor antibody). *Br J Dermatol* 2006;**155**: 617–620.
160. Lewis DJ, Haun PL, Samimi SS, *et al.* Brentuximab vedotin for relapsed or refractory Sézary syndrome. *JAMA Dermatol* 2021;**157**:317–321.
161. Shen K, Liu Y, Cao X, *et al.* Successful treatment of refractory Sezary syndrome by anti-PD-1 antibody (nivolumab). *Ann Hematol* 2017;**96**:687–688.
162. Kamstrup MR, Rahbek Gjerdrum LM, Biskup E, *et al.* Notch1 as a potential therapeutic target in cutaneous T-cell lymphoma. *Blood* 2010;**116**:2504–2512.
163. van der Fits L, Qin Y, Out-Luiting JJ, *et al.* NOTCH1 signaling as a therapeutic target in Sézary syndrome. *J Invest Dermatol* 2012;**132**:2810–2817.
164. French LE, Huard B, Wysocka M, *et al.* Impaired CD40L signaling is a cause of defective IL-12 and TNF-alpha production in Sézary syndrome: circumvention by hexameric soluble CD40L. *Blood* 2005;**105**:219–225.
165. Wysocka M, Zaki MH, French LE, *et al.* Sézary syndrome patients demonstrate a defect in dendritic cell populations: effects of CD40 ligand and treatment with GM-CSF on dendritic cell numbers and the production of cytokines. *Blood* 2002;**100**:3287–3294.
166. Boonstra PS, Polk A, Brown N, *et al.* A single center phase II study of ixazomib in patients with relapsed or refractory cutaneous or peripheral T-cell lymphomas. *Am J Hematol* 2017;**92**:1287–1294.
167. Bagot M, Porcu P, Marie-Cardine A, *et al.* IPH4102, a first-in-class anti-KIR3DL2 monoclonal antibody, in patients with relapsed or refractory cutaneous T-cell lymphoma: an international, first-in-human, open-label, phase 1 trial. *Lancet Oncol* 2019;**20**:1160–1170.
168. Bliss-Moreau M, Coarfa C, Gunaratne PH, *et al.* Identification of p38b as a therapeutic target for the treatment of Sézary syndrome. *J Invest Dermatol* 2015;**135**:599–608.
169. Giustiniani J, Ta VA, Belkhelouat S, *et al.* Targeting TGF-β activation in cutaneous T-cell lymphomas. *J Invest Dermatol* 2024;**144**:2329–2332.
170. Kohnken R, Mishra A. MicroRNAs in cutaneous T-cell lymphoma: the future of therapy. *J Invest Dermatol* 2019;**139**: 528–534.
171. Maronas-Jimenez L, Estrach T, Gallardo F, *et al.* Aprepitant improves refractory pruritus in primary cutaneous T-cell lymphomas: experience of the Spanish Working Group on Cutaneous Lymphomas. *Br J Dermatol* 2018;**178**:e273–e274.
172. Watanabe K, Gomez AM, Kuramitsu S, *et al.* Identifying highly active anti-CCR4 CAR T cells for the treatment of T-cell lymphoma. *Blood Adv* 2023;**7**:3416–3430.
173. Kubica AW, Davis MDP, Weaver AL, *et al.* Sézary syndrome: a study of 176 patients at Mayo Clinic. *J Am Acad Dermatol* 2012;**67**:1189–1199.
174. Vonderheid EC, Pena J, Nowell P. Sézary cell counts in erythrodermic cutaneous T-cell lymphoma: implications for prognosis and staging. *Leukem Lymph* 2006;**47**:1841–1856.
175. Haththotuwa R, Zilinskiene L, Oliff J, *et al.* Biopsy correlation of surface area vs. single-axis measurements on computed tomography scan of lymph nodes in patients with erythrodermic mycosis fungoides and Sezary syndrome. *Br J Dermatol* 2017;**177**:877–878.
176. Beylot-Barry M, Sibaud V, Thiebaut R, *et al.* Evidence that an identical T cell clone in skin and peripheral blood lymphocytes is an independent prognostic factor in primary cutaneous T cell lymphoma. *J Invest Dermatol* 2001;**117**:920–926.
177. Kim YH, Liu HL, Mraz-Gernhard S, *et al.* Long-term outcome of 525 patients with mycosis fungoides and Sézary syndrome. *Arch Dermatol* 2003;**139**:857–866.
178. Diamandidou E, Colome M, Fayad L, *et al.* Prognostic factor analysis in mycosis fungoides/Sézary syndrome. *J Am Acad Dermatol* 1999;**40**:914–924.
179. Scarisbrick JJ, Whittaker S, Evans AV, *et al.* Prognostic significance of tumor burden in the blood of patients with erythrodermic primary cutaneous T-cell lymphoma. *Blood* 2001;**97**:624–630.
180. Stevens SR, Baron ED, Masten S, Cooper KD. Circulating $CD4^+$ $CD7^-$ lymphocyte burden and rapidity of response. Predictors of outcome in the treatment of Sézary syndrome and erythrodermic mycosis fungoides with extracorporeal photopheresis. *Arch Dermatol* 2002;**138**:1347–1350.
181. Talpur R, Singh L, Daulat S, *et al.* Long-term outcomes of 1,263 patients with mycosis fungoides and Sézary syndrome from 1982 to 2009. *Clin Cancer Res* 2012;**18**:5051–5060.
182. Mundy-Bosse B, Denlinger N, McLaughlin E, *et al.* Highly cytotoxic natural killer cells are associated with poor prognosis in patients with cutaneous T-cell lymphoma. *Blood Adv* 2018;**2**:1818–1827.
183. Di Raimondo C, Rubio-Gonzalez B, Palmer J, *et al.* Expression of immune checkpoint molecules programmed death protein 1, programmed death-ligand 1 and inducible T-cell co-stimulator in mycosis fungoides and Sèzary syndrome: association with disease stage and clinical outcome. *Br J Dermatol* 2022;**187**:234–243.
184. (a)Benton EC, Crichton S, Talpur R, *et al.* A cutaneous lymphoma international prognostic index (CLIPi) for mycosis fungoides and Sézary syndrome. *Eur J Cancer* 2013;**49**:2859–2868.(b) Scarisbrick JJ, Quaglino P, Whittaker SJ, *et al.* A new prognostic index (CLIPI) for advanced cutaneous lymphoma enables precise patient risk stratification. *Blood* 2025. doi: 10.1182/blood.2025029628. Online ahead of print.
185. Laharanne E, Chevret E, Idrissi Y, *et al.* CDKN2A–CDKN2B deletion defines an aggressive subset of cutaneous T-cell lymphoma. *Mod Pathol* 2010;**23**:547–558.
186. Litvinov IV, Jones DA, Sasseville D, *et al.* Transcriptional profiles predict disease outcome in patients with cutaneous T-cell lymphoma. *Clin Cancer Res* 2010;**16**:2106–2114.

# CHAPTER 5

# Primary cutaneous CD30$^+$ lymphoproliferative disorders

Lymphomatoid papulosis and cutaneous anaplastic large cell lymphoma are included in the group of the "primary cutaneous CD30$^+$ T-cell lymphoproliferative disorders" in the International Consensus Classification (ICC) *of Myeloid and Lymphoid Neoplasms*, the 2019 and 2024 updates of classification of cutaneous lymphomas by the European Organization of Research and Treatment of Cancer (EORTC) – Cutaneous Lymphoma Histopathology Group, and the World Health Organization (WHO) *Classification of Haematolymphoid Tumours* [1–5]. These entities represent two ends of a spectrum without clear-cut boundaries, and "borderline" cases may be difficult to classify precisely as either lymphomatoid papulosis or cutaneous anaplastic large cell lymphoma.

The CD30 antigen is a cytokine receptor belonging to the tumor necrosis factor receptor superfamily. The antigen was initially described within Reed–Sternberg and Hodgkin cells of Hodgkin lymphoma and subsequently identified within neoplastic cells of a new group of non-Hodgkin lymphomas (anaplastic large cell lymphoma). Soon after the first description, it became clear that anaplastic large cell lymphoma could occur as a primary skin tumor, where it was characterized by a good prognosis [6]. The term "cutaneous CD30$^+$ lymphoproliferative disorders" has been subsequently proposed to denote a group of primary cutaneous T-cell lymphoproliferative disorders characterized by expression of the CD30 antigen and favorable prognosis, including lymphomatoid papulosis and primary cutaneous anaplastic large cell lymphoma [7, 8]. Cases described in the past as "regressing atypical histiocytosis" or "pseudo-Hodgkin disease" are part of the spectrum of primary cutaneous CD30$^+$ lymphoproliferative disorders [9]. In addition, most, if not all, cases reported as "primary cutaneous Hodgkin lymphoma" [10] represent, in my view, examples of either lymphomatoid papulosis or cutaneous anaplastic large cell lymphoma (see Chapter 27). Interestingly, cases of CD30$^+$ lymphoproliferative disorders arising in the mucosal region of the oral cavity (including lip and tongue), of the orbit and conjunctiva, or of the nasal cavity and sinuses share many similarities to the cutaneous lesions, thus probably representing a mucosal variant of the cutaneous disease [11].

It should be underlined that CD30 is a very important marker for diagnosis and classification of cutaneous lymphomas, but interpretation of the staining cannot be made without knowledge of full histopathologic and phenotypic features, as well as complete clinical information. I have observed cases of aggressive cytotoxic lymphomas or even B-cell lymphomas (not to mention the many pseudolymphomas) that had been erroneously classified as cutaneous anaplastic large cell lymphoma because of CD30 positivity. These mistakes can have disastrous consequences for patients. Several similar cases with incomplete phenotypic features and possibly erroneous diagnoses have been published in the literature. In this context, it must be clearly understood that a histopathological diagnosis of lymphomatoid papulosis or cutaneous anaplastic large cell lymphoma should be made only upon compelling evidence, particularly in cases that present with clinical features that are not typical of these disorders.

Several studies attempted to elucidate the reason(s) for the frequent partial or complete spontaneous resolution of the lesions and the good prognosis of cutaneous CD30$^+$ lymphoproliferative disorders. It has been suggested that CD30 and CD30-ligand are involved in the control of apoptosis and that activation of the CD30 signaling pathway plays a role in tumor regression [12]. Resistance to CD30-mediated growth inhibition provides a possible mechanism for escape from tumor regression in cases with more aggressive behavior. A higher expression of apoptotic-related proteins has been observed in lymphomatoid papulosis as compared to cutaneous anaplastic large cell lymphoma, suggesting that the apoptosis index may play a role in the spontaneous resolution of the lesions and better prognosis of lymphomatoid papulosis [13]. However, this difference alone cannot explain the clinical dissimilarities between the two disorders, as in most instances, lymphomatoid papulosis is characterized by recurrent crops of generalized papules and small nodules, and cutaneous anaplastic large cell lymphoma by solitary tumors.

As already mentioned, there is no clear-cut boundary between lymphomatoid papulosis and primary cutaneous anaplastic large cell lymphoma. The term "borderline lymphomatoid

*Skin Lymphoma: The Illustrated Guide*, Sixth Edition. Lorenzo Cerroni.

papulosis – anaplastic large cell lymphoma" has been used by some authors for cases where a definitive diagnosis is not possible. In this group are included uncommon cases with clinical aspects of lymphomatoid papulosis and histopathologic features of primary cutaneous anaplastic large cell lymphoma and vice versa (see the section on borderline cases in this chapter).

Several studies investigated the relationship and differential features of lymphomatoid papulosis and cutaneous anaplastic large cell lymphoma. *IRF4* gene rearrangements are found in both conditions, although more commonly in cutaneous anaplastic large cell lymphoma [14–16]. Increased expression of the Toll-like receptors (TLRs) 2, 4, 7, and 9 has been detected in the keratinocytes overlying infiltrates of lymphomatoid papulosis type C as well as of cutaneous anaplastic large cell lymphoma [17]. Higher numbers of forkhead box protein P3 (FOXP3)+ T-regulatory (Treg) lymphocytes were observed in lymphomatoid papulosis as compared to cutaneous anaplastic large cell lymphoma [18]. The inhibitor of differentiation 2 (Id2, located on 2p25) and the oncogenic transcription factor Fra2 (located on 2p23) are aberrantly expressed both in anaplastic large cell lymphoma and in lymphomatoid papulosis [19]. Deregulation of the *ID2* and *FRA2* genes may be involved in the reorganization of chromosome 2 prior to the t(2;5) translocation. This genetic feature may represent an important step also for cases of translocation-positive anaplastic large cell lymphoma [19], possibly representing a common molecular background of both anaplastic large cell lymphomas and lymphomatoid papulosis. In this context, the level of Fra2 and Id2 is lower in lymphomatoid papulosis than in anaplastic large cell lymphoma, suggesting that gene dosage may be involved in the progression and invasiveness of these diseases [19].

## Lymphomatoid Papulosis

Lymphomatoid papulosis is defined as a chronic, recurrent, self-healing eruption of papules and small nodules with the histopathologic features of a cutaneous T-cell lymphoma ("rhythmic paradoxical eruption") [20]. The etiology of the disease is unknown. No repeatable association with in flammatory skin disorders or viral infections has been demonstrated, but a study suggested a link to atopic diathesis and staphylococcal superantigens [21]. As the self-resolution of the lesions without specific treatment is part of the definition of the disease, and as the histopathological features are protean and not pathognomonic, it follows as a consequence that *a diagnosis of lymphomatoid papulosis cannot be made without complete and precise clinical information*. This should be kept in mind by all dermatopathologists attempting to make the diagnosis on histopathological grounds alone. Another thing to keep in mind is that the so-called "subtypes" of lymphomatoid papulosis do not have any diagnostic or prognostic implication and should not be included in the clinical or histopathological report (see below and Table 5.1).

In 10–20% of patients, lymphomatoid papulosis is preceded by, concomitant with, or followed by another type of lymphoma (usually mycosis fungoides, Hodgkin lymphoma, or anaplastic large cell lymphoma, but other malignant hematologic disorders have also been observed) (see also Chapter 3) [22–27]. The percentage was higher (40%) in one study [28], possibly due to referral bias. A second lymphoma has been observed in a similar proportion of patients, also in children with lymphomatoid papulosis [29, 30]. Although the prognosis of most patients with lymphomatoid papulosis and a second hematological malignancy is usually excellent, those developing extracutaneous anaplastic large cell lymphoma may show an aggressive course [31]. In some of the patients with lymphomatoid papulosis and associated lymphomas, the same clone of neoplastic T lymphocytes has been identified in lesions of the two lymphoproliferative disorders, raising the question of a common origin of the diseases [32–35]. In this context, it has been suggested that nodal anaplastic large cell lymphomas arising in the context of lymphomatoid papulosis should be considered as a form of transformation or progression rather than as a second lymphoma [36]. However, response to treatment may be different, and lesions of lymphomatoid papulosis may continue to appear while the second lymphoma is in complete remission [37]. Coexistence of lesions of different disorders with a common clonal origin but with different genetic abnormalities may be due to early divergence of cells arising from a common precursor. In two patients with lymphomatoid papulosis associated with a B-cell malignancy, exacerbation of lymphomatoid papulosis was observed during therapy with rituximab, suggesting that the B lymphocytes may play a role in the control of the disease [38].

In patients with mycosis fungoides, self-healing papules with CD30+ lymphoid infiltrates may develop during the course of the disease, possibly suggesting a diagnosis of lymphomatoid papulosis associated with mycosis fungoides. In these patients, it is of crucial importance to rule out a large cell transformation of mycosis fungoides. In fact, one case that our group published in 1991 as "PUVA-induced lymphomatoid papulosis in a patient with mycosis fungoides" [39] died with large cell transformation of mycosis fungoides 48 months after the onset of the "lymphomatoid papulosis" (see also Chapter 3). As a matter of fact, differentiation of mycosis fungoides with CD30+ large cell transformation from lymphomatoid papulosis or cutaneous anaplastic large cell lymphoma is extremely difficult and may be impossible in given cases. Useful information may be obtained by molecular analyses of *IRF4* translocations. Most cases of mycosis fungoides with CD30+ large cell transformation are negative for *IRF4* translocations, whereas cutaneous large cell anaplastic lymphoma is positive [14, 16]. The fluorescence in situ hybridization (FISH) analysis is of less value for the

**Table 5.1** The "alphabet soup" of variants of lymphomatoid papulosis*

| Type | Histopathological features | Main phenotype | Main histopathological differential diagnosis | Comment |
|---|---|---|---|---|
| A | Wedge-shaped infiltrate with several large, atypical cells admixed with small lymphocytes, eosinophils, and neutrophils. | $CD4^+$ | Arthropod bite reactions. | This is the most common histopathological subtype of lymphomatoid papulosis |
| B | Band-like or wedge-shaped infiltrate of small/medium-sized atypical cells with epidermotropism. | $CD4^+$ | Mycosis fungoides. | $CD30^-$ cases are reported in the literature but should be evaluated critically; in my experience, type B lymphomatoid papulosis is always $CD30^+$ |
| C | Large nodules or sheets of large, atypical cells. | $CD4^+$ | Anaplastic large cell lymphoma. | Differentiation from anaplastic large cell lymphoma is possible only upon clinical correlation |
| D | Band-like or wedge-shaped infiltrate with prominent (pagetoid reticulosis-like) epidermotropism of cytotoxic atypical cells. | $CD8^+$ | Aggressive epidermotropic $CD8^+$ cytotoxic T-cell lymphoma. | Differentiation from aggressive epidermotropic $CD8^+$ cytotoxic T-cell lymphoma is possible only upon clinical correlation |
| E | Presence of angiotropism/angiodestruction with perivascular and intraluminal infiltrates of atypical cells. | $CD4^+$ or $CD8^+$ | Aggressive "angiotropic" lymphomas (e.g., extranodal NK/T-cell lymphoma, nasal-type). | Angiotropism is sometimes present in lesions of other histopathological variants |
| F | Infiltrate centered around a hair follicle with pilotropism (with or without mucin deposition within the follicle). | $CD4^+$ | Follicular mycosis fungoides. | In some cases, it may represent a chance finding (i.e., lymphomatoid papulosis arising in the vicinity of a hair follicle) |
| G | Gamma/delta cytotoxic phenotype. | $CD8^+$ | Cutaneous gamma/delta T-cell lymphoma and other T-cell lymphomas with gamma/delta phenotype. | Differentiation from cutaneous gamma/delta T-cell lymphoma or other T-cell lymphomas with gamma/delta phenotype is possible only upon clinical correlation |
| H | Presence of Hodgkin and Reed-Sternberg-like cells. | $CD4^+$ | Hodgkin lymphoma. | Similar cells may also be encountered in cutaneous anaplastic large cell lymphoma |
| I | Presence of intralymphatic complexes of atypical cells. | $CD4^+$ | Intravascular lymphoma is, benign intralymphatic proliferation of blasts. | Staining for podoplanin is crucial for a precise classification |
| K | Presence of "keratoacanthoma-like" pseudoepitheliomatous epidermal hyperplasia. | $CD4^+$ | Keratoacanthoma. | In some cases, association with genuine keratoacanthomas has been documented |
| R | Regional lymphomatoid papulosis: lesions are localized to one area of the body; recurrences occur at the same site. | $CD4^+$ or $CD8^+$ | Arthropod bite reactions, anaplastic large cell lymphoma. | Clinically should be differentiated from cutaneous anaplastic large cell lymphoma with satellites |
| 6 | Presence of a chromosomal rearrangement of the *DUSP22–IRF4* locus on 6p25.3. | $CD4^-$ $CD8^+$ or $CD4^-$ $CD8^-$ | Anaplastic large cell lymphoma, transformed mycosis fungoides. | Often a "biphasic" pattern with epidermotropism of small lymphocytes and larger cells in the dermis |

* All of these variants are described in the literature, but at present letters defining specific variants are accepted only for 5 of them (A to E). There is no need to classify cases of lymphomatoid papulosis according to any of these "variants" (see text for details).

discrimination of mycosis fungoides-associated lymphomatoid papulosis, however, as only a minority of cases of lymphomatoid papulosis are positive [16].

In addition to these hematologic malignancies, patients with lymphomatoid papulosis are also at higher risk of developing other lymphoid or non-lymphoid second malignancies [40]. I have observed cases of lymphomatoid papulosis in patients with B-cell chronic lymphocytic leukemia (B-CLL), and others have been published [41, 42], suggesting that this association is not rare. Association with hepatitis E viral (HEV) infection has been reported in one case [43]. In this case, complete remission of lymphomatoid papulosis was observed with antiviral treatment, achieving sustained virological response, and HEV was detected within dermal microvascular endothelial cells by immunofluorescence staining, in situ hybridization, and electron microscopy.

In the absence of specific symptoms of other associated diseases, complete staging investigations are not necessary in patients with lymphomatoid papulosis. As well as in some healthy individuals, T-cell clonality may be detected within the peripheral blood or the bone marrow of patients with lymphomatoid papulosis or cutaneous anaplastic large cell lymphoma, but the clones are not related to those of the cutaneous disorder and do not have clinical significance [44].

## Clinical features

Young adults are usually affected, but lymphomatoid papulosis has been reported in children and in the elderly as well [30, 45–51]. As already mentioned, the hallmark of the disease and a pre-requisite for the diagnosis is the spontaneous resolution of the lesions, which is observed within a few weeks or, rarely, months. The time interval between two episodes (i.e., between the resolution of lesions and the onset of new ones) is variable: some patients may experience several eruptions within short periods of time, whereas others may have only a few lesions over several years. Rarely, patients may have a single eruption of otherwise typical lymphomatoid papulosis and do not experience recurrences. Frequency and number of recurrences have no prognostic meaning.

Clinically, lymphomatoid papulosis presents in most patients with a generalized eruption of reddish-brown papules or small nodules on the trunk and proximal extremities, but in some cases, only a few lesions may be present (Figs. 5.1 and 5.2). Oral or other mucosal involvement may be observed rarely, as well as involvement of the palms and soles (Figs. 5.3 and 5.4). Lesions on the hands should be distinguished from those of milker's nodule and orf, which may present with similar clinical and histopathological features (see Chapter 31). The size of the lesions is variable, but they are usually smaller than 1 cm. In a few patients, large, rapidly growing nodules, sometimes with ulceration, may be the first manifestation of lymphomatoid papulosis (Fig. 5.5) [7]. The onset of large tumors with complete spontaneous resolution has also been observed during the

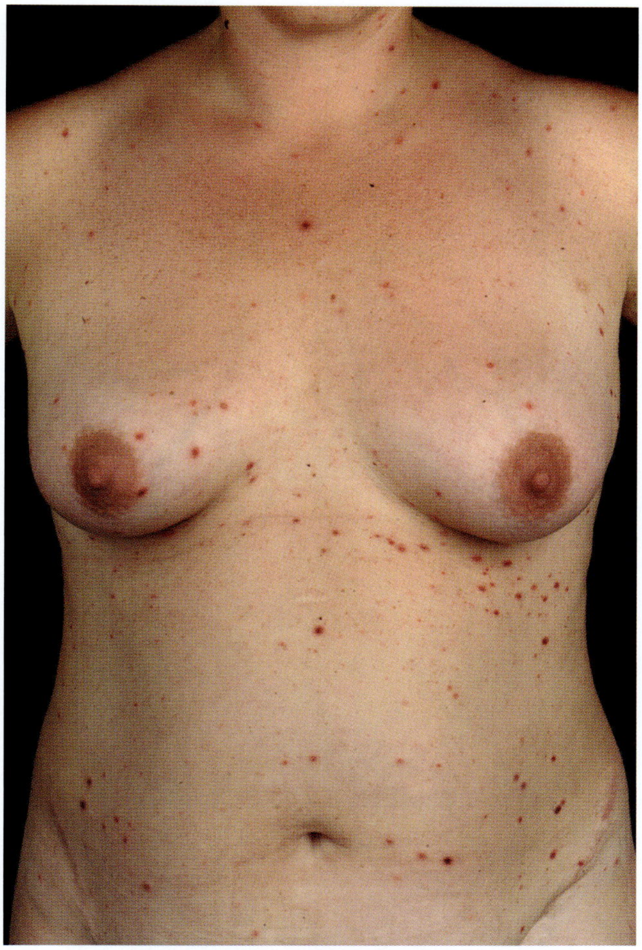

**Figure 5.1** Lymphomatoid papulosis. Generalized papular eruption, with some lesions showing partial necrosis.

course of the disease (Fig. 5.6). In these cases, the prognosis is not affected, suggesting that large tumors that regress spontaneously represent a morphologic variation of lymphomatoid papulosis rather than a transformation into a more aggressive lymphoma [7]. The clinical picture is usually polymorphic due to the presence of lesions in different stages of evolution (Fig. 5.7). Ulceration is common and sometimes is followed by prominent scarring (Fig. 5.8).

I have observed only in children a peculiar clinical presentation with perilesional depigmentation surrounding livid, flat resolving plaques, usually in the context of more conventional papules and small nodules of the disease (Fig. 5.9). Another uncommon presentation, seen both in children and adults, is related to angiodestruction and shows clinically deep red or livid hemorrhagic lesions that may be misinterpreted as a vasculitic process or a purpura (Fig. 5.10) [52, 53]. This presentation often corresponds to the histopathological subtype E (see below). Sometimes small papules may be clustered with a herpetiform arrangement (Fig. 5.11), or tiny clustered papules may

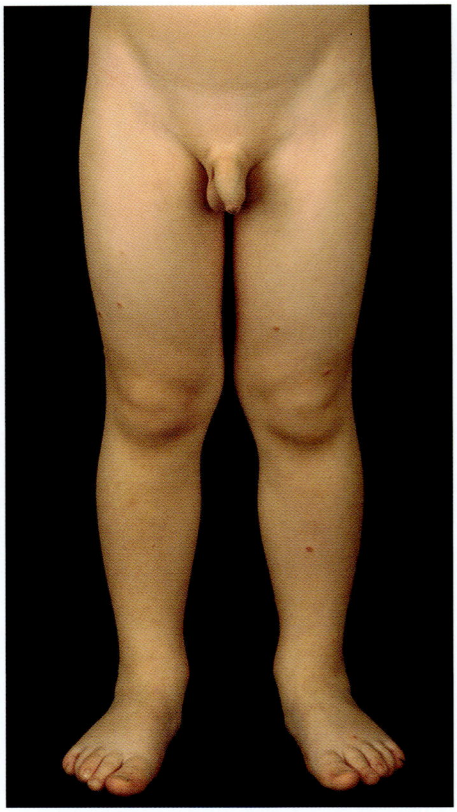

Figure 5.2 Lymphomatoid papulosis. Few papules in a 4-year-old child.

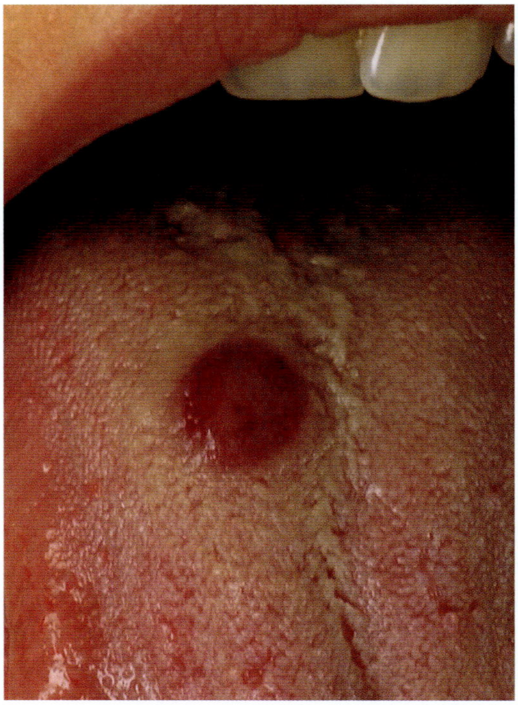

Figure 5.3 Lymphomatoid papulosis. Nodule on the tongue. (*Courtesy of Prof. Andreas Chott, Vienna, Austria.*).

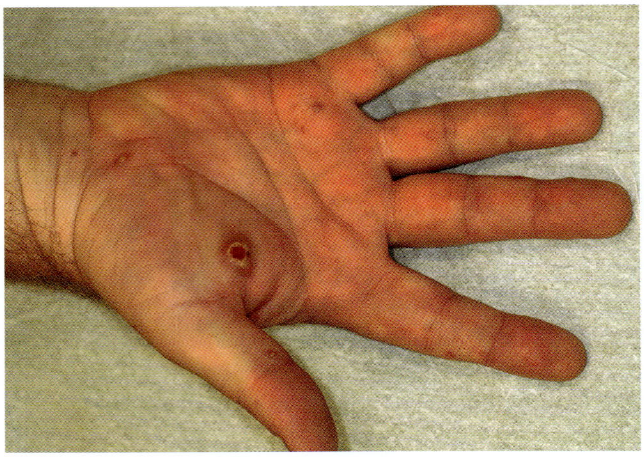

Figure 5.4 Lymphomatoid papulosis. Few papules, pustules, and a small ulcerated nodule on the palm. (*Courtesy of Prof. Robert Müllegger, Wiener Neustadt, Austria.*)

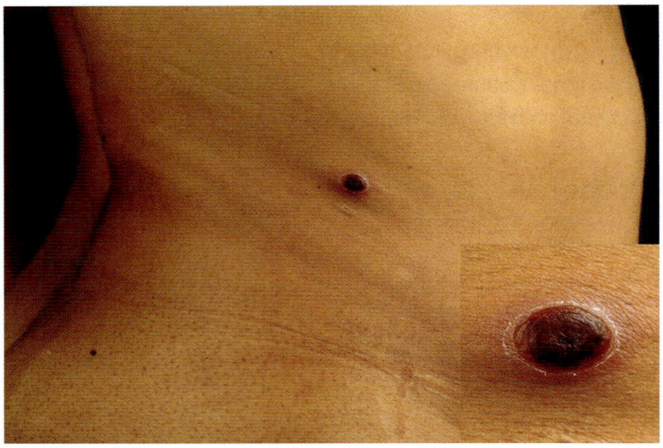

Figure 5.5 Lymphomatoid papulosis. Large, solitary, crusted tumor on the flank, resembling the clinical picture of cutaneous anaplastic large cell lymphoma (detail in the inset). The patient subsequently developed several papules of lymphomatoid papulosis on the trunk.

convey the impression of a large, flat plaque that deviates from the conventional clinical presentation (Fig. 5.12). In some patients, continuous recurrences of clustered lesions on a given body area are associated with post-lesional hyperpigmentation. Such lesions may be misinterpreted as large, infiltrated plaques and may suggest a clinical diagnosis of mycosis fungoides, but careful clinical examination and follow-up data allow them to be classified properly (Fig. 5.13). Another unusual clinical variant of lymphomatoid papulosis clinically resembles hydroa vacciniforme [54].

The onset of lymphomatoid papulosis has been observed after allogeneic stem cell transplantation, during pregnancy, and in patients with severe hypereosinophilic syndrome [55–57].

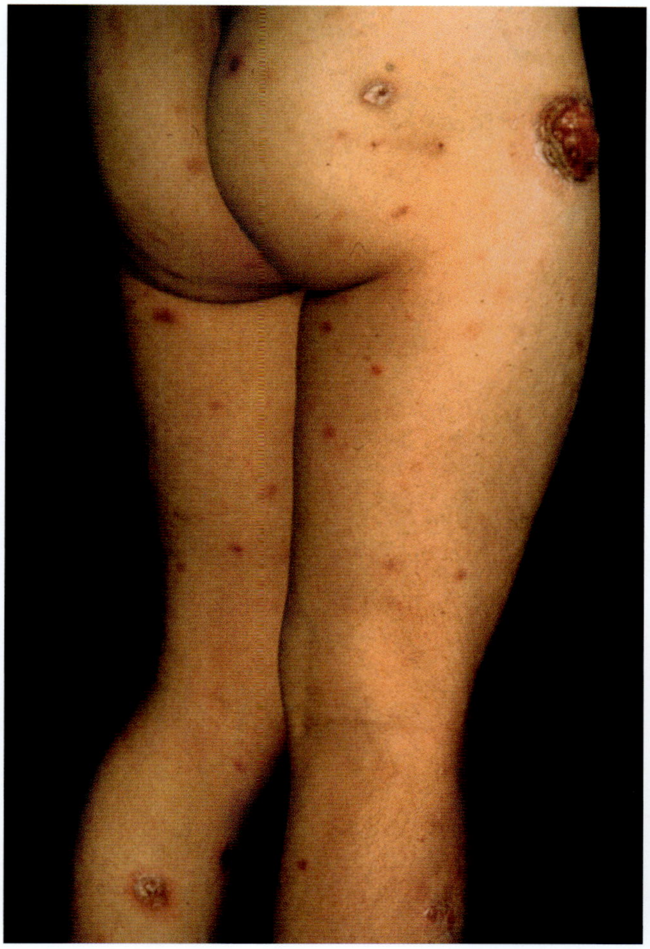

Figure 5.6 Lymphomatoid papulosis. Large, ulcerated tumor on the right flank, as well as several papules and small ulcerated nodules on both legs and buttocks. Larger, ulcerated tumors may rarely arise in the context of lymphomatoid papulosis.

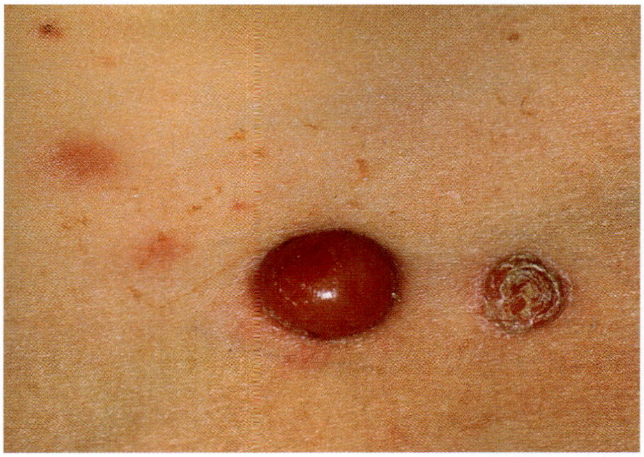

Figure 5.7 Lymphomatoid papulosis. Small erythematous nodule. Note a resolving lesion on the right side of the nodule and two early papules on the left side.

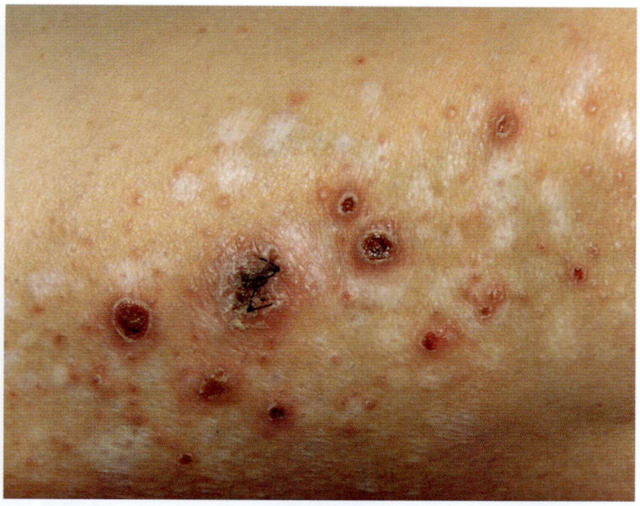

Figure 5.8 Lymphomatoid papulosis. Ulcerated erythematous papules and small nodules with scarring after resolution of previous lesions.

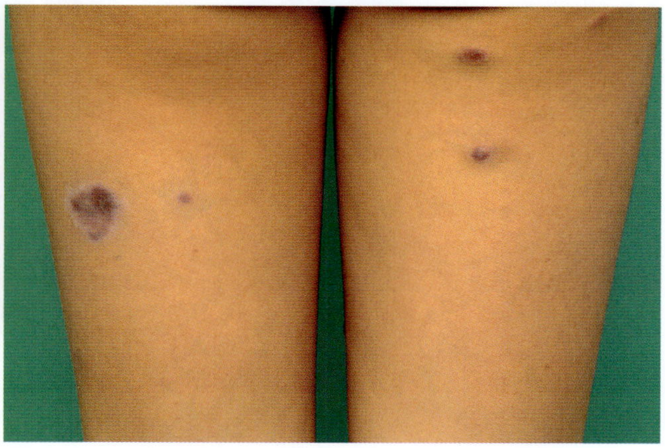

Figure 5.9 Lymphomatoid papulosis. Livid papules, plaques, and small nodules with irregular perilesional hypopigmentation. (*Courtesy of Dr. Cornelia Müller, Homburg am Saar, Germany.*)

### Regional lymphomatoid papulosis ("type R")

In some patients, lesions of lymphomatoid papulosis are localized to just one area of the body, and recurrences always occur in the same area (regional lymphomatoid papulosis) (Fig. 5.14; see Table 5.1) [58–60]. Such cases have also been reported as "persistent agmination" of lymphomatoid papulosis [59, 61]. A peculiar type of regional lymphomatoid papulosis was localized to the skin site of a Becker nevus [62]. I have also observed a rare case of regional lymphomatoid papulosis localized only to the oral mucosa, with recurrent lesions restricted to this site for a period of 7 years (Fig. 5.15).

Differentiation of regional lymphomatoid papulosis from cutaneous anaplastic large cell lymphoma can be extremely difficult because the last can present with nodules surrounded by satellite lesions of smaller dimensions, clinically similar to those observed in lymphomatoid papulosis. Although *IRF4* translocations are

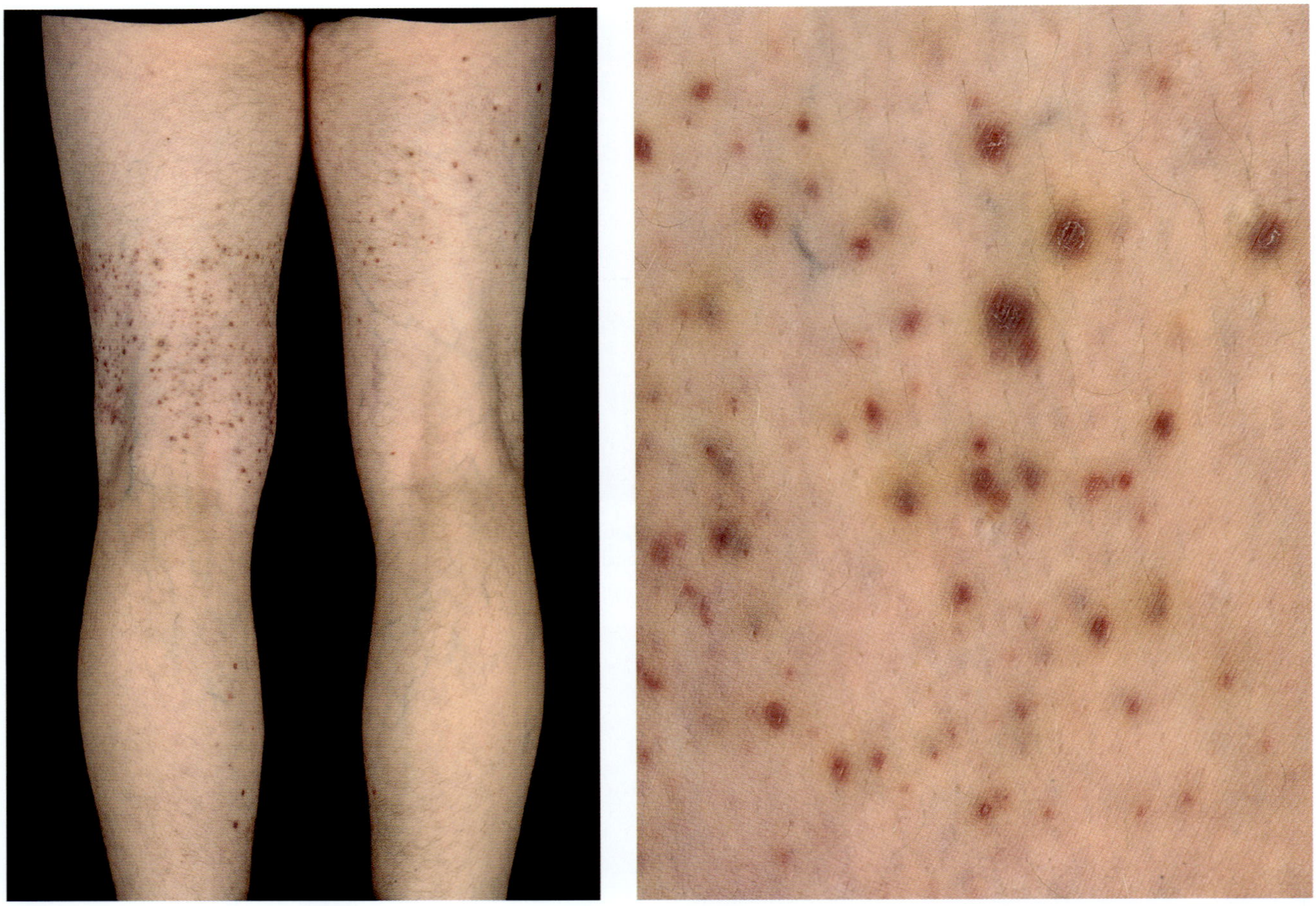

(a) (b)

Figure 5.10 Lymphomatoid papulosis. (a) Hemorrhagic ("angiomatoid") features are a characteristic clinical presentation of lymphomatoid papulosis with angiodestruction (type E). (b) Details of the lesions with clinical features that may be misconstrued as those of a vasculitis.

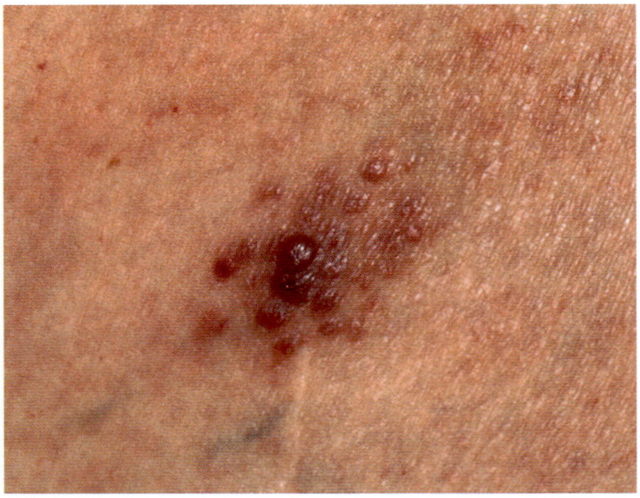

Figure 5.11 Lymphomatoid papulosis. Small clustered papules with a herpetiform arrangement.

more common in cutaneous anaplastic large-cell lymphoma than in lymphomatoid papulosis [16], a positive or negative result cannot be considered completely diagnostic. On the other hand, lesions of regional lymphomatoid papulosis may resolve completely without treatment between two episodes, unlike those of cutaneous anaplastic large cell lymphoma (in this context, a pitfall is represented by cases in which spontaneous resolution of some lesions is concomitant with the onset of new ones, thus never showing complete clearance in the affected area).

## Histopathology, immunophenotype, and molecular genetics

### Histopathology

The histopathologic features of lymphomatoid papulosis are variable. Five main histologic subtypes (types A, B, C, D, and E) and several other variants have been described (Table 5.1). It is important to recognize that these variants can all be observed in one patient at the same time or during the course of the disease

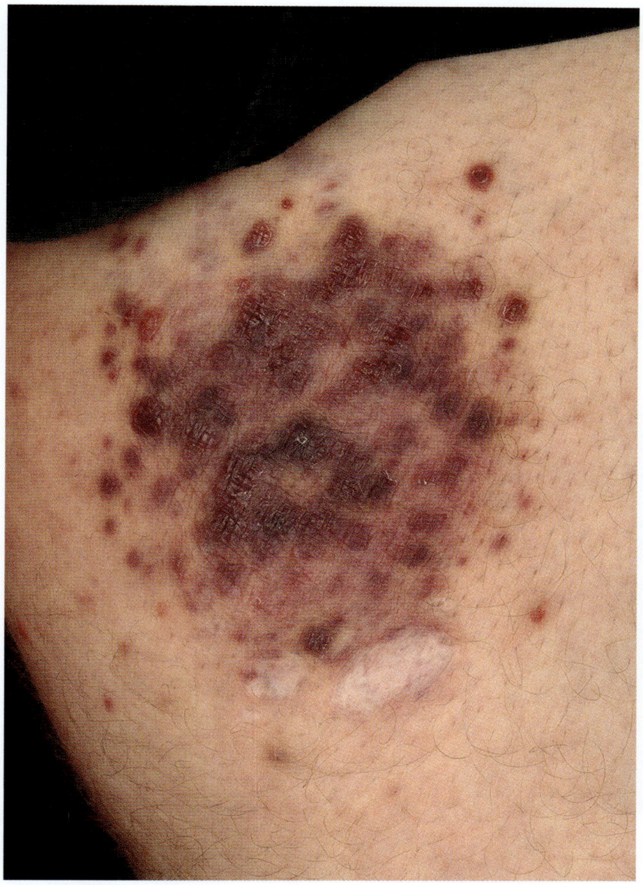

Figure 5.12 Lymphomatoid papulosis. Several confluent papules form a large, violaceous plaque.

and that the histopathologic "subtype" does not have any diagnostic or prognostic implications. Sometimes, features of different histological subtypes may be found even in a single lesion. In short, it must be clearly stated that the histopathological "subtypes" of lymphomatoid papulosis do not represent a real "variant" of the disease and should not be mentioned in the histopathology report; they are useful to dermatopathologists only as a reminder that the disease has a protean appearance and that it may mimic histopathologically several, often aggressive lymphomas.

### *Type A ("conventional" or "histiocytic" type)*

This is the most frequent histopathologic type of lymphomatoid papulosis, characterized by wedge-shaped lesions with the presence of scattered or clustered large, atypical, anaplastic cells admixed with small lymphocytes, histiocytes, neutrophils, and eosinophils (Figs. 5.16 and 5.17). In past publications, it was referred to as the "histiocytic" type because the large, atypical cells bear some morphologic resemblance to histiocytes (and were believed to be of histiocytic origin as well; some older reports on lymphomatoid papulosis were published under the diagnosis of "regressing atypical histiocytosis"). Epidermotropism is variable. Necrosis may be present and is related to the age of the lesion. Scattered intraepidermal necrotic keratinocytes may be observed as well, but are an uncommon finding. Large, atypical lymphocytes resembling Hodgkin and Reed–Sternberg cells are found in some of the cases.

### *Type B (mycosis fungoides-like)*

This is a rare type of lymphomatoid papulosis that reveals a wedge-shaped or, more rarely, band-like infiltrate of CD4+, small- to medium-sized pleomorphic cells with epidermotropism (Fig. 5.18). Small intraepidermal collections resembling Darier nests may be observed (Fig. 5.19a) and can be highlighted with a staining for CD30 (Fig. 5.19b). Some large cells are usually found within the dermal infiltrate. Although the epidermotropic cells are positive for CD4 by definition, cytotoxic proteins may be expressed in this type of lymphomatoid papulosis, too (Figs. 5.19c and d).

It is crucial to understand that differentiation of lymphomatoid papulosis type B from mycosis fungoides can be achieved only by clinicopathologic correlation and that a diagnosis of lymphomatoid papulosis type B should never be established without a complete clinical history. While epidermotropism is a characteristic feature of both type B and type D lymphomatoid papulosis (and, parenthetically, can be observed in variable degrees in all other types as well), neoplastic cells in type D are strongly positive for CD8, and the epidermotropism is more pronounced ("pagetoid"), simulating the picture of cutaneous aggressive epidermotropic CD8+ cytotoxic T-cell lymphoma (see below).

Although large atypical cells are the hallmark of lymphomatoid papulosis and the existence of a "small cell" variant may seem a morphologic contradiction, cases of lymphomatoid papulosis type B with a predominance of small/medium-sized lymphocytes may be conceptually compared to the small/medium cell variant of cutaneous anaplastic large cell lymphoma, which is a well-recognized morphologic subtype of that lymphoma (a small/medium cell variant of anaplastic large cell lymphoma is well known in the lymph nodes, too).

### *Type C (anaplastic large cell lymphoma-like)*

Lymphomatoid papulosis type C is characterized by a nodular infiltrate with sheets of cohesive, large atypical cells admixed with a few small lymphocytes, neutrophils, and eosinophils (Fig. 5.20). The histopathologic features are indistinguishable from those of cutaneous anaplastic large cell lymphoma, and a definitive diagnosis can be achieved only upon clinicopathologic correlation [63].

### *Type D (cutaneous aggressive epidermotropic CD8+ cytotoxic T-cell lymphoma-like)*

Our group described a variant of lymphomatoid papulosis characterized by marked epidermotropism of CD8+ cytotoxic T lymphocytes, simulating histopathologically the features of

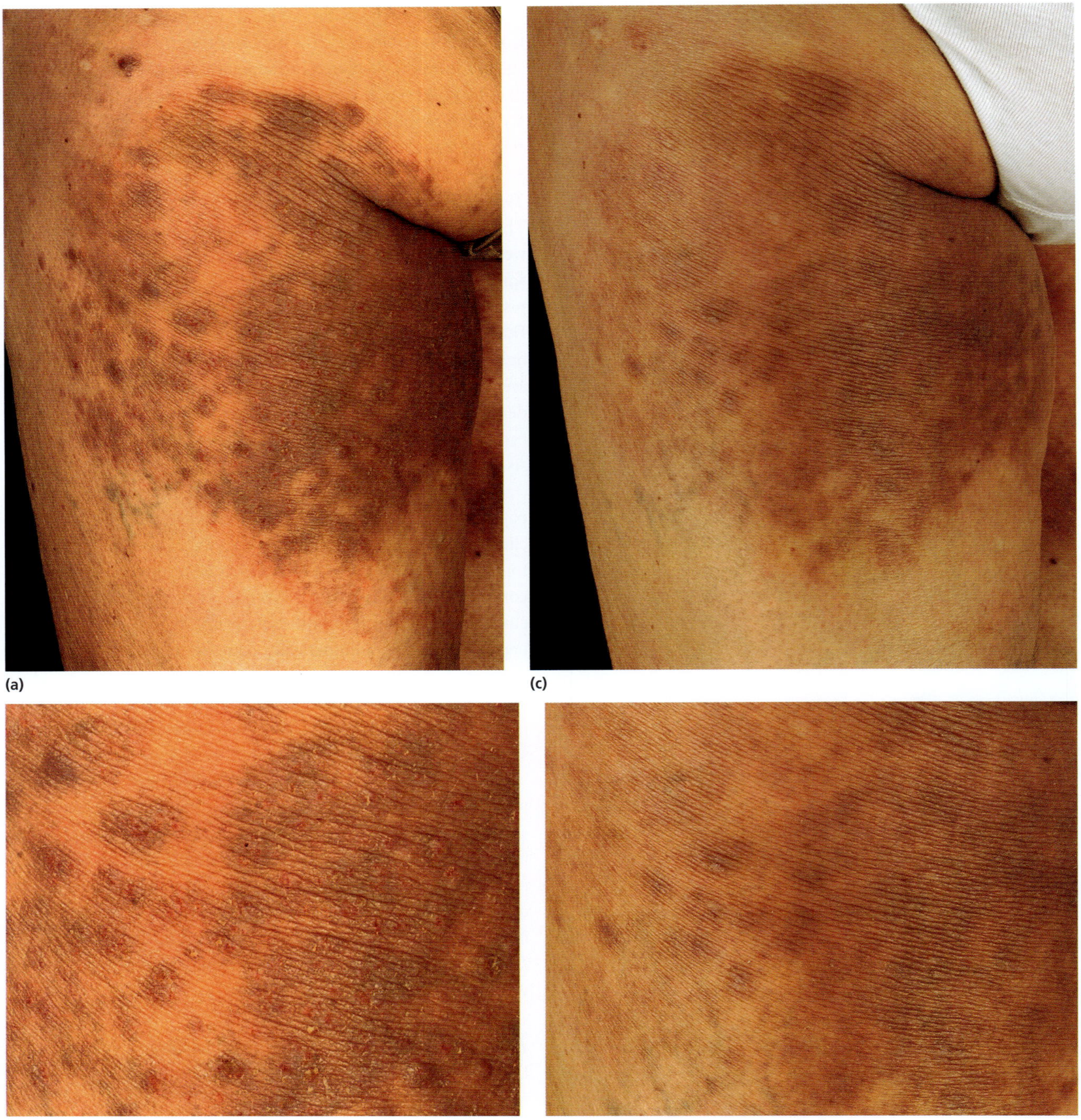

(a) (c) (b) (d)

**Figure 5.13** Lymphomatoid papulosis in a patient with a 38-year history of the disease. (a) Many confluent, partly ulcerated, small papules in an area with post-inflammatory hyperpigmentation, conveying the impression of a very large plaque that would be inconsistent with a diagnosis of lymphomatoid papulosis. The patient had a generalized eruption with conventional lesions at other body sites as well. (b) Detail of the confluent, partly eroded papules. (c) A picture of the same area taken 5 months later shows unchanged hyperpigmentation, but no active lesions of lymphomatoid papulosis. (d) Detail of the hyperpigmentation without active lesions.

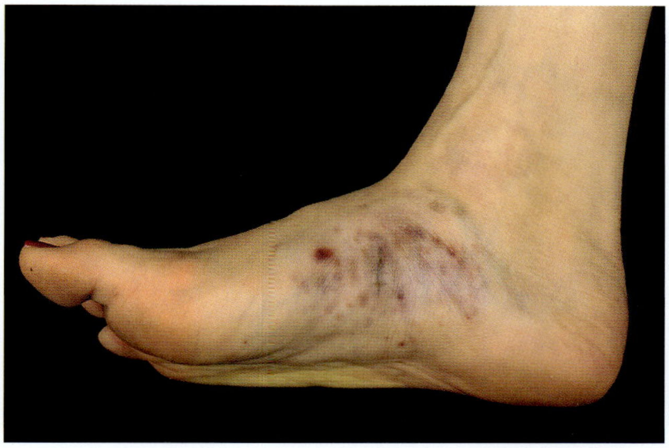

Figure 5.14 Regional lymphomatoid papulosis. Cluster of reddish, flat papules restricted to one foot.

cutaneous aggressive epidermotropic CD8+ cytotoxic T-cell lymphoma [64]. Several similar cases have been subsequently reported [65–67]. The lymphoid infiltrate is either superficial and band-like or wedge-shaped (Fig. 5.21a). Epidermotropism is prominent (Fig. 5.21b). In some cases, the combination of marked epidermotropism and hyperplastic epidermis conveys an overall similarity to pagetoid reticulosis. Neoplastic lymphocytes strongly express CD8 (Fig. 5.22a). Demonstration of CD30 positivity is a prerequisite for the diagnosis (Fig. 5.22b). It must be underlined, though, that CD30 expression may be weak in some cases (Fig. 5.23). I have seen biopsies with negative staining in one laboratory and positivity on repeated staining in our laboratory. As in these cases, evaluation of CD30 is paramount for diagnosis; care should be taken to get reliable results. In this context, external

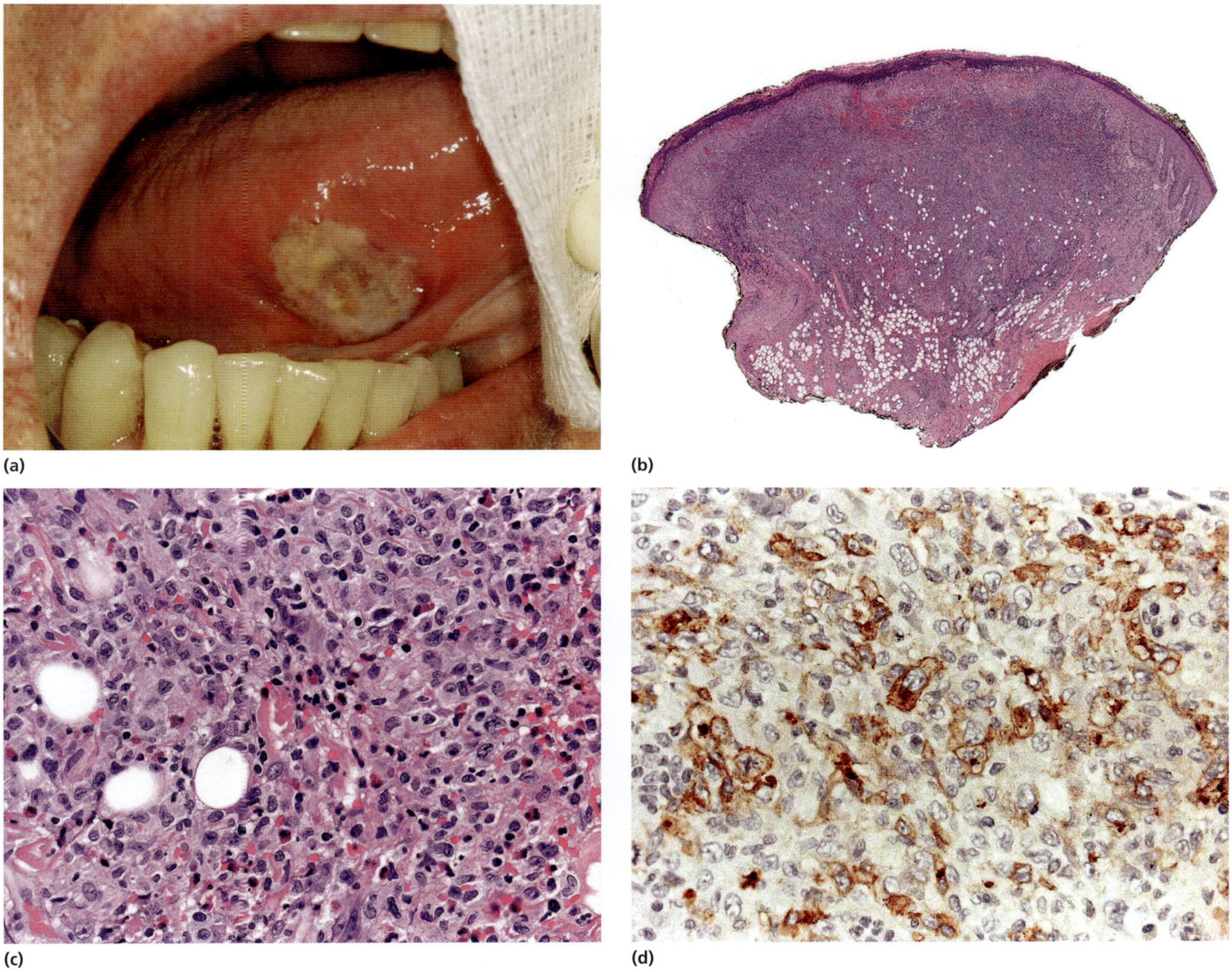


Figure 5.15 Regional lymphomatoid papulosis restricted to the oral mucosa. (a) A 78-year-old man presented with recurrent, self-healing, ulcerative lesions located only on the oral mucosa for the last 7 years. (*Clinical picture courtesy of Dr. Ben Tallon, Tauranga, New Zealand.*) (b) Histology showed dense infiltrates within the lamina propria, (c) characterized by a predominance of medium-sized and large, atypical lymphocytes admixed with several eosinophils. Large cells were positive for pan-T-cell markers, (d) CD30, and TIA-1, with double expression of CD4 and CD8. The in situ hybridization for EBV (EBER-1) was negative. The clinicopathological differential diagnosis in this case is with mucocutaneous ulcer, a rare low-grade B-cell lymphoproliferative disorder associated with EBV. Although the clinical presentation may be indistinguishable and histological features may be overlapping, complete phenotypic analyses allow us to clearly separate the two entities.

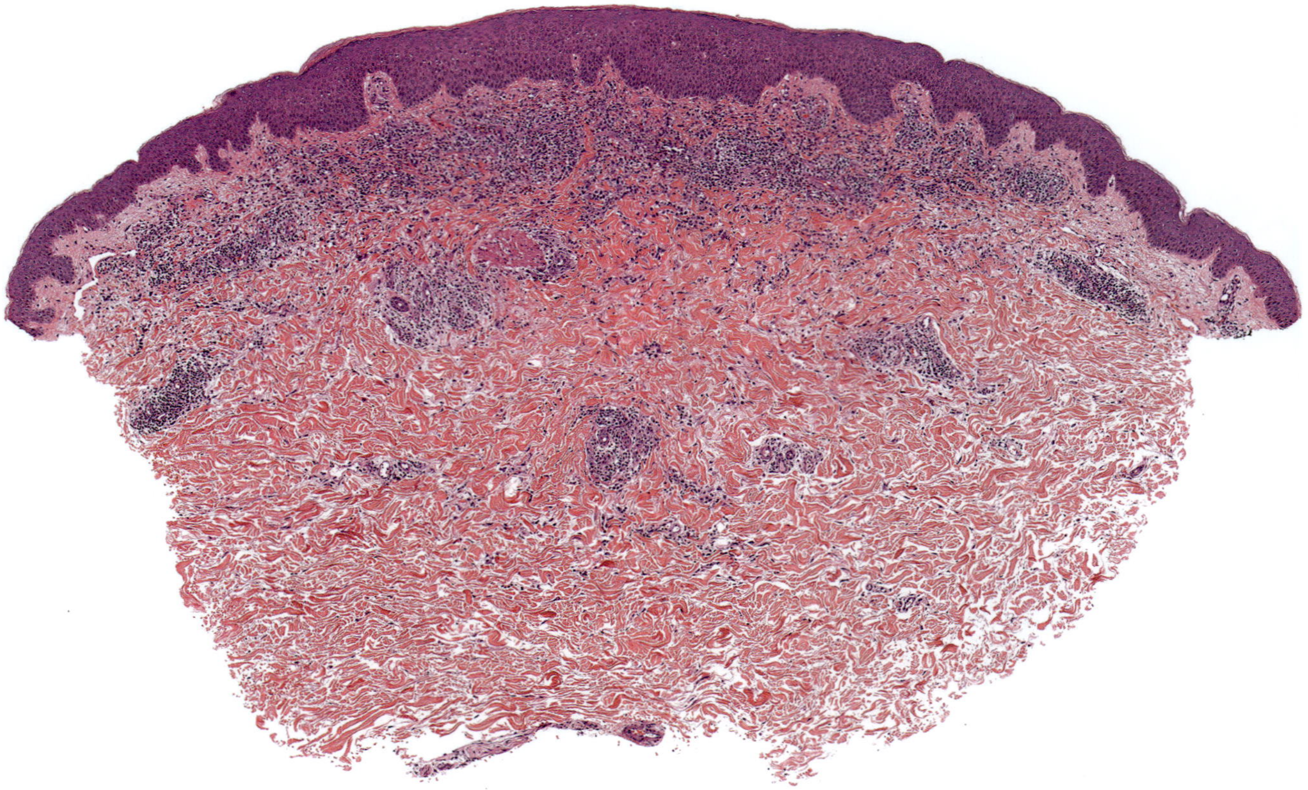

**Figure 5.16** Lymphomatoid papulosis, type A. Wedge-shaped infiltrate in the dermis.

controls (i.e., staining of reference sections such as tonsil or other lymphoid tissues) do not provide any meaningful information, as the level of the antigen may be low in tumoral cells but high in positive controls. As a general rule, most antibodies used in the diagnosis of cutaneous lymphoproliferative disorders have good internal controls (i.e., normal skin structures or inflammatory cells) that can be used in order to judge the quality of the staining. In suspect cases, we routinely perform two CD30 stainings with different protocols on separate, different automatic immunostainers.

The clinical features in all of these patients are typical of lymphomatoid papulosis. Follow-up data do not reveal relevant differences from other variants of lymphomatoid papulosis, but some studies suggested that association with other cutaneous lymphomas may be more common [68, 69].

### *Type E (angiocentric/angiodestructive)*

In some cases of lymphomatoid papulosis, prominent angiotropism with angiodestruction can be observed (Fig. 5.24a). The term "angioinvasive" lymphomatoid papulosis has been proposed for this variant by the group of Dr. Kempf and coworkers [70]. CD30 and sometimes CD56 are expressed by the neoplastic cells (Fig. 5.24b) [53]. Some of the affected vessels may show intraluminal thrombi (Fig. 5.25).

The histopathologic presentation of lymphomatoid papulosis type E may mimic that of aggressive cytotoxic lymphomas, thus representing a pitfall in the diagnosis. In situ hybridization for Epstein-Barr virus (EBV) is constantly negative, allowing extranodal natural killer T (NK/T)-cell lymphoma, nasal-type, to be ruled out. Clinically, these cases are usually necrotic and often characterized by hemorrhagic lesions that may be misinterpreted as necrotizing vasculitis (Fig. 5.10).

It should be underlined that focal angiotropism/angiodestruction may be rarely observed in other types of lymphomatoid papulosis as well. As for all "variants" of the disease, classification of a given lesion into a specific category may be subjective.

### *Follicular lymphomatoid papulosis ("type F")*

A variant of lymphomatoid papulosis characterized by infiltrates located around a hair follicle has been termed "follicular lymphomatoid papulosis" (since types A to E have been described, this variant may be denominated "type F" for "follicular") [71–74]. Lesions are centered around the hair follicles, and these may be partially destructed by the infiltrate (Fig. 5.26). Mucin deposition may be observed within the affected follicles [75]. Some cases show prominent eosinophils, mimicking a fungal or eosinophilic folliculitis [76]. One case of

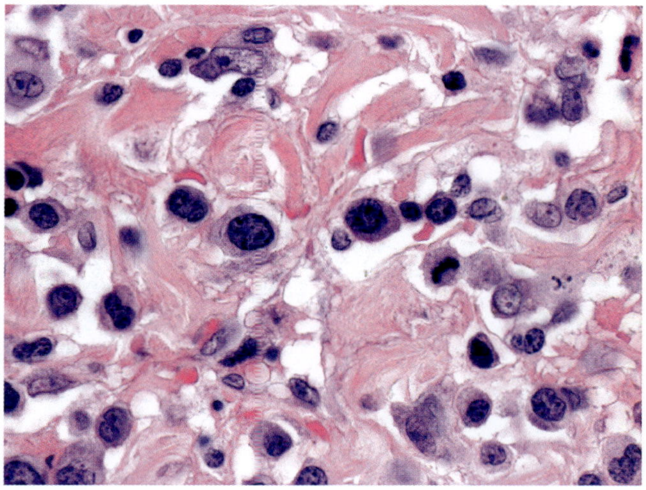

(a)

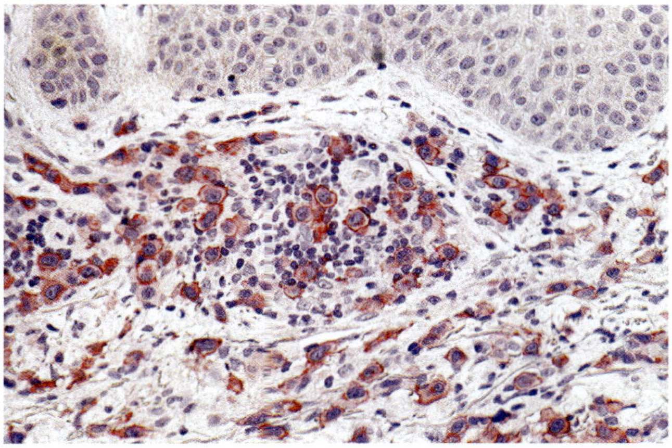

(b)

**Figure 5.17** Lymphomatoid papulosis, type A. (a) Large, atypical cells are usually arranged in solitary units between the collagen bundles or in small perivascular clusters. (b) Staining for CD30 shows many positive atypical cells in small clusters and as solitary units between the collagen bundles.

folliculotropic lymphomatoid papulosis also showed eccrinotropism and neurotropism [77]. A diagnosis of follicular lymphomatoid papulosis should be made only when pilotropism is found besides a perifollicular infiltrate (Fig. 5.27). Staining for CD30 in these cases highlights the perifollicular distribution of the infiltrate and confirms the presence of positive cells within the hair follicle (Fig. 5.28).

It may be that at least some of the cases reported as follicular lymphomatoid papulosis represented conventional variants of the disease (type A) and that involvement of the hair follicle is not due to a particular pilotropism of tumor cells (this is especially true for cases arising in areas of the body with high numbers of hair follicles). On the other hand, true pilotropism is present in genuine cases, and in rare instances, mucin deposition can be observed within the hair follicles as well, thus suggesting analogies with follicular (pilotropic) mycosis fungoides [74].

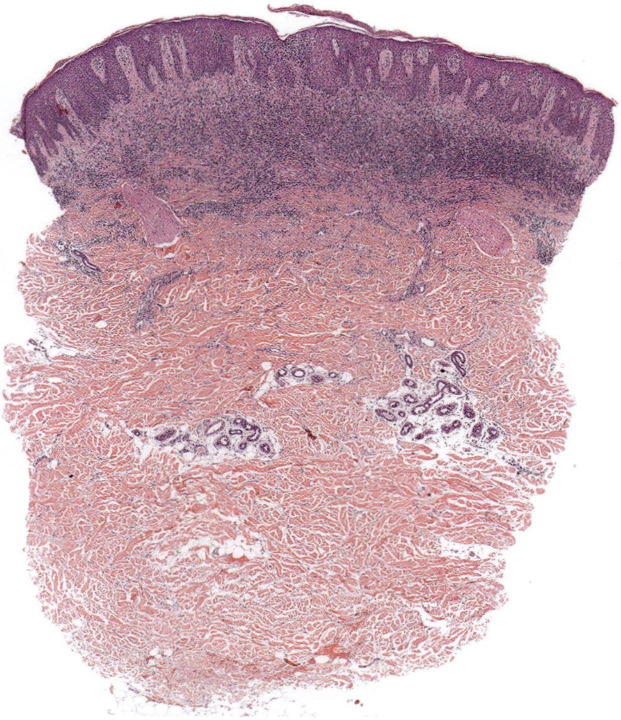

**Figure 5.18** Lymphomatoid papulosis, type B. Dense, band-like infiltrate of lymphocytes within the superficial and mid dermis.

### *Other "variants" of lymphomatoid papulosis*

Other unusual histopathologic findings in lymphomatoid papulosis include the presence of myxoid changes, subepidermal blisters, and syringotropic/eccrinotropic or neurotropic infiltrates (Fig. 5.29) [44, 78, 79]. One case with a *DUSP22–IRF4* rearrangement was associated with lesions that were clinically partially vesicular [80]. Presence of Hodgkin and Reed-Sternberg-like cells can be observed in some cases (*type H, "Hodgkin-like"*).

A peculiar variant of lymphomatoid papulosis is characterized by intralymphatic complexes of tumor cells (*type I, "intralymphatic"*) (Fig. 5.30) [81, 82]. This variant is conceptually similar to intralymphatic anaplastic large cell lymphoma (see below in this chapter). There is no prognostic implication in the finding of intralymphatic complexes of neoplastic cells and no need for different staging procedures.

In some cases of lymphomatoid papulosis (and of anaplastic large cell lymphoma as well), a pseudoepitheliomatous hyperplasia of the epidermis can be observed (*type K, "keratoacanthomatous"*) [83–85] (Fig. 5.31). The association with multiple keratoacanthomas has been documented in a few cases [86]. I have rarely observed patients with multiple lesions that were in

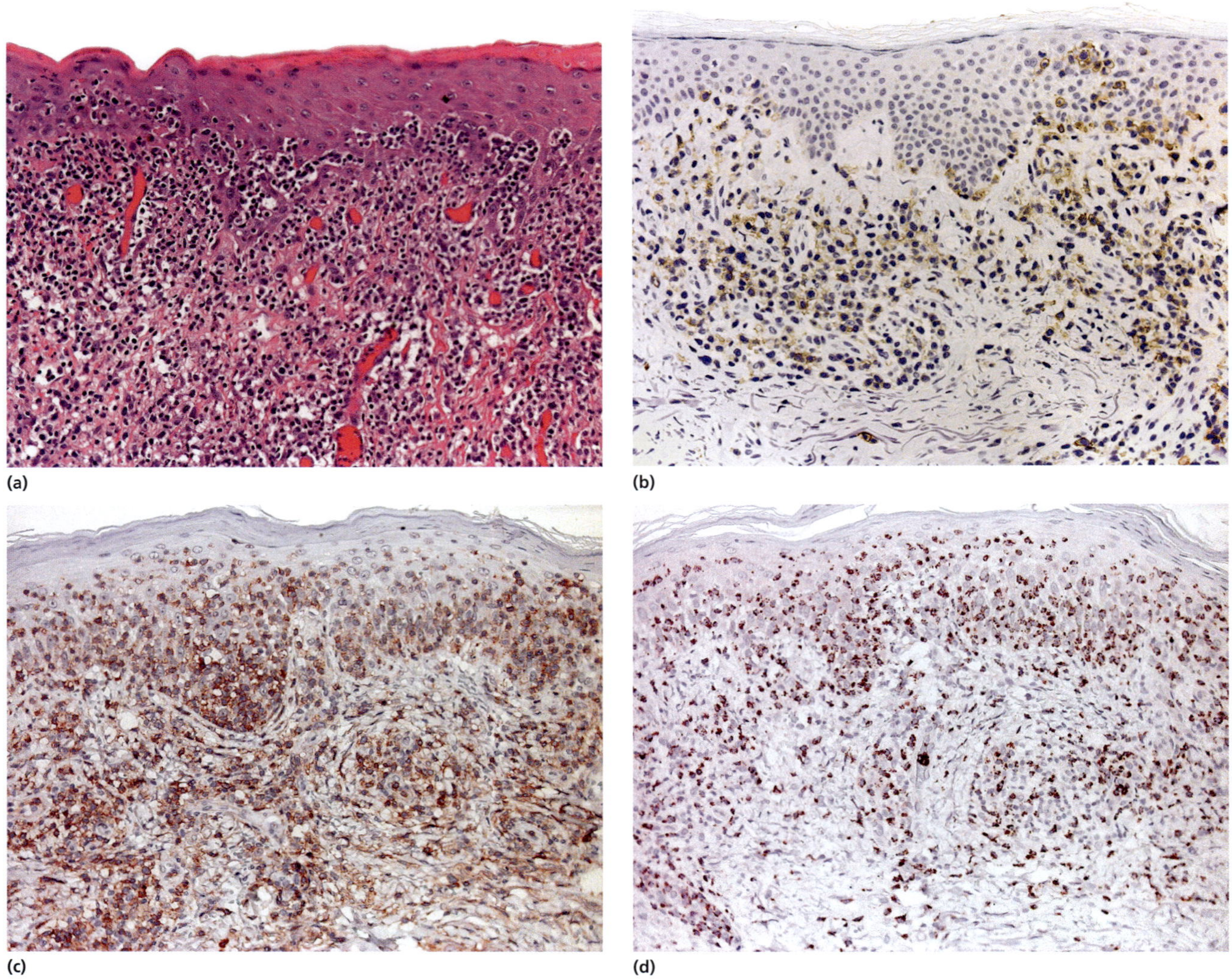


**Figure 5.19** Lymphomatoid papulosis, type B. (a) Epidermotropism of lymphocytes with small intraepidermal collections resembling the histopathologic features of mycosis fungoides. (b) Staining for CD30 highlights the intraepidermal positive cells. (c) Another case showing positivity for CD4 of intraepidermal lymphocytes, which are also positive for (d) TIA-1.

part conventional papules of lymphomatoid papulosis, in part conventional keratoacanthomas devoid of $CD30^+$ cells, and in part typical "collision tumors" of lymphomatoid papulosis and keratoacanthoma (Fig. 5.32).

One reported case of lymphomatoid papulosis presented with a peculiar spindle cell morphology of $CD30^+$ cells [87]. However, the published pictures also showed the presence of conventional, large cells without spindle cell morphology.

As already mentioned, one peculiar type of lymphomatoid papulosis shows nodules of large cells with epidermotropism of smaller cells and is characterized at the genetic level by a chromosomal rearrangement of the *DUSP22–IRF4* locus on 6p25.3 [15, 88]. This type of lymphomatoid papulosis is characterized by nodular lesions with a biphasic pattern, showing epidermotropism of small lymphocytes and dermal infiltrates with many large cells (Figs. 5.33a to c). Both components are positive for CD30 (Figs. 5.33d and e). FISH analysis with a dual-color break-apart probe can confirm the presence of a *DUSP22–IRF4* chromosomal rearrangement (Fig. 5.33f).

Finally, lymphomatoid papulosis can express a cytotoxic $\gamma/\delta$ phenotype (Fig. 5.34), and such cases should be differentiated from cutaneous $\gamma/\delta$ T-cell lymphoma and from mycosis fungoides with cytotoxic phenotype [89–91]. In keeping with other "variants" of the disease, $\gamma/\delta^+$ lymphomatoid papulosis may be denominated "*type G*."

Once again, the "alphabet soup" of lymphomatoid papulosis does not have any diagnostic or prognostic implication and should only be considered as a useful reminder of the protean

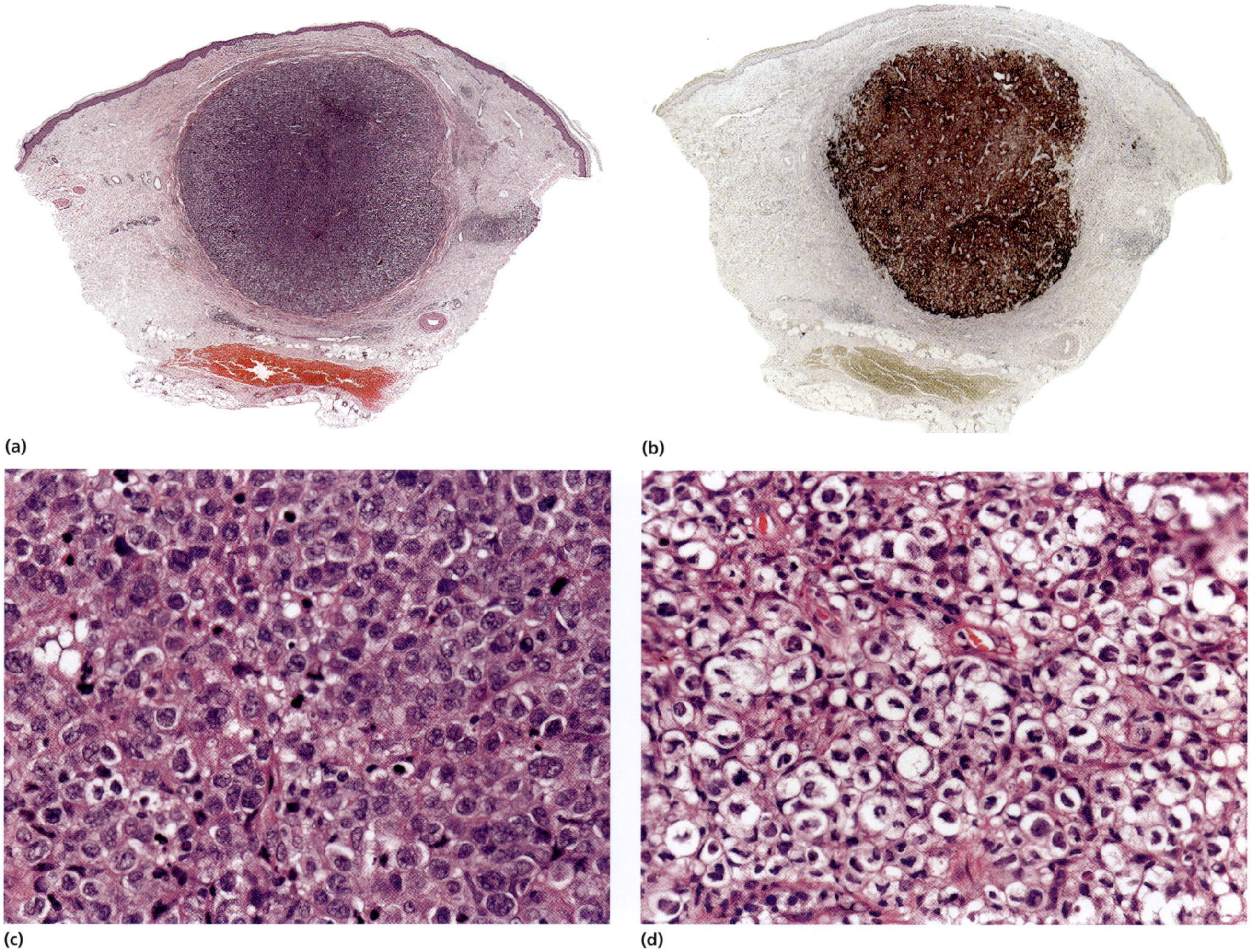

Figure 5.20 Lymphomatoid papulosis, type C. (a) Dense infiltrate of atypical lymphocytes arranged in a large dermal nodule. (b) Positivity of all cells for CD30. (c) Details of large, atypical cells, (d) some showing a clear cytoplasm. The histopathologic and phenotypic features are indistinguishable from those of cutaneous anaplastic large cell lymphoma.

clinicopathological features of the disease (Table 5.1). There is no need to mention the "type" of lymphomatoid papulosis in the histopathological report.

## Immunophenotype

The hallmark of lymphomatoid papulosis is the expression of CD30 by neoplastic cells. The different patterns of CD30 expression in various types of lymphomatoid papulosis are depicted in Figs. 5.17b, 5.19b, 5.20c, 5.22b, 5.23, 5.24e, 5.28, and 5.33d and e. $CD30^+$ lymphocytes are arranged as solitary units between the collagen bundles or in small perivascular clusters. Sheets of $CD30^+$ cells are observed only in the histopathologic type C and in the variant with *DUSP22–IRF4* chromosomal rearrangement. In some cases, most $CD30^+$ cells are in the superficial part of the lesion, immediately below the epidermis. When epidermotropic neoplastic lymphocytes are present, they are invariably positive for CD30. The arrangement of $CD30^+$ cells is useful in the differential diagnosis of lymphomatoid papulosis from benign inflammatory skin diseases, where $CD30^+$ cells are usually (but not always!) scattered and isolated. Another useful differential diagnostic criterion is the ratio between positive and negative cells, which is higher in lymphomatoid papulosis than in reactive inflammatory disorders (the ratio, however, varies remarkably in lymphomatoid papulosis depending on the age of the lesion).

Although the infiltrate of type B lymphomatoid papulosis in the past has often been reported as being CD30-negative, all cases do in fact express the antigen, and such a diagnosis should not be made by CD30-negativity. Negativity in old reports was probably due to low levels of intracellular CD30 and, at the same time, a lack of antigen demasking techniques, and it may have a similar background as the weak positivity observed in some

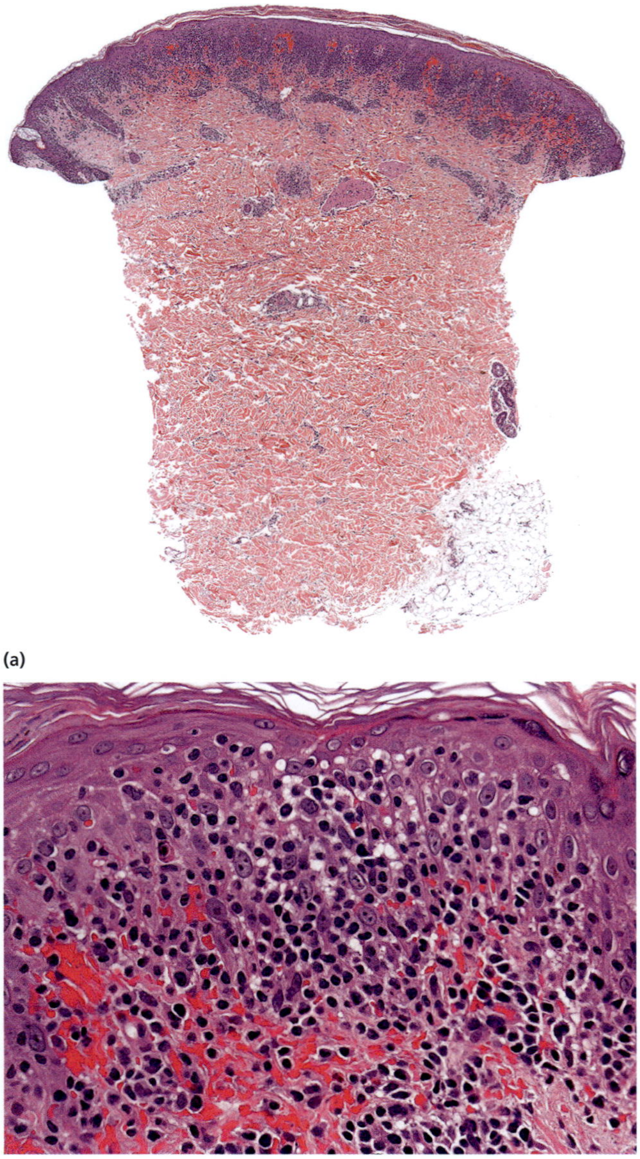

(a)

(b)

**Figure 5.21** Lymphomatoid papulosis, type D. (a) Superficial, band-like lymphoid infiltrate with hemorrhage. Note hyperplastic epidermis. (b) Marked epidermotropism of pleomorphic lymphocytes mimicking the histopathologic picture of pagetoid reticulosis or of cutaneous aggressive epidermotropic CD8$^{+}$ cytotoxic T-cell lymphoma.

cases of type D of the disease. In this context, care should be taken to avoid misinterpreting the papular variant of mycosis fungoides (which is always CD30-negative and does not show spontaneous resolution) as type B lymphomatoid papulosis (see also Chapter 3).

Neoplastic cells express the phenotypic markers of T-helper lymphocytes (CD3$^{+}$, CD4$^{+}$) in some cases and of T cytotoxic cells (CD3$^{+}$, CD8$^{+}$, and TIA-1$^{-}$) in others [92, 93]. CD4$^{+}$ cases may express cytotoxic proteins as well [93]. Expression of CD56 can be observed only rarely [94–96]. Pan-T-cell antigens may be partially lost, but the pronounced aberrations observed often in cutaneous anaplastic large cell lymphoma are usually not found in lymphomatoid papulosis. Most lesions of lymphomatoid papulosis are characterized by a T-cell receptor (TCR) $\alpha/\beta$ phenotype, but expression of $\gamma/\delta$ can be observed in some cases (see above) [89–91].

Although lymphomatoid papulosis type D may mimic the histopathological presentation of cutaneous aggressive epidermotropic CD8$^{+}$ cytotoxic T-cell lymphoma and shares with it the same positivity for CD8, neoplastic cells in type D lymphomatoid papulosis are usually positive for CD45Ra [97], and most cases of cutaneous aggressive epidermotropic CD8$^{+}$ cytotoxic T-cell lymphoma are CD30-negative. A differential diagnosis between the two entities, however, can only be achieved by correlation with the clinical picture.

The anaplastic lymphoma kinase (ALK) is not expressed by neoplastic cells. Positivity for JunB and c-Jun is found frequently in lymphomatoid papulosis [98, 99], whereas expression of fascin, survivin, and Bcl-2 is present in a minority of cases only [100, 101]. It has been suggested that CD56 or fascin expression by neoplastic cells may be helpful in the distinction between lymphomatoid papulosis and anaplastic large cell lymphoma [100], but in my experience, the usefulness of these markers is very limited, and they do not play any role in the differential diagnosis between the two diseases.

TRAF1 and MUM-1 are expressed in the vast majority of cases of lymphomatoid papulosis. In contrast to previous reports, stainings for MUM-1 and TRAF1 do not provide any helpful information in the differentiation of lymphomatoid papulosis from anaplastic large cell lymphoma [102, 103]. Expression of SATB1, a thymocyte-specific chromatin organizer that plays a crucial role in T-cell development, seems to be more common in lymphomatoid papulosis than in cutaneous anaplastic large cell lymphoma [104].

## Molecular genetics

Rearrangement of the TCR is found in the majority of lesions [105], but some authors pointed to a less frequent presence of clonality in pediatric patients [106]. Studies on single cells after microdissection of the specimens showed that the atypical CD30$^{+}$ large cells have a common clonal origin [107]. The interchromosomal (2;5) translocation is absent [108, 109].

*IRF4* gene rearrangements are found commonly in cutaneous anaplastic large cell lymphoma, but only in some cases of lymphomatoid papulosis in the same studies [14, 16]. However, chromosomal rearrangement of the *DUSP22–IRF4* locus on 6p25.3 is observed in a subset of cases of lymphomatoid papulosis with peculiar histopathologic features, characterized by epidermotropism and the presence of large dermal nodules of atypical cells (see above) [15]. The rearrangement can be detected by fluorescence in situ hybridization using a dual-color

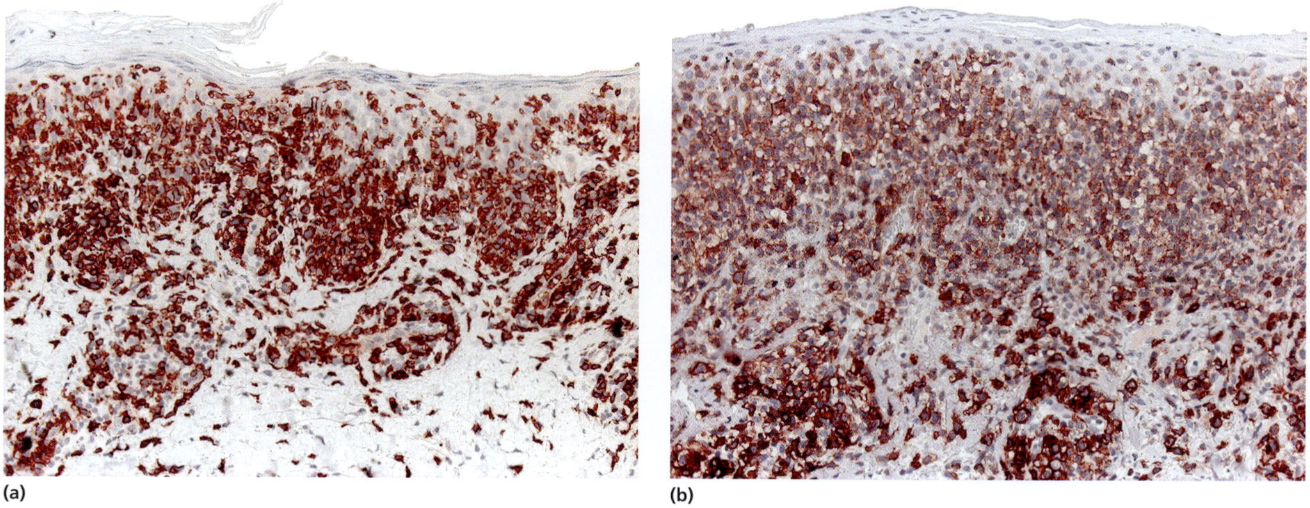

Figure 5.22 Lymphomatoid papulosis, type D. Stainings for (a) CD8 and (b) CD30 reveal uniform positivity of epidermotropic lymphocytes.

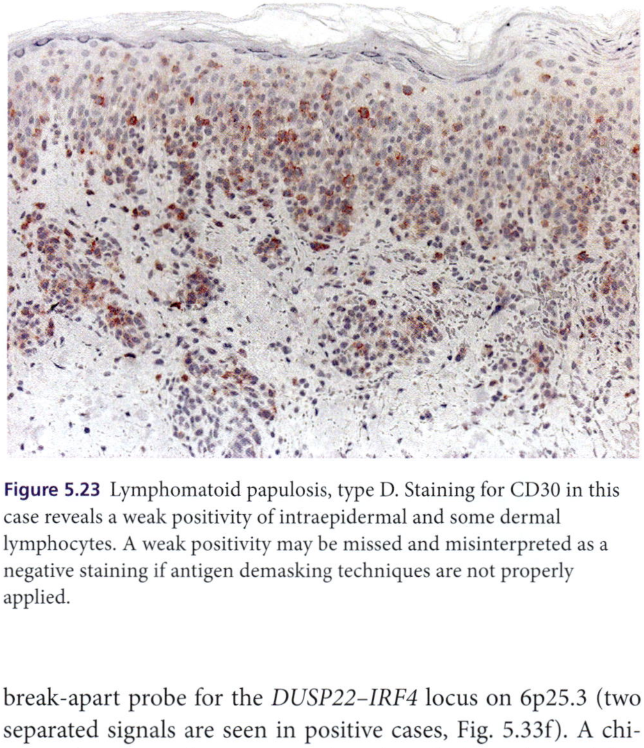

Figure 5.23 Lymphomatoid papulosis, type D. Staining for CD30 in this case reveals a weak positivity of intraepidermal and some dermal lymphocytes. A weak positivity may be missed and misinterpreted as a negative staining if antigen demasking techniques are not properly applied.

break-apart probe for the *DUSP22–IRF4* locus on 6p25.3 (two separated signals are seen in positive cases, Fig. 5.33f). A chimeric fusion involving *NPM1* (5q35) and *TYK2* (19p13) has been observed in one case of lymphomatoid papulosis [110]. Similar to what can be observed in other cutaneous T-cell lymphomas, activation of the Janus kinase-signal transducer and activator of transcription signaling (JAK–STAT) pathway has been detected in a subset of cases, due either to pathogenic *STAT* mutations or to oncogenic fusion transcripts comprising effector domains of *JAK* [111].

## Clinicopathologic differential diagnosis

Besides cutaneous anaplastic large cell lymphoma, the differential diagnosis of lymphomatoid papulosis includes other cutaneous papulonecrotic eruptions, and particularly pityriasis lichenoides (pityriasis lichenoides et varioliformis acuta or pityriasis lichenoides chronica – personally I don't think that the two "variants" of the disease can reliably be distinguished from one another and refer to both as "pityriasis lichenoides"). The distinction between the two diseases can be particularly difficult, as they share overlapping clinicopathologic features. However, in the differentiation of pityriasis lichenoides from lymphomatoid papulosis, the presence of large atypical $CD30^+$ cells, in my opinion, is almost always diagnostic of lymphomatoid papulosis, although rare examples of $CD30^+$ pityriasis lichenoides may indeed exist (see also Chapter 31). Cases reported as "pityriasis lichenoides et varioliformis with atypical $CD30^+$ cells" [112, 113] most likely represent examples of lymphomatoid papulosis. A report on $CD30^+$ pityriasis lichenoides associated with parvovirus B19 infection has been published [114]. However, many of the cases had phenotypic aberrations such as loss of pan-T-cell markers and/or double CD4/CD8 positivity, features that are very unusual in genuine pityriasis lichenoides. On the other hand, a relationship between pityriasis lichenoides and lymphomatoid papulosis, or the existence of transition forms, cannot be excluded a priori, and rare examples of lymphomatoid papulosis followed by pityriasis lichenoides have been reported [115]. In a recent study, we demonstrated that lymphomatoid papulosis can be reliably distinguished from pityriasis lichenoides and atypical cases of pityriasis lichenoides (defined as pityriasis lichenoides with phenotypic aberrations) (see Chapter 31) [116]. Some cases of atypical pityriasis lichenoides progressed to mycosis fungoides, but there was no overlap with lymphomatoid papulosis [116].

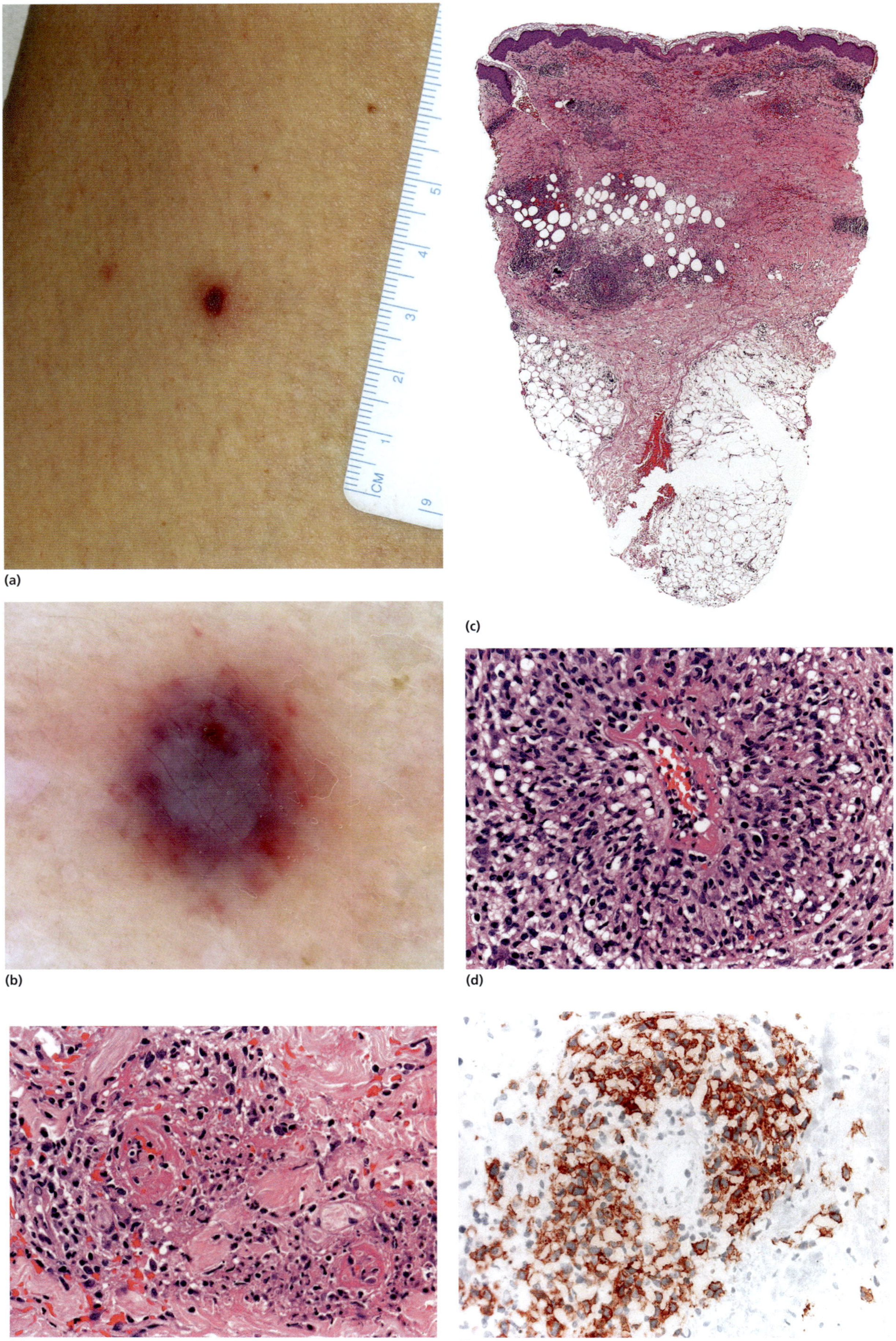


**Figure 5.24** Lymphomatoid papulosis, type E. (a) The clinical picture resembles a vasculitic process. (b) Dermatoscopic features of the lesion. (c) Lymphoid infiltrates with hemorrhage and with (d) angiocentric/angiodestructive pattern of atypical lymphocytes. (e) Some small vessels show intraluminal thrombi. (f) Staining for CD30 highlights positive, angiocentric, large lymphocytes.

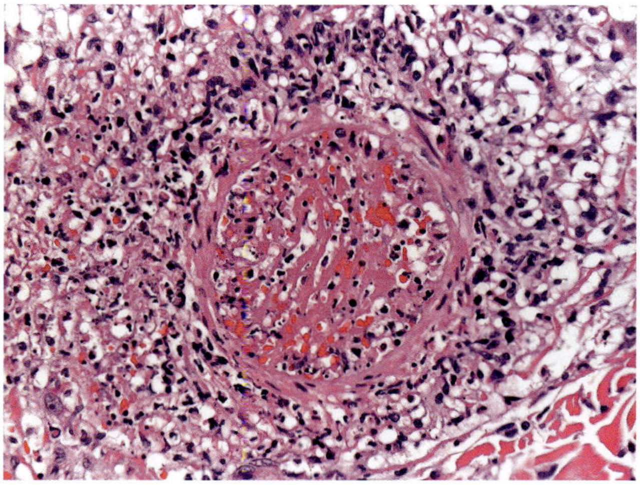

Figure 5.25 Lymphomatoid papulosis, type E. Angiotropic lymphocytes with intraluminal thrombus.

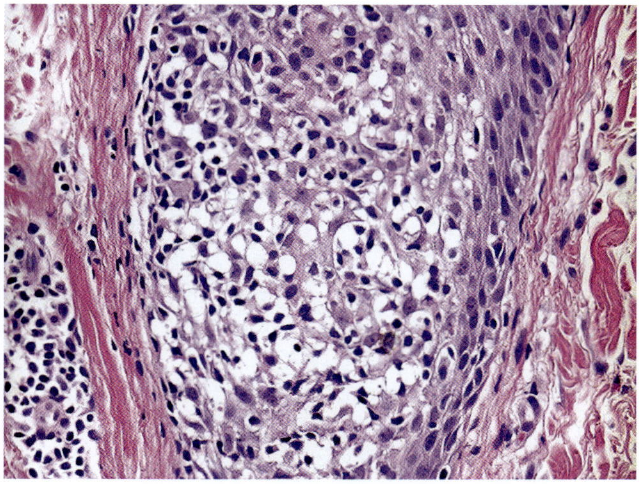

Figure 5.27 Follicular lymphomatoid papulosis. Note the pilotropic lymphocytes.

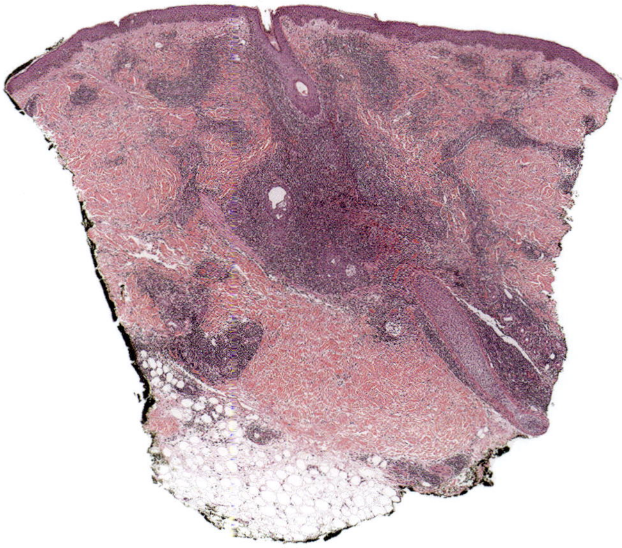

Figure 5.26 Follicular lymphomatoid papulosis. Wedge-shaped infiltrate arranged around a hair follicle with partial destruction of the follicle.

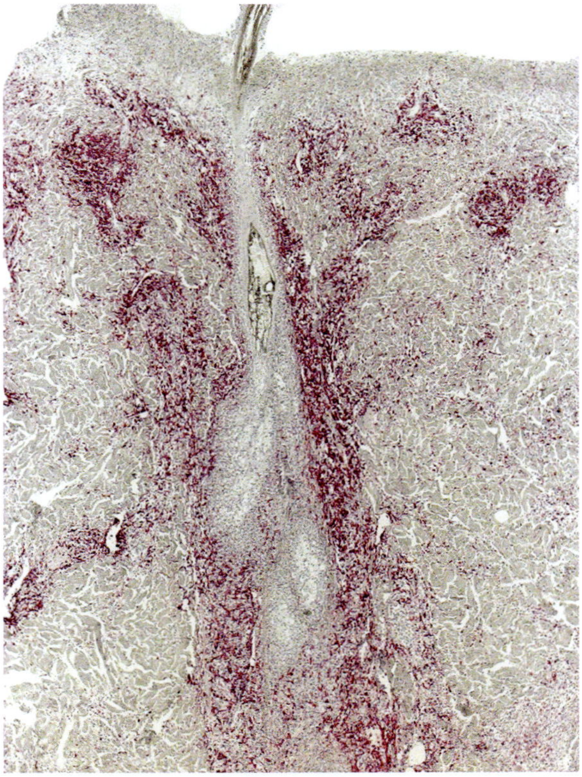

Figure 5.28 Follicular lymphomatoid papulosis. Staining for CD30 shows the perifollicular distribution of the infiltrate, with some intraepithelial lymphocytes positive cells.

One study suggested that the presence of a wedge-shaped infiltrate represents a helpful feature for distinction of type D lymphomatoid papulosis from primary cutaneous aggressive epidermotropic $CD8^+$ cytotoxic T-cell lymphoma and from other $CD8^+$ cutaneous T-cell lymphomas [68]. Although this is true for some cases, I would caution against trying to distinguish epidermotropic infiltrates of $CD8^+$ T-cells based on histopathological features alone, as correlation with the clinical picture is mandatory for establishing a precise diagnosis.

Clustering expression, originally thought to be specific for systemic anaplastic large cell lymphoma as opposed to cutaneous cases, was found in half of tested examples of lymphomatoid papulosis in a study, as well as in tumor cells of cutaneous anaplastic large cell lymphoma and in $CD30^+$ large cell transformation of mycosis fungoides, but only in a small minority of cases of reactive infiltrates with $CD30^+$ cells, thus representing a

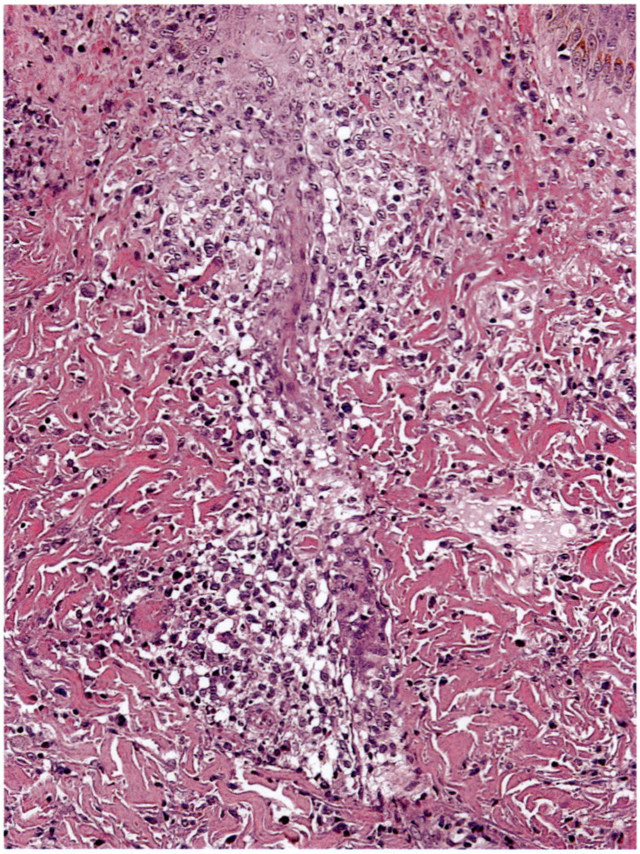

**Figure 5.29** Syringotropic lymphomatoid papulosis. Atypical cells are arranged around and within an eccrine duct.

potential tool in differential diagnosis of lymphomatoid papulosis from CD30+ pseudolymphomas [117]. As with all other small studies, however, these results should not be overemphasized unless confirmed on larger numbers of cases.

## Treatment

Since the disease is self-limiting, many patients with lymphomatoid papulosis will not require specific treatment [7]. Therapy should be directed mainly at controlling symptoms in widespread eruptions or at slowing down the frequency of recurrences [7, 118]. There are no data to support the efficacy of any given treatment scheme in diminishing the number and frequency of recurrences, and cutaneous relapses after discontinuation of any type of treatment are the rule. Even more important, there is no therapy that has demonstrated a preventive effect on the development of a second lymphoma.

Local steroids may be used in many cases, particularly when lesions are few and/or localized. Local steroids, psoralen + plus ultraviolet A (PUVA), and low-dose methotrexate are the treatments that have been used more often in patients with generalized lesions [7, 119]. Methotrexate has also been administered topically. A better response to methotrexate and interferon treatment was observed in cases of lymphomatoid papulosis with high levels of SATB1 expression [104]. A further treatment possibility is represented by bexarotene, either systemically or topically.

Many other options have been tested with partial success, including systemic steroids, UV-A1, interferon–α2a, interferon–γ, and retinoids (alone or in combination) [7, 119]. Some patients have been treated with imiquimod cream or 308 nm excimer laser. Only a few cases have been managed with the anti-CD30 antibody (brentuximab vedotin) [120], and this option should be used only in exceptional cases, after failure of other first-line agents [121]. One patient with lymphomatoid papulosis associated with mycosis fungoides has been successfully treated with topical chlormethine gel [122]; however, the lesions of lymphomatoid papulosis cleared within 3 weeks, thus it cannot be excluded that the resolution was independent of the local treatment.

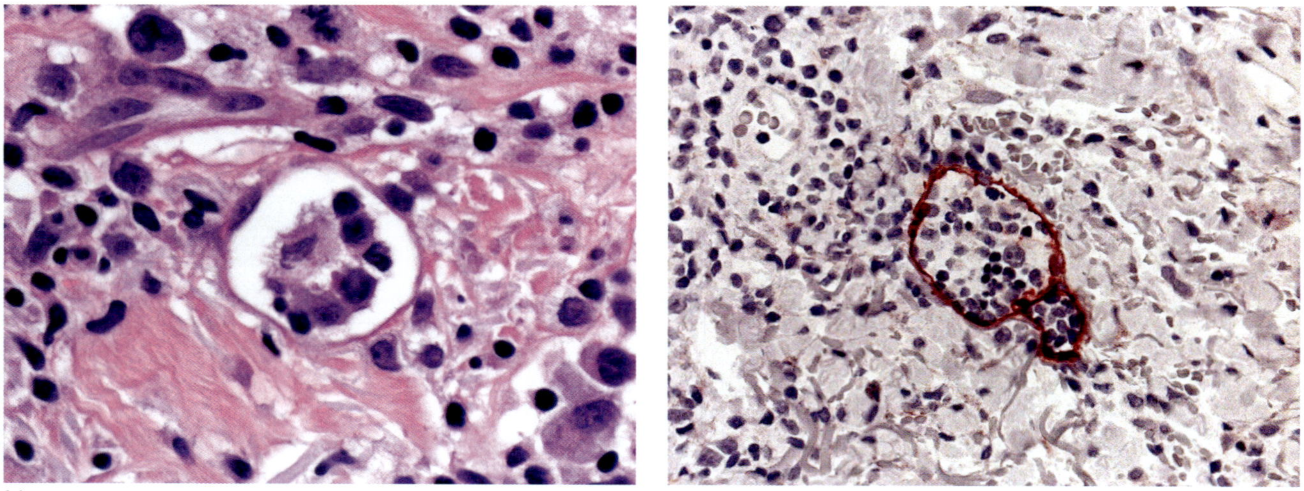

(a) (b)

**Figure 5.30** Intralymphatic lymphomatoid papulosis. (a) Atypical cells within and around a small dermal vessel. (b) Staining for podoplanin shows that the vessel is of lymphatic origin.

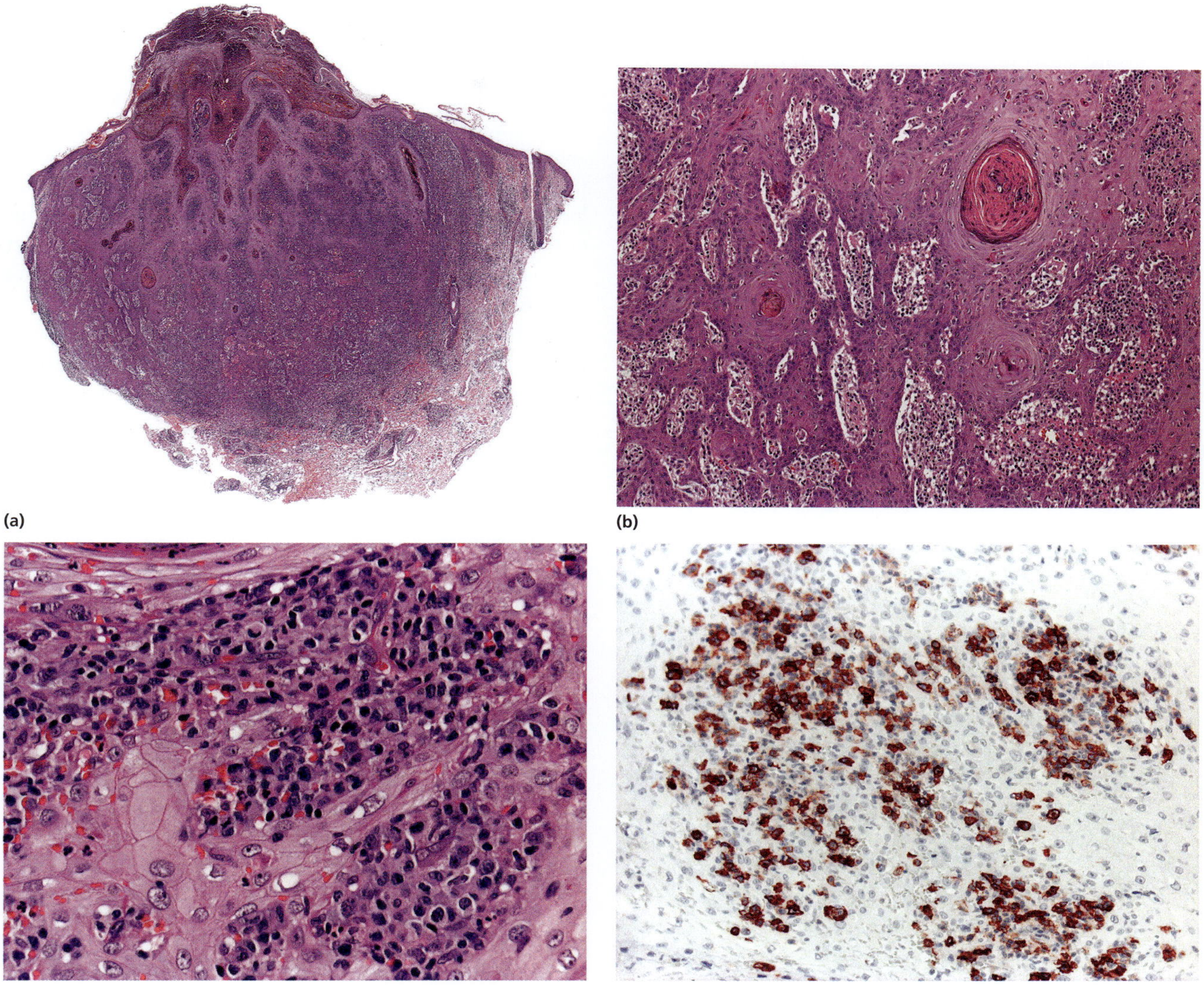


**Figure 5.31** Lymphomatoid papulosis with pseudoepitheliomatous hyperplasia. (a) Partly exophytic, crusted lesion characterized by (b) prominent, pseudoepitheliomatous epithelial hyperplasia; (c) the hyperplastic epithelium is in tight connection with aggregates of medium-sized and large, atypical lymphocytes, (d) which are positive for CD30.

Multiagent chemotherapy should be avoided, as it does not provide any protection from recurrences and/or progression to higher-grade lymphoma, and it may be associated with severe short-term and long-term side effects. Radiotherapy has been advocated for the treatment of large tumors that may be slower to regress. However, all lesions of lymphomatoid papulosis eventually resolve, and local aggressive treatment such as radiotherapy should be administered only if the clinical setting is appropriate (e.g., large plantar lesions that may render walking impossible, or disfiguring lesions).

Finally, it should be mentioned that the analysis of data on different treatment modalities in lymphomatoid papulosis is hindered by the fact that lesions resolve spontaneously by definition. Usually, a "shorter" time to resolution and/or a decrease in the frequency of the eruptions are considered significant in judging the value of a given treatment. However, resolution time is variable in the absence of any therapy, and it may be very subjective to establish whether a given lesion has resolved earlier because of treatment or not. In addition, the number of eruptions that a single patient experiences is also variable. A consensus statement of the EORTC–Cutaneous Lymphoma Task Force, the International Society of Cutaneous Lymphoma (ISCL), and the United States Cutaneous Lymphoma Consortium (USCLC) defined complete remission as the disappearance of 100% of the lesions and partial remission as a 50–99% clearance of skin disease from baseline without new larger (>2 cm in diameter) and persistent nodules (persistency being defined as no spontaneous regression after 12 weeks) in those with papular disease only [119].

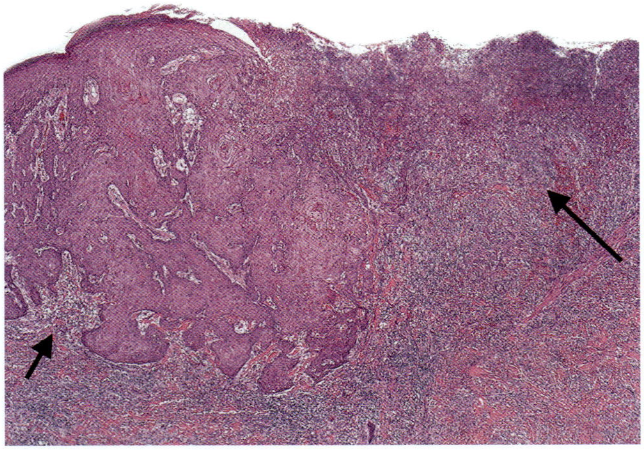

**Figure 5.32** Lymphomatoid papulosis associated with multiple keratoacanthomas. The remnant of a keratoacanthoma is visible on the left side of this lesion (short arrow), whereas most atypical cells of the lymphomatoid papulosis are located on the right part of it (long arrow). The patient, a 79-year-old male, had concomitant typical lesions of keratoacanthoma without infiltrating CD30 atypical cells, as well as conventional lesions of lymphomatoid papulosis without epidermal hyperplasia.

## Prognosis

Lymphomatoid papulosis is characterized by an excellent prognosis, and the expected 5-year survival is 100% [1–5, 45, 123]. Some patients may experience very few recurrences of the disease over the years, whereas others may have lesions appearing almost continuously. There are no features that can help predict the course of the disease in a given patient. The presence of a monoclonal TCR gene rearrangement or of different histopathologic subtypes in the same patient has been suggested as a prognostic indicator of possible progression to other lymphomas [124]. In my experience, however, these features do not allow the identification of patients with different disease behavior.

It is still unclear whether long-standing, complete remissions may be achieved in lymphomatoid papulosis. In one study, 9/21 patients were in complete remission after a follow-up time variable between 1 and 18 years (median 6 years) [125]. However, the authors did not specify whether the patients experienced long-standing remissions or were just symptom-free at the time of the last follow-up control. In my experience, genuine lymphomatoid papulosis may show very long periods of clinical remission, but recurrences are common.

As already discussed, the occurrence of large CD30⁺ tumors limited to the skin at the onset of lymphomatoid papulosis or during the course of the disease does not affect the prognosis of these patients [7]. Large tumors may take longer to regress, but do invariably so; on the other hand, patients with large lesions should be carefully monitored in order to rule out progression to a higher-grade lymphoma. Absence of any sign of regression after a period of 12 weeks should be regarded as suspicious, and the possibility of evolution into a second lymphoma should be seriously taken into account.

The knowledge that 10–20% of the patients develop an associated malignant lymphoma means that regular follow-up is important. A similar rate of association with hematological malignancies (10%) has been observed in a large study of lymphomatoid papulosis in children and adolescents, suggesting that long-term follow-up should be recommended for these patients as well [30]. Unfortunately, clinicopathologic, phenotypic, or molecular features do not provide clues for the early identification of patients who will progress to a more aggressive lymphoma. In addition, as already mentioned, there are no data to support a preventive effect of any given treatment on the progression or transformation of lymphomatoid papulosis into high-grade lymphoma.

### Résumé

**Lymphomatoid papulosis**

| | | |
|---|---|---|
| **Clinical** | Adults. Children may be affected. Chronic, recurrent eruption of papules and nodules that heal mostly within 3–6 weeks without treatment *(essential criterion)*. Excellent prognosis. | |
| **Morphology** | Several histopathologic types and several other histopathologic variants. The "alphabet soup" of lymphomatoid papulosis subtypes does not have any diagnostic or prognostic implications. | |
| **Immunohistochemistry** | CD2, CD3, CD5 | + (−) |
| | CD30 | + *(essential criterion)* |
| | CD15 | − |
| | CD4 | + (−) (depending on the subtype) |
| | CD8, TIA-1 | − (+) (depending on the subtype) |
| | TCR-β | + (−) (depending on the subtype) |
| | TCR-γ, TCR-δ | − (+) (depending on the subtype) |
| | CD56 | − (+) |
| | MUM-1 | + |
| | SATB1 | + |
| **Genetics** | Monoclonal rearrangement of the TCR genes was detected in the majority of the cases. Chromosomal rearrangement of the *DUSP22–IRF4* locus on 6p25.3 was observed in a subset of cases. | |
| **Treatment guidelines** | Topical steroids; PUVA; low-dose methotrexate; bexarotene. Watchful waiting (spontaneous resolution is the rule). | |

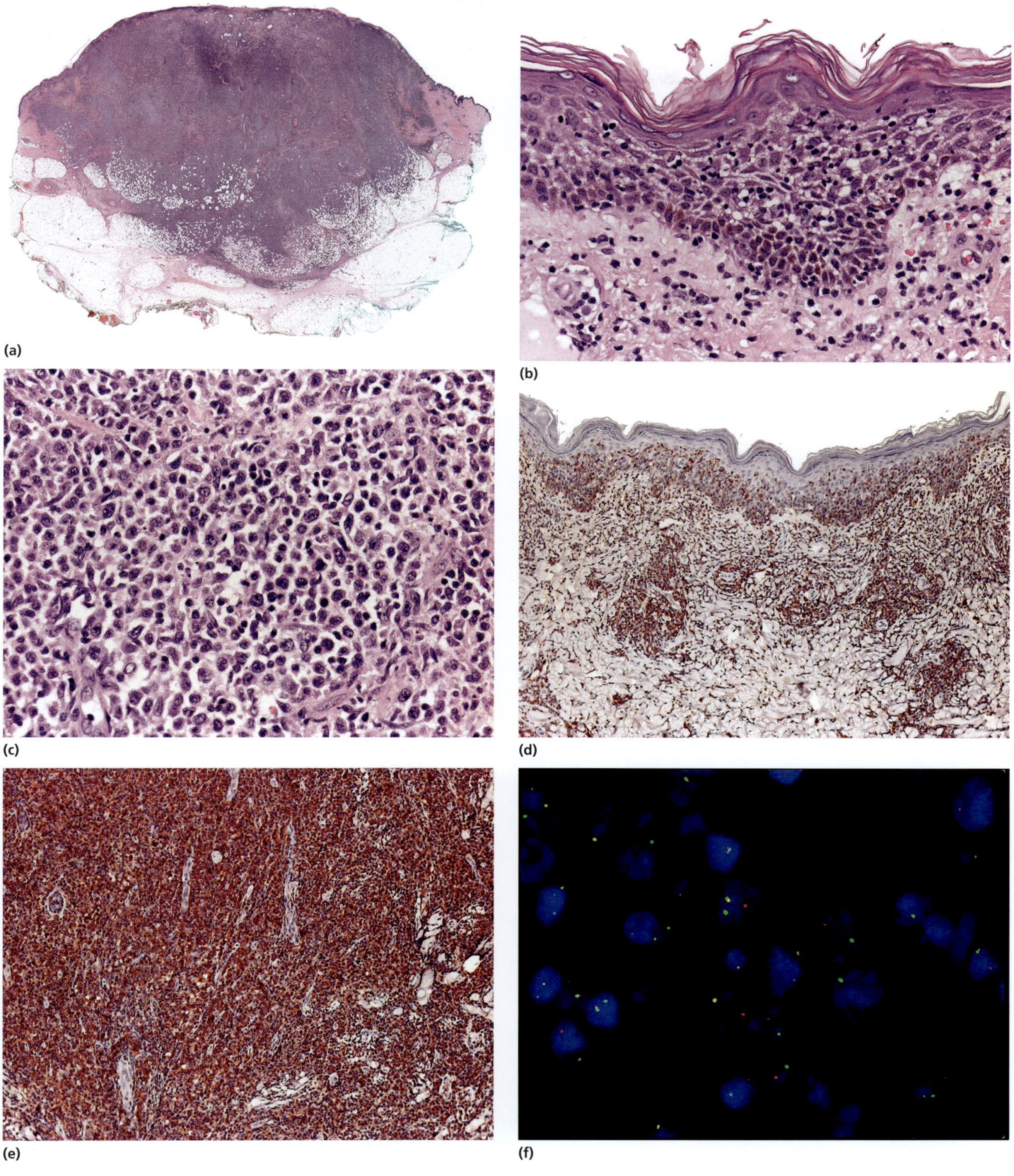

**Figure 5.33** Lymphomatoid papulosis with chromosomal rearrangement of the *DUSP22–IRF4* locus on 6p25.3. (a) Large nodule with involvement of the entire dermis and subcutaneous fat. (b) Epidermotropism of small lymphocytes. (c) The dermal component is composed of larger cells. CD30 positivity can be observed both in the (d) epidermotropic cells and (e) the dermal component. (f) FISH analysis with a dual-color break-apart probe confirms the presence of a *DUSP22–IRF4* chromosomal rearrangement. (*Courtesy of Prof. Fabio Facchetti, Brescia, Italy.*)

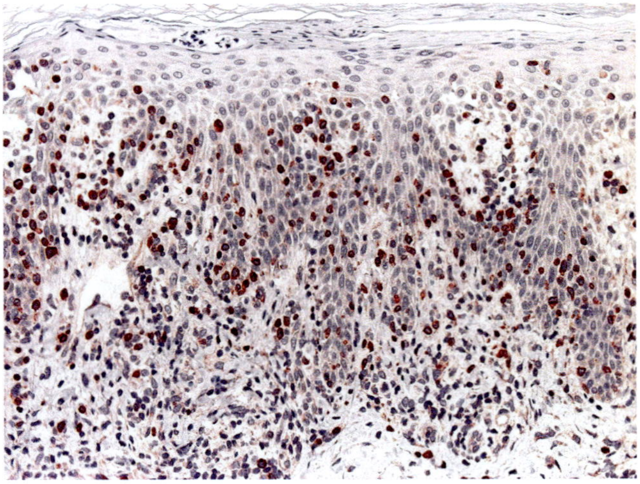

Figure 5.34 Lymphomatoid papulosis with a γ/δ phenotype. Positivity for TCR-γ.

## Cutaneous Anaplastic Large Cell Lymphoma

Cutaneous anaplastic large cell lymphoma is defined as a CD30+ large T-cell lymphoma presenting primarily in the skin and characterized by a good prognosis and response to treatment [1, 2].

The differences in biologic behavior and prognosis between primary cutaneous and nodal anaplastic large cell lymphomas have been known for some time, and both the ICC *of Myeloid and Lymphoid Neoplasms* and the WHO *Classification of Haematolymphoid Tumours* list the primary cutaneous form as a distinct entity, separate from the nodal counterpart and from other subtypes [3, 5]. The interchromosomal (2;5) translocation and the related ALK-1 positivity, typical of a subset of nodal anaplastic large cell lymphoma, are absent in most primary cutaneous cases [1, 108, 109]. However, ALK-1 negativity cannot be interpreted as synonymous with primary cutaneous disease, and staging investigations are mandatory before a definitive diagnosis is made.

A tumor, nodes and metastases (TNM) staging system for cutaneous lymphomas other than mycosis fungoides and Sézary syndrome has been proposed by the EORTC and ISCL (Table 5.2) [126], and has been validated by a study on more than 100 patients [127], and subsequently slightly modified in conjunction with the USCLC [128, 129].

It should be emphasized that CD30+ tumors with anaplastic large cell morphology may be seen in patients with mycosis fungoides as a consequence of large cell transformation (see also Chapter 3). Thus, a diagnosis of primary cutaneous anaplastic large cell lymphoma should be made only when accurate clinical history and clinical examination exclude the presence of mycosis fungoides. As already mentioned, useful information may be obtained by FISH analysis of *IRF4* translocations. Most cases of mycosis fungoides with CD30+ large cell transformation are negative for *IRF4* translocations, whereas primary

Table 5.2 TNM classification system for cutaneous lymphomas other than mycosis fungoides and Sézary syndrome (adapted from [128])

| Classification | Description |
|---|---|
| $T_1$ | Solitary skin involvement<br>$T_{1a}$: Solitary lesion <5 cm in diameter<br>$T_{1b}$: Solitary lesion ≥5 cm in diameter |
| $T_2$ | Regional involvement of skin: multiple lesions limited to 1 body region or 2 contiguous body regions<br>$T_{2a}$: All disease encompassing a <15-cm-diameter circular area<br>$T_{2b}$: All disease encompassing a ≥15 to <30-cm-diameter circular area<br>$T_{2c}$: All disease encompassing a ≥30-cm-diameter circular area |
| $T_3$ | Generalized skin involvement<br>$T_{3a}$: Multiple lesions involving 2 noncontiguous body regions<br>$T_{3b}$: Multiple lesions involving ≥3 body regions |
| $N_0$ | No clinical or pathologic involvement of lymph nodes |
| $N_1$ | Involvement of 1 peripheral lymph node region that drains an area of current or previous skin involvement; biopsy positive for lymphoma |
| $N_2$ | Involvement of ≥2 peripheral lymph node regions or involvement of any lymph node region that does not drain an area of current or previous skin involvement; biopsy positive for lymphoma |
| $N_3$ | Involvement of central lymph nodes; biopsy positive for lymphoma |
| $N_X$ | Clinically abnormal peripheral or central LN but no pathologic determination. |
| $M_0$ | No visceral involvement |
| $M_1$ | Visceral involvement |
| $M_X$ | Visceral involvement is neither confirmed nor refuted by available pathologic or imaging assessment |

cutaneous large cell anaplastic lymphomas are positive in a proportion of cases [14, 16]. Expression of GATA3 is usually acquired in CD30+ mycosis fungoides with large cell transformation but is not found in cutaneous anaplastic large cell lymphoma, thus representing a possible helpful staining for this differential diagnosis [130]. The most important feature to separate the two entities, however, is correlation with the clinical picture.

The association of cutaneous anaplastic large cell lymphoma and lymphomatoid papulosis has been observed in several instances. The distinction between the two entities may be very difficult, as clinical, histologic, and immunophenotypic features may overlap. In this context, in 1995 LeBoit wrote: ". . . if one could line up 100 patients with lymphomatoid papulosis, primary cutaneous anaplastic large cell lymphoma, and cutaneous dissemination of Hodgkin's disease, a skilled clinician could more accurately sort the patients into diagnostic groups than a pathologist could by looking only at the immunophenotype of the large atypical cells" [131]. Although cutaneous dissemination of Hodgkin lymphoma (at least of the classical variant of it) can be confirmed by immunohistochemical analyses (see Chapter 24), the sentence holds true for what concerns the differentiation of lymphomatoid papulosis from anaplastic large cell lymphoma. In this context, it must be underlined that large, ulcerated tumors may be the presenting sign of lymphomatoid papulosis or may arise during the course of the disease, and that these lesions should not be misinterpreted as tumors of cutaneous anaplastic large cell lymphoma. In fact, it may be that at least some of the cases reported previously as "progression" of lymphomatoid papulosis to cutaneous anaplastic large cell lymphoma without systemic involvement represented indeed variants of lymphomatoid papulosis.

CD30 expression can be observed in a variety of cutaneous and extracutaneous lymphoproliferative (and even non-lymphoid) disorders and cannot be regarded as specific for any entity. In this context, it should be noted that expression of CD30 and anaplastic large cell morphology can be observed rarely in diffuse large B-cell lymphomas (see Chapter 15), and that complete phenotypic and genotypic analyses are necessary before classifying any given case.

Cutaneous anaplastic large cell lymphoma has been observed in patients with severe immunodeficiency due to both human immunodeficiency virus (HIV) infection and iatrogenic immune suppression. A detailed discussion of these cases is presented in Chapter 18. An intralymphatic variant of the disease has also been described (see below in this chapter).

Anaplastic large cell lymphoma with ALK-1 positivity has been observed at the skin site of insect bites and/or within draining lymph nodes [132]. The authors hypothesize that the antigenic stimulation may influence the T lymphocytes, some of which are positive for the t(2;5), and that the release of cytokines at the skin site of the bite could then act as a "second hit," causing expression of the oncogenic *NPM–ALK* protein and uncontrolled proliferation. Interestingly, a conceptually similar case occurred on the glans penis in the absence of an arthropod bite, suggesting that a concomitant cutaneous/nodal presentation of ALK+ anaplastic large cell lymphoma may be related to different types of antigenic stimulation [133]. In addition, it seems that ALK+ cases are more common in children and adolescents [132, 134–137]. It is still a matter of discussion whether in the skin ALK+ cases should be considered as a phenotypic variation of cutaneous anaplastic large cell lymphoma or a different entity ("ALK+ anaplastic large cell lymphoma presenting exclusively with cutaneous disease"). At present, there are no data supporting a different behavior of ALK+ primary cutaneous cases, but it seems prudent to follow up carefully with these patients.

## Clinical features

Cutaneous anaplastic large cell lymphoma occurs mostly in adults of both sexes, but cases in children have been reported. Clinically, patients usually present with variably large, solitary, mostly ulcerated plaques or tumors (Fig. 5.35). Non-ulcerated lesions show a smooth surface, often with prominent telangiectatic vessels (Fig. 5.36), but the rapid neoplastic growth is

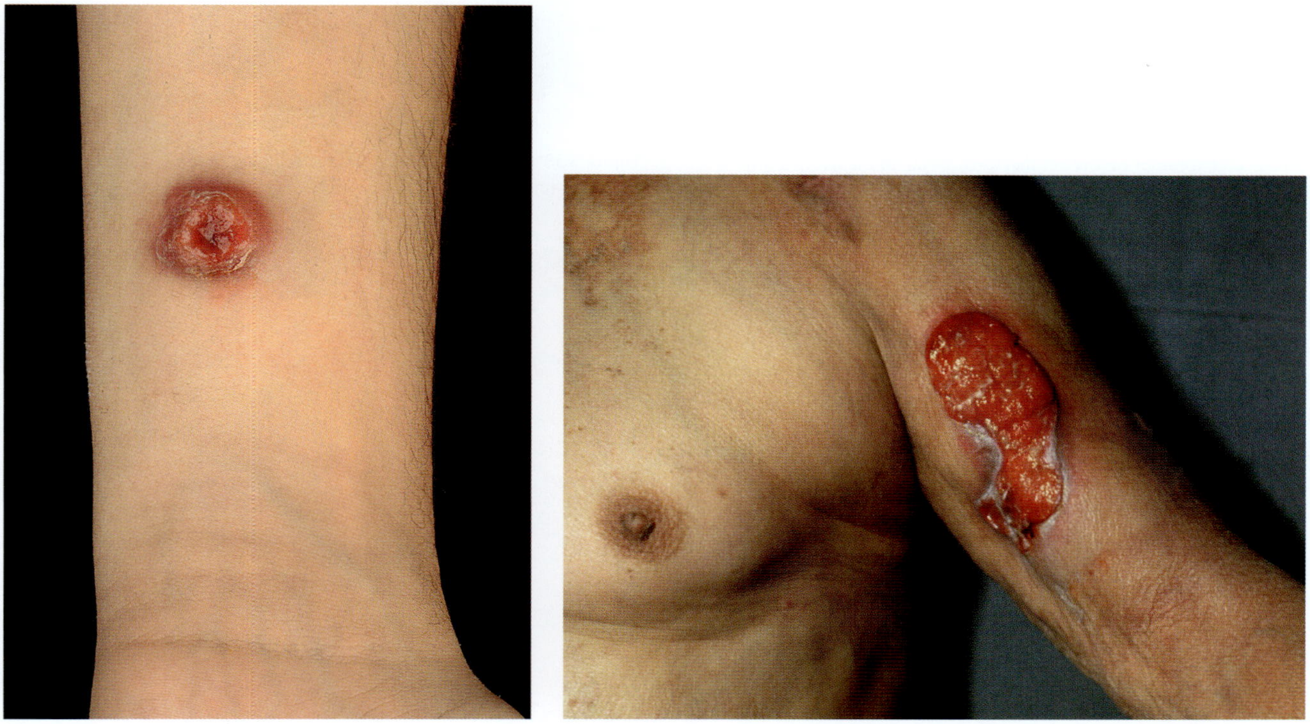

(a) (b)

**Figure 5.35** Cutaneous anaplastic large cell lymphoma. (a) Solitary, small, ulcerated tumor on the lower arm. (b) Large, ulcerated tumor on the upper arm.

commonly followed by ulceration of the lesion (Fig. 5.37). Clustered lesions may give rise to large, multinodular tumors (Fig. 5.38). As already mentioned for lymphomatoid papulosis, lesions located on the hands may be misdiagnosed clinically as orf or milker's nodule (Fig. 5.39) (see also Chapter 31), and both the histopathological features and the pattern of CD30 expression in orf and milker's nodule may be indistinguishable from those observed in lymphomatoid papulosis or anaplastic large cell lymphoma. Besides the relevant history (no contact with infected cattle), a useful diagnostic feature, when present, is represented by loss of pan-T-cell markers in lymphomatoid papulosis (observed uncommonly) or anaplastic large cell lymphoma (observed commonly) (Figs. 5.39b, c). Mucosal regions can be affected (Fig. 5.40). Complete spontaneous regression has been observed in a few cases [138], but regression is more commonly partial (see Fig. 5.61a). Sometimes the combination of radial growth and partial

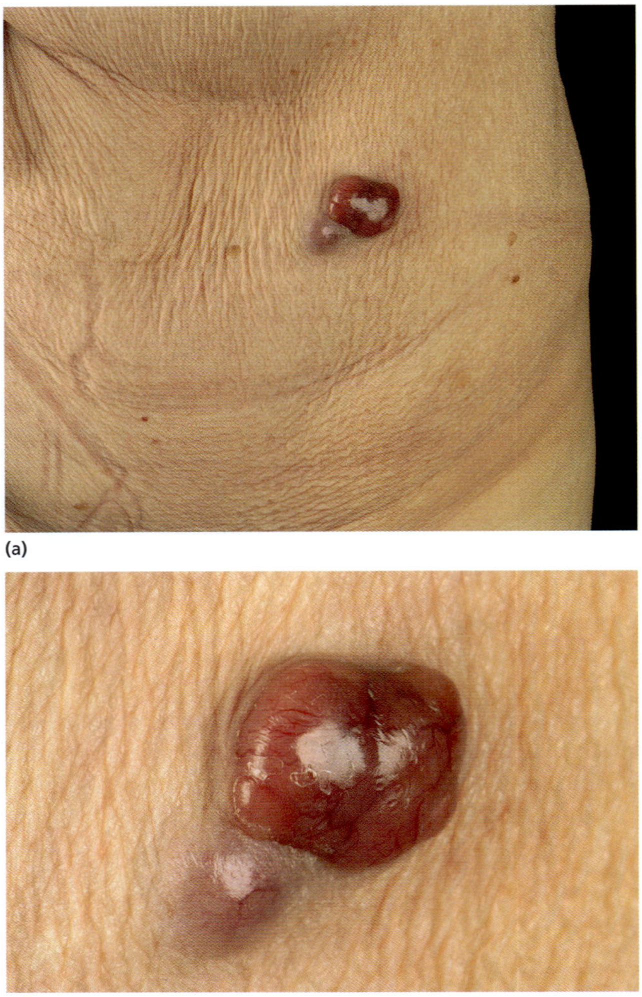

(a)

(b)

**Figure 5.36** Cutaneous anaplastic large cell lymphoma. (a) Solitary, non-ulcerated tumor on the left flank. (b) Detail of the lesion showing a smooth surface with prominent telangiectatic vessels.

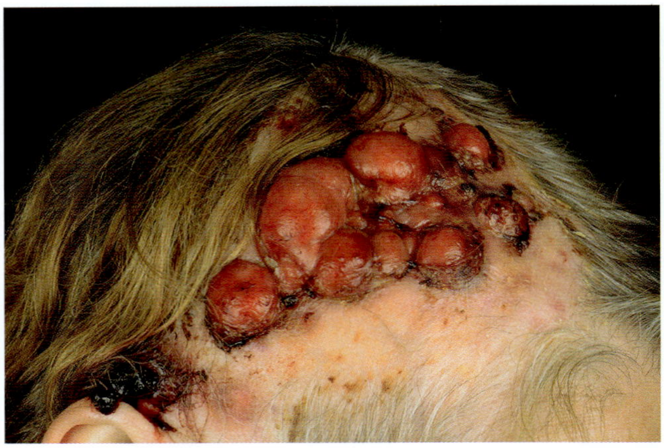

**Figure 5.38** Cutaneous anaplastic large cell lymphoma. Clustered, large, ulcerated tumors on the scalp.

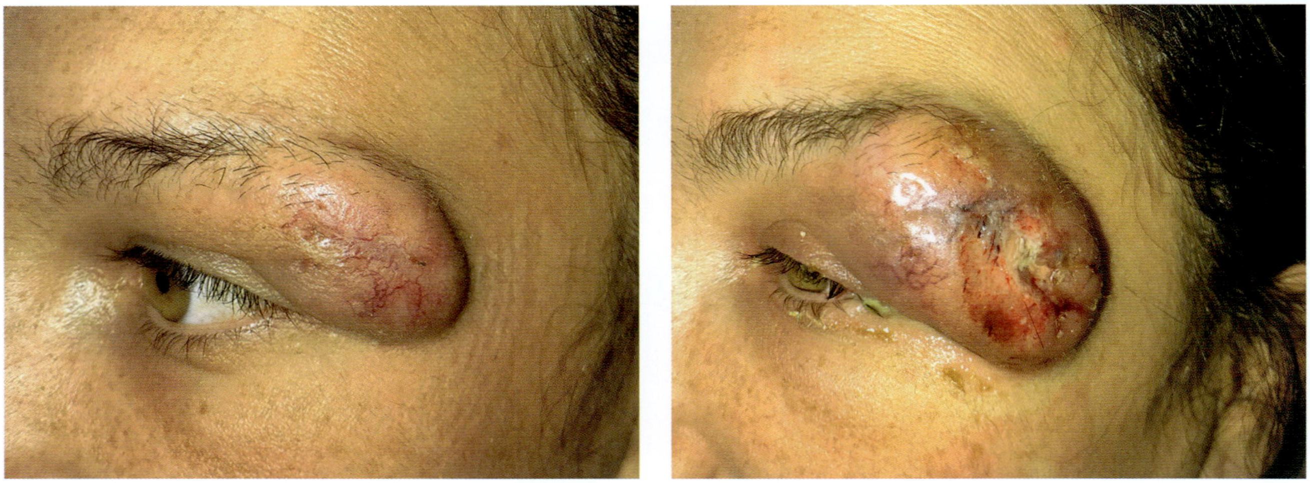

(a) (b)

**Figure 5.37** Cutaneous anaplastic large cell lymphoma. (a) A picture taken at the first presentation shows a non-ulcerated tumor on the left eyebrow. (b) A second picture taken 18 days later shows considerable growth and superficial ulcerations. (*Courtesy of Dr. Carlo Cota, Rome, Italy.*)

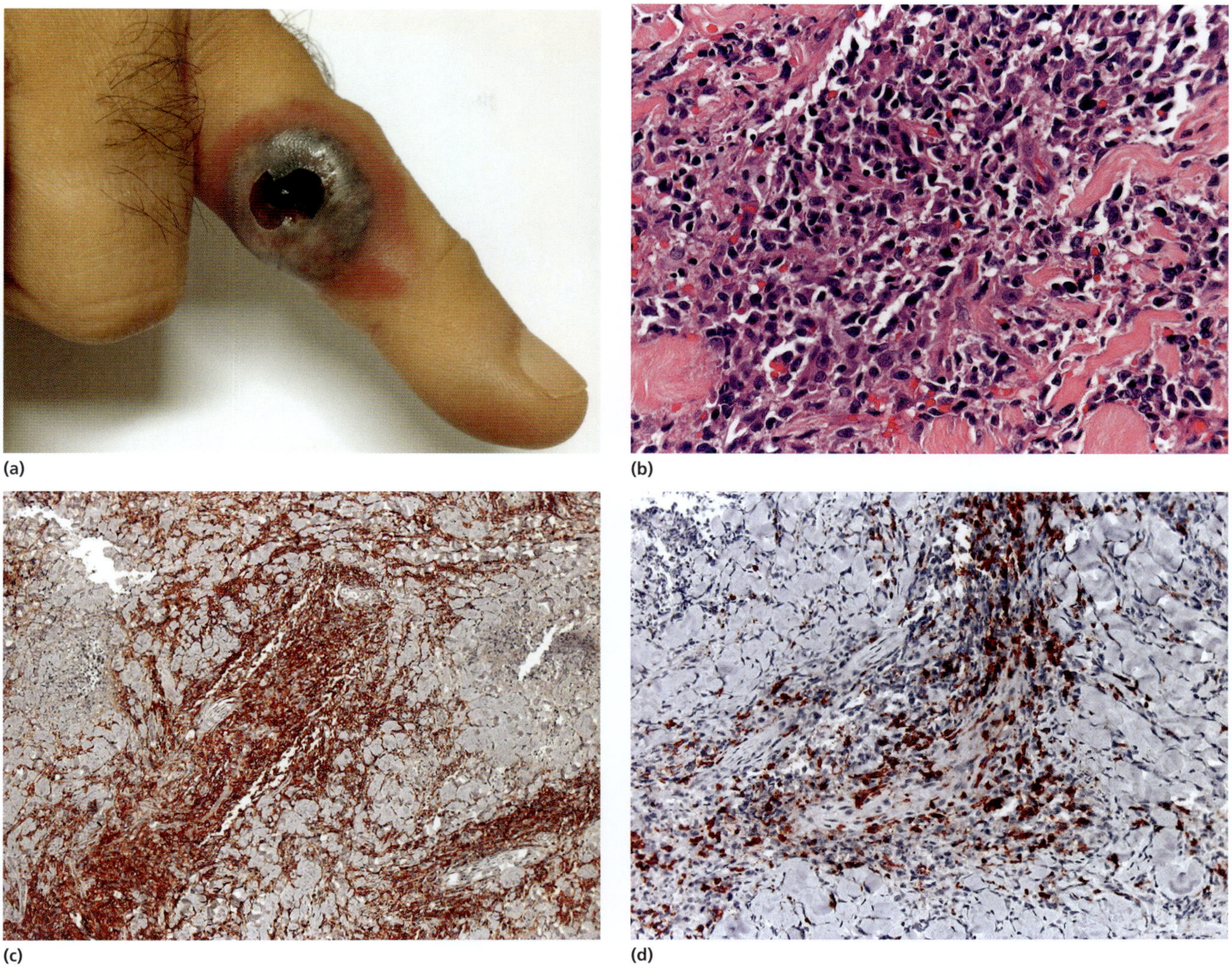

Figure 5.39 Cutaneous anaplastic large cell lymphoma. (a) Hemorrhagic, ulcerated tumor on the finger resembling the clinical presentation of milker's nodule or orf. (*Courtesy of Drs. Isabella Viana and Esmeralda Vale, Lisbon, Portugal.*) (b) Dermal infiltrate of atypical lymphocytes with (c) strong expression of CD30, (d) but negativity of most large cells for CD5.

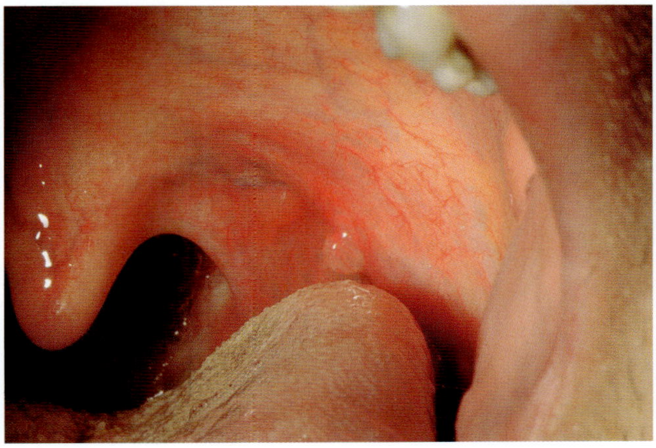

Figure 5.40 Cutaneous anaplastic large cell lymphoma. Involvement of the palate with ulceration and clustered papules.

regression with re-epithelization may confer unusual, "geographical" features to the clinical aspect (Fig. 5.41). Recurrent lesions are commonly localized on the scar or in the immediate vicinity of it (Fig. 5.42). The presence of multiple, localized lesions may simulate the clinical picture of regional lymphomatoid papulosis (Fig. 5.43). In some cases, several lesions may involve an entire limb (Fig. 5.44). These cases are referred to as "extensive limb disease" and are characterized by a worse prognosis [139, 140].

As already described in the section on lymphomatoid papulosis, T-cell clonality may be detected within the peripheral blood or the bone marrow of patients with cutaneous anaplastic large cell lymphoma, but the clones are not related to those of the cutaneous disorder, and the finding has no clinical significance [44].

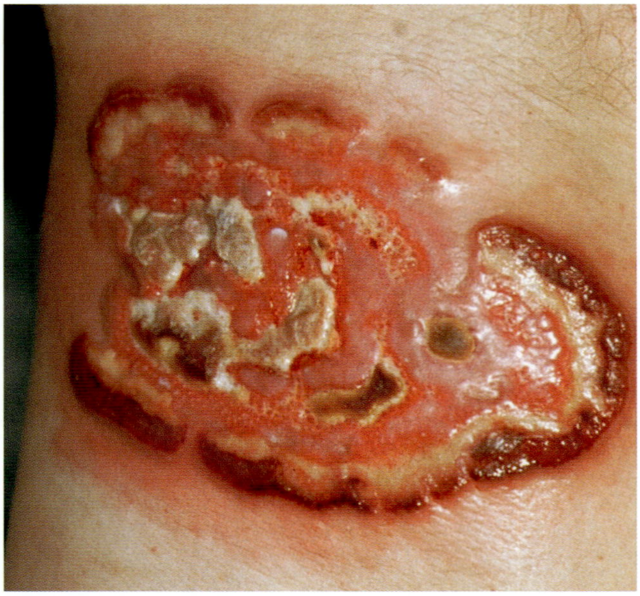

Figure 5.41 Cutaneous anaplastic large cell lymphoma. Large, irregular, ulcerated plaque with radial growth and small areas of regression conveying a "geographical" aspect to the lesion.

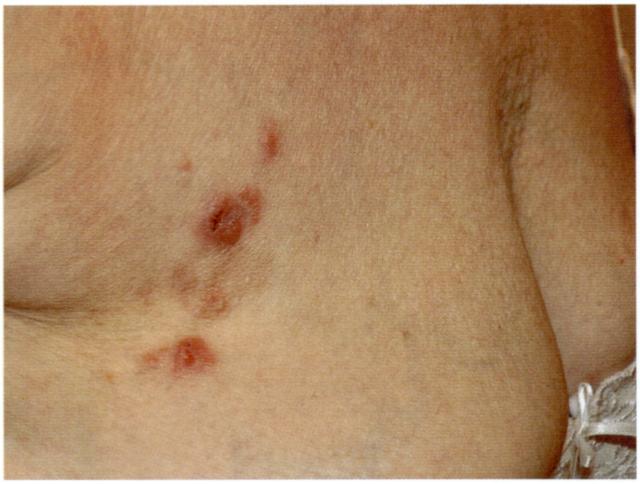

Figure 5.43 Cutaneous anaplastic large cell lymphoma. Small, partly ulcerated tumors on the breast with a "sporotrichoid" arrangement.

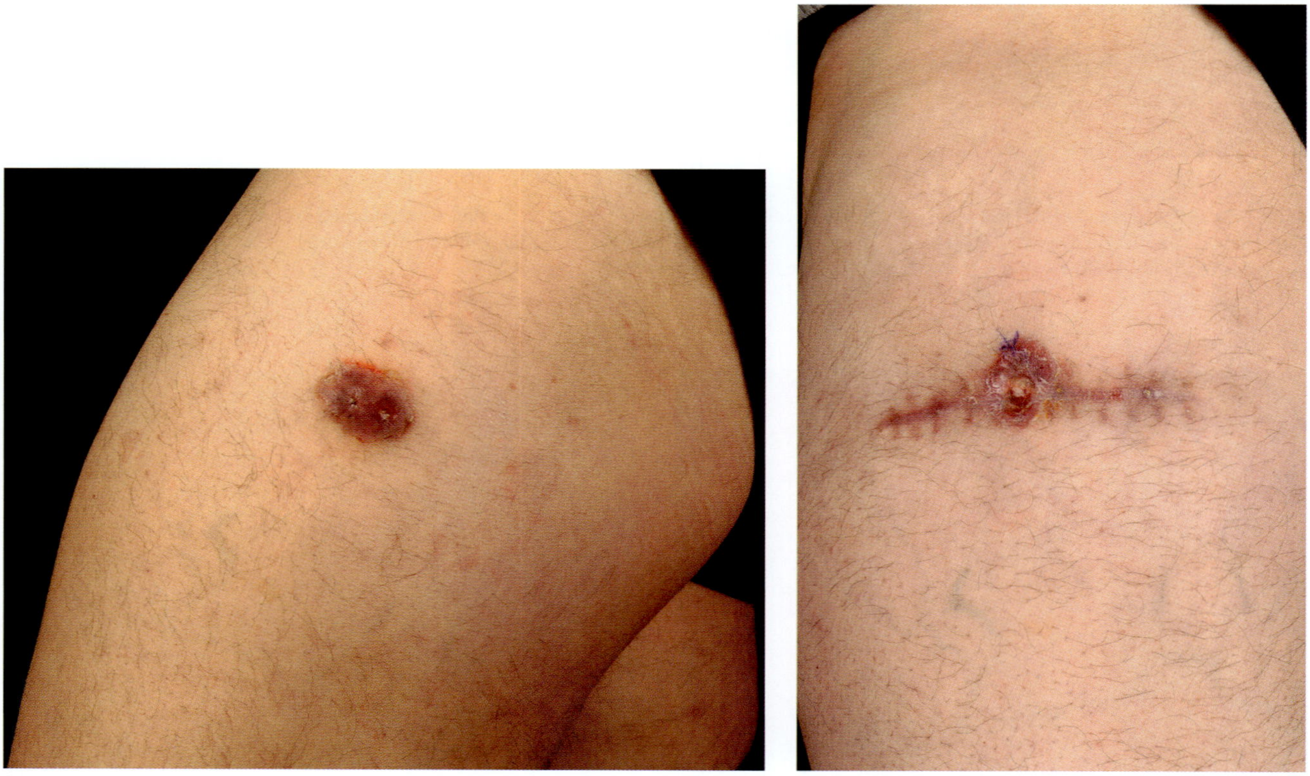

(a) (b)

Figure 5.42 Cutaneous anaplastic large cell lymphoma. (a) Erosive plaque on the left thigh. (b) Recurrent lesion on the scar three months after surgical excision.

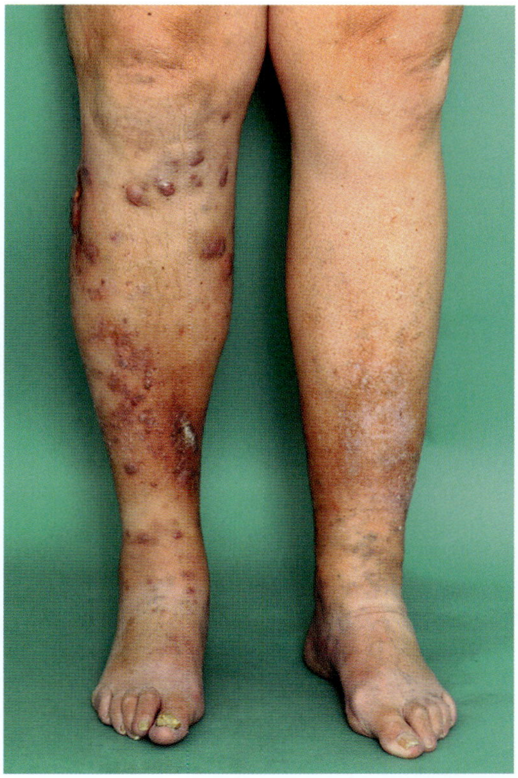

**Figure 5.44** Extensive limb disease in cutaneous anaplastic large cell lymphoma. Several papules, nodules, and tumors involving the entire distal part of one leg. *(Courtesy of Dr. Cornelia Müller, Homburg/Saar, Germany.)*

## Histopathology, immunophenotype, and molecular genetics

### Histopathology

Several patterns and cell morphologies may be observed in lesions of cutaneous anaplastic large cell lymphoma [141]. In most cases, at scanning magnification, there is a nodular or diffuse infiltrate within the entire dermis and superficial part of the subcutis, composed of sheets of cohesive, large CD30+ atypical cells (Fig. 5.45). Some degree of epidermotropism is often present, and in some cases may be prominent (Figs. 5.46a and b). Adnexal structures, too, may be infiltrated by neoplastic lymphocytes (Fig. 5.46c). Epidermotropic and adnexotropic lymphocytes are usually of smaller size than the dermal ones, but both populations are positive for CD30 (Fig. 5.46d). This peculiar presentation is mostly found in cases with t(6;7)(p25.3;q32.3) translocation involving the *DUSP22–IRF4* locus. Cytomorphologic features are variable, and in my experience, cases composed of large anaplastic cells (large, rounded, or irregularly shaped nuclei with prominent nucleoli and abundant cytoplasm; giant cells with features of Reed–Sternberg cells) are as frequent as those composed of large pleomorphic cells (Figs. 5.47a and b). Immunoblast-like cells with abundant cytoplasm can also be observed (Fig. 5.47c). Rare cases are characterized by a predominant small/medium-sized pleomorphic cell morphology (Fig. 5.47d). Although a "small-to-medium-cell" variant of a large-cell lymphoma is an oxymoron, similar cases are also well known in the lymph nodes [142]. Sometimes, anaplastic cells show epithelioid-like cytomorphologic features resembling undifferentiated carcinoma, and at other times have a sarcomatous aspect (Figs. 5.47e and f) [143]. Rarely, a signet-ring morphology can be observed (Fig. 5.48), and a unique case with morphological features mimicking clear-cell morphology has been reported [144].

Besides nodular and diffuse infiltrates, the second most common histopathologic presentation of cutaneous anaplastic large cell lymphoma is characterized by prominent, sometimes geographical, necrosis. In some cases, peripheral palisading of neoplastic cells around necrotic areas may mimic the picture of a palisading granuloma (Fig. 5.49a). However, the cellular infiltrate is much more dense than in palisading granulomas, and many eosinophils are almost invariably present in the inflammatory infiltrate, features unusual for skin diseases in the spectrum of the palisading granulomas (Fig. 5.49b). Positivity for CD30 and for T-cell markers in palisading cells allows one to make a correct diagnosis in these cases (Fig. 5.49c). In some cases, the necrotic areas may be surrounding vessels with angiocentric and/or angiotropic infiltrates of CD30+ cells (Fig. 5.50). In general, the presence of prominent necrosis in the context of an infiltrate rich in eosinophils should always prompt consideration of the differential diagnosis of a cutaneous anaplastic large cell lymphoma.

Ulcerated lesions, and sometimes also lesions without ulceration, may show epidermal hyperplasia and a prominent reactive infiltrate with small lymphocytes, neutrophils, and eosinophils (Fig. 5.51). Cases with a predominance of neutrophils have been referred to as "inflammatory," "neutrophil-rich," or "pyogenic" anaplastic large cell lymphoma [145, 146]. It has been suggested that this variant is more frequent in young persons or in immunocompromised individuals [146]. In my experience, cases with large numbers of eosinophils are more common than those with neutrophil-rich infiltrates and sometimes may be the reason for differential diagnostic concerns with reactive conditions (Fig. 5.52).

In some cases of cutaneous anaplastic large cell lymphoma, epithelial hyperplasia is prominent and confers a pseudoepitheliomatous aspect to the lesion, simulating the picture of a squamous cell carcinoma (Fig. 5.53) [147]. These cases are similar to those of lymphomatoid papulosis with "keratoacanthomatous" epithelial hyperplasia, demonstrating once again the overlapping clinicopathologic spectrum of cutaneous CD30+ lymphoproliferative disorders.

Other rare histopathologic variants include prominent involvement of the subcutaneous fat resembling subcutaneous panniculitis-like T-cell lymphoma and the presence of a myxoid stroma resembling a sarcomatous lesion [148–150]. The presence of many eosinophils is typical for subcutaneous lesions of anaplastic large cell lymphoma (Fig. 5.54), and neoplastic

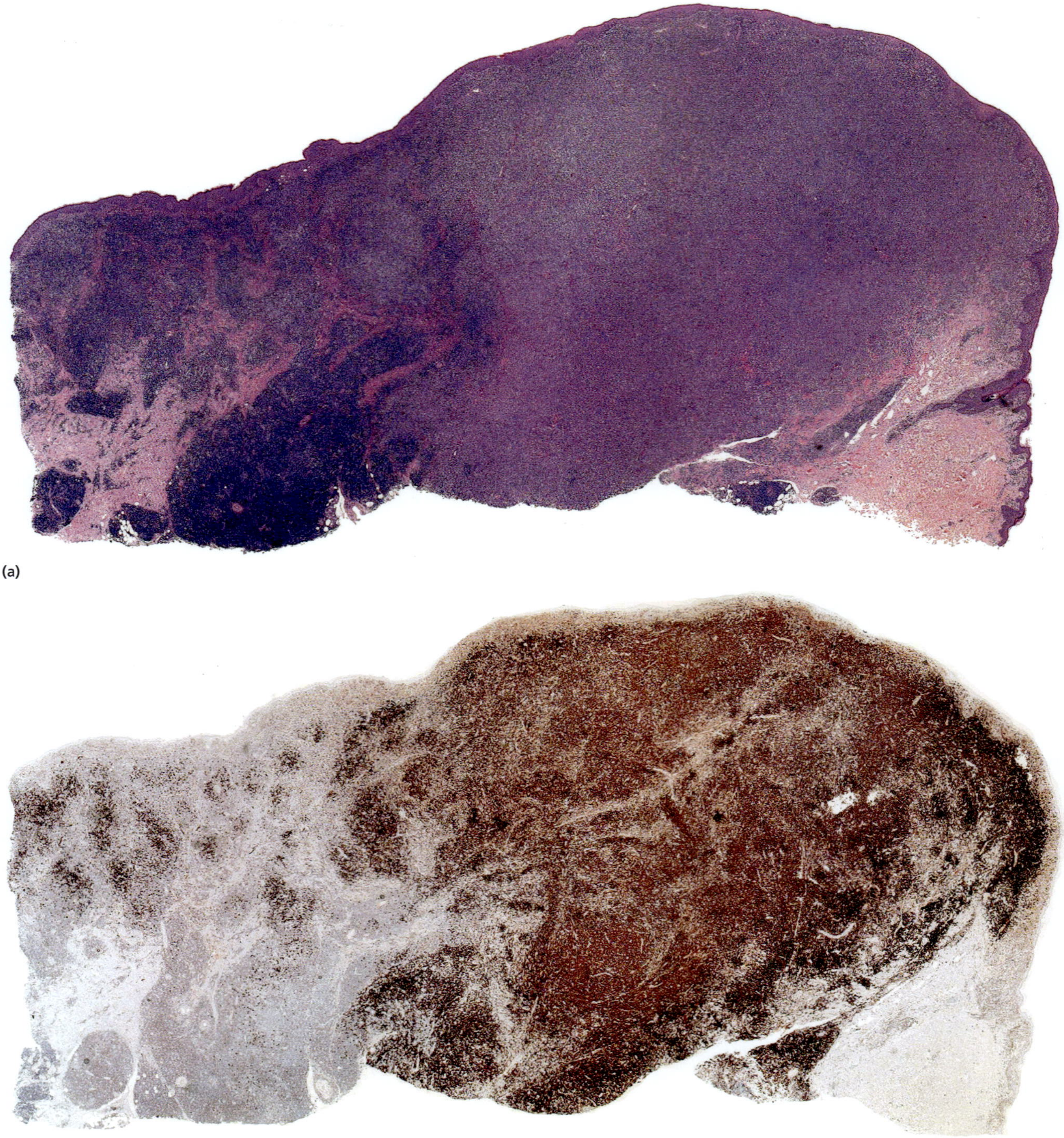

(a)

(b)

**Figure 5.45** Cutaneous anaplastic large cell lymphoma. (a) Large tumor with sheets of cells infiltrating the entire dermis and visible subcutis. (b) Most cells strongly express CD30.

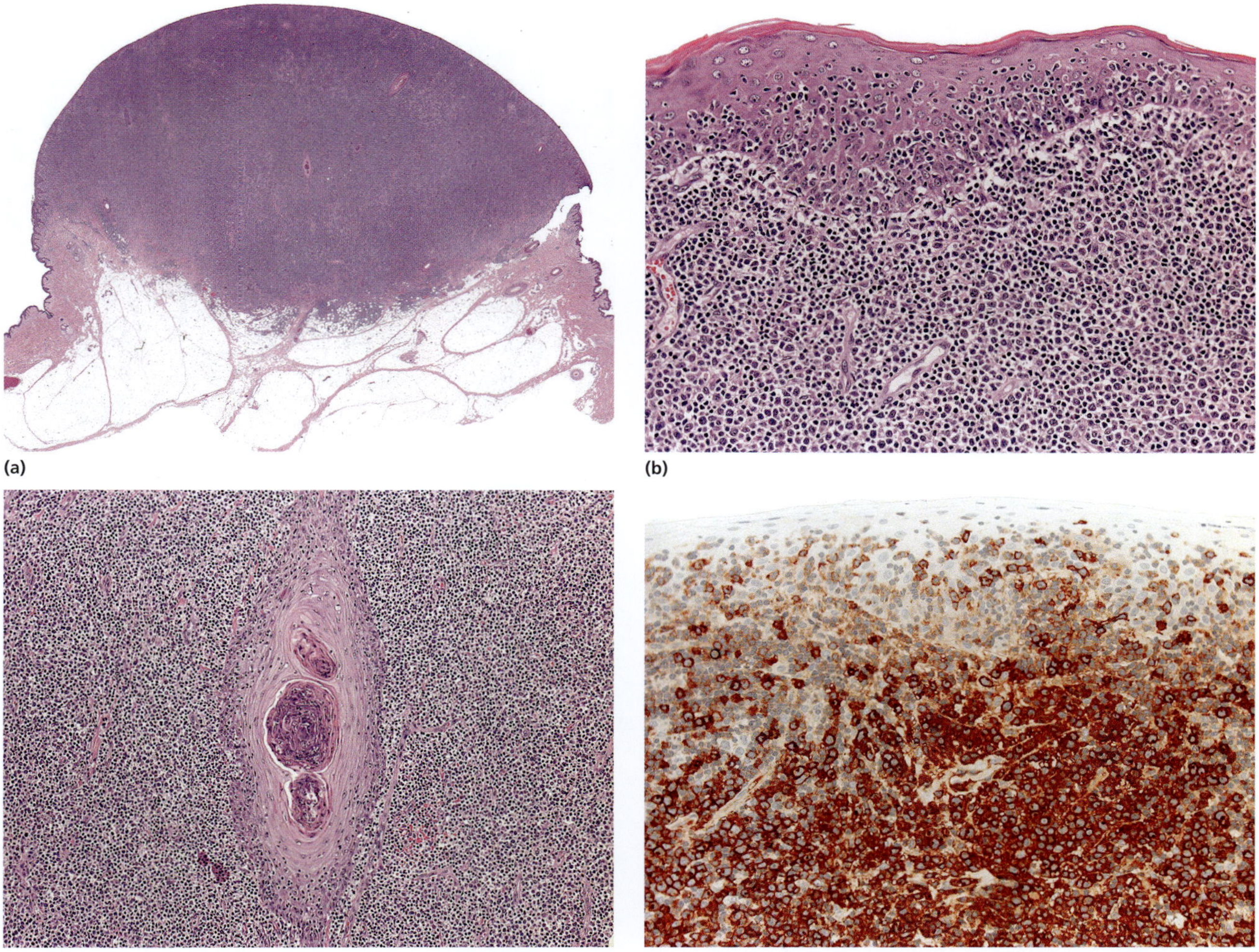

(a) (b) (c) (d)

Figure 5.46 Cutaneous anaplastic large cell lymphoma. (a) Large dermal nodule of atypical cells infiltrating the superficial part of the subcutaneous fat and with (b) prominent epidermotropism. (c) Adnexal structures are also infiltrated by neoplastic cells. (d) All cells express CD30. These histopathological features are typical of cases with a *DUSP22–IRF4* chromosomal rearrangement (see text for explanation).

cells usually demonstrate a T-helper phenotype rather than the T-cytotoxic one observed in subcutaneous panniculitis-like T-cell lymphoma. In addition, some of these cases show prominent necrosis surrounded by neoplastic infiltrates (usually corresponding to angiocentric/angiodestructive features), a pattern that is usually not found in subcutaneous panniculitis-like T-cell lymphoma (Fig. 5.55). Dystrophic calcifications may be observed in cases characterized by prominent necrosis of the subcutaneous tissues (Fig. 5.56). In contrast to true sarcomatous neoplasms, the myxoid and sarcomatoid variants of cutaneous anaplastic large cell lymphoma are characterized by solid aggregates of anaplastic or pleomorphic tumor cells that are strongly positive for CD30 (Fig. 5.57). As already mentioned, cases of cutaneous anaplastic large lymphoma characterized by the 6p25.3 rearrangement show peculiar histopathological features characterized by a "biphasic" pattern (diffuse dermal infiltrate of atypical medium- to large cells and marked epidermotropism of smaller, atypical lymphocytes) [151].

Angiocentricity with or without angiodestruction may be prominent in some cases of cutaneous anaplastic large cell lymphoma, sometimes with the formation of intraluminal thrombi mimicking the histopathologic picture of a necrotizing vasculitis (Figs. 5.50 and 5.58) [152]. In these cases, necrosis is usually prominent.

A peculiar histopathologic variant of anaplastic large cell lymphoma with predominant or exclusive intralymphatic arrangement of tumor cells is discussed in detail in a specific Section in this Chapter.

## Immunophenotype

Neoplastic cells express CD30 by definition (at least 75% of neoplastic cells must be positive for CD30 in order to meet

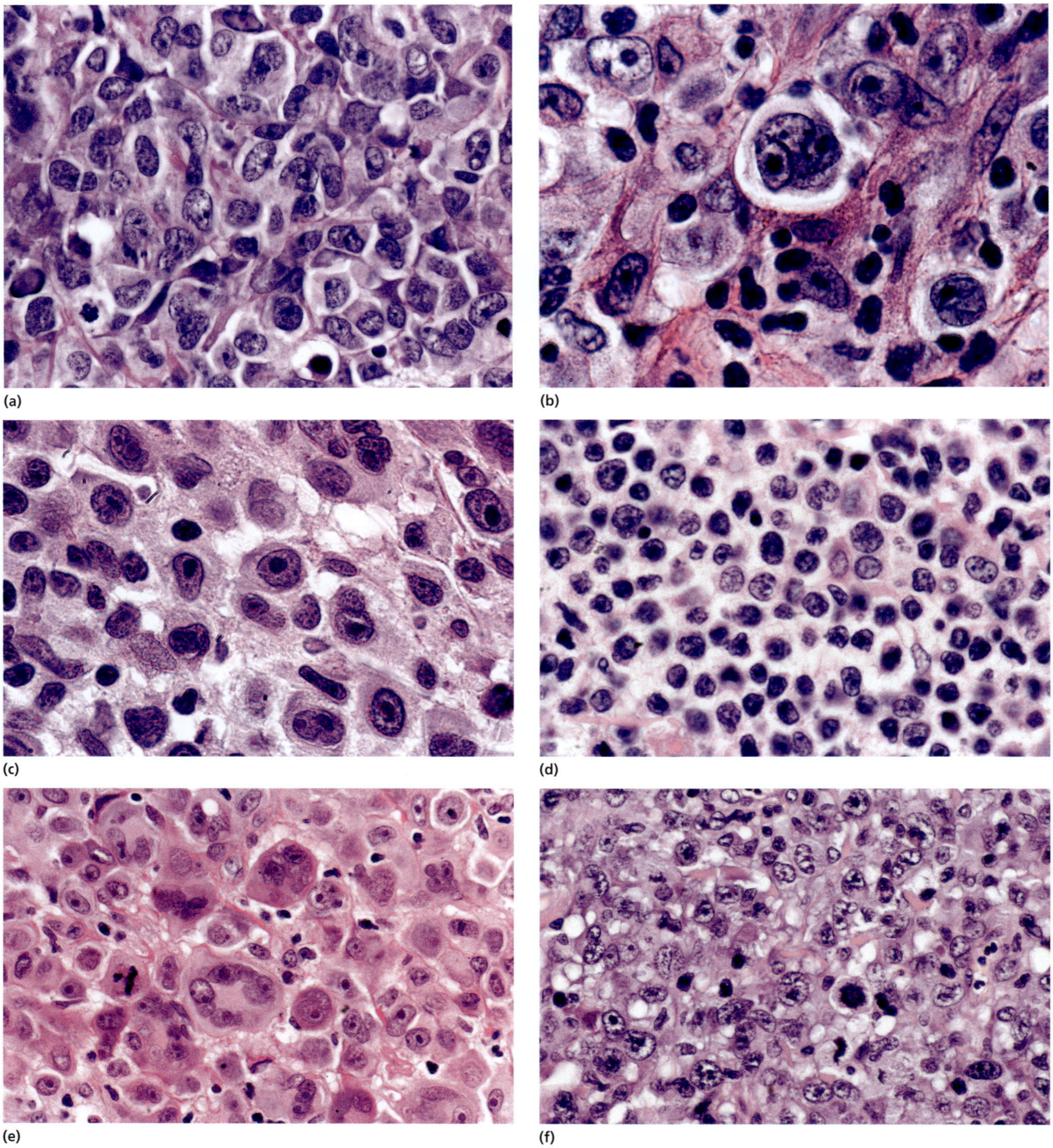

**Figure 5.47** Various cytomorphological features of cutaneous anaplastic large cell lymphoma. (a) Large pleomorphic and anaplastic cells. (b) Presence of multinucleated cells resembling Reed–Sternberg cells of Hodgkin lymphoma. (c) Immunoblast-like cells predominate in this case. (d) Predominance of small- to medium-sized pleomorphic lymphocytes (so-called "small cell variant" of anaplastic large cell lymphoma). (e) Predominance of "epithelioid" cells with abundant eosinophilic cytoplasm. Some multinucleated cells are present. (f) Sarcomatous aspect with large, atypical cells with vesicular nuclei.

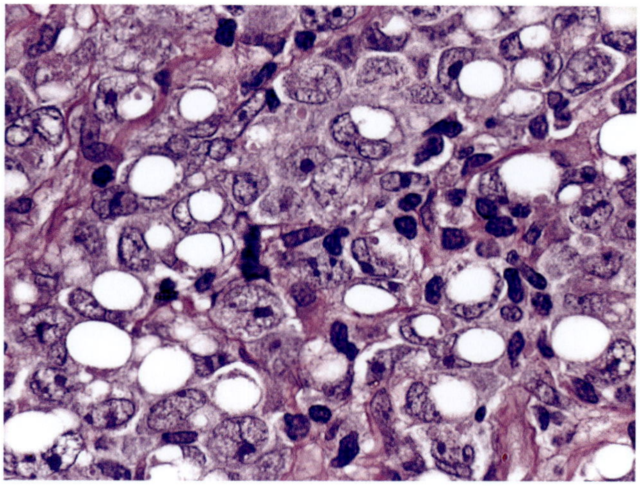

Figure 5.48 Cutaneous anaplastic large cell lymphoma with signet-ring cell morphology of neoplastic cells.

diagnostic criteria of cutaneous anaplastic large cell lymphoma [1]). The various patterns of CD30 positivity in different morphologic expressions of cutaneous anaplastic large cell lymphoma can be observed in Figs. 5.45b, 5.46d, 5.49c, 5.50c, 5.53b, 5.54c, 5.56c, and 5.57c. Particularly in cases with prominent necrosis, the pattern at low magnification may suggest expression of CD30 by less than 75% of the infiltrate (Fig. 5.49c), but many neoplastic lymphocytes are necrotic in such variants and many reactive cells are mixed with the neoplastic ones, thus conveying a false sense of only focal positivity of the specimen. Loss of CD30 expression has been described after therapy with anti-CD30 molecules (brentuximab vedotin) [153]. Expression of pan-T-cell antigens is often partially lost, and almost one-third of cases reveal profound phenotypic aberrations and positivity of only a few markers (Figs. 5.59a to d) [154]. Although a T-helper phenotype is considered typical for cutaneous anaplastic large cell lymphoma (CD3+, CD4+,

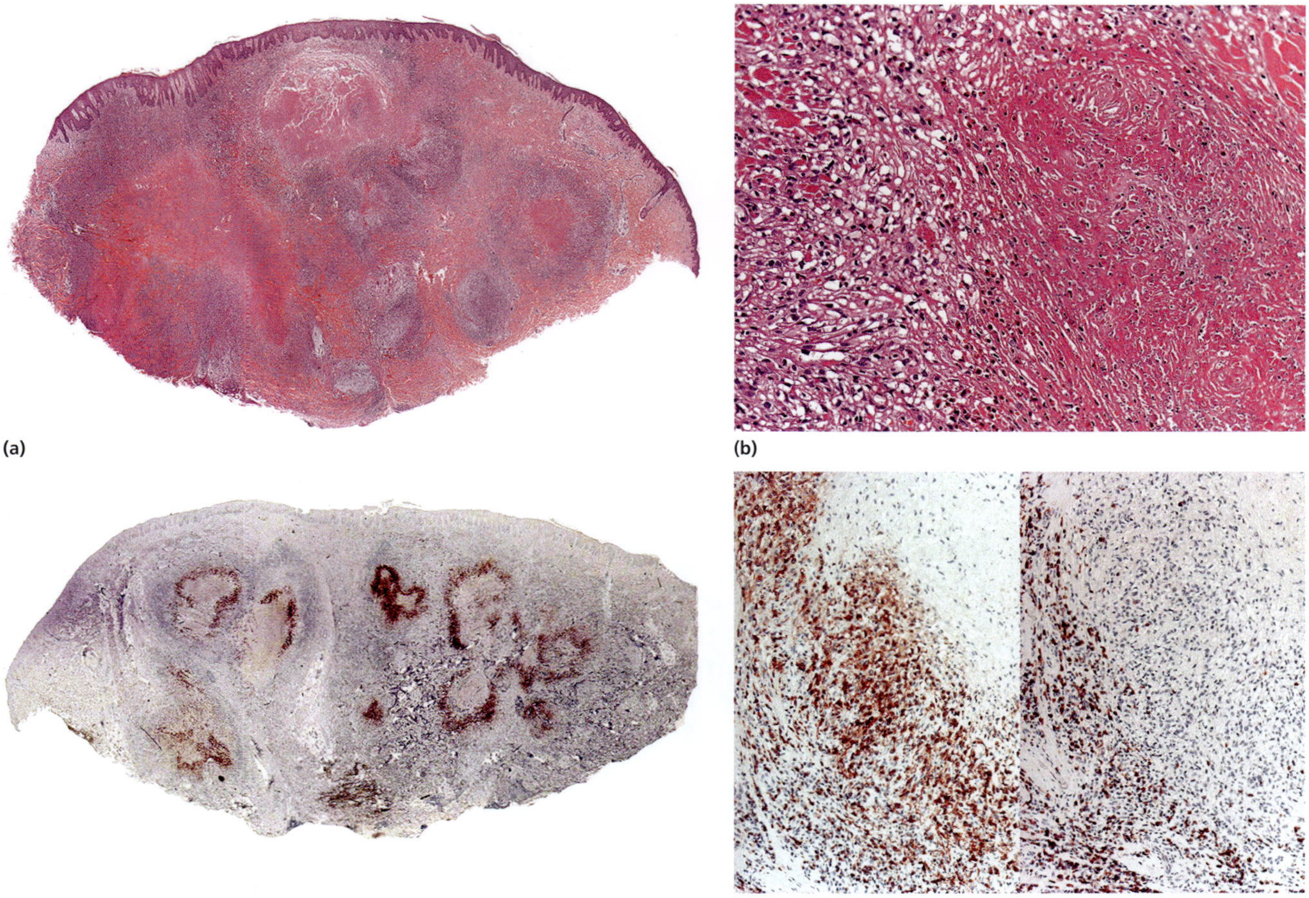

(a) (b) (c) (d)

Figure 5.49 Cutaneous anaplastic large cell lymphoma with prominent necrosis. (a) Large geographical areas of necrosis. (b) Atypical cells around areas of necrosis, admixed with several eosinophils. (c) Staining for CD30 highlights the palisading distribution of neoplastic cells around areas of necrosis. (d) Positivity of neoplastic cells for CD3 (left) with loss of CD5 expression (right).

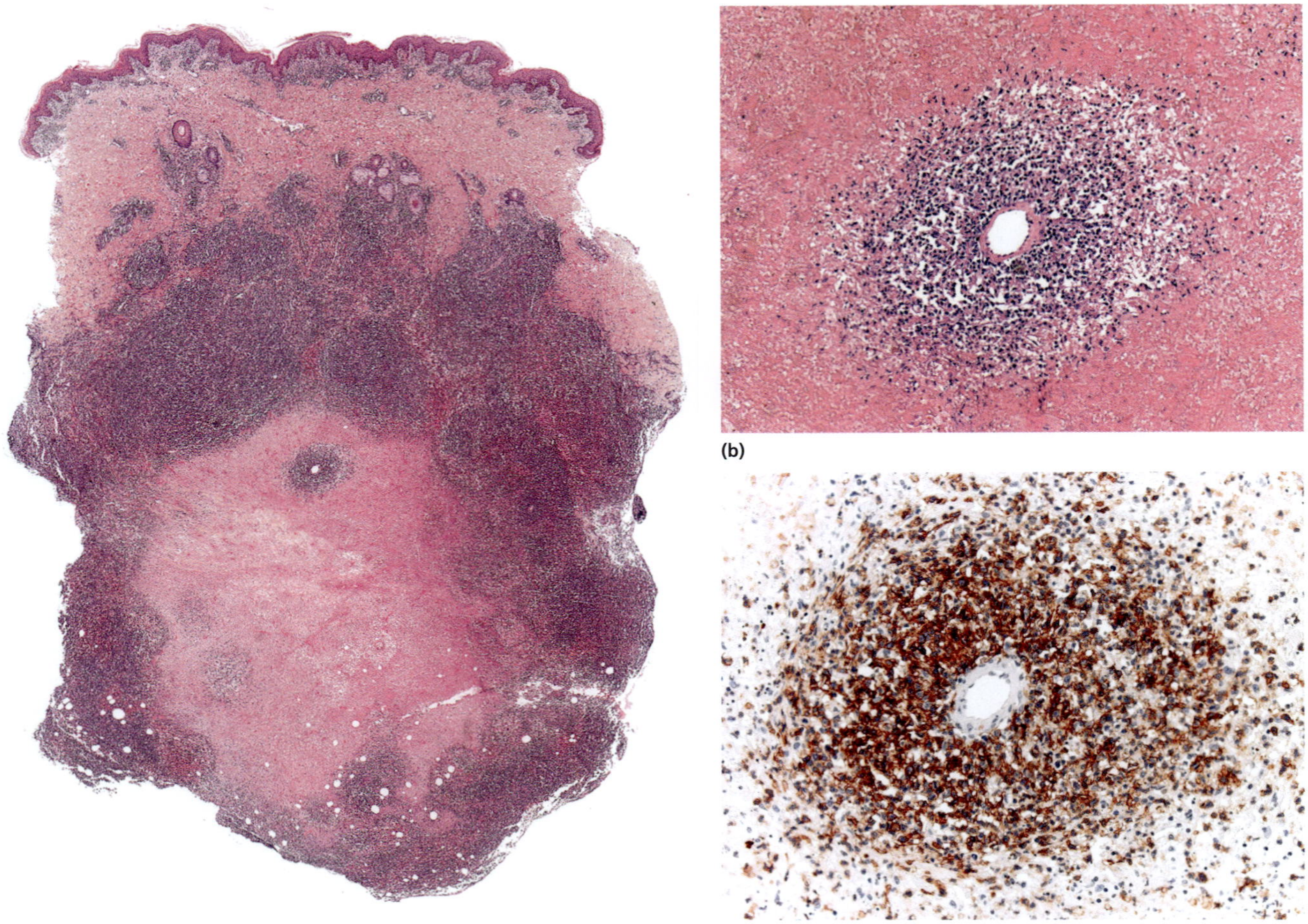


**Figure 5.50** Cutaneous anaplastic large cell lymphoma with prominent necrosis. (a) Large, well-circumscribed area of necrosis. (b) Angiocentricity with prominent necrosis of the surrounding tissues. (c) Staining for CD30 highlights angiocentric neoplastic cells.

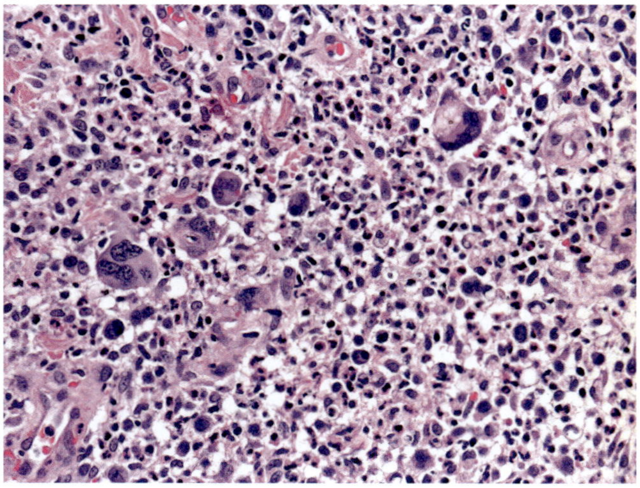

**Figure 5.51** Cutaneous anaplastic large cell lymphoma, "inflammatory type". Large anaplastic cells, some of which are multinucleated, admixed with several neutrophils.

$CD8^-$), cases with a cytotoxic profile are not uncommon [155], and a great degree of phenotypic variability exists (Figs. 5.59e and f) [154]. In fact, a study demonstrated that only one-third of cases are positive for CD4 and that the majority of the $CD4^+$ cases also express cytotoxic proteins [154]. In this study, positivity for both CD4 and CD8 or negativity for both markers was found in almost half of the cases [154], but in my experience it is less frequent. Some cases may show positivity for markers of T follicular helper (TFH) lymphocytes by neoplastic cells (Fig. 5.59g) [156a].

Most cases of primary scutaneous anaplastic large cell lymphoma express TCR-$\alpha/\beta$ receptors, but expression of TCR-$\gamma/\delta$ has been described [156b]. These cases are mostly $CD4^-/CD8^-$ and $ALK^-$, and are clinically similar to the TCR-$\alpha/\beta^+$ ones. The percentage of cases with *DUSP22* rearrangement, too, is similar to that observed in TCR-$\alpha/\beta^+$ cases.

Expression of lymphoid enhancer-binding factor 1 (LEF1), a transcription factor involved in the Wnt/$\beta$-catenin signaling

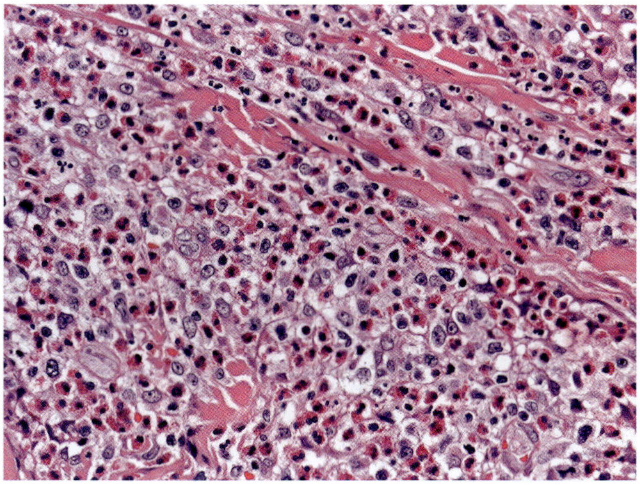

Figure 5.52 Cutaneous anaplastic large cell lymphoma, "inflammatory type". Neoplastic cells are admixed with large numbers of eosinophils.

pathway, has been observed in the majority of cases of ALK-negative systemic anaplastic large cell lymphoma with *DUSP22* rearrangement and only in a minimal fraction of *DUSP22* negative cases [157]. In cutaneous $CD30^+$ lymphoproliferative disorders, both lymphomatoid papulosis and cutaneous anaplastic large cell lymphoma, *DUSP22*-rearranged cases commonly show a phenotype characterized by positivity for LEF1 and negativity for TIA1 [158]. However, in a study on cutaneous anaplastic large cell lymphoma, the LEF1 expression pattern was not related to the presence of a *DUSP22* rearrangement, although a complete negativity for LEF1 was never observed in rearranged cases [159].

Expression of ALK protein is rare in primary cutaneous anaplastic large cell lymphoma, but it is present in secondary skin manifestations of nodal $ALK^+$ anaplastic large cell lymphoma (Fig. 5.59h) [160–163]. Primary cutaneous $ALK^+$ cases (with breaks within the *ALK* gene) have been observed in

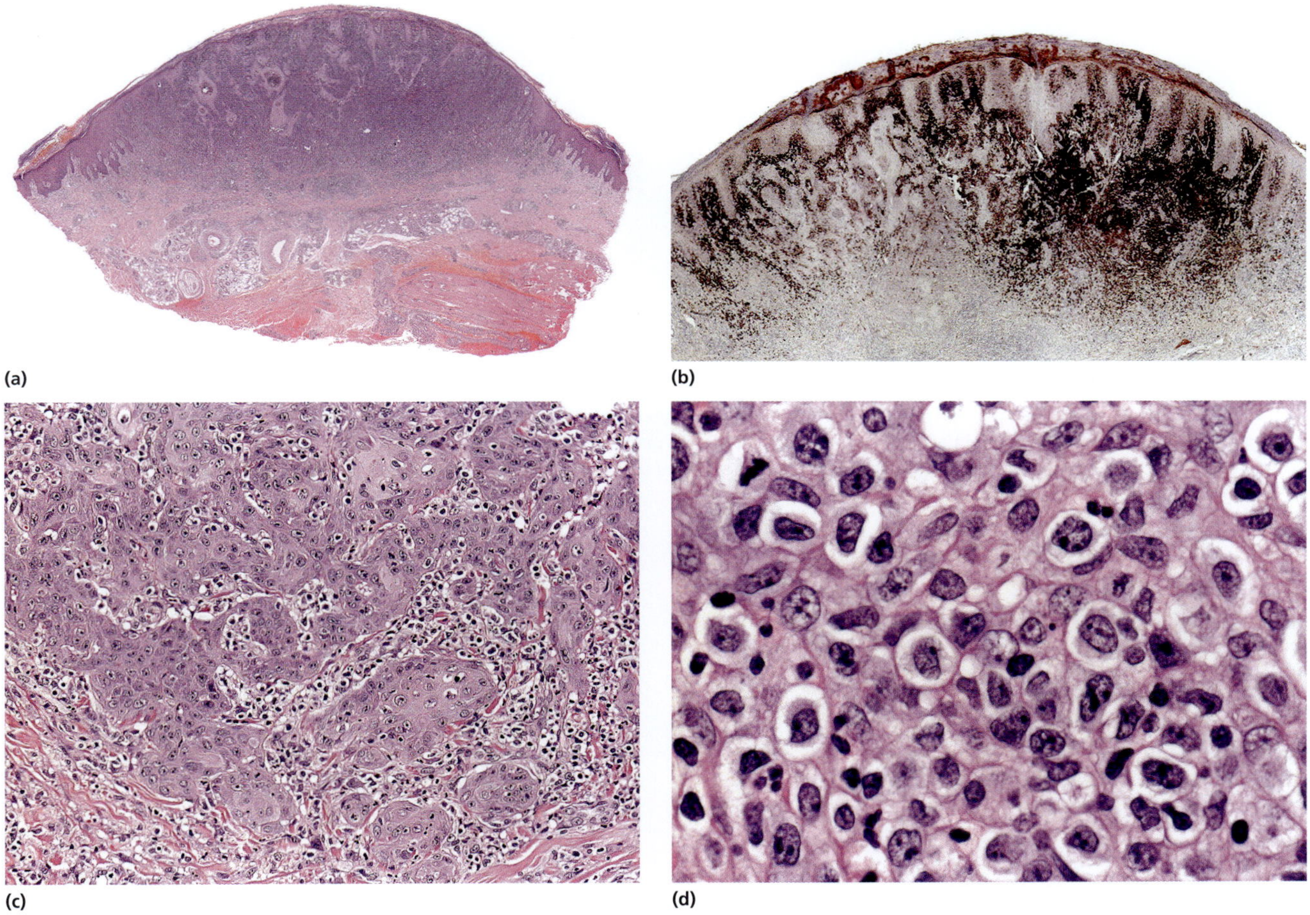

Figure 5.53 Cutaneous anaplastic large cell lymphoma. (a) Prominent pseudoepitheliomatous epithelial hyperplasia and dense dermal lymphoid infiltrates. (b) Positivity for CD30 highlights large numbers of neoplastic cells. (c) Detail of the pseudoepitheliomatous hyperplasia. (d) Detail of the lymphoid infiltrate with atypical, anaplastic cells.

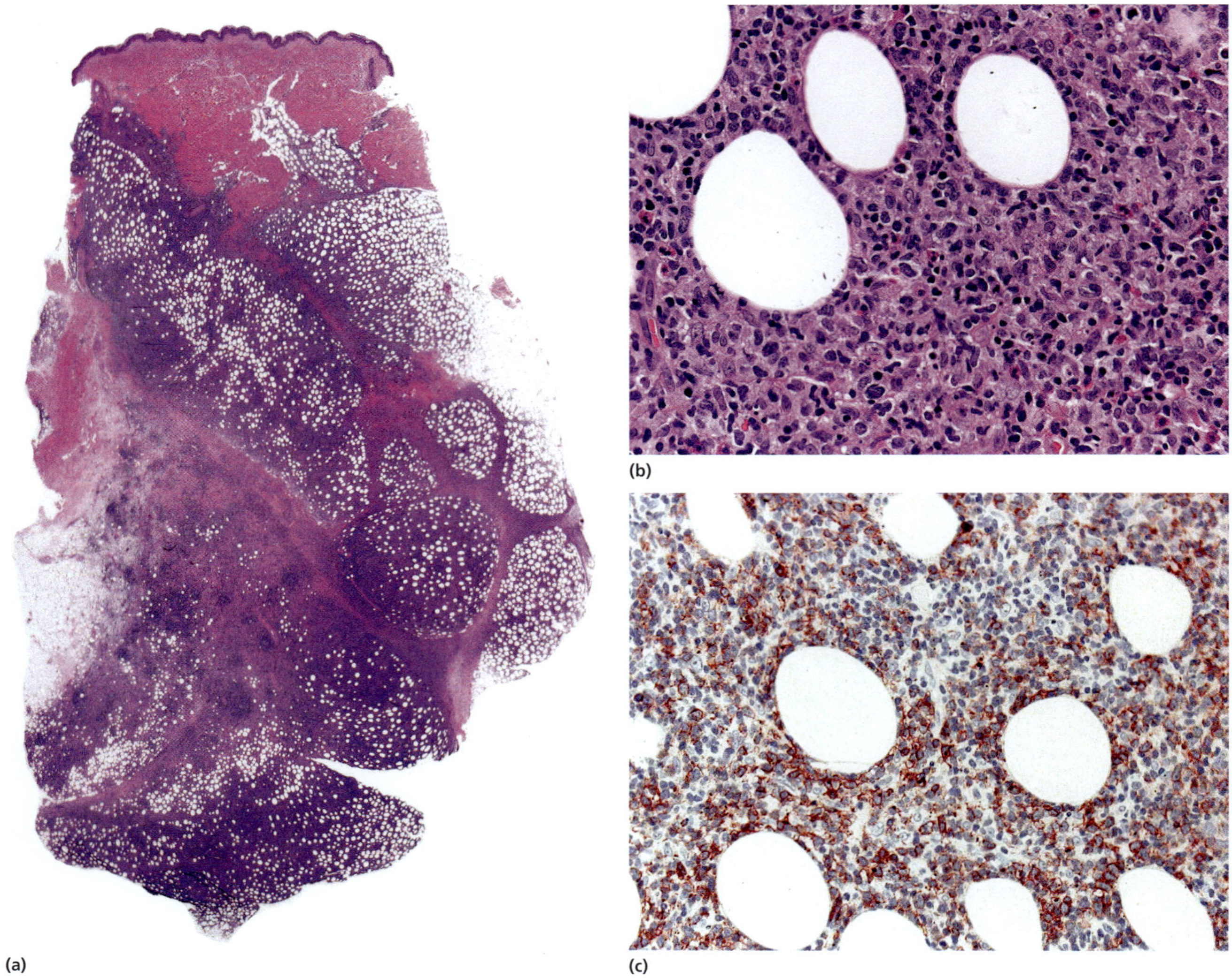

Figure 5.54 Cutaneous anaplastic large cell lymphoma confined to the subcutaneous fat. (a) At scanning magnification, the distribution of the infiltrate reminds that of a subcutaneous panniculitis-like T-cell lymphoma. (b) High magnification reveals large, atypical cells admixed with eosinophils. (c) Staining for CD30 shows positivity of most lymphocytes; note rimming of some adipocytes by CD30⁺ neoplastic cells.

pediatric patients, showing overlapping clinicopathologic and prognostic features with the more common ALK- ones [134–136], and rarely in adults, particularly in lesions arising following insect bites [132, 164]. In a small series including six cases of primary cutaneous ALK⁺ anaplastic large cell lymphoma, nuclear and cytoplasmic ALK expression was found in three cases with underlying *NPM1-ALK* fusions, while the other three cases with variant *ALK* fusion partners (*TRAF1*, *ATIC*, *TPM3*) showed only cytoplasmic ALK expression [165]. In the lymph nodes, different patterns of ALK positivity are associated with different genetic features of the neoplasm (both cytoplasmic and nuclear in cases harboring the t(2;5) *NPM–ALK*; membranous or cytoplasmic in cases with variant translocations; restricted to the nucleus in the small cell variant). It must be remembered that nodal ALK-negative cases exist and represent a specific entity in the WHO classification; thus, negativity for ALK in cutaneous cases cannot be considered synonymous with primary skin disease.

CD15 expression has been reported in 40% of cases [103], but in my experience, the percentage is lower. Epithelial membrane antigen (EMA) is usually negative but may be expressed in the rare ALK-1⁺ cases [132, 134]. MUM-1 is positive in almost all cases. Aberrant PAX-5 expression and extra copies of the *PAX5* gene locus have been observed in three nodal and one vertebral anaplastic large cell lymphomas, but not in cutaneous cases [166]. GATA3 is negative in cutaneous anaplastic large cell lymphoma (it is usually positive in CD30⁺ mycosis fungoides with large cell transformation) [130].

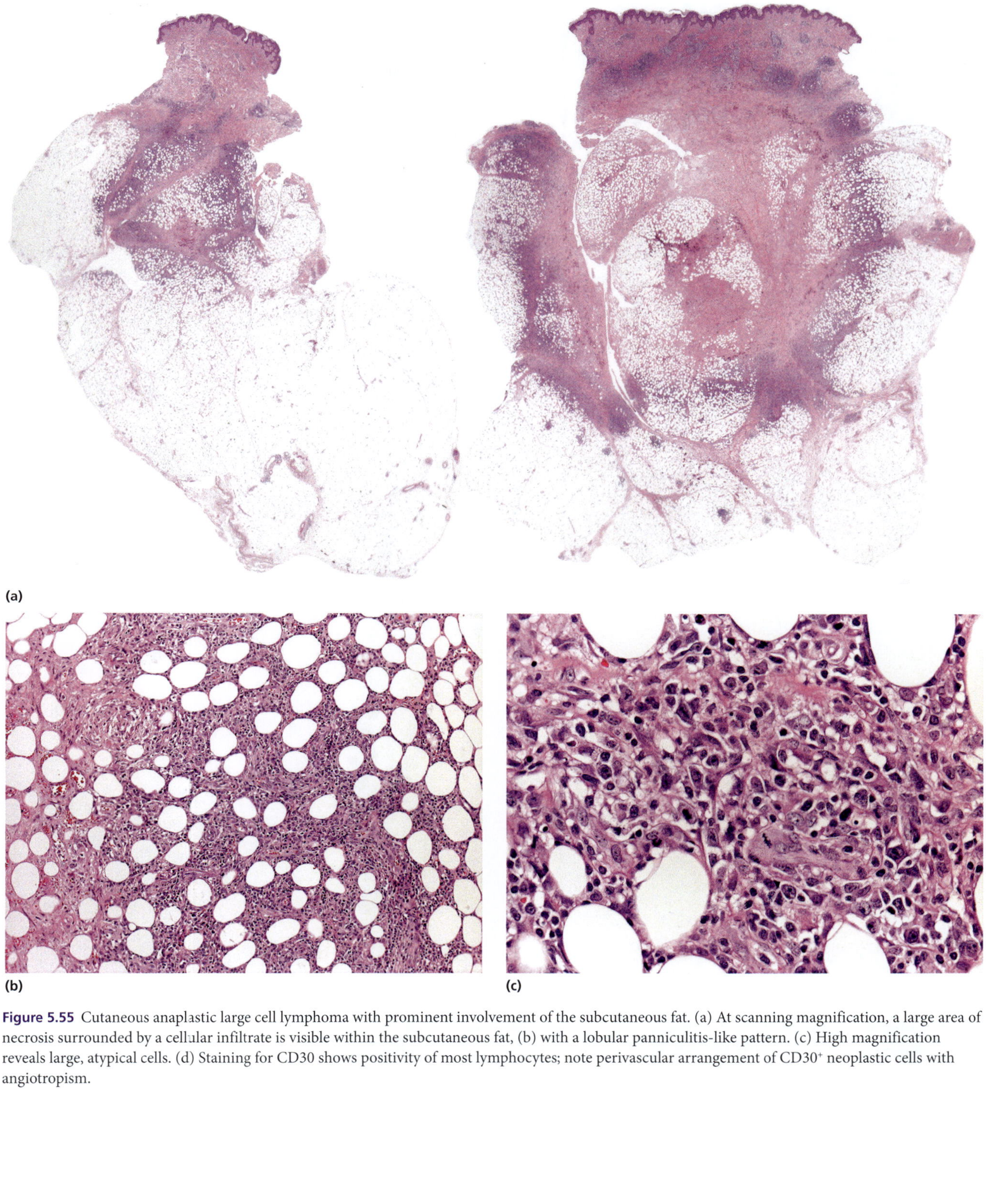


Figure 5.55 Cutaneous anaplastic large cell lymphoma with prominent involvement of the subcutaneous fat. (a) At scanning magnification, a large area of necrosis surrounded by a cellular infiltrate is visible within the subcutaneous fat, (b) with a lobular panniculitis-like pattern. (c) High magnification reveals large, atypical cells. (d) Staining for CD30 shows positivity of most lymphocytes; note perivascular arrangement of CD30+ neoplastic cells with angiotropism.

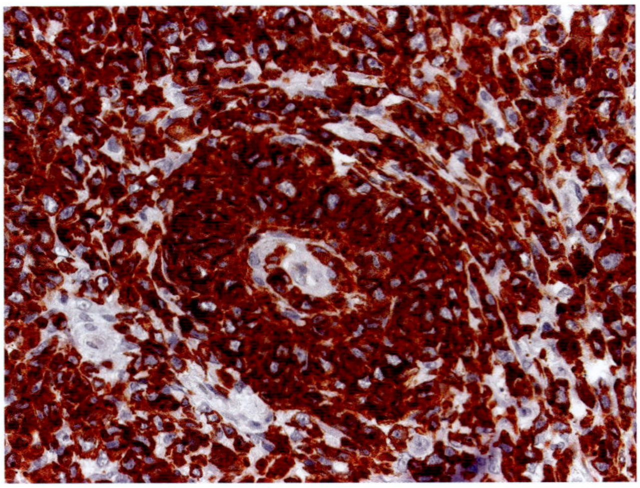

(d)

Figure 5.55 (Continued)

## Molecular genetics

Monoclonal rearrangement of the TCR genes is observed in most cases. Single-cell PCR analysis has demonstrated that most of the large CD30⁺ cells are monoclonal [167].

There is good evidence that the interchromosomal (2;5) translocation seen in the ALK⁺ nodal anaplastic large cell lymphoma is not present in most primary cutaneous lesions [109, 161]. However, as already mentioned, cutaneous pediatric cases with breaks in the *ALK* gene detected by FISH and with *NPM–ALK* transcripts detected by PCR have been described, and rare ALK-1⁺ cases showing the typical nuclear and cytoplasmic positivity are also highly suggestive of an *NPM–ALK* fusion [132].

Recurrent t(6;7)(p25.3;q32.3) translocations, involving the *DUSP22–IRF4* locus on 6p25.3, have been identified in ALK-negative anaplastic large cell lymphomas, including cutaneous cases [14, 168, 169]. The translocation is present in a distinct proportion of cases of cutaneous anaplastic large cell lymphomas

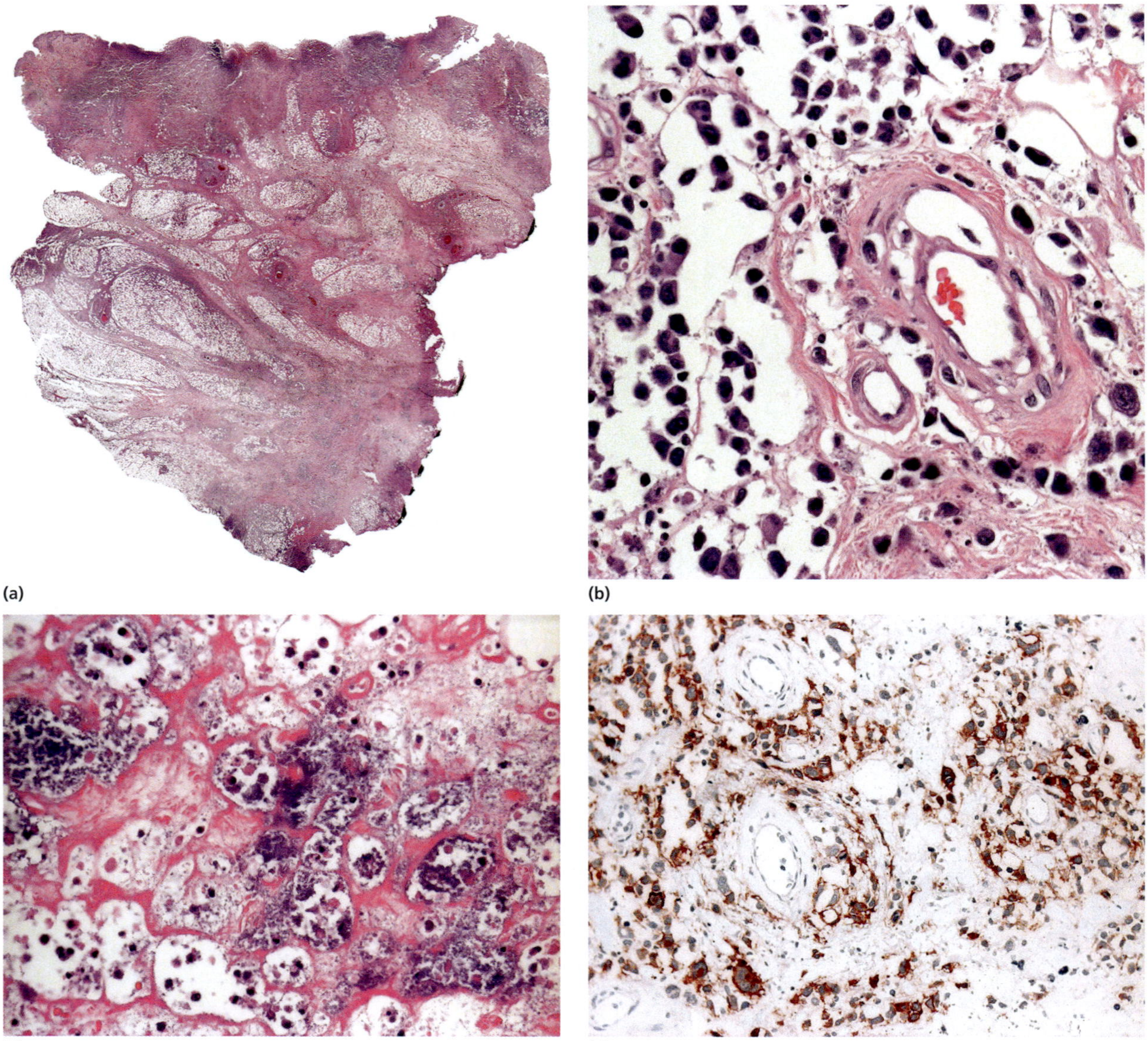

(a) (b) (c) (d)

Figure 5.56 Cutaneous anaplastic large cell lymphoma with prominent involvement of the subcutaneous fat. (a) Dense, diffuse infiltrates with focal, large areas of necrosis and with (b) several pleomorphic lymphocytes. (c) Focal necrosis and dystrophic calcifications. (d) Staining for CD30 shows positivity of large, atypical lymphocytes.

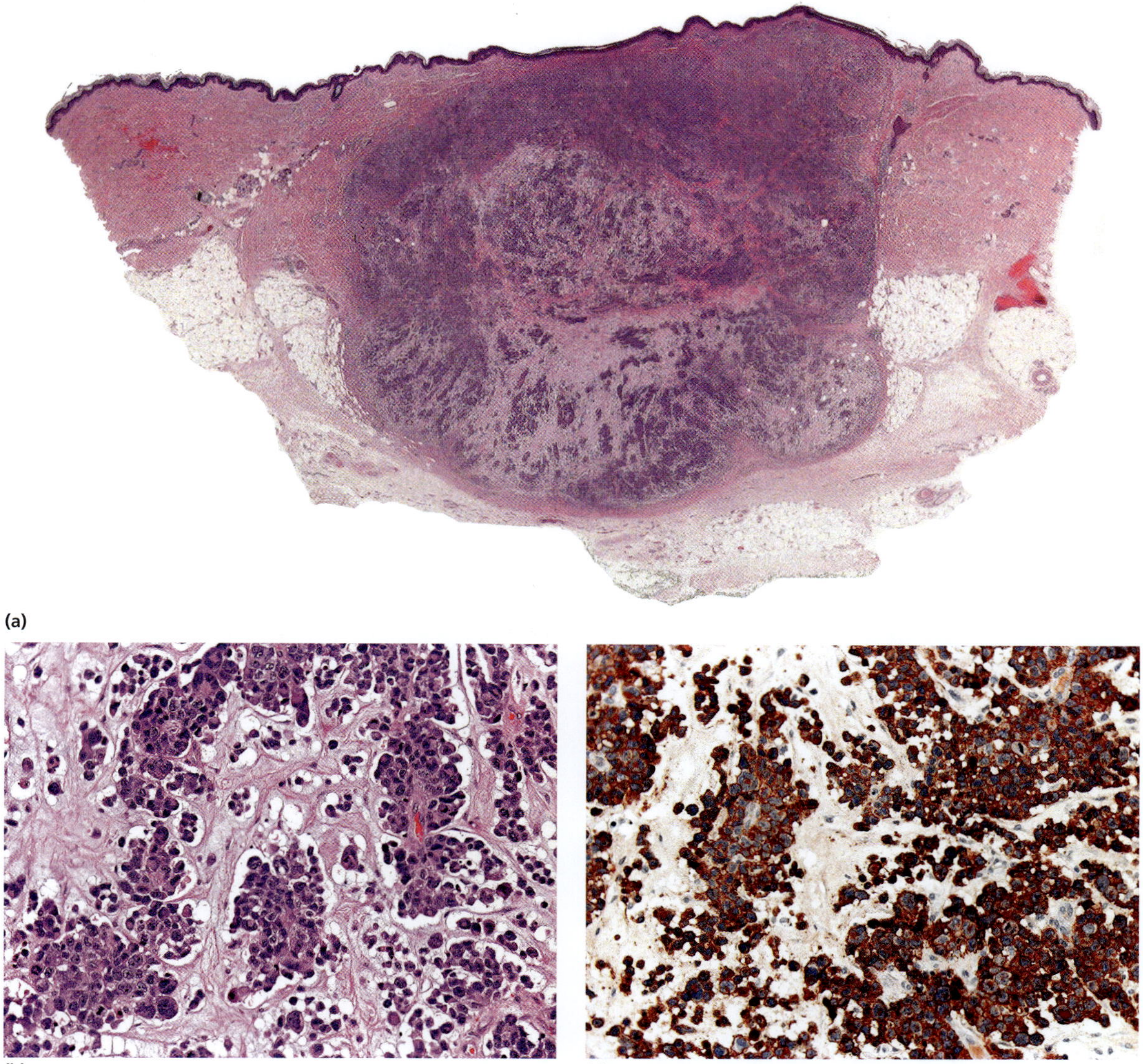

(a) (b) (c)

Figure 5.57 Cutaneous anaplastic large cell lymphoma with myxoid stroma. (a) Irregular tumor complexes within a myxoid stroma. (b) Detail of clusters of large atypical cells within a myxoid stroma. (c) Staining for CD30 strongly decorates the neoplastic cells.

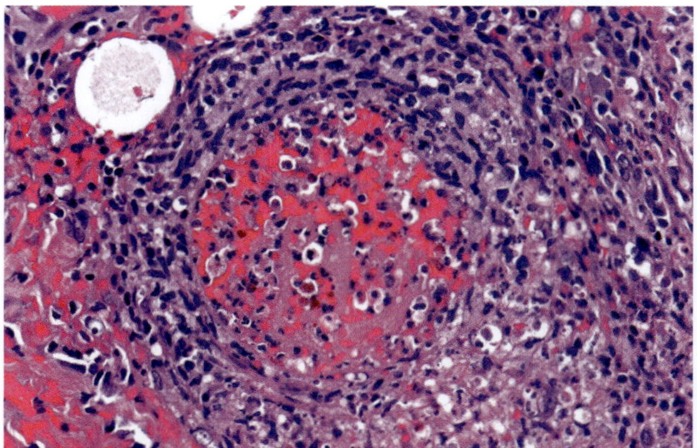

Figure 5.58 Cutaneous anaplastic large cell lymphoma. Angiocentric/angiodestructive infiltrate of large, atypical cells with intraluminal thrombotic occlusion.

and only rarely in lymphomatoid papulosis and transformed mycosis fungoides, thus representing a potential differential diagnostic criterion. Translocations involving *IRF4/MUM1* have also been detected by FISH studies [170].

Activating mutations of *JAK1* and/or *STAT* genes have been observed in approximately 20% of cases of cutaneous anaplastic large cell lymphoma [111, 171], leading to the constitutive activation of the JAK/STAT pathway. Activation of the JAK–STAT pathway is due to either pathogenic *STAT* mutations or oncogenic fusion transcripts comprising effector domains of *JAK* [111]; these last include a chimeric fusion involving *NPM1* (5q35) and *TYK2* (19p13) observed in a small minority of cases [110]. A recurrent $MSC^{E116K}$ mutation has been observed in some cases of ALK-negative anaplastic large cell lymphoma, including cutaneous ones [172]. The mutation affects the gene encoding musculin, a basic helix–loop–helix (bHLH) transcription factor likely involved in the CD30–IRF4–MYC axis and cell cycle progression in a subset of cases of ALK-negative anaplastic

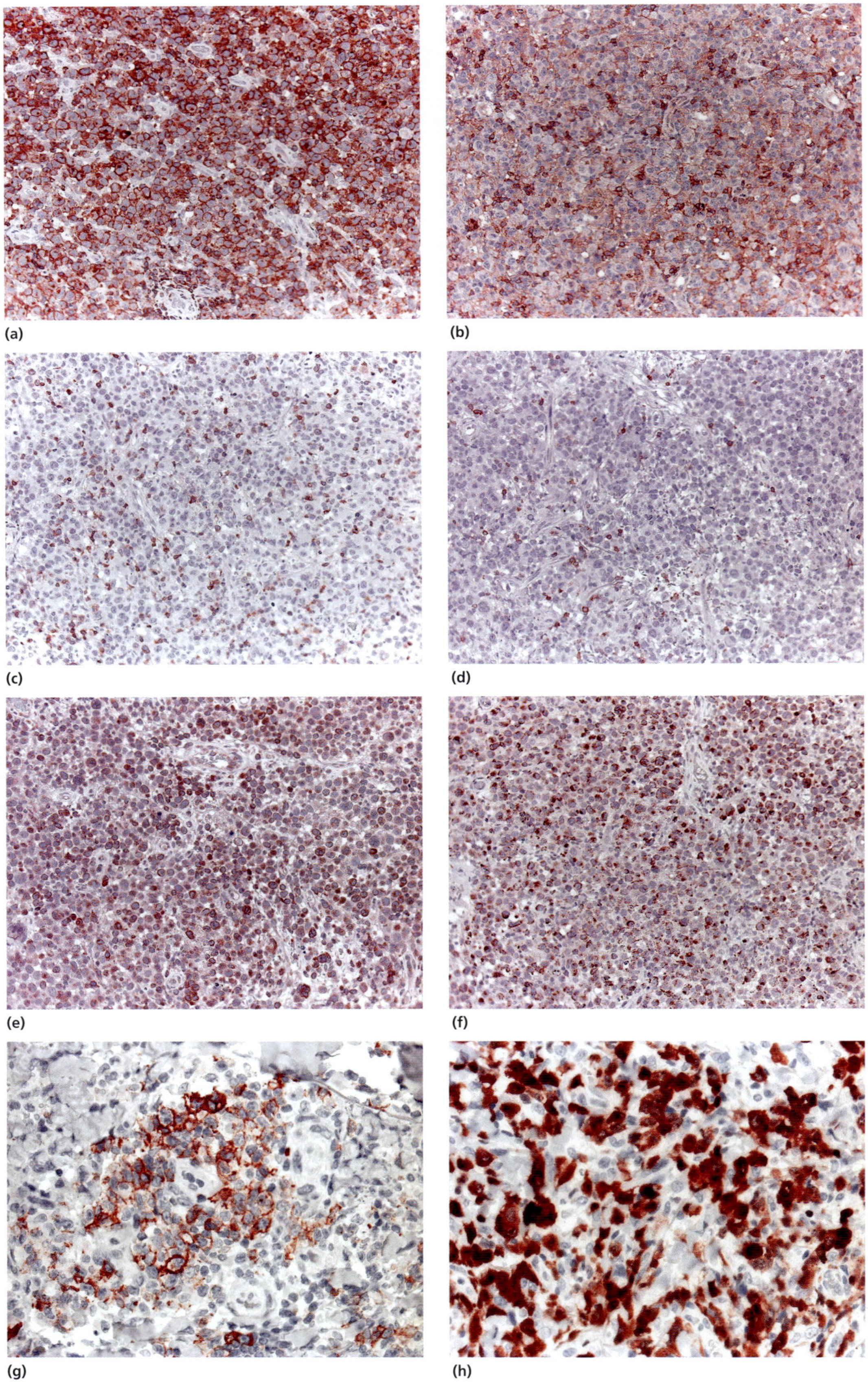


**Figure 5.59** Different phenotypic features of cutaneous anaplastic large cell lymphoma. (a) Positivity for CD2 and (b) CD4, with loss of (c) CD3 and (d) CD5 in one typical case. (e) Positivity for TCR-γ and (f) TIA-1 in a case with cytotoxic phenotype. (g) Positivity for ICOS-1 in a case with phenotype of T follicular helper cells, and (h) both nuclear and cytoplasmic positivity for ALK-1 in a case of secondary cutaneous anaplastic large cell lymphoma (this pattern of positivity is usually found in cases harboring the t(2;5) *NPM–ALK*).

large cell lymphomas. High expression of skin-homing chemokine receptor genes CCR10 and CCR8 may explain the tropism for the skin and the infrequent dissemination of cutaneous anaplastic large cell lymphoma to extracutaneous sites [173]. A recent study showed that common molecular alterations in primary cutaneous anaplastic large cell lymphoma involve the cell cycle and T-cell physiology regulation processes and the transcription and signaling via the PI-3-K, MAPK, and G-protein pathways [174].

Studies by aCGH showed that chromosomal aberrations in cutaneous anaplastic large cell lymphoma are heterogeneous and are characterized by gains on chromosomes 1p, 5, 7q, and 17q and losses on 6q, 7, 8, 13q, 16q, 17p13, 19, and 20q13 [173, 175, 176]. Particularly frequent are the gain of 7q31 and the losses on 6q16-6q21 and 13q34, each affecting almost half of the patients [177]. High expression of the skin-homing chemokine receptor genes *CCR8* and *CCR10* may explain the peculiar tropism for the skin, and aberrant expression of *IRF4/MUM1* and *PRKCQ*, involved in the apoptosis and proliferation pathways, may be responsible for the better prognosis [173].

An allelic deletion at the chromosome region 9p21, containing the tumor suppressor gene *P16*, has been shown in some cases of cutaneous anaplastic large cell lymphoma [178], but seems to be a rare event [179].

Studies on microRNA (miRNA) expression profiles demonstrated a differential expression of miR-155, miR-27b, miR-93, miR-29b, and miR-92a between tumor-stage mycosis fungoides and cutaneous anaplastic large cell lymphoma, thus being of possible help in the precise characterization of CD30+ tumors arising in patients with mycosis fungoides [180].

## Treatment

Solitary or localized lesions may be treated by surgical excision, radiotherapy, or a combination of the two [118, 119, 181]. Patients with concomitant involvement of skin and regional lymph nodes are usually offered treatment with brentuximab vedotin (anti-CD30 antibody) as first-line therapy (usually together with surgical excision) [121]. In fact, a large study showed that the response to brentuximab vedotin is good [182]; it may be used as an adjunctive treatment together with other modalities, particularly in more aggressive cases such as those with extensive limb disease. Patients presenting with extracutaneous involvement beyond the regional lymph nodes require systemic chemotherapy. The role of systemic chemotherapy in primary cutaneous lesions has been debated, but it is widely accepted that this treatment can be avoided in most patients with primary skin involvement [119, 121]. Patients with multifocal lesions may be treated by brentuximab vedotin, methotrexate, pralatrexate, retinoids, or interferon-α [119, 121], but management of these patients is not yet standardized [183]. A Dutch study suggested that patients with five or less lesions should be treated with low-dose radiotherapy (2 × 4 Gy), whereas maintenance low-dose methotrexate (20 mg weekly) is a suitable option in patients with more than five lesions [184]. Patients with extensive disease located on one limb ("extensive limb disease") may need a more aggressive therapy, as prognosis seems to be worse in this setting [139, 140]. Patients with involvement of non-regional lymph nodes and/or visceral sites are better managed with protocols for systemic anaplastic large cell lymphoma. Treatment of recurrences confined to the skin is similar to that of the primary tumors, as prognosis is not affected by cutaneous relapses.

It has been suggested that patients with primary cutaneous anaplastic large cell lymphoma with tumors extending to the fat, fascia, and/or skeletal muscles may require a more aggressive approach [121]. However, I would be very cautious if only the subcutaneous fat is involved, as this is not a rare finding in cutaneous anaplastic large cell lymphoma, and prognosis does not seem to be affected by involvement of the subcutaneous fat tissue.

Thalidomide has been used successfully in two patients presenting with multifocal cutaneous disease [185]. As Notch signaling is deregulated in cutaneous anaplastic large cell lymphoma, its targeting may represent a potential therapeutic approach [186]. In the subgroup of cutaneous anaplastic large cell lymphoma characterized by JAK–STAT activation, the use of JAK1/2/3 inhibitors may be a potential treatment strategy [187]. Finally, the rare patients with ALK+ cutaneous anaplastic large cell lymphoma could be managed with the ALK kinase inhibitors crizotinib, alectinib, or ceritinib.

## Prognosis

Although the morphologic features are those of a high-grade non-Hodgkin lymphoma, the prognosis of patients with primary cutaneous anaplastic large cell lymphoma is generally (but not always!) very favorable. The estimated 5-year survival is over 90% [1, 45, 123, 140, 188]. Older age seems to adversely affect prognosis, whereas patients with T1 disease, solitary lesions, or lesions showing spontaneous regression may have a more favorable course [119, 139]. Spontaneous regression and absence of extracutaneous spread have been associated with a better prognosis [189]. The presence of multiple lesions at presentation, early skin relapse, and nodal progression has been associated with a worse prognosis in a Spanish study [190].

As already mentioned, extensive limb disease represents an adverse prognostic factor, with a 2-year disease-specific survival of 50% as compared to 93% in conventional cutaneous anaplastic large cell lymphoma [139, 140, 191], and it has been suggested to include "lower limb disease" in T-stage subcategorization of TNM schemes [159].

Patients presenting with skin tumors and evidence of specific lesions within regional lymph nodes at staging (concomitant cutaneous and nodal anaplastic large cell lymphoma) have a prognosis similar to that of patients with disease confined to the skin [7, 192]. The prognosis of ALK+ primary cutaneous anaplastic large cell lymphoma has been reported to be similar to that of ALK-negative cases [165]; however, three of six patients (50%) in the Dutch series showed recurrence, two of which were extracutaneous (33.4%), and one patient (16.7%) died of disease progression [165]. Thus, in my opinion, ALK+ cases should be managed with greater concern than ALK-negative ones.

### Résumé

**Cutaneous anaplastic large cell lymphoma**

**Clinical**
Adults and younger patients. Solitary or regionally localized tumors, often ulcerated. Generally favorable prognosis. Patients with extensive limb disease may have a more aggressive course.

**Morphology**
Nodular or diffuse infiltrates characterized by cohesive sheets of large CD30+ cells. Cases with prominent necrosis are frequent. Variable cytomorphology: in most cases, large anaplastic cells or large pleomorphic cells; small/medium-sized cells and signet-ring cells may be observed.

**Immunohistochemistry**

| | |
|---|---|
| CD2, CD3, CD5 | +/– |
| CD30 | + (>75% of tumor cells by definition) *(essential criterion)* |
| CD4 | +/– |
| CD8 | –/+ |
| MUM-1 | + |
| CD15 | –/+ |
| EMA | –(+) |
| TIA-1, perforin, granzyme-B | +(–) |
| CD56 | –(+) |
| TCR-α/β | +(–) |
| TCR-γ/δ | –(+) |

**Genetics**
Monoclonal rearrangement of the TCR genes was detected in the majority of cases; t(6;7) involving the *DUSP22–IRF4* locus on 6p25.3.

**Treatment guidelines**
Solitary or localized lesions: surgical excision and/or radiotherapy, low-dose methotrexate.
Involvement of regional lymph nodes: brentuximab vedotin, low-dose methotrexate, pralatrexate, local radiotherapy.
Multifocal disease without extracutaneous involvement: brentuximab vedotin, low-dose methotrexate, pralatrexate.
Patients with extensive limb disease may require more aggressive options, including multiagent chemotherapy.
Non-locoregional and/or visceral involvement: multiagent chemotherapy, eventually with brentuximab vedotin.

## "Borderline" Cases

As mentioned before, lymphomatoid papulosis and cutaneous anaplastic large cell lymphoma represent two ends of a spectrum of cutaneous CD30+ lymphoproliferative disorders. In this spectrum, there are cases that do not fit clearly into one or the other entity and are classified as "borderline." Most of the cases diagnosed in the past as "regressing atypical histiocytosis" [9], as well as some "primary cutaneous Hodgkin lymphoma" [10], belong to this category.

I have seen patients presenting with solitary tumors diagnosed as cutaneous anaplastic large cell lymphoma who subsequently developed typical lesions of lymphomatoid papulosis, as well as patients with cutaneous anaplastic large cell lymphoma and small satellites in the surrounding skin, who did not develop further lesions of lymphomatoid papulosis. In these cases, at first presentation, a differentiation between regional lymphomatoid papulosis and cutaneous anaplastic large cell lymphoma is not possible on clinicopathologic grounds. It should be underlined that a precise distinction between the two entities is not always necessary for the proper management of the patients. In addition, it is important to mention that pathologists and dermatopathologists should avoid generating confusion by classifying cases without proper clinicopathologic correlation. When a precise classification is not possible on histopathologic grounds, I use the following phrasing: "cutaneous CD30+ lymphoproliferative disorder (spectrum lymphomatoid papulosis/cutaneous anaplastic large cell lymphoma) with histopathologic features more likely suggesting –" and then adding the most likely histologic diagnosis, that is, lymphomatoid papulosis or cutaneous anaplastic large cell lymphoma. In this way, clinicians know how to manage the patients, and any misunderstanding is avoided.

### Résumé

**"Borderline" lesions of cutaneous CD30+ lymphoproliferative disorders**

**Clinical**
Cases that at first presentation do not fit clearly into the categories of lymphomatoid papulosis or cutaneous anaplastic large cell lymphoma.

**Morphology**
Most cases show cohesive sheets of large CD30+ cells, thus resembling cutaneous anaplastic large cell lymphoma histopathologically.

**Immunohistochemistry**
As in lymphomatoid papulosis and cutaneous anaplastic large cell lymphoma. There are no immunohistologic stainings that allow a precise histopathologic differentiation between the two entities.

**Genetics**
As in lymphomatoid papulosis and anaplastic large cell lymphoma.

**Treatment guidelines**
Management should follow the guidelines for cutaneous anaplastic large cell lymphoma.

## Intralymphatic CD30+ Large T-Cell Lymphoma

Some cases of intralymphatic cutaneous anaplastic large cell lymphoma have been described [81, 193–201]. It may be that at least some of the CD30+ intravascular large T-cell lymphomas reported in the past belong to this group rather than to the intravascular large cell lymphomas *strictu sensu*, as precise characterization of the vessels was not provided (see also Chapter 19). In my experience and that of others [81, 194], a conventional anaplastic large cell lymphoma is invariably present in the vicinity of the intralymphatic complexes or in the regional lymph nodes, and the tumor is never primary or exclusively intralymphatic (Fig. 5.60). In fact, intralymphatic complexes of neoplastic cells are common in conventional tumors of cutaneous anaplastic large cell lymphoma (Fig. 5.61) [81, 201]. In some cases, however, the intralymphatic complexes may be observed at some distance from the main tumor, which may not be present on the sections of tissue (Fig. 5.62).

Patients present clinically with localized plaques or tumors, sometimes with small satellite lesions in the surrounding skin. Telangiectasia is not observed. Histology is characterized by variably large, irregular complexes of anaplastic cells filling dilated lymphatic vessels (Figs. 5.60b and 5.62b). Blood vessels are not involved. The histopathologic features are different from conventional intravascular lymphomas. The aggregates of neoplastic cells are large and irregular, conferring at low magnification the aspect of a multinodular dermal/subcutaneous infiltrate. Variably large

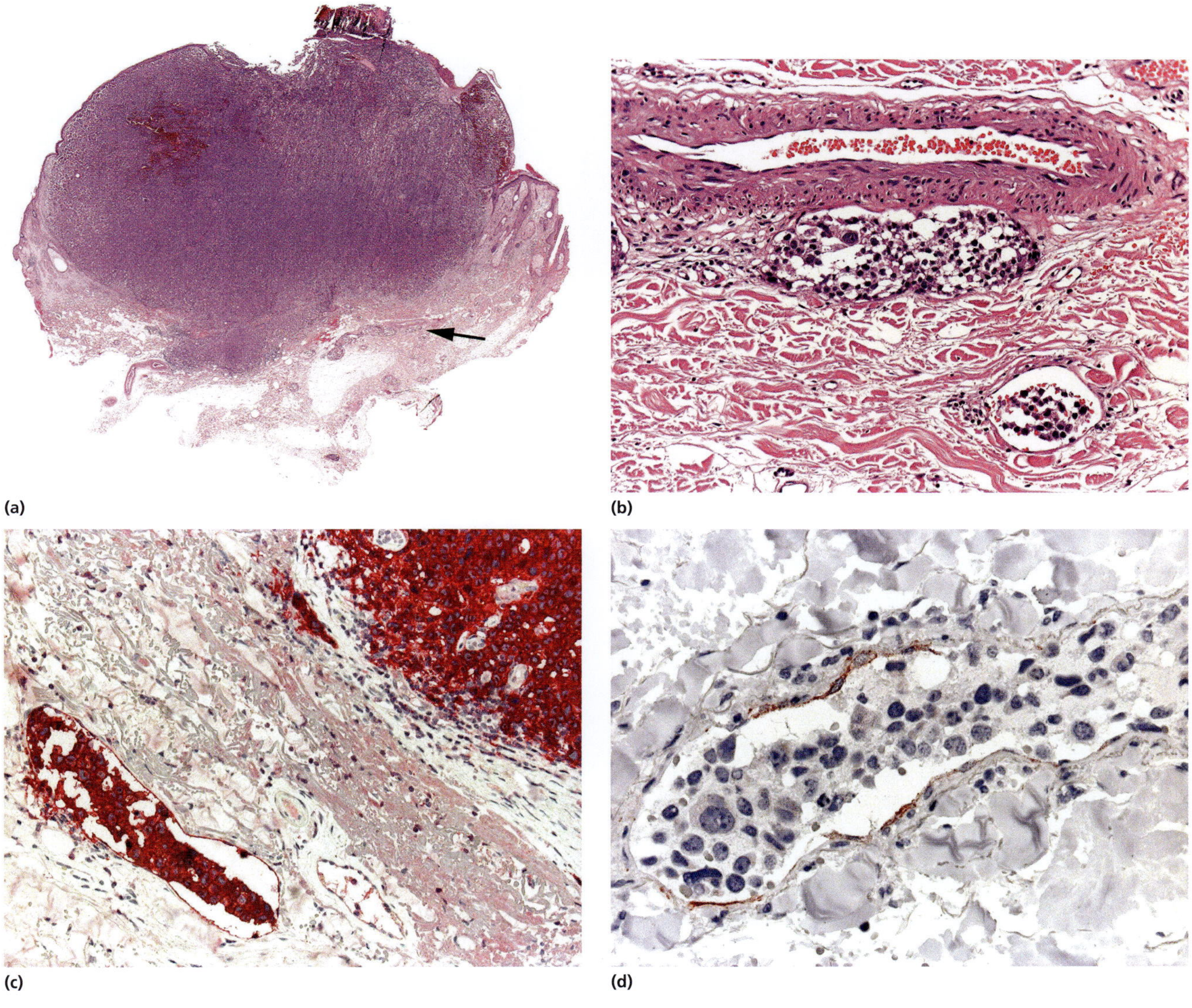

Figure 5.60 Cutaneous anaplastic large cell lymphoma with intralymphatic neoplastic cells. (a) Large, ulcerated tumor; the arrow corresponds to the site of (b) intralymphatic neoplastic cells. (c) Staining for CD30 shows intralymphatic complexes at the border of the main tumor. (d) Staining for podoplanin (D2–40) confirms the lymphatic origin of the affected vessels.

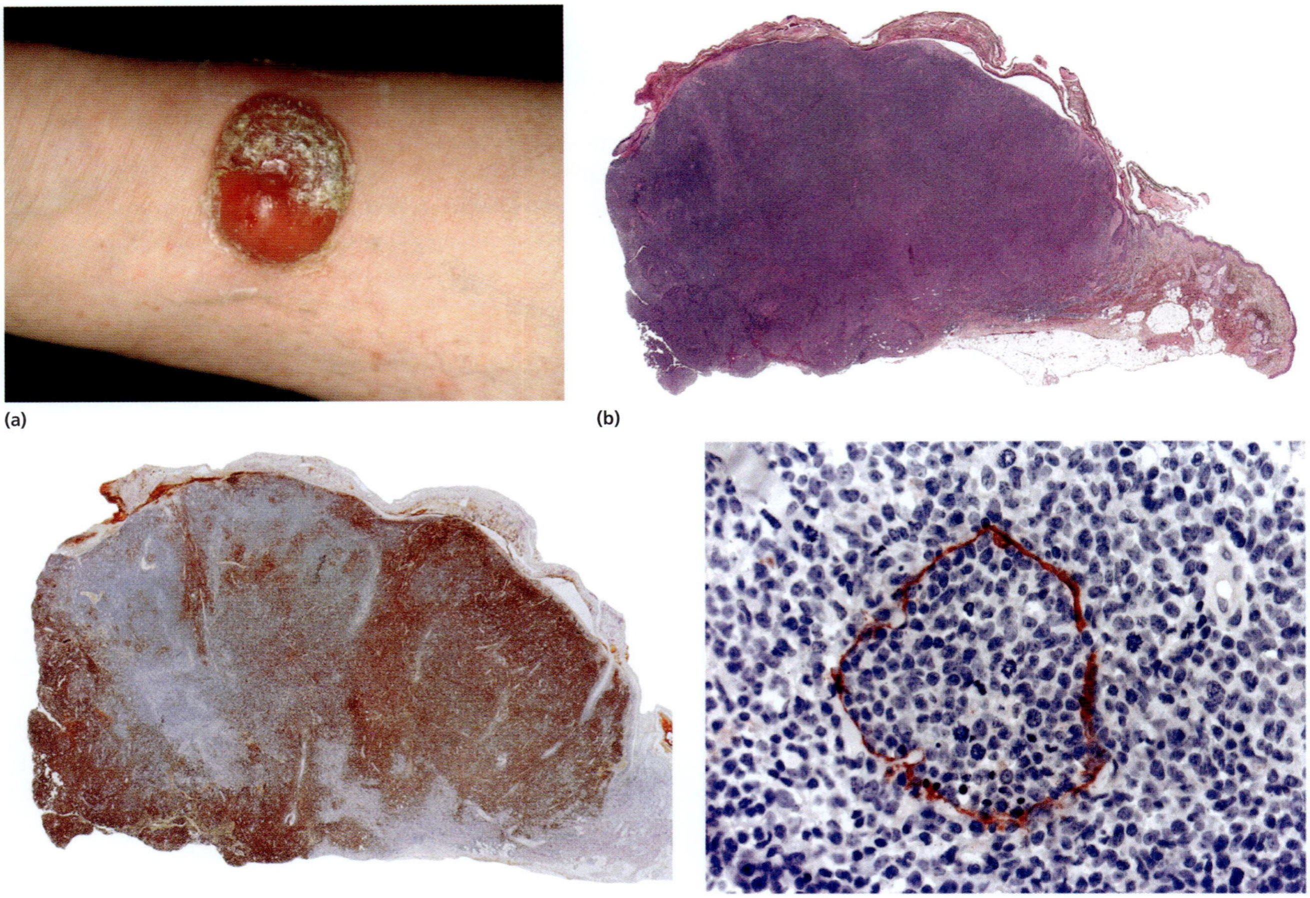


**Figure 5.61** Cutaneous anaplastic large cell lymphoma with intralymphatic neoplastic cells. (a) Large, partly regressed tumor on the left lower arm of a 70-year-old man. (*Courtesy of Dr. Irene Höpfel-Kreiner, Linz, Austria.*) (b) A biopsy revealed a dense, nodular lymphoid infiltrate occupying the entire dermis, (c) with strong positivity for CD30. (d) Staining for podoplanin (D2-40) showed several distended, enlarged lymphatic vessels filled with neoplastic cells.

extravascular aggregates of tumor cells and/or large "conventional" tumors can be found in deeper sections or in different biopsies from the same region. By contrast, in true intravascular large cell lymphoma, extravascular aggregates are never found.

Neoplastic cells in intralymphatic CD30$^+$ large T-cell lymphoma have the same phenotype as conventional cases of the disease. Cytotoxic proteins (TIA-1) are negative, and there is no association with EBV. ALK-1 is usually negative, but one positive case has been reported [194].

Intralymphatic cutaneous anaplastic large cell lymphoma should be clearly separated from genuine cases of intravascular large NK/T-cell lymphoma, since clinical, histopathologic, and prognostic features are completely different. Neoplastic cells in intralymphatic CD30$^+$ anaplastic large cell lymphoma are confined to lymphatic rather than blood vessels, a feature that allows differentiation from true intravascular large NK/T-cell lymphoma. As lymphatic vessels may be both CD31$^+$ and CD34$^+$, a staining for podoplanin (D2–40) is necessary in order to confirm the diagnosis (Figs. 5.60c and 5.61d). It must be underlined once more that rare cases of true intravascular CD30$^+$ large NK/T-cell lymphoma with an aggressive course have been documented [202, 203], clearly showing that determination of the exact nature of the involved vessels (blood versus lymphatic) is paramount for a proper classification.

Cases of intralymphatic CD30$^+$ large T-cell lymphoma should also be distinguished from a reactive condition called "benign intralymphatic proliferation of T-cell lymphoid blasts" (see Chapter 31). Benign intralymphatic proliferation of T-cell lymphoid blasts, like intralymphatic CD30$^+$ large T-cell lymphoma, is characterized by collections of large lymphocytes within lymphatic vessels. However, in benign intralymphatic proliferation of T-cell lymphoid blasts the aggregates of lymphocytes are surrounded by prominent inflammatory infiltrates comprising different cells types (i.e., small lymphocytes, histiocytes, eosinophils, neutrophils, plasma cells), and the finding is an incidental one in biopsies taken for different reasons, thus allowing an easy

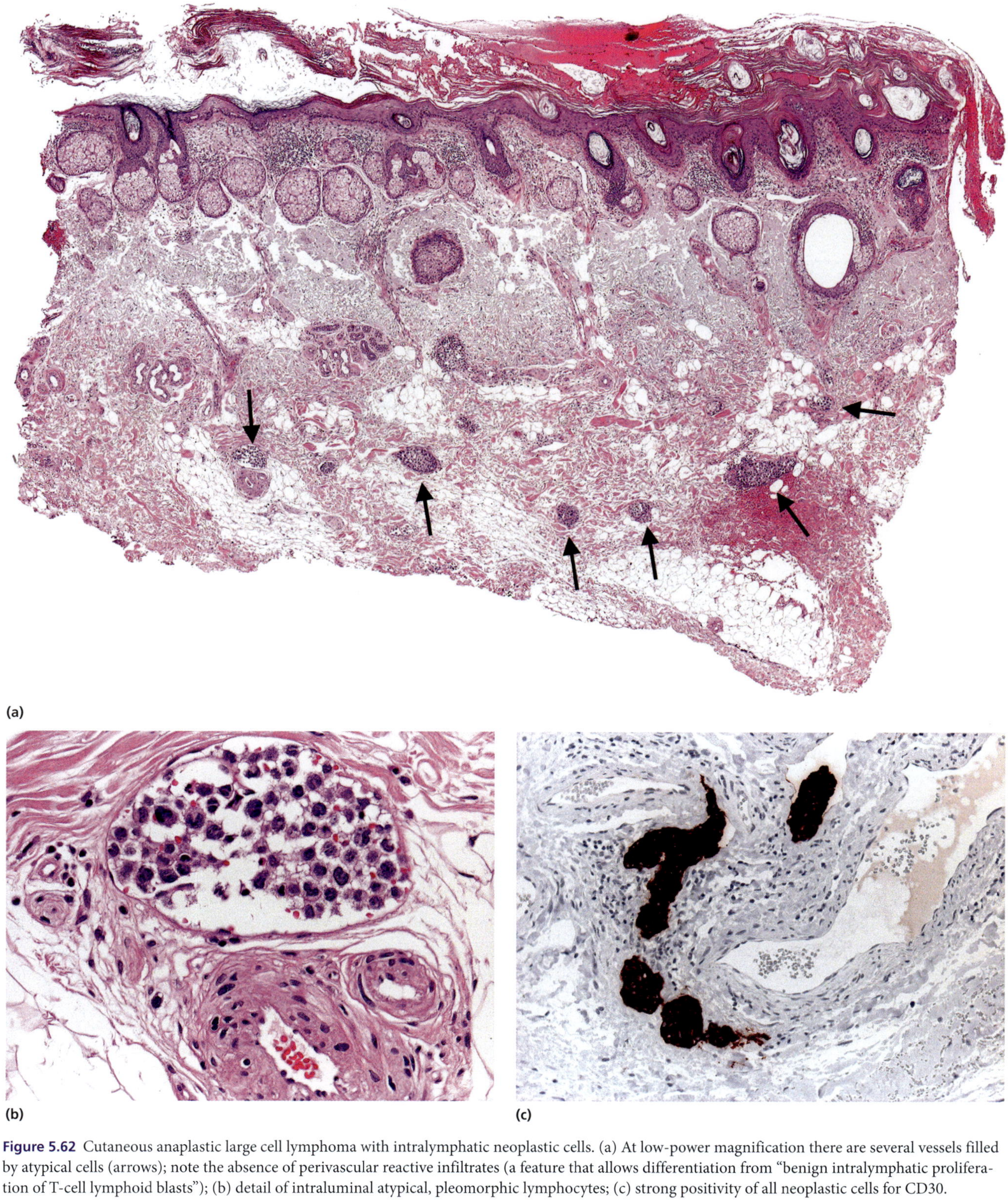

**Figure 5.62** Cutaneous anaplastic large cell lymphoma with intralymphatic neoplastic cells. (a) At low-power magnification there are several vessels filled by atypical cells (arrows); note the absence of perivascular reactive infiltrates (a feature that allows differentiation from "benign intralymphatic proliferation of T-cell lymphoid blasts"); (b) detail of intraluminal atypical, pleomorphic lymphocytes; (c) strong positivity of all neoplastic cells for CD30.

distinction of the two conditions. Analysis of the TCR gene rearrangement may be helpful in unclear cases. Differentiation of intralymphatic CD30$^+$ large T-cell lymphoma from intralymphatic lymphomatoid papulosis, too, is based on clinical presentation and histopathologic findings.

Cutaneous intralymphatic CD30$^+$ large cell lymphoma is characterized by an indolent course with good prognosis [81], similarly to conventional cases of cutaneous anaplastic large cell lymphoma. The frequent finding of intralymphatic complexes of neoplastic cells in conventional tumors of cutaneous anaplastic large cell lymphoma provides a plausible explanation for cases with "concomitant" skin and regional nodal involvement. As these "concomitant" cases have a prognosis similar to purely cutaneous ones, management of patients with intralymphatic complexes of cutaneous anaplastic large cell lymphoma should not differ from that of conventional cutaneous anaplastic large cell lymphoma, and these patients should not be treated aggressively.

**Résumé**

**Intralymphatic CD30$^+$ large T-cell lymphoma**

| | | |
|---|---|---|
| **Clinical** | Localized plaques or tumors, sometimes with small satellite lesions. It represents a variant of cutaneous anaplastic large cell lymphoma. | |
| **Morphology** | Irregular intralymphatic complexes of large, atypical lymphoid cells. | |
| **Immunohistochemistry** | CD3 | + |
| | CD4 | + |
| | ALK-1 | – (rarely +) |
| | CD20, CD79a | – |
| | TIA-1, granzyme B | – |
| | CD30 | + *(essential criterion)* |
| | EBER-1 | – |
| | D2-40 | + (involved vessels) *(essential criterion)* |
| **Genetics** | Monoclonal rearrangement of the TCR genes. | |
| **Treatment guidelines** | Localized primary cutaneous cases should be managed with non-aggressive options (similar to conventional primary cutaneous anaplastic large cell lymphomas). | |

## Implant-associated anaplastic large cell lymphoma

An increasing number of cases of CD30$^+$ anaplastic large cell lymphoma have been reported in association with breast implants [204], and "breast implant-associated anaplastic large cell lymphoma" has been introduced as an entity in the ICC *of Myeloid and Lymphoid Neoplasms* and in the 5th edition of the WHO *Classification of Haematolymphoid Tumours* [205, 206]. In some cases, the first diagnosis is made due to skin involvement by the underlying breast neoplasm [207]. Although earlier available data were considered as not being supportive of an increased risk of lymphoma in patients with breast implants [208, 209], the incidence in several European countries is increasing steadily [210], and a link with particular implants has been demonstrated [211]. In 2019, the French national agency for security of drugs and medical products (Agence nationale de sécurité du médicament et des produits de santé – ANSM) banned the use of some breast implant devices (textured breast implants but did not recommend explanting already mounted implants). In the same year, the United States Food and Drug Administration decided not to ban textured breast implants, but the largest producer of them has withdrawn them from the market, even though they are still available from other producers. Three highly textured breast implants have been banned in Australia. The European Scientific Committee on Health, Environmental and Emerging Risks (SCHEER) in 2020 reported that there is a moderate weight of evidence for a causal relationship between textured breast implants and anaplastic large cell lymphoma, particularly in relation to implants with an intermediate to high surface roughness [212]; the European Union did not ban the implants, but the largest producer of them decided to withdraw the supply of textured breast implants worldwide.

As rare cases have also been observed associated with implants located at sites different than the breast (e.g., buttocks), the entity should probably be better termed "implant-associated anaplastic large cell lymphoma" [213]. In fact, the breast does not play any role in the etiology and pathogenesis, and it is the implant material that is responsible for the chronic inflammation related to the lymphoma. In cases associated with non-breast implants, most lymphomas are fibrin-associated large B-cell lymphomas [214].

Breast implant-associated anaplastic large cell lymphoma presents as a unilateral expansion confined to the capsule of a breast implant (mostly textured breast implants), but bilateral cases may be observed. Skin manifestations are characterized by direct involvement *per continuitatem*, with swelling and possibly ulceration of the overlying skin. Regional lymph nodes may be affected. The median time of onset is approximately nine years after the implantation [204]. Histopathological and immunophenotypical features are indistinguishable from those of ALK-negative anaplastic large cell lymphoma, thus sharing similarities to primary cutaneous anaplastic large cell lymphoma [215]. Whole-exome sequencing in some cases of breast implant-associated anaplastic large cell lymphoma revealed activating *JAK1* and *STAT3* mutations as well as alterations in epigenetic modifiers and genes in the JAK/STAT pathway [216, 217], resulting in amplification of the JAK/STAT pathway in the majority of patients. In other cases, alterations of 9p24.1 resulting in PDL1 overexpression have been described [218]. Loss of 20q13.12-13.2 is highly specific for breast implant-associated anaplastic large cell lymphoma [219]. Point mutations in *TP53* and in epigenetic modifiers (*KMT2C*, *KMT2D*, *CHD2*, *CREBBP*, and *DNMT3A*) have also been described in breast implant-associated anaplastic large cell lymphoma [217].

Breast implant-associated anaplastic large cell lymphoma has an indolent behavior with excellent overall survival, although local growth may cause spread through the capsule into the breast parenchyma or soft tissue and/or to the regional lymph nodes [204, 220]. In most cases, surgical removal of the implant with complete capsulectomy is curative [220]. Chemotherapy is not needed in cases limited to the breast.

## Résumé

| Implant-associated anaplastic large cell lymphoma | |
|---|---|
| **Clinical** | Mostly reported in the breast, rarely at other sites (buttocks). Unilateral expansion confined to the capsule of a breast implant (almost exclusively textured breast implants); if present, skin involvement is characterized by direct extension with swelling and possible ulceration. |
| **Morphology** | Same as for primary cutaneous anaplastic large cell lymphoma. |
| **Immunohistochemistry** | As in cutaneous anaplastic large cell lymphoma. ALK is negative. |
| **Genetics** | Monoclonal rearrangement of the TCR genes. Recurrent activating *JAK1* and *STAT3* mutations; alterations of 9p24.1 resulting in PDL1 overexpression. |
| **Treatment guidelines** | Surgical removal of the implant with complete capsulectomy. |

## References


1. Willemze R, Cerroni L, Kempf W, *et al.* The 2018 update of the WHO-EORTC classification for primary cutaneous lymphomas. *Blood* 2019;**133**:1703–1714.
2. Kempf W, Mitteldorf C, Cerroni L, *et al.* Classifications of cutaneous lymphomas and lymphoproliferative disorders: an update from the EORTC cutaneous lymphoma histopathology group. *J Eur Acad Dermatol Venereol* 2024;**38**:1491–1503.
3. Feldman AL, Cerroni L. Primary cutaneous CD30-positive T-cell lymphoproliferative disorders. In: Arber DA, Borowitz MJ, Cook JR, *et al.*, eds. *The International Consensus Classification of myeloid and lymphoid neoplasms.* Philadelphia (US): Wolters Kluwer, 2025: 684–694.
4. Kempf W, Paulli M, Gujral S, *et al.* Primary cutaneous CD30-positive T-cell lymphoproliferative disorder: lymphomatoid papulosis. In: *WHO Classification of Tumours Editorial Board. Haematolymphoid Tumours.* 5th edition. Lyon (France): IARC, 2024: 694–697.
5. Jansen PM, Paulli M, Gujral S, *et al.* Primary cutaneous CD30-positive T-cell lymphoproliferative disorder: primary cutaneous anaplastic large cell lymphoma. In: *WHO Classification of Tumours Editorial Board. Haematolymphoid Tumours.* 5th edition. Lyon (France): IARC, 2024: 698–699.
6. Beljaards RC, Kaudewitz P, Berti E, *et al.* Primary cutaneous CD30-positive large cell lymphoma: definition of a new type of cutaneous lymphoma with a favorable prognosis. *Cancer* 1993;**71**:2097–2104.
7. Bekkenk MW, Geelen FAMJ, van Voorst-Vader PC, *et al.* Primary and secondary cutaneous CD30 lymphoproliferative disorders: a report from the Dutch Cutaneous Lymphoma Group on the long-term follow-up data of 219 patients and guidelines for diagnosis and treatment. *Blood* 2000;**95**:3653–3661.
8. Paulli M, Berti E, Rosso R, *et al.* CD30/Ki-1-positive lymphoproliferative disorders of the skin: clinicopathologic correlation and statistical analysis of 86 cases. A multicentric study from the European Organization for Research and Treatment of Cancer Cutaneous Lymphoma project group. *J Clin Oncol* 1995;**13**:1343–1354.
9. Flynn KJ, Dehner LP, Gajl-Peczalska KJ, *et al.* Regressing atypical histiocytosis: a cutaneous proliferation of atypical neoplastic histiocytes with unexpectedly indolent biologic behaviour. *Cancer* 1982;**49**:959–970.
10. Sioutos N, Kerl H, Murphy SB, Kadin ME. Primary cutaneous Hodgkin's disease. Unique clinical, morphologic, and immunophenotypic findings. *Am J Dermatopathol* 1994;**16**:2–8.
11. Sciallis AP, Law ME, Inwards DJ, *et al.* Mucosal CD30-positive T-cell lymphoproliferations of the head and neck show a clinicopathologic spectrum similar to cutaneous CD30-positive T-cell lymphoproliferative disorders. *Mod Pathol* 2012;**25**:983–992.

12. Mori M, Manuelli C, Pimpinelli N, *et al.* CD30–CD30 ligand interaction in primary cutaneous CD30 T-cell lymphomas: a clue to the pathophysiology of clinical regression. *Blood* 1999;**94**:3077–3083.
13. Greisser J, Doebbeling U, Roos M, *et al.* Apoptosis in CD30 positive lymphoproliferative disorders of the skin. *Exp Dermatol* 2005;**14**:380–385.
14. Pham-Ledard A, Prochazkova-Carlotti M, Laharanne E, *et al.* IRF4 gene rearrangements define a subgroup of CD30-positive cutaneous T-cell lymphoma: a study of 54 cases. *J Invest Dermatol* 2010;**130**:816–825.
15. Karai LJ, Kadin ME, Hsi ED, *et al.* Chromosomal rearrangements of 6p25.3 define a new subtype of lymphomatoid papulosis. *Am J Surg Pathol* 2013;**37**:1173–1181.
16. Wada DA, Law ME, Hsi ED, *et al.* Specificity of IRF4 translocations for primary cutaneous anaplastic large cell lymphoma: a multicenter study of 204 skin biopsies. *Mod Pathol* 2011;**24**:596–605.
17. Knol AC, Ehst BD, Dompmartin A, *et al.* Toll-like receptor 2, 4, 7 and 9 expression in primary cutaneous CD30$^+$ T-cell lymphoma. *Br J Dermatol* 2009;**161**:1414–1416.
18. Gjerdrum LM, Woetmann A, Odum N, *et al.* FOXP3 positive regulatory T-cells in cutaneous and systemic CD30 positive T-cell lymphoproliferations. *Eur J Haematol* 2008;**80**:483–489.
19. Mathas S, Kreher S, Meaburn KJ, *et al.* Gene deregulation and spatial genome reorganization near breakpoints prior to formation of translocations in anaplastic large cell lymphoma. *Proc Natl Acad Sci USA* 2009;**106**:5831–5836.
20. MacAulay WL. Lymphomatoid papulosis: a continuing self-healing eruption, clinically benign-histologically malignant. *Arch Dermatol* 1968;**97**:23–30.
21. Kadin ME, Hamilton RG, Vonderheid EC. Evidence linking atopy and staphylococcal superantigens to the pathogenesis of lymphomatoid papulosis, a recurrent CD30$^+$ cutaneous lymphoproliferative disorder. *PLoS One* 2020;**15**:e0228751.
22. Thomsen K, Lange WG. Lymphomatoid papulosis: a follow-up study of 30 patients. *J Am Acad Dermatol* 1987;**17**:632–636.
23. Weinman VF, Ackerman AB. Lymphomatoid papulosis: a critical review and new findings. *Am J Dermatopathol* 1981;**3**:129–162.
24. Kaudewitz P, Stein H, Plewig G, *et al.* Hodgkin's disease followed by lymphomatoid papulosis: immunophenotypic evidence for a close relationship between lymphomatoid papulosis and Hodgkin's disease. *J Am Acad Dermatol* 1990;**22**:999–1006.
25. Basarab T, Fraser-Andrews EA, Orchard G, *et al.* Lymphomatoid papulosis in association with mycosis fungoides: a study of 15 cases. *Br J Dermatol* 1998;**139**:630–638.
26. Cordel N, Tressieres B, D'Incan M, *et al.* Frequency and risk factors for associated lymphomas in patients with lymphomatoid papulosis. *Oncologist* 2016;**21**:1–8.
27. Wieser I, Oh CW, Talpur R, Duvic M. Lymphomatoid papulosis: treatment response and associated lymphomas in a study of 180 patients. *J Am Acad Dermatol* 2016;**74**:59–67.
28. Kunishige JH, McDonald H, Alvarez G, *et al.* Lymphomatoid papulosis and associated lymphomas: a retrospective case series of 84 patients. *Clin Exp Dermatol* 2009;**34**:576–581.
29. Nijsten T, Curiel-Lewandrowski C, Kadin ME. Lymphomatoid papulosis in children. A retrospective cohort study of 35 cases. *Arch Dermatol* 2004;**140**:306–312.
30. Blanchard M, Morren MA, Busschots AM, *et al.* Paediatric-onset lymphomatoid papulosis: results of a multicentre retrospective cohort study on behalf of the EORTC Cutaneous Lymphoma Tumours Group (CLTG). *Br J Dermatol* 2024;**191**:233–242.
31. Melchers RC, Willemze R, Bekkenk MW, *et al.* Frequency and prognosis of associated malignancies in 504 patients with lymphomatoid papulosis. *J Eur Acad Dermatol Venereol* 2020;**34**:260–266.
32. Chott A, Vonderheid EC, Olbricht S, *et al.* The same dominant T cell clone is present in multiple regressing skin lesions and associated T cell lymphomas of patients with lymphomatoid papulosis. *J Invest Dermatol* 1996;**106**:696–700.
33. Davis TH, Morton CC, Miller-Cassman R, *et al.* Hodgkin's disease, lymphomatoid papulosis, and cutaneous T-cell lymphoma derived from a common T-cell clone. *N Engl J Med* 1992;**326**:1115–1122.
34. Zackheim HS, Jones C, LeBoit PE, *et al.* Lymphomatoid papulosis associated with mycosis fungoides: a study of 21 patients including analyses for clonality. *J Am Acad Dermatol* 2003;**49**:620–623.
35. de la Garza Bravo MM, Patel KP, Loghavi S, *et al.* Shared clonality in distinctive lesions of lymphomatoid papulosis and mycosis fungoides occurring in the same patients suggests a common origin. *Hum Pathol* 2015;**46**:558–569.
36. Xerri L, Adélaïde J, Avenin M, *et al.* Common origin of sequential cutaneous CD30$^+$ lymphoproliferations with nodal involvement evidenced by genome-wide clonal evolution. *Histopathology* 2019;**74**:654–662.
37. Zackheim HS, LeBoit PE, Gordon BI, Glassberg AB. Lymphomatoid papulosis followed by Hodgkin's lymphoma: differential response to therapy. *Arch Dermatol* 1993;**129**:86–91.
38. McCurdy O, McCormack C, Ritchie D, Prince HM. Exacerbation of lymphomatoid papulosis during rituximab therapy. *Australas J Dermatol* 2014;**55**:e1–e3.
39. Wolf P, Cerroni L, Smolle J, Kerl H. PUVA-induced lymphomatoid papulosis in a patient with mycosis fungoides. *J Am Acad Dermatol* 1991;**25**:422–426.
40. Wang HH, Myers T, Lach LJ, *et al.* Increased risk of lymphoid and non-lymphoid malignancies in patients with lymphomatoid papulosis. *Cancer* 1999;**86**:1240–1245.
41. Hibler J, Salavaggione AL, Martin A, Gru AA. A unique case of concurrent chronic lymphocytic leukemia/small lymphocytic lymphoma and lymphomatoid papulosis in the same biopsy. *J Cutan Pathol* 2015;**42**:276–284.
42. Adamski H, Ingen-Housz-Oro S, Machet L, *et al.* Lymphomatoid papulosis associated with chronic lymphocytic leukaemia/small lymphocytic lymphoma: three cases. *Br J Dermatol* 2018;**178**:e5–e6.
43. Mallet V, Bruneau J, Zuber J, *et al.* Hepatitis E virus-induced primary cutaneous CD30(+) T cell lymphoproliferative disorder. *J Hepatol* 2017;**67**:1334–1339.
44. Humme D, Lukowsky A, Steinhoff M, *et al.* Dominance of nonmalignant T-cell clones and distortion of the TCR repertoire in the peripheral blood of patients with cutaneous CD30$^+$ lymphoproliferative disorders. *J Invest Dermatol* 2009;**129**:89–98.
45. Fink-Puches R, Zenahlik P, Bäck B, *et al.* Primary cutaneous lymphomas: applicability of current classification schemes (European Organization for Research and Treatment of Cancer, World Health Organization) based on clinicopathologic features observed in a large group of patients. *Blood* 2002;**99**:800–805.
46. el-Azhary RA, Gibson LE, Kurtin PJ, *et al.* Lymphomatoid papulosis: a clinical and histopathologic review of 53 cases with leukocyte immunophenotyping, DNA flow cytometry, and T-cell receptor gene rearrangement studies. *J Am Acad Dermatol* 1994;**30**:210–218.

47. Sanchez NP, Pittelkow MR, Muller SA, *et al.* The clinicopathologic spectrum of lymphomatoid papulosis: study of 31 cases. *J Am Acad Dermatol* 1983;**8**:81–94.
48. van Neer FJMA, Toonstra J, van Voorst Vader PC, *et al.* Lymphomatoid papulosis in children: a study of 10 children registered by the Dutch Cutaneous Lymphoma Working Group. *Br J Dermatol* 2001;**144**:351–354.
49. Willemze R, Meijer CJLM, van Vloten WA, Scheffer E. The clinical and histological spectrum of lymphomatoid papulosis. *Br J Dermatol* 1982;**107**:131–144.
50. Boccara O, Blanche S, de Prost Y, *et al.* Cutaneous hematologic disorders in children. *Pediatr Blood Cancer* 2012;**58**:226–232.
51. Miquel J, Fraitag S, Hamel-Teillac D, *et al.* Lymphomatoid papulosis in children: a series of 25 cases. *Br J Dermatol* 2014;**171**:1138–1146.
52. Garcias-Ladaria J, Fink-Puches R, Wolf I, Cerroni L. Acral lymphomatoid papulosis with hemorrhagic features mimicking a vasculitis. *Pathol Case Rev* 2014;**19**:191–194.
53. Ba W, Yin G, Yang J, *et al.* Lymphomatoid papulosis type E with a CD56+ immunophenotype presenting with purpura-like lesions. *J Cutan Pathol* 2019;**46**:542–545.
54. Tabata N, Aiba S, Ichinohazama R, *et al.* Hydroa vacciniforme-like lymphomatoid papulosis in a Japanese child: a new subset. *J Am Acad Dermatol* 1995;**32**:378–381.
55. Yamamoto O, Tajiri M, Asahi M. Lymphomatoid papulosis associated with pregnancy. *Clin Exp Dermatol* 1997;**22**:141–143.
56. Granel B, Serratrice J, Swiader L, *et al.* Lymphomatoid papulosis associated with both severe hypereosinophilic syndrome and CD30 positive large T-cell lymphoma: a case report. *Cancer* 2000;**89**: 2138–2143.
57. Kim SK, Kim YC. Lymphomatoid papulosis after allogenic stem cell transplantation. *Eur J Dermatol* 2009;**19**:520–521.
58. Scarisbrick JJ, Evans AV, Woolford AJ, *et al.* Regional lymphomatoid papulosis: a report of four cases. *Br J Dermatol* 1999;**141**: 1125–1128.
59. Heald P, Subtil A, Breneman D, Wilson LD. Persistent agmination of lymphomatoid papulosis: an equivalent of limited plaque mycosis fungoides type of cutaneous T-cell lymphoma. *J Am Acad Dermatol* 2007;**57**:1005–1011.
60. Thomas GJ, Conejo-Mir JS, Ruiz AP, *et al.* Lymphomatoid papulosis in childhood with exclusive acral involvement. *Pediatr Dermatol* 1998;**15**:146–147.
61. Torrelo A, Colmenero I, Hernandez A, *et al.* Persistent agmination of lymphomatoid papulosis. *Ped Dermatol* 2009;**26**:762–764.
62. Buder K, Wendel AM, Cerroni L, *et al.* A case of lymphomatoid papulosis limited to Becker's melanosis. *Dermatology* 2013;**226**: 124–127.
63. De Souza A, Carter JB, Harris NL, *et al.* Contribution of longitudinal follow up and clinical pathological correlation in the diagnosis CD30-positive skin infiltrates. *J Cutan Pathol* 2015;**42**:452–458.
64. Saggini A, Gulia A, Argenyi Z, *et al.* A variant of lymphomatoid papulosis simulating primary cutaneous aggressive epidermotropic CD8+ cytotoxic T-cell lymphoma. Description of 9 cases. *Am J Surg Pathol* 2010;**34**:1168–1175.
65. Bertolotti A, Pham-Ledard AL, Vergier B, *et al.* Lymphomatoid papulosis type D: an aggressive histology for an indolent disease. *Br J Dermatol* 2013;**169**:1157–1159.
66. Cardoso J, Duhra P, Thway Y, *et al.* Lymphomatoid papulosis type D: a newly described variant easily confused with cutaneous aggressive CD8-positive cytotoxic T-cell lymphoma. *Am J Dermatopathol* 2012;**34**:762–765.
67. Marschalkó M, Gyöngyösi N, Noll J, *et al.* Histopathological aspects and differential diagnosis of CD8 positive lymphomatoid papulosis. *J Cutan Pathol* 2016;**43**:963–973.
68. McQuitty E, Curry JL, Tetzlaff MT, *et al.* The differential diagnosis of CD8-positive ("type D") lymphomatoid papulosis. *J Cutan Pathol* 2014;**41**:88–100.
69. Bergqvist C, Beylot-Barry M, Ram-Wolff C, *et al.* Lymphomatoid papulosis types D and E: a multicentre series of the French Cutaneous Lymphomas Study Group. *Clin Exp Dermatol* 2021;**46**:1441–1451.
70. Kempf W, Kazakov DV, Schärer L, *et al.* Angioinvasive lymphomatoid papulosis: a new variant simulating aggressive lymphomas. *Am J Surg Pathol* 2013;**37**:1–13.
71. Pierard GE, Ackerman AB, Lapiere CM. Follicular lymphomatoid papulosis. *Am J Dermatopathol* 1980;**2**:173–180.
72. Requena L, Sanchez M, Coca S, Sanchez Yus E. Follicular lymphomatoid papulosis. *Am J Dermatopathol* 1990;**12**:67–75.
73. Kato N, Matsue K. Follicular lymphomatoid papulosis. *Am J Dermatopathol* 1997;**19**:189–196.
74. Kempf W, Kazakov DV, Baumgartner HP, *et al.* Follicular lymphomatoid papulosis revisited: a study of 11 cases, with new histopathologic findings. *J Am Acad Dermatol* 2013;**68**:809–816.
75. Dore E, Swick BL, Link BK, *et al.* Follicular lymphomatoid papulosis with follicular mucinosis: a clinicopathologic study of 3 cases with literature review and conceptual reappraisal. *J Cutan Pathol* 2017;**44**:360–366.
76. Ross NA, Truong H, Keller MS, *et al.* Follicular lymphomatoid papulosis: an eosinophilic-rich follicular subtype masquerading as folliculitis clinically and histologically. *Am J Dermatopathol* 2016;**38**:e1–e10.
77. Ba W, Yang Y, Zhang Z, *et al.* Lymphomatoid papulosis with folliculotropism, eccrinotropism and neurotropism. *J Cutan Pathol* 2018;**45**:530–534.
78. Atkins KA, Dahlem MM, Kohler S. A case of lymphomatoid papulosis with prominent myxoid change resembling a mesenchymal neoplasm. *Am J Dermatopathol* 2003;**25**:62–65.
79. Baschinsky D, Magro CM, Kovatich A, Crowson AN. Eccrinotropic and neurotropic lymphomatoid papulosis (LyP): a novel variant. *Mod Pathol* 2001;**14**:65.
80. Pan PY, Liao JB, Hsieh SM, Tseng HW. Vesicular lymphomatoid papulosis with DUSP22-IRF4 rearrangement on chromosome 6p25.3: a case report. *Am J Dermatopathol* 2023;**45**:391–396.
81. Ferrara G, Ena L, Cota C, Cerroni L. Intralymphatic spread is a common finding in cutaneous CD30+ lymphoproliferative disorders. *Am J Surg Pathol* 2015;**39**:1511–1517.
82. Samols MA, Su A, Ra S, *et al.* Intralymphatic cutaneous anaplastic large cell lymphoma/lymphomatoid papulosis. Expanding the spectrum of CD30-positive lymphoproliferative disorders. *Am J Surg Pathol* 2014;**38**:1203–1211.
83. Scarisbrick JJ, Calonje E, Orchard G, *et al.* Pseudocarcinomatous change in lymphomatoid papulosis and primary cutaneous CD30 lymphoma: a clinicopathologic and immunohistochemical study of 6 patients. *J Am Acad Dermatol* 2001;**44**:239–247.
84. Zayour M, Gilmore E, Heald P, *et al.* A distinct entity in the spectrum of the CD30+ cutaneous lymphoproliferative diseases: oligolesional nodules with pseudoepitheliomatous hyperplasia followed by spontaneous resolution. *Am J Dermatopathol* 2009;**31**:37–43.

85. Xiong J, Ma Y, Chen H, *et al.* Lymphomatoid papulosis with pseudocarcinomatous hyperplasia in a 7-year-old girl: a case report. *J Cutan Pathol* 2016;**43**:430–433.
86. Guitart J, Gordon K. Keratoacanthomas and lymphomatoid papulosis. *Am J Dermatopathol* 1998;**20**:430–432.
87. Martires KJ, Cohen BE, Cassarino DS. CD30+ lymphoproliferative disorder with spindle-cell morphology. *J Cutan Pathol* 2016;**43**:1041–1044.
88. Kluk J, Child F, Robson A. Lymphomatoid papulosis with 6p25.3 rearrangement: a further case of the newly described variant. *Br J Dermatol* 2014;**171**:1590–1592.
89. Rodrıguez-Pinilla SM, Ortiz-Romero PL, Monsalvez V, *et al.* TCR-gamma expression in primary cutaneous T-cell lymphomas. *Am J Surg Pathol* 2013;**37**:375–384.
90. King RL, Yan AC, Sekiguchi DR, Choi JK. Atypical cutaneous gamma/delta T cell proliferation with morphologic features of lymphoma but with clinical features and course of PLEVA or lymphomatoid papulosis. *J Cutan Pathol* 2015;**42**:1012–1017.
91. Martinez-Escala ME, Sidiropoulos M, Deonizio J, *et al.* Gamma/delta T-cell-rich variants of pityriasis lichenoides and lymphomatoid papulosis: benign cutaneous disorders to be distinguished from aggressive cutaneous gamma/delta T-cell lymphomas. *Br J Dermatol* 2015;**172**:372–379.
92. Kadin ME, Nasu K, Sako D, *et al.* Lymphomatoid papulosis: a cutaneous proliferation of activated helper T cells expressing Hodgkin's disease-associated antigens. *Am J Pathol* 1985;**119**: 315–325.
93. Kummer JA, Vermeer MH, Dukers D, *et al.* Most primary cutaneous CD30-positive lymphoproliferative disorders have a CD4-positive cytotoxic T-cell phenotype. *J Invest Dermatol* 1997;**109**:636–640.
94. Harvell JD, Vaseghi M, Natkunam Y, *et al.* Large atypical cells of lymphomatoid papulosis are CD56-negative: a study of 18 cases. *J Cutan Pathol* 2002;**29**:88–92.
95. Flann S, Orchard GE, Wain EM, Russell-Jones R. Three cases of lymphomatoid papulosis with a CD56+ immunophenotype. *J Am Acad Dermatol* 2006;**55**:903–906.
96. Natkunam Y, Warnke RA, Haghighi B, *et al.* Co-expression of CD56 and CD30 in lymphomas with primary presentation in the skin: clinicopathologic, immunohistochemical and molecular analyses of seven cases. *J Cutan Pathol* 2000;**27**:392–399.
97. Plaza JA, Feldman AL, Magro C. Cutaneous CD30-positive lymphoproliferative disorders with CD8 expression: a clinicopathologic study of 21 cases. *J Cut Pathol* 2013;**40**:236–247.
98. Rassidakis GZ, Thomaides A, Atwell C, *et al.* JunB expression is a common feature of CD30+ lymphomas and lymphomatoid papulosis. *Mod Pathol* 2005;**18**:1365–1370.
99. Drakos E, Leventaki V, Schlette EJ, *et al.* c-Jun expression and activation are restricted to CD30+ lymphoproliferative disorders. *Am J Surg Pathol* 2007;**31**:447–453.
100. Kempf W, Levi E, Kamarashev J, *et al.* Fascin expression in CD30-positive cutaneous lymphoproliferative disorders. *J Cut Pathol* 2002;**29**:295–300.
101. Goteri G, Simonetti O, Rupoli S, *et al.* Differences in survivin location and Bcl-2 expression in CD30+ lymphoproliferative disorders of the skin compared with systemic anaplastic large cell lymphomas: an immunohistochemical study. *Br J Dermatol* 2007;**157**:41–48.
102. Wasco MJ, Fullen D, Su L, Ma L. The expression of MUM1 in cutaneous T-cell lymphoproliferative disorders. *Hum Pathol* 2008;**39**:557–563.
103. Benner MF, Jansen PM, Meijer CJ, Willemze R. Diagnostic and prognostic evaluation of phenotypic markers TRAF1, MUM1, BCL2 and CD15 in cutaneous CD30-positive lymphoproliferative disorders. *Br J Dermatol* 2009;**161**:121–127.
104. Sun J, Yi S, Qiu L, *et al.* SATB1 defines a subtype of cutaneous CD30+ lymphoproliferative disorders associated with a T-helper 17 cytokine profile. *J Invest Dermatol* 2018;**138**:1795–1804.
105. Weiss LM, Wood GS, Trela M, *et al.* Clonal T-cell populations in lymphomatoid papulosis: evidence for a lymphoproliferative origin for a clinically benign disease. *N Engl J Med* 1986;**315**: 475–479.
106. de Souza A, Camilleri MJ, Wada DA, *et al.* Clinical, histopathologic, and immunophenotypic features of lymphomatoid papulosis with CD8 predominance in 14 pediatric patients. *J Am Acad Dermatol* 2009;**61**:993–1000.
107. Steinhoff M, Hummel M, Anagnostopoulos I, *et al.* Single-cell analysis of CD30 cells in lymphomatoid papulosis demonstrates a common clonal T-cell origin. *Blood* 2002;**100**:578–584.
108. Wood GS, Hardman DL, Boni R, *et al.* Lack of the t(2;5) or other mutations resulting in expression of anaplastic lymphoma kinase catalytic domain in CD30 primary cutaneous lymphoproliferative disorders and Hodgkin's disease. *Blood* 1996;**88**:1765–1770.
109. DeCoteau JF, Butmarc JR, Kinney MC, Kadin ME. The t(2;5) chromosomal translocation is not a common feature of primary cutaneous CD30 lymphoproliferative disorders: comparison with anaplastic large-cell lymphoma of nodal origin. *Blood* 1996;**87**:3437–3441.
110. Velusamy T, Kiel MJ, Sahasrabuddhe AA, *et al.* A novel recurrent *NPM1-TYK2* gene fusion in cutaneous CD30-positive lymphoproliferative disorders. *Blood* 2014;**124**:3768–3771.
111. Maurus K, Appenzeller S, Roth S, *et al.* Recurrent oncogenic *JAK* and *STAT* alterations in cutaneous CD30-positive lymphoproliferative disorders. *J Invest Dermatol* 2020;**140**:2023–2031.
112. Panhans A, Bodemer C, Macinthyre E, *et al.* Pityriasis lichenoides of childhood with atypical CD30-positive cells and clonal T-cell receptor gene rearrangements. *J Am Acad Dermatol* 1996;**35**:489–490.
113. Herron MD, Bohnsack JF, Vanderhooft SL. Septic, CD-30 positive febrile ulceronecrotic pityriasis lichenoides et varioliformis acuta. *Ped Dermatol* 2005;**22**:360–365.
114. Kempf W, Kazakov DV, Palmedo G, *et al.* Pityriasis lichenoides et varioliformis acuta with numerous CD30+ cells. A variant mimicking lymphomatoid papulosis and other cutaneous lymphomas. A clinicopathologic, immunohistochemical, and molecular biological study of 13 cases. *Am J Surg Pathol* 2012;**36**:1021–1029.
115. Vonderheid EC, Kadin ME, Gocke CD. Lymphomatoid papulosis followed by pityriasis lichenoides: a common pathogenesis? *Am J Dermatopathol* 2011;**33**:835–840.
116. Borra T, Custrin A, Saggini A, *et al.* Pityriasis lichenoides, atypical pityriasis lichenoides, and related conditions: a study of 66 cases. *Am J Surg Pathol* 2018;**42**:1101–1112.
117. Olsen SH, Ma L, Schnitzer B, Fullen DR. Clusterin expression in cutaneous CD30-positive lymphoproliferative disorders and their histologic simulants. *J Cut Pathol* 2009;**36**:302–307.

118. Willemze R, Hodak E, Zinzani PL, *et al.* Primary cutaneous lymphomas: ESMO Clinical Practice Guidelines for diagnosis, treatment and follow-up. *Ann Oncol* 2018;**29**(Supplement 4): iv30–iv40.
119. Kempf W, Pfaltz K, Vermeer MH, *et al.* EORTC, ISCL, and USCLC consensus recommendations for the treatment of primary cutaneous CD30-positive lymphoproliferative disorders: lymphomatoid papulosis and primary cutaneous anaplastic large-cell lymphoma. *Blood* 2011;**118**:4024–4035.
120. Lewis DJ, Talpur R, Huen AO, *et al.* Brentuximab vedotin for patients with refractory lymphomatoid papulosis: an analysis of phase 2 results. *JAMA Dermatol* 2017;**153**:1302–1306.
121. Shinohara MM, Shustov A. How I treat primary cutaneous CD30+ lymphoproliferative disorders. *Blood* 2019;**134**:515–524.
122. Dege T, Netzer I, Strobel K, *et al.* Successful treatment of lymphomatoid papulosis with chlormethine gel. *J Deutsch Dermatol Ges* 2024;**22**:826–828.
123. Yu JB, Blitzblau RC, Decker RH, *et al.* Analysis of primary CD30 cutaneous lymphoproliferative disease and survival from the surveillance, epidemiology, and end results database. *J Clin Oncol* 2008;**26**:1483–1488.
124. De Souza A, el-Azhary RA, Camilleri MJ, *et al.* In search of prognostic indicators for lymphomatoid papulosis: a retrospective study of 123 patients. *J Am Acad Dermatol* 2012;**66**:928–937.
125. Gruber R, Sepp NT, Fritsch PO, Schmuth M. Prognosis of lymphomatoid papulosis. *Oncologist* 2006;**11**:955–957.
126. Kim YH, Willemze R, Pimpinelli N, *et al.* TNM classification system for primary cutaneous lymphomas other than mycosis fungoides and Sézary syndrome: a proposal of the International Society for Cutaneous Lymphomas (ISCL) and the Cutaneous Lymphoma Task Force of the European Organization of Research and Treatment of Cancer (EORTC). *Blood* 2007;**110**:479–484.
127. Benner MF, Willemze R. Applicability and prognostic value of the new TNM classification system in 135 patients with primary cutaneous anaplastic large cell lymphoma. *Arch Dermatol* 2009;**145**:1399–1404.
128. Olsen EA, Whittaker S, Willemze R, *et al.* Primary cutaneous lymphoma: recommendations for clinical trial design and staging update from the ISCL, USCLC, and EORTC. *Blood* 2022;**140**:419–437.
129. National Comprehensive Cancer Network. Primary Cutaneous Lymphomas (Version 3.2025). Accessed September 20, 2025. https://www.nccn.org/professionals/physician_gls/pdf/primary_cutaneous.pdf.
130. Hsi AC, Lee SJ, Rosman IS, *et al.* Expression of helper T cell master regulators in inflammatory dermatoses and primary cutaneous T-cell lymphomas: diagnostic implications. *J Am Acad Dermatol* 2015;**72**:159–167.
131. LeBoit PE. Hodgkin's disease, anaplastic large cell lymphoma, and lymphomatoid papulosis. Another scalpel blunted. *Am J Clin Pathol* 1995;**104**:3–4.
132. Lamant L, Pileri S, Sabattini E, *et al.* Cutaneous presentation of ALK-positive anaplastic large cell lymphoma following insect bites: evidence for an association in five cases. *Haematologica* 2010;**95**:449–455.
133. Calista D, Valenzano F, Riccioni L. Unusual cutaneous presentation of ALK+ anaplastic large cell lymphoma mimicking syphilis on the glans penis. *Eur J Dermatol* 2009;**19**:76–77.
134. Oschlies I, Lisfeld J, Lamant L, *et al.* ALK-positive anaplastic large cell lymphoma limited to the skin: clinical, histopathological and molecular analysis of 6 pediatric cases. A report from the ALCL99 study. *Haematologica* 2013;**98**:50–56.
135. Gould JW, Eppes RB, Gilliam AC, *et al.* Solitary primary cutaneous CD30+ large cell lymphoma of natural killer cell phenotype bearing the t(2;5)(p23;q35) translocation and presenting in a child. *Am J Dermatopathol* 2000;**22**:422–428.
136. Pulitzer M, Ogunrinade O, Lin O, Steinherz P. ALK-positive (2p23 rearranged) anaplastic large cell lymphoma with localization to the skin in a pediatric patient. *J Cutan Pathol* 2015;**42**:182–187.
137. Hinshaw M, Trowers AB, Kodish E, *et al.* Three children with CD30+ cutaneous anaplastic large cell lymphomas bearing the t(2;5)(q23;q35) translocation. *Ped Dermatol* 2004;**21**:212–217.
138. Bernier M, Bagot M, Broyer M, *et al.* Distinctive clinicopathologic features associated with regressive primary CD30 positive cutaneous lymphomas: analysis of 6 cases. *J Cutan Pathol* 1997;**24**: 157–163.
139. Woo DK, Jones CR, Vanoli-Storz MN, *et al.* Prognostic factors in primary cutaneous anaplastic large cell lymphoma. Characterization of clinical subset with worse outcome. *Arch Dermatol* 2009;**145**:667–674.
140. Liu HL, Hoppe RT, Kohler S, *et al.* CD30+ cutaneous lymphoproliferative disorders: the Stanford experience in lymphomatoid papulosis and primary cutaneous anaplastic large cell lymphoma. *J Am Acad Dermatol* 2003;**49**:1049–1058.
141. Massone C, El Shabrawi-Caelen L, Kerl H, Cerroni L. The morphologic spectrum of primary cutaneous anaplastic large T-cell lymphoma: a histopathologic study on 66 biopsy specimens from 47 patients with report of rare variants. *J Cutan Pathol* 2008;**35**:46–53.
142. Magro CM, Momtahen S, Kiuru M. Primary cutaneous small cell variant of anaplastic large cell lymphoma: a case series and review of the literature. *Am J Dermatopathol* 2017;**39**:877–889.
143. Chen H, Xiong JS, Sheng N, *et al.* Primary cutaneous sarcomatoid anaplastic lymphoma kinase-positive anaplastic large-cell lymphoma with linear distributional lesions. *Am J Dermatopathol* 2017;**39**:863–866.
144. Ronen S, Rothschild M, Ollague J, Suster S. Clear cell primary cutaneous anaplastic large cell lymphoma. *Am J Dermatopathol* 2019;**41**:e111–e115.
145. Kong YY, Dai B, Kong JC, *et al.* Neutrophil/eosinophil-rich type of primary cutaneous anaplastic large cell lymphoma: a clinicopathological, immunophenotypic and molecular study of nine cases. *Histopathology* 2009;**55**:189–196.
146. Papalas JA, Van Mater D, Wang E. Pyogenic variant of primary cutaneous anaplastic large-cell lymphoma: a lymphoproliferative disorder with a predilection for the immunocompromised and the young. *Am J Dermatopathol* 2010;**32**:821–827.
147. Kreuter A, Pantelaki I, Michalowitz AL, *et al.* CD30-positive primary cutaneous anaplastic large cell lymphoma with coexistent pseudocarcinomatous hyperplasia. *Clin Exp Dermatol* 2018;**43**:585–588.
148. Monterroso V, Bujan W, Jaramillo O, Medeiros LJ. Subcutaneous tissue involvement by T-cell lymphoma. A report of 2 cases. *Arch Dermatol* 1996;**132**:1345–1350.
149. Chan JKC, Buchanan R, Fletcher CDM. Sarcomatoid variant of anaplastic large cell Ki1 lymphoma. *Am J Surg Pathol* 1990;**14**: 983–988.

150. Gru AA, Bhagat G, Subtil A, *et al.* Spindle-cell (sarcomatoid) variant of cutaneous anaplastic large-cell lymphoma (C-ALCL) an unusual mimicker of cutaneous malignant mesenchymal tumors—a series of 11 cases. *Am J Surg Pathol* 2021;**45**:796–802.
151. Onaindia A, Montes-Moreno S, Rodrıguez-Pinilla SM, *et al.* Primary cutaneous anaplastic large cell lymphomas with 6p25.3 rearrangement exhibit particular histological features. *Histopathology* 2015;**66**:846–855.
152. Nambudiri VE, Aboutalebi A, Granter SR, Saavedra A. Recurrent ALK-negative anaplastic large T-cell lymphoma presenting as necrotizing vasculitis. *Am J Dermatopathol* 2013;**35**:512–516.
153. Al-Rohil RN, Torres-Cabala CA, Patel A, *et al.* Loss of CD30 expression after treatment with brentuximab vedotin in a patient with anaplastic large cell lymphoma: a novel finding. *J Cutan Pathol* 2016;**43**:1161–1166.
154. Massone C, Cerroni L. Phenotypic variability in primary cutaneous anaplastic large T-cell lymphoma: a study on 35 patients. *Am J Dermatopathol* 2014;**36**:153–157.
155. Plaza JA, Ortega P, Lynott J, *et al.* CD8-positive primary cutaneous anaplastic large T-cell lymphoma (PCALCL): case report and review of this unusual variant of PCALCL. *Am J Dermatopathol* 2010;**32**:489–491.
156. (a)Bosisio FM, Cerroni L. Expression of T-follicular helper markers in sequential biopsies of progressive mycosis fungoides and other primary cutaneous T-cell lymphomas. *Am J Dermatopathol* 2015;**37**:115–121.(b)Erem AS, Kempf W, Mitteldorf C, *et al.* Primary cutaneous anaplastic large cell lymphoma with TCR-γδ expression: a case series of eleven patients of a rare immunophenotypic variant. *J Cutan Pathol* 2025;**52**:487–496.
157. Ravindran A, Feldman AL, Ketterling RP, *et al.* Striking association of lymphoid enhancing factor (LEF1) overexpression and *DUSP22* rearrangements in anaplastic large cell lymphoma. *Am J Surg Pathol* 2021;**45**:550–557.
158. Chen BJ, Hsieh SM, Hsieh TH, *et al.* *DUSP22*-rearranged primary cutaneous CD30-positive T-cell lymphoproliferative disorders and adult T-cell leukemia/lymphoma frequently share the $LEF1^+$/$TIA1^-$ immunophenotype. *Hum Pathol* 2024;**150**:58–66.
159. Miyagaki T, Inoue N, Kamijo H, *et al.* Prognostic factors for primary cutaneous anaplastic large-cell lymphoma: a multicentre retrospective study from Japan. *Br J Dermatol* 2023;**189**:612–620.
160. Herbst H, Sander C, Tronnier M, *et al.* Absence of anaplastic lymphoma kinase (ALK) and Epstein–Barr virus gene products in primary cutaneous anaplastic large cell lymphoma and lymphomatoid papulosis. *Br J Dermatol* 1997;**137**:680–686.
161. Beylot-Barry M, Groppi A, Vergier B, *et al.* Characterization of t(2;5) reciprocal transcripts and genomic breakpoints in $CD30^+$ cutaneous lymphoproliferations. *Blood* 1998;**91**:4668–4676.
162. ten Berge RL, Oudejans JJ, Ossenkoppele GJ, *et al.* ALK expression in extranodal anaplastic large cell lymphoma favours systemic disease with (primary) nodal involvement and a good prognosis and occurs before dissemination. *J Clin Pathol* 2000;**53**:445–450.
163. Su LD, Schnitzer B, Ross CW, *et al.* The t(2;5)-associated p80 NPM/ALK fusion protein in nodal and cutaneous $CD30^+$ lymphoproliferative disorders. *J Cutan Pathol* 1997;**24**:597–603.
164. Chan DV, Summers P, Tuttle M, *et al.* Anaplastic lymphoma kinase expression in a recurrent primary cutaneous anaplastic large cell lymphoma with eventual systemic involvement. *J Am Acad Dermatol* 2011;**65**:671–673.
165. Melchers RC, Willemze R, van de Loo M, *et al.* Clinical, histologic, and molecular characteristics of anaplastic lymphoma kinase-positive primary cutaneous anaplastic large cell lymphoma. *Am J Surg Pathol* 2020;**44**:776–781.
166. Feldman AL, Law ME, Inwards DJ, *et al.* PAX5-positive T-cell anaplastic large cell lymphomas associated with extra copies of the PAX5 gene locus. *Mod Pathol* 2010;**23**:593–602.
167. Gellrich S, Wilks A, Lukowsky A, *et al.* T cell receptor-g gene analysis of $CD30^+$ large atypical individual cells in $CD30^+$ large primary cutaneous T cell lymphomas. *J Invest Dermatol* 2003; **120**:670–675.
168. Feldman AL, Dogan A, Smith DI, *et al.* Discovery of recurrent t(6;7)(p25.3;q32.3) translocations in ALK-negative anaplastic large cell lymphomas by massively parallel genomic sequencing. *Blood* 2011;**117**:915–919.
169. Csikesz CR, Knudson RA, Greipp PT, *et al.* Primary cutaneous CD30-positive T-cell lymphoproliferative disorders with Biallelic rearrangements of *DUSP22*. *J Invest Dermatol* 2013;**133**:1680–1682.
170. Feldman AL, Law M, Remstein ED, *et al.* Recurrent translocations involving the *MUM1* oncogene locus in peripheral T-cell lymphomas. *J Haematopathol* 2008;**1**:191.
171. Crescenzo R, Abate F, Lasorsa E, *et al.* Convergent mutations and kinase fusions lead to oncogenic STAT3 activation in anaplastic large cell lymphoma. *Cancer Cell* 2015;**27**:516–532.
172. Luchtel RA, Zimmermann MT, Hu G, *et al.* Recurrent $MSC^{E116K}$ mutations in ALK-negative anaplastic large cell lymphoma. *Blood* 2019;**133**:2776–2789.
173. van Kester MS, Tensen CP, Vermeer MH, *et al.* Cutaneous anaplastic large cell lymphoma and peripheral T-cell lymphoma NOS show distinct chromosomal alterations and differential expression of chemokine receptors and apoptosis regulators. *J Invest Dermatol* 2010;**130**:563–575.
174. Bastidas Torres AN, Melchers RC, van Grieken L, *et al.* Whole-genome profiling of primary cutaneous anaplastic large cell lymphoma. *Haematologica* 2022;**107**:1619–1632.
175. Mao X, Orchard G, Lillington DM, *et al.* Genetic alterations in primary cutaneous $CD30^+$ anaplastic large cell lymphoma. *Gene Chromos Cancer* 2003;**37**:176–185.
176. Sanchez-Schmidt JM, Salgado R, Servitje O, *et al.* Primary cutaneous $CD30^+$ anaplastic large-cell lymphomas show a heterogeneous genomic profile: an oligunucleotide arrayCGH approach. *J Invest Dermatol* 2011;**131**:269–271.
177. Szuhai K, van Doorn R, Tensen CP, Van Kester MS. Array-CGH analysis of cutaneous anaplastic large cell lymphoma. *Methods Mol Biol* 2013;**973**:197–212.
178. Böni R, Xin H, Kamarashev J, *et al.* Allelic deletion at 9p21-22 in primary cutaneous $CD30^+$ large cell lymphoma. *J Invest Dermatol* 2000;**115**:1104–1107.
179. Laharanne E, Chevret E, Idrissi Y, *et al.* *CDKN2A–CDKN2B* deletion defines an aggressive subset of cutaneous T-cell lymphoma. *Mod Pathol* 2010;**23**:547–558.
180. Benner MF, Ballabio E, van Kester MS, *et al.* Primary cutaneous anaplastic large cell lymphoma shows a distinct miRNA expression profile and reveals differences from tumor-stage mycosis fungoides. *Exp Dermatol* 2012;**21**:630–642.
181. Dippel E, Assaf C, Becker JC, *et al.* S2k-guidelines – cutaneous lymphomas (ICD10 C82-C86): update 2021. *J Dtsch Dermatol Ges* 2022;**20**:537–555.

182. Prince HM, Kim YH, Horwitz SM, *et al.* Brentuximab vedotin or physician's choice in CD30-positive cutaneous T-cell lymphoma (ALCANZA): an international, open-label, randomised, phase 3, multicentre trial. *Lancet* 2017;**390**:555–566.
183. Kempf W. Multifocal anaplastic large cell lymphoma - insight into its biology and treatment. *Br J Dermatol* 2018;**179**:565–566.
184. Melchers RC, Willemze R, Bekkenk MW, *et al.* Evaluation of treatment results in multifocal primary cutaneous anaplastic large cell lymphoma: report of the Dutch Cutaneous Lymphoma Group. *Br J Dermatol* 2018;**179**:724–731.
185. Lee JH, Cheng AL, Lin CW, *et al.* Multifocal primary cutaneous CD30+ anaplastic large cell lymphoma responsive to thalidomide: the molecular mechanism and the clinical application. *Br J Dermatol* 2009;**160**:887–889.
186. Kamstrup MR, Biskup E, Gniadecki R. Notch signaling in primary cutaneous CD30+ lymphoproliferative disorders: a new therapeutic approach? *Br J Dermatol* 2010;**163**:781–788.
187. Prieto-Torres L, Rodriguez-Pinilla SM, Onaindia A, *et al.* CD30-positive primary cutaneous lymphoproliferative disorders: molecular alterations and targeted therapies. *Haematologica* 2019;**104**:226–235.
188. Hapgood G, Pickles T, Sehn LH, *et al.* Outcome of primary cutaneous anaplastic large cell lymphoma: a 20-year British Columbia Cancer Agency experience. *Br J Haematol* 2017;**176**:234–240.
189. Vergier B, Beylot-Barry M, Pulford K, *et al.* Statistical evaluation of diagnostic and prognostic features of CD30+ cutaneous lymphoproliferative disorders. A clinicopathologic study of 56 cases. *Am J Surg Pathol* 1998;**22**:1192–1202.
190. Fernandez-de-Misa R, Hernandez-Machin B, Combalia A, *et al.* Prognostic factors in patients with primary cutaneous anaplastic large cell lymphoma: a multicentric, retrospective analysis of the Spanish Group of Cutaneous Lymphoma. *J Eur Acad Dermatol Venereol* 2020;**34**:762–768.
191. Lee WJ, Moon IJ, Lee SH, *et al.* Cutaneous anaplastic large-cell lymphoma (ALCL): a comparative clinical feature and survival outcome analysis of 52 cases according to primary tumor site. *J Am Acad Dermatol* 2016;**74**:1135–1143.
192. D'Incan M, Ingen-Housz-Oro S, Beylot-Barry M, *et al.* Locoregional nodal extension does not impair prognosis of primary cutaneous anaplastic lymphomas. *Br J Dermatol* 2021;**184**:356–358.
193. Iacobelli J, Spagnolo DV, Tesfai Y, *et al.* Cutaneous intravascular anaplastic large T-cell lymphoma: a case report and review of the literature. *Am J Dermatopathol* 2012;**34**:e133–e138.
194. Krishnan C, Moline S, Anders K, *et al.* Intravascular ALK-positive anaplastic large-cell lymphoma mimicking inflammatory breast carcinoma. *J Clin Oncol* 2009;**27**:2563–2565.
195. Metcalf RA, Bashey S, Wysong A, *et al.* Intravascular ALK-negative anaplastic large cell lymphoma with localized cutaneous involvement and an indolent clinical course. Toward recognition of a distinct clinicopathologic entity. *Am J Surg Pathol* 2013;**37**:617–623.
196. Rieger KE, Polidore T, Warnke R, *et al.* ALK-negative systemic intravascular anaplastic large cell lymphoma presenting in the skin. *J Cutan Pathol* 2011;**38**:216–220.
197. Wang L, Li C, Gao T. Cutaneous intravascular anaplastic large cell lymphoma. *J Cutan Pathol* 2011;**38**:221–226.
198. Deetz CO, Gilbertson KG II, Anadkat MJ, *et al.* A rare case of intravascular large T-cell lymphoma with an unusual T helper phenotype. *Am J Dermatopathol* 2011;**33**:e99–e102.
199. Zizi-Sermpetzoglou A, Petrakopoulou N, Tepelenis N, *et al.* Intravascular T-cell lymphoma of the vulva, CD30 positive: a case report. *Eur J Gynaecol Oncol* 2009;**30**:586–588.
200. Fan P, Nong L, Sun J, *et al.* Primary cutaneous anaplastic large cell lymphoma with intralymphatic involvement associated with chronic lymphedema. *J Cutan Pathol* 2017;**44**:616–619.
201. Gratzinger D, Million L, Kim YH. Occult dermal lymphatic involvement is frequent in primary cutaneous anaplastic large cell lymphoma. *Am J Dermatopathol* 2015;**37**:767–770.
202. Cerroni L, Massone C, Kutzner H, *et al.* Intravascular large T-cell or NK-cell lymphoma. A rare variant of intravascular large cell lymphoma with frequent cytotoxic phenotype and association with Epstein–Barr virus infection. *Am J Surg Pathol* 2008;**32**:891–898.
203. Takahashi E, Kajimoto K, Fukatsu T, *et al.* Intravascular large T-cell lymphoma: a case report of CD30-positive and ALK-negative anaplastic type with cytotoxic molecule expression. *Virchows Arch* 2005;**447**:1000–1006.
204. Quesada AE, Medeiros LJ, Clemens MW, *et al.* Breast implant-associated anaplastic large cell lymphoma: a review. *Mod Pathol* 2019;**32**:166–188.
205. Laurent C, Di Napoli A, Feldman AL, Horwitz SM. Breast implant-associated anaplastic large-cell lymphoma. In: Arber DA, Borowitz MJ, Cook JR, *et al.*, eds. *The International Consensus Classification of Myeloid and Lymphoid Neoplasms.* Philadelphia (US): Wolters Kluver, 2025: 749–751.
206. Miranda RN, de Jong D, Di Napoli A, *et al.* Breast implant-associated anaplastic large cell lymphoma. In: *WHO Classification of Tumours Editorial Board. Haematolymphoid Tumours.* 5th edition. Lyon (France): IARC, 2024: 738–741.
207. Alcalá R, Llombart B, Lavernia J, *et al.* Skin involvement as the first manifestation of breast implant-associated anaplastic large cell lymphoma. *J Cutan Pathol* 2016;**43**:602–608.
208. Lipworth L, Tarone RE, McLaughlin JK. Breast implants and lymphoma risk: a review of the epidemiologic evidence through 2008. *Plast ReconstrSurg* 2009;**123**:790–793.
209. Largent J, Oefelein M, Kaplan HM, *et al.* Risk of lymphoma in women with breast implants: analysis of clinical studies. *Eur J Cancer* 2012;**21**:274–280.
210. Stark B, Magneli M, van Heijningen I, *et al.* Considerations on the demography of BIA-ALCL in European countries based on an E(A)SAPS Survey. *Aesthetic Plast Surg* 2021;**45**:2639–2644.
211. de Jong WH, Panagiotakos D, Proykova A, *et al.* Final opinion on the safety of breast implants in relation to anaplastic large cell lymphoma: report of the scientific committee on health, emerging and environmental risks (SCHEER). *Regul Toxicol Pharmacol* 2021;**125**:104982.
212. SCHEER - Public consultation on the Preliminary Opinion on the safety of breast implants in relation to anaplastic large cell lymphoma (BIA-ALCL). Accessed February 20, 2025. https://health.ec.europa.eu/consultations/scheer-public-consultation-preliminary-opinion-safety-breast-implants-relation-anaplastic-large-cell_en.
213. Mendes J, Mendes Maykeh VA, Frascino LF, Zacchi FFS. Gluteal implant associated anaplastic large cell lymphoma. *Plast Reconstr Surg* 2019;**144**:610–613.
214. Di Napoli A, Fruscione S, Mazzola S, *et al.* Emerging non-breast implant-associated lymphomas: a systematic review. *Cancers (Basel)* 2024;**16**:4085.

215. Jones JL, Hanby AM, Wells C, *et al.* Breast implant-associated anaplastic large cell lymphoma (BIA-ALCL): an overview of presentation and pathogenesis and guidelines for pathological diagnosis and management. *Histopathology* 2019;**75**:787–796.
216. Blombery P, Thompson ER, Jones K, *et al.* Whole exome sequencing reveals activating *JAK1* and *STAT3* mutations in breast implant-associated anaplastic large cell lymphoma. *Haematologica* 2016;**101**:e387–e390.
217. Laurent C, Nicolae A, Laurent C, *et al.* Gene alterations in epigenetic modifiers and JAK-STAT signaling are frequent in breast implant-associated ALCL. *Blood* 2020;**135**:360–370.
218. Tabanelli V, Corsini C, Fiori S, *et al.* Recurrent PDL1 expression and PDL1 (CD274) copy number alterations in breast implant-associated anaplastic large cell lymphomas. *Hum Pathol* 2019;**90**:60–69.
219. Los-de-Vries GT, de Boer M, van Dijk E, *et al.* Chromosome 20 loss is characteristic of breast implant-associated anaplastic large cell lymphoma. *Blood* 2020;**136**:2927–2932.
220. Miranda RN, Aladily TN, Prince HM, *et al.* Breast implant-associated anaplastic large-cell lymphoma: long-term follow-up of 60 patients. *J Clin Oncol* 2014;**32**:114–120.

## CHAPTER 6

# Subcutaneous panniculitis-like T-cell lymphoma

Subcutaneous panniculitis-like T-cell lymphoma is included as a distinct entity in the International Consensus Classification (ICC) *of Myeloid and Lymphoid Neoplasms*, the 2019 and 2024 updates of classification of cutaneous lymphomas by the European Organization of Research and Treatment of Cancer (EORTC) – Cutaneous Lymphoma Histopathology Group, and the World Health Organization (WHO) *Classification of Haematolymphoid Tumours* [1–4]. Subcutaneous panniculitis-like T-cell lymphoma is very rare, and it seems to be more common in Asiatic patients, and in females [5]. As a degree of involvement of subcutaneous fat by neoplastic lymphocytes is common in many primary or secondary cutaneous T- and B-cell lymphomas, it is necessary to strictly separate true subcutaneous panniculitis-like T-cell lymphoma from other lymphomas involving the subcutaneous fat. Interestingly, although the description of subcutaneous panniculitis-like T-cell lymphoma is relatively recent, cases published in the past may have been examples of this entity misdiagnosed as a "persistent erythema nodosum" (Fig. 6.1) [6]. In his article, Pick described two young female patients (17-year and 19-year old, respectively), with long-standing (6 months and 1 year) panniculitic lesions located on the lower extremities (unilateral in the first case and bilateral in the second case).

Neoplastic cells in subcutaneous panniculitis-like T-cell lymphoma are located exclusively within the subcutaneous fat and display an $\alpha/\beta$ cytotoxic T-cell phenotype [3, 4, 7, 8]. Cases with a prominent subcutaneous involvement by $\gamma/\delta^+$ T-cells do not belong to this group and should be classified separately (see Chapter 7). Since neoplastic cells in cutaneous $\gamma/\delta$ T-cell lymphoma may express CD8, a positive staining for the $\alpha/\beta$ receptor as well as a negative staining for $\gamma/\delta$ are mandatory for the diagnosis of subcutaneous panniculitis-like T-cell lymphoma (neoplastic cells in cutaneous $\gamma/\delta$ T-cell lymphoma may coexpress $\alpha/\beta$ receptors, thus both stainings are necessary in order to confirm the lineage). When properly used, the term "subcutaneous panniculitis-like T-cell lymphoma" encompasses a group of patients with relatively homogeneous clinicopathologic, phenotypic, and prognostic features.

As in the former times, different entities were included in this group, dermatologists and dermatopathologists should understand that criteria used in the past differ from those that are required today for a diagnosis of subcutaneous panniculitis-like T-cell lymphoma [7, 8]. In the past, cases of subcutaneous panniculitis-like T-cell lymphoma were classified as malignant histiocytosis or histiocytic cytophagic panniculitis [9, 10]. Soon after the first description, it became clear that many cases of histiocytic cytophagic panniculitis showed a monoclonal population of T lymphocytes, proving the lymphoid origin of the disease [11]. It subsequently became clear that histiocytic cytophagic panniculitis was not always fatal, as previously thought, and that cases with a good prognosis could be observed [12]. Not all of the cases formerly classified as histiocytic cytophagic panniculitis belong to the group of subcutaneous panniculitis-like T-cell lymphoma, and some probably represent examples of cutaneous $\gamma/\delta$ T-cell lymphoma or of Epstein–Barr virus (EBV)-associated extranodal natural killer (NK)/T-cell lymphoma, nasal type. In fact, involvement of the subcutis is common in these types of lymphoma (see Chapters 8 and 9) [7, 13, 14]. It has also been demonstrated that some cases classified in the past as Weber–Christian panniculitis represent in truth examples of subcutaneous panniculitis-like T-cell lymphoma [15, 16].

A precise definition of subcutaneous panniculitis-like T-cell lymphoma is available for several years, but the old literature (and sometimes recent reports as well) is extremely confusing and misleading. In the past, based only on the involvement of the subcutis, many types of lymphoma with different clinicopathologic features and prognostic behavior have been lumped together in this group, and the exact definition and diagnostic criteria were unclear [13, 14, 16]. Moreover, any comprehensive review of the literature is hindered by the fact that in many of the earlier cases, and in some recent reports as well, phenotypic investigations were incomplete or not carried out at all. It must be clearly underlined that a purely subcutaneous pattern ("lobular panniculitis-like") can be observed rarely in various cutaneous lymphomas of T- and B-cell phenotype and that a prominent involvement of the subcutis *per se* is not a sufficient criterion for the diagnosis of subcutaneous panniculitis-like T-cell lymphoma [7, 17–20]. In this context, it should be remembered also that many overlapping features can be observed in the group of so-called "cytotoxic lymphomas," including subcutaneous

*Skin Lymphoma: The Illustrated Guide*, Sixth Edition. Lorenzo Cerroni.

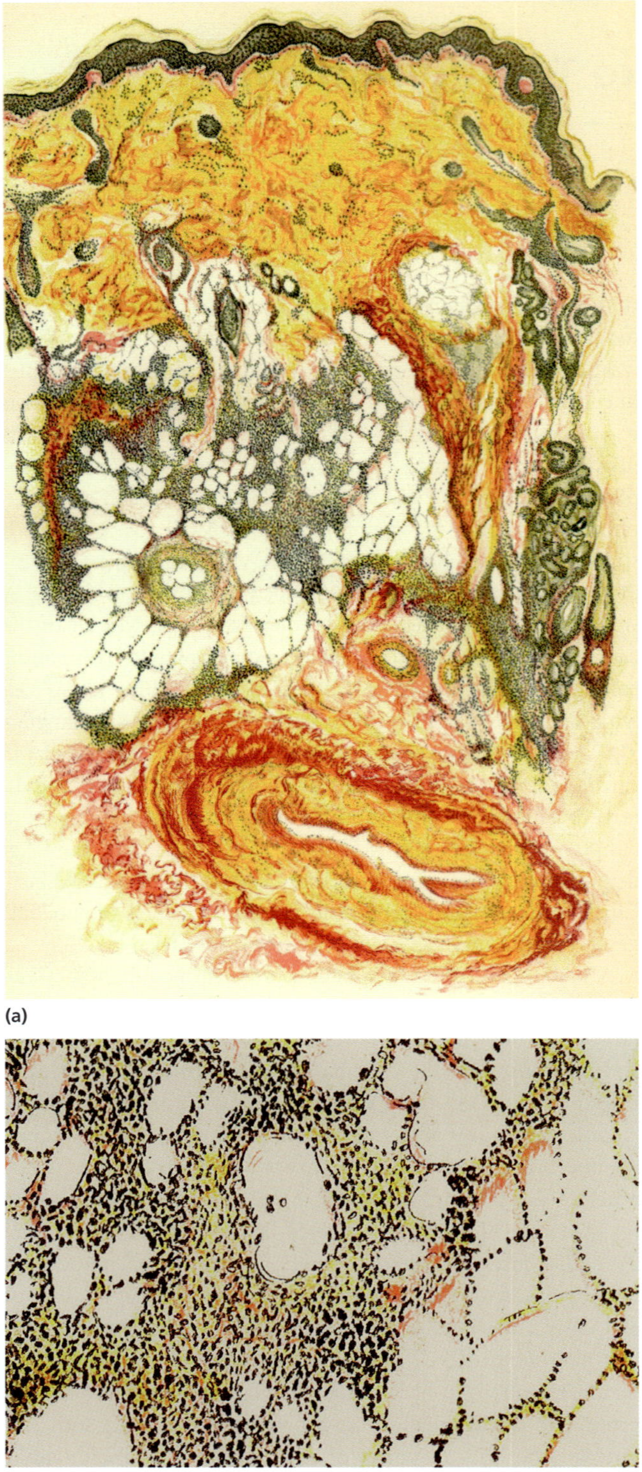

(a)

(b)

Figure 6.1 [6]/Dr. Walther Pick, showing (a) a lobular panniculitis-like pattern without any involvement of the dermis or epidermis, characterized (b) by a mononuclear cell infiltrate with rimming of the adipocytes. These histopathological features were considered diagnostic of a "persistent form of erythema nodosum," but may represent in truth an example of subcutaneous panniculitis-like T-cell lymphoma.

involvement by neoplastic lymphocytes, and that multiple parameters are required to classify a given case into a precise category (see Chapters 7 to 9) [7, 21]. Finally, lesions with exclusive subcutaneous involvement have also been observed in patients with mycosis fungoides [22]. An accurate clinical history should always be obtained in patients with a putative subcutaneous panniculitis-like T-cell lymphoma, and any skin lesions clinically suspicious of mycosis fungoides (e.g., superficial patches) should be biopsied.

It seems likely that some of the cases reported in the literature as lupus panniculitis (lupus erythematosus profundus) or "benign panniculitis evolving into overt lymphoma" represent in truth examples of slowly progressing subcutaneous panniculitis-like T-cell lymphoma that had been misdiagnosed at the beginning [16]. In this context, it has been proposed that lupus panniculitis and subcutaneous panniculitis-like T-cell lymphoma may represent two ends of a spectrum of the same entity, and the term "panniculitic T-cell dyscrasia" has been introduced in order to classify unclear cases [23]. The relationship between these two entities, if any, is still unclear. Although in previous editions of this book, I mentioned that "overlapping" cases may exist, I think that such cases represent most likely examples of atypical lupus panniculitis, and that subcutaneous panniculitis-like T-cell lymphoma and lupus panniculitis represent two distinct entities which in most cases can be differentiated precisely, and do not belong to a spectrum (see also below the paragraph on differential diagnosis with lupus panniculitis).

The etiology and pathogenesis of subcutaneous panniculitis-like T-cell lymphoma are still unknown. Autoimmune disorders, particularly lupus erythematous, are present in a distinct proportion of patients [8], and onset of the disease has been observed also in patients receiving immune modulatory drugs such as etanercept [24]. Transmission of the disease by allogeneic bone marrow transplantation has been documented in a single case [25], as well as onset in an immunosuppressed individual after cardiac transplantation [26]. A study showed that neoplastic lymphocytes express CCL5, a ligand for the C-chemokine receptor 5 (CCR5), which is expressed by adipocytes, thus providing a possible explanation for the peculiar tropism of neoplastic T lymphocytes for the adipose tissues [27].

## Clinical features

Patients are adults of both sexes [1, 8, 28], often with a variably long history of "benign panniculitis" (particularly lupus panniculitis). There is a slight predominance for females [29]. Reports in children exist [30–33], and aggressive pediatric cases with hemophagocytic syndrome have been described as well [34, 35]. In this context, it should be remembered that a lobular panniculitis with monoclonal $CD8^{+}$ T-lymphocytes may be observed in children with congenital immune deficiency syndromes and that in this setting, the diagnosis of

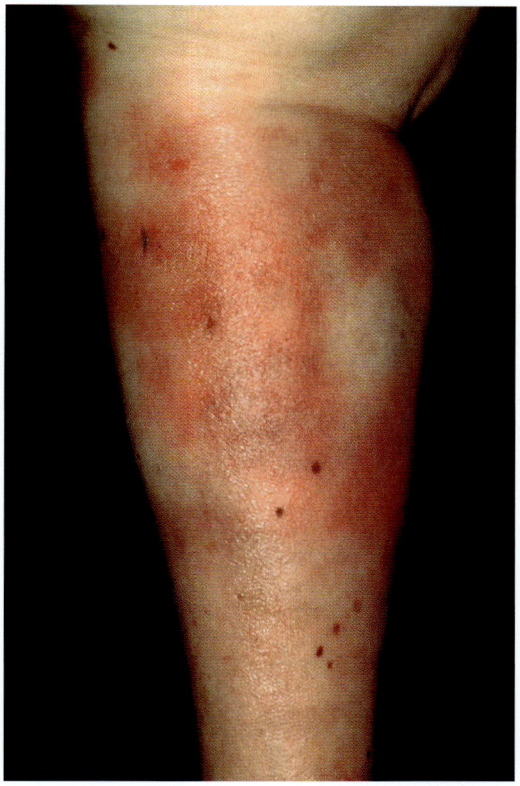

Figure 6.2 Subcutaneous panniculitis-like T-cell lymphoma. Infiltrated erythematous plaques ("panniculitis-like") on the leg.

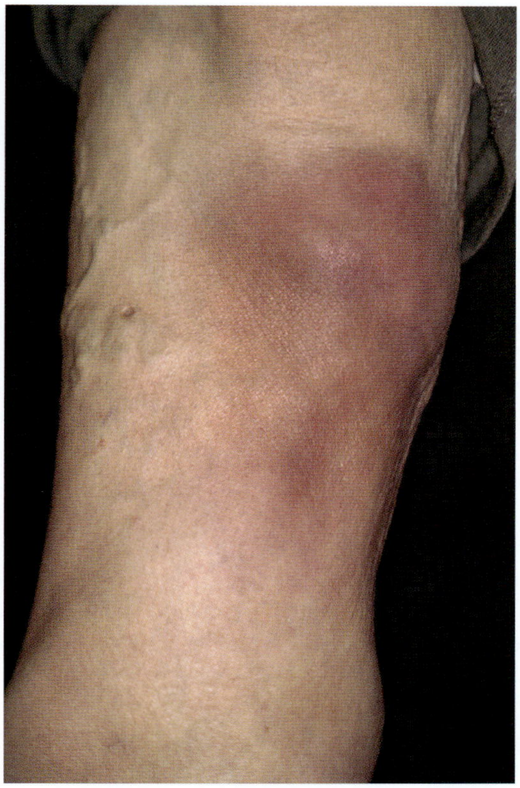

Figure 6.3 Subcutaneous panniculitis-like T-cell lymphoma. Large, infiltrated lesion on the thigh.

subcutaneous panniculitis-like T-cell lymphoma should be made with extreme caution (see also Chapter 31).

Staging investigations should be performed in cases of subcutaneous panniculitis-like T-cell lymphoma, and the bone marrow can be rarely involved [36]. There is no dedicated tumor, node, metastasis (TNM) staging system; the one devised for cutaneous lymphomas other than mycosis fungoides or Sézary syndrome may be used (see Chapter 1, Table 1.3), but in my opinion, it is not well suited for subcutaneous panniculitis-like T-cell lymphoma.

Clinically, patients present with solitary or multiple, infiltrated, "panniculitis-like" plaques or subcutaneous tumors. The lesions are usually not ulcerated and are located most commonly on the extremities, especially the lower ones (Figs. 6.2 to 6.4). Other sites of the body, including the head, may be affected (Fig. 6.5). Skin lesions reveal nonspecific clinical features of panniculitis and may simulate erythema nodosum, lupus panniculitis, or other panniculitic diseases. One patient with alopecic lesions on the scalp has also been described, and one with a lesion on the leg resembling venous stasis ulceration [37, 38]. Spontaneous resolution of some of the lesions may be observed [14, 39]. It must be underlined that some of the clinical variants described in the past may in truth represent examples of other cytotoxic lymphomas with subcutaneous involvement, as in many reported

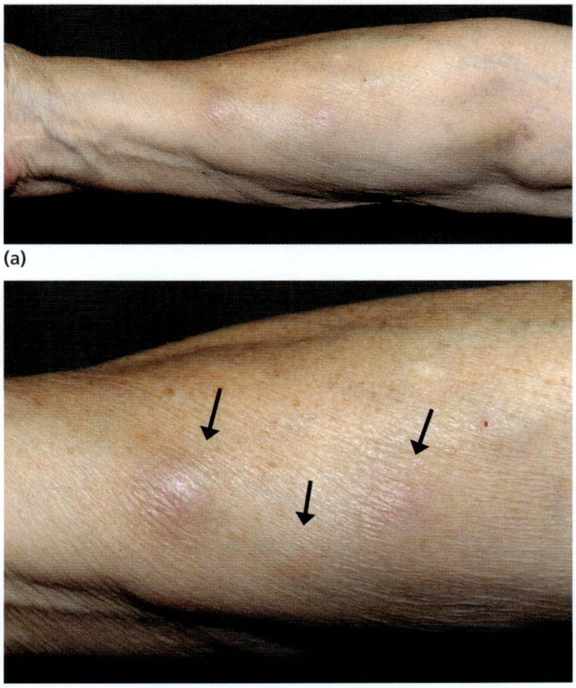

(a)

(b)

Figure 6.4 Subcutaneous panniculitis-like T-cell lymphoma. (a) Three subcutaneous nodules on the arm; (b) detail of the nodules (arrows).

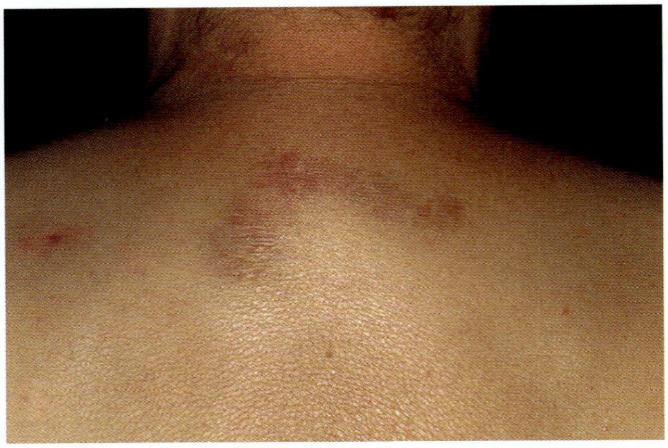

Figure 6.5 Subcutaneous panniculitis-like T-cell lymphoma. Subcutaneous tumor on the upper back.

cases, phenotypic details were not sufficient to classify them precisely. In addition, some of the reported cases may be examples of lupus panniculitis with atypical histopathological features. In one patient, neoplastic T lymphocytes have been detected in the peripheral blood [40], but the clinical relevance of this finding, if any, has not been elucidated.

In a subset of patients (only a small minority), there are accompanying symptoms such as fever, malaise, fatigue, and weight loss, sometimes mimicking those of rheumatic diseases [41], and a history of autoimmune disorders is present in about 20% of patients [8]. Clinical features of lupus erythematosus may be coexistent with those of subcutaneous panniculitis-like T-cell lymphoma in a small minority of patients [42]. These features include positivity for antinuclear antibodies and subsets, hematologic changes (e.g., anemia and neutropenia), renal changes, and positive immunofluorescence test on lesional skin. In this context, it should be noted that some of these patients may have in truth an atypical presentation of lupus panniculitis rather than a genuine subcutaneous panniculitis-like T-cell lymphoma, and the number of cases showing a true association between the two diseases may be smaller.

A hemophagocytic syndrome may be seen in advanced stages or rarely at first presentation, and can be the cause of death [8]. The onset of an hemophagocytic syndrome has been observed frequently in patients showing *HAVCR2* mutations [43, 44]. It should be underlined that the hemophagocytic syndrome is more common in the aggressive cytotoxic lymphomas with a γ/δ T-cell or NK-cell phenotype (see also Chapters 8 and 9) [45].

## Histopathology, immunophenotype, and molecular genetics

### Histopathology

Histopathology reveals dense, nodular, or diffuse infiltrates of small, medium, and (rarely) large pleomorphic lymphocytes confined to the subcutaneous fat with the pattern of a lobular panniculitis (Figs. 6.6 and 6.7). Small perivascular aggregates of non-neoplastic cells may be located within the reticular dermis, but clusters of neoplastic T lymphocytes are almost never situated outside of the subcutaneous fat. In fact, in typical cases, the reticular dermis is completely devoid of any infiltrate. Epidermotropism is never found. In many areas, neoplastic cells within the subcutaneous fat are arranged in small clusters or as solitary units around the single adipocytes (so-called "rimming" of the adipocytes) (Fig. 6.8). Necrosis is often a prominent feature and may completely mask the specific histopathologic features. In such cases, clues to the diagnosis, if present, are the finding of small aggregates of atypical cells within the areas of necrosis (Fig. 6.9a) and of "ghost cells" (Fig. 6.9b), representing necrotic lymphocytes still showing the original distribution of the infiltrate. Angiocentricity/angiodestruction is uncommon,

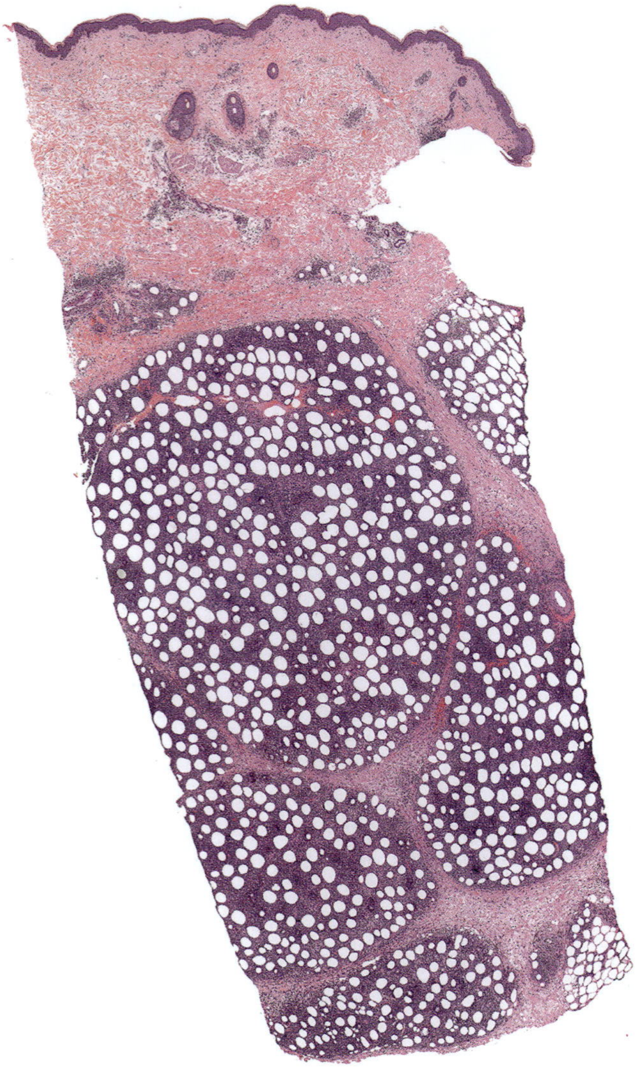

Figure 6.6 Subcutaneous panniculitis-like T-cell lymphoma. Dense lymphoid infiltrates showing exclusive involvement of the subcutaneous fat with a lobular panniculitis-like pattern.

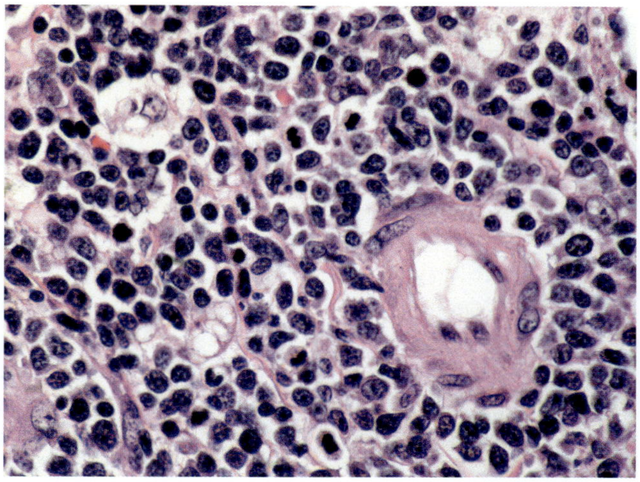

**Figure 6.7** Subcutaneous panniculitis-like T-cell lymphoma. Infiltration of subcutaneous fat by small- to medium-sized pleomorphic lymphocytes.

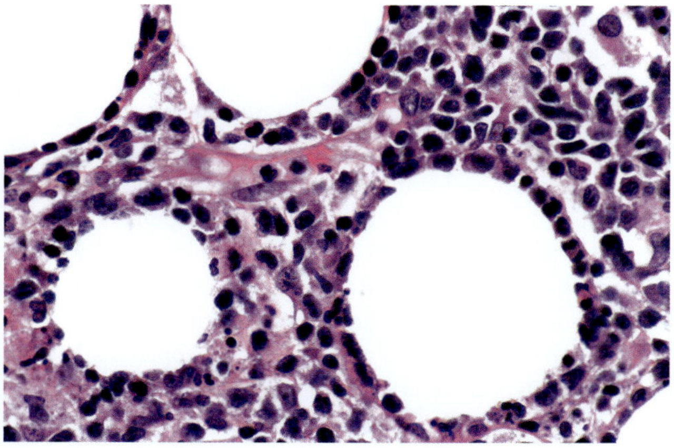

**Figure 6.8** Subcutaneous panniculitis-like T-cell lymphoma. "Rimming" of adipocytes by neoplastic lymphocytes. Note pleomorphism of the nuclei.

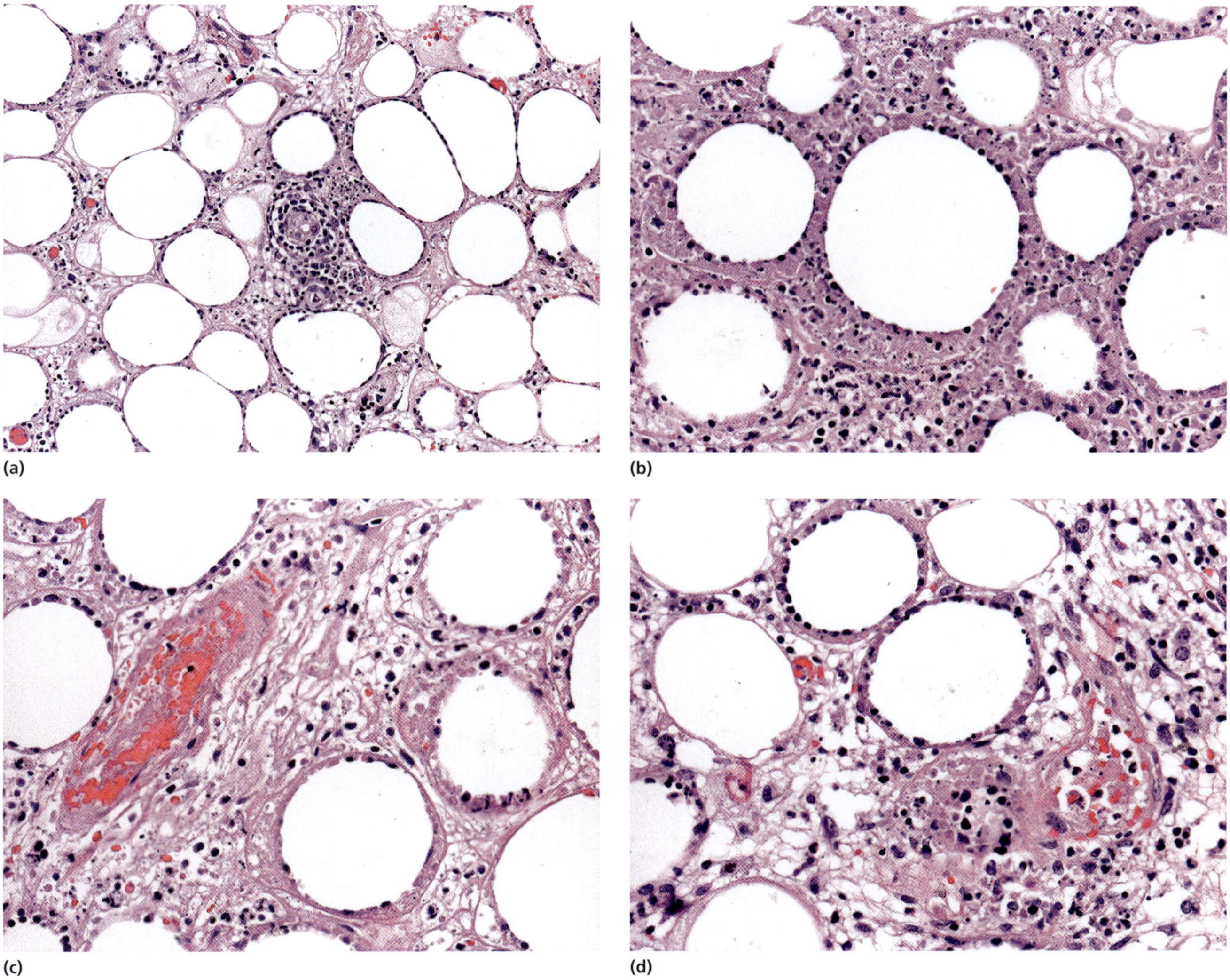


**Figure 6.9** Subcutaneous panniculitis-like T-cell lymphoma. (a) Small cluster of atypical lymphocytes on the background of prominent necrosis; (b) degenerative features of the subcutaneous fat with atypical lymphocytes admixed with "ghost cells" representing necrotic neoplastic lymphocytes; (c) necrotic vessel with intraluminal fibrin thrombus. (d) Pleomorphic lymphocytes, some of which necrotic, admixed with cellular debris.

but necrotic vessels with intraluminal thrombi may be observed in the areas of necrosis (Fig. 6.9c). Pleomorphic lymphocytes may be observed in necrotic areas (Fig. 6.9d). A histiocytic infiltrate, often with the formation of granulomas, is also frequent, particularly in late stages. In addition, reactive small lymphocytes can be admixed with the neoplastic cells, but plasma cells and eosinophils are rare. Membranocystic (lipomembranous) fat necrosis has been described in some cases [46]. The presence of a genuine "interface dermatitis" should prompt to consider the differential diagnosis of lupus erythematosus.

Although "rimming" of adipocytes by neoplastic lymphocytes has often been described as a histopathologic feature diagnostic of subcutaneous panniculitis-like T-cell lymphoma, a similar phenomenon can be observed in virtually all lymphomas with prominent involvement of the subcutaneous fat, as well as in reactive subcutaneous infiltrates [47]. In fact, I have observed B-cell lymphomas showing both clinical and histopathologic features indistinguishable from those of subcutaneous panniculitis-like T-cell lymphoma [17]. Necrosis and degenerative changes within the subcutaneous fat, which are often remarkable in subcutaneous panniculitis-like T-cell lymphoma, are only rarely found in subcutaneous infiltration of B-cell lymphomas.

In early lesions of subcutaneous panniculitis-like T-cell lymphoma, the specific findings are confined to a small portion of the subcutaneous fat, thus rendering the examination of small biopsies (i.e., punch biopsies) problematic (Fig. 6.10). In this context, it must be underlined that for a diagnosis of subcutaneous panniculitis-like T-cell lymphoma large, deep biopsies should be performed.

Subcutaneous panniculitis-like T-cell lymphoma has been observed in an exceptional case of primary cutaneous composite lymphoma, associated to a diffuse large B-cell lymphoma, leg-type (see also Chapter 28) [48].

## Immunohistology

Immunohistologic analyses show an α/β T-cytotoxic phenotype of neoplastic cells (βF1$^+$, CD3$^+$, CD4$^-$, CD8$^+$, T-cell receptor [TCR]γ$^-$, TCRδ$^-$) with positivity for cytotoxic proteins (TIA-1, granzyme-B, perforin) and negativity for CD56 (Figs. 6.11a to c) [8]. Proliferation markers (i.e., Ki-67) highlight a characteristic pattern of positive neoplastic cells arranged in small clusters and around the adipocytes (Fig. 6.11d). As already mentioned, a positive staining for βF1, a marker of TCRβ, as well as a negative staining for TCRγ or TCRδ, are necessary in order to confirm the diagnosis. Particularly in recurrent lesions, the βF1 expression may get partially lost by neoplastic cells, but it is usually retained by at least a proportion of them (Fig. 6.12). It should be reminded that variable numbers of reactive γ/δ T lymphocytes may be observed in otherwise typical cases of subcutaneous panniculitis-like T-cell lymphoma [49]. Staining for CD30 is consistently negative in subcutaneous panniculitis-like T-cell lymphoma.

However, EBV has been detected only in very rare cases of subcutaneous panniculitis-like T-cell lymphoma [50]. I have

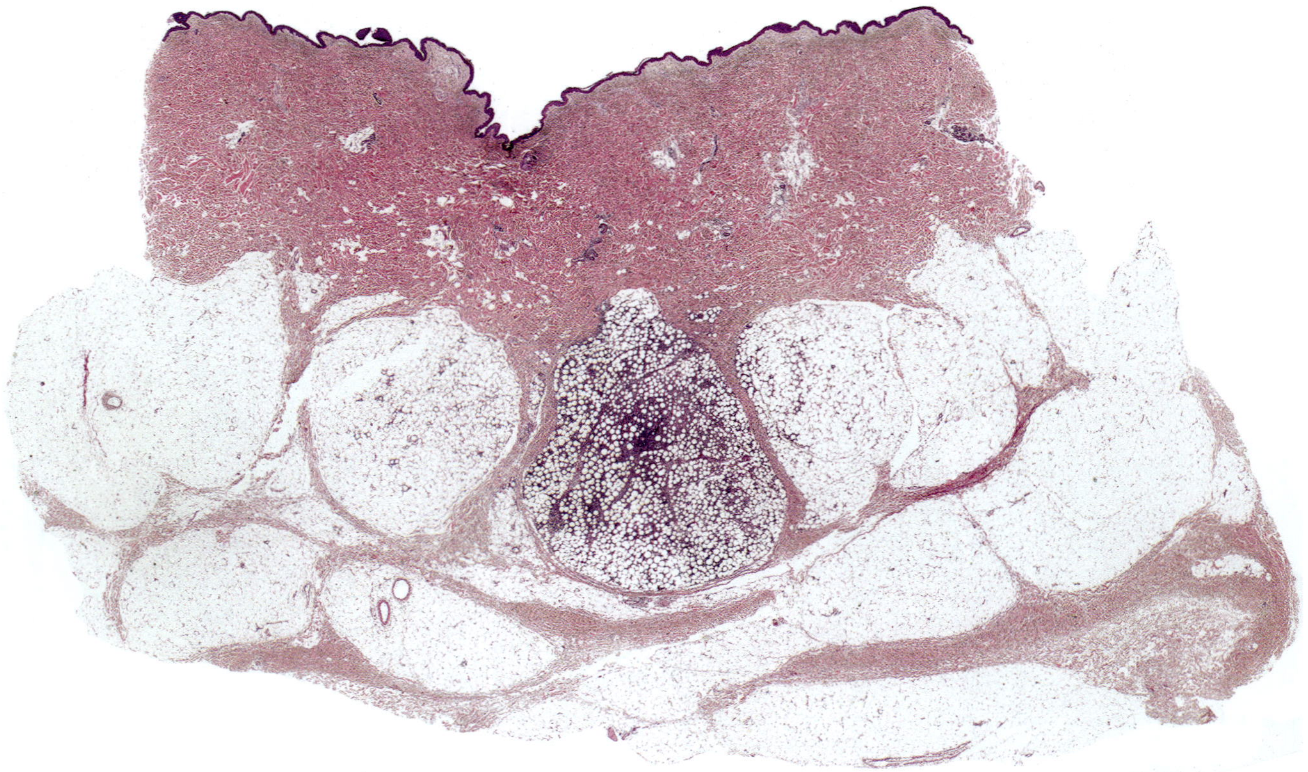

Figure 6.10 Subcutaneous panniculitis-like T-cell lymphoma. Focal involvement restricted to one part of the subcutaneous fat.

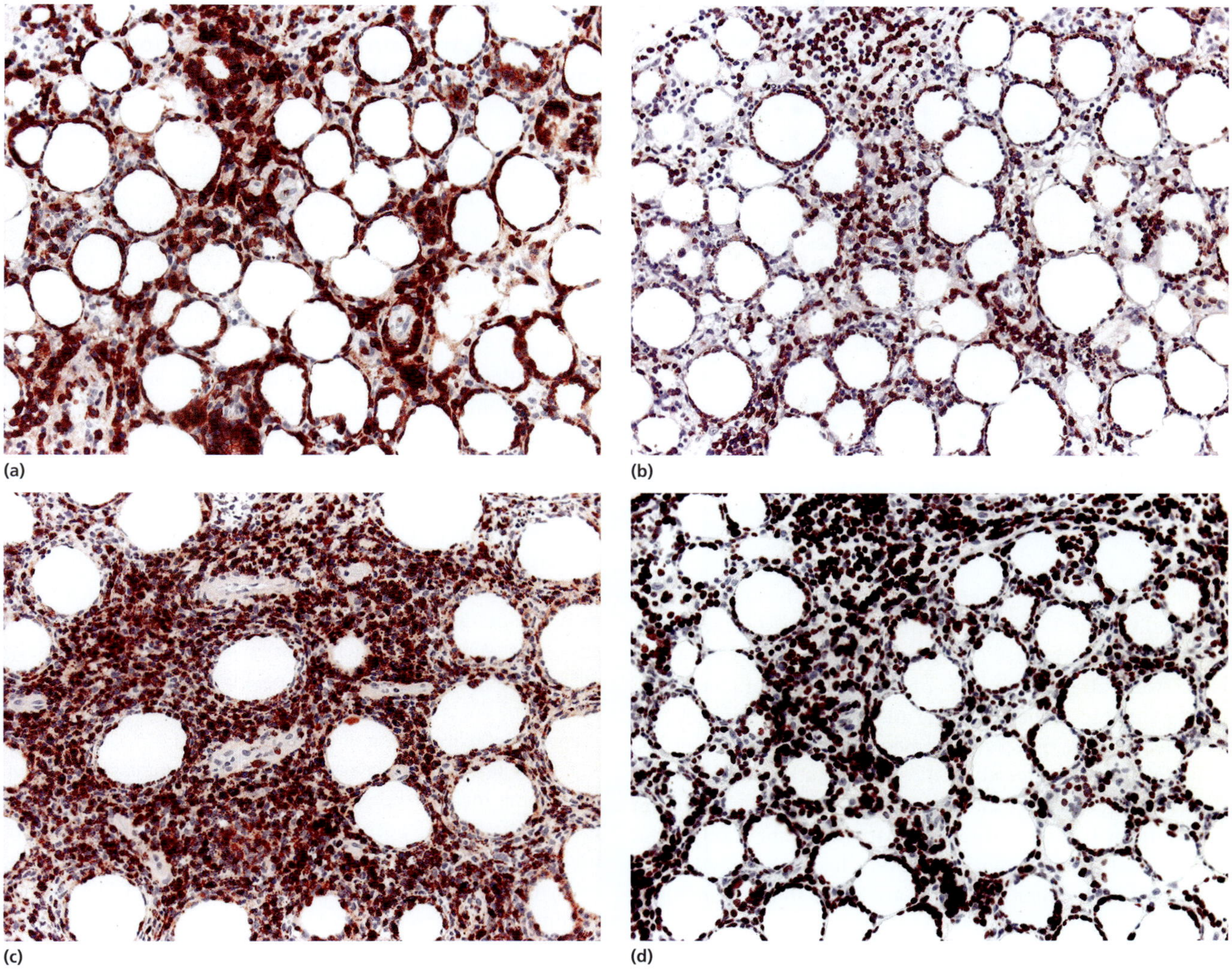


**Figure 6.11** Subcutaneous panniculitis-like T-cell lymphoma. (a) Staining for CD8 demonstrates positivity of neoplastic lymphocytes in small clusters and around the adipocytes. (b) Staining for βF1 shows positivity of neoplastic cells. (c) Positivity of all cells for granzyme B. (d) Staining for Ki-67 is a helpful diagnostic tool, highlighting proliferating neoplastic lymphocytes in small clusters and around the adipocytes.

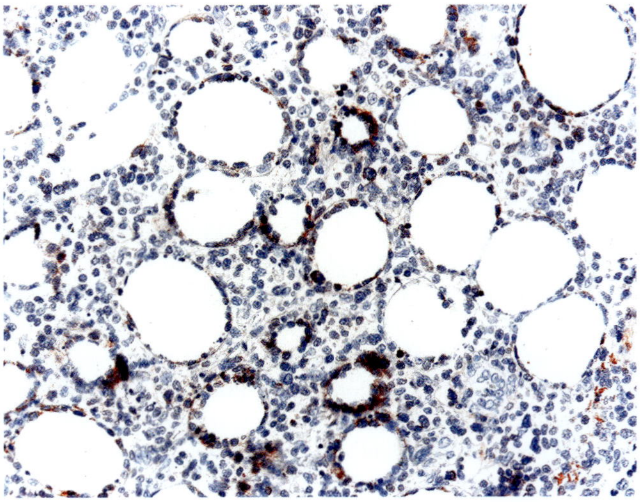

**Figure 6.12** Subcutaneous panniculitis-like T-cell lymphoma. Partial loss of expression of βF1 by neoplastic cells.

observed EBER-1$^+$ cells only in very rare cases, which had otherwise conventional clinicopathologic features of the disease and were not associated with immune deficiency (Fig. 6.13). In cases positive for EBV, the presence of an immune deficiency (iatrogenic or noniatrogenic) should be investigated.

## Molecular genetics

The molecular analysis of the TCR genes shows a monoclonal rearrangement in the majority of cases [1, 3, 4, 8].

Germline loss-of-function, missense variants altering highly conserved residues of T-cell immunoglobulin mucin 3 (TIM3), a modulator of immune responses expressed on subgroups of T and innate immune cells, have been observed in approximately 60% of cases of subcutaneous panniculitis-like T-cell lymphoma in one study [51]. These variants lead to persistent immune activation and increased production of inflammatory cytokines, and are associated with the onset of

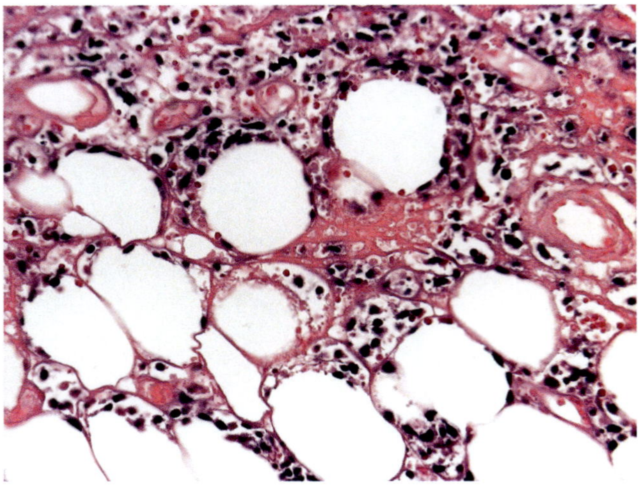

**Figure 6.13** Subcutaneous panniculitis-like T-cell lymphoma associated with EBV infection. In situ hybridization for EBV (EBER-1) shows positivity of most neoplastic cells.

hemophagocytic syndrome in patients with subcutaneous panniculitis-like T-cell lymphoma [51]. Consistent with this observation, germline mutations in *HAVCR2*, encoding TIM3, were identified in 85% of cases in a recent study, suggesting that individuals with germline mutations of *HAVCR2* are at risk of developing subcutaneous panniculitis-like T-cell lymphoma [52]. Indeed, *HAVCR2* mutations have been observed in a subset of patients (24.5–51% in different studies from French and Korean patients, respectively), and are frequently associated with severe hemophagocytic syndrome [43, 44]. Other mutations are found in genes involved in immune response, epigenetic modifications, and cell signaling, and are more frequently observed in *HAVCR2* mutated patients [44]. In a study on T- and NK-cell lymphomas, somatic mutations in the FAS pathway were associated with the development of an hemophagocytic syndrome (but cases of subcutaneous panniculitis-like T-cell lymphoma were not included) [53].

Compared to other T-cell lymphomas, low numbers of somatic mutations are observed, suggesting that germline *HAVCR2* mutations play an important role in the pathogenesis of the disease [54]. Single-cell comparative genomic hybridization of laser-microdissected specimens revealed gains of chromosomes 2q and 4q and losses of chromosomes 1pter, 2pter, 10qter, 11qter, 12qter, 16, 19, 20, and 22 [55]. In the same study, allelic *NAV3* aberrations were found by loss of heterozygosity and fluorescence in situ hybridization analyses in almost half of the cases [55]. Recurrent mutations involved in the phosphoinositide 3-kinase (PI3K)/AKT/mechanistic/mammalian target of rapamycin (mTOR) and the Janus kinase-signal transducer and activator of transcription (JAK–STAT) signaling pathways have been reported [56]. It seems that alterations of the JAK–STAT signaling pathway as well as upregulation of *CCR4* are a feature of *HAVCR2* mutated cases [44].

## Differential diagnosis with other cutaneous NK/T-cell lymphomas with prominent involvement of the subcutaneous tissue

Rare cases of mycosis fungoides presenting with subcutaneous lesions can only be excluded by an accurate clinical history and by clinicopathologic correlation. In addition, mycosis fungoides usually shows a $CD4^+$ phenotype, in contrast to the $CD8^+$ one of subcutaneous panniculitis-like T-cell lymphoma. Examination of more than one skin biopsy usually is sufficient for a precise classification, as purely subcutaneous infiltration is only an occasional finding in mycosis fungoides.

The following features favor a histopathological diagnosis of cutaneous $\gamma/\delta$ T-cell lymphoma: involvement of the dermis and/or epidermis (sometimes with marked epidermotropism) in the same biopsy or in sequential biopsies taken at the same time or over time; negativity for $\alpha/\beta$ and positivity for $\gamma/\delta$ T-cell markers; and positivity for CD56.

Features that favor the histopathological diagnosis of extranodal NK/T-cell lymphoma, nasal type, are marked involvement of the dermis, more rarely also of the epidermis in the same biopsy or in sequential biopsies taken at the same time or over time; NK-cell phenotype; positivity for CD56; positive signal for EBV upon in situ hybridization (EBER-1); and lack of monoclonal rearrangement of the TCR genes.

Finally, features that favor a subcutaneous anaplastic large cell lymphoma include the presence of large pleomorphic or anaplastic cells strongly positive for CD30 and for CD4. It should be underlined, however, that purely subcutaneous anaplastic large cell lymphomas are exceedingly rare and that the CD30 expression may be observed in neoplastic cells of other T- and B-cell lymphomas, thus implying that such a diagnosis should be made only upon compelling evidence and after careful exclusion of other lymphoproliferative disorders.

## Differential diagnosis with lupus panniculitis

Clinically, both lupus panniculitis and subcutaneous panniculitis-like T-cell lymphoma present with panniculitic lesions located mostly on the limbs, thus not allowing a differential diagnosis. In typical cases of either condition, histology shows features that allow a precise diagnosis (see also Chapter 31). In this context, it should be reminded that small biopsies may fail to show diagnostic aspects, and that in both diseases, biopsies of older lesions may be characterized by necrosis and degenerative changes and be not diagnostic. The role of molecular investigations in the differentiation of the two diseases has been addressed in a comparative study showing that subcutaneous panniculitis-like T-cell lymphoma was characterized by mutations in *TP53* in 40% of cases, whereas all cases of lupus erythematosus were negative [57]. Only one out of 10 cases of subcutaneous panniculitis-like T-cell lymphoma in this study showed a *HAVCR2* mutation.

Although both entities are characterized by the pattern of a lobular panniculitis, many differences exist that allow in most cases a precise classification:

1. Presence of an "interface dermatitis" with prominent vacuolization of basal keratinocytes is a feature observed in several cases of lupus panniculitis [58], but should be considered as a very unusual feature (and prompt a reconsideration of the diagnosis) in subcutaneous panniculitis-like T-cell lymphoma;
2. Cellular atypia in most of the infiltrate is not observed in all cases of subcutaneous panniculitis-like T-cell lymphoma, but when present is a feature arguing against lupus panniculitis [59];
3. Nodules of B lymphocytes, sometimes with germinal centers, as well as plasma cells are a feature of many cases of lupus panniculitis but not of subcutaneous panniculitis-like T-cell lymphoma [60];
4. $CD8^+$ cells may be observed in lupus panniculitis, but $CD4^+$ cells are also present and represent a consistent part of the infiltrate (unlike the situation in subcutaneous panniculitis-like T-cell lymphoma);
5. The proliferation rate is much lower in lupus panniculitis, and "Ki-$67^+$ hot-spots" are not observed [59]; in addition, the cells around the adipocytes are never homogeneously positive for Ki-67, unlike what can be observed in many areas in subcutaneous panniculitis-like T-cell lymphoma ("periadipocytic cell proliferation index") [61];
6. Clusters of plasmacytoid dendritic cells positive for CD123 are common in lupus panniculitis, but very rare if ever observed in subcutaneous panniculitis-like T-cell lymphoma (a few positive cells may be present, but never large clusters) [59, 60, 62, 63];
7. Cells positive for c-myc on immunohistology have been observed more often in subcutaneous panniculitis-like T-cell lymphoma than in lupus panniculitis [64];
8. Clusters of dermal cells expressing interferon regulatory factor 8 (IRF8) were observed in lupus panniculitis but not in subcutaneous panniculitis-like T-cell lymphoma in one study [60];
9. Finally, evidence of a clonal rearrangement of the TCR genes strongly supports a diagnosis of subcutaneous panniculitis-like T-cell lymphoma.

Notwithstanding the criteria just mentioned, in a small number of cases, features of both diseases may be present in one and the same specimen (Fig. 6.14) [65]. These specimens show focally areas that are characteristics of subcutaneous panniculitis-like T-cell lymphoma, and in other parts of the biopsy areas with histopathological features that are characteristics of lupus panniculitis, and pose a formidable diagnostic problem. These cases represent a conceptual as well as a practical problem, since besides diagnostic difficulties, they raise the question as to whether the two diseases may be indeed related. Patients with lupus erythematosus are at a higher risk of developing hematologic malignancies, but these are mostly of B-cell lineage, and the true risk of developing subcutaneous panniculitis-like T-cell lymphoma is unclear. On the other hand, it has been reported that about 20% of patients with subcutaneous panniculitis-like T-cell lymphoma have a history of autoimmune disorders, particularly lupus erythematosus [8]. I have never observed a patient with these "overlapping" features progressing to extracutaneous lymphoma. In this context, in my opinion, these cases represent most likely examples of "atypical" lupus panniculitis, that is, lupus panniculitis with atypical histopathological features (Fig. 6.15). In these cases, cellular atypia may be focally prominent with the presence of medium-sized cells admixed also with some large pleomorphic lymphocyte. On the other hand, these findings are only focal, and other areas of the specimen show typical features of lupus panniculitis. Although it is conceptually possible that in some cases of lupus panniculitis, a $CD8^+$ clone arises which may eventually progress over time to a true lymphoma, a convincing case has not been reported yet. However, diagnosis of such cases is very difficult, and dermatologists and dermatopathologists should be careful and mention that a subcutaneous panniculitis-like T-cell lymphoma cannot be ruled out with certainty (currently, I use the phrasing: "atypical lymphoid proliferation with overlapping features of lupus panniculitis and subcutaneous panniculitis-like T-cell lymphoma, most likely to be interpreted as an atypical lupus panniculitis"). In this context, it must be mentioned that there is no need to perform staging investigations in patients with "atypical" lupus panniculitis or to treat them differently than it is usually done, but careful follow-up controls should be performed.

## Treatment

The evaluation of different treatment schemes reported in the literature reflects the confusion concerning the classification of the disease in older publications. In fact, extremely aggressive treatment modalities mentioned in some publications are not necessary for cases of subcutaneous panniculitis-like T-cell lymphoma as defined in this chapter and in modern classification schemes. Many patients can be controlled for long periods of time with systemic steroids [8, 16, 66]. Monotherapy with systemic steroids is recommended as a treatment of choice for uncomplicated cases (i.e., those without hemophagocytic syndrome) [67]. Combinations of steroids with cyclosporine or methotrexate, or cyclosporine alone, have also been used [68–70], and in general, immunosuppressive drugs are considered better than systemic chemotherapy as the first treatment option [71]. Radiotherapy may be used for solitary lesions [72]. Complete remission has been achieved in one of the two children treated by cyclosporine A followed by chemotherapy [31], and immunosuppressive treatment (systemic steroids, cyclosporine A) has been used in pediatric patients with good results in two studies [73, 74]. A "watchful waiting" strategy has been suggested by other authors

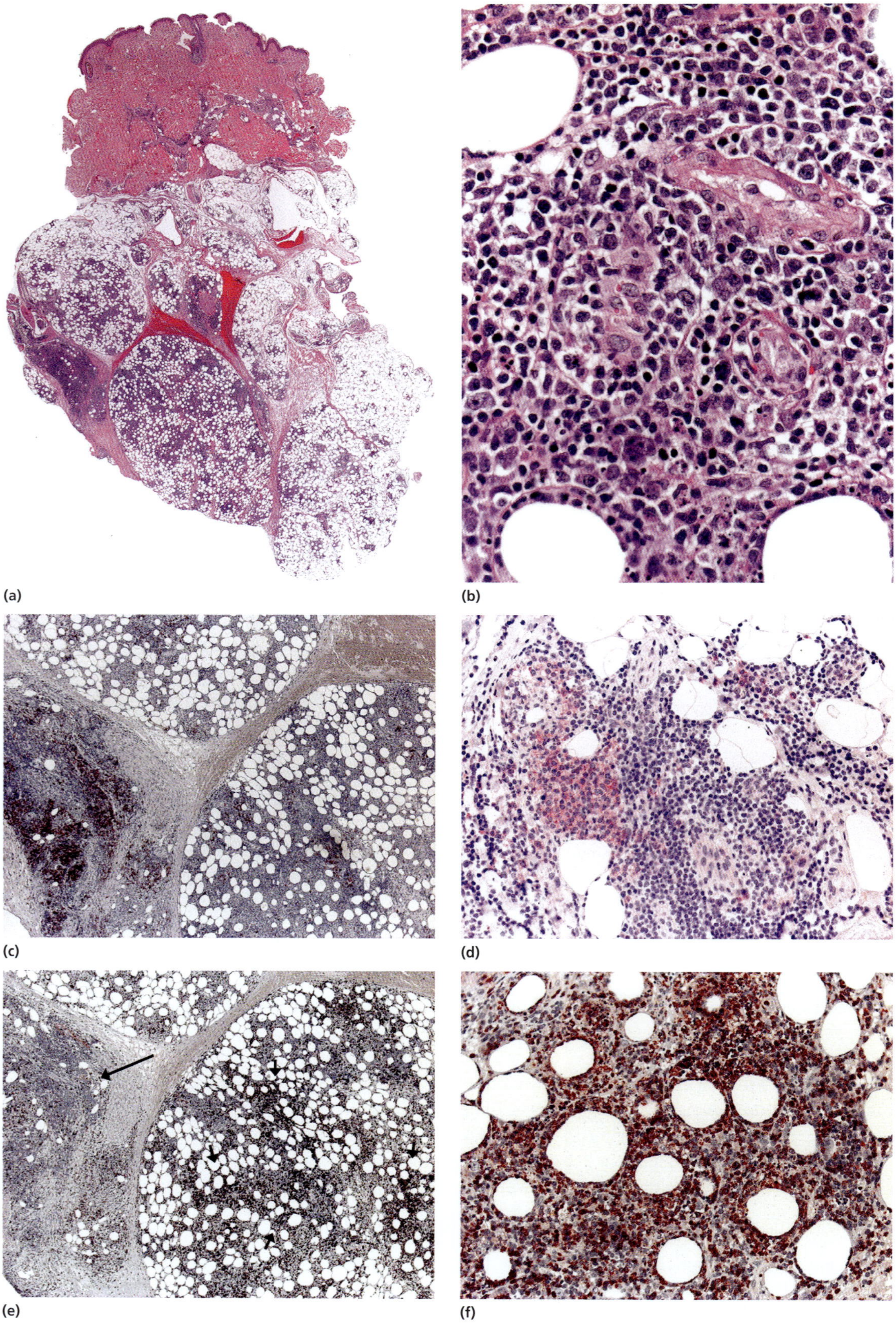

**Figure 6.14** Overlapping histopathological features of subcutaneous panniculitis-like T-cell lymphoma and lupus panniculitis. (a) Dense lymphoid infiltrates within the subcutaneous tissues. (b) Detail showing clusters of atypical, pleomorphic lymphocytes consistent with a diagnosis of subcutaneous panniculitis-like T-cell lymphoma. (c) Staining for CD20 shows several clusters of positive cells, a finding typical of lupus panniculitis. (d) Staining for CD123 reveals clusters of positive plasmacytoid dendritic cells, again consistent with lupus panniculitis. (e) Staining for Ki-67 shows areas with high proliferation and proliferating rimming lymphocytes (short arrows), and another area with low proliferation (long arrow). (f) Staining for TIA-1 confirms the cytotoxic phenotype in the area with high proliferation.

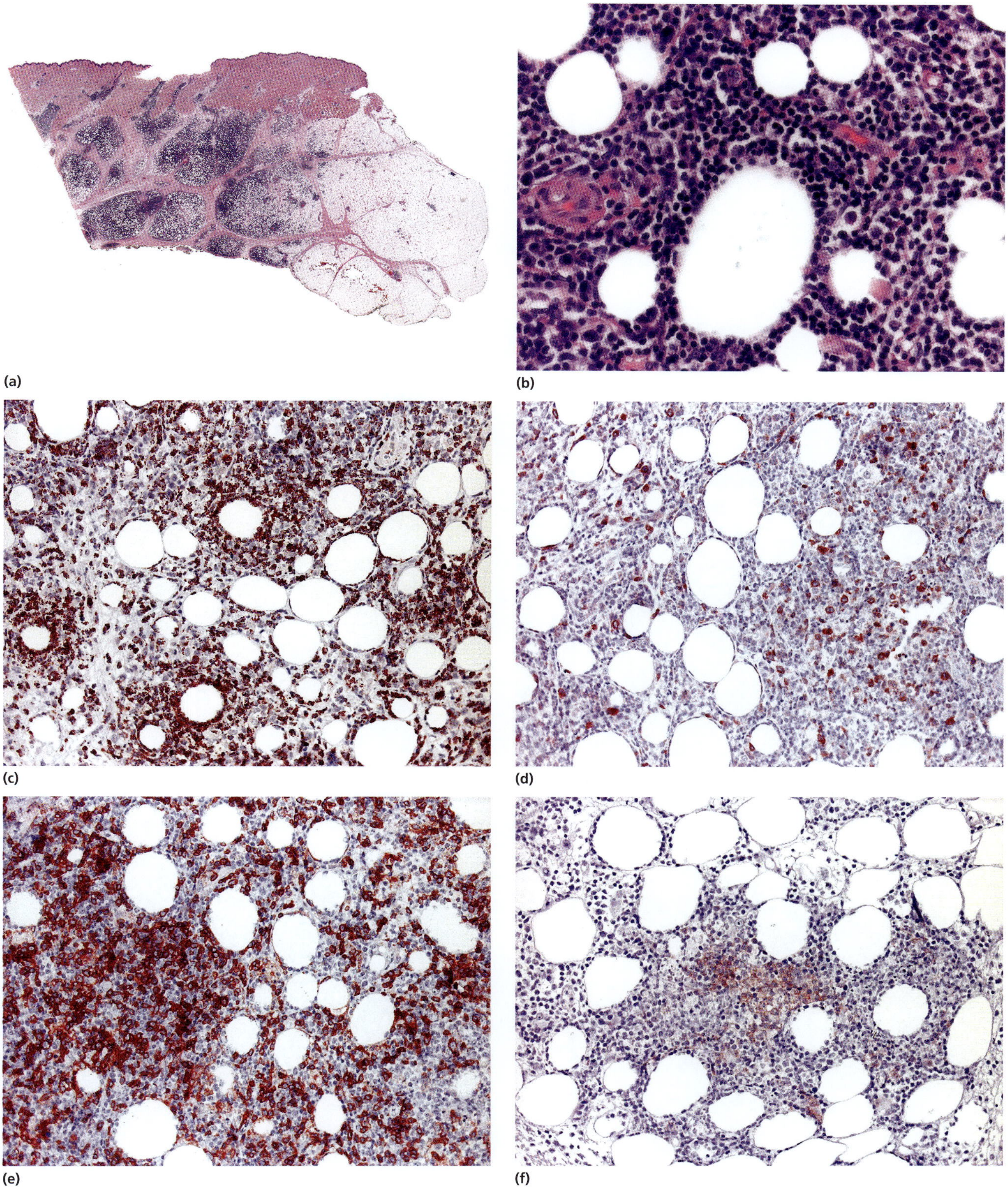

**Figure 6.15** A 45-year-old woman presented with a solitary subcutaneous nodule on the right arm for the last few months. There was neither relevant history nor any associated disease. Histology showed (a) a "panniculitic-like" infiltrate with few aggregates of dermal lymphocytes, (b) consisting mostly of small lymphocytes with "rimming" of adipocytes. Many cells were positive for CD8 and βF1, and (c) expressed TIA1. (d) A few cells positive for TCR-γ were also present, as well as (e) several $CD4^+$ T lymphocytes and (f) small clusters of $CD123^+$ plasmacytoid dendritic cells. A diagnosis of atypical lobular panniculitis was made. Staging investigations were negative. According to patient's wish, a complete surgical excision was performed. She presented again 14, 16, and 17 years later with new nodules on the upper extremities, which she always let be managed surgically. The biopsy performed 17 years after the first one revealed again (g) a lobular panniculitis-like lymphocytic infiltrate with (h) morphologic features similar to the original biopsy. Repeated immunohistologic investigations showed a similar phenotype as that of 17 years before with (i) strong positivity for CD8, and presence of $CD4^+$ T cells and (j) of large clusters of $CD123^+$ plasmacytoid dendritic cells. This time clusters of $CD20^+$ B lymphocytes (k) could be observed as well. The proliferation rate (Ki-67) (l) was focally increased. Repeated staging did not reveal extracutaneous involvement. Comment: This case exemplifies the characteristic history of "atypical lobular panniculitis" showing overlapping histopathological features of lupus panniculitis and subcutaneous panniculitis-like T-cell lymphoma. I consider such cases as examples of "atypical" lupus panniculitis, supported by (a) focal involvement of the dermis; (b) presence of clusters of $CD123^+$ plasmacytoid dendritic cells; (c) presence of many $CD4^+$ T lymphocytes, and (d) presence of clusters of B lymphocytes. However, patients presenting with similar lesions should be followed-up regularly, as the potential for progression into overt lymphoma is yet uncertain.

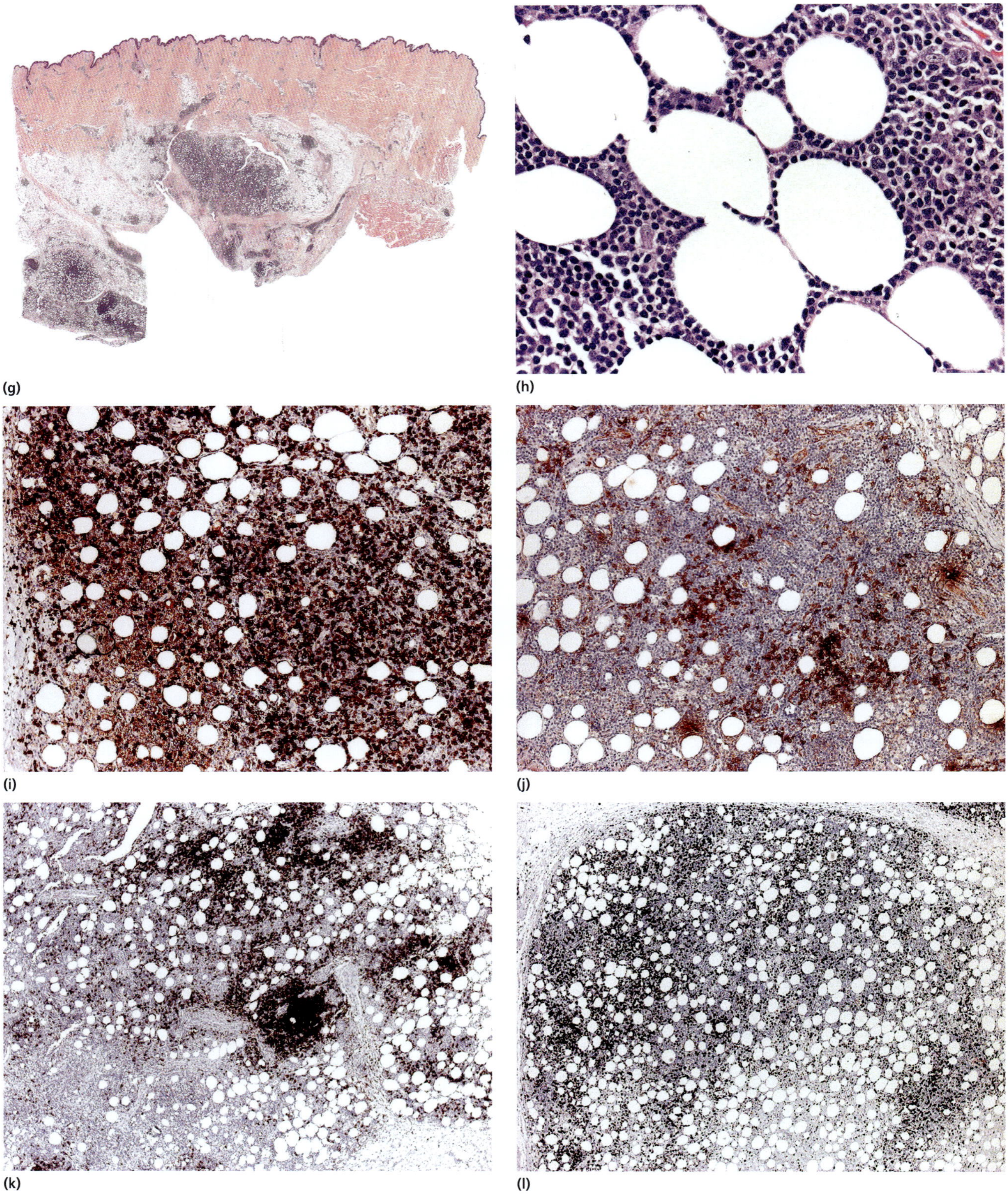


Figure 6.15 (Continued)

as an option for pediatric cases [75]. Treatment with ruxolitinib, a selective JAK1/JAK2 inhibitor, has showed promising results in cases characterized by hemophagocytic syndrome [76].

Systemic chemotherapy (CHOP or other schemes) has been used, but should be considered only for recalcitrant lesions that do not respond to less aggressive treatments, for progressive disease, or for cases associated with hemophagocytic syndrome [8, 14]. A study reported that systemic chemotherapy was necessary in 80% of cases in Japanese patients [77], but this percentage seems very high based on my own experience and on survey of the literature. Some reports have highlighted the efficacy of autologous or allogeneic bone marrow/stem cell transplantation [78–81]. Such an aggressive therapeutic option should be considered only for the management of patients with progressive disease and extracutaneous involvement.

## Prognosis

Subcutaneous panniculitis-like T-cell lymphoma is an indolent lymphoma with good prognosis and a five-year overall survival of over 80% [1, 8, 28, 82]. The onset of a hemophagocytic syndrome is a bad prognostic sign [8], and the presence of angiotropism has been recognized as a bad prognostic marker in one Chinese study [83].

Once again, it should be remembered that exact appreciation of the prognosis of cases reported in the past as "subcutaneous T-cell lymphoma" is hindered by the lack of proper phenotypic investigations and by the inclusion in the group of subcutaneous panniculitis-like T-cell lymphoma of cases that in modern classifications would be placed in different categories.

### Résumé

| | | |
|---|---|---|
| **Subcutaneous panniculitis-like T-cell lymphoma** | | |
| **Clinical** | Adults, rarely children. Localized or generalized subcutaneous ("panniculitic") erythematous plaques and tumors arising preferentially on the extremities. Usually protracted course. In some patients, a hemophagocytic syndrome occurs (more frequent in Asiatic patients). | |
| **Morphology** | Dense, nodular, or diffuse infiltrates within the subcutaneous fat. "Rimming" of adipocytes by neoplastic lymphocytes. Cytomorphology characterized by small- to medium-sized and (rarely) large pleomorphic cells. Necrosis may be present in late lesions. | |
| **Immunohistochemistry** | CD2, CD3, CD5 | + |
| | CD8 | + ***(essential criterion)*** |
| | TIA-1, granzyme-B, perforin | + |
| | βF1 | + ***(essential criterion)*** |
| | TCR-γ, TCR-δ | – ***(essential criterion)*** |
| | CD4, CD30, CD56 | – |
| | Ki-67 | "hot-spots," periadipocyte positivity |
| | CD123 | – |
| **Genetics** | Monoclonal rearrangement of the TCR genes detected in the majority of the cases. Germline mutations in *HAVCR2* are frequently associated with hemophagocytic syndrome. | |
| **Treatment guidelines** | Systemic steroids; immunosuppressive regimens; systemic chemotherapy only in cases with extracutaneous involvement or in cases with hemophagocytic syndrome. | |

## References

1. Willemze R, Cerroni L, Kempf W, *et al.* The 2018 update of the WHO-EORTC classification for primary cutaneous lymphomas. *Blood* 2019;**133**:1703–1714.
2. Kempf W, Mitteldorf C, Cerroni L, *et al.* Classifications of cutaneous lymphomas and lymphoproliferative disorders: an update from the EORTC cutaneous lymphoma histopathology group. *J Eur Acad Dermatol Venereol* 2024;**38**:1491–1503.
3. Gaulard P, Goodlad JR, Pro B. Subcutaneous panniculitis-like T-cell lymphoma. In: Arber DA, Borowitz MJ, Cook JR, *et al.*, eds. *The International Consensus Classification of Myeloid and Lymphoid Neoplasms.* Philadelphia (US): Wolters Kluwer, 2025: 697–701.
4. Guitart J, Jeon YK, Pulitzer M, Willemze R. Subcutaneous panniculitis-like T-cell lymphoma. In: *WHO Classification of Tumours Editorial Board. Haematolymphoid Tumours.* 5th edition. Lyon (France): IARC, 2024: 700–701.
5. Pruksaeakanan C, Teyateeti P, Patthamalai P, *et al.* Primary cutaneous lymphomas in Thailand: a 10-year retrospective study. *Biomed Res Int* 2021;**2021**:4057661.
6. Pick W. Über die persistierende Form des Erythema nodosum. *Arch Dermatol Syphil* 1904;**72**:361–372.
7. Massone C, Lozzi GP, Egberts F, *et al.* The protean spectrum of non-Hodgkin lymphomas with prominent involvement of subcutaneous fat. *J Cutan Pathol* 2006;**33**:418–425.
8. Willemze R, Jansen PM, Cerroni L, *et al.* Subcutaneous panniculitis like T-cell lymphoma: definition, classification, and prognostic

factors: an EORTC Cutaneous Lymphoma Group Study of 83 cases. *Blood* 2008;**111**:838–845.

9. Winkelmann RK, Bowie EJW. Hemorrhagic diathesis associated with benign histiocytic, cytophagic panniculitis and systemic histiocytosis. *Arch Intern Med* 1980;**140**:1460–1463.
10. Alegre VA, Winkelmann RK. Histiocytic cytophagic panniculitis. *J Am Acad Dermatol* 1989;**20**:177–185.
11. Hytiroglou P, Phelps RG, Wattenberg DJ, Strauchen JA. Histiocytic cytophagic panniculitis: molecular evidence for a clonal T-cell disorder. *J Am Acad Dermatol* 1992;**27**:333–336.
12. Craig AJ, Cualing H, Thomas G, *et al.* Cytophagic histiocytic panniculitis: a syndrome associated with benign and malignant panniculitis – case comparison and review of the literature. *J Am Acad Dermatol* 1998;**39**:721–736.
13. Kim YC, Kim SC, Yang WI, *et al.* Extranodal NK/T-cell lymphoma with extensive subcutaneous involvement, mimicking subcutaneous panniculitis-like T cell lymphoma. *Int J Dermatol* 2002;**41**:919–921.
14. Santucci M, Pimpinelli N, Massi D, *et al.* Cytotoxic natural killer cell cutaneous lymphomas: report of the EORTC cutaneous lymphoma task force workshop. *Cancer* 2003;**97**:610–627.
15. White JW Jr, Winkelmann RK. Weber–Christian panniculitis: a review of 30 cases with this diagnosis. *J Am Acad Dermatol* 1998;**39**:56–62.
16. Hoque SR, Child FJ, Whittaker SJ, *et al.* Subcutaneous panniculitis-like T-cell lymphoma: a clinicopathological, immunophenotypic and molecular analysis of six patients. *Br J Dermatol* 2003;**148**:516–525.
17. Cerroni L. Subcutaneous immunocytoma. *Dermatopathol Pract Concept* 2000;**6**:87–88.
18. Marzano AV, Alessi E, Berti E. CD30-positive multilobated peripheral T-cell lymphoma primarily involving the subcutaneous tissue. *Am J Dermatopathol* 1997;**19**:284–288.
19. Salhany KE, MacOn WR, Choi JK, *et al.* Subcutaneous panniculitis-like T-cell lymphoma: clinicopathologic, immunophenotypic, and genotypic analysis of alpha/beta and gamma/delta subtypes. *Am J Surg Pathol* 1998;**22**:881–893.
20. Laggis C, Miles R, Stephens DM, *et al.* Cutaneous mantle cell lymphoma histomorphologically mimicking subcutaneous panniculitis-like T-cell lymphoma: case report. *J Cutan Pathol* 2019;**46**:538–541.
21. Kinney MC. The role of morphologic features, phenotype, genotype, and anatomic site in defining extranodal T-cell or NK-cell neoplasms. *Am J Clin Pathol* 1999;**111**:S104–S118.
22. Proctor MS, Price NM, Cox AJ, Hoppe RT. Subcutaneous mycosis fungoides. *Arch Dermatol* 1978;**114**:1326–1328.
23. Magro CM, Crowson AN, Kovatich AJ, Burns F. Lupus profundus, indeterminate lymphocytic lobular panniculitis and subcutaneous T-cell lymphoma: a spectrum of subcuticular T-cell lymphoid dyscrasia. *J Cutan Pathol* 2001;**28**:235–247.
24. Michot C, Costes V, Gerard-Dran D, *et al.* Subcutaneous panniculitis-like T-cell lymphoma in a patient receiving etanercept for rheumatoid arthritis. *Br J Dermatol* 2009;**160**:889–890.
25. Berg KD, Brinster NK, Huhn KM, *et al.* Transmission of a T-cell lymphoma by allogeneic bone marrow transplantation. *N Engl J Med* 2001;**345**:1458–1463.
26. Bragman SG, Yeaney GA, Greig BW, *et al.* Subcutaneous panniculitic T-cell lymphoma in a cardiac allograft recipient. *J Cutan Pathol* 2005;**32**:366–370.
27. Magro CM, Wang X. CCL5 expression in panniculitic T-cell dyscrasias and its potential role in adipocyte tropism. *Am J Dermatopathol* 2013;**35**:332–337.
28. Fink-Puches R, Zenahlik P, Bäck B, *et al.* Primary cutaneous lymphomas: applicability of current classification schemes (European Organization for Research and Treatment of Cancer, World Health Organization) based on clinicopathologic features observed in a large group of patients. *Blood* 2002;**99**:800–805.
29. Rutnin S, Porntharukcharoen S, Boonsakan P. Clinicopathologic, immunophenotypic, and molecular analysis of subcutaneous panniculitis-like T-cell lymphoma: a retrospective study in a tertiary care center. *J Cutan Pathol* 2019;**46**:44–51.
30. Taniguchi S, Kono T. Subcutaneous T-cell lymphoma in a child with eosinophilia. *Br J Dermatol* 2000;**142**:183–184.
31. Shani-Adir A, Lucky AW, Prendiville J, *et al.* Subcutaneous panniculitic T-cell lymphoma in children: response to combination therapy with cyclosporine and chemotherapy. *J Am Acad Dermatol* 2004;**50**:s18–s22.
32. Huppmann AR, Xi L, Raffeld M, *et al.* Subcutaneous panniculitis-like T-cell lymphoma in the pediatric age group: a lymphoma of low malignant potential. *Pediatr Blood Cancer* 2013;**60**:1165–1170.
33. Hu ZL, Sang H, Deng L, Li ZH. Subcutaneous panniculitis-like T-cell lymphoma in children: a review of the literature. *Ped Dermatol* 2015;**32**:526–532.
34. Koh MJA, Sadarangani SP, Chan YC, *et al.* Aggressive subcutaneous panniculitis-like T-cell lymphoma with hemophagocytosis in two children (subcutaneous panniculitis-like T-cell lymphoma). *J Am Acad Dermatol* 2009;**61**:875–881.
35. Oschlies I, Simonitsch-Klupp I, Maldyk J, *et al.* Subcutaneous panniculitis-like T-cell lymphoma in children: a detailed clinicopathological description of 11 multifocal cases with a high frequency of haemophagocytic syndrome. *Br J Dermatol* 2015;**172**:793–797.
36. Gao J, Gauerke SJ, Martinez-Escala ME, *et al.* Bone marrow involvement by subcutaneous Panniculitis-like T-cell lymphoma: a report of three cases. *Mod Pathol* 2014;**27**:800–807.
37. Török L, Gurbity TP, Kirschner A, Krenacs L. Panniculitis-like T-cell lymphoma clinically manifested as alopecia. *Br J Dermatol* 2002;**147**:785–788.
38. Weenig RH, Su WPD. Subcutaneous panniculitis-like T-cell lymphoma presenting as venous stasis ulceration. *Int J Dermatol* 2006;**45**:1083–1085.
39. Perniciaro C, Zalla MJ, White JW Jr, Menke DM. Subcutaneous T cell lymphoma: report of two additional cases and further observations. *Arch Dermatol* 1993;**129**:1171–1176.
40. Nishie W, Yokota K, Sawamura D, *et al.* Detection of circulating lymphoma cells in subcutaneous panniculitis-like T-cell lymphoma. *Br J Dermatol* 2003;**149**:1081–1082.
41. Yi L, Qun S, Wenjie Z, *et al.* The presenting manifestations of subcutaneous panniculitis-like T-cell lymphoma and T-cell lymphoma and cutaneous $\gamma/\delta$ T-cell lymphoma may mimic those of rheumatic diseases: a report of 11 cases. *Clin Rheumatol* 2013;**32**:1169–1175.
42. Pincus LB, LeBoit PE, McCalmont TH, *et al.* Subcutaneous panniculitis-like T-cell lymphoma with overlapping clinicopathologic features of lupus erythematosus: coexistence of 2 entities? *Am J Dermatopathol* 2009;**31**:520–526.

43. Sonigo G, Battistella M, Beylot-Berry M, *et al.* HAVCR2 mutations are associated with severe hemophagocytic syndrome in subcutaneous panniculitis-like T-cell lymphoma. *Blood* 2020;**135**:1058–1061.
44. Koh J, Jang I, Moon S, *et al.* Genetic profiles of subcutaneous panniculitis-like T-cell lymphoma and clinicopathological impact of *HAVCR2* mutations. *Blood Adv* 2021;**5**:3919–3930.
45. Lee DE, Martinez-Escala ME, Serrano LM, *et al.* Hemophagocytic lymphohistiocytosis in cutaneous T-cell lymphoma. *JAMA Dermatol* 2018;**154**:828–831.
46. Weenig RH, Ng CS, Perniciaro C. Subcutaneous panniculitis-like T-cell lymphoma. An elusive case presenting as lipomembranous panniculitis and a review of 72 cases in the literature. *Am J Dermatopathol* 2001;**23**:206–215.
47. Lozzi GP, Massone C, Citarella L, *et al.* Rimming of adipocytes by neoplastic lymphocytes. A histopathologic feature not restricted to subcutaneous T-cell lymphoma. *Am J Dermatopathol* 2006; **28**:9–12.
48. Szablewski V, Costes-Martineau V, René C, *et al.* Composite cutaneous lymphoma of diffuse large B-cell lymphoma-leg type and subcutaneous panniculitis-like T-cell lymphoma. *J Cutan Pathol* 2018;**45**:716–720.
49. Guitart J, Martinez-Escala ME. Gamma/delta T-cell in cutaneous and subcutaneous lymphoid infiltrates: malignant or not? *J Cutan Pathol* 2016;**43**:1242–1244.
50. Soylui S, Gul U, Kilic A, *et al.* A case with an indolent course of subcutaneous panniculitis-like T-cell lymphoma demonstrating Epstein–Barr virus positivity and simulating dermatitis artefacta. *Am J Clin Dermatol* 2010;**11**:147–150.
51. Gayden T, Sepulveda FE, Khuong-Quang DA, *et al.* Germline HAVCR2 mutations altering TIM-3 characterize subcutaneous panniculitis-like T cell lymphomas with hemophagocytic lymphohistiocytic syndrome. *Nat Genet* 2018;**50**:1650–1657.
52. Polprasert C, Takeuchi Y, Kakiuchi N, *et al.* Frequent germline mutations of HAVCR2 in sporadic subcutaneous panniculitis-like T-cell lymphoma. *Blood Adv* 2019;**3**:588–595.
53. Liu L, Sardana R, Nemirovsky D, *et al.* Somatic mutations in FAS pathway increase hemophagocytic lymphohistiocytosis risk in patients with T- and/or NK-cell lymphoma. *Blood Adv* 2024;**8**: 3064–3075.
54. Okamura Y, Makishima K, Suehara Y, *et al.* Genetic profiles and clinical features in subcutaneous panniculitis-like T-cell lymphomas. *Cancer Sci* 2024;**115**:3788–3794.
55. Hahtola S, Burghart E, Jeskanen L, *et al.* Clinicopathological characterization and genomic aberrations in subcutaneous panniculitis-like T-cell lymphoma. *J Invest Dermatol* 2008;**128**:2304–2309.
56. Li Z, Lu L, Zhou Z, *et al.* Recurrent mutations in epigenetic modifiers and the PI3K/AKT/mTOR pathway in subcutaneous panniculitis-like T-cell lymphoma. *Br J Haematol* 2018;**181**: 406–410.
57. Machan S, Rodríguez M, Manso R, *et al.* Different mutational profiles of subcutaneous panniculitis-like T-cell lymphoma and lupus panniculitis: an additional case series. *Actas Dermosifiliogr* 2025;**116**(3):210–217.
58. Massone C, Kodama K, Salmhofer W, *et al.* Lupus erythematosus panniculitis (lupus profundus): clinical, histopathological, and molecular analysis of nine cases. *J Cutan Pathol* 2005;**32**:396–404.
59. LeBlanc RE, Tavallaee M, Kim YH, Kim J. Useful parameters for distinguishing subcutaneous panniculitis-like T-cell lymphoma from lupus erythematosus panniculitis. *Am J Surg Pathol* 2016;**40**:745–754.
60. Wong J, Roy SF, McNiff JM, Xu ML. IRF8 in conjunction with CD123 and CD20 to distinguish lupus erythematosus panniculitis from subcutaneous panniculitis-like T-cell lymphoma. *Am J Surg Pathol* 2023;**47**:1425–1431.
61. Sitthinamsuwan P, Pattanaprichakul P, Treetipsatit J, *et al.* Subcutaneous panniculitis-like T-cell lymphoma versus lupus erythematosus panniculitis: distinction by means of the periadipocytic cell proliferation index. *Am J Dermatopathol* 2018;**40**:567–574.
62. Liau JY, Chuang SS, Chu CA, *et al.* The presence of clusters of plasmacytoid dendritic cells is a helpful feature for differentiating lupus panniculitis from subcutaneous panniculitis-like T-cell lymphoma. *Histopathology* 2013;**62**:1057–1066.
63. Chen SJT, Tse JY, Harms PW, *et al.* Utility of CD123 immunohistochemistry in differentiating lupus erythematosus from cutaneous T cell lymphoma. *Histopathology* 2019;**74**:908–916.
64. Fernandez-Pol S, De Stefano D, Kim J. Immunohistochemistry reveals an increased proportion of MYC-positive cells in subcutaneous panniculitis-like T-cell lymphoma compared with lupus panniculitis. *J Cutan Pathol* 2017;**44**:925–930.
65. Bosisio F, Boi S, Caputo V, *et al.* Lobular panniculitic infiltrates with overlapping histopathologic features of lupus panniculitis (lupus profundus) and subcutaneous T-cell lymphoma A conceptual and practical dilemma. *Am J Surg Pathol* 2015; **39**:206–211.
66. Guenova E, Schanz S, Hoetzenecker W, *et al.* Systemic corticosteroids for subcutaneous panniculitis-like T-cell lymphoma. *Br J Dermatol* 2014;**171**:891–894.
67. Dippel E, Assaf C, Becker JC, *et al.* S2k-guidelines – cutaneous lymphomas (ICD10 C82-C86): update 2021. *J Dtsch Dermatol Ges* 2022;**20**:537–555.
68. Tsukamoto Y, Katsumobu Y, Omura Y, *et al.* Subcutaneous panniculitis-like T-cell lymphoma: successful initial treatment with prednisolone and cyclosporin A. *Intern Med* 2006;**45**:21–24.
69. Briki H, Bouaziz JD, Molinier-Frenkel V, *et al.* Subcutaneous panniculitis-like T-cell lymphoma α/β: complete sustained remission with corticosteroids and methotrexate. *Br J Dermatol* 2010; **163**:1136–1138.
70. Tauro S, MacCallum S, Groves MJ, *et al.* Immunohistochemical localization of cellular NFATc1 does not predict clinical responses to cyclosporine in subcutaneous panniculitis-like T-cell non-Hodgkin lymphoma. *Br J Dermatol* 2010;**162**:887–889.
71. Michonneau D, Petrella T, Ortonne N, *et al.* Subcutaneous panniculitis-like T-cell lymphoma: immunosuppressive drugs induce better response than polychemotherapy. *Acta Derm Venereol* 2017;**97**:358–364.
72. Willemze R, Hodak E, Zinzani PL, *et al.* Primary cutaneous lymphomas: ESMO Clinical Practice Guidelines for diagnosis, treatment and follow-up. *Ann Oncol* 2018;**29**(Supplement 4):iv30–iv40.
73. Duan Y, Gao H, Zhou C, *et al.* A retrospective study of 18 children with subcutaneous panniculitis-like T-cell lymphoma: multidrug combination chemotherapy or immunomodulatory therapy? *Orphanet J Rare Dis* 2022;**17**:432.
74. Koh YK, Yoon SH, Kang SH, *et al.* Immunosuppressive therapy as first-line and relapse treatment in paediatric subcutaneous panniculitis-like T-cell lymphoma. *Br J Haematol* 2025;**206**(4):1233–1236.

75. Johnston EE, LeBlanc RE, Kim J, *et al.* Subcutaneous panniculitis-like T-cell lymphoma: pediatric case series demonstrating heterogeneous presentation and option for watchful waiting. *Pediatr Blood Cancer* 2015;**62**:2025–2028.
76. Levy R, Fusaro M, Guerin F, *et al.* Efficacy of ruxolitinib in subcutaneous panniculitis-like T-cell lymphoma and hemophagocytic lymphohistiocytosis. *Blood Adv* 2020;**4**:1383–1387.
77. Ohtsuka M, Miura T, Yamamoto T. Clinical characteristics, differential diagnosis, and treatment outcome of subcutaneous panniculitis-like T-cell lymphoma: a literature review of published Japanese cases. *Eur J Dermatol* 2017;**27**:34–41.
78. Alaibac M, Berti E, Pigozzi B, *et al.* High-dose chemotherapy with autologous blood stem cell transplantation for aggressive subcutaneous panniculitis-like T-cell lymphoma. *J Am Acad Dermatol* 2005;**52**:s121–s123.
79. Ichii M, Hatanaka K, Imakita M, *et al.* Successful treatment of refractory subcutaneous panniculitis-like T-cell lymphoma with allogeneic peripheral blood stem cell transplantation from HLA-mismatched sibling donor. *Leukem Lymph* 2006;**47**:2250–2252.
80. Perez-Persona E, Mateos-Mazon JJ, Lopez-Villar O, *et al.* Complete remission of subcutaneous panniculitic T-cell lymphoma after allogeneic transplantation. *Bone Marrow Transpl* 2006;**38**:821–822.
81. Nakahashi H, Tsukamoto N, Yamane A, *et al.* Autologous peripheral blood stem cell transplantation to treat CHOP-refractory aggressive subcutaneous panniculitis-like T cell lymphoma. *Acta Haematol* 2009;**121**:239–242.
82. López-Lerma I, Peñate Y, Gallardo F, *et al.* Subcutaneous panniculitis-like T-cell lymphoma: clinical features, therapeutic approach, and outcome in a case series of 16 patients. *J Am Acad Dermatol* 2018;**79**:892–898.
83. Kong YY, Dai B, Kong JC, *et al.* Subcutaneous panniculitis-like T-cell lymphoma. A clinicopathologic, immunophenotypic, and molecular study of 22 Asian cases according to WHO-EORTC classification. *Am J Surg Pathol* 2008;**32**:1495–1502.

## CHAPTER 7

# Primary cutaneous aggressive epidermotropic CD8⁺ cytotoxic T-Cell lymphoma

Primary cutaneous aggressive epidermotropic $CD8^+$ cytotoxic T-cell lymphoma is included as a distinct entity in the International Consensus Classification (ICC) *of Myeloid and Lymphoid Neoplasms*, the 2019 and 2024 updates of classification of cutaneous lymphomas by the European Organization of Research and Treatment of Cancer (EORTC) – Cutaneous Lymphoma Histopathology Group, and the World Health Organization (WHO) *Classification of Haematolymphoid Tumours* [1–4].

Primary cutaneous aggressive epidermotropic $CD8^+$ cytotoxic T-cell lymphoma is a disease characterized by aggressive behavior clinically and proliferation of epidermotropic $CD8^+$ T lymphocytes histopathologically [4–6]. In the past, these cases were classified as either aggressive mycosis fungoides (mycosis fungoides "a tumeur d'emblée") or as generalized pagetoid reticulosis (Ketron–Goodman type). A set of diagnostic criteria for primary cutaneous aggressive epidermotropic $CD8^+$ cytotoxic T-cell lymphoma has been proposed, summarizing clinical, histopathologic, and phenotypic features [7].

Staging of primary cutaneous aggressive epidermotropic $CD8^+$ cytotoxic T-cell lymphoma is performed according to criteria for cutaneous lymphomas other than mycosis fungoides or Sézary syndrome (see Table 1.3 in Chapter 1).

## Clinical features

The disease occurs in adults of both sexes with a slight male predominance [5, 8]. Only a few reports in children exists [9, 10]. Patients present with generalized patches, plaques, and tumors, almost invariably ulcerated (Figs. 7.1 and 7.2). The clinical features are indistinguishable from those observed in patients with cutaneous $\gamma/\delta$ T-cell lymphoma or with advanced mycosis fungoides, and are identical to those reported in the past as "generalized pagetoid reticulosis" (Fig. 7.3). Large ulcerations may resemble clinically pyoderma gangrenosum [11], or at some sites an infectious process (Fig. 7.4). Involvement of the mucosal regions is common [5]. The tumor often spreads to unusual sites such as the lung, testis, and central nervous system, whereas rarely involves the lymph nodes [5].

Early lesions of the disease may show erythema multiforme-like features both clinically and histopathologically, thus representing a pitfall in the diagnosis, but concomitant presence of larger, ulcerated lesions is almost invariable (Fig. 7.5) [12]. A small percentage of patients may present with a "prodromic" phase characterized by psoriasiform skin lesions [13], and cases of cutaneous aggressive epidermotropic $CD8^+$ cytotoxic T-cell lymphoma presenting as "ulcerative psoriasis" have been reported [14]. It should be underlined that, although psoriasis may present rarely with dense, band-like inflammatory infiltrates (see Chapter 31), the presence of atypical cells in a "psoriasiform dermatitis" must always be a reason for great concern and prompt a differential diagnosis with a cutaneous T-cell lymphoma. In some patients, facial lesions may resemble those of adnexotropic mycosis fungoides (Fig. 7.6).

## Histopathology, immunophenotype, and molecular genetics

### Histopathology

Histology reveals a band-like, nodular or diffuse proliferation of lymphocytes with epidermotropism. In biopsies from flat lesions, the infiltrate is superficial, and at scanning, magnification may be misinterpreted as a patch of mycosis fungoides (Fig. 7.7) or even as a lesion of pagetoid reticulosis (Fig. 7.8), but neoplastic cells are usually large and pleomorphic. Spongiosis and intraepidermal vesiculation may be observed (Fig. 7.9). The epidermotropism is variable and may be pagetoid (Fig. 7.10) or only focal (Fig. 7.11). In addition, in spite of the name of this lymphoma, the epidermotropism may be minimal or even be missing in some lesions, especially in advanced stages (Fig. 7.12). In such cases, in order to confirm the diagnosis, a previous or concomitant biopsy with typical features of cutaneous aggressive epidermotropic $CD8^+$ cytotoxic T-cell lymphoma is necessary. As in all aggressive cutaneous lymphomas, invasion and destruction of adnexal skin structures are common, but angiocentricity and angiodestruction are infrequent. In one study, mycosis fungoides-like adnexotropism was found in a distinct proportion of cases, rarely combined with mucin

*Skin Lymphoma: The Illustrated Guide*, Sixth Edition. Lorenzo Cerroni.

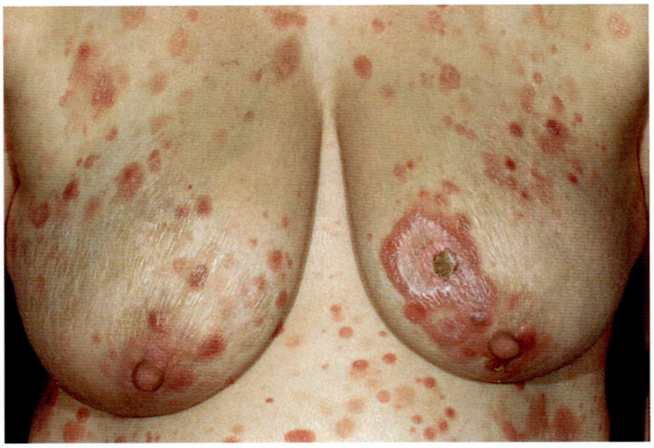

**Figure 7.1** Cutaneous aggressive epidermotropic CD8⁺ cytotoxic T-cell lymphoma. Multiple papules, plaques, and flat tumors, partly ulcerated.

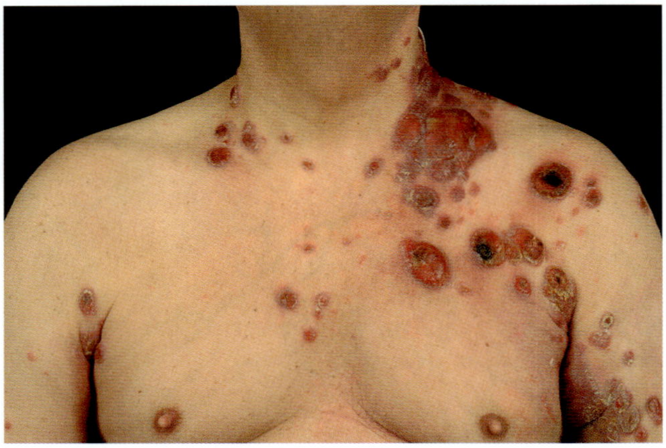

**Figure 7.2** Cutaneous aggressive epidermotropic CD8⁺ cytotoxic T-cell lymphoma. Multiple, partly ulcerated papules, plaques, and tumors on the trunk, neck, and upper extremities.

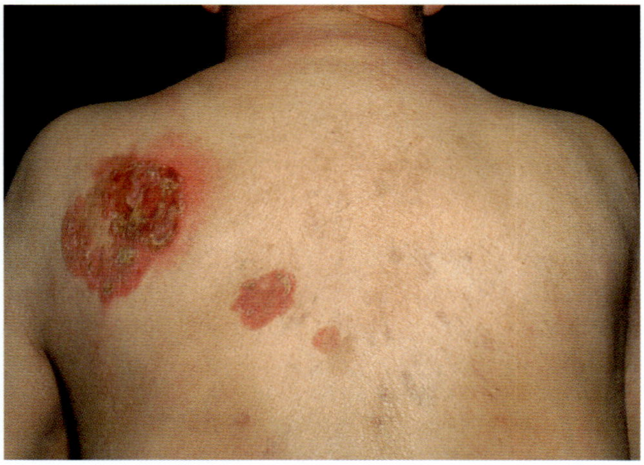

**Figure 7.3** Cutaneous aggressive epidermotropic CD8⁺ cytotoxic T-cell lymphoma. Multiple plaques with large erosions. The clinical presentation was described in the past as generalized pagetoid reticulosis (Ketron–Goodman type).

deposition within the hair follicles (follicular mucinosis) [15], but in my experience, I have never observed classical features of follicular mucinosis similar to pilotropic mycosis fungoides. Cytomorphology is variable and can be characterized by small-, medium-, or large-sized pleomorphic cells. Rare cases may show a predominance of immunoblasts.

One case occurring in a pediatric patient showed marked involvement of the subcutaneous fat mimicking subcutaneous panniculitis-like T-cell lymphoma, in addition to the conventional epidermotropism of $CD8^+$ cells [10].

## Immunophenotype

Immunohistology reveals a characteristic phenotypic profile of neoplastic lymphocytes ($\beta F1^+$, $CD2^-/^+$, $CD3^+$, $CD4^-$, $CD7^+$, $CD8^+$, TIA-$1^+$, granzyme-$B^+$, $perforin^+$, $CD45RA^+$, and $CD45RO^-$) (Figs. 7.13 and 7.14) [5]. Some pan-T-cell markers may be lost. CD30 is usually negative, providing a differential diagnostic clue from lymphomatoid papulosis, type D. I have observed rare cases showing weak positivity of some neoplastic cells for CD30; in these cases, CD30-negativity of many atypical cells, as well as correlation with the clinical picture, are features that allow to rule out lymphomatoid papulosis (Fig. 7.15). In the original description by Berti *et al.*, CD56 was consistently negative [5], but $CD56^+$ cases classified as cutaneous aggressive epidermotropic $CD8^+$ cytotoxic T-cell lymphoma have been described by Santucci *et al.* [16]. However, in this study, cutaneous γ/δ T-cell lymphoma was not included as a specific category, and it may be that these cases represented $CD8^+$ examples of this type of lymphoma. On the other hand, a small percentage of cases reported by Guitart *et al.* were positive for CD56 [13]. In cases with pagetoid epidermotropism, staining for pan-cytokeratins may be helpful in order to highlight the remnants of the epidermis (Fig. 7.16). The Epstein–Barr virus (EBV) is not detectable in neoplastic cells.

In spite of the name of this lymphoma, the CD8 expression may be lacking in some biopsies that show otherwise typical features of cutaneous aggressive epidermotropic $CD8^+$ cytotoxic T-cell lymphoma [13]. In my experience, in some cases, the CD8 expression may be weak rather than really negative (Fig. 7.17), and repeated stainings may show a dim but recognizable positivity; however, exceptional cases characterized by genuine CD8-negativity may be observed (Fig. 7.18). In such cases, diagnosis relies on histopathological features (prominent epidermotropism), expression of cytotoxic proteins, positivity for βF1 and other typical markers of cutaneous aggressive epidermotropic $CD8^+$ cytotoxic T-cell lymphoma, and absence of markers typical of other cutaneous cytotoxic lymphomas (e.g., negativity for TCRγ, TCRδ, and EBV).

## Molecular genetics

Molecular biology shows a monoclonal rearrangement of the T-cell receptor (TCR) genes. Recurrent *JAK2* fusions, leading to activation of the JAK/STAT pathway, were found in a majority

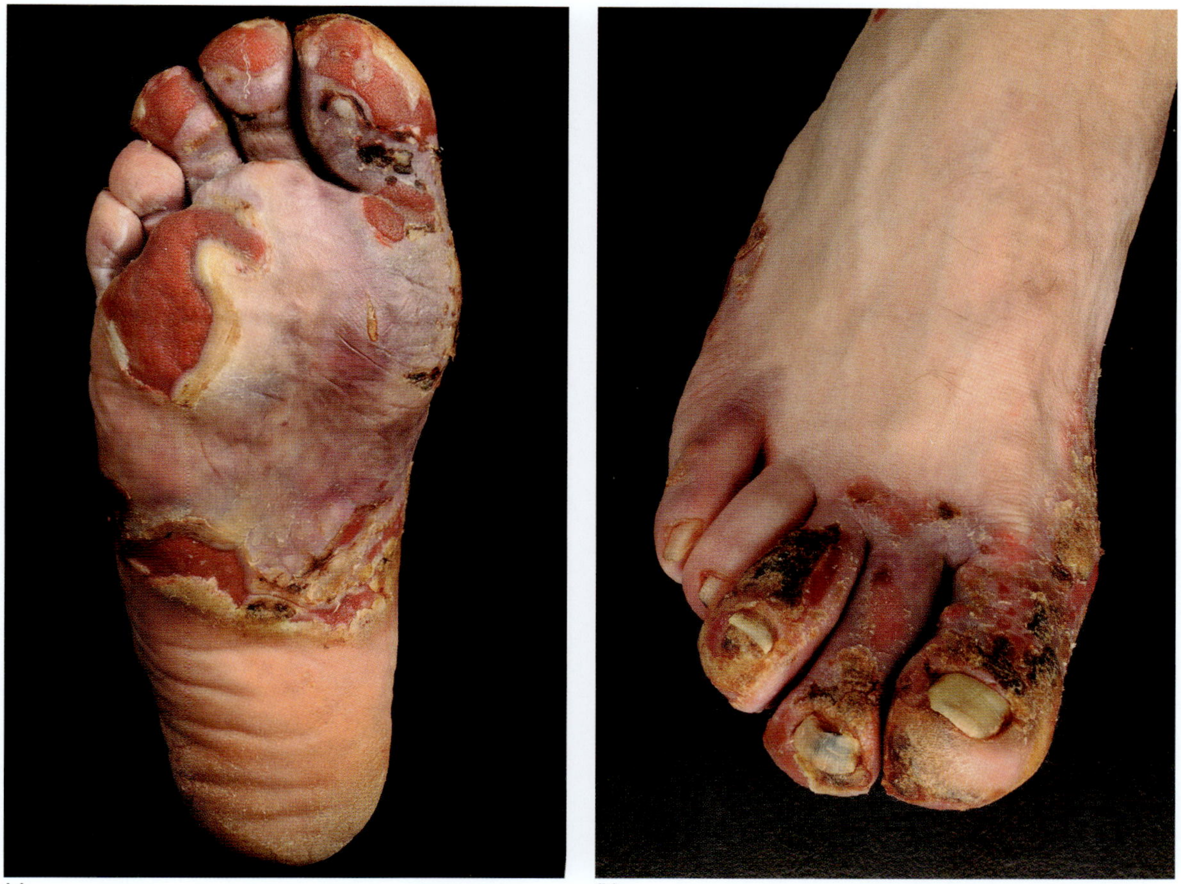

(a) (b)

Figure 7.4 Cutaneous aggressive epidermotropic CD8+ cytotoxic T-cell lymphoma. Large, erosive lesions on the foot involving (a) the sole and (b) most toes, bearing some resemblance to an infectious disorder.

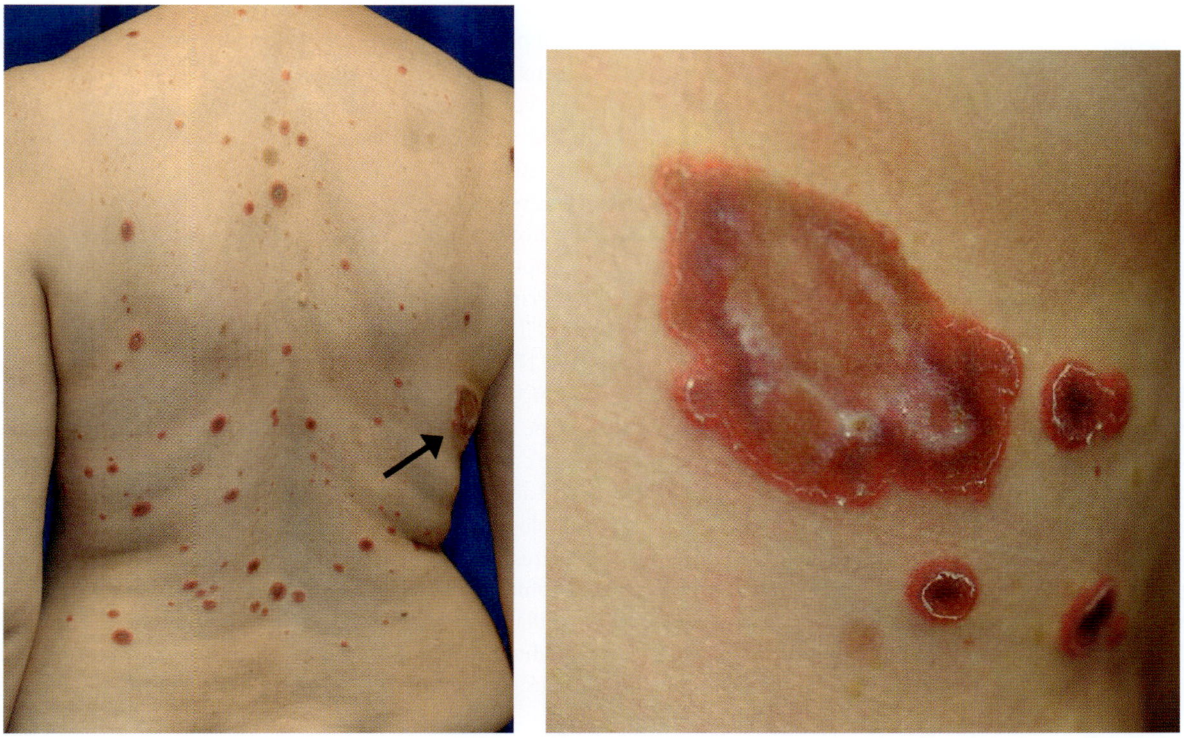

(a) (b)

Figure 7.5 Cutaneous aggressive epidermotropic CD8+ cytotoxic T-cell lymphoma. (a) Early lesions bearing clinically some resemblance to erythema multiforme; note large erosive flat tumor (arrow). (b) Detail of the large lesion surrounded by multiforme-like lesions.

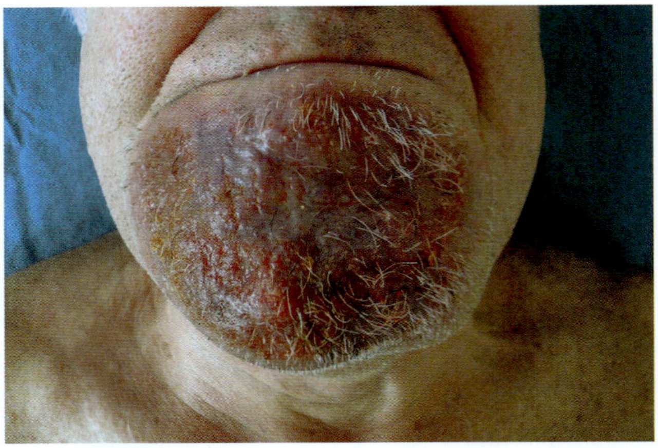

Figure 7.6 Cutaneous aggressive epidermotropic CD8+ cytotoxic T-cell lymphoma. Lesions on the chin mimicking the clinical presentation of adnexotropic mycosis fungoides.

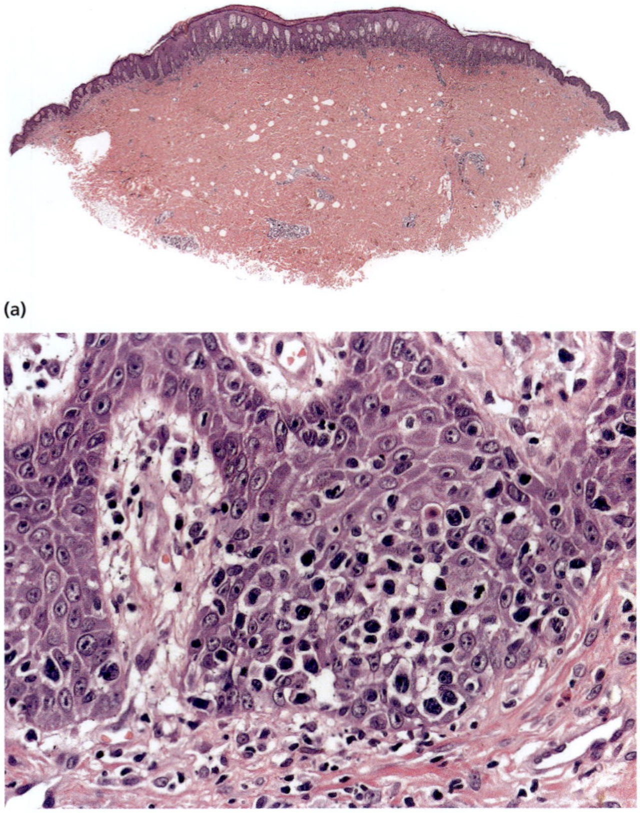

(a)

(b)

Figure 7.7 Cutaneous aggressive epidermotropic CD8+ cytotoxic T-cell lymphoma. (a) Biopsy from an early lesion shows a superficial infiltrate, characterized by (b) prominent epidermotropism of large, pleomorphic lymphocytes.

of cases [17, 18]. The presence of kinase fusions seems to be restricted to primary cutaneous aggressive epidermotropic CD8+ cytotoxic T-cell lymphoma and is not found in other aggressive cutaneous lymphomas with cytotoxic phenotype, potentially implying a role for ruxolitinib or other JAK2 inhibitors in the treatment of the disease [18, 19]. Cases without JAK2 fusions may present other deregulating alterations of JAK2, such as gain-of-function mutations in *JAK2*, *STAT3*, and *STAT5B*, and loss of negative regulators of the JAK/STAT pathway, particularly *SH2B3* [17].

Array comparative genomic hybridization (aCGH) investigations reveal that gains (particularly in 7q, 8q24.3, and 17q) are more frequent than losses (these last being found particularly in chromosome 9p21.3 [*CDKN2A–CDKN2B*], suggesting a role of p16) [20].

## Differential diagnosis from other cutaneous cytotoxic lymphomas

Distinction of primary cutaneous CD8+ epidermotropic aggressive cytotoxic T-cell lymphoma from cases of CD8+ mycosis fungoides and from lymphomatoid papulosis type D is made mainly on the basis of the clinical presentation and behavior. In contrast to mycosis fungoides, patients with primary cutaneous aggressive epidermotropic CD8+ cytotoxic T-cell lymphoma present with plaques and tumors, often ulcerated, at the onset of their disease [5, 7, 21]. Lymphomatoid papulosis type D is characterized by the typical "waxing and waning" of papules and small nodules (see Chapter 5). Primary cutaneous aggressive epidermotropic CD8+ cytotoxic T-cell lymphoma should also be distinguished from acral CD8+ T-cell lymphoma, which is a lymphoproliferative condition showing no epidermotropism and characterized by an indolent behavior (see Chapter 12), and from subcutaneous panniculitis-like T-cell lymphoma, characterized by exclusive involvement of the subcutis by CD8+ neoplastic cells (see Chapter 6). On the other hand, histopathological distinction from CD8+ mycosis fungoides and from lymphomatoid papulosis type D may be impossible on a given biopsy, and correlation with the clinical features is necessary; in general, unlike lymphomatoid papulosis type D, primary cutaneous CD8+ epidermotropic aggressive cytotoxic T-cell lymphoma is negative for CD30. Pediatric patients with a clinical presentation resembling hydroa vacciniforme should be better classified as hydroa vacciniforme-like lymphoproliferative disorder (see Chapter 15).

Primary cutaneous CD8+ epidermotropic aggressive cytotoxic T-cell lymphoma, cutaneous γ/δ T-cell lymphoma, and extranodal NK/T-cell lymphoma, nasal type, show many overlapping clinicopathologic features, and classification may be subjective in some cases. It is important to underline that in cutaneous aggressive cytotoxic lymphomas, cytomorphologic features are variable and are not related to the clinical outcome. In addition, cytomorphological features of primary cutaneous CD8+ epidermotropic aggressive cytotoxic T-cell lymphoma, cutaneous γ/δ T-cell lymphoma, and extranodal NK/T-cell lymphoma, nasal type are similar, and may be characterized by predominance of small-, medium-, or large-sized cells (usually with pleomorphic nuclei). Thus, cytomorphologic aspects are neither useful for a specific

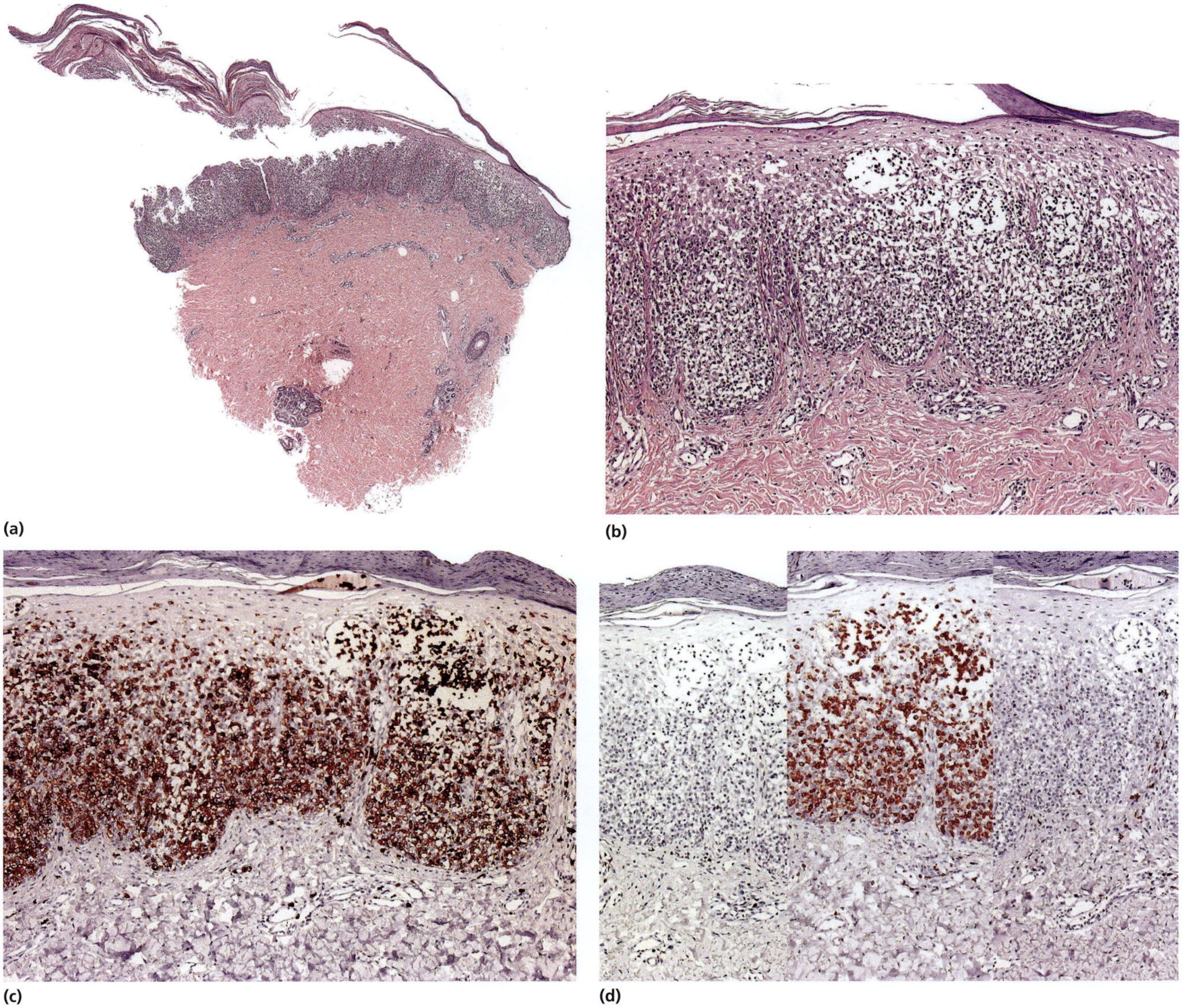

**Figure 7.8** Cutaneous aggressive epidermotropic CD8+ cytotoxic T-cell lymphoma. (a) Epidermotropic infiltrate with (b) histopathological features of pagetoid reticulosis; (c) staining for CD8 shows positivity of all neoplastic cells; (d) expression of CD3 (middle) with loss of CD2 (left) and CD5 (right).

diagnosis and classification of the lymphoma nor are a feature associated with the biologic behavior, and should always be evaluated together with all other clinical, histopathologic, phenotypic, and molecular genetic features.

In most cases, synthesis of all clinicopathologic features allows a precise classification. On the other hand, in spite of extensive phenotypic and genotypic studies, a few cases may defy precise classification. Particularly, the distinction of primary cutaneous aggressive epidermotropic CD8+ cytotoxic T-cell lymphoma from cutaneous γ/δ T-cell lymphoma may be difficult. Cutaneous γ/δ T-cell lymphoma usually shows a more prominent involvement of the subcutaneous fat, and in some cases only limited epidermal involvement. Another differential diagnostic feature is represented by the presence of a marked interface dermatitis-like pattern in some cases of cutaneous γ/δ T-cell lymphoma. With the exception of the expression of α/β T-cell receptors in cutaneous CD8+ epidermotropic aggressive cytotoxic T-cell lymphoma in contrast to γ/δ T-cell receptors in cutaneous γ/δ T-cell lymphoma, other phenotypic features may be overlapping, thus staining for TCR α/β and TCR γ/δ is a prerequisite for the diagnosis. As already mentioned, recurrent *JAK2* fusions seem to be restricted to primary cutaneous CD8+ epidermotropic aggressive cytotoxic T-cell lymphoma [18], thus molecular features may also be useful for the differential diagnosis.

Aggressive cutaneous cytotoxic lymphomas must be distinguished also from secondary cutaneous involvement by primary extracutaneous cytotoxic lymphomas. On the other hand, it should be emphasized that distinguishing between primary and secondary cutaneous involvement is less important for these

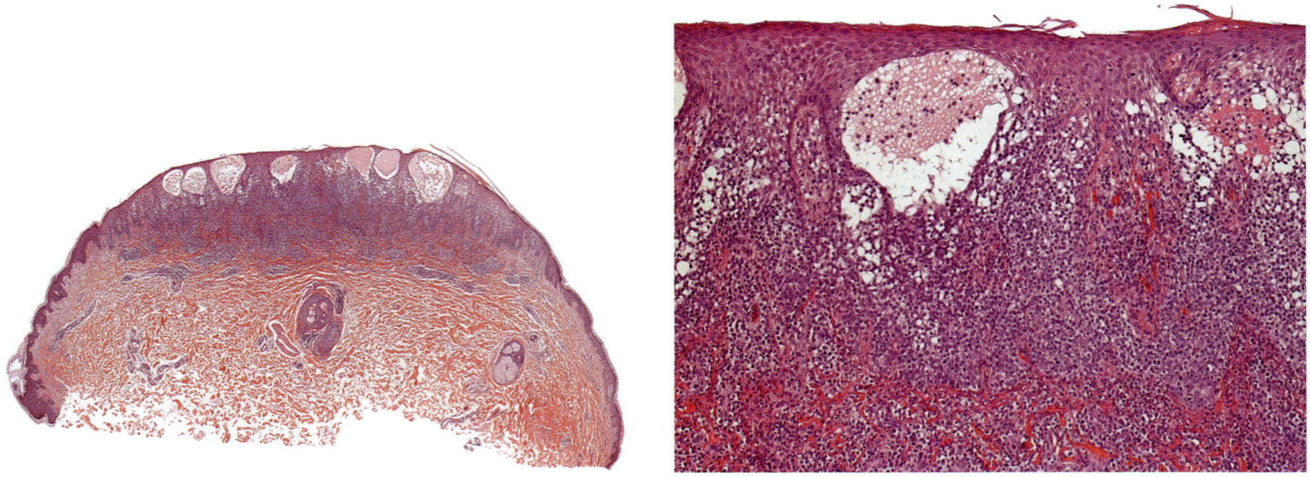

(a) (b)

**Figure 7.9** Cutaneous aggressive epidermotropic CD8⁺ cytotoxic T-cell lymphoma. (a) Epidermotropic infiltrate with prominent intraepidermal vesiculation; (b) detail of the infiltrate with only a few neoplastic cells within the vesicles.

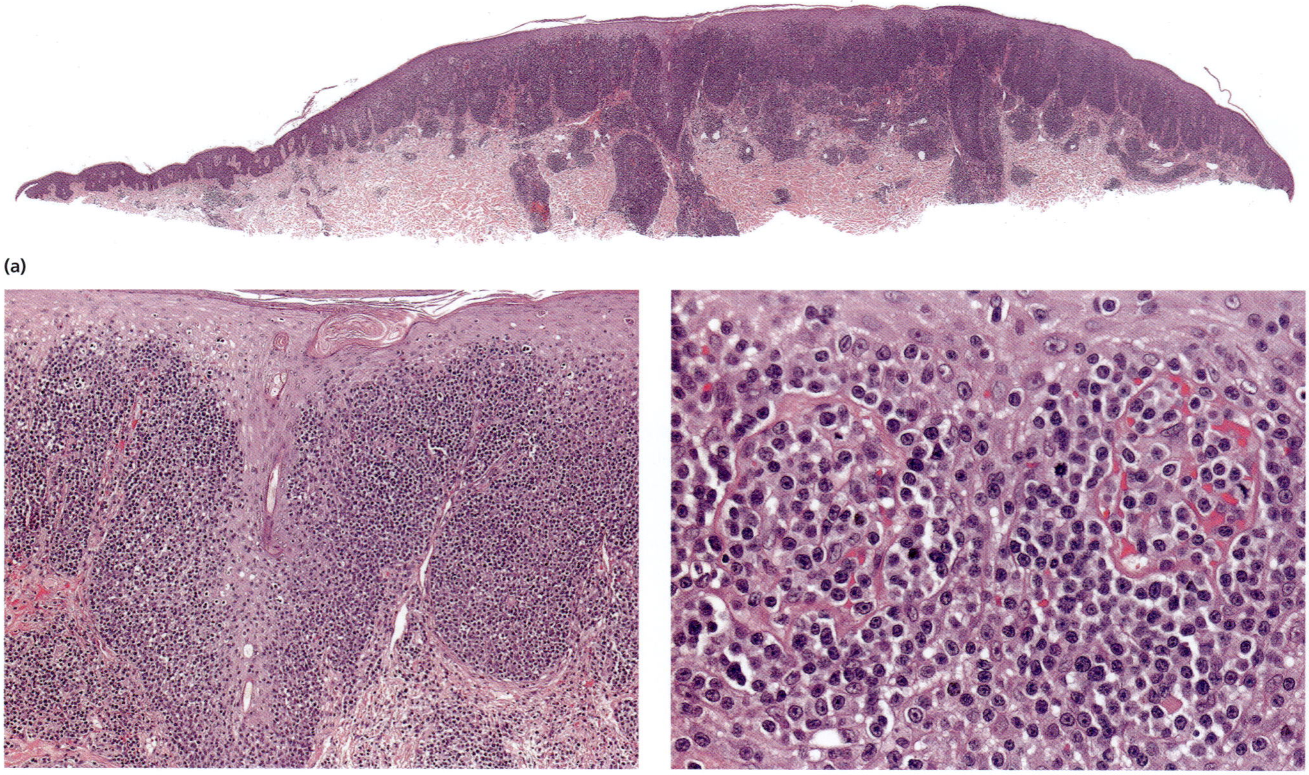

(a) (b) (c)

**Figure 7.10** Cutaneous aggressive epidermotropic CD8⁺ cytotoxic T-cell lymphoma. (a) Dense, band-like infiltrate of lymphocytes. (b) The epidermis is hyperplastic and shows (c) a pagetoid epidermotropism of lymphocytes.

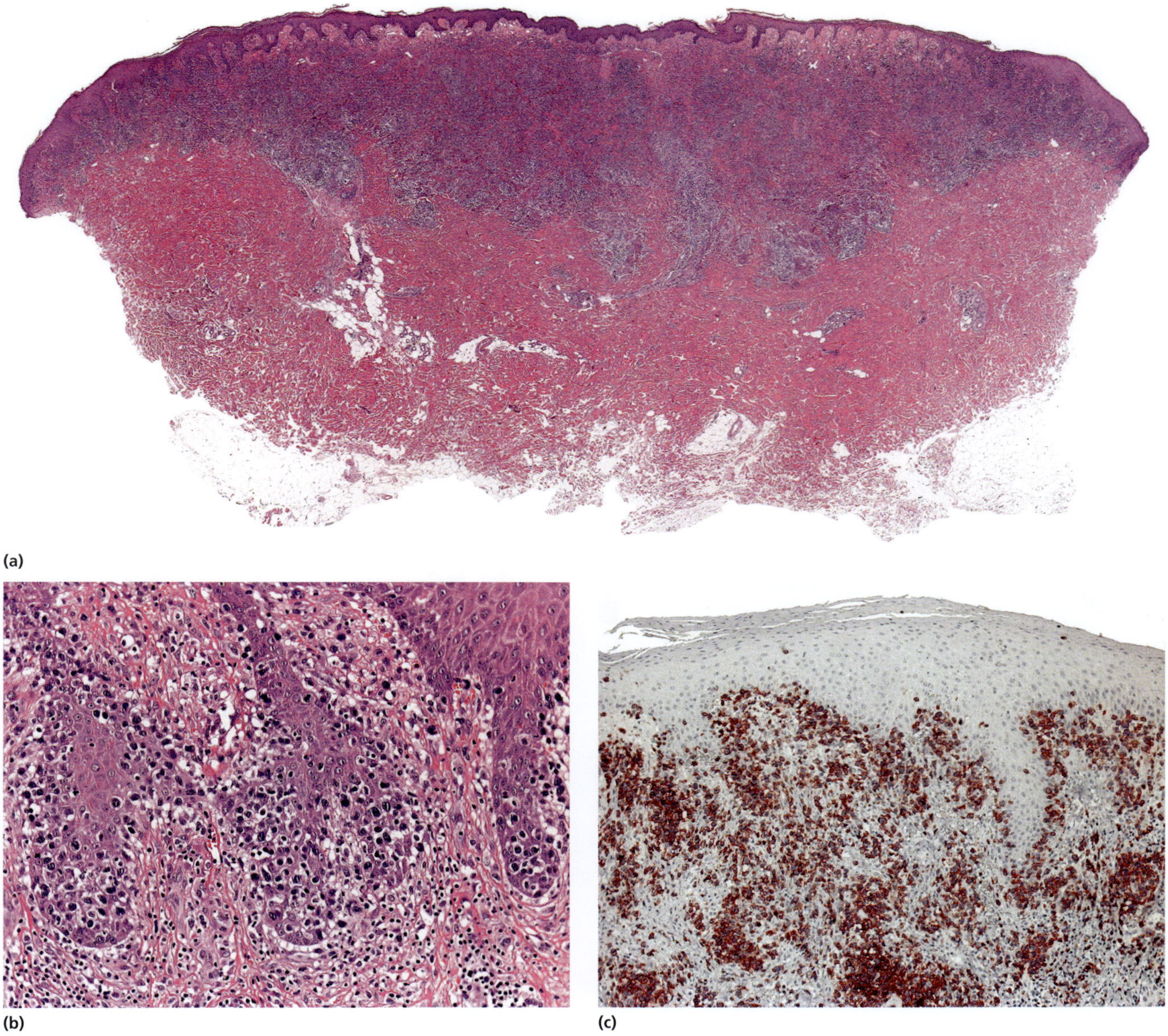

Figure 7.11 Cutaneous aggressive epidermotropic CD8+ cytotoxic T-cell lymphoma. (a) Diffuse infiltrate in the superficial and mid-dermis. (b) Epidermotropic lymphocytes are found only focally on both lateral edges of the lesion, whereas the entire central part is devoid of epidermotropism. (c) Neoplastic cells are strongly positive for CD8.

entities than it is for most other skin lymphomas [8, 22, 23]. In fact, primary cutaneous cases often develop extracutaneous dissemination within a short period of time, and prognosis is usually very poor regardless of the results of staging investigations at presentation. Thus, although staging investigations are mandatory in all of these patients, treatment should be aggressive even in cases with disease limited to the skin.

## Treatment

As the disease is very rare, data on therapy are lacking, and double-blinded studies have not been carried out. At present, the treatment of choice is systemic chemotherapy. Due to the common presence of *JAK2* fusions, *JAK2* inhibitors such as ruxolitinib may be used [19]. One patient with a FGFR1 fusion

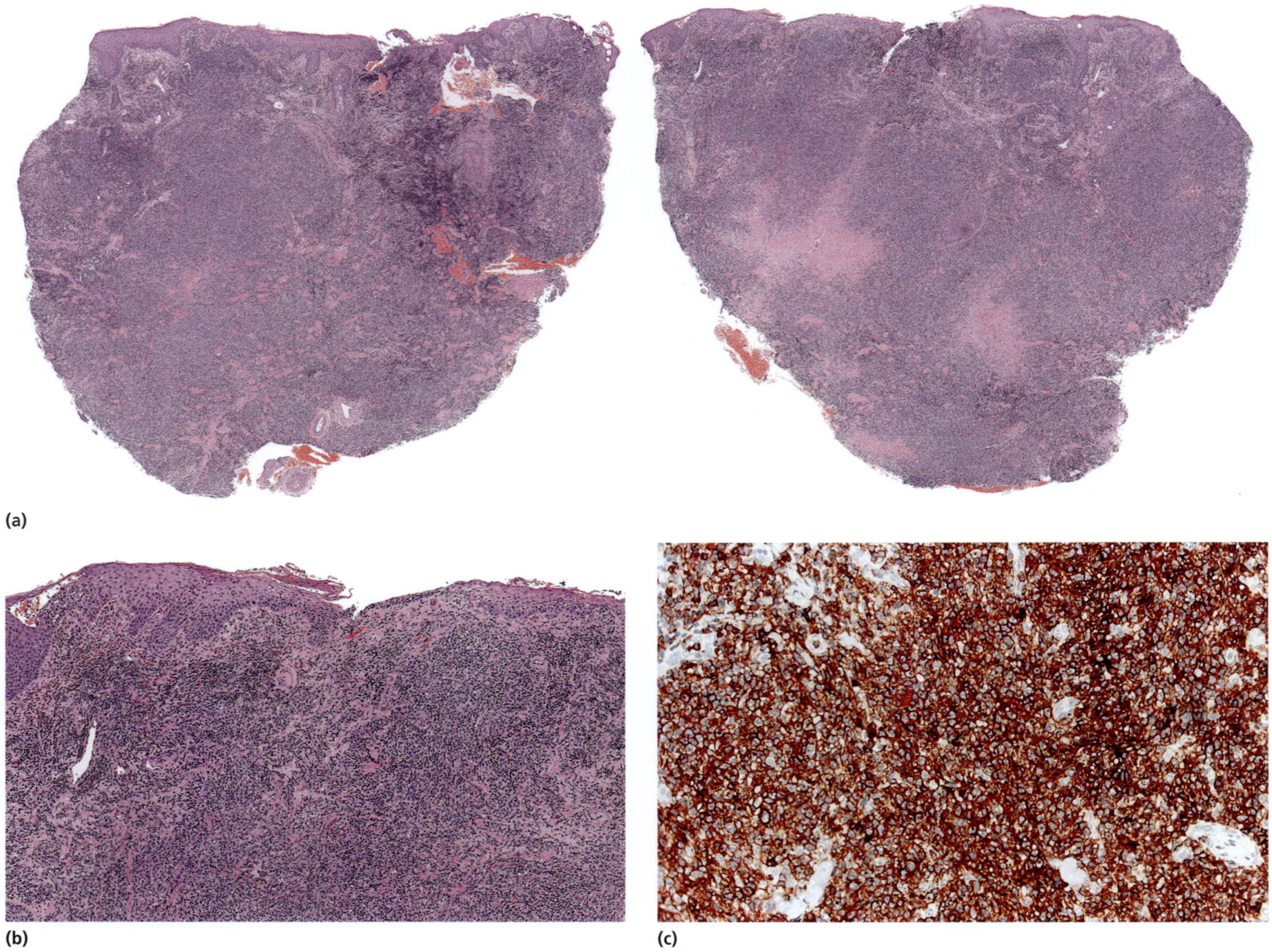

Figure 7.12 Cutaneous aggressive epidermotropic CD8+ cytotoxic T-cell lymphoma. (a) Diffuse infiltrate within the entire dermis with (b) only a few epidermotropic lymphocytes; (c) all cells are positive for CD8.

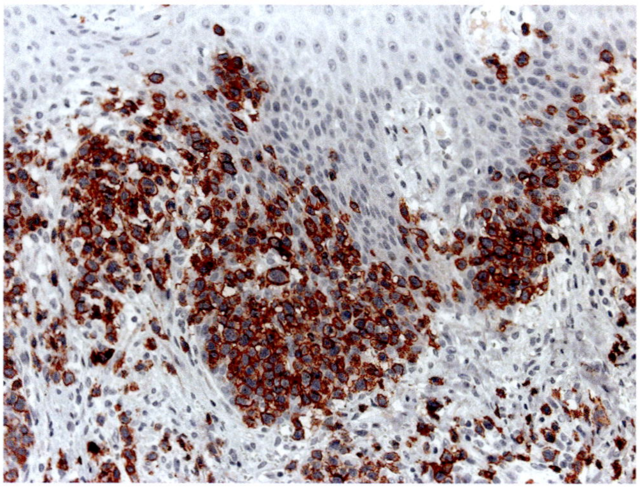

Figure 7.13 Cutaneous aggressive epidermotropic CD8+ cytotoxic T-cell lymphoma. Staining for CD8 highlights the epidermotropic lymphocytes.

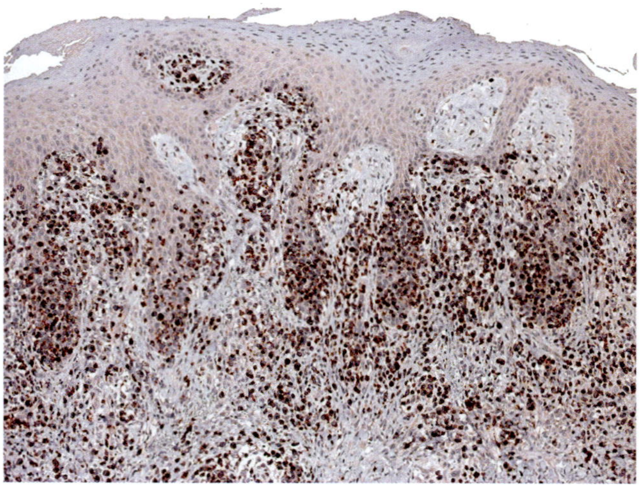

Figure 7.14 Cutaneous aggressive epidermotropic CD8+ cytotoxic T-cell lymphoma. Positivity for TIA-1.

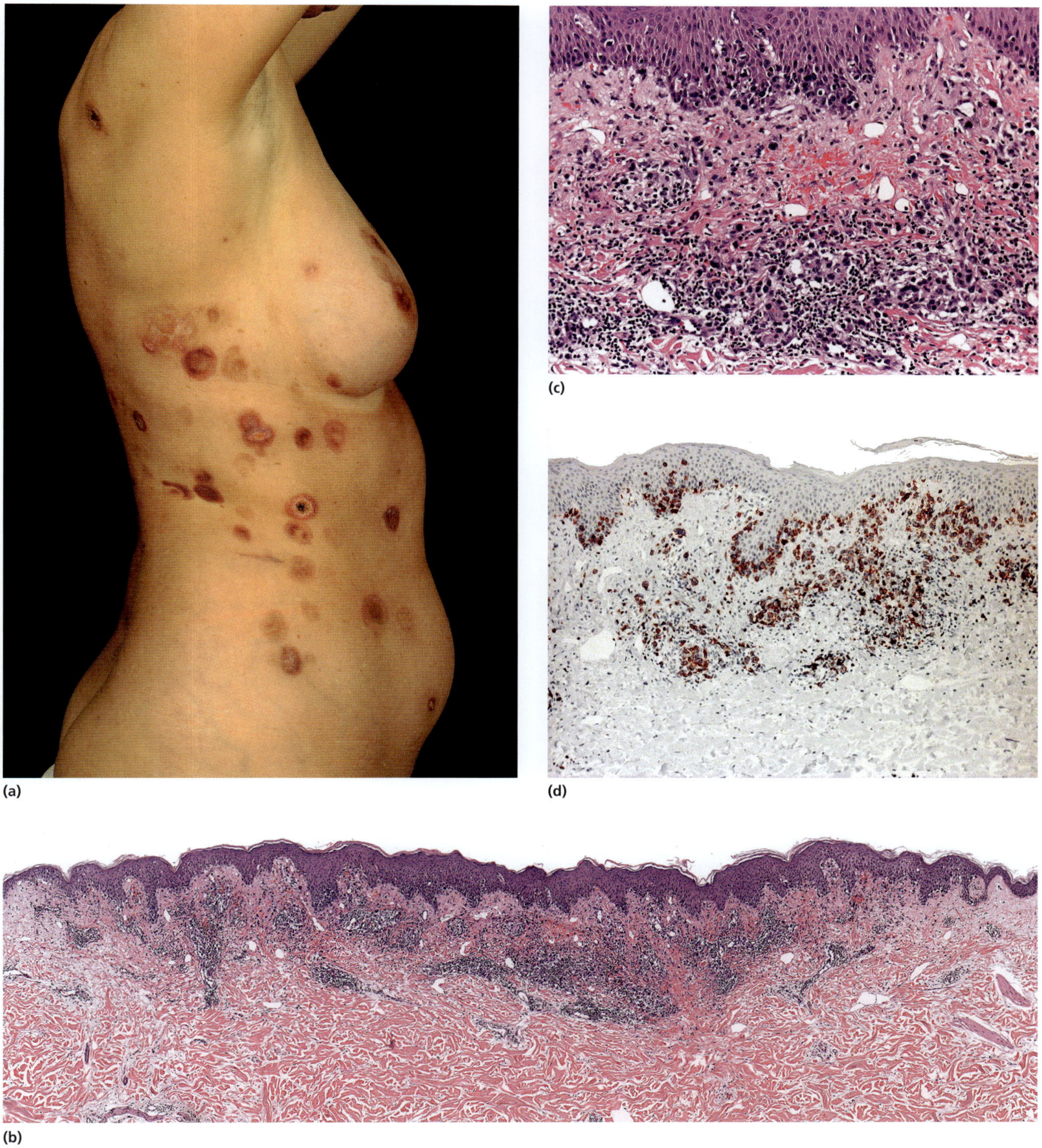


**Figure 7.15** Cutaneous aggressive epidermotropic $CD8^+$ cytotoxic T-cell lymphoma. (a) Clinical features showing irregular, confluent, partly erosive lesions on the trunk; hyperpigmented areas represent partial resolution after treatment with methotrexate. (b) Histology shows a band-like infiltrate characterized by (c) many epidermotropic and dermal large, pleomorphic lymphocytes. (d) Immunohistochemistry confirms positivity for (d) CD8 and (e) βF1, and reveals also (f) weak positivity for CD30 in some, but not all atypical cells. Correlation with the clinical picture and lack of CD30 positivity in many neoplastic cells allows to rule out lymphomatoid papulosis.

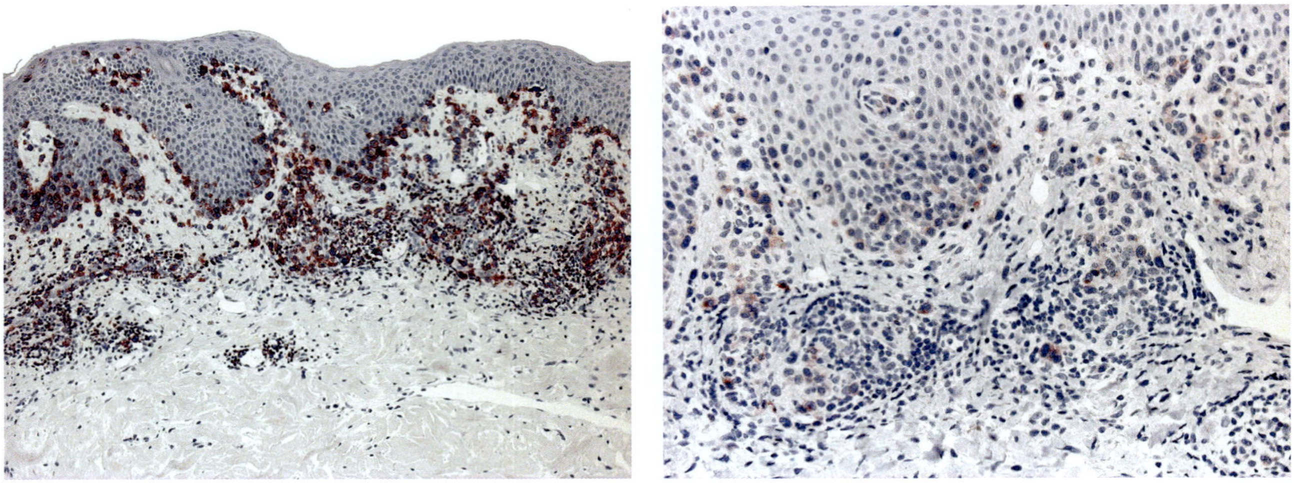

(e) (f)

Figure 7.15 (Continued)

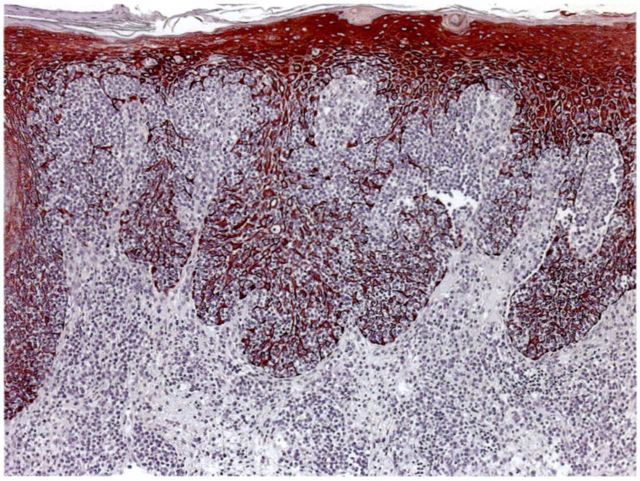

Figure 7.16 Cutaneous aggressive epidermotropic CD8⁺ cytotoxic T-cell lymphoma. Staining for pan-cytokeratin highlights the remnants of a hyperplastic epidermis.

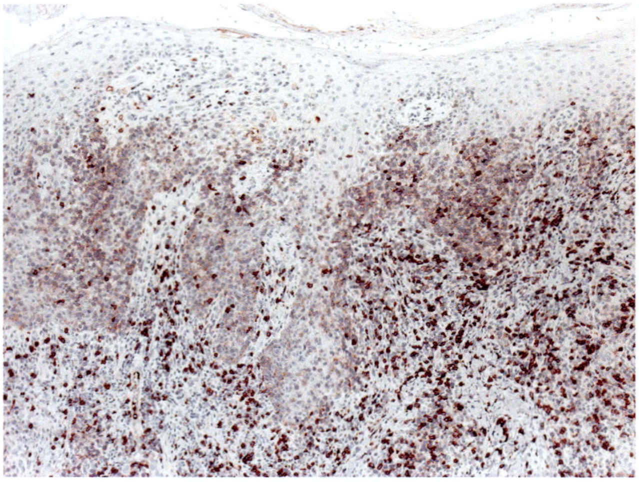

Figure 7.17 Cutaneous aggressive epidermotropic $CD8^+$ cytotoxic T-cell lymphoma. Dim positivity of neoplastic cells for CD8; note strong positivity in some reactive lymphocytes. Good internal controls are crucial in order to evaluate cases with weak positivity.

was managed with pemigatinib (an FGFR inhibitor) with partial remission lasting for 4 months, but subsequent relapse [24]. Allogeneic stem cell transplantation has been performed in some patients with promising results [13, 25, 26].

## Prognosis

The prognosis of patients with primary cutaneous aggressive epidermotropic $CD8^+$ cytotoxic T-cell lymphoma is poor, and the estimated 5-year survival is <1% [5, 8]. The median survival is 12 months [6].

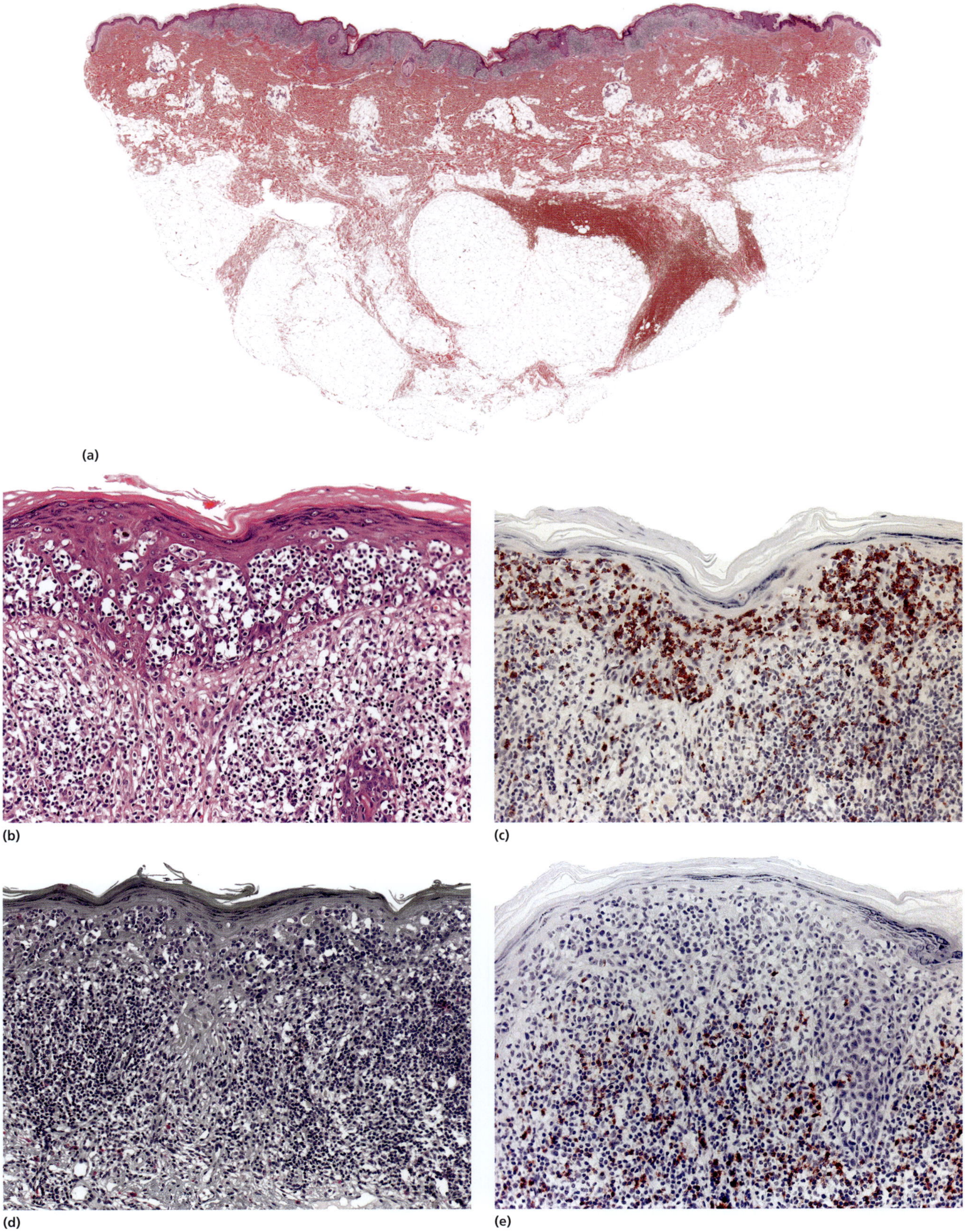

**Figure 7.18** Cutaneous aggressive epidermotropic CD8⁺ cytotoxic T-cell lymphoma in a 73-year-old woman with generalized, partly ulcerated plaques and tumors of recent onset and without history of mycosis fungoides. (a) Histology shows superficial lymphoid infiltrates with (b) prominent epidermotropism, resembling the pattern of pagetoid reticulosis. The cells were positive for CD3, βF1, TIA-1, perforin, and (c) granzyme B, with loss of CD2 and CD5 and with negativity for both (d) CD4 and (e) CD8. Stainings for CD30, TCR-γ, and TCR-δ as well as in situ hybridization for EBV (EBER-1) were negative. Mycosis fungoides could be ruled out by the absence of pertinent history; lymphomatoid papulosis by negativity for CD30; cutaneous γ/δ T-cell lymphoma by positivity for βF1 and negativity for TCR-γ and TCR-δ; and extranodal NK/T-cell lymphoma by negativity for EBER-1. The clinical presentation, histopathological pattern, and positivity for cytotoxic proteins of this case are consistent with a diagnosis of cutaneous aggressive $CD8^+$ cytotoxic T-cell lymphoma, but histology displayed negativity for CD8. Such rare cases of CD8-negative cutaneous aggressive $CD8^+$ cytotoxic T-cell lymphoma represent a pitfall in the histopathological diagnosis.

## Résumé

**Primary cutaneous aggressive epidermotropic CD8+ cytotoxic T-cell lymphoma**

| | | |
|---|---|---|
| **Clinical** | Adults, rarely children. Generalized plaques and tumors, frequently ulcerated. Aggressive course. Involvement of mucosal sites common. Absence of previous history of mycosis fungoides or of lymphomatoid papulosis mandatory for the diagnosis. | |
| **Morphology** | Band-like, nodular, or diffuse infiltrates characterized by small-, medium-, or large-sized pleomorphic cells or immunoblasts. Prominent epidermotropism (may be minimal or lacking in some lesions, particularly in late stages). | |
| **Immunohistochemistry** | CD8 | + *(essential criterion, yet CD8 may rarely be negative in given biopsies)* |
| | CD3, CD7, CD45RA | + |
| | βF1 | + *(essential criterion)* |
| | TCR-γ, TCR-δ | – *(essential criterion)* |
| | CD4, CD30 | – |
| | CD56 | – (+) |
| | TIA-1, Granzyme B, Perforin | + |
| | EBER-1 | – |
| **Genetics** | Monoclonal rearrangement of the TCR genes detected in the majority of the cases. Activation of the JAK/STAT pathway due to *JAK2* fusions or other molecular alterations. | |
| **Treatment guidelines** | Systemic chemotherapy. Allogeneic stem cell transplantation. Ruxolitinib (or other JAK2 inhibitors) may represent a novel therapeutic option. | |

## References


1. Willemze R, Cerroni L, Kempf W, *et al.* The 2018 update of the WHO-EORTC classification for primary cutaneous lymphomas. *Blood* 2019;**133**:1703–1714.
2. Kempf W, Mitteldorf C, Cerroni L, *et al.* Classifications of cutaneous lymphomas and lymphoproliferative disorders: an update from the EORTC cutaneous lymphoma histopathology group. *J Eur Acad Dermatol Venereol* 2024;**38**:1491–1503.
3. Goodlad JR, Cerroni L, Pro B. Primary cutaneous CD8-positive aggressive epidermotropic cytotoxic T-cell lymphoma. In: Arber DA, Borowitz MJ, Cook JR, *et al.*, eds. *The International Consensus Classification of Myeloid and Lymphoid Neoplasms.* Philadelphia (US): Wolters Kluwer, 2025: 709–711.
4. Berti E, Guitart J, Nardi V, *et al.* Primary cutaneous CD8-positive aggressive epidermotropic cytotoxic T-cell lymphoma. In: *WHO Classification of Tumours Editorial Board. Haematolymphoid Tumours.* 5th edition. Lyon (France): IARC, 2024: 705–707.
5. Berti E, Tomasini D, Vermeer MH, *et al.* Primary cutaneous CD8-positive epidermotropic cytotoxic T cell lymphomas. A distinct clinicopathological entity with an aggressive clinical behaviour. *Am J Pathol* 1999;**155**:483–492.
6. Robson A, Assaf C, Bagot M, *et al.* Aggressive epidermotropic cutaneous CD8+ lymphoma: a cutaneous lymphoma with distinct clinical and pathological features Report of an EORTC Cutaneous Lymphoma Task Force Workshop. *Histopathology* 2015;**67**:425–441.
7. Nofal A, Abdel-Mawla Y, Assaf M, *et al.* Primary cutaneous aggressive epidermotropic CD8+ T-cell lymphoma: proposed diagnostic criteria and therapeutic evaluation. *J Am Acad Dermatol* 2012;**67**: 748–759.
8. Fink-Puches R, Zenahlik P, Bäck B, *et al.* Primary cutaneous lymphomas: applicability of current classification schemes (European Organization for Research and Treatment of Cancer, World Health Organization) based on clinicopathologic features observed in a large group of patients. *Blood* 2002;**99**:800–805.
9. Kikuchi Y, Kashii Y, Gunji Y, *et al.* Six-year-old girl with primary cutaneous aggressive epidermotropic CD8+ T-cell lymphoma. *Ped Internat* 2011;**53**:393–396.
10. Wang L, Gao T, Wang G. Primary cutaneous CD8+ cytotoxic T-cell lymphoma involving the epidermis and subcutis in a young child. *J Cutan Pathol* 2015;**42**:271–275.
11. Deenen NJ, Koens L, Jaspars EH, *et al.* Pitfalls in diagnosing primary cutaneous aggressive epidermotropic CD8+ T-cell lymphoma. *Br J Dermatol* 2019;**180**:411–412.
12. Tomasini C, Novelli M, Fanoni D, *et al.* Erythema multiforme-like lesions in primary cutaneous aggressive cytotoxic epidermotropic CD8+ T-cell lymphoma: a diagnostic and therapeutic challenge. *J Cutan Pathol* 2017;**44**:867–873.
13. Guitart J, Martinez-Escala ME, Subtil A, *et al.* Primary cutaneous aggressive epidermotropic cytotoxic T-cell lymphomas: reappraisal of a provisional entity in the 2016 WHO classification of cutaneous lymphomas. *Mod Pathol* 2017;**30**:761–772.
14. Weenig RH, Comfere NI, Gibson LE, *et al.* Fatal cytotoxic cutaneous lymphoma presenting as ulcerative psoriasis. *Arch Dermatol* 2009;**145**:801–808.
15. Walker CJ, Martinez-Escala ME, Tan TL, *et al.* High incidence of adnexotropism in cytotoxic cutaneous lymphomas. *J Cut Pathol* 2021;**48**:1231–1238.
16. Santucci M, Pimpinelli N, Massi D, *et al.* Cytotoxic natural killer cell cutaneous lymphomas: report of the EORTC Cutaneous Lymphoma Task Force Workshop. *Cancer* 2003;**97**:610–627.
17. Bastidas Torres AN, Cats D, Out-Luiting JJ, *et al.* Deregulation of JAK2 signaling underlies primary cutaneous CD81 aggressive epidermotropic cytotoxic T-cell lymphoma. *Haematologica* 2022; **107**:702–714.

18. Lee K, Evans MG, Yang L, *et al.* Primary cytotoxic T-cell lymphomas harbor recurrent targetable alterations in the JAK-STAT pathway. *Blood* 2021;**138**:2435–2440.
19. Buus TB, Koralov SB. Oncogenic fusions JAK up $CD8^+$ cytotoxic CTCL. *Blood* 2021;**138**:2311–2312.
20. Fanoni D, Corti L, Alberti-Violetti S, *et al.* Array-based CGH of primary cutaneous $CD8^+$ aggressive EPIDERMO-tropic cytotoxic T-cell lymphoma. *Genes Chromosomes Cancer* 2018;**57**:622–629.
21. Gormley RH, Hess SD, Anand D, *et al.* Primary cutaneous aggressive epidermotropic $CD8^+$ T-cell lymphoma. *J Am Acad Dermatol* 2010;**62**:300–307.
22. Massone C, Chott A, Metze D, *et al.* Subcutaneous, blastic natural killer (NK) NK/T-cell and other cytotoxic lymphomas of the skin: a morphologic, immunophenotypic and molecular study of 50 patients. *Am J Surg Pathol* 2004;**28**:719–735.
23. Bekkenk MW, Vermeer MH, Jansen PM, *et al.* Peripheral T-cell lymphomas unspecified presenting in the skin: analysis of prognostic factors in a group of 82 patients. *Blood* 2003;**102**:2213–2219.
24. Torres-Cabala CA, Yescas J, Zhang Y, *et al.* Primary cutaneous $CD8^+$ aggressive epidermotropic cytotoxic T-cell lymphoma with novel FGFR1 fusion treated with pemigatinib. *Blood Adv* 2025;**9**(8): 1786–1790.
25. Moritz RKC, Ditschkowski M, Klemke CD, *et al.* Allogeneic stem cell transplantation in patients with aggressive primary cutaneous T-cell lymphoma – a case series of the ADF working group "cutaneous lymphomas". *J Dtsch Dermatol Ges* 2014;**12**:39–46.
26. Wehkamp U, Glaeser D, Oschlies I, *et al.* Successful stem cell transplantation in a patient with primary cutaneous aggressive cytotoxic epidermotropic $CD8^+$ T-cell lymphoma. *Br J Dermatol* 2015;**173**:869–871.

## CHAPTER 8

# Primary cutaneous γ/δ T-cell lymphoma

Primary cutaneous γ/δ T-cell lymphoma is included as a specific entity in the International Consensus Classification (ICC) *of Myeloid and Lymphoid Neoplasms*, the 2019 and 2024 updates of the classification of cutaneous lymphomas by the European Organization of Research and Treatment of Cancer (EORTC) – Cutaneous Lymphoma Histopathology Group, and the World Health Organization (WHO) *Classification of Haematolymphoid Tumours* [1–4], and should be distinguished from other γ/δ T-cell lymphomas involving the skin [5].

Primary cutaneous γ/δ T-cell lymphoma is a tumor of cytotoxic γ/δ T lymphocytes with specific tropism for the skin. This lymphoma shows many overlapping features with other cutaneous lymphoma entities, especially with subcutaneous panniculitis-like T-cell lymphoma and with primary cutaneous aggressive epidermotropic $CD8^+$ cytotoxic T-cell lymphoma. The availability of markers for γ/δ T-lymphocytes on routinely fixed, paraffin-embedded sections of tissue (TCR-γ and TCR-δ) facilitate the diagnosis of this cytotoxic lymphoma [6], and staining for both TCR α/β and TCR γ/δ allows a proper classification. In fact, in T-cell lymphomas, lack of the α/β expression *per se* is not synonymous with γ/δ differentiation, as "TCR silent" ("null-cell") cases negative for both α/β and γ/δ may be observed [7]. In addition, the double expression of α/β and γ/δ receptors may be observed in cutaneous γ/δ T-cell lymphomas [8, 9], thus emphasizing the need for complete phenotypic analyses in order to properly classify these cases. Recent studies showed that two distinct classes of neoplastic lymphocytes are found within the epidermal/dermal and subcutaneous compartments, namely, Vδ1 T-lymphocytes in the epidermis and dermis, and Vδ2 T-lymphocytes in the subcutaneous tissue, reflecting the distribution of normal γ/δ T lymphocytes within the skin [10].

Besides cutaneous and hepatosplenic cases, γ/δ T-cell lymphomas can be observed rarely also at other nodal or extranodal sites [7], thus underlying the need for careful staging investigations. It is also important to remember that a γ/δ phenotype is not unique to primary cutaneous γ/δ T-cell lymphoma, as it can be observed in several cutaneous (and extracutaneous) lymphoma types, including mycosis fungoides and lymphomatoid papulosis among others [9].

In the past, cases of cutaneous γ/δ T-cell lymphoma were classified as either generalized pagetoid reticulosis (Ketron–Goodman type) or mycosis fungoides "a tumeur d'emblée." Distinction from rare cases of conventional mycosis fungoides with γ/δ T-cell phenotype is made on the basis of the clinical presentation and behavior. In contrast to mycosis fungoides, patients with cutaneous γ/δ T-cell lymphoma present at the onset with rapidly growing, disseminated patches, plaques, and tumors that are often ulcerated.

Due to the frequent prominent involvement of subcutaneous tissues, in the past, many cases of cutaneous γ/δ T-cell lymphoma were incorrectly classified as subcutaneous panniculitis-like T-cell lymphoma (see also Chapter 6). However, γ/δ T-cell lymphoma invariably shows also prominent involvement of the dermis, and epidermal involvement can be commonly found either in the same biopsy specimen or in other biopsies taken at the same time or during the course of the disease. A typical example is represented by the patient pictured in Fig. 8.1, whose picture was included in the chapter on subcutaneous T-cell lymphomas in the first edition of this book published in 1998. The patient died in 1976 of "histiocytic medullary reticulosis." The case was included as an example of "malignant histiocytosis" in the book on cutaneous lymphomas published in 1983 by Burg and Braun-Falco, who had received the case courtesy of Helmut Kerl [11], and then reclassified as "histiocytic cytophagic panniculitis" in 1985. All previous classifications made perfect sense at the time when they had been proposed. On the other hand, this case clearly shows how these unusual lymphomas are reclassified over time, thanks to new phenotypic and molecular studies that allow definition of more specific categories. As a matter of fact, staining with the antibody specific for TCR-δ allowed the diagnosis of cutaneous γ/δ T-cell lymphoma to be confirmed more than 36 years after the patient had succumbed to his disease. In fact, although it was previously thought that the epidermotropic and subcutaneous variants may be distinct and characterized by different prognosis, there are data suggesting that they probably represent morphological variations of the same entity [12, 13].

Finally, it should be reminded that the presence of γ/δ T-lymphocytes in the skin or subcutaneous tissues is not synonymous with γ/δ T-cell lymphoma, as variable numbers of such

*Skin Lymphoma: The Illustrated Guide*, Sixth Edition. Lorenzo Cerroni.

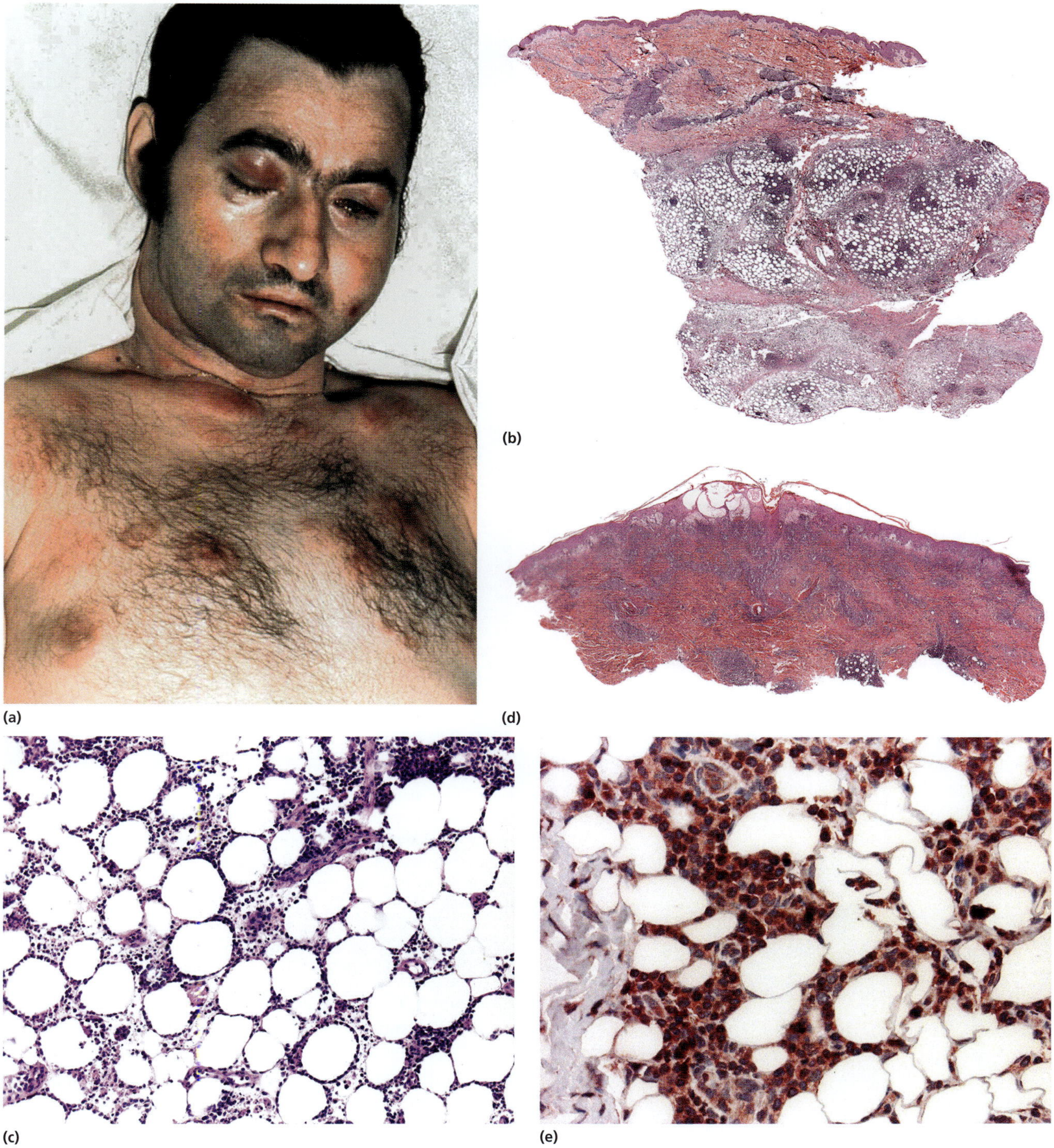

Figure 8.1 Cutaneous γ/δ T-cell lymphoma. (a) Multiple erythematous plaques and tumors on the trunk and face. (b) The first biopsy showed prominent involvement of the subcutaneous fat tissue with (c) rimming of adipocytes, whereas (d) the second biopsy showed also prominent involvement of the epidermis and dermis. This case was included within the “subcutaneous T-cell lymphomas” in the first edition of this book; (e) staining for TCR-γ, performed more than 36 years after the patient had succumbed to his disease, allowed reclassification of the case as cutaneous γ/δ T-cell lymphoma.

lymphocytes may be observed in other lymphoma types (including subcutaneous panniculitis-like T-cell lymphoma) [14], and prominent populations of $\gamma/\delta$ T-lymphocytes may be observed also in a subset of cases of pityriasis lichenoides (atypical pityriasis lichenoides, see also Chapters 3 and 31) [15, 16]. In addition, an inflammatory reaction with a predominant population of $\gamma/\delta$ T lymphocytes has been observed at the site of a tick bite [17], and the finding of a population of $\gamma/\delta$-positive T lymphocytes alone does not convey any information concerning the diagnosis in any given case.

## Clinical features

Cutaneous $\gamma/\delta$ T-cell lymphoma occurs in adults, with an equal distribution of males and females. Rare cases in children are well documented [18, 19]. Patients present with localized or generalized patches, plaques, and tumors, which are frequently ulcerated (Fig. 8.2). Localized lesions are often found on the lower extremities. Large, solitary tumors may also be seen. In some patients, the clinical features are similar to those observed in patients with mycosis fungoides or with diseases characterized by interface dermatitis (Fig. 8.3). In most of these cases, besides patches and plaques similar to those observed in mycosis fungoides, variably large tumors are observed at other sites of the body (Fig. 8.4). Involvement of the mucosal regions and of other locations unusual for mycosis fungoides is common (Figs. 8.5 and 8.6).

Staging investigations are mandatory and usually show the presence of tumor masses within the soft tissues and/or the lymph nodes. Lactate dehydrogenase (LDH) is elevated in the majority of patients [20]. Bone marrow involvement is uncommon. A hemophagocytic syndrome is a frequent complication in subcutaneous cases [21], and may be related to enrichment in interferon-$\gamma$ and other inflammatory cytokines [10]. B symptoms (fever, night sweat, and weight loss) occur in most patients.

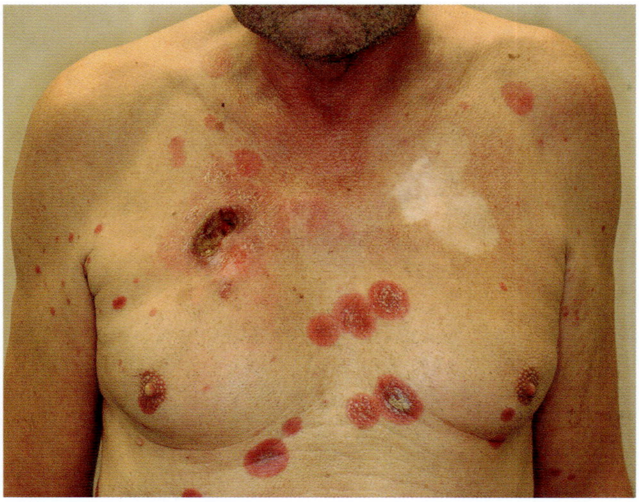

**Figure 8.2** Cutaneous $\gamma/\delta$ T-cell lymphoma. Multiple, partly erosive, infiltrated plaques on the trunk. (*Courtesy of Dr. Martin Laimer, Salzburg, Austria.*)

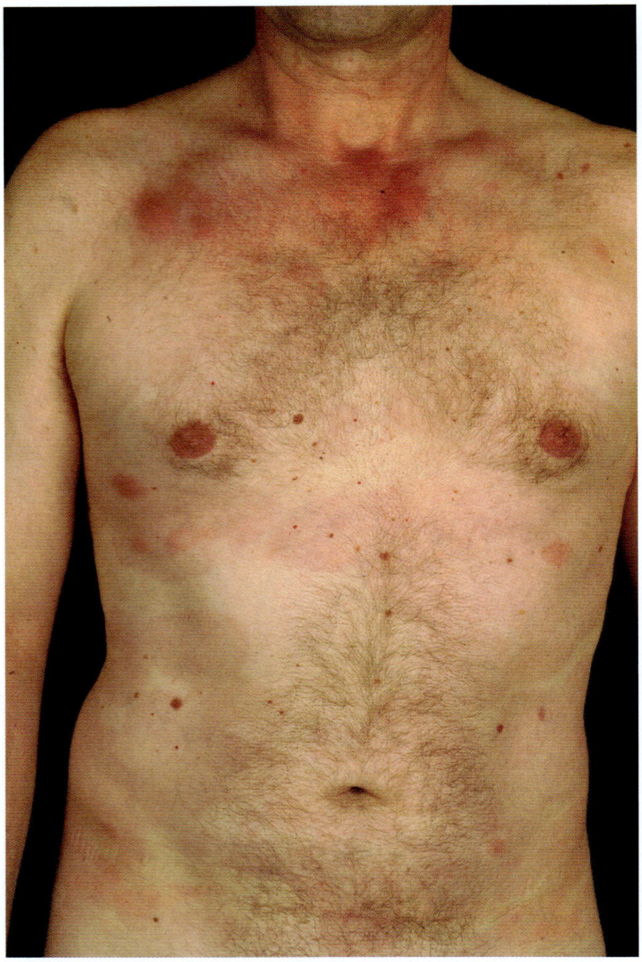

**Figure 8.3** Cutaneous $\gamma/\delta$ T-cell lymphoma. Generalized erythematous patches and some plaques mimicking the clinical presentation of mycosis fungoides. Differently from mycosis fungoides, there are neither scales nor atrophic lesions. The less infiltrated lesions resemble morphologically those seen in diseases presenting with features of interface dermatitis.

Almost one-fourth of the patients had an associated autoimmune disorder in one study [20], and onset of cutaneous $\gamma/\delta$ T-cell lymphoma has been observed also during treatment with etanercept for rheumatoid arthritis [22]. In such cases, it is difficult to ascertain whether the lymphoma arises in the setting of the autoimmune disorder or as a consequence of the immunomodulatory treatment.

As well as for other aggressive cytotoxic lymphomas, for a diagnosis of cutaneous $\gamma/\delta$ T-cell lymphoma, it is crucial to exclude a history of mycosis fungoides.

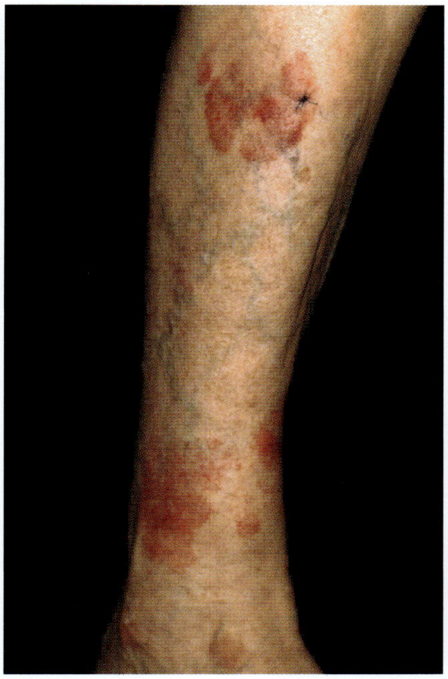

(a)

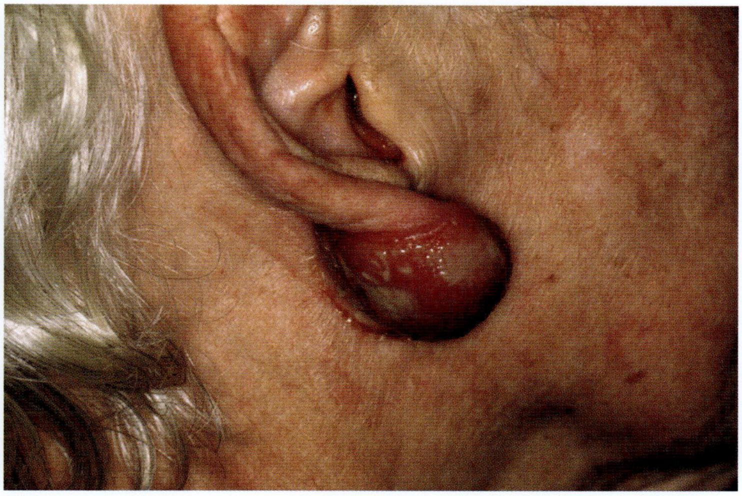

(b)

Figure 8.4 Cutaneous γ/δ T-cell lymphoma. (a) Patches and plaques on the right arm mimicking the clinical features of mycosis fungoides; at the same time, the patient had (b) an ulcerated small tumor on the right earlobe.

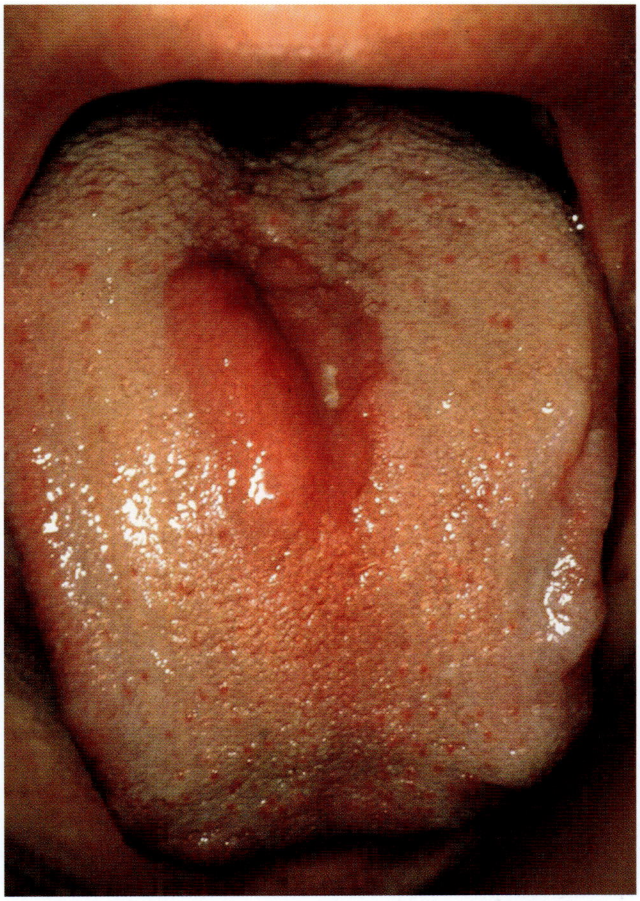

Figure 8.5 Cutaneous γ/δ T-cell lymphoma. Large tumor on the tongue.

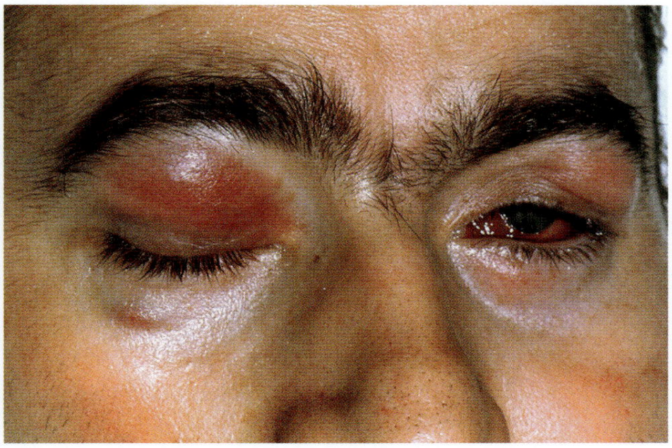

Figure 8.6 Cutaneous γ/δ T-cell lymphoma. Infiltration of the palpebra and of the conjunctiva (same patient of Fig. 8.1).

## Histopathology, immunophenotype, and molecular genetics

### Histopathology

Histology reveals a diffuse proliferation of lymphocytes, usually with prominent involvement of the subcutaneous tissues with a lobular panniculitis-like pattern (Fig. 8.7). Cases with prominent involvement of the subcutaneous tissue show also dermal and often epidermal involvement, allowing differentiation from subcutaneous panniculitis-like T-cell lymphoma where the dermis is spared as a rule. In late lesions, subcutaneous infiltrates may be present only focally and degenerative features of

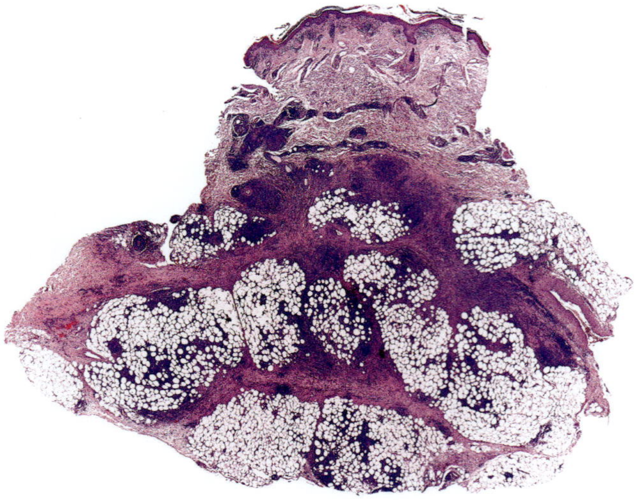

**Figure 8.7** Cutaneous γ/δ T-cell lymphoma. Prominent involvement of the subcutaneous fat with lymphoid infiltrates also in the dermis and subepidermal area.

the fat may be prominent, akin to what is observed in subcutaneous panniculitis-like T-cell lymphoma, but the presence of dermal involvement is usually discriminatory between the two entities (Fig. 8.8). In some cases, the infiltrate is almost only confined to the epidermis with prominent, pagetoid epidermotropism, mimicking the histopathological features of mycosis fungoides and pagetoid reticulosis; negativity or only very weak positivity for CD4 and CD8 and strong positivity for TCRγ/δ represent diagnostic clues (Fig. 8.9). In other cases, the epidermotropism may be moderate or even absent. As for other aggressive cutaneous cytotoxic lymphomas, cytomorphology is variable and can be characterized by small-, medium-, or large-sized pleomorphic cells. Involvement of the hair follicles (pleiotropism) may be observed but is uncommon (Fig. 8.10). In some cases, edema of the papillary dermis and pronounced hemorrhage may be observed as signs of an acute lesion (Fig. 8.11), and in other intraepidermal vesiculation with only scant infiltrates may mimic the pattern of a spongiotic dermatitis (Fig. 8.12). Vacuolization of basal keratinocytes may be prominent, even in the absence of marked epidermotropism (interface dermatitis-like features) (Fig. 8.13). Necrosis can be seen, and angiocentricity and/or angiodestruction is a common finding (Fig. 8.14). Abundant deposition of dermal mucin may prompt one to consider lupus erythematosus in the differential diagnosis, but an infiltrate composed almost exclusively of TCRγ/δ lymphocytes allows one to make the correct diagnosis (Fig. 8.15). The presence of large macrophages engulfing neoplastic lymphocytes or other blood cells is a typical feature of cases associated with a hemophagocytic syndrome (Fig. 8.16).

Differential diagnostic criteria for distinction of cutaneous γ/δ T-cell lymphoma from primary cutaneous aggressive epidermotropic CD8$^+$ cytotoxic T-cell lymphoma are summarized in Chapter 7. Morphologically, lesions of cutaneous γ/δ T-cell lymphoma show a more prominent involvement of the subcutaneous fat than those of primary cutaneous aggressive epidermotropic CD8$^+$ cytotoxic T-cell lymphoma. Another differential feature is the presence of a marked interface dermatitis in some cases of cutaneous γ/δ T-cell lymphoma, but not in those of primary cutaneous aggressive epidermotropic CD8$^+$ cytotoxic T-cell lymphoma. In cases with marked epidermotropism and positivity for CD8, positive staining for TCR α/β and γ/δ allows the two conditions to be distinguished, and represents an essential diagnostic feature.

## Immunophenotype

Immunohistology reveals a characteristic phenotypic profile of neoplastic lymphocytes (TCR-γ$^+$, TCR-δ$^+$, βF1$^-$, CD2$^+$, CD3$^+$, TIA-1$^+$, granzyme-B$^+$, perforin$^+$, CD56$^+$, and CD57$^-$) (Fig. 8.17). CD5 is frequently lost. CD4 is usually (not invariably) negative, and CD8 may be expressed (CD8-positivity has been observed in up to 40% of cases in the series by Guitart *et al.*) [14]. The proliferation rate (Ki-67) is high, usually >50% and sometimes nearly 100%.

Although positivity for γ/δ should be considered a prerequisite to establish the diagnosis, rare cases of cutaneous γ/δ T-cell lymphoma may have a silent phenotype with negativity for both α/β and γ/δ markers [23]. In this context, it must be remembered that the double expression of α/β and γ/δ can be observed as well [8]. In addition, immunophenotypic shift of one or more antigens (including TCR-αβ and TCR-γδ) may be observed in sequential biopsies of cutaneous γ/δ T-cell lymphoma [24]. Cases with these phenotypic features may be very difficult to classify precisely, as they show overlapping aspects with other cutaneous cytotoxic NK/T-cell lymphomas.

EBV is not present in the neoplastic cells. The classification of rare cases of cutaneous T-cell lymphoma with a γ/δ phenotype and positivity for EBV is a matter of discussion [20, 25, 26]. As already mentioned, the group of cutaneous aggressive cytotoxic lymphomas presents several overlapping features and sometimes classification of a given case may be subjective.

## Molecular genetics

Molecular biology shows a monoclonal rearrangement of the TCR genes. Cutaneous γ/δ T-cell lymphoma reveals oncogenic mutations in the JAK/STAT with activation of the JAK/STAT pathway similarly to what is observed in other cytotoxic lymphomas [10, 27], as well as oncogenic mutations in the mitogen-activated protein kinase (MAPK), MYC, and chromatin modification pathways [10]. Ultraviolet (UV)-associated mutations are more common in epidermotropic cases with a Vδ1 phenotype, whereas senescence-related molecular features can be observed in subcutaneous cases with a Vδ2 phenotype. Chromosomal aberrations suggesting the involvement of a *WWOX–TCL* gene cluster and *BCL11B* have been observed in one study [28]. The γ/δ T-cell lymphomas (including both cutaneous and extracutaneous forms) have a different molecular

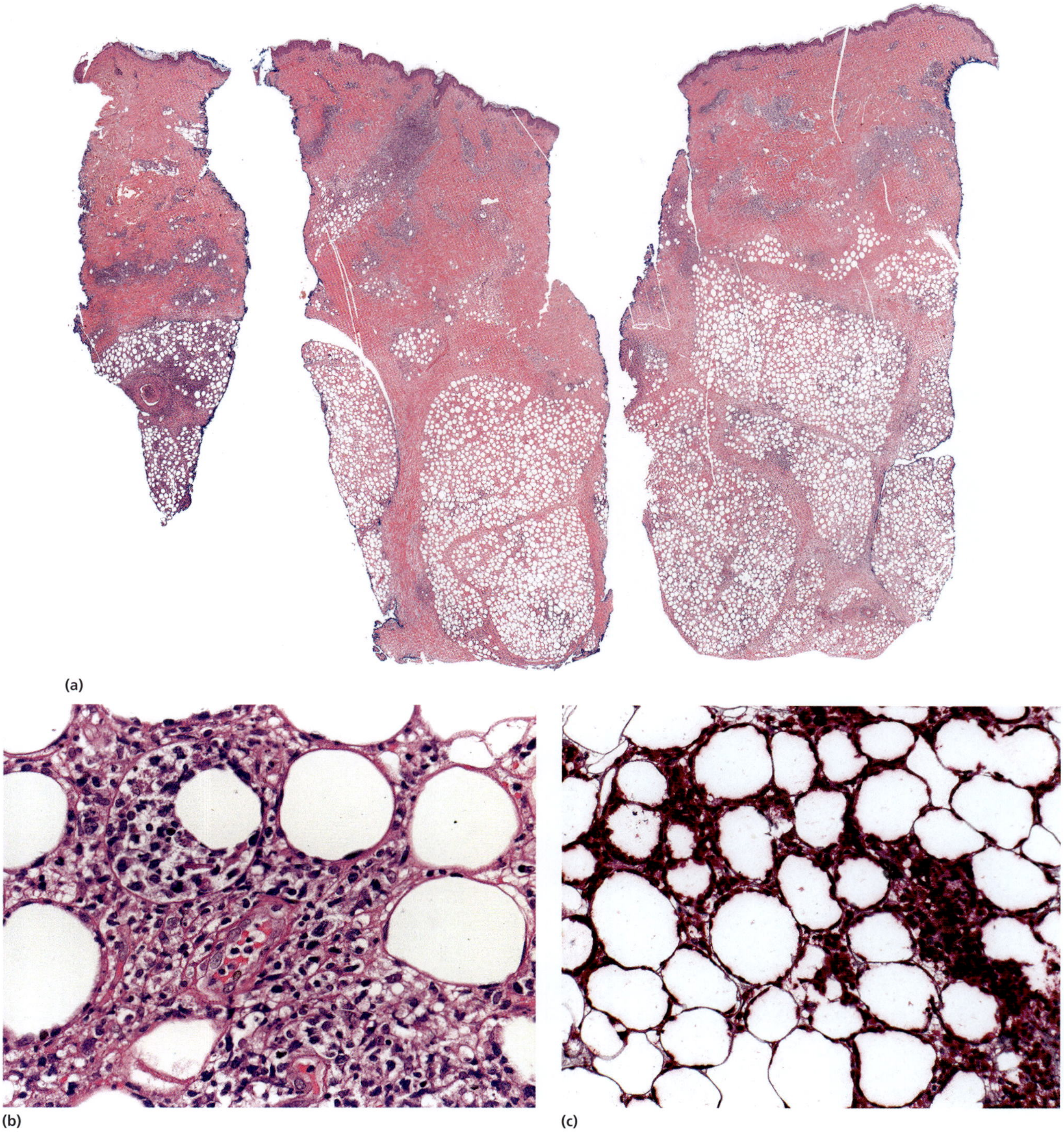


Figure 8.8 Cutaneous γ/δ T-cell lymphoma. (a) Subcutaneous involvement is only focal and degenerative changes of the subcutaneous fat predominate. (b) Detail of pleomorphic subcutaneous lymphocytes in the infiltrated area. (c) Neoplastic cells are positive for TCR-δ. Dense infiltrates within the dermis allow differentiation from subcutaneous panniculitis-like T-cell lymphoma.

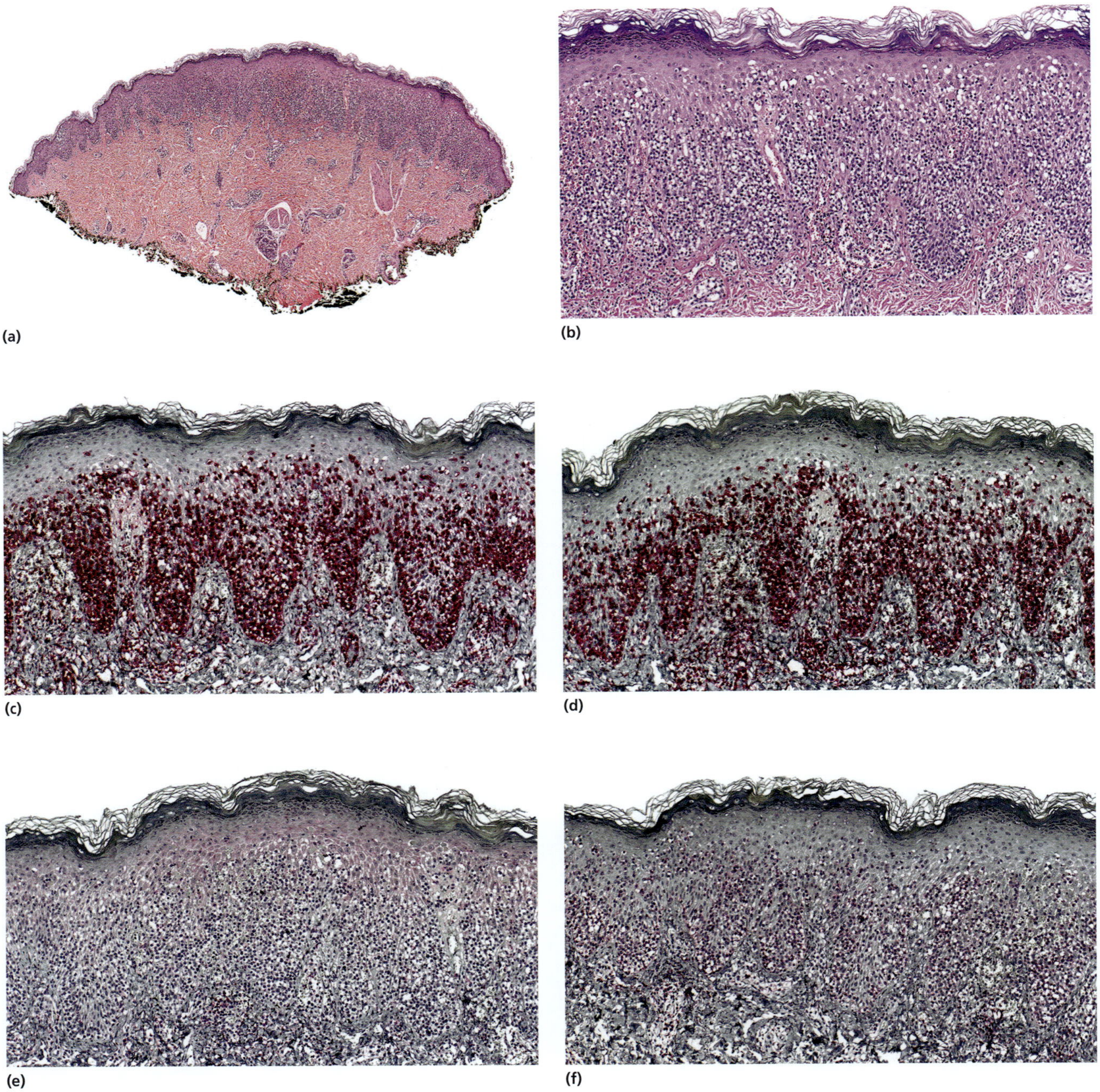

Figure 8.9 Cutaneous γ/δ T-cell lymphoma. (a) Superficial infiltrate confined almost exclusively to the epidermis with (b) pagetoid epidermotropism of (c) TCRδ+ neoplastic cells which are also (d) positive for CD3, (e) negative for CD4, and (f) weakly positive for CD8.

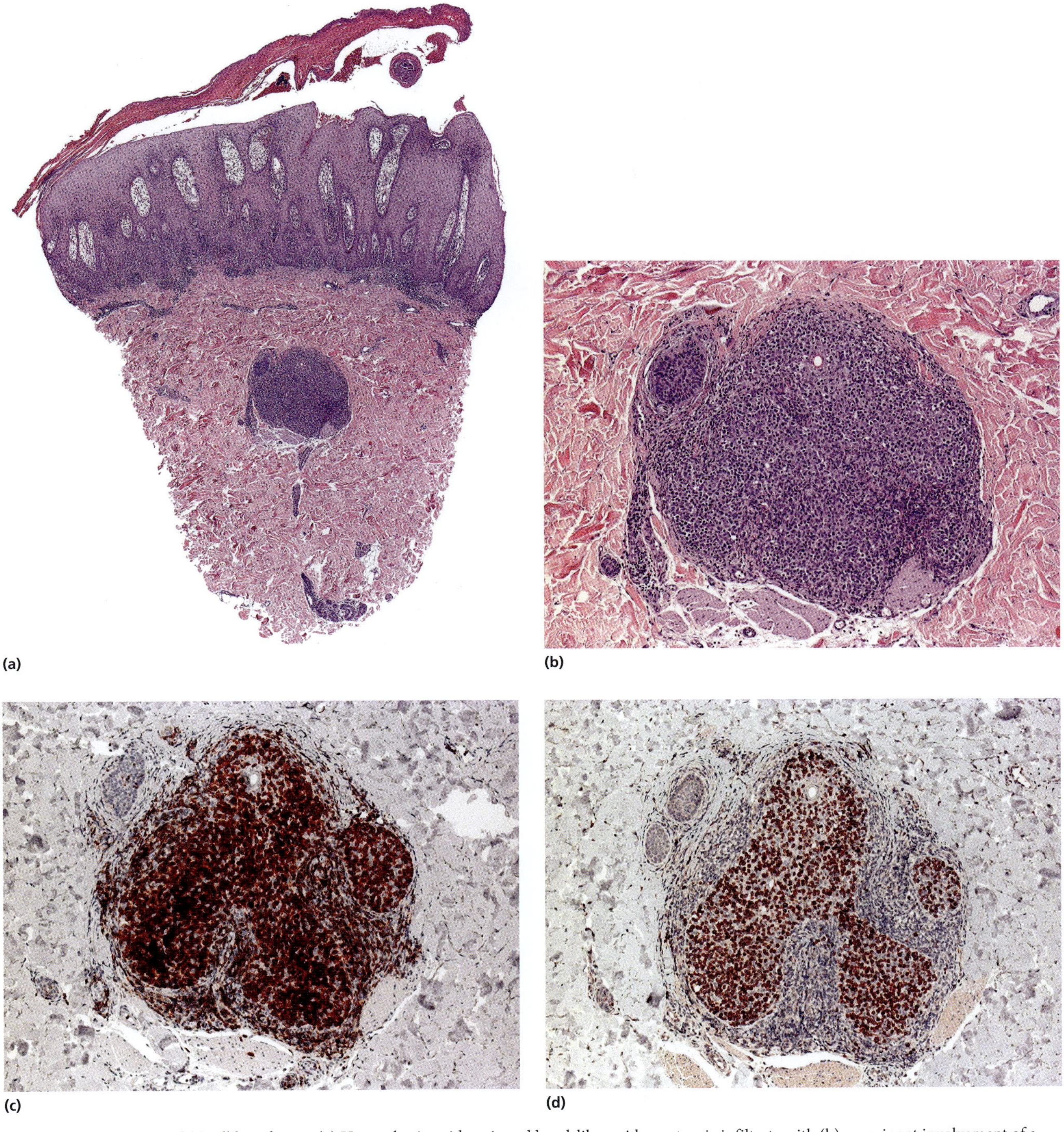

**Figure 8.10** Cutaneous γ/δ T-cell lymphoma. (a) Hyperplastic epidermis and band-like, epidermotropic infiltrate with (b) prominent involvement of a hair follicle; the pilotropic lymphocytes are positive for (c) CD3 and (d) TCRδ, and negative for (e) CD4 and (f) CD8.

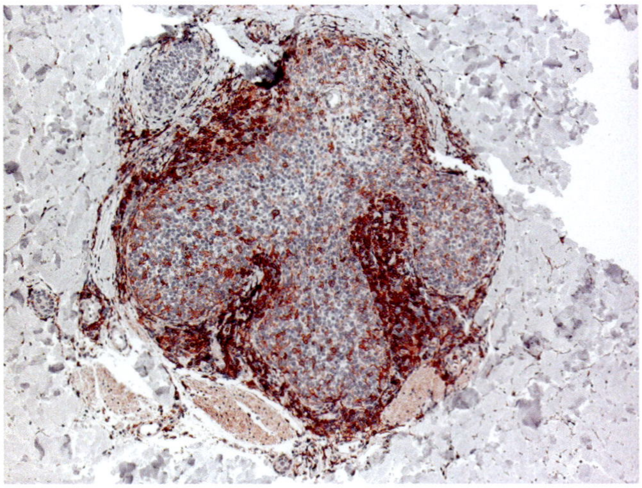

(e)

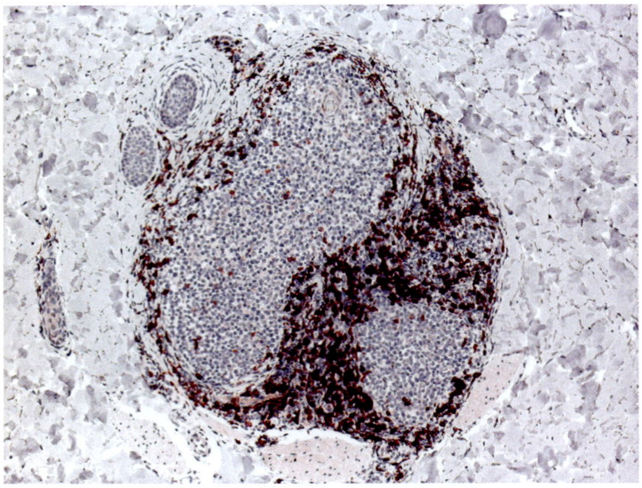

(f)

Figure 8.10 (Continued)

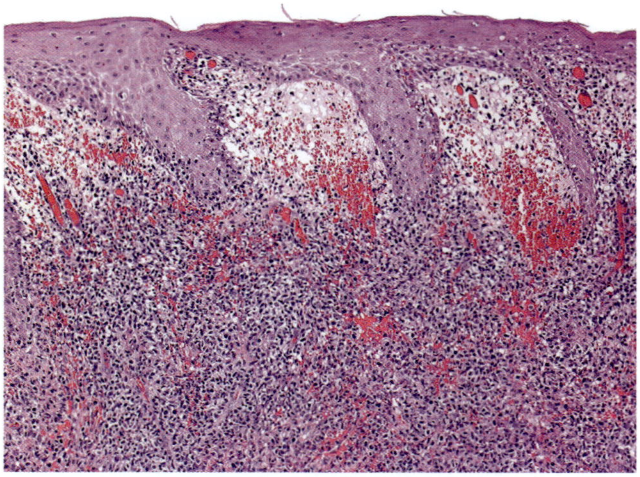

Figure 8.11 Cutaneous γ/δ T-cell lymphoma. Edema and hemorrhage within the papillary dermis are signs of an acute lesion, contrasting with the fibrotic papillary dermis observed in long-standing lesions of mycosis fungoides.

profile than α/β T-cell lymphomas and reveal overexpression of genes of NK-cell-associated molecules such as killer cell immunoglobulin-like receptor (KIR) genes (*KIR3DL1*, *KIR2DL4*, and *KIR2DL2*) and killer cell lectin-like receptor genes (*KLRC4*, *KLRD1*, and *KLRC2*) [29]. In the same study, it was shown that hepatosplenic γ/δ T-cell lymphoma represents a tumor distinct from other γ/δ T-cell lymphomas arising at other sites including the skin [29], thus confirming the need for separating different entities of γ/δ T-cell lymphoma.

### Treatment

Data on therapy are lacking, and double-blinded studies have not been carried out. The treatment of choice is systemic chemotherapy. Stem cell transplantation may represent a curative option [30–32].

## Prognosis

The prognosis of patients with cutaneous γ/δ T-cell lymphoma is poor [2], but occasional patients may show a prolonged course [33, 34]. Involvement of the subcutaneous fat tissues has been related to a bad prognosis [35, 36]. When evaluating prognosis of cutaneous γ/δ T-cell lymphoma, the current, somewhat dogmatic approach is that cases with indolent course represent examples of mycosis fungoides with a γ/δ phenotype. This may be true for many cases, but probably not for all of them. I have seen several patients with conventional mycosis fungoides clinically and a γ/δ phenotype histopathologically, thus fitting within the "dogmatic" approach, but also others presenting with features different from early mycosis fungoides clinically (e.g., eroded plaques, infiltrated panniculitic-like lesions) and yet showing an indolent behavior. In fact, in my opinion, some cases defy a precise classification and should be managed carefully but probably not aggressively from the outset.

As already mentioned, in the group of aggressive cutaneous cytotoxic NK/T-cell lymphomas, prognostic features of cases reported in the literature, even in recent studies, may be related to an incorrect classification rather than to genuine

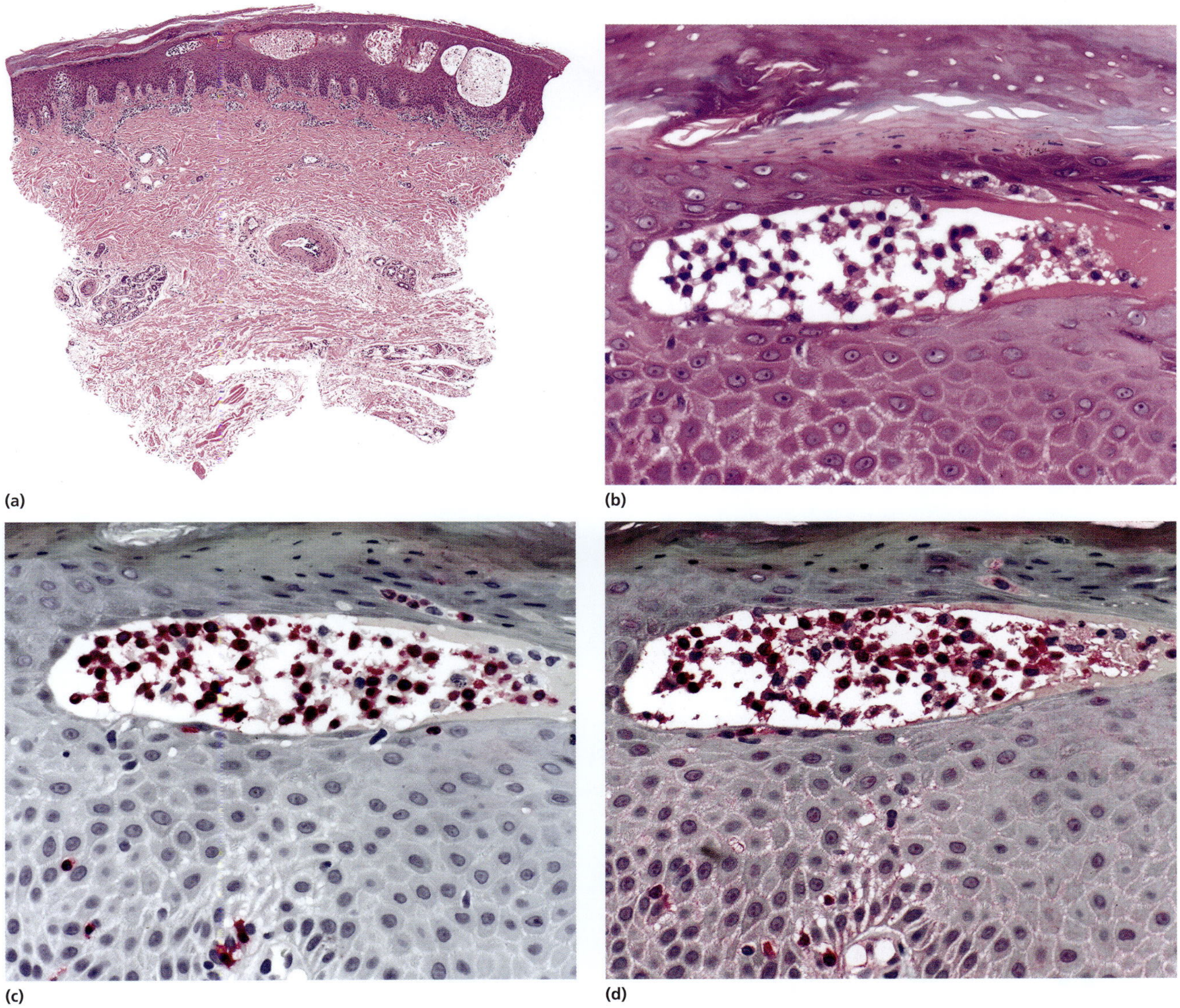


**Figure 8.12** Cutaneous $\gamma/\delta$ T-cell lymphoma. (a) Intraepidermal vesiculation in the context of a sparse infiltrate, mimicking the histopathological features of a spongiotic dermatitis; (b) the cells within a vesicle may be misconstrued as keratinocytes and Langerhans cells, but are uniformly positive for (c) CD3 and (d) TCR$\delta$; note also TCR$\delta^+$ lymphocytes within the epidermis.

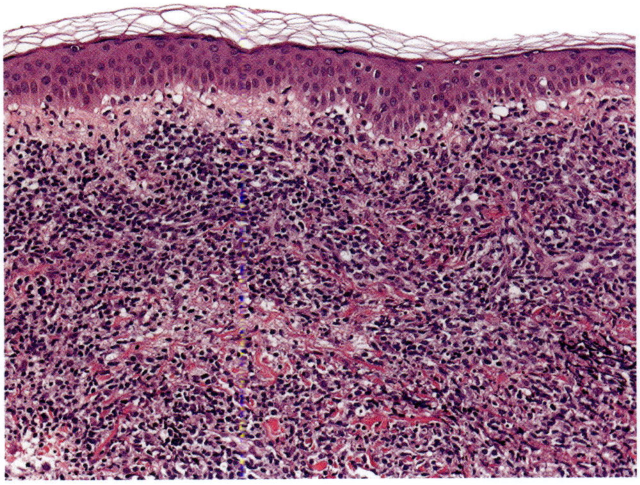

**Figure 8.13** Cutaneous $\gamma/\delta$ T-cell lymphoma. Vacuolization of basal keratinocytes (interface dermatitis-like) in the absence of epidermotropism.

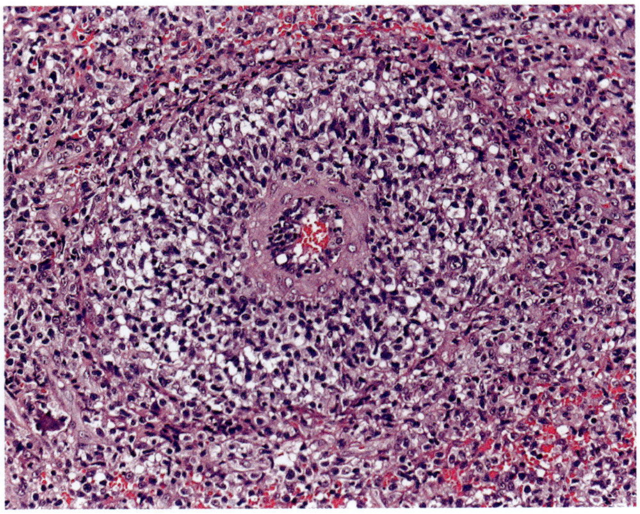

**Figure 8.14** Cutaneous $\gamma/\delta$ T-cell lymphoma. Prominent angiocentricity with early angiodestruction. Note pleomorphic lymphocytes.

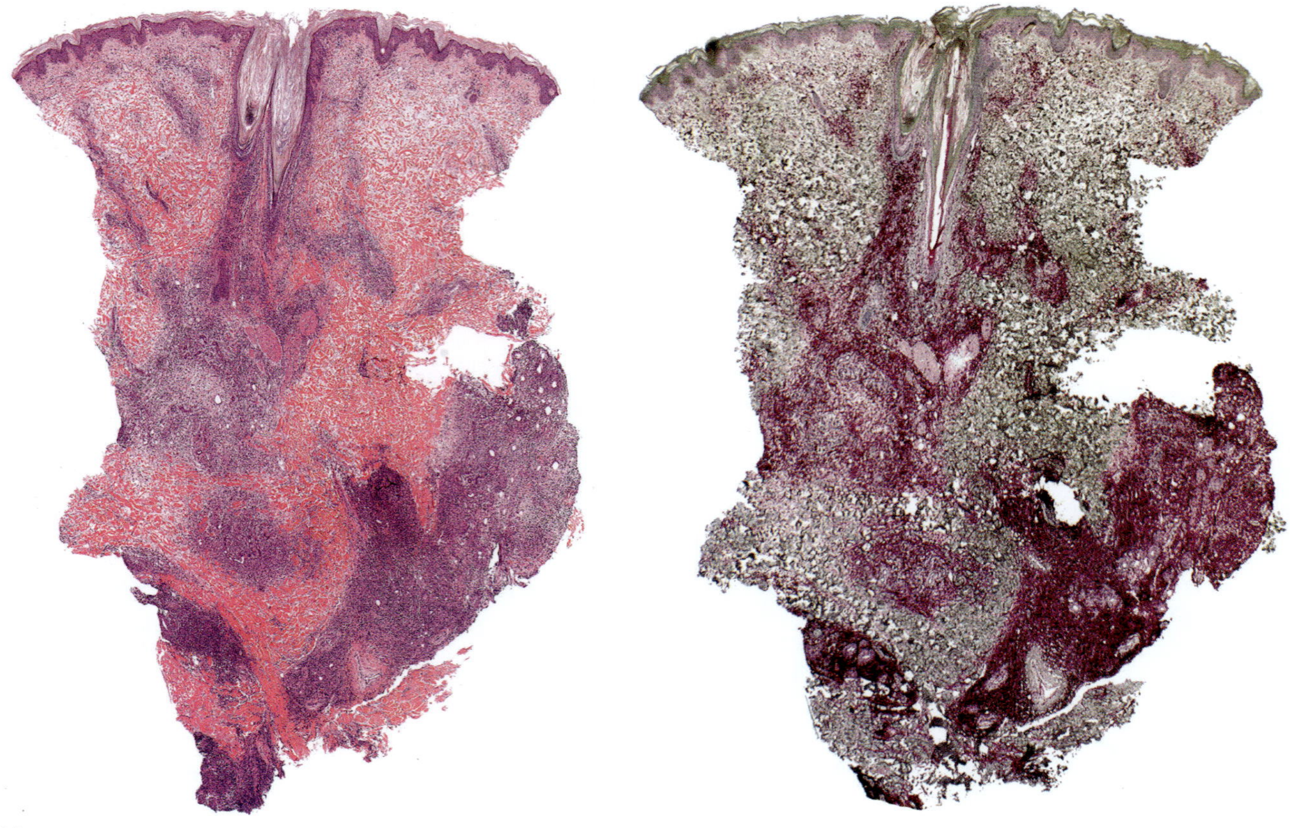

**Figure 8.15** Cutaneous γ/δ T-cell lymphoma. (a) Prominent dermal deposition of mucin and dense lymphoid infiltrate within the dermis and subcutaneous fat, (b) composed almost exclusively of TCRδ⁺ lymphocytes.

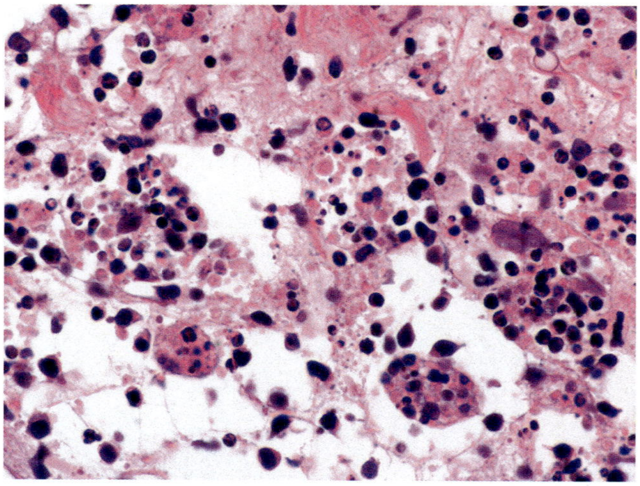

**Figure 8.16** Cutaneous γ/δ T-cell lymphoma. Hemophagocytosis characterized by large histiocytes engulfing leukocytes. This histopathologic feature is usually associated with clinical signs of hemophagocytic syndrome.

features of the neoplasms described. Particularly for cutaneous γ/δ T-cell lymphoma, overlapping clinicopathological features with benign (atypical pityriasis lichenoides), indolent malignant (mycosis fungoides, lymphomatoid papulosis, and subcutaneous panniculitis-like T-cell lymphoma), and aggressive malignant conditions (aggressive epidermotropic $CD8^+$ cytotoxic T-cell lymphoma) may be the source of confusion and of debatable classification of given cases. In this context, it has been suggested that the expression of the γ/δ phenotype is a bad prognostic indicator in cutaneous T-cell lymphomas irrespective of the classification [35]. However, in my experience, a cytotoxic phenotype does not have any prognostic implication in mycosis fungoides or lymphomatoid papulosis (see also Chapters 3 and 5) [37].

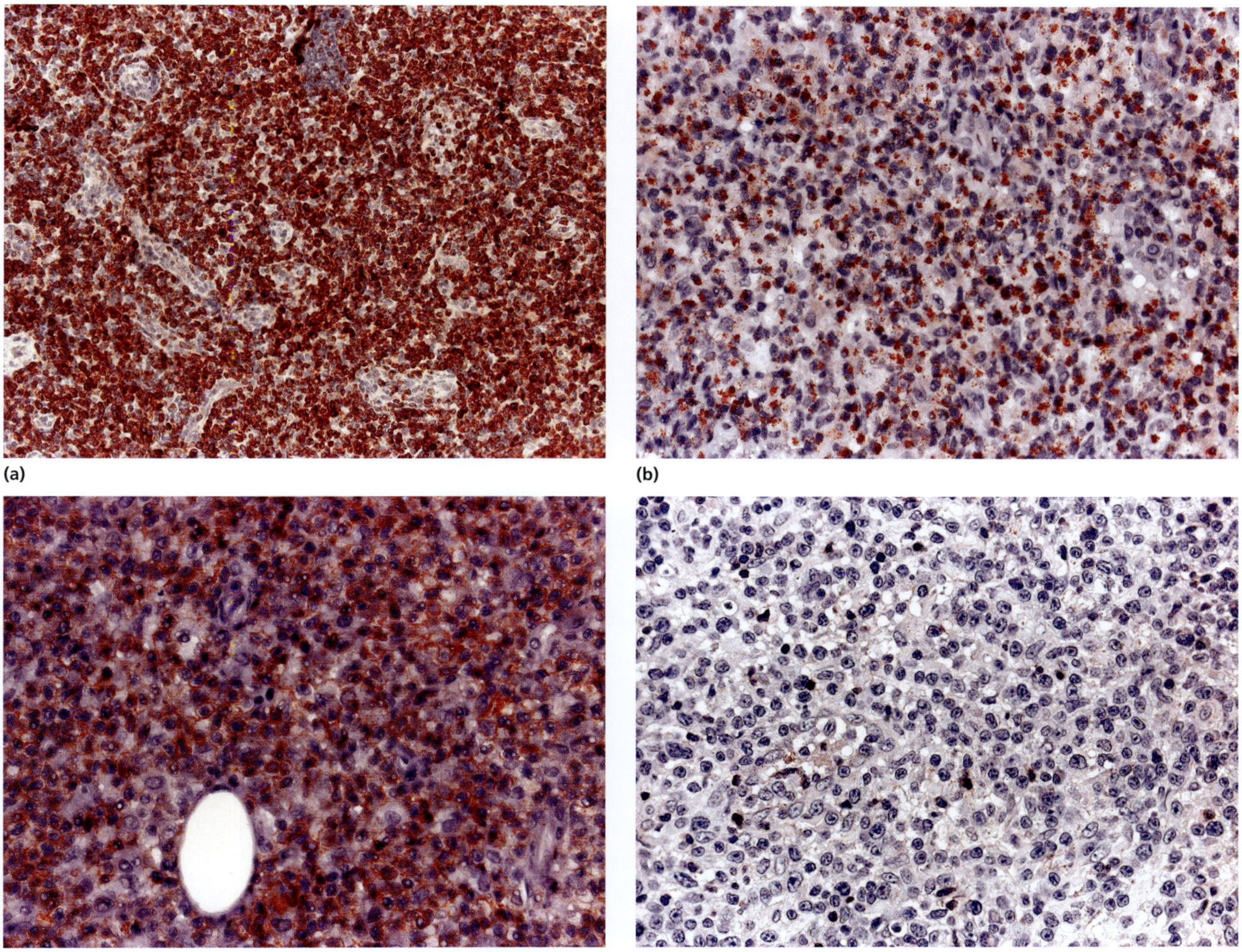


**Figure 8.17** Cutaneous γ/δ T-cell lymphoma. Neoplastic cells positive for (a) TCR-γ, (b) granzyme B and (c) CD56, and (d) negative for βF1.

## Résumé

**Cutaneous γ/δ T-cell lymphoma**

| | | |
|---|---|---|
| **Clinical** | Adults, rarely children. Generalized patches, plaques, and tumors, commonly ulcerated. Aggressive course. No previous history of mycosis fungoides. | |
| **Morphology** | Nodular or diffuse infiltrates characterized by small-, medium-, or large-sized pleomorphic cells. Subcutaneous fat commonly involved. Features of interface dermatitis at the dermoepidermal junction are frequent; epidermotropism may be prominent. | |
| **Immunohistochemistry** | CD2, CD3 | + |
| | CD5 | − (+) |
| | TCR-γ, TCR-δ | + (*essential criterion*) |
| | CD4, βF1 | − |
| | CD8 | − (+) |
| | CD30 | − (+) |
| | TIA-1, granzyme B, perforin | + |
| | CD56 | + (−) |
| | EBER-1 | − |
| **Genetics** | Monoclonal rearrangement of the TCR genes detected in the majority of the cases. Genetic differences from α/β T-cell lymphomas and from γ/δ T-cell lymphomas arising at organs other than the skin. Activation of the JAK/STAT pathway in some cases. | |
| **Treatment guidelines** | Systemic chemotherapy. Allogeneic stem cell transplantation. | |

## References


1. Rodriguez-Pinilla SM, Pro B. Primary cutaneous gamma-delta T-cell lymphoma. In: Arber DA, Borowitz MJ, Cook JR, *et al*., eds. *The International Consensus Classification of Myeloid and Lymphoid Neoplasms*. Philadelphia (US): Wolters Kluwer, 2025: 702–705.
2. Willemze R, Cerroni L, Kempf W, *et al*. The 2018 update of the WHO-EORTC classification for primary cutaneous lymphomas. *Blood* 2019;**133**:1703–1714.
3. Kempf W, Mitteldorf C, Cerroni L, *et al*. Classifications of cutaneous lymphomas and lymphoproliferative disorders: an update from the EORTC cutaneous lymphoma histopathology group. *J Eur Acad Dermatol Venereol* 2024;**38**:1491–1503.
4. Pulitzer M, Berti E, Guitart J, *et al*. Primary cutaneous gamma-delta T-cell lymphoma. In: *WHO Classification of Tumours Editorial Board. Haematolymphoid Tumours*. 5th edition. Lyon (France): IARC, 2024: 702–704.
5. Arnulf B, Copie-Bergman C, Delfau-Larue MH, *et al*. Non-hepatosplenic γ/δ T-cell lymphoma: a subset of cytotoxic lymphomas with mucosal or skin localization. *Blood* 1998;**91**:1723–1731.
6. Pulitzer M, Geller S, Kumar E, *et al*. T-cell receptor-δ expression and $\gamma/\delta^+$ T-cell infiltrates in primary cutaneous γδ T-cell lymphoma and other cutaneous T-cell lymphoproliferative disorders. *Histopathology* 2018;**73**:653–662.
7. Garcia-Herrera A, Song JY, Chuang SS, *et al*. Nonhepatosplenic γ/δ T-cell lymphomas represent a spectrum of aggressive cytotoxic T-cell lymphomas with a mainly extranodal presentation. *Am J Surg Pathol* 2011;**35**:1214–1225.
8. Omland SH, Gjerdrum LM, Walter L, *et al*. Primary cutaneous gamma-delta T-cell lymphoma positive for both T-cell receptor gamma and T-cell receptor beta. *Pathol Case Rev* 2014;**19**:216–220.
9. Rodrıguez-Pinilla SM, Ortiz-Romero PL, Monsalvez V, *et al*. TCR-gamma expression in primary cutaneous T-cell lymphomas. *Am J Surg Pathol* 2013;**37**:375–384.
10. Daniels J, Doukas PG, Martinez Escala ME, *et al*. Cellular origins and genetic landscape of cutaneous gamma delta T cell lymphomas. *Nat Commun* 2020;**11**:1806.
11. Burg G, Braun-Falco O. *Cutaneous Lymphomas*. Berlin: Springer Verlag, 1983: 391–392.
12. Alberti-Violetti S, Maronese CA, Venegoni L, *et al*. Primary cutaneous gamma-delta T cell lymphomas: a case series and overview of the literature. *Dermatopathology* 2021;**8**:515–524.
13. Goyal A, O'Leary D, Duncan LM. The significance of epidermal involvement in primary cutaneous gamma/delta (γδ) T-cell lymphoma: a systematic review and meta-analysis. *J Cutan Pathol* 2021;**48**:1449–1454.
14. Guitart J, Martinez-Escala ME. Gamma/delta T-cell in cutaneous and subcutaneous lymphoid infiltrates: malignant or not? *J Cutan Pathol* 2016;**43**:1242–1244.
15. Borra T, Custrin A, Saggini A, *et al*. Pityriasis lichenoides, atypical pityriasis lichenoides, and related conditions: a study of66 cases. *Am J Surg Pathol* 2018;**42**:1101–1112.
16. Martinez-Escala ME, Sidiropoulos M, *et al*. Gamma/delta T-cell-rich variants of pityriasis lichenoides and lymphomatoid papulosis: benign cutaneous disorders to be distinguished from aggressive cutaneous gamma/delta T-cell lymphomas. *Br J Dermatol* 2015;**172**:372–379.
17. Martin SM, Flowers R, Saavedra AP, Gru AA. A reactive peripheral gamma-delta T-cell lymphoid proliferation after a tick bite. *Am J Dermatopathol* 2019;**41**:e73–e75.
18. Boccara O, Blanche S, de Prost Y, *et al*. Cutaneous hematologic disorders in children. *Pediatr Blood Cancer* 2012;**58**:226–232.
19. Kerbout M, Mekouar F, Bahadi N, *et al*. A rare pediatric case of cutaneous gamma/delta T-cell lymphoma. *Ann Biol Clin (Paris)* 2014;**72**:483–485.
20. Guitart J, Weisenburger DD, Subtil A, *et al*. Cutaneous gamma/delta T-cell lymphomas. A spectrum of presentations with overlap with other cytotoxic lymphomas. *Am J Surg Pathol* 2012;**36**:1656–1665.
21. Lee DE, Martinez-Escala ME, Serrano LM, *et al*. Hemophagocytic lymphohistiocytosis in cutaneous T-cell lymphoma. *JAMA Dermatol* 2018;**154**:828–831.
22. Koens L, Senff NJ, Vermeer MH, *et al*. Cutaneous gamma/delta T-cell lymphoma during treatment with etanercept for rheumatoid arthritis. *Acta Derm Venereol (Stockh)* 2009;**89**:653–654.
23. Patsatsi A, Koletsa T, Sotiriadis D, *et al*. Silent T-cell lymphoma of gamma/delta T-cell origin initially presented as panniculitis. *J Eur Acad Dermatol Venereol* 2015;**29**:1244–1245.
24. Agbay RLMC, Torres-Cabala CA, Patel KP, *et al*. Immunophenotypic shifts in primary cutaneous gamma/delta T-cell lymphoma suggest antigenic modulation: a study of sequential biopsy specimens. *Am J Surg Pathol* 2017;**41**:431–445.
25. Schieke SM, Sharaf MA, Lerner A, *et al*. Primary cutaneous CD56 positive lymphoma: a diagnostic conundrum in an unusual case of lymphoma. *J Cut Pathol* 2012;**39**:540–544.
26. Yu WW, Hsieh PP, Chuang SS. Cutaneous EBV-positive γ/δ T-cell lymphoma vs. extranodal NK/T-cell lymphoma: a case report and literature review. *J Cutan Pathol* 2013;**40**:310–316.
27. Küçük C, Jiang B, Hu X, *et al*. Activating mutations of STAT5B and STAT3 in lymphomas derived from y5-T or NK cells. *Nat Commun* 2015;**6**:6025.
28. Yamamoto-Sugitani M, Kuroda J, Shimura Y, *et al*. Comprehensive cytogenetic study of primary cutaneous gamma-delta T-cell lymphoma by means of spectral karyotyping and genome-wide single nucleotide polymorphism array. *Cancer Genet* 2012;**205**:459–464.
29. Miyazaki K, Yamaguchi M, Imai H, *et al*. Gene expression profiling of peripheral T-cell lymphoma including gamma-delta T-cell lymphoma. *Blood* 2009;**113**:1071–1074.
30. Moritz RKC, Ditschkowski M, Klemke CD, *et al*. Allogeneic stem cell transplantation in patients with aggressive primary cutaneous T-cell lymphoma – a case series of the ADF working group "cutaneous lymphomas". *J Dtsch Dermatol Ges* 2014;**12**:39–46.
31. Gibson JF, Alpdogan O, Subtil A, *et al*. Hematopoietic stem cell transplantation for primary cutaneous γδ T-cell lymphoma and refractory subcutaneous panniculitis-like T-cell lymphoma. *J Am Acad Dermatol* 2015;**72**:1010–1015.
32. Isufi I, Seropian S, Gowda L, *et al*. Outcomes for allogeneic stem cell transplantation in refractory mycosis fungoides and primary cutaneous gamma delta T cell lymphomas. *Leuk Lymphoma* 2020;**61**:2955–2961.
33. Hosler GA, Liegeois N, Anhalt GJ, Moresi JM. Transformation of cutaneous gamma/delta T-cell lymphoma following 15 years of indolent behavior. *J Cutan Pathol* 2008;**35**:1063–1067.

34. Endly DC, Weenig RH, Peters MS, *et al.* Indolent course of cutaneous gamma-delta T-cell lymphoma. *J Cutan Pathol* 2013;**40**: 896–902.
35. Toro JR, Liewehr DJ, Pabby N, *et al.* Gamma-delta T-cell phenotype is associated with significantly decreased survival in cutaneous T-cell lymphoma. *Blood* 2003;**101**:3407–3412.
36. Merrill ED, Agbay R, Miranda RN, *et al.* Primary cutaneous T-cell lymphomas showing gamma-delta phenotype and predominantly epidermotropic pattern are clinicopathologically distinct from classic primary cutaneous gamma/delta T-cell lymphomas. *Am J Surg Pathol* 2017;**41**:204–215.
37. Massone C, Crisman G, Kerl H, Cerroni L. The prognosis of early mycosis fungoides is not influenced by phenotype and T-cell clonality. *Br J Dermatol* 2008;**159**:881–886.

CHAPTER 9

# Cutaneous extranodal NK/T-cell lymphoma, nasal type

Primary cutaneous extranodal natural killer (NK)/T-cell lymphoma, nasal type is not listed as a specific entity in the 2019 and 2024 updates of classification of cutaneous lymphomas by the European Organization of Research and Treatment of Cancer (EORTC) – Cutaneous Lymphoma Histopathology Group [1, 2], and is included within the group of extranodal NK/T-cell lymphoma, nasal type in the International Consensus Classification (ICC) *of Myeloid and Lymphoid Neoplasms* and the World Health Organization (WHO) *Classification of Haematolymphoid Tumours* [3, 4].

Extranodal NK/T-cell lymphoma, nasal type, is a well-defined cytotoxic lymphoma commonly located in the upper respiratory tract, especially the nasal cavity [4]. Involvement of other organs, particularly the skin, is frequent. The disease may be primary cutaneous, that is, staging investigations can be negative at presentation [5–9]. Staging in these patients is performed according to the Lugano classification (see Chapter 1, Table 1.3). It is more common in particular areas of the globe such as Asia, Mexico, and Central and South America. Immune senescence due to advanced age may be related to a proportion of primary cutaneous cases [10].

In the past, similar cases were reported as "lethal midline granuloma" or "granuloma gangrenescens" [11]. Over many years, it has become recognized that lethal midline granuloma is a term encompassing various diseases with different etiologies and pathogeneses, and that the majority of cases have a lymphoid differentiation, are associated with EBV, and are characterized by an aggressive course. Lethal midline granuloma represents direct extension of the lymphoma from the nasal cavity to the overlying skin, with destruction of the bone and soft tissues. Some cases of extranodal NK/T-cell lymphoma, nasal type, were also included in the past in the groups of angiocentric lymphoma and polymorphic reticulosis.

The majority of cases of cutaneous extranodal NK/T-cell lymphoma, nasal type, have an NK phenotype and are associated with EBV infection. Negativity for T-cell markers and germline rearrangement of T lymphocytes, together with positivity for EBV in neoplastic cells, should be interpreted as a strong diagnostic hint. Positivity for EBV represents an essential diagnostic criterion, and in negative cases, alternative diagnoses should be considered.

## Clinical features

Patients are adults with a predominance of males. Children are rarely affected [12]. In this age group, extranodal NK/T-cell lymphoma, nasal type, shows overlapping features with systemic $EBV^+$ T-cell lymphoproliferative disease of childhood and may be part of a spectrum including also aggressive NK-cell leukemia [13]. As in other cytotoxic lymphomas, an hemophagocytic syndrome is a possible, potentially lethal complication.

Skin lesions are characterized by nonspecific erythematous or violaceous plaques and tumors, which are sometimes ulcerated (Fig. 9.1). Irregular, infiltrated patches may be found as well, particularly on the trunk, and skin lesions at presentation may be clinically indistinguishable from those of mycosis fungoides (Fig. 9.2). The oral cavity and upper respiratory tract should be checked carefully at presentation and during follow-up, as involvement of these regions is common (Fig. 9.3). Symptoms of nasal obstruction and/or epistaxis should be thoroughly investigated for evidence of nasal lymphoma. The variant described in the past as lethal midline granuloma is associated with large ulcers of the nose and adjacent tissues, representing secondary spread from the nasal mucosa to the skin (Fig. 9.4).

Some patients present with marked, persistent swelling of the head and neck area that histopathologically reveals a specific infiltrate of extranodal NK/T-cell lymphoma, nasal type (Fig. 9.5). This lymphoma should be considered as a serious differential diagnosis in patients with persistent facial swelling that do not respond to conventional treatment (a similar clinical presentation can be observed also in systemic hydroa vacciniforme lymphoproliferative disorder – see Chapter 15).

A case of "lethal midline granuloma" in a patient with lymphomatoid papulosis has been described in the past [14]. In this case, the nasal lesion had a $CD30^+$ phenotype and showed the same monoclonal rearrangement of the TCR genes as the skin lesions of the lymphomatoid papulosis, thus probably representing

*Skin Lymphoma: The Illustrated Guide*, Sixth Edition. Lorenzo Cerroni.

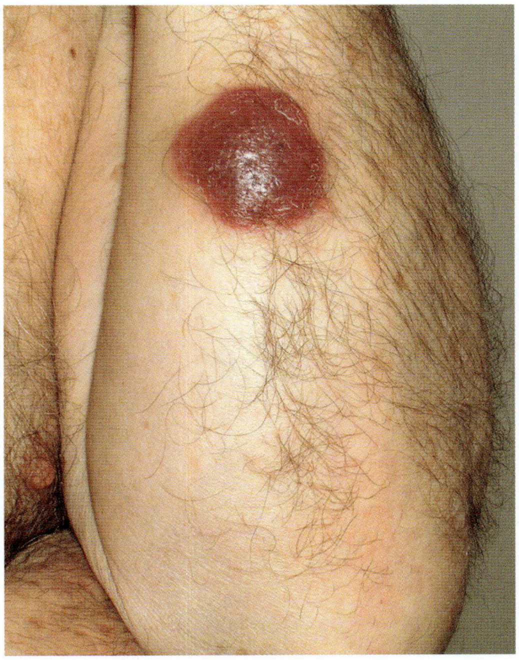

Figure 9.1 Cutaneous extranodal NK/T-cell lymphoma, nasal type. Large tumor on the arm. (*Courtesy of Dr. Esmeralda Vale, Lisboa, Portugal.*)

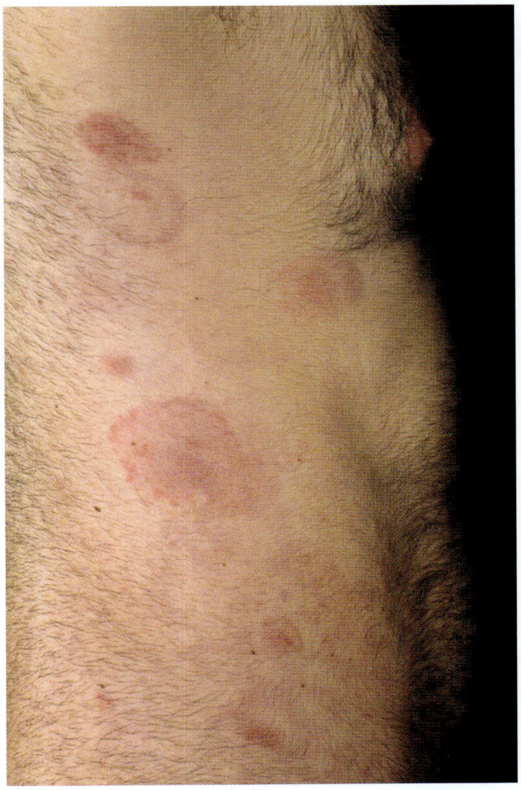

Figure 9.2 Cutaneous extranodal NK/T-cell lymphoma, nasal type. Erythematous patches on the trunk with morphologic features similar to those of mycosis fungoides. Differently from early mycosis fungoides scaling is minimal, suggesting lack of epidermal involvement. (*Courtesy of Dr. Carlo Cota, Rome, Italy.*)

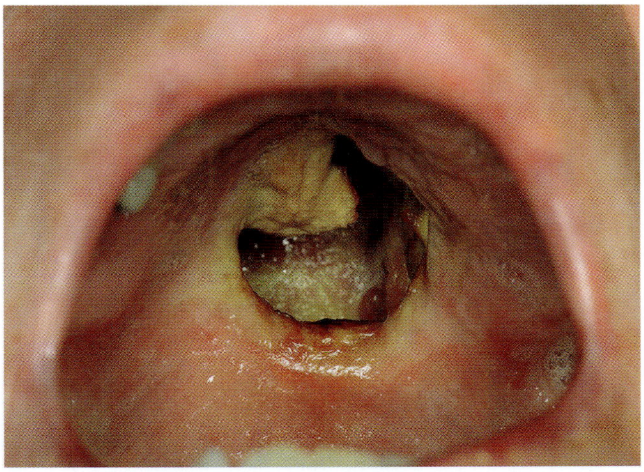

Figure 9.3 Cutaneous extranodal NK/T-cell lymphoma, nasal type. Large ulceration of the palate due to direct tumor extension from the nasopharyngeal cavity.

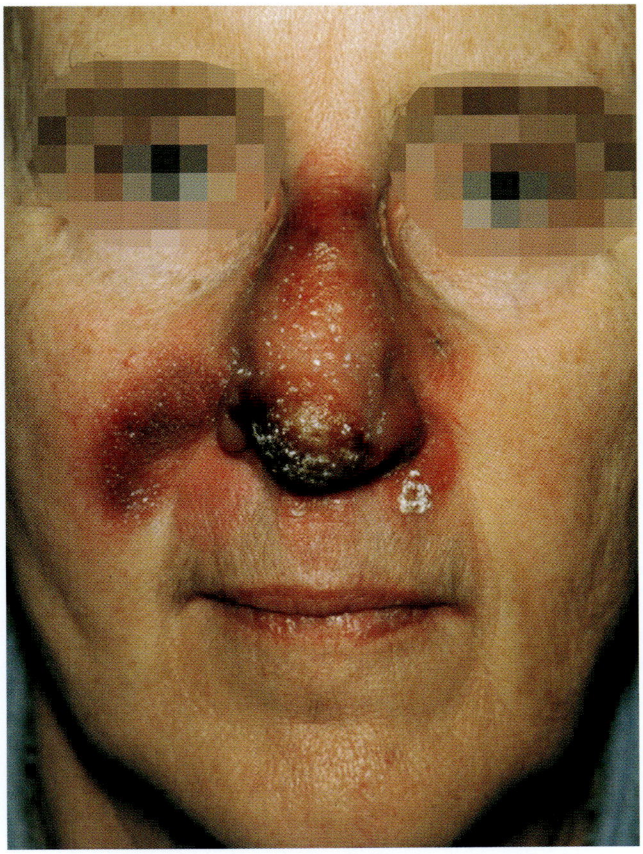

Figure 9.4 Cutaneous extranodal NK/T-cell lymphoma, nasal type. Erythematous, partly necrotic plaques on the nose and cheek (so-called "lethal midline granuloma"), due to direct extension of the lymphoma from the nasal mucosa.

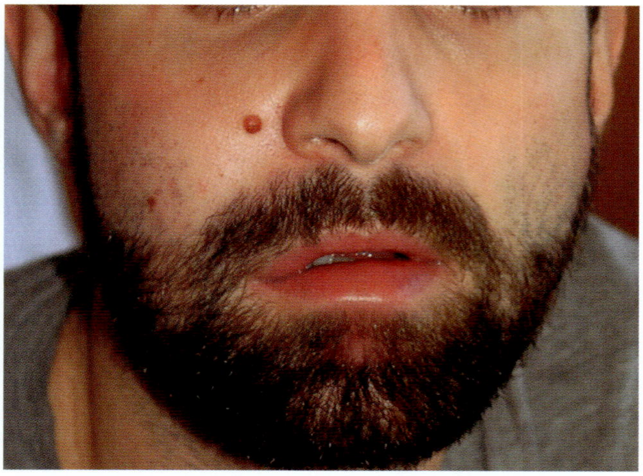

**Figure 9.5** Cutaneous extranodal NK/T-cell lymphoma, nasal type. Prominent, persistent swelling of the right cheek. (*Courtesy of Dr. Carlo Cota, Rome, Italy.*)

progression of the lymphomatoid papulosis to an anaplastic large cell lymphoma rather than association with a true extranodal NK/T-cell lymphoma, nasal type. In this context, it should be underlined that different lymphomas of both B- and T-cell lineage can develop in the mucosa of the nasal and upper respiratory tract.

## Histopathology, immunophenotype, and molecular genetics

### Histopathology

Histology reveals a diffuse proliferation of lymphocytes involving the dermis and, often, the subcutaneous tissues (Fig. 9.6). Although the pattern may be identical to that observed in cutaneous $\gamma/\delta$ T-cell lymphoma, positivity for EBV allows to distinguish the two entities (Fig. 9.7). Epidermotropism may be present, even with the formation of intraepidermal collections indistinguishable from Darier nests (Fig. 9.8). An interface dermatitis at the dermoepidermal junction may be observed in some cases, though not as frequently as in cutaneous $\gamma/\delta$ T-cell lymphoma. Cases with exclusive involvement of the subcutaneous fat may be morphologically indistinguishable from subcutaneous panniculitis-like T-cell lymphoma, but positivity for EBV allows to distinguish the two conditions (Fig. 9.9). In some cases, there is focal angiocentricity and/or angiodestruction (Fig. 9.10), but I have seen many biopsies without any hint of angiodestruction in the entire specimen. In some cases, however, angiotropism may be masked by the density of the infiltrate, and be visible only with specific stainings for the vessels (Fig. 9.11). When angiotropism is present, some of the affected vessels may show intraluminal fibrin thrombi. Necrosis may also be found. As in the other cutaneous aggressive cytotoxic

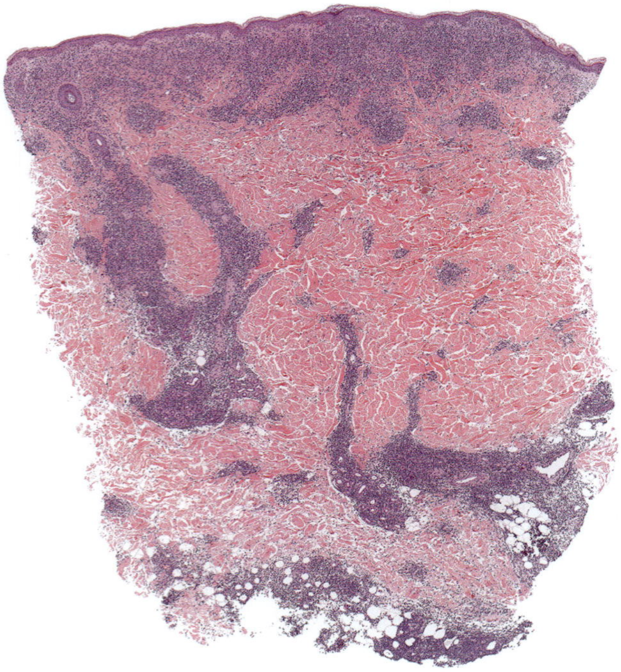

(a)

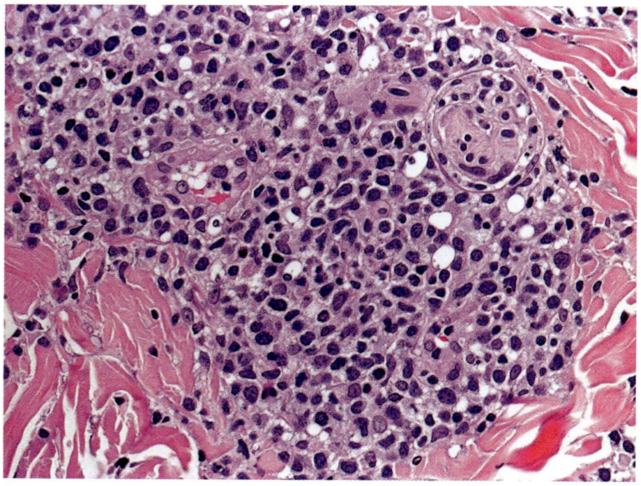

(b)

**Figure 9.6** Cutaneous extranodal NK/T-cell lymphoma, nasal type. (a) Neoplastic infiltrate in the entire dermis with involvement of the epidermis and of the subcutaneous fat; (b) small-, medium-, and large-sized neoplastic lymphocytes with pleomorphic nuclei.

lymphomas, the cytomorphologic features are variable (and unrelated to the prognosis): some cases show a predominance of small, some of medium-sized, and some of large pleomorphic lymphocytes. Azurophilic granules are commonly observed in Giemsa-stained sections of the tissue. In some cases, the infiltration of subcutaneous tissues resembles the morphologic picture of subcutaneous panniculitis-like T-cell lymphoma. However, the same biopsy or other biopsies invariably show involvement of the dermis, and sometimes of the epidermis as well.

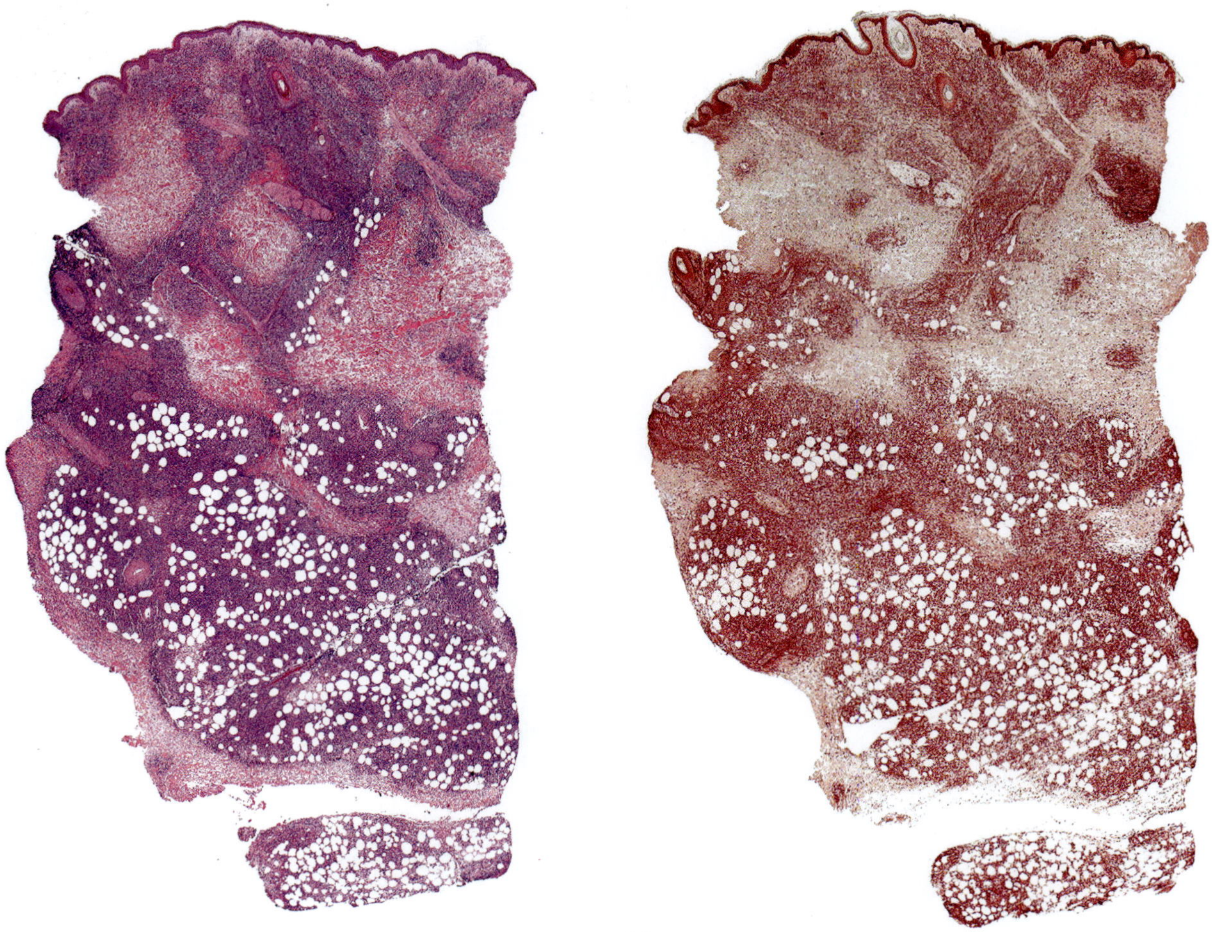

(a) (b)

Figure 9.7 Cutaneous extranodal NK/T-cell lymphoma, nasal type. (a) The distribution of the neoplastic infiltrate is identical to that observed in many cases of cutaneous $\gamma/\delta$ T-cell lymphoma, but (b) positivity for EBER-1 allows to distinguish the two conditions.

Non-infiltrated patches reveal perivascular lymphoid aggregates that on morphologic grounds may be indistinguishable from inflammatory infiltrates, representing a diagnostic pitfall (Fig. 9.12) [15]. Phenotypic studies and in situ hybridization for EBV allow a precise diagnosis in these cases.

Reactive cells, including small lymphocytes, histiocytes, and eosinophils, may be admixed with the neoplastic lymphocytes. A granulomatous reaction may also be present, as well as pseudo-epitheliomatous epidermal hyperplasia.

Differential diagnostic features from other aggressive cutaneous cytotoxic NK/T-cell lymphomas are summarized in Chapter 7. In general, in immune competent patients, positivity for EBER-1 in the context of a primary cutaneous cytotoxic NK/T-cell lymphoma should be considered strongly suggestive (if not diagnostic) of cutaneous extranodal NK/T-cell lymphoma, nasal type. Cutaneous extranodal NK/T-cell lymphoma should also be differentiated from another EBV-associated condition, systemic hydroa vacciniforme lymphoproliferative disorder, an entity observed only in particular ethnical backgrounds (for details, see Chapter 15).

## Immunophenotype

Neoplastic cells are characterized in the majority of cases by negativity for T-cell markers such as TCR-β, TCR-γ, TCR-δ, CD3, CD4, CD5, and CD8 [3, 4, 16], consistent with an NK-cell phenotype, but approximately 40% of cases show a T-cell phenotype. Cytotoxic proteins (TIA-1, granzyme B, and perforin) are positive in all cases. CD2 and cytoplasmic expression of the ε chain of the CD3 molecule are observed in most cases with NK-cell phenotype, but CD5 is invariably negative (Fig. 9.13). CD56 is positive in the vast majority of cases, but CD57 is negative (Figs. 9.14a to c). It should be reminded that the expression of CD56 is not unique to cutaneous extranodal NK/T-cell lymphoma, nasal type, as it can be observed in cases of mycosis fungoides and lymphomatoid papulosis among other cutaneous T-cell lymphomas, as well as in peripheral T-cell lymphoma, NOS [17]. Cases with a

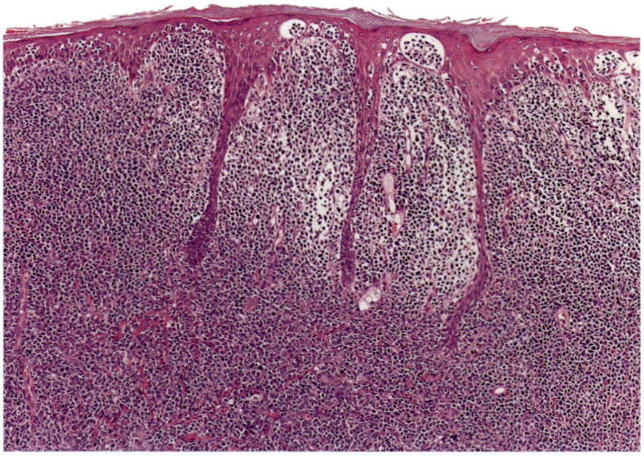

**Figure 9.8** Cutaneous extranodal NK/T-cell lymphoma, nasal type. Dense dermal infiltrates with epidermotropism and intraepidermal collections of cells indistinguishable from Darier nests.

true T-cell phenotype are positive for CD5 and variably positive for CD8, and may express α/β or, rarely, γ/δ T-cell receptors.

CD45RO, CD7, CD43, and CD25 are usually positive. PD-L1 is expressed in the majority of cases and PD-1 in a smaller number, providing a rationale for specific therapy. CD30 expression may be found in up to 40% of the cases. Aberrant expression of B-cell markers (CD79a) has been detected in one case, underlining the need for complete phenotypic investigations [18]. Increased MYC expression has been observed in cases with *BCOR* mutations [19]. In one study, using three immunohistochemical markers (FoxP3, PD-L1, and CD68), different disease stages of the disease have been linked to four different tumor immune microenvironments, termed "immune tolerance" (characterized by high-Treg counts and observed frequently in the early stage of nasal cases), "immune evasion-A and B" (characterized by high cytotoxic T-cell counts and high PD-L1 expression but low Treg counts), and "immune silenced" (characterized by exhaustion of almost all immune responses and advanced stage) [20].

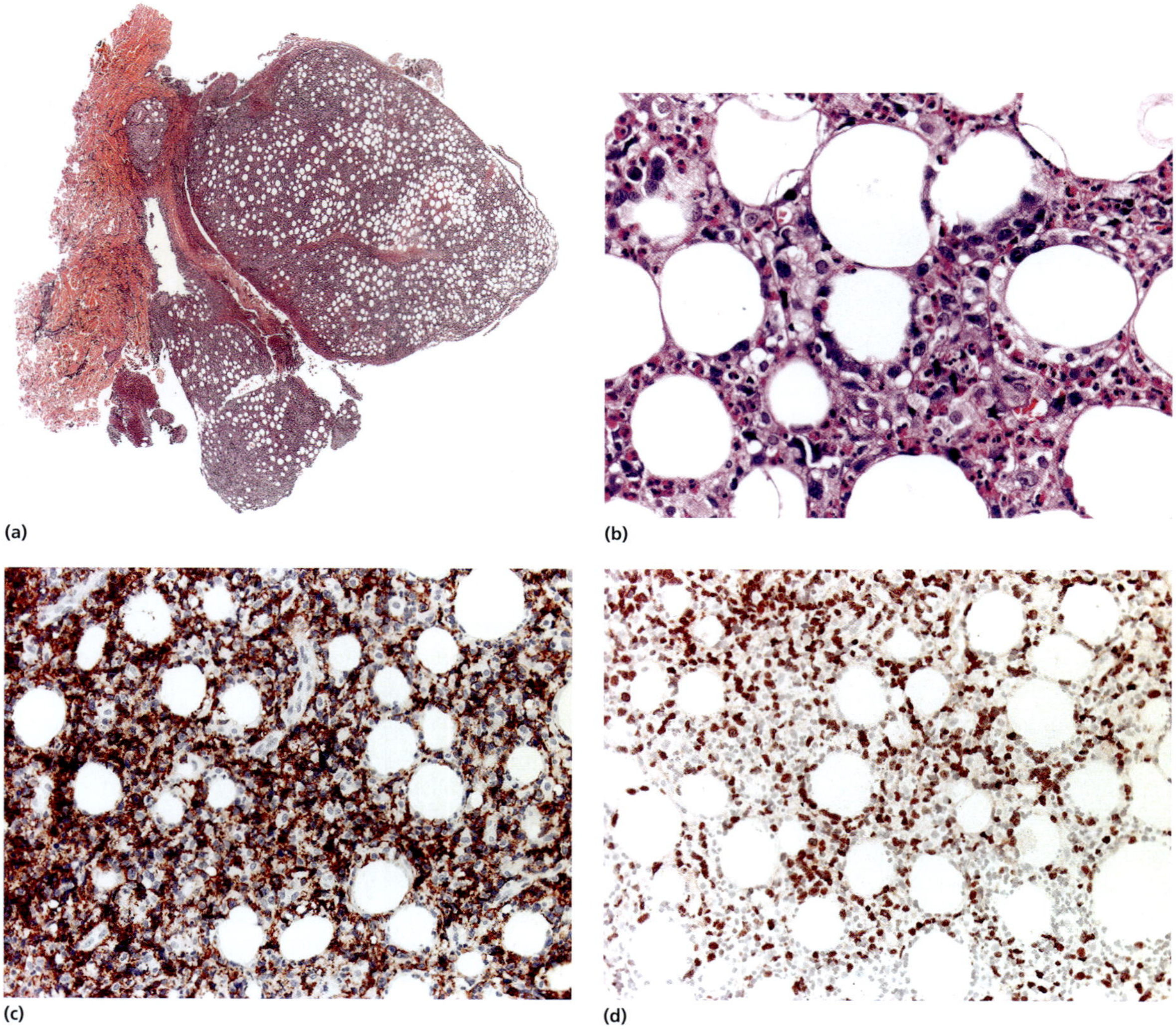


**Figure 9.9** Cutaneous extranodal NK/T-cell lymphoma, nasal type. (a) Exclusive involvement of the subcutaneous fat may be identical to the morphologic presentation of subcutaneous panniculitis-like T-cell lymphoma, even (b) with rimming of adipocytes by neoplastic lymphocytes (in this particular case admixed with numerous eosinophils), but (c) positivity for CD56 and (d) EBER-1 allows to distinguish the two conditions.

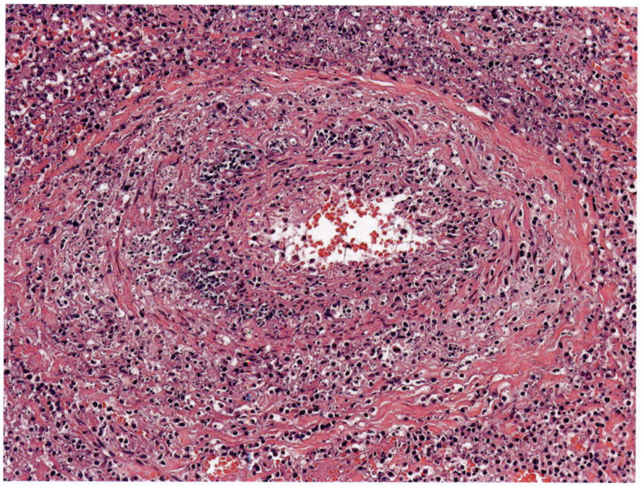

**Figure 9.10** Cutaneous extranodal NK/T-cell lymphoma, nasal type. Angiocentricity with angiotropic lymphocytes.

EBV can be demonstrated by in situ hybridization (EBER-1) in the majority of the neoplastic cells (Figs. 9.7b, 9.9c, 9.12d, 9.14d) and a negative result rules out the diagnosis. Immunohistochemical staining for EBV latent membrane protein (LMP) gives inconsistent results. The EBV strain subtype A is found more frequently than the subtype B [21].

## Molecular genetics

Molecular analyses reveal a germline configuration of the TCR genes in most of the cases of extranodal NK/T-cell lymphoma, nasal type, but a proportion of cases show a true T-cell phenotype with a monoclonal rearrangement of the TCR genes (it seems to be more common in primary cutaneous cases), and some authors even suggested that a T-cell lineage may be more frequent than an NK-cell one [22, 23]. A restricted killer cell immunoglobulin-like receptor repertoire has been found by the reverse transcriptase polymerase chain reaction (RT-PCR)

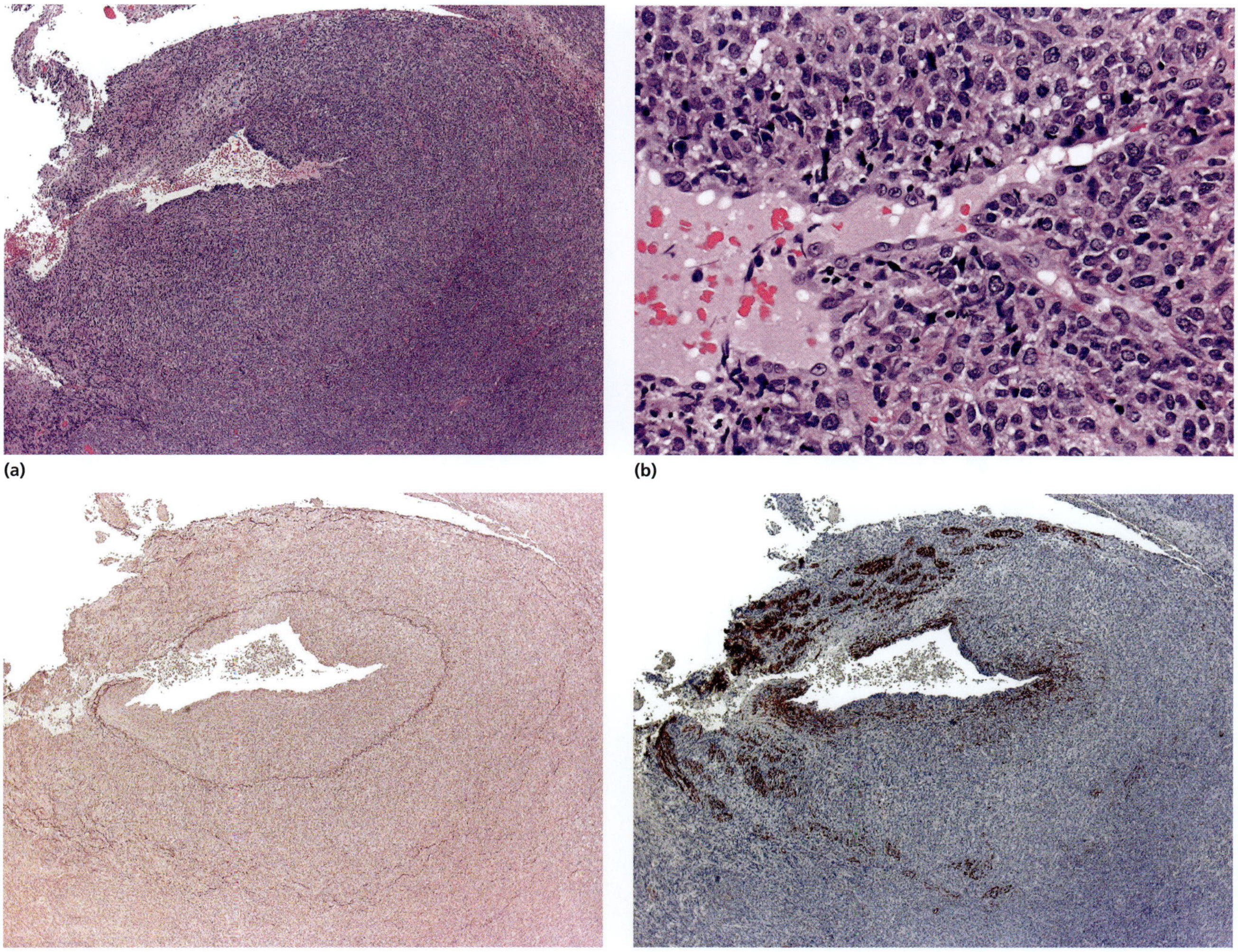

(a) (b) (c) (d)

**Figure 9.11** Cutaneous extranodal NK/T-cell lymphoma, nasal type. (a, b) Angiotropism is not visible on a section stained with hematoxylin and eosin, but appears evident with stainings for (c) elastic fibers (orcein) and (d) smooth muscle actin, highlighting the remnants of a large vein.

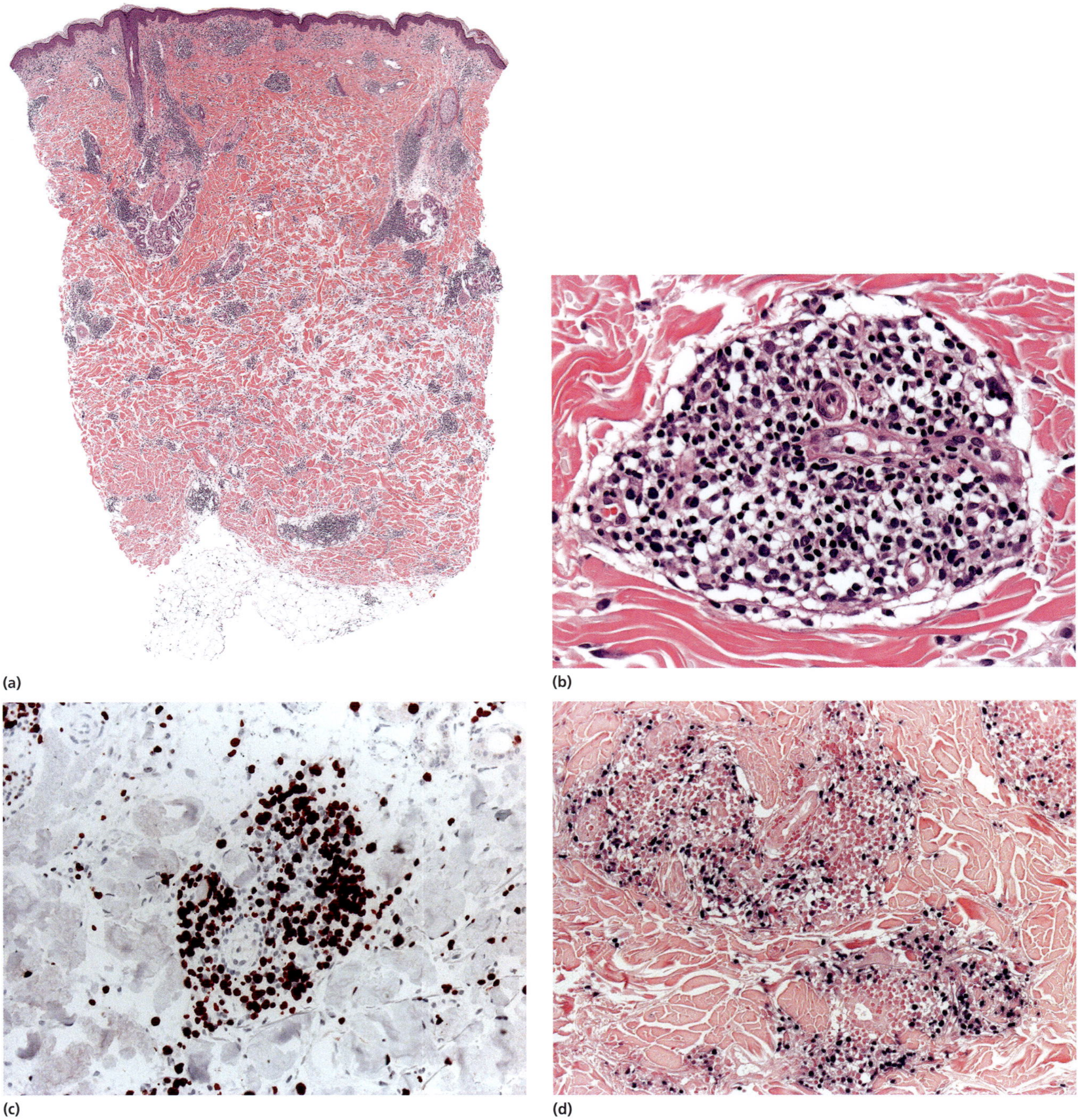

Figure 9.12 Cutaneous extranodal NK/T-cell lymphoma, nasal type. (a) Early lesion showing in the dermis mucin deposition with sparse perivascular aggregates composed of (b) small- and mid-sized lymphocytes, mimicking the picture of lupus erythematosus. (c) The proliferation rate (Ki-67) is >80%, and (d) many cells are positive for EBV (EBER-1), providing diagnostic clues. The patient subsequently developed involvement of the nasal mucosa and of a cervical lymph node.

technique, indicating the presence of a monoclonal or possibly oligoclonal NK cell proliferation [24]. As expected, given the association with EBV infection, neoplastic cells overexpress EBV-induced genes [25]. Gene expression profiling revealed a distinct molecular signature, confirming the origin from activated NK cells and showing the overexpression of genes with different functions, including cell–cell interactions (integrins, E-cadherin, and *VCAM1*), extracellular matrix degradation (*TIMP1*, *TIMP2*, and *TIMP3*), innate immune responses (Toll-like receptors), and chemokine encoding (*CXCL9/Mig*, *CXCL10/IP-10*,

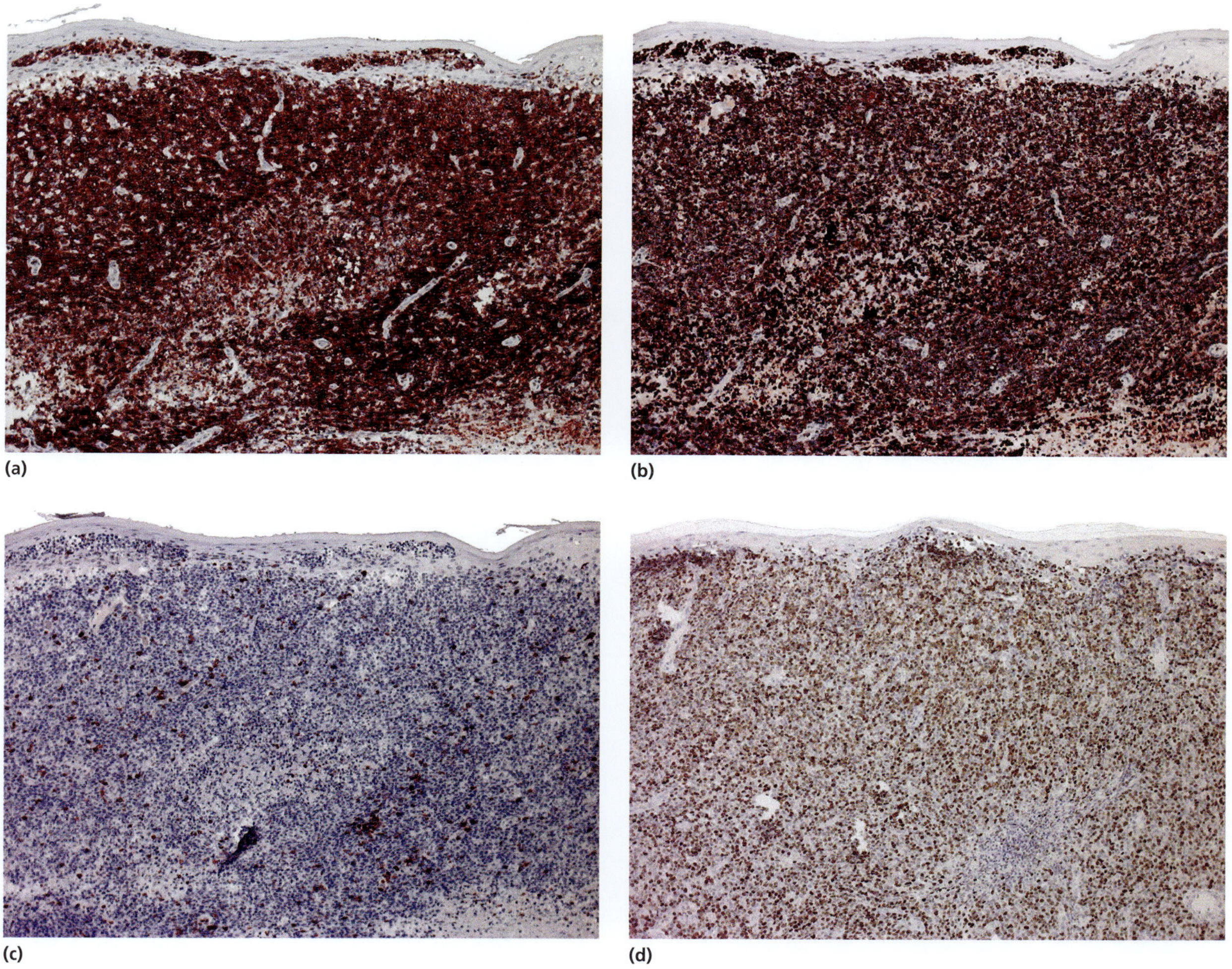

Figure 9.13 Cutaneous extranodal NK/T-cell lymphoma, nasal type. In cases with a true NK-cell phenotype, neoplastic cells are (a) positive for CD2 and (b) granzyme B, (c) negative for CD5, and (d) positive for EBER-1.

and *CXCL12/SDF-1*), as well as of oncogenes such as *C-MYC*, among others, and EBV-related genes (*EBI3*) [25]. Interestingly, it seems that different EBV-associated lymphomas, including extranodal NK/T-cell lymphoma and EBV-positive diffuse large B-cell lymphoma, share a common pathway observed in patients with chronic active EBV infection, characterized by disease originating from an EBV-infected lymphoid progenitor that acquires *DDX3X* and other mutations, causing clonal evolution in different cell lineages [26]. In extranodal NK/T-cell lymphoma, nasal type, deletions in BamHI A rightward transcript (*BART*) microRNA clusters and in other genes essential for the production of viral particles may be responsible for reactivation of the lytic cycle by upregulating the expression of *BZLF1* and *BRLF1*, and at the same time preventing viral production and cell lysis [26].

Recurrent mutations, deletions, and hypermethylation affect the JAK/STAT signaling pathway (*STAT3*, *STAT5B*, *JAK3*, and *PTPRK*) and other signaling pathways [27–29]. aCGH studies revealed recurrent abnormalities, namely, gains of 2q and losses of 6q16.1-q27, 11q22.3-q23.3, 5p14.1-p14.3, 5q34-q35.3, 1p36.23-p36.33, 2p16.1-p16.3, 4q12, and 4q31.3-q32.1 [30]. Especially, the loss of 6q21-25 has been frequently reported, and the transcription factors *PRDM1*, *FOXO3*, *PTPRK*, and *HACE1* have been identified as the most likely targets in this locus. In fact, the re-expression of *PRDM1* and *FOXO3* suppressed proliferation, and reconstitution of *PRDM1* led to G2/M cell cycle arrest, increased apoptosis, and a strong negative selection pressure in 6q-deleted NK cell lines, supporting their role as tumor suppressors. The tumor suppressor *HACE1* on 6q21 is also frequently deregulated [25].

Berti *et al.* have detected loss of 9p21 in one case of secondary cutaneous extranodal NK/T-cell lymphoma, nasal type, but in none of the three primary cutaneous cases, suggesting that *CDKN2A* loss could be useful to distinguish primary cutaneous from secondary cutaneous cases [31]. However, our group found *CDNK2A* loss in 3/5 cases of primary cutaneous extranodal NK/T-cell lymphoma, nasal type [32]. *CDNK2A* is an important gene for cell cycle G1 control, encoding the inhibitor of

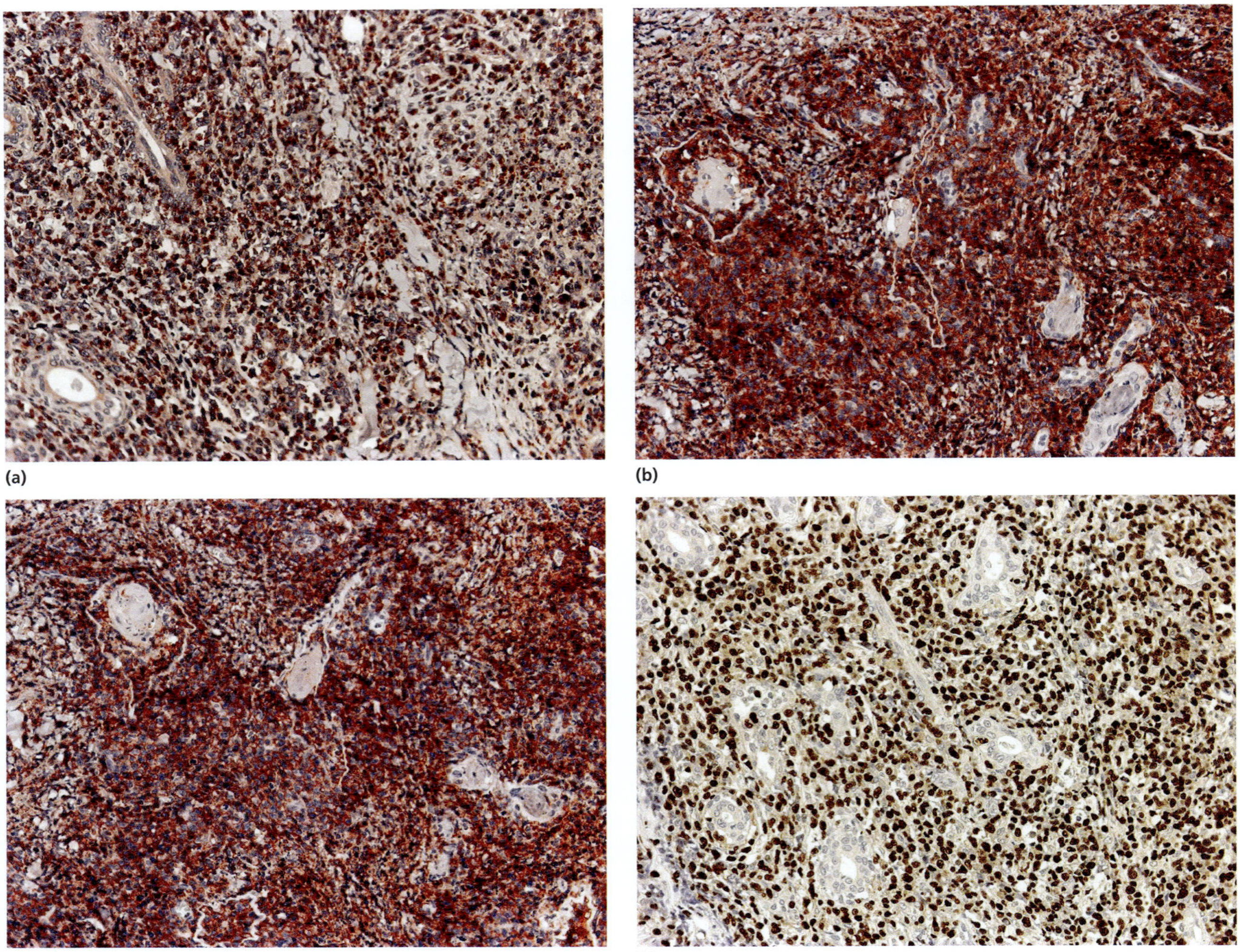

(a) (b) (c) (d)

**Figure 9.14** Cutaneous extranodal NK/T-cell lymphoma, nasal type. (a) Positivity of neoplastic cells for the cytotoxic marker TIA-1. (b) Strong positivity for CD2 and (c) CD56. (d) Positive signal of all neoplastic cells upon in situ hybridization for EBV (EBER-1).

cyclin D-dependent kinase, p16INK4a, and the unrelated ARF protein, which acts as a stabilizer of the tumor suppressor protein p53. *CDKN2A* loss may represent a late event in lymphomagenesis in extranodal NK/T-cell lymphoma, nasal type. Loss of 17p13.1, harboring the tumor suppressor gene *TP53*, can be observed in some cases [31]. Recurrent mutations have been identified also in epigenetic regulators (*BCOR*, *KMT2D*, *ARID1A*, and *EP300*) [19, 33].

Using the aCGH analysis, our group had the opportunity to study the genetic alterations in different biopsies taken over a 23-year period from a long-term survivor [32]. A less complex profile, with losses in 7p and gains in 6p, was observed in the first diagnostic biopsy. Only additional losses in 19 and gains in 7q could be observed in a second biopsy taken from a solitary recurrent lesion at the same site 22 years after the first one. By contrast, several new aberrations were present in the last biopsy taken one year afterwards when the patient had progressive disease, with additional gains in 1, 3, 4, 14, 16, and 20 and losses in 4, 6, 9, and 13, suggesting that in some cases of extranodal NK/T-cell lymphoma, nasal type, these alterations may represent late events in the lymphomagenesis.

## Treatment

Cases with involvement limited to the skin should be treated like those with extracutaneous involvement. The therapy of choice is systemic chemotherapy (L-asparaginase-containing chemotherapy, SMILE) [34]. Platinum anticancer agents are also used, whereas anthracycline-containing chemotherapy is not recommended [35]. Radiotherapy has been used for solitary lesions or for localized disease [36, 37], and is effective at a dose of 50 Gy to 54 Gy for nasal lesions [35]. Allogeneic stem-cell transplantation is efficacious, but there is a high transplant-related mortality [38]. Daratumumab (a naked anti-CD38 antibody) and brentuximab vedotin (anti-CD30 antibody) have been used in some cases. In the light of the PD-L1 expression, nivolumab, pembrolizumab, or other anti-PD-L1 antibodies represent further therapeutic options in patients with advanced or relapsed disease [39, 40]. The PD-L1 expression due to genetic alterations, such as *PD-L1*$^{MUT}$, may predict the response to immune checkpoint inhibitors (whereas the induced PD-L1 expression is likely a factor of resistance to immune checkpoint blockade), suggesting a potential role of *PD-L1*$^{MUT}$ as a biomarker to select patients for PD-1 blockade therapy [41]. Different microenvironments may be associated with different response to immunotherapy [20].

## Prognosis

The prognosis of cutaneous extranodal NK/T-cell lymphoma, nasal type, is poor and most patients die a few months after the diagnosis. The estimated five-year survival is <1% [42]. No histopathologic or clinical features are predictive of prognosis [43], but a better course has been described in patients who have primary skin involvement, as opposed to those with nasal lymphoma and secondary skin manifestations [12, 44]. The aberrant overexpression of the enhancer of zeste homolog 2 (EZH2, an H3K27-specific histone methyltransferase inducing H3K27 dimethylation and trimethylation) and underexpression of H3K27me3 were correlated with a worse prognosis in one study, showing also that pharmacologic suppression of the JAK3/STAT3 pathway effectively reduced the expression of EZH2 and enhanced expression of H3K27me3 in NK/T tumor cell lines [45]. The presence of *BCOR* mutations associated with increased MYC expression seems to be an independent indicator of poor prognosis, suggesting a possible role of immunohistochemistry for MYC in stratifying patients [19].

Prognosis is worse in patients with positive end-of-treatment plasma EBV DNA and/or PET-CT findings [46]. In secondary skin involvement from extranodal lymphoma, the extent of cutaneous lesions was related to prognosis [47]. In cases arising at various extranodal sites, a high proliferation rate was correlated with a more aggressive course [48]. Patients reported to have the coexpression of CD30 and CD56, and better prognosis may have had in truth a cutaneous anaplastic large cell lymphoma [49].

Patients with tumors of the $CD56^{dim/}$–$CD16^{+}$ phenotype had a poorer prognosis than patients with tumors of the other phenotypes in one study [50]. A correlation has been observed between vascular endothelial growth factor (VEGF) protein expression and worse prognosis in patients with cutaneous extranodal NK/T-cell lymphoma, suggesting a possible role for the VEGF monoclonal antibody bevacizumab in the therapy of cutaneous extranodal NK/T-cell lymphoma [51].

Although extranodal NK/T-cell lymphoma, nasal type, is considered to be a disease with aggressive behavior, rare patients experience a prolonged course over several years or even decades in spite of nonaggressive treatment (both at cutaneous and extracutaneous sites) [32, 52, 53]. The histologic and phenotypic features of the lesions are indistinguishable from those observed in more aggressive cases. Molecular genetic analyses show less complex aberrations (see the section on molecular genetics), but data are very limited and other patients with few aberrations at presentation had a conventional, aggressive course.

### Résumé

**Extranodal NK/T-cell lymphoma, nasal type**

| | | |
|---|---|---|
| **Clinical** | Adults; children rarely affected. Solitary, regionally localized or generalized patches, plaques, and tumors, sometimes ulcerated. Midline facial ulcerated plaques/tumors ("lethal midline granuloma") and persistent facial swelling are typical presentations. Usually aggressive course; prolonged survival reported in rare patients. | |
| **Morphology** | Nodular or diffuse infiltrates characterized by small-, medium-, or large-sized pleomorphic cells. Frequent involvement of subcutaneous fat. Variable epidermotropism. | |
| **Immunohistochemistry** | CD2, cytoplasmic CD3ε, CD56 | + |
| | CD3, CD4, CD5, CD8 | – (cases with T-cell phenotype $CD3^{+}$ may be $CD8^{+}$) |
| | CD30 | –/+ |
| | TIA-1, granzyme B, perforin | + |
| | PD-L1 | + (–) |
| | EBER-1 | + *(essential criterion)* |
| **Genetics** | TCR genes in germline configuration in the majority of the cases. Complex genetic aberrations. Common loss of 6q21-25. Frequent gains of 2q and 7q and losses of 7p. Recurrent mutations, deletions, and hypermethylation affect the JAK/STAT signaling pathway. | |
| **Treatment guidelines** | Systemic chemotherapy (L-asparaginase-containing chemotherapy, SMILE). Radiotherapy of localized disease. PD-1 blockade therapy in advanced and/or relapsed disease. | |

## References


1. Willemze R, Cerroni L, Kempf W, *et al.* The 2018 update of the WHO-EORTC classification for primary cutaneous lymphomas. *Blood* 2019;**133**:1703–1714.
2. Kempf W, Mitteldorf C, Cerroni L, *et al.* Classifications of cutaneous lymphomas and lymphoproliferative disorders: an update from the EORTC cutaneous lymphoma histopathology group. *J Eur Acad Dermatol Venereol* 2024;**38**:1491–1503.
3. Chan WC, Kim WS, Ko YH, Pittaluga S. Extranodal natural killer/T-cell lymphoma, nasal type. In: Arber DA, Borowitz MJ, Cook JR, *et al.*, eds. *The International Consensus Classification of Myeloid and Lymphoid Neoplasms*. Philadelphia (US): Wolters Kluwer, 2025: 627–634.
4. Chuang SS, Ng SB, Cheng CL, *et al.* Extranodal NK/T-cell lymphoma. In: *WHO Classification of Tumours Editorial Board. Haematolymphoid Tumours.* 5th edition. Lyon (France): IARC, 2024: 765–769.
5. Massone C, Chott A, Metze D, *et al.* Subcutaneous, blastic natural killer (NK) NK/T-cell and other cytotoxic lymphomas of the skin: a morphologic, immunophenotypic and molecular study of 50 patients. *Am J Surg Pathol* 2004;**28**:719–735.
6. Santucci M, Pimpinelli N, Massi D, *et al.* Cytotoxic natural killer cell cutaneous lymphomas: report of the EORTC Cutaneous Lymphoma Task Force Workshop. *Cancer* 2003;**97**:610–627.
7. Miyamoto T, Yoshino T, Takehisa T, *et al.* Cutaneous presentation of nasal/nasal type T/NK cell lymphoma: clinicopathological findings of four cases. *Br J Dermatol* 1998;**139**:481–487.
8. Natkunam Y, Smoller BR, Zehnder JL, *et al.* Aggressive cutaneous NK and NK-like T-cell lymphomas. Clinicopathologic, immunohistochemical, and molecular analyses of 12 cases. *Am J Surg Pathol* 1999;**23**:571–581.
9. Yu JB, Zuo Z, Tang Y, *et al.* Extranodal nasal-type natural killer/T-cell lymphoma of the skin: a clinicopathologic study of 16 cases in China. *Hum Pathol* 2009;**40**:807–816.
10. Wu CC, Takahashi E, Asano N, *et al.* Primary cutaneous NK/T-cell lymphoma of nasal type: an age-related lymphoproliferative disease? *Hum Pathol* 2017;**68**:61–68.
11. Chott A, Rappersberger K, Schlossarek W, Radaszkiewicz T. Peripheral T cell lymphoma presenting primarily as lethal midline granuloma. *Hum Pathol* 1988;**19**:1093–1101.
12. Boccara O, Blanche S, de Prost Y, *et al.* Cutaneous hematologic disorders in children. *Pediatr Blood Cancer* 2012;**58**:226–232.
13. Takahashi E, Ohshima K, Kimura H, *et al.* Clinicopathological analysis of the age-related differences in patients with Epstein–Barr virus (EBV)-associated extranasal natural killer (NK). T-cell lymphoma with reference to the relationship with aggressive NK cell leukaemia and chronic active EBV infection-associated lymphoproliferative disorders. *Histopathology* 2011;**59**:660–671.
14. Harabuchi Y, Kataura A, Kobayashi K, *et al.* Lethal midline granuloma (peripheral T-cell lymphoma) after lymphomatoid papulosis. *Cancer* 1992;**70**:835–839.
15. Lee WJ, Kang HJ, Won CH, *et al.* Cutaneous extranodal natural killer/T-cell lymphomas histopathologically mimicking benign inflammatory disease. *Am J Dermatopathol* 2017;**39**:171–176.
16. Schwartz EJ, Molina-Kirsch H, Zhao S, *et al.* Immunohistochemical characterization of nasal-type extranodal NK/T-cell lymphoma using a tissue microarray. An analysis of 84 cases. *Am J Clin Pathol* 2008;**130**:343–351.
17. Takata K, Hong M, Sitthinamsuwan P, *et al.* Primary cutaneous NK/T-cell lymphoma, nasal type and CD56-positive peripheral T-cell lymphoma. A cellular lineage and clinicopathologic study of 60 patients from Asia. *Am J Surg Pathol* 2015;**39**:1–12.
18. Blakolmer K, Vesely M, Kummer JA, *et al.* Immunoreactivity of B-cell markers (CD79a, L26) in rare cases of extranodal cytotoxic peripheral T (NK/T-) cell lymphomas. *Mod Pathol* 2000;**13**:766–772.
19. Oishi N, Satou A, Miyaoka M, *et al.* Genetic and immunohistochemical profiling of NK/T-cell lymphomas reveals prognostically relevant BCOR-MYC association. *Blood Adv* 2023;**7**:178–189.
20. Cho J, Kim SJ, Park WY, *et al.* Immune subtyping of extranodal NK/T-cell lymphoma: a new biomarker and an immune shift during disease progression. *Mod Pathol* 2020;**33**:603–615.
21. Gualco G, Domeny-Duarte P, Chioato L, *et al.* Clinicopathologic and molecular features of 122 Brazilian cases of nodal and extranodal NK/T-cell lymphoma, nasal type, with EBV subtyping analysis. *Am J Surg Pathol* 2011;**35**:1195–1203.
22. Hong M, Lee T, Kang SY, *et al.* Nasal-type NK/T-cell lymphomas are more frequently T rather than NK lineage based on T-cell receptor gene, RNA, and protein studies: lineage does not predict clinical behavior. *Mod Pathol* 2016;**29**:430–443.
23. Jhuang JY, Chang ST, Weng SF, *et al.* Extranodal natural killer/T-cell lymphoma, nasal type in Taiwan: a relatively higher frequency of T-cell lineage and poor survival for extranasal tumors. *Hum Pathol* 2015;**46**:313–321.
24. Lin CW, Lee WH, Chang CL, *et al.* Restricted killer cell immunoglobulin-like receptor repertoire without T-cell receptor g rearrangement supports a true natural killer-cell lineage in a subset of sinonasal lymphomas. *Am J Pathol* 2001;**159**:1671–1679.
25. Huang Y, de Reynies A, de Leval L, *et al.* Gene expression profiling identifies emerging oncogenic pathways operating in extranodal NK/T-cell lymphoma, nasal type. *Blood* 2010;**115**:1225–1237.
26. Okuno Y, Murata T, Sato Y, *et al.* Defective Epstein-Barr virus in chronic active infection and haematological malignancy. *Nat Microbiol* 2019;**4**:404–413.
27. Küçük C, Jiang B, Hu X, *et al.* Activating mutations of STAT5B and STAT3 in lymphomas derived from y5-T or NK cells. *Nat Commun* 2015;**6**:6025.
28. Coppo P, Gouilleux-Gruart V, Huang Y, *et al.* STAT3 transcription factor is constitutively activated and is oncogenic in nasal-type NK/T-cell lymphoma. *Leukemia* 2009;**23**:1667–1678.
29. Lee S, Park HY, Kang SY, *et al.* Genetic alterations of JAK/STAT cascade and histone modification in extranodal NK/T-cell lymphoma nasal type. *Oncotarget* 2015;**6**:17764–17776.
30. Nakashima Y, Tagawa H, Suzuki R, *et al.* Genome-wide array-based comparative genomic hybridization of natural killer cell lymphoma/leukemia: different genomic alteration patterns of aggressive NK-cell leukemia and extranodal NK/T-cell lymphoma, nasal type. *Genes Chromosomes Cancer* 2005;**44**:247–255.
31. Berti E, Recalcati S, Girgenti V, *et al.* Cutaneous extranodal NK/T-cell lymphoma: a clinicopathologic study of 5 patients with array-based comparative genomic hybridization. *Blood* 2010;**116**:165–170.
32. Fried I, Artl M, Cota C, *et al.* Clinicopathologic and molecular features in cutaneous extranodal natural killer-/T-cell lymphoma, nasal type, with aggressive and indolent course. *J Am Acad Dermatol* 2014;**70**:716–723.

33. Dobashi A, Tsuyama N, Asaka R, *et al.* Frequent *BCOR* aberrations in extranodal NK/T-cell lymphoma, nasal type. *Genes Chromosomes Cancer* 2016;**55**:460–471.
34. Willemze R, Hodak E, Zinzani PL, *et al.* Primary cutaneous lymphomas: ESMO Clinical Practice Guidelines for diagnosis, treatment and follow-up. *Ann Oncol* 2018;**29**(Supplement 4):iv30–iv40.
35. Yamaguchi M, Suzuki R, Oguchi M. Advances in the treatment of extranodal NK/T-cell lymphoma, nasal type. *Blood* 2018;**131**: 2528–2540.
36. Ahn HK, Suh C, Chuang SS, *et al.* Extranodal natural killer/T-cell lymphoma from skin or soft tissue: suggestion of treatment from multinational retrospective analysis. *Ann Oncol* 2012;**23**:2703–2707.
37. Kim TM, Heo DS. Extranodal NK/T-cell lymphoma, nasal type: new staging system and treatment strategies. *Cancer Science* 2009;**100**:2242–2248.
38. Liang R. Advances in the management and monitoring of extranodal NK/T-cell lymphoma, nasal type. *Br J Haematol* 2009;**147**:13–21.
39. Kwong YL, Chan TSY, Tan D, *et al.* PD1 blockade with pembrolizumab is highly effective in relapsed or refractory NK/T-cell lymphoma failing l-asparaginase. *Blood* 2017;**129**:2437–2442.
40. Kim SJ, Lim JQ, Laurensia Y, *et al.* Avelumab for the treatment of relapsed or refractory extranodal NK/T-cell lymphoma: an open-label phase 2 study. *Blood* 2020;**136**:2754–2763.
41. Lim JQ, Huang D, Tang T, *et al.* Whole-genome sequencing identifies responders to pembrolizumab in relapse/refractory natural-killer/T cell lymphoma. *Leukemia* 2020;**34**:3413–3419.
42. Fink-Puches R, Zenahlik P, Bäck B, *et al.* Primary cutaneous lymphomas: applicability of current classification schemes (European Organization for Research and Treatment of Cancer, World Health Organization) based on clinicopathologic features observed in a large group of patients. *Blood* 2002;**99**:800–805.
43. Au WY, Weisenburger DD, Intragumtomchai T, *et al.* Clinical differences between nasal and extranasal natural killer/T-cell lymphoma: a study of 136 cases from the International Peripheral T-Cell Lymphoma Project. *Blood* 2009;**113**:3931–3937.
44. Choi YL, Park JH, Namkung JH, *et al.* T-cell lymphoma with cutaneous involvement: "nasal" vs. "nasal-type" subgroups – a retrospective study of 18 patients. *Br J Dermatol* 2009;**160**:333–337.
45. Liu J, Liang L, Huang S, *et al.* Aberrant differential expression of EZH2 and H3K27me3 in extranodal NK/T-cell lymphoma, nasal type, is associated with disease progression and prognosis. *Hum Pathol* 2019;**83**:166–176.
46. Kim SJ, Choi JY, Hyun SH, *et al.* Risk stratification on the basis of Deauville score on PET-CT and the presence of Epstein-Barr virus DNA after completion of primary treatment for extranodal natural killer/T-cell lymphoma, nasal type: a multicentre, retrospective analysis. *Lancet Haematol* 2015;**2**:e66–e74.
47. Qi SN, Li YX, Wang WH, *et al.* The extent of cutaneous lesions predicts outcome in extranodal nasal-type NK/T-cell lymphoma of the upper aerodigestive tract with secondary cutaneous involvement. *Leuk Lymphoma* 2012;**53**:855–861.
48. Li S, Feng X, Li T, *et al.* Extranodal NK/T-cell lymphoma, nasal type. A report of 73 cases at MD Anderson Cancer Center. *Am J Surg Pathol* 2013;**37**:14–23.
49. Mraz-Gernhard S, Natkunam Y, Hoppe RT, *et al.* Natural killer/natural killer-like T-cell lymphoma, $CD56^{+}$, presenting in the skin: an increasingly recognized entity with an aggressive course. *J Clin Oncol* 2001;**19**:2179–2188.
50. Yu JB, Zuo Z, Zhang WY, *et al.* Identification of immunophenotypic subtypes with different prognoses in extranodal natural killer/T-cell lymphoma, nasal type. *Hum Pathol* 2014;**45**: 2255–2262.
51. Lee WJ, Kim YJ, Lee YJ, *et al.* Vascular endothelial growth factor protein expression is associated with a poor prognosis in patients with cutaneous extranodal natural killer/T-cell lymphoma. *Br J Dermatol* 2018;**178**:e11–e12.
52. Zuriel D, Fink-Puches R, Cerroni L. A case of primary cutaneous extranodal natural killer/T-cell lymphoma, nasal-type, with a 22-year indolent clinical course. *Am J Dermatopathol* 2012;**34**: 194–197.
53. Watabe D, Kanno H, Inoue-Narita T, *et al.* A case of primary cutaneous natural killer T-cell lymphoma, nasal type, with indolent clinical course: monoclonal expansion of Epstein–Barr virus genome correlating with the terminal aggressive behaviour. *Br J Dermatol* 2009;**160**:205–207.

CHAPTER 10

# Cutaneous peripheral T-cell lymphoma, not otherwise specified (NOS)

Cutaneous peripheral T-cell lymphoma, not otherwise specified (NOS) represents a sort of "waste basket" of all cases that cannot be put into another of the categories of mature cutaneous T-cell lymphoma. In this sense, it is a diagnosis of exclusion. Occurrence in the skin represents in most instances a secondary involvement by extracutaneous disease (usually nodal), but primary cutaneous cases exist. In the past, cutaneous peripheral T-cell lymphoma, NOS was lumped in the group of "CD30$^-$ medium/large pleomorphic T-cell lymphoma" [1–3]. In my experience, many cutaneous cases, even those with a CD4$^+$ phenotype, express one or more cytotoxic proteins, thus belonging conceptually to the group of cytotoxic natural killer (NK)/T-cell lymphomas.

In the World health Organization (WHO) *Classification of Haematolymphoid Tumours*, peripheral T-cell lymphoma, NOS, is defined as "a heterogeneous category of nodal and extranodal mature T-cell lymphomas that cannot be assigned to a specific peripheral T-cell lymphoma entity" [4], thus representing a diagnosis of exclusion also at extracutaneous sites. The cutaneous variant is included as a specific entity in the WHO classification [5], but not in the International Consensus Classification (ICC) *of Myeloid and Lymphoid Neoplasms* [6]. Primary cutaneous peripheral T-cell lymphoma, NOS represents a distinct entity in the 2018 and 2024 updates of the European Organization for Research and Treatment of Cancer (EORTC)/WHO classification of cutaneous lymphomas [7, 8]. In the skin, cutaneous peripheral T-cell lymphoma, NOS should be distinguished from other cutaneous aggressive cytotoxic lymphomas and also from cases of cutaneous CD4$^+$ small–medium pleomorphic T-cell lymphoproliferative disorder. In fact, cutaneous CD4$^+$ small/medium T-cell lymphoproliferative disorder may present with histopathological and phenotypical features similar to those of cutaneous peripheral T-cell lymphoma, NOS, and differentiation of these two entities may be difficult. For a detailed discussion on differential diagnostic features, see Chapter 11. Cutaneous peripheral T-cell lymphoma, NOS should also be distinguished from acral CD8$^+$ T-cell lymphoma (see Chapter 12).

As for other rare types of cutaneous T-cell lymphoma, mycosis fungoides should be ruled out before a diagnosis of cutaneous peripheral T-cell lymphoma, NOS, can be accepted. Complete staging investigations are mandatory, and in my experience, they often reveal the presence of extracutaneous disease. Treatment, on the other hand, is independent from staging results, for even if no extracutaneous disease is found, aggressive options should be selected. Staging of cutaneous peripheral T-cell lymphoma, NOS is made according to the TNM staging system for cutaneous lymphomas other than mycosis fungoides and Sézary syndrome proposed by the EORTC and ISCL, slightly modified in conjunction with the US Cutaneous Lymphoma Consortium (USCLC) (see Chapter 1, Tables 1.2 and 1.3) [9, 10].

For a diagnosis of cutaneous peripheral T-cell lymphoma, NOS, the following criteria should be fulfilled:

- The absence of clinical history of mycosis fungoides or Sézary syndrome.
- The absence of extracutaneous disease at the first presentation.
- $\alpha/\beta$ phenotype of neoplastic cells ($\gamma/\delta^+$ cases should be classified as cutaneous $\gamma/\delta$ T-cell lymphoma).
- The absence of prominent epidermotropism of CD8$^+$ lymphocytes (cases showing this feature should be classified as cutaneous aggressive epidermotropic CD8$^+$ cytotoxic T-cell lymphoma, keeping in mind that cutaneous peripheral T-cell lymphoma, NOS may be positive for CD8, but usually lacks prominent epidermotropism).
- Negativity for CD30 or positivity in a minority of cells (in cases with >70% of CD30$^+$ cells a diagnosis of cutaneous anaplastic large cell lymphoma should be considered).
- The absence of Epstein–Barr virus (EBV) within neoplastic cells (rare positive cases may occur, but positivity should prompt careful evaluation of the differential diagnosis with cutaneous extranodal NK/T-cell lymphoma, nasal type).
- The absence of HTLV-1 infection (positive cases should be classified as cutaneous adult T-cell lymphoma/leukemia)

*Skin Lymphoma: The Illustrated Guide*, Sixth Edition. Lorenzo Cerroni.

## Clinical features

Patients are adults of both genders. There are reports on children and adolescents with cutaneous peripheral T-cell lymphoma, NOS, but it is unclear whether the neoplasm was primary cutaneous or represented secondary skin involvement from a nodal lymphoma [11]. Patients present usually with regionally localized or generalized, rapidly growing plaques and tumors (Fig. 10.1). In some cases, clinical features may be inconspicuous at the first presentation, but rapidly worsening within a few weeks (Fig. 10.2). Ulceration may be present. The clinical picture may be indistinguishable from that of advanced mycosis

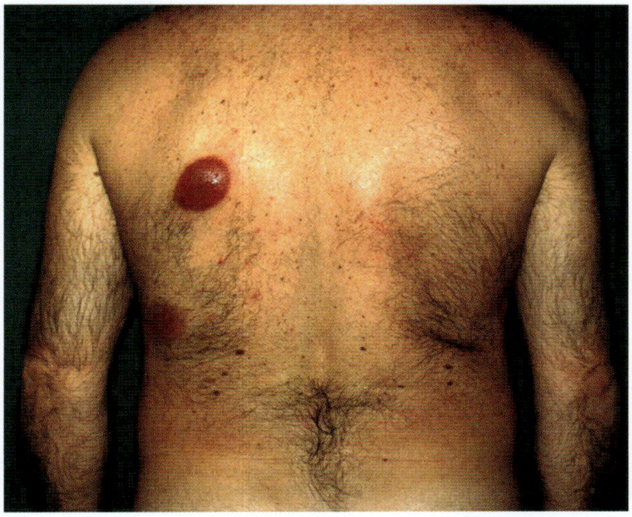

(a)

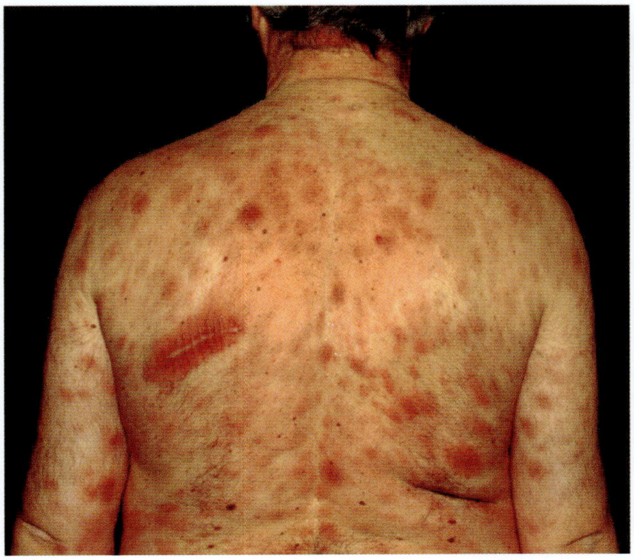

(b)

**Figure 10.1** Cutaneous peripheral T-cell lymphoma, NOS. (a) Large tumor, infiltrated plaque and small papules on the back; (b) generalized papules, plaques, and tumors after a few months. Note the scar of the excision of the large tumor.

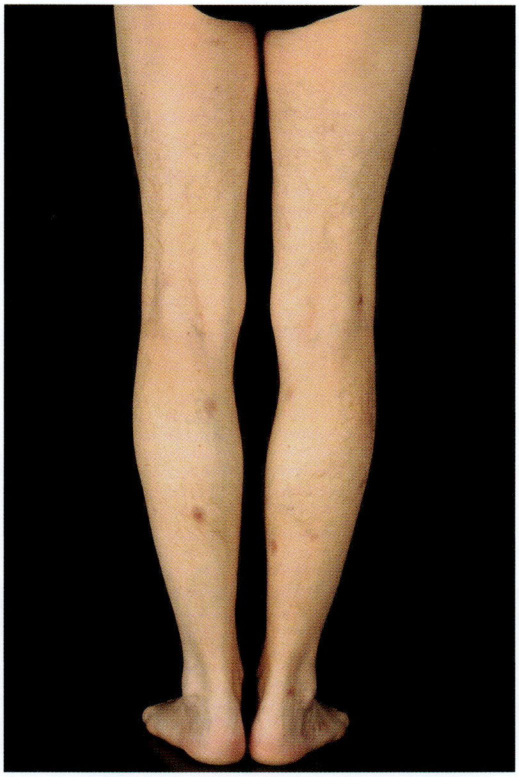

(a)

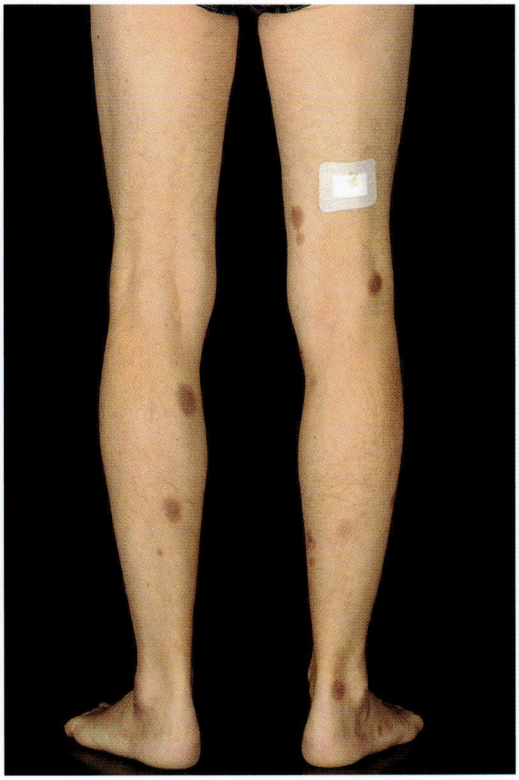

(b)

**Figure 10.2** Cutaneous peripheral T-cell lymphoma, NOS. (a) Small patches on both lower extremities; (b) After 6 weeks, the same lesions became more infiltrated, and new lesions appeared.

fungoides or other aggressive cutaneous T-cell lymphomas (Fig. 10.3). Sometimes, multiple localized papules may resemble clinically persistent arthropod bite reactions (Fig. 10.4). In patients with secondary skin involvement, I have observed rarely infiltrated, large flat erythematous lesions (Fig. 10.5a) or purpuric, partly necrotic papules mimicking a necrotizing vasculitis (Fig. 10.5b). It may be that these cases represent specific cutaneous involvement at the site of skin inflammation, akin to other systemic hematological disorders (e.g., myeloid leukemia and B-cell chronic lymphocytic leukemia). In fact, I have observed in one patient specific skin manifestations of peripheral T-cell lymphoma, NOS at the site of a cutaneous squamous cell carcinoma.

Rare cases presenting with solitary lesions on the head and neck area represent a particular differential diagnostic problem with cutaneous CD4$^+$ small–medium pleomorphic lymphoproliferative disorder (Fig. 10.6a); histopathological features, however, are different and allow a proper diagnosis to be made (Fig. 10.6b to d).

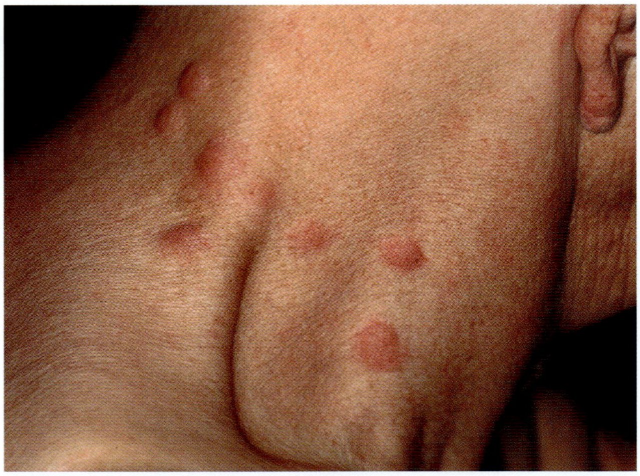

**Figure 10.4** Cutaneous peripheral T-cell lymphoma, NOS. Several small erythematous nodules with a linear arrangement resembling clinically persistent arthropod bite reactions.

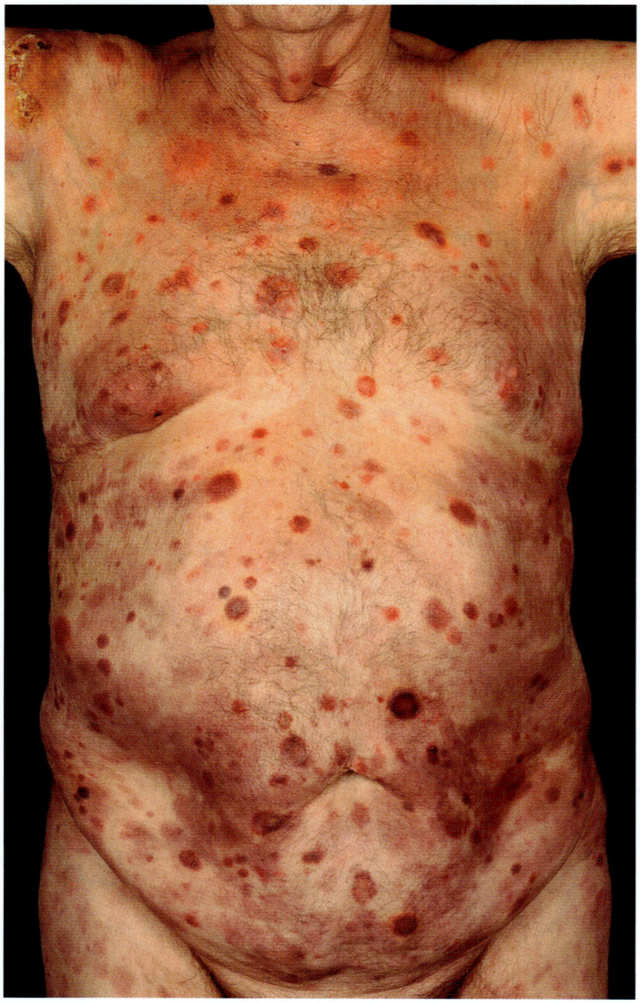

**Figure 10.3** Cutaneous peripheral T-cell lymphoma, NOS. Generalized patches, plaques, and tumors, some ulcerated, similar to the clinical features of advanced mycosis fungoides or of other aggressive cutaneous T-cell lymphomas.

As in other aggressive cutaneous T-cell lymphomas, particularly in cases of peripheral T-cell lymphoma, NOS with cytotoxic phenotype mucosal sites and conjunctiva may be involved (Fig. 10.7).

## Histopathology, immunophenotype, and molecular genetics

### Histopathology

Histology shows nodular or diffuse infiltrates involving the entire dermis and subcutaneous fat (Fig. 10.8). Small-, medium-, and large-sized pleomorphic cells may all be observed in variable proportions (Fig. 10.9). Epidermotropism may be present but it is not a constant feature (Fig. 10.10). A high mitotic rate is found, particularly in tumoral infiltrates. Prominent necrosis, presence of angiocentricity and/or angiodestruction, or predominant involvement of the subcutaneous tissues are uncommon. In some cases, immunohistochemical stainings highlight lymphocytes within the walls of medium-sized vessels (Fig. 10.11a) or within the nerves (Fig. 10.11b). In some cases, the histopathological presentation may be similar to that of cutaneous $\gamma/\delta$ T-cell lymphoma, with a panniculitis-like involvement of the subcutaneous fat and rimming of adipocytes by neoplastic lymphocytes (Fig. 10.12).

Early lesions may show only moderately dense, perivascular and periadnexal lymphoid infiltrates of small- and medium-sized lymphocytes (Fig. 10.13). If present, infiltration and/or destruction of adnexal structures is a helpful diagnostic clue in such

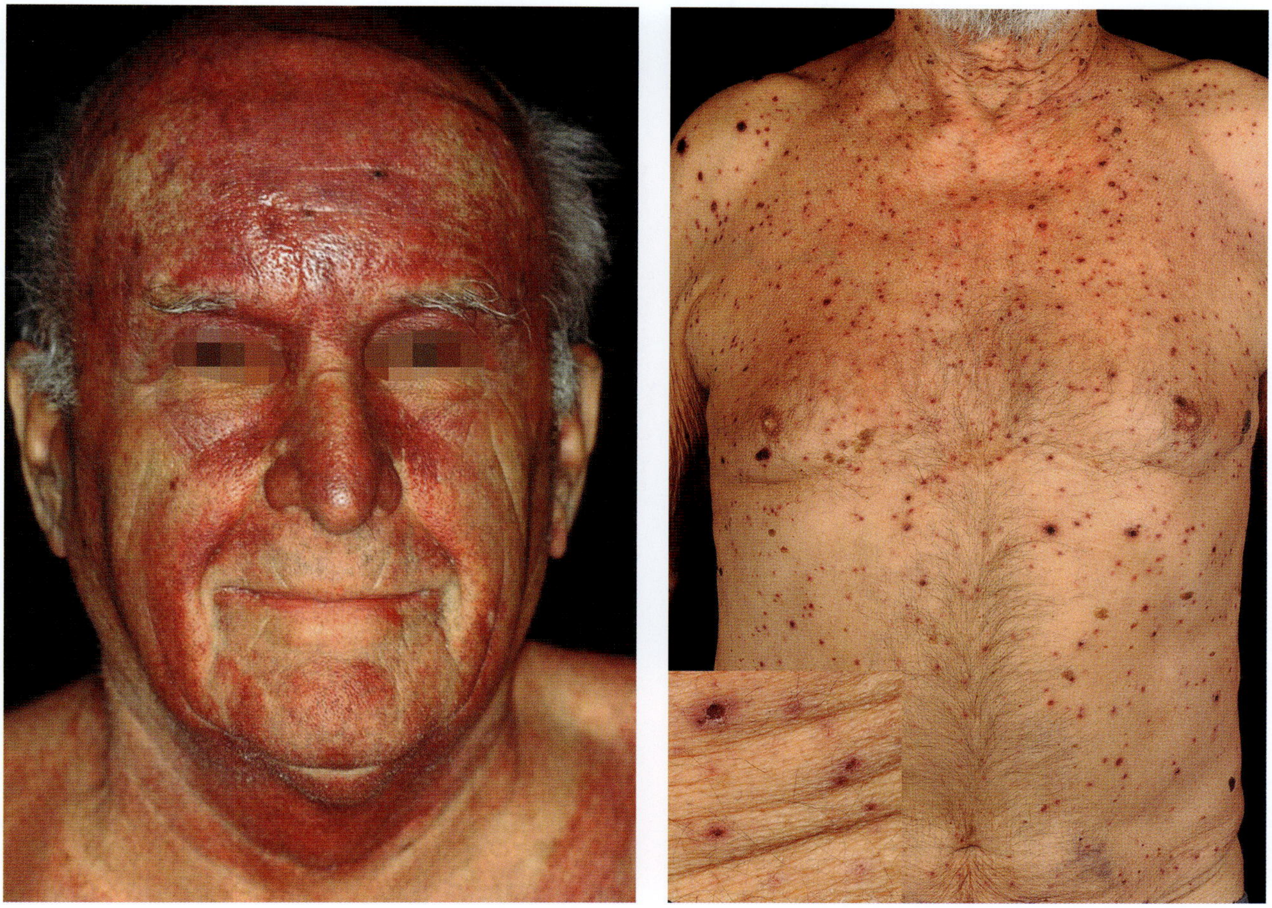

(a) (b)

**Figure 10.5** Cutaneous peripheral T-cell lymphoma, NOS. (a) Infiltrated erythematous patches and plaques on the head and neck in a secondary cutaneous case. (b) Another patient showing small purpuric, partly necrotic lesions resembling a vasculitic process (detail of the lesions in the inset).

cases. Edema may be observed (Fig. 10.14a). Pseudoepitheliomatous epithelial hyperplasia has been reported in one case [12].

## Immunophenotype

Immunohistology reveals a variable phenotype of neoplastic cells ($CD4^{+/-}$ and $CD8^{-/+}$) with common loss of one or more pan-T-cell antigens and in some cases with double CD4/CD8 negativity (Fig. 10.15a to c). A phenotype switch may be observed in recurrent lesions [13]. The cells are negative for γ/δ receptors by definition and are usually positive for ßF1. CD30 is negative or expressed in a minority of cells. Anaplastic lymphoma kinase (ALK) is negative, whereas CD52 and CD56 may be positive in some cases. CD52 positivity may get lost after treatment with alemtuzumab [14]. Cytotoxic proteins (TIA-1, granzyme B, and perforin) are expressed in the majority of cutaneous cases, even those with a $CD4^{+}$ phenotype (Fig. 10.15d) [15, 16]. Aberrant positivity for CD20 can be observed in a minority of cases [17]. The proliferation rate is usually high. Cutaneous cases are negative for EBER-1, and positivity should prompt to consider a differential diagnosis of extranodal NK/T-cell lymphoma, nasal type.

Sporadic cutaneous cases may express the phenotype of TFH (Fig. 10.14b) [18]. Rare cases with strong, diffuse positivity for CD10 probably belong to this group (Fig. 10.16). In the last update of the WHO *Classification of Haematolymphoid Tumours*, cases with a TFH phenotype are classified within the group of nodal T follicular helper cell lymphomas [19]. As this category does not exist for cases arising primary in the skin, at present, the most appropriate diagnosis of such cases seems to be "peripheral T-cell lymphoma, NOS" with an addendum concerning the TFH phenotype.

A few reported cases of cutaneous peripheral T-cell lymphoma, NOS had the phenotype of T regulatory cells ($T_{reg}$) with positivity for FOX-P3 [20, 21].

## Molecular genetics

Molecular analysis of the T-cell receptor (TCR) genes reveals a monoclonal rearrangement in most cases. Genomic alterations

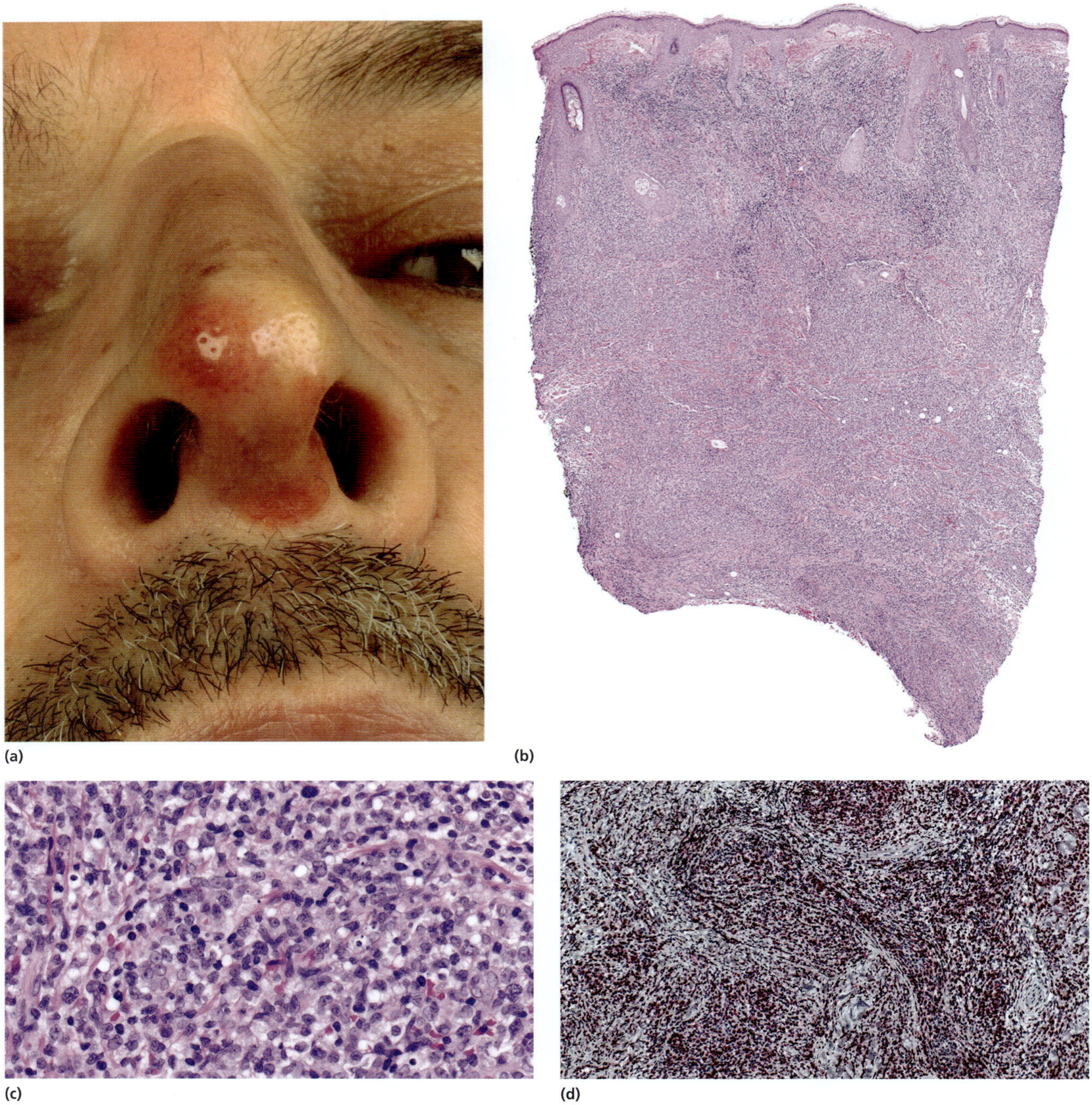

**Figure 10.6** Cutaneous peripheral T-cell lymphoma, NOS. (a) Solitary, infiltrated, red-livid lesion on the nose. (b) Histology shows diffuse infiltrates composed of (c) large pleomorphic lymphocytes; (d) staining for Ki-67 shows positivity of >70% of cells. Similar cases must be distinguished from cutaneous small–medium pleomorphic $CD4^+$ lymphoproliferative disorder, but predominance of large cells and high Ki-67 index are incompatible with such a diagnosis.

affecting the NF-κB pathway and the cell-cycle control are found in a distinct proportion of cases. Data from cutaneous cases are very limited, and most molecular features have been studied in extracutaneous cases. The genetic signature allows a clear distinction from cases of peripheral T-cell lymphoma, angioimmunoblastic type, and from cases formerly classified as peripheral T-cell lymphoma, NOS with TFH phenotype [22, 23]. Nodal cases show frequent gains of 1q, 3p, 5p, 7q, 7p, 8q, 9p,

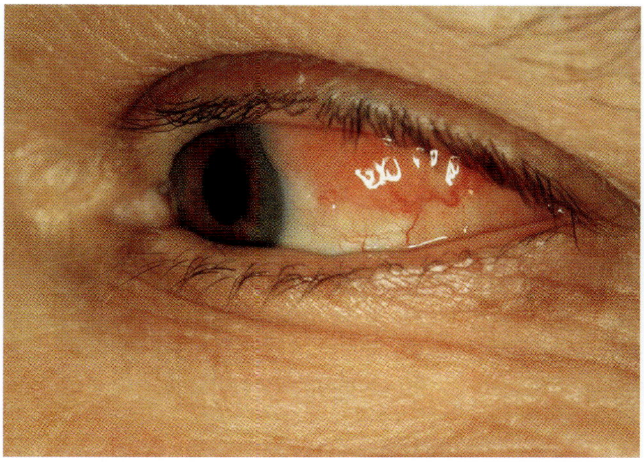

**Figure 10.7** Cutaneous peripheral T-cell lymphoma, NOS. Specific manifestation in the conjunctiva.

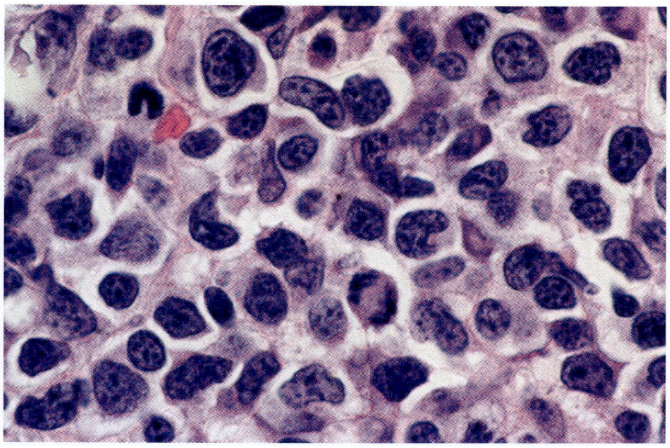

**Figure 10.9** Cutaneous peripheral T-cell lymphoma, NOS. Medium-sized and large pleomorphic lymphocytes predominate in this example.

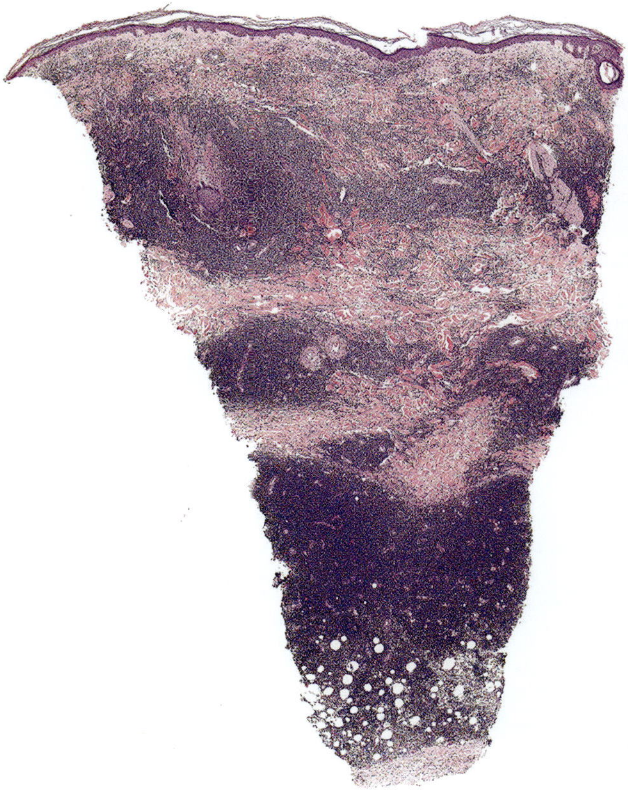

**Figure 10.8** Cutaneous peripheral T-cell lymphoma, NOS. Dense, bottom-heavy infiltrates of lymphocytes extending throughout the dermis into the subcutaneous fat.

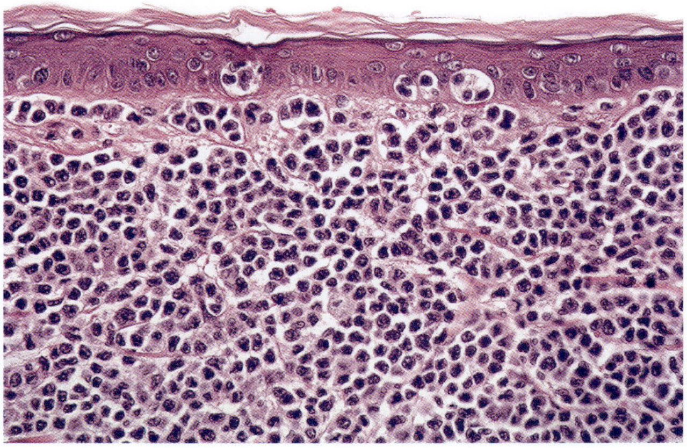

**Figure 10.10** Cutaneous peripheral T-cell lymphoma, NOS. Dense infiltrate with focal, small clusters of epidermotropic lymphocytes.

and 19q and losses of 3q, 6q, 9p, and 10p [24, 25]. A few cutaneous cases were characterized by gains of 7q, 8, and 17q, and loss of 9p21 [26]. In nodal cases, next-generation sequencing showed frequent aberrations in tumour suppressor genes, including rearrangements of *TP63* and mutations and deletions of *CDKN2A*, *PTEN*, and *TP53* [27].

The TBX21 and GATA3 expression (two regulators of gene expression profiles in T helper cells, skewing T helper cell polarization into T helper-1 cell and T helper-2 cell differentiation pathways, respectively) can be observed in subsets of peripheral T-cell lymphoma, NOS [28], suggesting that these subsets may evolve by distinct genetic pathways. GATA3$^{+}$ cases showed frequent loss or mutation of tumor suppressor genes targeting the *CDKN2A/B-TP53* and *PTEN-PI3K* pathways, with additional gains/amplifications of *STAT3* and *MYC* [28]. The TBX21$^{+}$ subgroup had fewer copy number abnormalities targeting mostly cytotoxic effector genes, and was characterized by mutations of genes regulating DNA methylation [28]. Consistent with these data, some cases characterized by the expression of TBX21 by gene expression profiling have a cytotoxic profile phenotypically [29], but data on cutaneous cases, where the cytotoxic profile is common, are lacking. At extracutaneous sites, the two distinct subgroups can be

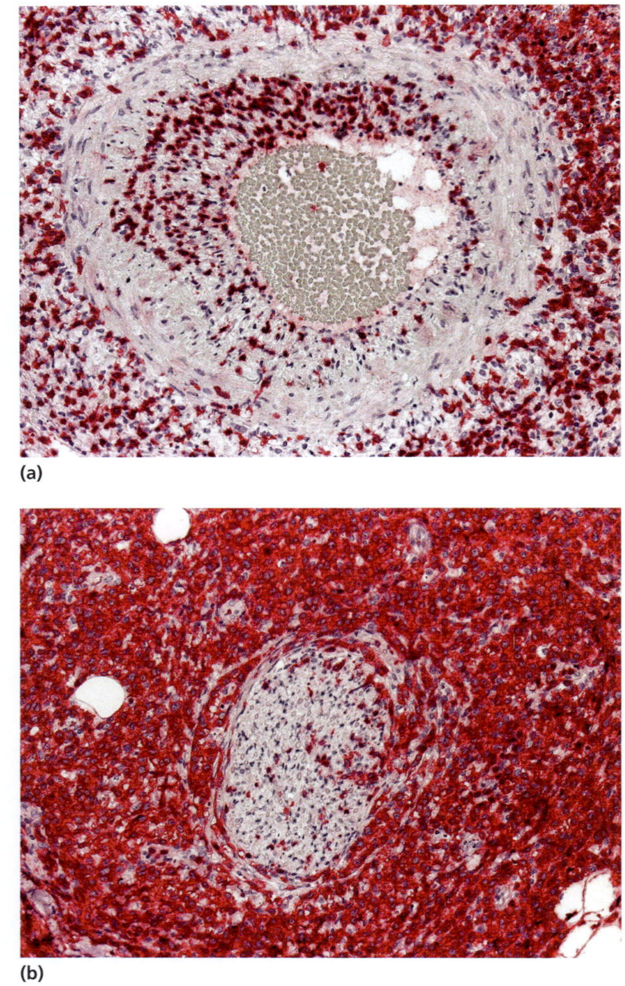

Figure 10.11 Cutaneous peripheral T-cell lymphoma, NOS. Staining for CD5 highlights (a) lymphocytes within the wall of a medium-sized vessel and (b) within a nerve.

identified by immunohistochemical stainings using antibodies to GATA3, TBX21, and their target proteins CCR4 and CXCR3 [27].

## Treatment

Patients should be managed in a hematologic setting. The treatment of choice is systemic chemotherapy using regimens for high-grade T-cell non-Hodgkin lymphoma. Autologous stem cell transplantation significantly improves survival. Cases expressing CD30 and/or CD52 may be additionally treated by brentuximab vedotin or alemtuzumab, respectively [30, 31].

## Prognosis

The prognosis of cutaneous peripheral T-cell lymphoma, NOS, is very poor and most patients die within a few months from the onset of the disease. The estimated five-year survival is less than 20% [7]. In nodal cases, a cytotoxic profile is a poor prognostic sign [4]. The role of this phenotype in cutaneous cases has not been elucidated.

Cases expressing the chemokines CXCR3 and CCR4 may have a worse prognosis [32], as well as those expressing GATA3 [33]. In a large number of primary cutaneous cases, however, the expression of GATA3 did not correlate with the prognosis [17]. Other prognostic factors identified in nodal cases (but not verified in cutaneous ones) are the presence of >70% transformed blasts, proliferation rate of >70% (detected by staining with Ki-67), CD56 expression, and background of >10% $CD8^+$ cells [32].

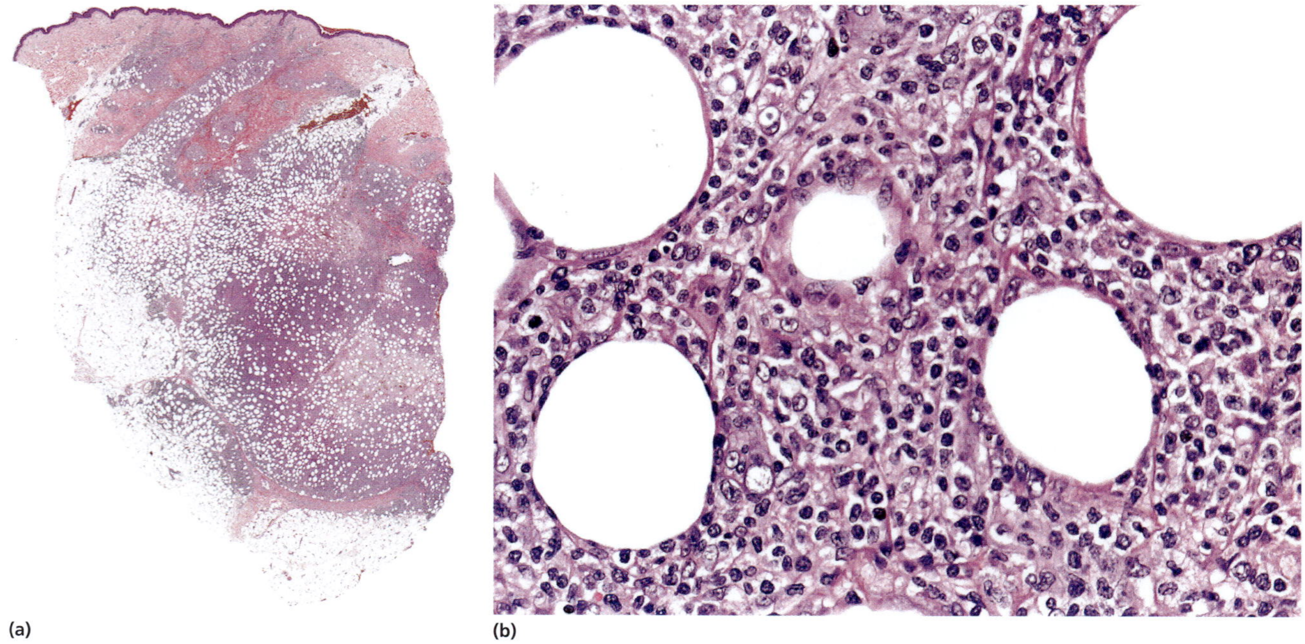

Figure 10.12 Cutaneous peripheral T-cell lymphoma, NOS. (a) Diffuse infiltrate with a "panniculitis-like" pattern, characterized also by (b) rimming of adipocytes by neoplastic lymphocytes.

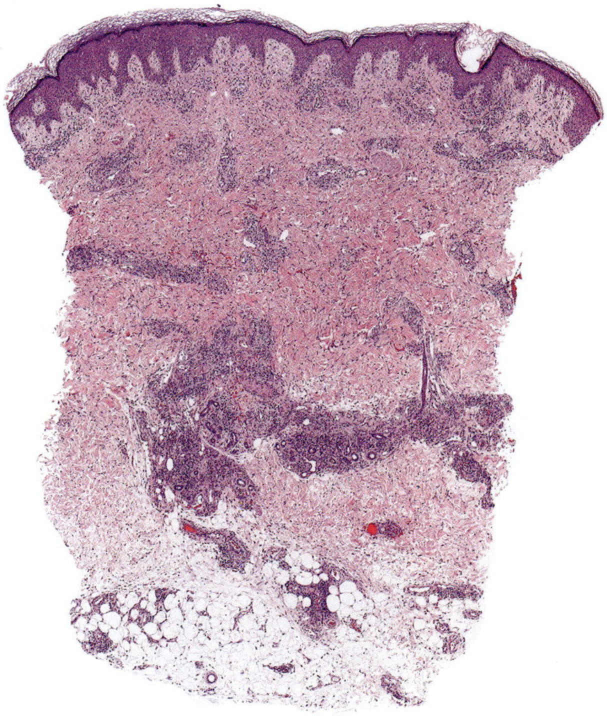

(a)

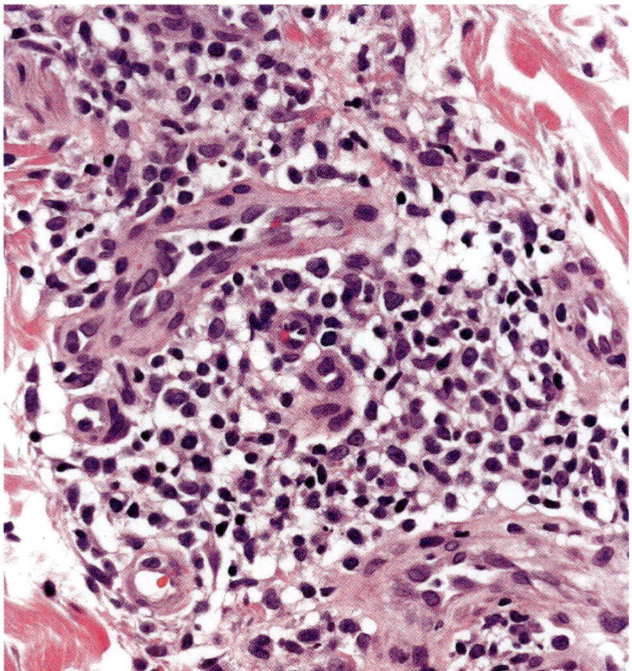

(b)

**Figure 10.13** Early lesion of cutaneous peripheral T-cell lymphoma, NOS. (a) Perivascular and periadnexal infiltrates composed predominantly of (b) small- and medium-sized lymphocytes.

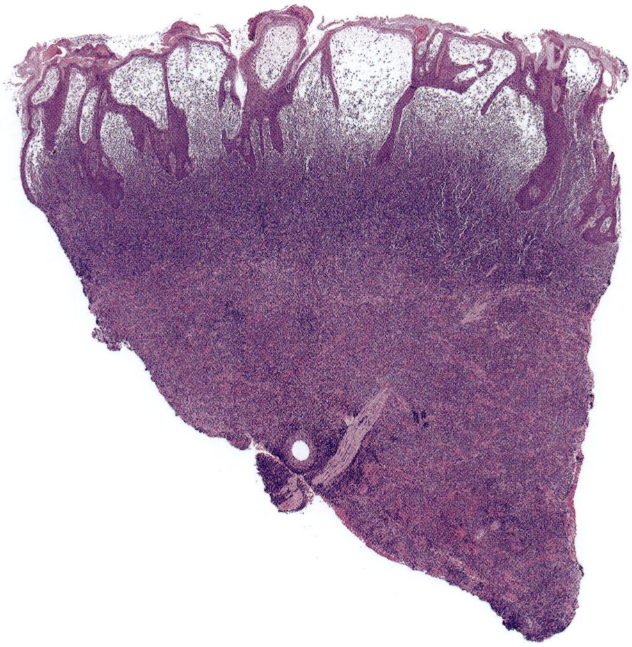

(a)

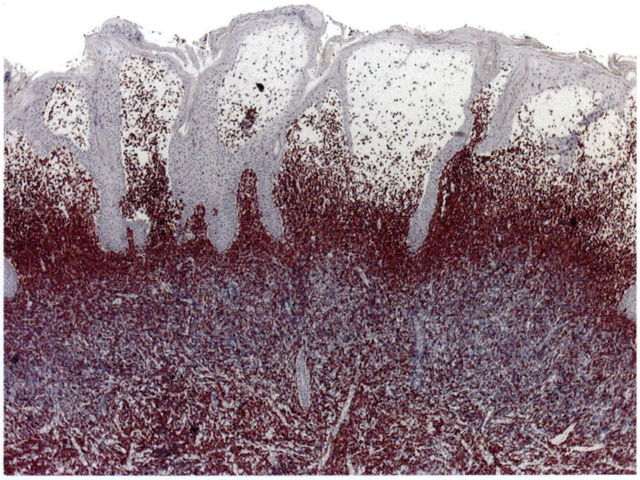

(b)

**Figure 10.14** Cutaneous peripheral T-cell lymphoma, NOS. (a) Tumoral infiltrate consisting of sheets of neoplastic cells; note prominent subepidermal edema. (b) Most tumor cells express PD-1.

Notwithstanding the aggressive behaviour of this lymphoma, exceptional cases show a prolonged course with cutaneous recurrences but without extracutaneous spread. I have observed a few such cases that fulfil all criteria for a primary cutaneous T-cell lymphoma, NOS, but are characterized by an indolent course (Fig. 10.17).

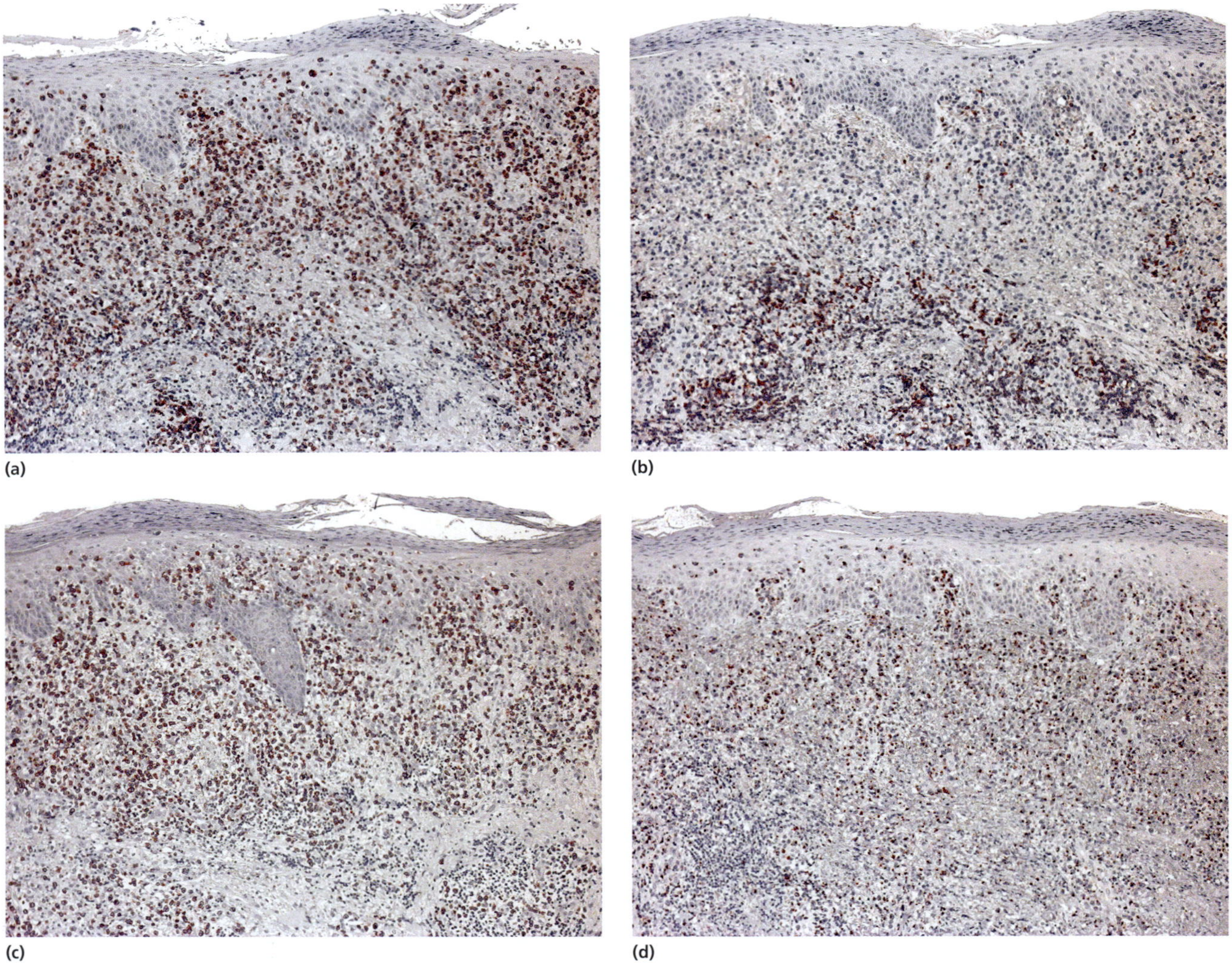

Figure 10.15 Cutaneous peripheral T-cell lymphoma, NOS. (a) Neoplastic cells express CD3 but (b) show a partial loss of CD5. (c) Positivity for βF1 and (d) for TIA-1.

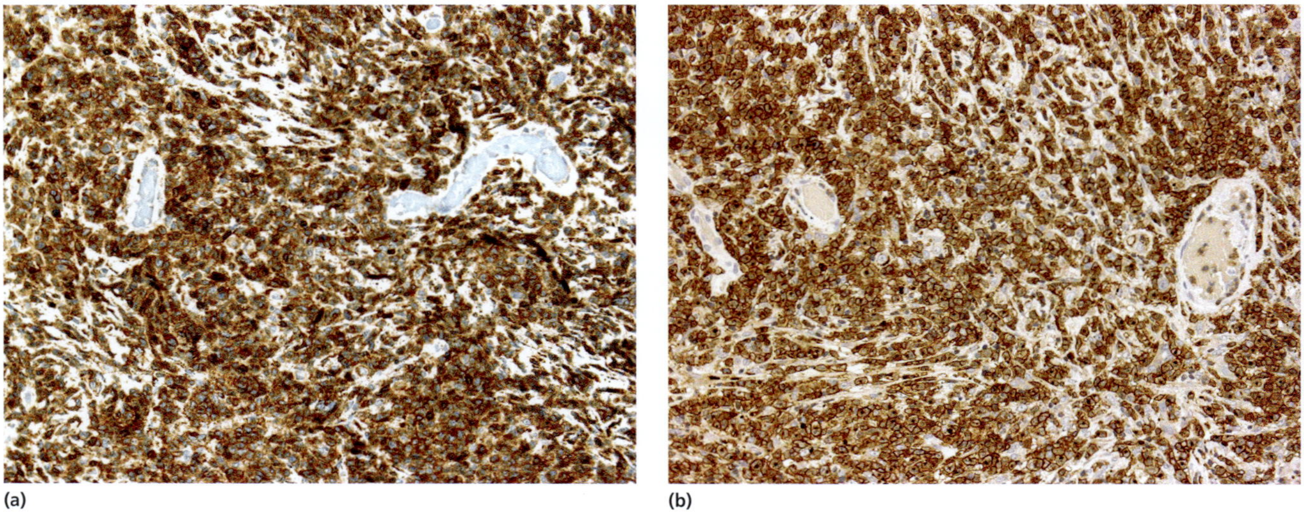

Figure 10.16 Cutaneous peripheral T-cell lymphoma, NOS. (a) Neoplastic cells in this case express CD3 and (b) CD10.

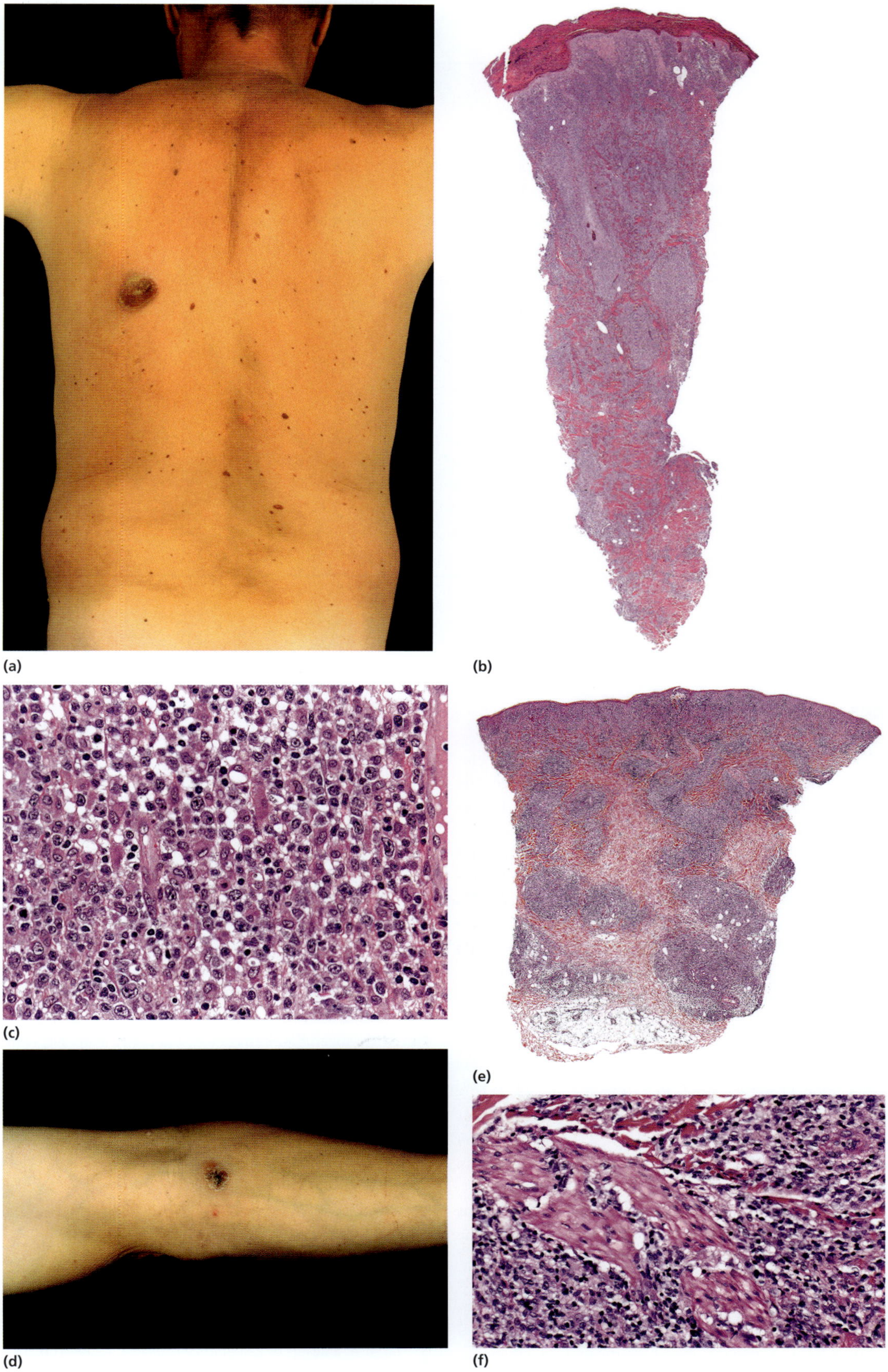

**Figure 10.17** Cutaneous peripheral T-cell lymphoma, NOS. (a) First presentation with a solitary, ulcerated tumor on the back, characterized histologically by (b) a diffuse infiltrate within the entire specimen with (c) predominance of large, pleomorphic lymphocytes. Immunohistochemical stainings and in situ hybridization for EBV allowed to rule out other entities such as cutaneous anaplastic large cell lymphoma, cutaneous aggressive epidermotropic CD8$^+$ cytotoxic T-cell lymphoma, cutaneous γ/δ T-cell lymphoma, and cutaneous extranodal NK/T-cell lymphoma, nasal-type. The patient was treated by local radiotherapy but got several recurrences over the years. (d) Last recurrence, 13 years after the first presentation, with an ulcerated lesion on the arm characterized again by (e) a diffuse infiltrate within the entire dermis with (f) predominance of medium-large lymphocytes. The phenotype of the two lesions (and of the previous recurrences) was completely overlapping.

## Résumé

**Primary cutaneous peripheral T-cell lymphoma, NOS**

| | | |
|---|---|---|
| **Clinical** | Adults. Solitary, regionally localized or generalized plaques and tumors, sometimes ulcerated. No previous history of mycosis fungoides. | |
| **Morphology** | Nodular or diffuse infiltrates characterized by small-, medium-, and/or large-sized cells. | |
| **Immunohistochemistry** | CD2, CD3, CD5 | (+) |
| | CD4 | +(−) |
| | CD8 | − |
| | βF1 | + |
| | TCR-γ/δ | − |
| | CD30 | − |
| | TIA-1 | +/− |
| | EBER-1 | − |
| **Genetics** | Monoclonal rearrangement of the TCR genes detected in the majority of cases. Data on cutaneous cases are limited. Genomic alterations affecting the NF-kB pathway and the cell-cycle control are found in a distinct proportion of nodal cases. In the lymph nodes, different genetic profile from lymphomas expressing a TFH phenotype. | |
| **Treatment guidelines** | Systemic chemotherapy. Autologous stem cell transplantation. Cases expressing CD30 and/or CD52 may be additionally treated by brentuximab vedotin or alemtuzumab, respectively. | |

## References


1. Beljaards RC, Meijer CJLM, van der Putte SCJ, *et al.* Primary cutaneous T cell lymphoma: clinicopathological features and prognostic parameters of 35 cases other than mycosis fungoides and CD30-positive large cell lymphoma. *J Pathol* 1994;**172**:53–60.
2. Joly P, Vasseur E, Esteve E, *et al.* Primary cutaneous medium and large cell lymphomas other than mycosis fungoides. An immunohistological and follow-up study on 54 cases. *Br J Dermatol* 1995; **132**:506–512.
3. Sterry W, Siebel A, Mielke V. HTLV-I-negative pleomorphic T-cell lymphoma of the skin: the clinicopathological correlations and natural history of 15 patients. *Br J Dermatol* 1992;**126**:456–462.
4. Amador C, Iqbal J, Tan SY, *et al.* Peripheral T-cell lymphoma NOS. In: *WHO Classification of Tumours Editorial Board. Haematolymphoid Tumours.* 5th edition. Lyon (France): IARC, 2024: 757–761.
5. Mitteldorf C, Berti E, Pulitzer M, Willemze R. Primary cutaneous peripheral T-cell lymphoma NOS. In: *WHO Classification of Tumours Editorial Board. Haematolymphoid Tumours.* 5th edition. Lyon (France): IARC, 2024: 708–709.
6. Campo E, Jaffe ES, Cook JR, *et al.* The International Consensus Classification of Mature Lymphoid Neoplasms: a report from the Clinical Advisory Committee. *Blood* 2022;**140**:1229–1253.
7. Willemze R, Cerroni L, Kempf W, *et al.* The 2018 update of the WHO-EORTC classification for primary cutaneous lymphomas. *Blood* 2019;**133**:1703–1714.
8. Kempf W, Mitteldorf C, Cerroni L, *et al.* Classifications of cutaneous lymphomas and lymphoproliferative disorders: an update from the EORTC cutaneous lymphoma histopathology group. *J Eur Acad Dermatol Venereol* 2024;**38**:1491–1503.
9. Olsen EA, Whittaker S, Willemze R, *et al.* Primary cutaneous lymphoma: recommendations for clinical trial design and staging update from the ISCL, USCLC, and EORTC. *Blood* 2022;**140**: 419–437.
10. National Comprehensive Cancer Network. Primary Cutaneous Lymphomas (Version 1.2025). Accessed February 15, 2025. https://www.nccn.org/professionals/physician_gls/pdf/primary_cutaneous.pdf
11. Kobayashi R, Yamato K, Tanaka F, *et al.* Retrospective analysis of non-anaplastic peripheral T-cell lymphoma in pediatric patients in Japan. *Pediatr Blood Cancer* 2010;**54**:212–215.
12. Ginsberg D, Hill H, Wilson B, *et al.* Pseudocarcinomatous hyperplasia mimicking squamous cell carcinoma in a case of CD56-positive cytotoxic T-cell lymphoma. *J Cutan Pathol* 2015;**42**:194–198.
13. Al-Ibraheemi A, Kanagal-Shamanna R, Patel KP, *et al.* Phenotypic evolution in a case of peripheral T-cell lymphoma suggests the presence of tumor heterogeneity. *J Cutan Pathol* 2013;**40**:573–579.
14. Dhandha MM, Sufficool KE, Vidal CI, *et al.* Immunophenotype expression change from CD52+ to CD52− on erythrodermic peripheral T-cell lymphoma, not otherwise specified after treatment with alemtuzumab. *Am J Dermatopathol* 2018;**40**:547–550.
15. Massone C, Chott A, Metze D, *et al.* Subcutaneous, blastic natural killer (NK) NK/T-cell and other cytotoxic lymphomas of the skin: a morphologic, immunophenotypic and molecular study of 50 patients. *Am J Surg Pathol* 2004;**28**:719–735.
16. Hagiwara M, Takata K, Shimoyama Y, *et al.* Primary cutaneous T-cell lymphoma of unspecified type with cytotoxic phenotype: clinicopathological analysis of 27 patients. *Cancer Sci* 2009;**100**: 33–41.
17. Kempf W, Mitteldorf C, Battistella M, *et al.* Primary cutaneous peripheral T-cell lymphoma, not otherwise specified: results of a multicentre European Organization for Research and Treatment of

Cancer (EORTC) cutaneous lymphoma taskforce study on the clinico-pathological and prognostic features. *J Eur Acad Dermatol Venereol* 2021;**35**:658–668.

18. Le Tourneau A, Audouin J, Molina T, *et al.* Primary cutaneous follicular variant of peripheral T-cell lymphoma NOS. *A report of two cases Histopathology* 2010;**56**:548–551.
19. Attygalle AD, Alaggio R, Du MQ. Nodal T follicular helper cell lymphoma: Introduction. In: *WHO Classification of Tumours Editorial Board. Haematolymphoid Tumours.* 5th edition. Lyon (France): IARC, 2024: 742–743.
20. Marzano AV, Vezzoli P, Fanoni D, *et al.* Primary cutaneous T-cell lymphoma expressing FOXP3: a case report supporting the existence of malignancies of regulatory T cells. *J Am Acad Dermatol* 2009;**61**:348–355.
21. Satou A, Asano N, Kato S, *et al.* FoxP3-positive T cell lymphoma arising in non-HTLV1 carrier: clinicopathological analysis of 11 cases of PTCL-NOS and 2 cases of mycosis fungoides. *Histopathology* 2016;**68**:1099–1108.
22. Vallois D, Dobay MPD, Morin RD, *et al.* Activating mutations in genes related to TCR signaling in angioimmunoblastic and other follicular helper T-cell–derived lymphomas. *Blood* 2016;**128**:1490–1502.
23. Pileri SA. Follicular helper T-cell–related lymphomas. *Blood* 2015;**126**:1733–1734.
24. Foss FM, Zinzani PL, Vose JM, *et al.* Peripheral T-cell lymphoma. *Blood* 2011;**117**:6756–6767.
25. Nelson M, Horsman DE, Weisenburger DD, *et al.* Cytogenetic abnormalities and clinical correlations in peripheral T-cell lymphoma. *Br J Haematol* 2008;**141**:461–469.
26. van Kester MS, Tensen CP, Vermeer MH, *et al.* Cutaneous anaplastic large cell lymphoma and peripheral T-cell lymphoma NOS show distinct chromosomal alterations and differential expression of chemokine receptors and apoptosis regulators. *J Invest Dermatol* 2010;**130**:563–575.
27. Amador C, Greiner TC, Heavican TB, *et al.* Reproducing the molecular subclassification of peripheral T-cell lymphoma-NOS by immunohistochemistry. *Blood* 2019;**134**:2159–2170.
28. Heavican TB, Bouska A, Yu J, *et al.* Genetic drivers of oncogenic pathways in molecular subgroups of peripheral T-cell lymphoma. *Blood* 2019;**133**:1664–1676.
29. Iqbal J, Wright G, Wang C, *et al.* Gene expression signatures delineate biological and prognostic subgroups in peripheral T-cell lymphoma. *Blood* 2014;**123**:2915–2923.
30. Berger GK, McBride A, Lawson S, *et al.* Brentuximab vedotin for treatment of non-Hodgkin lymphomas: a systematic review. *Crit Rev Oncol Hematol* 2017;**109**:42–50.
31. Buckstein R, Fraser G, Cheung M, *et al.* Alemtuzumab and CHOP chemotherapy for the treatment of aggressive histology peripheral T cell lymphomas: a multi-center phase I study. *Clin Lymphoma Myeloma Leuk* 2016;**16**:18–28.
32. Savage KJ, Ferreri AJ, Zinzani PL, Pileri SA. Peripheral T-cell lymphoma – not otherwise specified. *Crit Rev Oncol Hematol* 2011;**79**:321–329.
33. Zhang W, Wang Z, Luo Y, *et al.* GATA3 expression correlates with poor prognosis and tumor-associated macrophage infiltration in peripheral T cell lymphoma. *Oncotarget* 2016;**7**: 65284–65294.

**CHAPTER 11**

# Cutaneous CD4$^+$ small–medium T-cell lymphoproliferative disorder

Cutaneous CD4$^+$ small–medium T-cell lymphoproliferative disorder represents a distinct entity in the 2018 and 2024 updates of the European Organization for Research and Treatment of Cancer (EORTC)/World Health Organization (WHO) classification of cutaneous lymphomas, and is included as a specific entity in the International Consensus Classification (ICC) *of Myeloid and Lymphoid Neoplasms* [1–3]. In the 5th edition of the WHO, *Classification of Haematolymphoid Tumours* is listed as a distinct entity within the group of "primary cutaneous T-cell lymphoid proliferations and lymphomas" [4].

Since the first description in 1995 by Friedmann *et al.* [5], the existence of this entity has been the subject of numerous debates and controversial interpretations, and probably, a heterogeneous group of patients has been included in some studies [6–8]. In fact, in spite of more than three decades of discussion, since the first description, there is still no consensus on the existence, definition, and classification of cutaneous CD4$^+$ small–medium T-cell lymphoproliferative disorder as a distinct entity. Cases similar on clinical and histopathologic grounds to those reported as cutaneous CD4$^+$ small–medium T-cell lymphoproliferative disorder have been published under different diagnoses, including "idiopathic pseudo T-cell lymphoma," "pseudolymphomatous folliculitis," "cutaneous lymphoid hyperplasia," "solitary lymphomatoid papule, nodule or tumor," "primary cutaneous follicular helper T-cell lymphoma," "primary cutaneous peripheral T-cell lymphoma, unspecified," and "monoclonal atypical T-cell hyperplasia," among others [9–14]. In addition, cases of aggressive cutaneous cytotoxic lymphomas may show a small–medium pleomorphic cytomorphology (see Chapters 7–9), and cases of peripheral T-cell lymphoma, not otherwise specified (NOS) may be indistinguishable from CD4$^+$ small–medium T-cell lymphoproliferative disorder as well (see Chapter 10), thus generating more disarray in an already confused field. The term "small–medium pleomorphic T-cell nodule of undetermined significance" has been proposed for these lesions [14, 15], and the benign behavior observed in cases with a bona fide diagnosis of cutaneous CD4$^+$ small–medium T-cell "lymphoma" prompted reclassification of this entity as a lymphoproliferative disorder, thus avoiding the term lymphoma. Finally, it must be underlined that in the WHO classifications, it is stated that cutaneous CD4$^+$ small–medium T-cell lymphoproliferative disorder and reactive lymphoid hyperplasia exist on a spectrum [4], thus casting doubts on the classification of cutaneous CD4$^+$ small–medium T-cell lymphoproliferative disorder as a true entity distinct from other T-cell pseudolymphomas (see also the section on final considerations at the end of this chapter).

Since mycosis fungoides is a cutaneous T-cell lymphoma characterized by the predominance of small–medium pleomorphic CD4$^+$ T lymphocytes, the diagnosis of cutaneous CD4$^+$ small–medium T-cell lymphoproliferative disorder can only be accepted if mycosis fungoides is excluded by a complete clinical examination. In fact, a careful re-examination of the clinical pictures of the first cases reported as cutaneous small–medium pleomorphic T-cell lymphoproliferative disorder suggests that at least some of them were actually examples of mycosis fungoides. Even series published later mentioned the presentation of patients with "MF-like plaques" [16]. Recently, a "superficial pattern" of cutaneous CD4$^+$ small–medium T-cell lymphoproliferative disorder characterized by band-like, often epidermotropic infiltrates similar to mycosis fungoides has been described [17]. Personally, I think that cases reported as "superficial pattern" of cutaneous CD4$^+$ small–medium T-cell lymphoproliferative disorder represent examples of superficial T-cell pseudolymphoma, thus will not discuss them in detail in this chapter (see also Chapter 31 on pseudolymphomas).

In the context of the controversies mentioned above, in my opinion, the diagnosis of cutaneous CD4$^+$ small–medium T-cell lymphoproliferative disorder should be restricted to cases characterized by the following features:

- The absence of other lesions and/or clinical history of mycosis fungoides;
- Solitary lesion;
- Nodular or diffuse infiltrate of small–medium pleomorphic (monoclonal) T lymphocytes admixed with many reactive cells, with large cells not exceeding 30% of the infiltrate;
- The absence of marked epitheliotropism of neoplastic cells;

*Skin Lymphoma: The Illustrated Guide*, Sixth Edition. Lorenzo Cerroni.

- Low proliferation rate (not exceeding 30%, as detected by Ki-67 staining)
- α/β $CD4^+$ phenotype;
- The absence of CD30 expression, or expression restricted to scattered cells not arranged in clusters.

Staging investigations are not necessary for patients presenting with typical features of primary cutaneous $CD4^+$ small–medium T-cell lymphoproliferative disorder; cases characterized by either multiple, rapidly growing lesions, or high proliferation rate, or many large cells (>30% of the infiltrate) should be classified as cutaneous peripheral T-cell lymphoma, (NOS) [1], and staging investigations are necessary in these cases.

A relationship between cutaneous $CD4^+$ small–medium T-cell lymphoproliferative disorder and T follicular helper (TFH) lymphocytes has been postulated [12, 18], although the complete phenotype of TFH lymphocytes is not always expressed. In this context, in the literature, some publications reported on an entity of cutaneous T-cell lymphoma characterized by the proliferation of TFH lymphocytes [12, 18, 19]. Some of these cases were classified as "cutaneous $CD4^+$ small–medium T-cell lymphoma" in the original publication [18], and the existence of a genuine "primary cutaneous TFH-cell lymphoma" distinct from other, well-defined entities is questionable; in fact, a primary cutaneous TFH-cell lymphoma has not been included in modern classifications. Besides cutaneous $CD4^+$ small–medium T-cell lymphoproliferative disorder, in the skin, neoplastic TFH cells may be observed in three main situations:

1. Specific cutaneous manifestations of nodal angioimmunoblastic T-cell lymphoma (see chapter 14) [20];
2. Specific cutaneous manifestations of other nodal T-cell lymphomas with the phenotype of TFH-cells [21–23];
3. Primary cutaneous peripheral T-cell lymphoma, NOS with TFH cells [24].

In addition, TFH cells may be observed in the setting of several cutaneous T-cell lymphomas [25]. Most reported cases of "primary cutaneous T-follicular helper-cell lymphoma" showed overlapping clinicopathological features with cutaneous $CD4^+$ small–medium T-cell lymphoproliferative disorder. In addition, it must be underlined that, in many of these reports, confirmation of the TFH phenotype was based on the expression of PD-1 only, a marker that is not unique to TFH-cells (Fig. 11.1a) [26, 27]. Other TFH markers such as ICOS, CXCL-13, and Bcl-6 are usually positive only in a few cells (Fig. 11.1b), thus casting doubts on the real meaning of the PD-1 positivity in these cases. In this context, it has been suggested that the expression of at least three specific markers is necessary in order to confirm differentiation toward TFH lymphocytes [28]. In addition, positivity for PD-1 has been observed frequently in Sézary syndrome and in mycosis fungoides, as well as in other lymphoma types [25, 27, 29], and a complete TFH-cell phenotype has been observed in some cases of Sézary syndrome [30].

In short, cases positive for PD-1 alone do not show sufficient evidence of TFH-cell differentiation, and a TFH-cell phenotype can be observed in well-known cutaneous lymphomas, thus questioning the validity of a "primary cutaneous TFH-cell lymphoma" as a distinct entity. Personally, I don't make the diagnosis of primary cutaneous TFH-cell lymphoma. Although $CD4^+$ small–medium T-cell lymphoproliferative disorder is considered as a cutaneous lymphoproliferative disease with TFH phenotype [1, 2, 4], in my experience, positivity of at least three TFH markers in the majority of the cells is the exception rather than the rule, and a genuine TFH phenotype can be confirmed only in a subset of cases (without any distinguishing

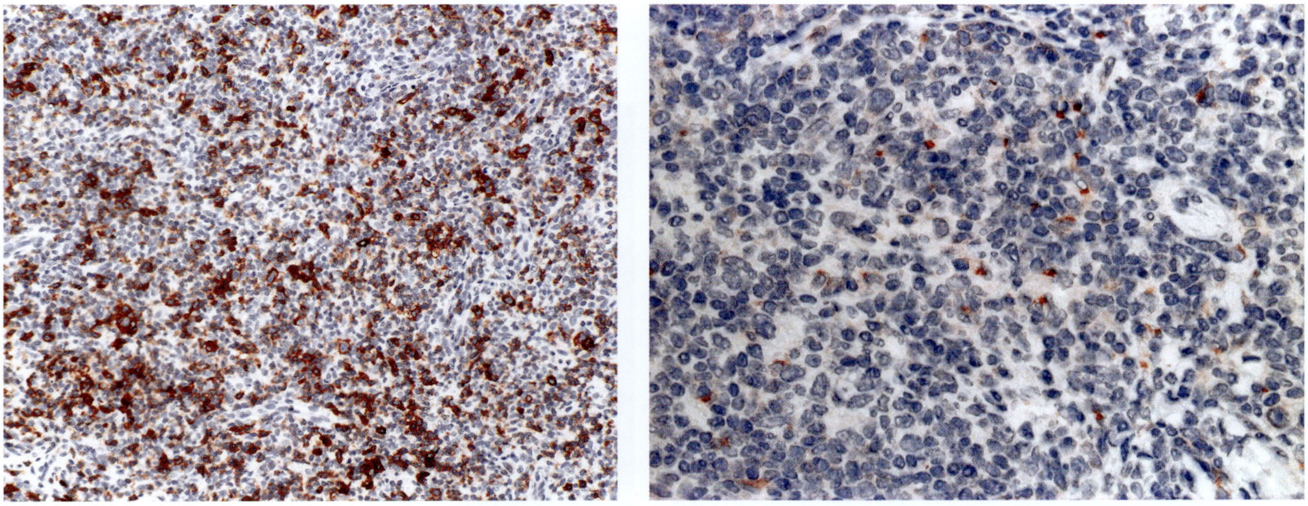

(a) (b)

**Figure 11.1** Cutaneous $CD4^+$ small–medium T-cell lymphoproliferative disorder. (a) Staining for PD-1 shows positivity of approximately half of the cells; (b) in the same case, staining for CXCL-13 reveals only scattered positive cells, suggesting that neoplastic lymphocytes do not express a genuine T-follicular helper (TFH) phenotype.

clinical and/or pathological features). In this context, genetic alterations typical of nodal T-follicular helper cell lymphoma, angioimmunoblastic type, are exceptional in cutaneous CD4$^+$ small–medium T-lymphoproliferative disorder [17].

## Clinical features

Patients are adults or elderly without a clear-cut gender predilection. Children may be affected rarely [31]. They present usually with solitary tumors located in the vast majority of cases on the head and neck area (Fig. 11.2). The lesions are usually symmetrical, dome-shaped, well circumscribed, and with a smooth surface (Figs. 11.3–11.5). The presence of tiny scales is usually due to mechanic irritation (Fig. 11.6). In some patients, lesions may arise outside of the head and neck area (Fig. 11.7), but

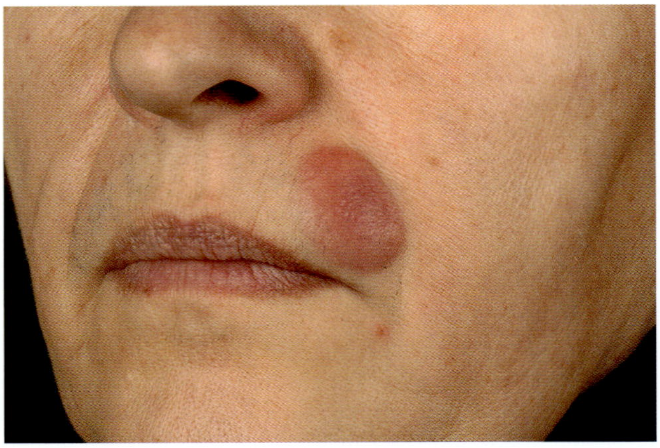

**Figure 11.4** Cutaneous CD4$^+$ small–medium T-cell lymphoproliferative disorder. Solitary tumor on the left side of the upper lip.

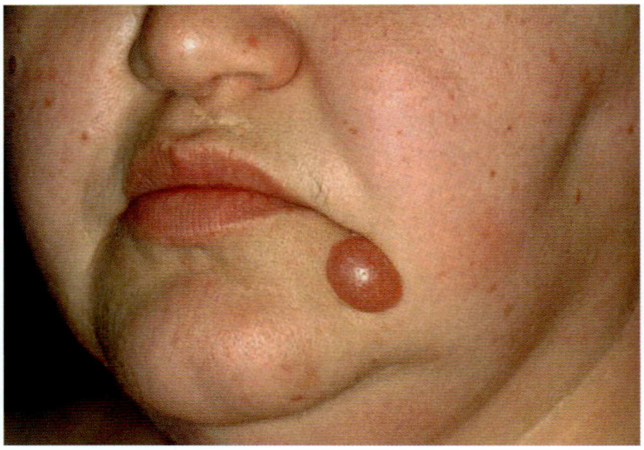

**Figure 11.2** Cutaneous CD4$^+$ small–medium T-cell lymphoproliferative disorder. Solitary tumor on the face.

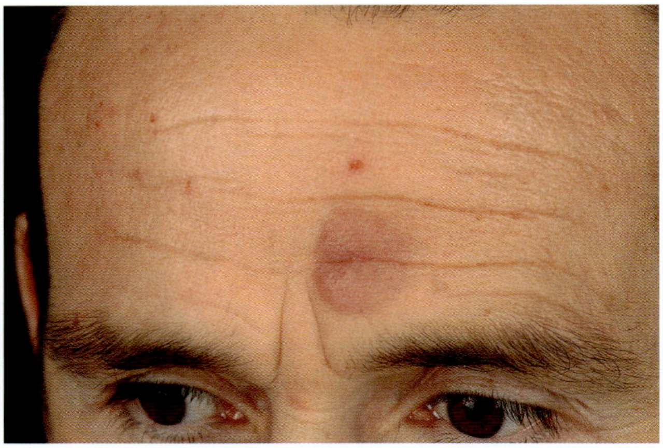

**Figure 11.5** Cutaneous CD4$^+$ small–medium T-cell lymphoproliferative disorder. Solitary, flat tumor on the forehead.

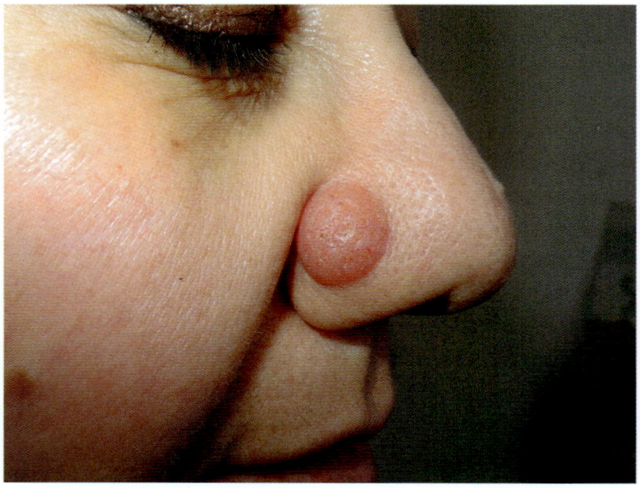

**Figure 11.3** Cutaneous CD4$^+$ small–medium T-cell lymphoproliferative disorder. Solitary tumor on the nose. The nose represents a common site of involvement.

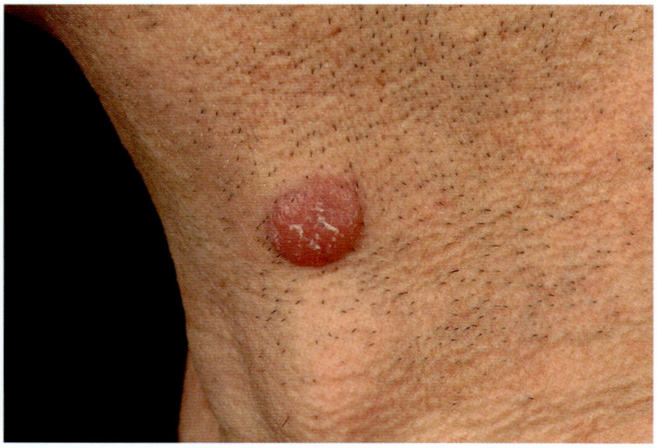

**Figure 11.6** Cutaneous CD4$^+$ small–medium T-cell lymphoproliferative disorder. Solitary tumor on the neck with tiny, small scales as a sign of mechanic irritation.

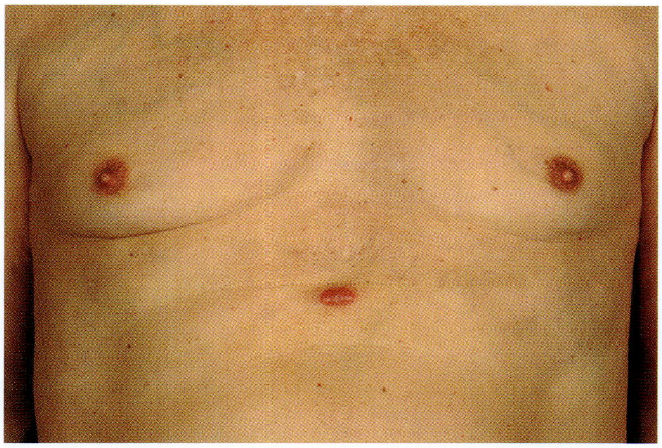

Figure 11.7 Cutaneous CD4+ small–medium T-cell lymphoproliferative disorder. Solitary tumor on the trunk.

diagnosis in these cases should be made only when the lesions are solitary, and the histopathological and phenotypic features are compelling. Patients with multiple tumors have been reported in the literature, but many of these cases may represent a different entity. The surface of the tumors is erythematous or purplish. Ulceration is very uncommon.

A reported case presenting with "acneiform" lesions and marked necrosis [32] in my opinion does not represent an example of cutaneous CD4+ small–medium T-cell lymphoproliferative disorder. In fact, once again it should be reminded that the published literature should be analyzed with a very critical eye.

## Histopathology, immunophenotype, and molecular genetics

### Histopathology

Histology reveals dense, nodular, or diffuse lymphoid infiltrates within the entire dermis, often involving the superficial part of the subcutaneous fat (Fig. 11.8). Cytomorphology shows a predominance of small–/medium-sized lymphocytes with pleomorphic nuclei (Fig. 11.9). Large cells, when present, do not exceed 30% of the neoplastic infiltrate [1, 33]. Epidermotropism is usually completely absent or restricted to a few lymphocytes (some lymphocytes may be found within the hair follicles). When present, intraepidermal cells represent an epiphenomenon restricted to areas of spongiosis and parakeratosis, i.e., of local irritation (Fig. 11.10). Many reactive cells are commonly found admixed with the neoplastic ones. A granulomatous reaction can be observed in a proportion of the cases and may sometimes be the cause of diagnostic problems [34]. Reactive germinal centers can be found, but are uncommon.

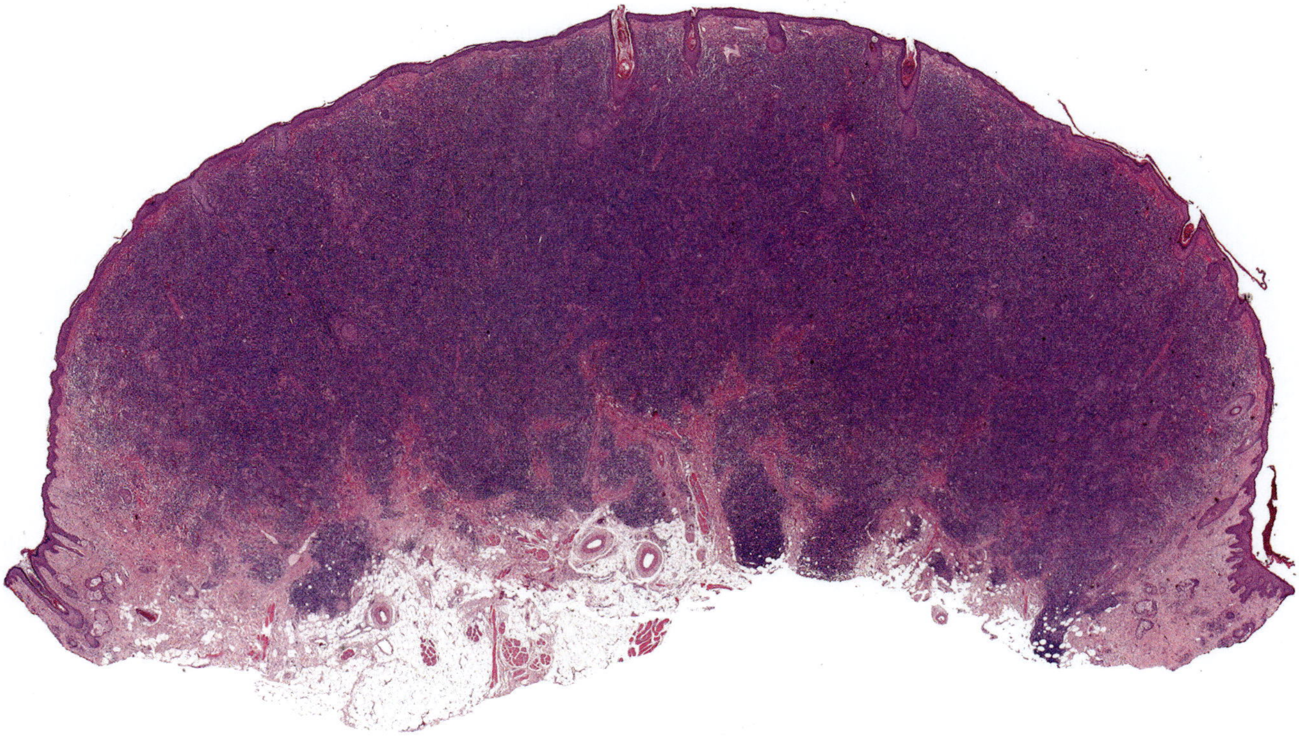

Figure 11.8 Cutaneous CD4+ small–medium T-cell lymphoproliferative disorder. Dense infiltrate of lymphocytes extending throughout the dermis into the superficial part of the subcutaneous fat.

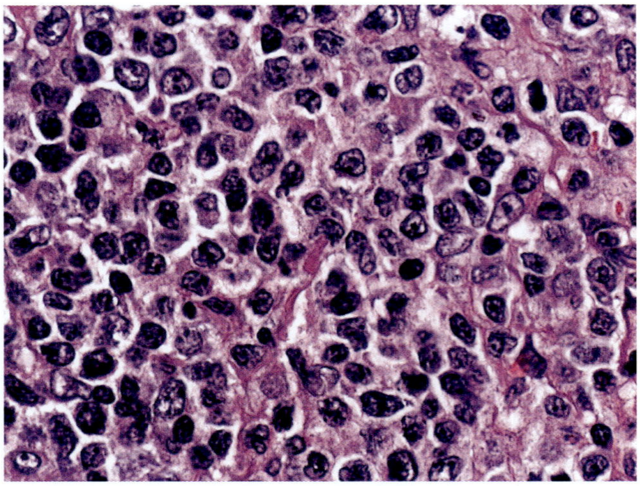

**Figure 11.9** Cutaneous CD4$^+$ small–medium T-cell lymphoproliferative disorder. Small- and medium-sized pleomorphic lymphocytes predominate, admixed with a few larger cells.

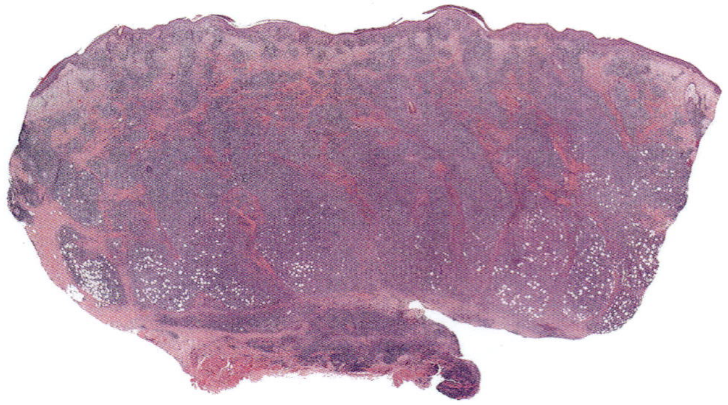

(a)

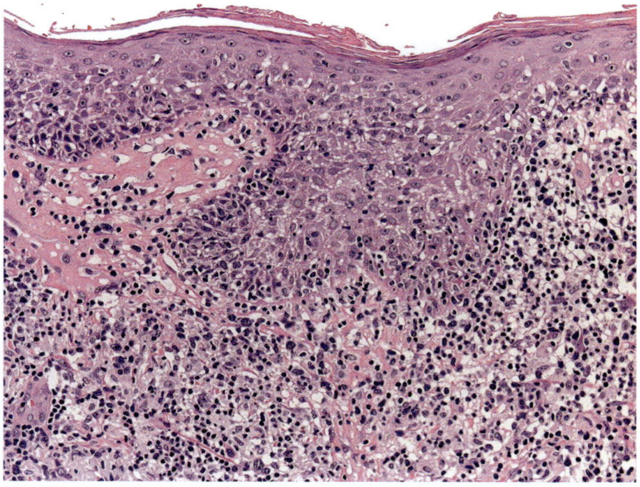

(b)

**Figure 11.10** Cutaneous CD4$^+$ small–medium T-cell lymphoproliferative disorder. (a) Diffuse infiltrate within the entire dermis involving also the visible portion of the subcutaneous fat. (b) Focal intraepidermal lymphocytes in areas of epidermal spongiosis with parakeratosis as a sign of mechanic irritation.

As already mentioned, cases presenting with a band-like infiltrate ("superficial pattern") have been described [17], but I do not consider them as a genuine examples of cutaneous CD4$^+$ small–medium T-cell lymphoproliferative disorder. It must be underlined, however, that the presence of two histopathological patterns, nodular and superficial, has been included in the last edition of the WHO classification [4].

## Immunophenotype

The neoplastic cells show a T-helper phenotype, rarely with loss of pan-T-cell antigens (Fig. 11.11a–d). CD8$^+$ cells expressing TIA-1 are constantly observed but represent a reactive, minor population. Staining for CD30 is negative or, more commonly, limited to scattered cells without formation of clusters. A variably large, reactive infiltrate of B lymphocytes is commonly found (Fig. 11.11e), sometimes with large, activated lymphocytes. The proliferation rate is usually increased but should not exceed 30% (Ki-67 staining) (Fig. 11.11f). Cases with higher proliferation may be rarely observed, but should be judged with great caution. There are reports of cases presenting with a monotypic plasma cell component [35], but in my experience, I have never observed genuine cases of cutaneous CD4$^+$ small–medium T-cell lymphoproliferative disorder presenting with a distinct population of monotypic plasma cells (a few monotypic plasma cells in the context of a dense, nodular/diffuse infiltrate do not represent a differential diagnostic concern with cutaneous marginal zone lymphoproliferative disorder; in addition, germinal centers are not found in cutaneous CD4$^+$ small–medium T-cell lymphoproliferative disorder).

A proportion of cells of cutaneous CD4$^+$ small–medium T-cell lymphoproliferative disorder express PD-1, and less frequently Bcl-6, ICOS, and CXCL-13 [12, 18], in some areas with a typical "rosetting" of CD4$^+$/PD-1$^+$ cells around B lymphocytes (Fig. 11.1a). The programmed death-1 (PD-1) expression can get lost in follow-up biopsies [36]. The cyclin D1 expression associated with increased proliferation has been reported in one study [37], but these findings in my opinion are uncertain and need validation in independent studies.

## Molecular genetics

The molecular analysis of the T-cell receptor (TCR) genes rearrangement shows monoclonality of T lymphocytes in the majority of the cases. Rarely, a concomitant B-cell clone has been observed [38].

Somatic mutations in *DNMT3A*, *ARID1A*, *EP300*, *SETD2*, *TP53*, *SH2B3*, and *NF1* have been described in cutaneous CD4$^+$ small–medium T-cell lymphoproliferative disorder [17, 39, 40], and more recently mutations in *ATM* and *DDX3X* (42% and 33% of cases, respectively), and less frequently in *JAK3*, *STAT5B*,

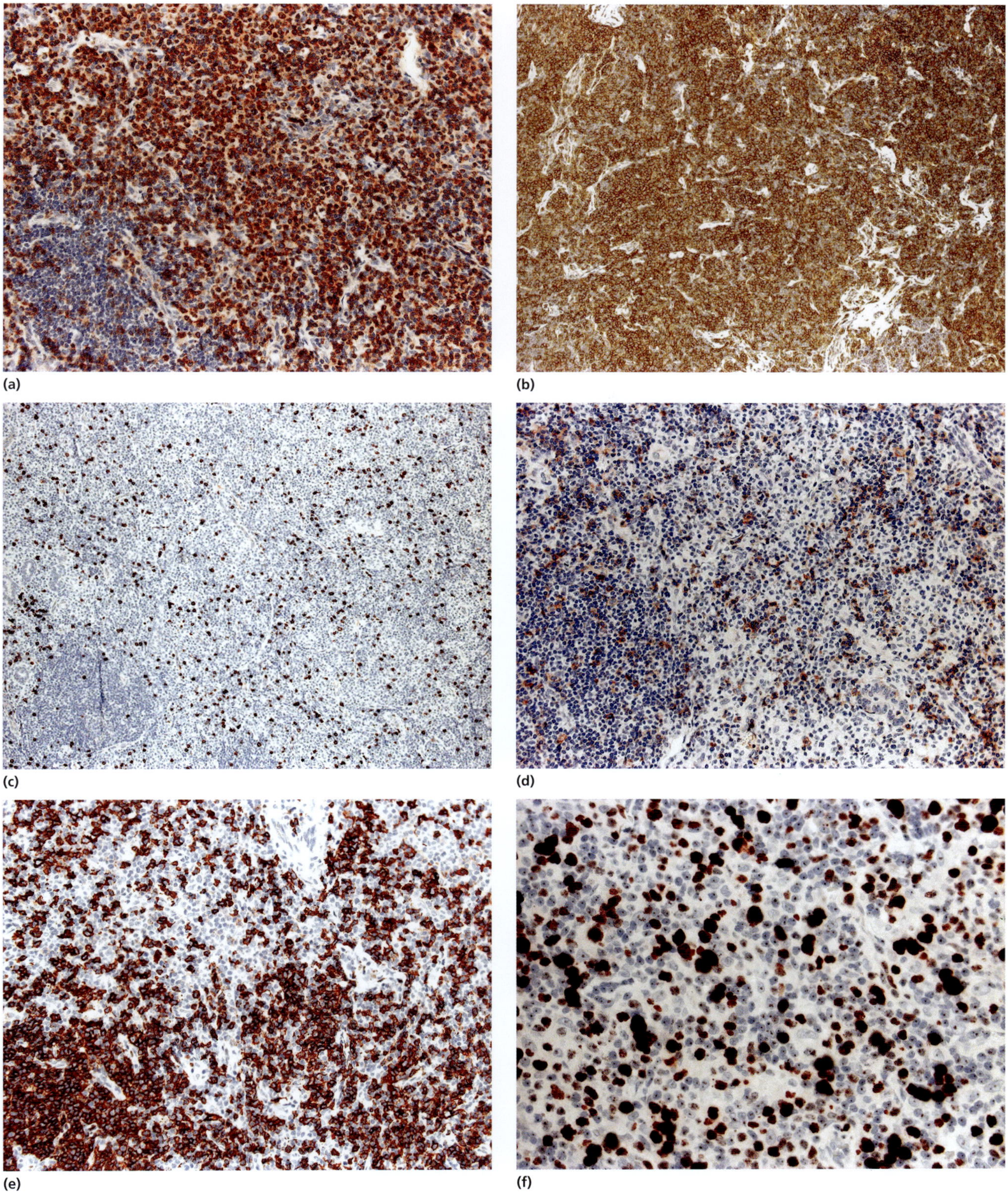

Figure 11.11 Cutaneous CD4$^+$ small–medium T-cell lymphoproliferative disorder. Neoplastic cells express (a) CD3 and (b) CD4, but (c) show negativity for CD8 and (d) loss of CD5 expression; (e) note several CD20$^+$ B lymphocytes and (f) an increased proliferation rate (Ki-67).

*NOTCH1*, *SMARCA4*, and *IDH2*, and rarely in *ARID1B*, *CARD11*, *CDKN2B*, *DNMT3A*, *HRAS*, *MAPK1*, *SMARCB1*, *TP53*, *TSC1*, and *ZEB1* [41]. In spite of positivity for PD-1, cutaneous CD4$^+$ small–medium T-cell lymphoproliferative disorder does not present molecular features typical of follicular helper nodal T-cell lymphomas [41].

The presence of Epstein–Barr virus (EBV) deoxyribonucleic acid (DNA) has been detected by polymerase chain reaction (PCR) techniques in two cases of cutaneous CD4$^+$ small–medium T-cell lymphoproliferative disorder [42], but this was most likely a false-positive finding. In my experience, the virus does not play any role in the pathogenesis of the disease.

## Treatment

Most patients present with solitary tumors that can be treated by surgical excision alone, local radiotherapy, or a combination of the two. Intralesional steroids represent a further option. We have rarely seen patients showing spontaneous regression of the lesions after incisional biopsy [15], and similar cases have been reported [43]. A watchful waiting strategy may be adopted before other measures are considered.

In one study, cyclophosphamide or interferon-α has been used for patients with generalized skin lesions [5]. It must be underlined that the analysis of treatment modalities reported in the literature is hindered by the inclusion of different entities in the various studies published. Multi-agent systemic chemotherapy is never needed for genuine cases of cutaneous CD4$^+$ small–medium T-cell lymphoproliferative disorder.

## Prognosis

Cutaneous CD4$^+$ small–medium T-cell lymphoproliferative disorder has an excellent prognosis, and cases classified according to the criteria listed in this chapter have a 5-year disease-specific survival of 100% [6, 14, 15, 31, 44–47]. Patients with lesions confined to the legs should be managed cautiously, as they may show a more aggressive course [48]. Cases that in the past were classified as cutaneous CD4$^+$ small–medium T-cell lymphoproliferative disorder and showed that progressive diseases were almost invariably those showing multiple lesions at presentation [7]. In fact, the old controversies concerning the prognosis were due to the difficulties in diagnosis and classification mentioned at the beginning of this chapter, and to the inclusion in this group of cases belonging to different entities, particularly peripheral T-cell lymphoma, NOS.

## Final considerations

In spite of over 30 years of discussion, CD4$^+$ small–medium T-cell lymphoproliferative disorder is still an unclear entity, and its precise nosology is yet uncertain. Following the "downgrading" from a true lymphoma to a lymphoproliferative disorder in previous editions of the WHO classification of tumors of hematopoietic and lymphoid tissues, in the last edition of this classification, it is mentioned that this entity exists on a spectrum with reactive lymphoid proliferations (i.e., pseudolymphomas) [4], suggesting a reactive nature of at least some of the cases; at the same time, some studies showed distinct molecular alterations, suggesting a true neoplastic nature of the disease [17, 39–41]. However, criteria for clearly distinguishing reactive from neoplastic cases have never been established, and to my eyes, the confusion remains. The main problem in the proper understanding of these lesions is represented by the considerable confusion existing in the literature, with several names given to the same disease, and the same name given to what may well be different entities. Most of the cases reported in the literature as "cutaneous CD4$^+$ small–medium T-cell lymphoma" (the former name of the entity) are characterized by solitary lesions, but patients presenting with virtually identical solitary tumors have been classified as cutaneous pseudolymphoma (under many different names) in the past. On the other hand, rapidly progressive cases characterized by multiple tumors, classified in the past as cutaneous "CD4$^+$ small–medium T-cell lymphoma," represent most likely examples of cutaneous peripheral T-cell lymphoma, NOS.

In this context, differentiation of cutaneous CD4$^+$ small–medium T-cell lymphoproliferative disorder from peripheral T-cell lymphoma, NOS, may be extremely difficult. There are no intrinsic morphological and/or phenotypical differences, as peripheral T-cell lymphoma, NOS, may present with the predominance of small–medium pleomorphic CD4$^+$ T lymphocytes (see also Chapter 10). Of particular concern are those cases presenting with unusual features (i.e., rapidly growing tumors and/or multiple tumors arising outside of the head and neck region, proliferation rate >30%, numbers of large cells exceeding 30% of the infiltrate, and profound phenotypic aberrations with loss of several pan-T-cell markers). Such cases should not be included in the group of CD4$^+$ small–medium T-cell lymphoproliferative disorder and rather classified as cutaneous peripheral T-cell lymphoma, NOS.

For practical purposes, patients presenting with solitary tumors on the head and neck area and with typical histopathological features never show progression to an aggressive disease, and should be managed in a conservative way; personally, I consider these cases as examples of cutaneous pseudolymphoma. On the other hand, patients presenting with multiple tumors at different skin sites require a more careful approach, and may show an aggressive course.

## Résumé

**Cutaneous CD4⁺ small–medium T-cell lymphoproliferative disorder**

| | | |
|---|---|---|
| **Clinical** | Adults. Children may be affected. Solitary tumors. Preferential location: head and neck. | |
| **Morphology** | Nodular-diffuse infiltrate within the entire dermis, sometimes involving the subcutaneous fat. Small–medium pleomorphic lymphocytes (large cells do not exceed 30% of the infiltrate). A second pattern characterized by superficial, band-like infiltrates has been described, but to my eyes, these cases do not represent genuine examples of cutaneous CD4⁺ small–medium T-cell lymphoproliferative disorder. | |
| **Immunohistochemistry** | CD2, CD3, CD4 | + |
| | CD5 | + (−) |
| | PD1, ICOS, Bcl-6, CXCL13 | + (proportion of cells) (PD1 > Bcl-6 > ICOS > CXCL13) |
| | CD10 | − |
| | βF1 | + |
| | TCR-γ, TCR-δ | − |
| | CD8 TIA-1 | − (positive in a proportion of the accompanying infiltrate) |
| | CD30 | − (positive in scattered cells, some of which B lymphocytes) |
| | CD20 | − (positive in a proportion of the accompanying infiltrate) |
| **Genetics** | Monoclonal rearrangement of the TCR genes is present in most cases. Mutations detected in some cases in *DNMT3A, ARID1A, EP300, SETD2, TP53, SH2B3, NF1, ATM,* and *DDX3X*. | |
| **Treatment** | Surgical excision, local radiotherapy, or a combination of the two. Intralesional steroids. Watchful waiting. Spontaneous regression may be observed after partial biopsy. | |

## References


1. Willemze R, Cerroni L, Kempf W, *et al.* The 2018 update of the WHO-EORTC classification for primary cutaneous lymphomas. *Blood* 2019;**133**:1703–1714.
2. Kempf W, Mitteldorf C, Cerroni L, *et al.* Classifications of cutaneous lymphomas and lymphoproliferative disorders: An update from the EORTC cutaneous lymphoma histopathology group. *J Eur Acad Dermatol Venereol* 2024;**38**:1491–1503.
3. Rodriguez-Pinilla SM, Cerroni L. Primary cutaneous CD4-positive small/medium T-cell lymphoproliferative disorder. In: Arber DA, Borowitz MJ, Cook JR, *et al.*, eds. *The International Consensus Classification of Myeloid and Lymphoid Neoplasms*. Philadelphia (US): Wolters Kluver, 2025: 695–696.
4. Vergier B, Jansen PM, Mitteldorf C, *et al.* Primary cutaneous CD4-positive small or medium T-cell lymphoproliferative disorder. In: *WHO Classification of Tumours Editorial Board. Haematolymphoid Tumours*. 5th edition. Lyon (France): IARC, 2024: 682–684.
5. Friedmann D, Wechsler J, Delfan MH, *et al.* Primary cutaneous pleomorphic small T-cell lymphoma: a review of 11 cases. *Arch Dermatol* 1995;**131**:1009–1015.
6. Grogg KL, Jung S, Erickson LA, *et al.* Primary cutaneous CD4-positive small/medium-sized pleomorphic T-cell lymphoma: a clonal T-cell lymphoproliferative disorder with indolent behavior. *Mod Pathol* 2008;**21**:708–715.
7. Garcia-Herrera A, Colomo L, Camos M, *et al.* Primary cutaneous small/medium CD4 T-cell lymphomas: A heterogeneous group of tumors with different clinicopathologic features and outcome. *J Clin Oncol* 2008;**26**:1–11.
8. Williams VL, Torres-Cabala CA, Duvic M. Primary cutaneous small- to medium-sized CD4⁺ pleomorphic T-cell lymphoma: a retrospective case series and review of the provisional cutaneous lymphoma category. *Am J Clin Dermatol* 2011;**12**:389–401.
9. Arai E, Okubo H, Tsuchida T, *et al.* Pseudolymphomatous folliculitis: a clinicopathologic study of 15 cases of cutaneous pseudolymphoma with follicular invasion. *Am J Surg Pathol* 1999;**23**:1313–1319.
10. Rijlaarsdam JU, Willemze R. Cutaneous pseudo-T-cell lymphomas. *Semin Diagn Pathol* 1991;**8**:102–108.
11. Kazakov DV, Belousova IE, Kacerovska D, *et al.* Hyperplasia of hair follicles and other adnexal structures in cutaneous lymphoproliferative disorders. A study of 53 cases, including so-called pseudolymphomatous folliculitis and overt lymphomas. *Am J Surg Pathol* 2008;**32**:1468–1478.
12. Battistella M, Beylot-Barry M, Bachelez H, *et al.* Primary cutaneous follicular helper T-cell lymphoma. *Arch Dermatol* 2012;**148**:832–839.
13. Ryan AJA, Robson A, Hayes BD, *et al.* Primary cutaneous peripheral T-cell lymphoma, unspecified with an indolent clinical course: a distinct peripheral T-cell lymphoma? *Clin Exp Dermatol* 2010;**35**:892–896.
14. Leinweber B, Beltraminelli H, Kerl H, Cerroni L. Solitary small–medium pleomorphic T-cell nodules of undetermined significance: clinical, histopathological, immunohistochemical, and molecular analysis of 26 cases. *Dermatology* 2009;**219**:42–47.
15. Beltraminelli H, Leinweber B, Kerl H, Cerroni L. Primary cutaneous CD4+ small/medium-sized pleomorphic T cell lymphoma: a cutaneous nodular proliferation of pleomorphic T lymphocytes of undetermined significance? A study of 136 cases. *Am J Dermatopathol* 2009;**31**:317–322.
16. Alberti-Violetti S, Torres-Cabala CA, Talpur R, *et al.* Clinicopathological and molecular study of primary cutaneous CD4+ small/medium-sized pleomorphic T-cell lymphoma. *J Cutan Pathol* 2016;**43**:1121–1130.
17. Beltzung F, Ortonne N, Pelletier L, *et al.* Primary cutaneous CD4+ small/medium T-cell lymphoproliferative disorders: a clinical,

pathologic, and molecular study of 60 cases presenting with a single lesion: a multicenter study of the French Cutaneous Lymphoma Study Group. *Am J Surg Pathol* 2020;**44**:862–872.
18. Rodriguez-Pinilla SM, Roncador G, Rodriguez-Peralto JJ, *et al.* Primary cutaneous CD4+ small/medium-sized pleomorphic T-cell lymphoma expresses follicular T-cell markers. *Am J Surg Pathol* 2009;**33**:81–90.
19. Wang JY, Nguyen GH, Ruan J, *et al.* Primary cutaneous follicular helper T-cell lymphoma: a case series and review of the literature. *Am J Dermatopathol* 2017;**39**:374–383.
20. Attygalle AD, Sekata-Yamagimoto M, Amador C, *et al.* Nodal T follicular helper cell lymphoma, angioimmunoblastic type. In: *WHO Classification of Tumours Editorial Board. Haematolymphoid Tumours.* 5th edition. Lyon (France): IARC, 2024: 744–751.
21. Hu S, Young KH, Konoplev SN, *et al.* Follicular T-cell lymphoma: a member of an emerging family of follicular helper T-cell derived T-cell lymphomas. *Hum Pathol* 2012;**43**:1789–1798.
22. Odejide O, Weigert O, Lane AA, *et al.* A targeted mutational landscape of angioimmunoblastic T-cell lymphoma. *Blood* 2014;**123**:1293–1296.
23. Vallois D, Dobay MPD, Morin RD, *et al.* Activating mutations in genes related to TCR signaling in angioimmunoblastic and other follicular helper T-cell–derived lymphomas. *Blood* 2016;**128**: 1490–1502.
24. Mitteldorf C, Berti E, Pulitzer M, Willemze R. Primary cutaneous peripheral T-cell lymphoma NOS. In: *WHO Classification of Tumours Editorial Board. Haematolymphoid Tumours.* 5th edition. Lyon (France): IARC, 2024: 708–709.
25. Bosisio FM, Cerroni L. Expression of T-follicular helper markers in sequential biopsies of progressive mycosis fungoides and other primary cutaneous T-cell lymphomas. *Am J Dermatopathol* 2015;**37**:115–121.
26. Guitart J, Gammon B. The difficulties in defining follicular T helper phenotype in cutaneous lymphomas. *Am J Dermatopathol* 2013;**35**:691.
27. Mitteldorf C, Bieri M, Wey N, *et al.* Expression of PD-1 (CD279) in cutaneous B-cell lymphomas with correlation to lymphoma entities and biologic behaviour. *Br J Dermatol* 2013;**169**:1212–1218.
28. Gaulard P, de Leval L. Follicular helper T cells: implications in neoplastic hematopathology. *Semin Diagn Pathol* 2011; **28**:202–213.
29. Cetinözman F, Jansen PM, Vermeer MH, *et al.* Differential expression of programmed death-1 (PD-1) in Sézary syndrome and mycosis fungoides. *Arch Dermatol* 2012;**148**:1379–1385.
30. Meyerson HJ, Awadallah A, Pavlidakey P, *et al.* Follicular center helper T-cell (TFH) marker positive mycosis fungoides/Sézary syndrome. *Mod Pathol* 2013;**26**:32–43.
31. Baum CL, Link BK, Neppalli VT, *et al.* Reappraisal of the provisional entity primary cutaneous $CD4^+$ small/medium pleomorphic T-cell lymphoma: a series of 10 adult and pediatric patients and review of the literature. *J Am Acad Dermatol* 2011;**65**:739–748.
32. Wang L, Wang G, Gao T. Acneiform primary cutaneous CD4-positive small/medium pleomorphic T-cell lymphoma with prominent necrosis. *J Cutan Pathol* 2015;**42**:265–270.
33. Beljaards RC, Meijer CJLM, van der Putte SCJ, *et al.* Primary cutaneous T-cell lymphoma: clinicopathological features and prognostic parameters of 35 cases other than mycosis fungoides and CD30-positive large cell lymphoma. *J Pathol* 1994;**172**:53–60.
34. Scarabello A, Leinweber B, Ardigó M, *et al.* Cutaneous lymphomas with prominent granulomatous reaction: a potential pitfall in the histopathologic diagnosis of cutaneous T- and B-cell lymphomas. *Am J Surg Pathol* 2002;**26**:1259–1268.
35. Magro CM, Ruan J, Grossman M, Hedayat AA. Monoclonal plasma cell infiltrates in the setting of cutaneous follicular helper T cell lymphoproliferative disorders. *Ann Diagn Pathol* 2019;**40**:94–104.
36. Buder K, Poppe LM, Bröcker EB, *et al.* Primary cutaneous follicular helper T-cell lymphoma: diagnostic pitfalls of this new lymphoma subtype. *J Cutan Pathol* 2013;**40**:903–908.
37. Oschlies I, Kock K, Wüseke T, *et al.* Cyclin D1 expression, cell proliferation, and clonal persistence characterize primary cutaneous CD4(+) small or medium T-cell lymphoproliferative disorder. *Histopathology* 2023;**82**:485–494.
38. Bakr F, Wain EM, Wong S, *et al.* Prominent blasts in primary cutaneous CD4+ small/medium T-cell lymphoproliferative disorder. A reconsideration of diagnostic criteria. *Am J Dermatopathol* 2021; **43**:e190–e196.
39. Richter J, Oschlies I, Kock K, *et al.* CD27/CD70 pathway activation in primary cutaneous CD4+ small/medium T-cell lymphoproliferative disorder. *J Pathol* 2024;**262**:189–197.
40. Soderquist CR, Hsiao S, Pang J, *et al.* Whole exome sequencing of primary cutaneous CD4+ small/medium T-cell lymphoproliferative disorders. *Hematol Oncol* 2023;**41**:768–770.
41. Rodriguez M, Rebollo-Gonzalez M, Diaz-Alejo JF, *et al.* Mutational profiling of primary cutaneous CD4+ small/medium T-cell lymphoproliferative disorder does not resemble nodal peripheral T-cell lymphomas with a follicular helper T-cell phenotype. *Br J Dermatol* 2024;**191**:456–458.
42. Nagore E, Ledesma E, Collado C, *et al.* Detection of Epstein–Barr virus and human herpesvirus 7 and 8 genomes in primary cutaneous T- and B-cell lymphomas. *Br J Dermatol* 2000;**143**:320–323.
43. Cetinözman F, Jansen PM, Willemze R. Expression of programmed death-1 in primary cutaneous CD4-positive small/medium-sized pleomorphic T-cell lymphoma, cutaneous pseudo-T-cell lymphoma, and other types of cutaneous T-cell lymphoma. *Am J Surg Pathol* 2012;**36**:109–116.
44. von den Driesch P, Coors EA. Localized cutaneous small to medium-sized pleomorphic T-cell lymphoma: a report of 3 cases stable for years. *J Am Acad Dermatol* 2002;**46**:531–535.
45. Sterry W, Siebel A, Mielke V. HTLV-I-negative pleomorphic T-cell lymphoma of the skin: the clinicopathological correlations and natural history of 15 patients. *Br J Dermatol* 1992;**126**:456–462.
46. Bekkenk MW, Vermeer MH, Jansen PM, *et al.* Peripheral T-cell lymphomas unspecified presenting in the skin: analysis of prognostic factors in a group of 82 patients. *Blood* 2003;**102**:2213–2219.
47. Fink-Puches R, Zenahlik P, Bäck B, *et al.* Primary cutaneous lymphomas: applicability of current classification schemes (European Organization for Research and Treatment of Cancer, World Health Organization) based on clinicopathologic features observed in a large group of patients. *Blood* 2002;**99**:800–805.
48. Poligone B, Wilson LD, Subtil A, Heald P. Primary cutaneous T-cell lymphoma localized to the lower leg. A distinct, locally aggressive cutaneous T-cell lymphoma. *Arch Dermatol* 2009;**145**:677–682.

## CHAPTER 12

# Primary cutaneous acral $CD8^+$ T-cell lymphoproliferative disorder

Primary cutaneous acral $CD8^+$ T-cell lymphoproliferative disorder was originally described by Petrella *et al.* as "indolent $CD8^+$ lymphoid proliferation of the ear" [1]. Several other cases have been reported subsequently by other groups under several terms, including "indolent $CD8^+$ lymphoid proliferation of the face" and "indolent $CD8^+$ lymphoid proliferation of acral sites" among others [2–11]. Although it was previously suggested that acral $CD8^+$ cutaneous T-cell lymphoproliferative disorder may represent a phenotypic variant of the cutaneous $CD4^+$ small–medium T-cell lymphoproliferative disorder, and a case had been reported as "pleomorphic $CD8^+$ small/medium size cutaneous T-cell lymphoma" prior to the publication by Petrella *et al.* [12], the histopathological differences between the two conditions prompted their classification as separate entities. Cutaneous acral $CD8^+$ T-cell lymphoproliferative disorder was still listed as a lymphoma (provisional entity) in the 2018 European Organization for Research and Treatment of Cancer (EORTC)/World Health Organization (WHO) classification of cutaneous lymphomas [13], and it has now been included as a distinct entity but downgraded to lymphoproliferative disorder in the 2024 update of it [14]. Cutaneous acral $CD8^+$ T-cell lymphoproliferative disorder represents a distinct entity in the International Consensus Classification (ICC) *of Myeloid and Lymphoid Neoplasms* [15]. In the 5th edition of the WHO *Classification of Haematolymphoid Tumours* is listed as a distinct entity within the group of "primary cutaneous T-cell lymphoid proliferations and lymphomas" [16].

The change in the name of this entity in recent classification schemes reflects the benign prognosis, and only one case with extracutaneous dissemination has been reported to date [17]. In this context, Rein Willemze recently wrote: "(. . .) acral $CD8^+$ T-cell lymphoproliferative disorder can best be considered and managed as a benign process and that the question of whether $CD8^+$ T-cell lymphoproliferative disorder is benign or malignant is more of academic than of clinical interest" [18].

Care should be taken to distinguish cutaneous acral $CD8^+$ T-cell lymphoproliferative disorder from primary cutaneous $CD8^+$ aggressive epidermotropic cytotoxic T-cell lymphoma and from $CD8^+$ mycosis fungoides, as they represent completely distinct entities with different clinical presentation and behavior. In typical cases arising in otherwise asymptomatic and immunocompetent patients, staging investigations are not recommended [1, 7, 13]. One case has been observed in an immunosuppressed patient after renal transplantation [19].

## Clinical features

Patients are adults of both genders with a male predominance. Lesions arise most frequently on the head and neck area (particularly ear[s] and nose) (Fig. 12.1), but extrafacial lesions may be observed rarely, particularly on the feet [8]. Lesions are commonly solitary, but bilateral involvement of the ears has been observed [3]. Ulceration is not present.

## Histopathology, immunophenotype, and molecular genetics

### Histopathology

Histology reveals dense, monomorphous, nodular, or diffuse lymphoid infiltrates within the entire dermis, often involving the superficial part of the subcutaneous fat (Fig. 12.2a). There is a clear grenz zone between the uninvolved epidermis and the dermis. Cytomorphology shows a predominance of medium-sized lymphocytes with pleomorphic nuclei (Fig. 12.2b,c). Epidermotropism is absent as a rule, but a few intraepithelial lymphocytes may be observed [7, 20]. Signet-ring cells have been observed in one case [21].

### Immunophenotype

Neoplastic cells are positive for CD3 and CD8 (Fig. 12.3a), negative for CD4 (Fig. 12.3b), CD30, and CD56, and may show variable loss of pan-T-cell antigens (CD2, CD5, and CD7). TIA-1 is positive, but granzyme B and perforin are negative (nonactivated cytotoxic phenotype). A peculiar and repeatable staining pattern is observed with CD68, showing positive dots located in the Golgi area (Fig. 12.3c) [22]. Markers of T follicular helper (TFH) lymphocytes are negative [7]. The proliferation rate (Ki-67) is low (Fig. 12.3d). A unique case showing a double expression

*Skin Lymphoma: The Illustrated Guide*, Sixth Edition. Lorenzo Cerroni.

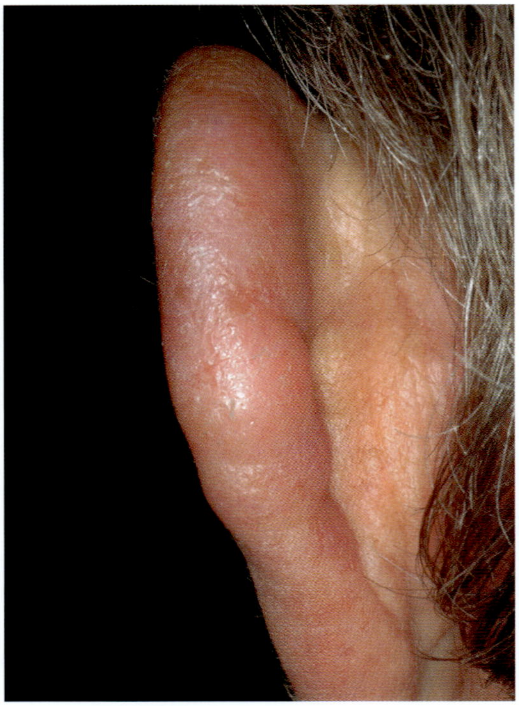

**Figure 12.1** Acral CD8⁺ cutaneous T-cell lymphoproliferative disorder. Erythematous, infiltrated lesions on the helix. (*Courtesy of Dr. Robert Müllegger, Wiener Neustadt, Austria*).

of both CD4 and CD8 but with otherwise typical clinical presentation has been reported [23].

## Molecular genetics

The molecular analysis of the T-cell receptor (TCR) genes rearrangement shows monoclonality of T lymphocytes in the majority of the cases. *PTEN* deletion on chromosome 10 may represent an acquired somatic mutation. Alterations in the killer immunoglobulin-like receptor (*KIR3DL1*) gene have been described in two out of five cases in a study, leading 14 to a loss of the KIR3DL1-expression at the protein level [24].

## Treatment

Patients should be managed conservatively (i.e., surgical excision alone, local radiotherapy, or a combination of the two). As the disease has been downgraded from lymphoma to a lymphoproliferative disorder, intralesional injection of steroids may be considered as an alternative option, akin to cutaneous $CD4^+$ small–medium T-cell lymphoproliferative disorder, but there are no reported cases at present.

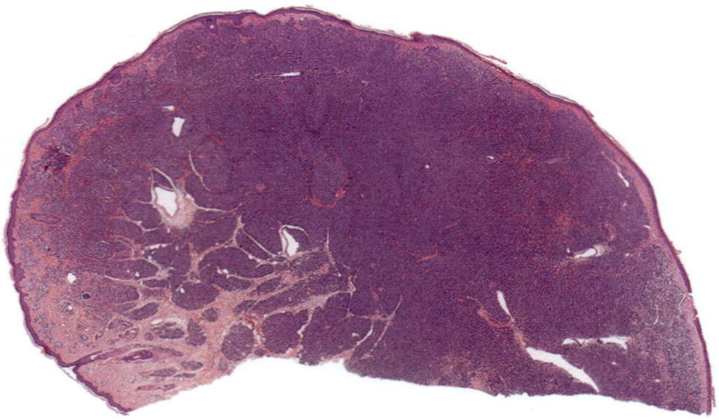

(a)

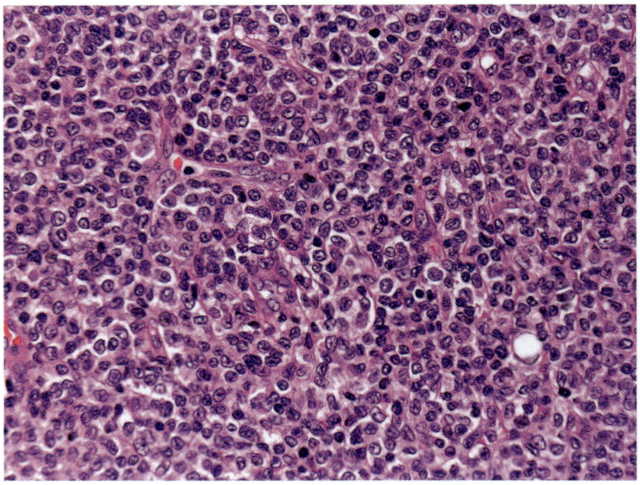

(b)

**Figure 12.2** Acral $CD8^+$ cutaneous T-cell lymphoproliferative disorder. (a) Dense, diffuse lymphoid infiltrates within the entire dermis. (b) Predominance of small- and mid-sized lymphocytes.

## Prognosis

Cutaneous acral $CD8^+$ T-cell lymphoproliferative disorder has an indolent behavior with excellent prognosis [13, 25]. Cutaneous recurrences may be observed [21], sometimes with a multifocal pattern [26], but systemic involvement is exceedingly rare and only one case with extracutaneous dissemination many years after the initial presentation has been reported [17].

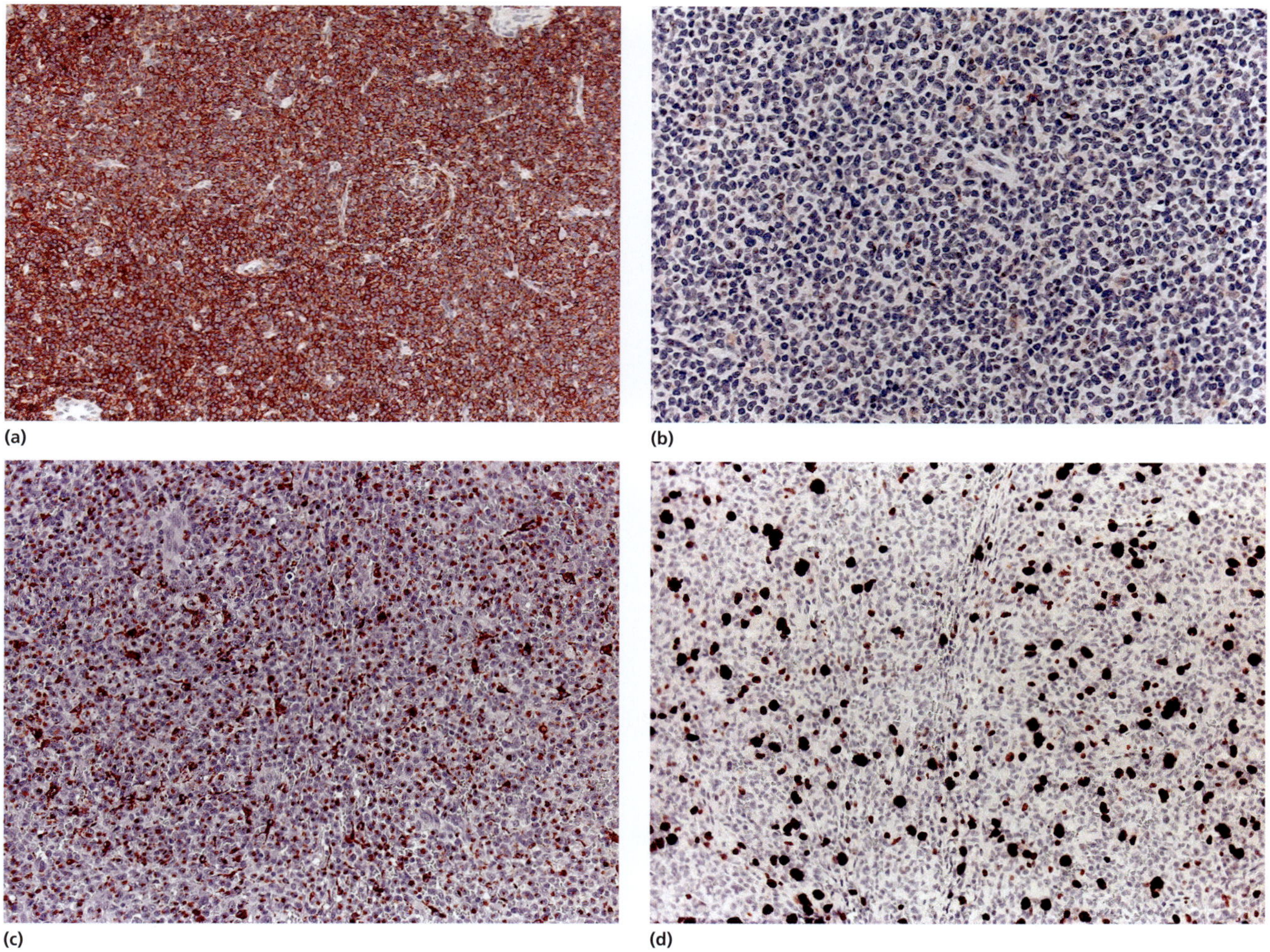


**Figure 12.3** Acral CD8+ cutaneous T-cell lymphoproliferative disorder. (a) Positivity for CD8 and (b) negativity for CD4. (c) Characteristic dot-like positivity for CD68. (d) Low proliferation detected by staining for Ki-67.

## Résumé

| | | |
|---|---|---|
| **Cutaneous acral CD8+ T-cell lymphoproliferative disorder** | | |
| **Clinical** | Solitary tumors located mostly on the ear or nose; sometimes bilateral ear involvement. Location at other acral sites less frequent. | |
| **Morphology** | Monomorphous, nodular, or diffuse infiltrate of small–medium pleomorphic lymphocytes. | |
| **Immunohistochemistry** | CD3, CD8 | + |
| | CD4 | – (one case with a double expression of CD4 and CD8 has been reported) |
| | CD2, CD5, CD7 | + (–) |
| | βF1 | + |
| | TCR-γ, TCR-δ | – |
| | TIA-1 | + |
| | Granzyme B, perforin | – |
| | CD30, CD56 | – |
| | CD68 | + (dot in the Golgi area) |
| | PD1, ICOS, CXCL13, Bcl-6, CD10 | – |
| **Genetics** | Monoclonal rearrangement of the TCR genes is present in most cases. Alterations in the *KIR3DL1* gene described in a few cases. | |
| **Treatment** | Surgical excision, local radiotherapy, or a combination of the two. | |

## References

1. Petrella T, Maubec E, Cornillet-Lefebvre P, *et al.* Indolent CD8-positive lymphoid proliferation of the ear. A distinct primary cutaneous T-cell lymphoma? *Am J Surg Pathol* 2007;**31**:1887–1892.
2. Suchak R, O'Connor S, McNamara C, *et al.* Indolent CD8-positive lymphoid proliferation on the face: part of the spectrum of primary cutaneous small-/medium-sized pleomorphic T-cell lymphoma or a distinct entity? *J Cutan Pathol* 2010;**37**:977–981.
3. Beltraminelli H, Müllegger R, Cerroni L. Indolent CD8+ lymphoid proliferation of the ear: a phenotypic variant of the small-medium pleomorphic cutaneous T-cell lymphoma? Report of three cases. *J Cutan Pathol* 2010;**37**:81–84.
4. Kempf W, Kazakov DV, Cozzio A, *et al.* Primary cutaneous CD8+ small- to medium-sized lymphoproliferative disorder in extrafacial sites: clinicopathologic features and concept on their classification. *Am J Dermatopathol* 2013;**35**:159–166.
5. Swick BL, Baum CL, Venkat AP, Liu V. Indolent CD8+ lymphoid proliferation of the ear: report of two cases and review of the literature. *J Cutan Pathol* 2011;**38**:209–215.
6. Geraud C, Goerdt S, Klemke CD. Primary cutaneous CD8+ small/medium-sized pleomorphic T-cell lymphoma, ear-type: a unique cutaneous T-cell lymphoma with a favourable prognosis. *Br J Dermatol* 2011;**164**:456–458.
7. Greenblatt D, Ally M, Child F, *et al.* Indolent CD8+ lymphoid proliferation of acral sites: a clinicopathologic study of six patients with some atypical features. *J Cutan Pathol* 2013;**40**:248–258.
8. Wobser M, Petrella T, Kneitz H, *et al.* Extrafacial indolent CD8-positive cutaneous lymphoid proliferation with unusual symmetrical presentation involving both feet. *J Cutan Pathol* 2013;**40**: 955–961.
9. Zeng W, Nava VE, Cohen P, *et al.* Indolent CD8-positive T-cell lymphoid proliferation of the ear: a report of two cases. *J Cutan Pathol* 2012;**39**:696–700.
10. Tjahjono LA, Davis MDP, Witzig TE, Comfere NI. Primary cutaneous acral CD8+ T-cell lymphoma – a single center review of 3 cases and recent literature review. *Am J Dermatopathol* 2019;**41**:644–648.
11. Kutlubay Z, Engin B, Kote E, *et al.* A case of CD8+ small/medium-sized pleomorphic T-cell lymphoma: clinical and histopathological differential diagnosis. *Br J Dermatol* 2014;**170**:204–206.
12. Khamaysi Z, Ben-Arieh Y, Epelbaum R, Bergman R. Pleomorphic CD8+ small/medium size cutaneous T-cell lymphoma. *Am J Dermatopathol* 2006;**28**:434–437.
13. Willemze R, Cerroni L, Kempf W, *et al.* The 2018 update of the WHO-EORTC classification for primary cutaneous lymphomas. *Blood* 2019;**133**:1703–1714.
14. Kempf W, Mitteldorf C, Cerroni L, *et al.* Classifications of cutaneous lymphomas and lymphoproliferative disorders: An update from the EORTC cutaneous lymphoma histopathology group. *J Eur Acad Dermatol Venereol* 2024;**38**:1491–1503.
15. Petrella T, Goodlad JR, Pro B. Primary cutaneous acral CD8-positive T-cell lymphoproliferative disorder. In: Arber DA, Borowitz MJ, Cook JR, *et al.*, eds. *The International Consensus Classification of Myeloid and Lymphoid Neoplasms.* Philadelphia (US): Wolters Kluver, 2025: 706–708.
16. Kempf W, Mitteldorf C, Pulitzer M, Robson A. Primary cutaneous acral CD8-positive T-cell lymphoproliferative disorder. In: *WHO Classification of Tumours Editorial Board. Haematolymphoid Tumours.* 5th edition. Lyon (France): IARC, 2024: 685–687.
17. Alberti-Violetti S, Fanoni D, Provasi M, *et al.* Primary cutaneous acral CD8 positive T-cell lymphoma with extra-cutaneous involvement: a long-standing case with an unexpected progression. *J Cutan Pathol* 2017;**44**:964–968.
18. Willemze R. Primary cutaneous acral CD8+ T-cell lymphoproliferative disorder: a benign or malignant process? *Br J Dermatol* 2024;**191**:659–660.
19. Baykal C, Büyükbabani N, Seçkin D, *et al.* Cutaneous atypical papular CD8+ lymphoproliferative disorder at acral sites in a renal transplant patient. *Clin Exp Dermatol* 2017;**42**:902–905.
20. Hagen JW, Magro CM. Indolent CD8+ lymphoid proliferation of the face with eyelid involvement. *Am J Dermatopathol* 2014;**36**: 137–141.
21. Li XQ, Zhou XY, Sheng WQ, *et al.* Indolent CD8+ lymphoid proliferation of the ear: a new entity and possible occurrence of signet ring cells. *Histopathology* 2009;**55**:468–470.
22. Wobser M, Roth S, Reinartz T, *et al.* CD68 expression is a discriminative feature of indolent cutaneous CD8-positive lymphoid proliferation and distinguishes this lymphoma subtype from other CD8-positive cutaneous lymphomas. *Br J Dermatol* 2015;**172**:1573–1580.
23. Toberer F, Christopoulos P, Lasitschka F, *et al.* Double-positive CD8/CD4 primary cutaneous acral T-cell lymphoma. *J Cutan Pathol* 2019;**46**:231–233.
24. Wobser M, Appenzeller S, Roth S, *et al.* Oncogenic alterations in *KIR3DL1* in cutaneous acral CD8+ lymphoproliferative disorder. *Br J Dermatol* 2024;**191**:816–822.
25. Li JY, Guitart J, Pulitzer MP, *et al.* Multicenter case series of indolent small/medium-sized CD8+ lymphoid proliferations with predilection for the ear and face. *Am J Dermatopathol* 2014; **36**:402–408.
26. Kluk J, Kai A, Koch D, *et al.* Indolent CD8-positive lymphoid proliferation of acral sites: three further cases of a rare entity and an update on a unique patient. *J Cutan Pathol* 2016;**43**:125–136.

CHAPTER 13

# Cutaneous adult T-cell leukemia/lymphoma

Adult T-cell leukemia/lymphoma (ATLL) is a malignant lymphoproliferative disease associated with a retrovirus infection caused by the human T-cell lymphotropic virus I (HTLV-1). The disease is endemic in the south of Japan, in the Caribbean Islands, and in parts of Central Africa, and is rare in other regions, but reports on its occurrence have come from many different countries besides the endemic ones. Cutaneous manifestations and histopathologic features are identical to those of mycosis fungoides; thus, demonstration of retroviral infection is mandatory for the diagnosis.

Four variants of ATLL are recognized in the International Consensus Classification (ICC) *of Myeloid and Lymphoid Neoplasms* and in the WHO *Classification of Haematolymphoid Tumours* [1, 2]: acute, chronic, lymphomatous, and smoldering. Although skin manifestations are usually considered as a smoldering form of the disease, it has been suggested that patients with purely cutaneous lesions may have a better prognosis and should be classified separately from those with smoldering ATLL [3, 4]. Cutaneous ATLL is included as a specific entity in the World Health Organization (WHO)–European Organization for Research and Treatment of Cancer (EORTC) classification of primary cutaneous lymphomas [5]. It should be reminded that infection with HTLV-1 may also be associated with non-neoplastic skin conditions (HTLV-1-associated infective dermatitis, lichenoid dermatitis).

The latency between infection with HTLV-1 and onset of ATLL is long, and most patients have been infected early in life. In this context, besides transmission through blood and blood products, the virus can also be transmitted by breast feeding of infants. Although exposure to HTLV-1 is a prerequisite for developing ATLL, infection alone is not sufficient for the malignant transformation of the cells, and additional genetic alterations are necessary for the development of the disease. In fact, it is estimated that only a small percentage of infected patients (3–5%) will develop the disease [6].

## Clinical features

Patients are adults or elderly with a prevalence of males. Adolescents may be affected rarely [7]. Specific skin manifestations can be observed in about half of the patients, especially those presenting with indolent forms of the disease [8–10]. Primary cutaneous involvement may also be seen [10]. Anti-HTLV-1 antibodies can be demonstrated in the serum of affected individuals. Onset of ATLL has been observed in three patients who received organs from an HTLV-1$^+$ donor [11], as well as in patients with human immunodeficiency virus (HIV) infection [12].

The clinical presentation of the cutaneous form is indistinguishable from that of mycosis fungoides. Cutaneous lesions are localized or generalized macules, papules, patches, plaques, and tumors (Figs. 13.1 to 13.4) [8, 9, 13, 14]. Erythroderma may also develop. Rarely, the disease may present with large solitary nodules [15]. A leukemic blood picture and involvement of the bone marrow are found in more than half of the patients. Spontaneous regression of skin lesions has been observed rarely [16].

Patients with ATLL have an impaired immune response and may develop atypical cutaneous mycotic infections characterized by little or no inflammation, due to downmodulation of skin immunity against dermatophytes. Besides cutaneous infections, a higher risk of systemic infections is also present in these patients [17].

## Histopathology

Histology shows an infiltrate of small/medium or medium/large pleomorphic lymphocytes with prominent epidermotropism (Fig. 13.5). The histopathologic picture is often indistinguishable from that of mycosis fungoides, and rarely, follicular mucinosis may be observed within the skin infiltrates as well [18, 19]. Perineural infiltrates may be observed (Fig. 13.6). Variants of ATLL with angiocentricity and/or angiodestruction or with bullous lesions have been reported [20–22].

## Immunophenotype

Immunohistology usually reveals a T-helper (CD3$^+$, CD4$^+$, and CD8$^-$) phenotype, but some cases may be CD4$^-$/CD8$^+$ or CD4$^+$/CD8$^+$ [22]. The tumor cells are positive for CD25, in most cases for CCR4 and, in a subset of cases, for the T regulatory (T*reg*)

*Skin Lymphoma: The Illustrated Guide*, Sixth Edition. Lorenzo Cerroni.

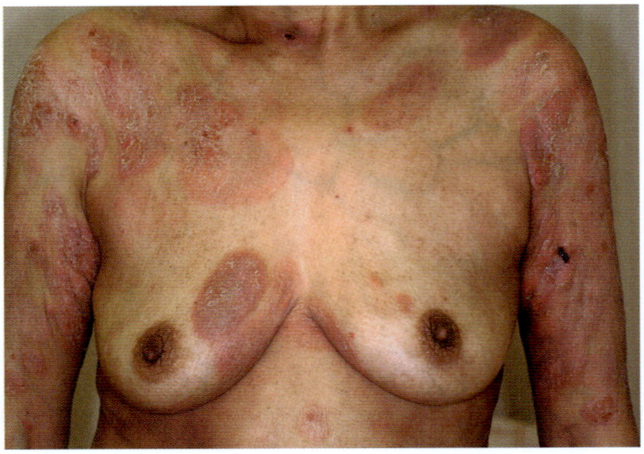

**Figure 13.1** Adult T-cell leukemia/lymphoma. Disseminated patches, plaques, and flat tumors. The clinical picture is indistinguishable from that of mycosis fungoides. (*Courtesy of Dr Tatsushi Shiomi, Okayama, Japan.*)

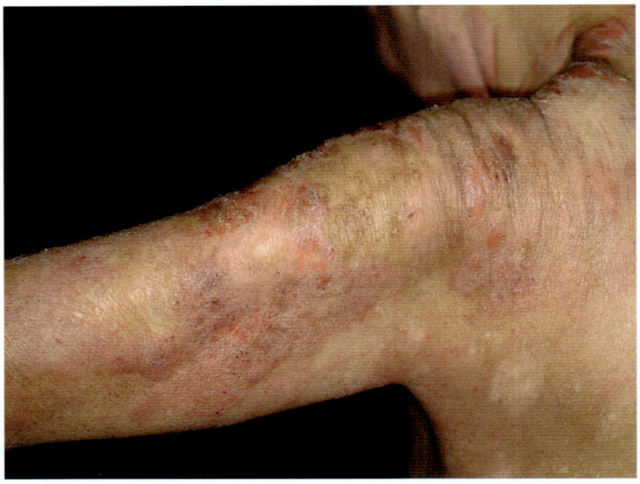

**Figure 13.2** Adult T-cell leukemia/lymphoma. Detail of erosive, infiltrated patches and plaques identical to those seen in mycosis fungoides. (*Courtesy of Dr Tatsushi Shiomi, Okayama, Japan.*)

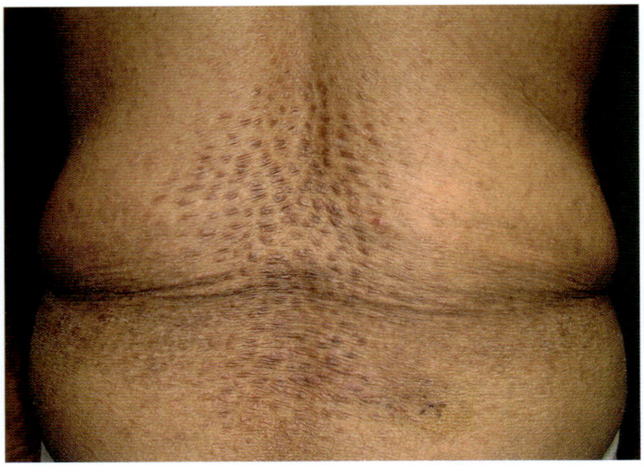

**Figure 13.3** Adult T-cell leukemia/lymphoma. Multiple, partly atrophic papules and small plaques on the back with a "cobblestone" appearance. (*Courtesy of Prof. Hiroshi Shimizu, Sapporo, Japan.*)

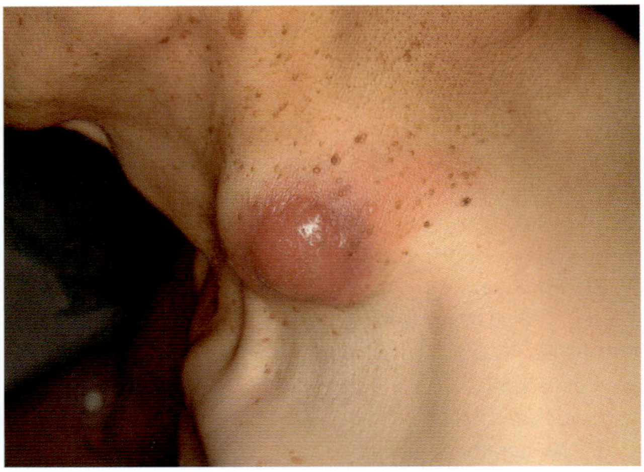

**Figure 13.4** Adult T-cell leukemia/lymphoma. Large tumor on the neck. (*Courtesy of Prof. Hiroshi Shimizu, Sapporo, Japan.*)

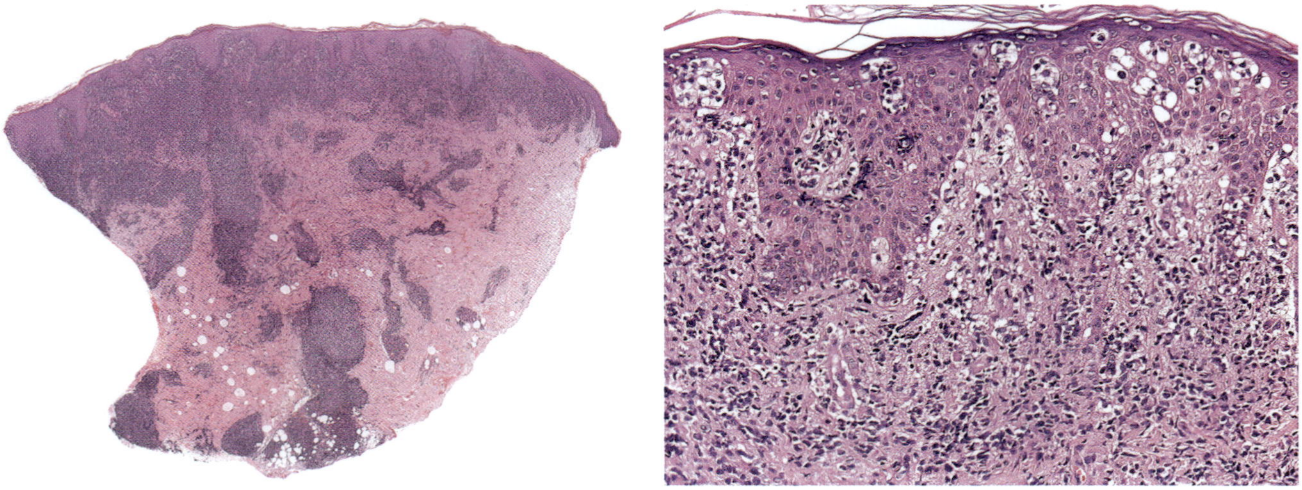

(a) (b)

**Figure 13.5** Adult T-cell leukemia/lymphoma. (a) Dense lymphoid infiltrate in the entire dermis. (b) Epidermotropism with the formation of Darier nests. (*Courtesy of Dr. Tatsushi Shiomi, Okayama, Japan.*)

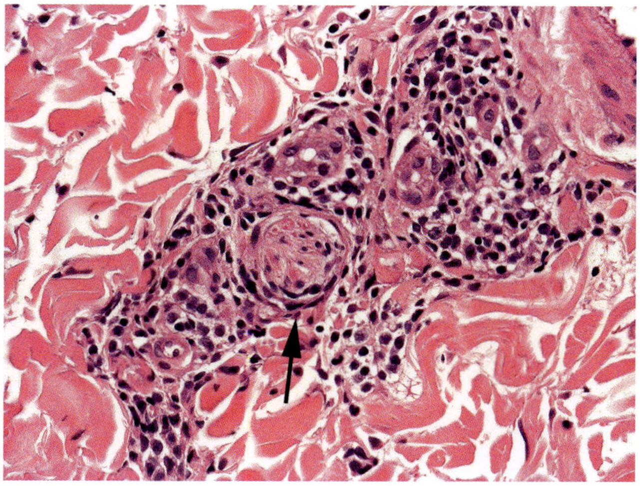

**Figure 13.6** Adult T-cell leukemia/lymphoma. Perineural infiltrates with focal neurotropism. (*Courtesy of Dr. Tatsushi Shiomi, Okayama, Japan.*)

molecule forkhead box protein P3 (FOX-P3) [23–25]; the T*reg* phenotype in these cases, however, is usually restricted to a proportion of tumor cells. Although the FOX-P3 expression by neoplastic cells is observed only in a minority of cases of mycosis fungoides [26], positivity or negativity for this marker cannot be considered as reliable differential diagnostic clues. Programmed cell death 1 (PD-1) is strongly expressed by neoplastic cells [27], as well as the intestinal homing receptor CD103 [28].

In a large study, most cases were negative for both TCR-ß and TCR-δ, and cases with anaplastic morphology were positive for CD30 and CD15 and negative for CD3 and FOX-P3 [29]. In the same study, some cases expressed T follicular helper markers, whereas cytotoxic proteins were positive only in a minimal proportion of cases.

## Molecular genetics

Molecular analyses show a monoclonal rearrangement of the T-cell receptor (TCR) genes, as well as the presence of the clonally integrated genome of HTLV-1 [30]. In this context, it should be underlined that, prompted by the clinicopathologic similarities to ATLL, several investigators have looked for the presence of HTLV-1 DNA in cases of mycosis fungoides and Sézary syndrome. There is no convincing evidence of the involvement of HTLV-1 in these diseases, thus demonstration of monoclonal integration of HTLV-1 DNA in neoplastic cells may be used as a reliable means to distinguish ATLL from mycosis fungoides and Sézary syndrome, and represents an essential diagnostic criterion for ATLL.

However, ATLL is characterized by marked genomic instability with frequent mutations in several genes including, among others, *IRF4*, *PLCG1*, *PRKCB*, *VAV1*, *FYN*, *TP53*, *CARD11*, and *STAT3*. Cases of ATLL with indolent behavior showed more common *STAT3* mutations, whereas cases with aggressive behavior were associated with an increased burden of genetic and epigenetic alterations, higher frequencies of *TP53* and *IRF4* mutations, and many copy number alterations including PD-L1 amplifications and *CDKN2A* deletions [31].

A recent report described the identification of the oncogenes *AK4* and *RHOC* as target genes of the tumor-suppressive microRNA miR-455-3p in ATLL, resulting in the activation of oncogenic pathways such as Myc targets and the deregulation of lipid metabolism, including an increased production of sphingomyelin, a tumor-promoting lipid [32]. ATLL is sensitive to sphingomyelin inhibition and *AK4* or *RHOC* depletion, suggesting that these may represent potential therapeutic targets.

## Treatment

The treatment of choice for ATLL is usually systemic chemotherapy, eventually followed by allogeneic stem cell transplantation. Cases with an indolent behavior and restricted to the skin may be managed with less aggressive therapeutic options such as psoralen and ultraviolet A (UV-A) (PUVA) or combination schemes [8, 9, 33, 34]. However, it has been emphasized that even the smoldering type of ATLL is not truly indolent, and a watchful waiting strategy may not be adequate [35]. Interferon alfa is a main option for smoldering cases, eventually associated to the antiviral drug zidovudine [35]. The Japanese Skin Cancer Society–Lymphoma Study Group has issued recommendations for treatment of cases with disease limited to the skin [36]. Besides PUVA, other useful options include radiation therapy, retinoids, interferon, and single-agent chemotherapy [36].

## Prognosis

The prognosis of ATLL is generally poor, but indolent variants have been described. The smoldering type seems to have a better prognosis [37]. The type of skin eruption may be an independent prognostic factor, as patients presenting with patches and plaques have a better prognosis than those showing erythroderma, multipapular, nodulotumoral, or purpuric lesions [38]. Among patients with cutaneous manifestations of the disease, median overall survival was significantly shorter in the acute and lymphoma types compared to the smoldering and chronic types [39].

**Résumé**

Adult T-cell lymphoma/leukemia

| | | |
|---|---|---|
| **Clinical** | Adults, rarely younger patients. Four variants recognized: acute, chronic, lymphomatous, and smoldering types. Primary cutaneous involvement may be seen. Clinically, there are patches, plaques, and tumors morphologically similar to those observed in mycosis fungoides. | |
| **Morphology** | Histopathologic features similar to those observed in mycosis fungoides. | |
| **Immunohistochemistry** | CD3, CD4 | + |
| | CD7, CD8 | − |
| | CD25, CCR4 | + |
| | CD103 | + |
| | FOX-P3 | +/− |
| | PD-1 | + |
| | TCR-ß, TCR-δ | − |
| **Genetics** | Monoclonal integration of HTLV-1 DNA. Monoclonal rearrangement of the TCR genes. Marked genomic instability. | |
| **Treatment guidelines** | Systemic chemotherapy, allogeneic stem cell transplantation. Interferon alfa, eventually associated to zidovudine in indolent cases. PUVA and retinoids may be used for cases restricted to the skin. | |


## References

1. Ohshima K, Gaulard P, Horwitz M, Nakamura S. Adult T-cell leukemia/lymphoma. In: Arber DA, Borowitz MJ, Cook JR, *et al.*, eds. *The International Consensus Classification of Myeloid and Lymphoid neoplasms*. Philadelphia (US): Wolters Kluver, 2025: 604–612.
2. Karube K, Miyoshi H, Cook LB, *et al.* Adult T-cell leukaemia/lymphoma. In: *WHO Classification of Tumours Editorial Board. Haematolymphoid Tumours*. 5th edition. Lyon (France): IARC, 2024: 667–673.
3. Amano M, Kurokawa M, Ogata K, *et al.* New entity, definition and diagnostic criteria of cutaneous adult T-cell leukemia/lymphoma: human T-lymphotropic virus type 1 proviral DNA load can distinguish between cutaneous and smoldering types. *J Dermatol* 2008;**35**:270–275.
4. Tsukasaki K, Imaizumi Y, Tokura Y, *et al.* Meeting report on the possible proposal of an extranodal primary cutaneous variant in the lymphoma type of adult T-cell leukemia-lymphoma. *J Dermatol* 2014;**41**:26–28.
5. Willemze R, Cerroni L, Kempf W, *et al.* The 2018 update of the WHO-EORTC classification for primary cutaneous lymphomas. *Blood* 2019;**133**:1703–1714.
6. Iwanaga M, Watanabe T, Yamaguchi K. Adult T-cell leukemia: a review of epidemiological evidence. *Front Microbiol* 2012;**3**:322.
7. Lucas CT, Gillis KJ, Ness JM, *et al.* Adult T-cell leukemia/lymphoma in an adolescent presenting with skin lesions. *Ped Dermatol* 2008;**25**:373–377.
8. DiCaudo DJ, Perniciaro C, Worrell JT, *et al.* Clinical and histologic spectrum of human T-cell lymphotropic virus type I-associated lymphoma involving the skin. *J Am Acad Dermatol* 1996;**34**:69–76.
9. Nagatani T, Miyazawa M, Matsuzaki T, *et al.* Adult T-cell leukemia–lymphoma (ATLL): clinical, histopathological, immunological and immunohistochemical characteristics. *Exp Dermatol* 1992;**1** :248–252.
10. Shimoyama M. Diagnostic criteria and classification of clinical subtypes of adult T-cell leukaemia–lymphoma: a report from the Lymphoma Study Group (1984–87). *Br J Haematol* 1991;**79**:428–437.
11. Glowacka I, Korn K, Potthoff SA, *et al.* Delayed seroconversion and rapid onset of lymphoproliferative disease after transmission of HTLV-1 from a multi organ donor. *Clin Infect Dis* 2013;**57**:1417–1424.
12. Richey JD, Chen BJ, Deng AC. Indolent, waxing and waning cutaneous presentation of HTLV-1-associated adult T-cell leukemia/lymphoma in an HIV-1-positive patient. *J Cutan Pathol* 2018;**45**:171–175.
13. Yamaguchi T, Ohshima K, Karube K, *et al.* Clinicopathological features of cutaneous lesions of adult T-cell leukaemia/lymphoma. *Br J Dermatol* 2005;**152**:76–81.
14. Pezeshkpoor F, Yazdanpanah MJ, Shirdel A. Specific cutaneous manifestations in adult T-cell leukemia/lymphoma. *Int J Dermatol* 2008;**47**:359–362.
15. Shimizu S, Yasui C, Koizumi K, *et al.* Cutaneous-type adult T-cell leukemia/lymphoma presenting as a solitary large skin nodule: a review of the literature. *J Am Acad Dermatol* 2007;**57**:s115–s117.
16. Kawabata H, Setoyama M, Fukushige T, Kanzaki T. Spontaneous regression of cutaneous lesions in adult T-cell leukaemia–lymphoma. *Br J Dermatol* 2001;**144**:434–435.
17. Miyashiro D, Sanches JA. Cutaneous manifestations of adult T-cell leukemia/lymphoma. *Semin Diagn Pathol* 2020;**37**:81–91.
18. Camp B, Horwitz S, Pulitzer MP. Adult T-cell leukemia/lymphoma with follicular mucinosis: an unusual histopathological finding and a commentary. *J Cutan Pathol* 2012;**39**:861–865.
19. Khanlari M, Ramos JC, Sanchez SP, *et al.* Adult T-cell leukemia/lymphoma can be indistinguishable from other more common T-cell lymphomas. The University of Miami experience with a large cohort of cases. *Mod Pathol* 2018;**31**:1046–1063.
20. Manabe T, Hirokawa M, Sugihara K, Kohda M. Angiocentric and angiodestructive infiltration of adult T-cell leukemia–lymphoma (ATLL) in the skin: report of two cases. *Am J Dermatopathol* 1988;**10**:487–496.
21. Michael EJ, Shaffer JJ, Collins HE, Grossman ME. Bullous adult T-cell lymphoma–leukemia and human T-cell lymphotropic virus-1 associated myelopathy in a 60-year-old man. *J Am Acad Dermatol* 2002;**46**:S137–S141.

22. Kamath P, Abrahams J, Cho-Vega JH. Bullous CD4+ CD8+ adult T-cell leukemia/lymphoma, a rare diagnostically challenging cutaneous variant. *J Cutan Pathol* 2018;**45**:964–965.
23. Kohno T, Yamada Y, Akamatsu N, *et al.* Possible origin of adult T-cell leukemia/lymphoma cells from human T lymphotropic virus type-1-infected regulatory T cells. *Cancer Sci* 2005;**96**: 527–533.
24. Karube K, Aoki R, Sugita Y, *et al.* The relationship of FOXP3 expression and clinicopathological characteristics in adult T-cell leukemia/lymphoma. *Mod Pathol* 2008;**21**:617–625.
25. Abe M, Uchihashi K, Kazuto T, *et al.* Foxp3 expression on normal and leukemic CD4+CD25+ T cells implicated in human T-cell leukemia virus type-1 is inconsistent with Treg cells. *Eur J Haematol* 2008;**81**:209–217.
26. Fried I, Cerroni L. FOXP3 in sequential biopsies of progressive mycosis fungoides. *Am J Dermatopathol* 2012;**34**:263–265.
27. Tokura Y, Sawada Y, Shimauchi T. Skin manifestations of adult T-cell leukemia/lymphoma: Clinical, cytological and immunological features. *J Dermatol* 2014;**41**:19–25.
28. Ishibashi H, Nimura S, Ishitsuka K, *et al.* High expression of intestinal homing receptor CD103 in adult T-cell leukemia/lymphoma, similar to 2 other CD8+ T-cell lymphomas. *Am J Surg Pathol* 2016;**40**:462–470.
29. Tamaki T, Karube K, Sakihama S, *et al.* A comprehensive study of the immunophenotype and its clinicopathologic significance in adult T-cell leukemia/lymphoma. *Mod Pathol* 2023;**36**:100169.
30. Kato N, Sugawara H, Aoyagi S, Mayuzumi M. Lymphoma-type adult T-cell leukemia–lymphoma with a bulky cutaneous tumour showing multiple human T-lymphotropic virus-1 DNA integration. *Br J Dermatol* 2001;**144**:1244–1248.
31. Kataoka K, Iwanaga M, Yasunaga JI, *et al.* Prognostic relevance of integrated genetic profiling in adult T-cell leukemia/lymphoma. *Blood* 2018;**131**:215–225.
32. Liu B, Yasunaga JI, Liang Y, *et al.* Identification of *AK4* and *RHOC* as potential oncogenes addicted by adult T cell leukemia. *Proc Natl Acad Sci USA* 2025;**122**:e2416412122.
33. Chan EF, Dowdy YG, Lee B, *et al.* A novel chemotherapeutic regimen (interferon-α, zidovudine, and etretinate) for adult T-cell lymphoma resulting in rapid tumor destruction. *J Am Acad Dermatol* 1999;**40**:116–121.
34. Takemori N, Hirai K, Onodera R, *et al.* Satisfactory remission achieved by PUVA therapy in a case of crisis-type adult T-cell leukemia–lymphoma with generalized cutaneous leukaemic cell infiltration. *Br J Dermatol* 1995;**133**:955–960.
35. Stuver R, Horwitz SM, Epstein-Peterson ZD. Treatment of adult T-cell leukemia/lymphoma: established paradigms and emerging directions. *Curr Treat Options in Oncol* 2023;**24**:948–964.
36. Sugaya M, Hamada T, Kawai K, *et al.* Guidelines for the management of cutaneous lymphomas (2011): a consensus statement by the Japanese Skin Cancer Society–Lymphoma Study Group. *J Dermatol* 2013;**40**:2–14.
37. Ishitsuka K, Ikeda S, Utsonomiya A, *et al.* Smouldering adult T-cell leukaemia/lymphoma: a follow-up study in Kyushu. *Br J Haematol* 2008;**143**:442–444.
38. Sawada Y, Hino R, Hama K, *et al.* Type of skin eruption is an independent prognostic indicator for adult T-cell leukemia/lymphoma. *Blood* 2011;**117**:3961–3967.
39. Hurabielle C, Battistella M, Ram-Wolff C, *et al.* Cutaneous presentation of adult T-cell leukemia/lymphoma (ATLL). Single-center study on 37 patients in metropolitan France between 1996 and 2016. *Ann Dermatol Venereol* 2018;**145**:405–412.

CHAPTER 14

# Specific cutaneous manifestations of nodal T-follicular helper cell lymphoma, angioimmunoblastic type, and of other nodal T-follicular helper cell lymphomas

A peculiar group of nodal lymphomas expressing the phenotype of T follicular helper (TFH) lymphocytes has been described, with nodal TFH cell lymphoma, angioimmunoblastic type (formerly angioimmunoblastic T-cell lymphoma) being the best characterized entity in this group. In the International Consensus Classification (ICC) *of Myeloid and Lymphoid Neoplasms* and in the new World Health Organization (WHO) *Classification of Haematolymphoid Tumours*, nodal TFH cell lymphoma, angioimmunoblastic type has been included in a group of nodal TFH cell lymphoma including also nodal TFH cell lymphoma, follicular type, and nodal TFH cell lymphoma, NOS [1, 2]. It is still unclear whether these three conditions represent distinct entities or, as it appears more likely, variants of a single lymphoma type with TFH phenotype. In this context, a TFH phenotype is defined as positivity of neoplastic cells for two TFH markers (including CD10, CXCL13, BCL6, ICOS, PD-1, and CXCR5) *and* for CD4. None of the TFH markers is specific for TFH lymphocytes; CXCL13 is more specific, whereas ICOS and PD-1 are more sensitive. Besides cases of nodal TFH cell lymphoma, angioimmunoblastic type arising secondary in the skin, and cases of primary cutaneous T-cell lymphoproliferative disorders with a similar TFH phenotype are well characterized. In particular, several cases of cutaneous $CD4^+$ small–medium T-cell lymphoproliferative disorder show a TFH phenotype (see Chapter 11). A more detailed discussion on cutaneous entities with TFH phenotype other than cutaneous manifestations of nodal TFH cell lymphoma, angioimmunoblastic type is presented in Chapter 11. It must be underlined that cases of primary cutaneous or primary nodal T-cell lymphoma, NOS, may show positivity for PD-1 and ICOS, but not for other markers of TFH cells. In the skin, however, differentiation of specific manifestations of nodal T-follicular helper cell lymphoma, angioimmunoblastic type from other lymphomas with a similar phenotype may be very difficult. In this context, a diagnosis of specific manifestations of nodal TFH cell lymphoma, angioimmunoblastic type can be accepted only in cases with confirmed nodal disease. Data on skin involvement by nodal TFH cell lymphomas are mainly available for the angioimmunoblastic type; thus, in this chapter, I will concentrate on this condition only.

Nodal TFH cell lymphoma, angioimmunoblastic type, formerly called angioimmunoblastic T-cell lymphoma or angioimmunoblastic lymphadenopathy, is a peripheral T-cell lymphoma of TFH lymphocytes with a peculiar proliferation of high endothelial venules [2]. Nonspecific skin manifestations have been described in several patients, including maculopapular eruptions, purpura, and erythroderma. Specific skin involvement is uncommon but it may be observed [3a, 3b], and a diagnosis of cutaneous angioimmunoblastic T-cell lymphoma should be made only in cases with extracutaneous disease (known or found at first staging). Development of a second, Epstein–Barr virus (EBV)-associated B-cell lymphoma may occur in nodal cases. In the skin, a clonal plasma cell proliferation coinciding with disease progression has been reported [4]. Coexistence of angioimmunoblastic T-cell lymphoma and chromic myelomonocytic leukemia may be observed, as both may harbor *TET2* mutations and may arise from clonal hematopoiesis of indeterminate potential.

## Clinical features

Patients are elderly adults, though cutaneous involvement in children has been reported [5]. Skin lesions may be the first manifestation of the disease, but primary cutaneous involvement does not occur [6, 7]. Thus, evidence of nodal disease is necessary for the diagnosis. Specific cutaneous involvement in nodal TFH cell lymphoma, angioimmunoblastic type is characterized by nondescript erythematous papules, plaques, and tumors (Figs. 14.1 and 14.2). In some instances, due to the small number of infiltrating cells, the clinical picture may resemble that of an inflammatory condition (Fig. 14.3).

## Histopathology

Histology shows nodular or rarely diffuse dermal infiltrates consisting of small-, medium-, or large-sized pleomorphic lymphocytes intermingled with reactive cells (plasma cells, eosinophils, and histiocytes) (Fig. 14.4). Same cases present

*Skin Lymphoma: The Illustrated Guide*, Sixth Edition. Lorenzo Cerroni.

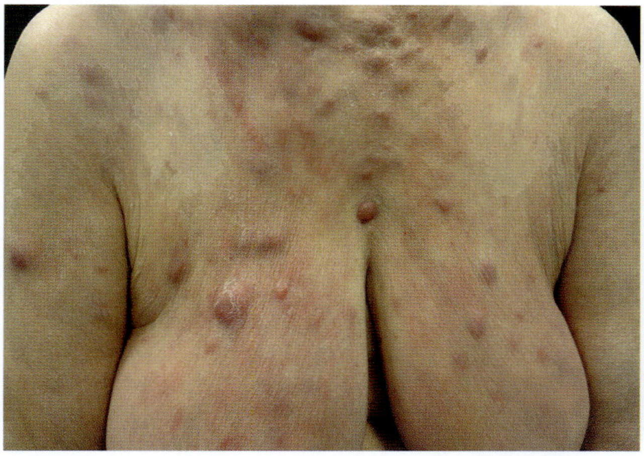

Figure 14.1 Cutaneous infiltrate of nodal T-follicular helper cell lymphoma, angioimmunoblastic type. Generalized patches, papules, plaques, and tumors. The clinical features are not distinctive and resemble other cutaneous lymphomas. (*Courtesy of Prof. Luis Requena, Madrid, Spain*).

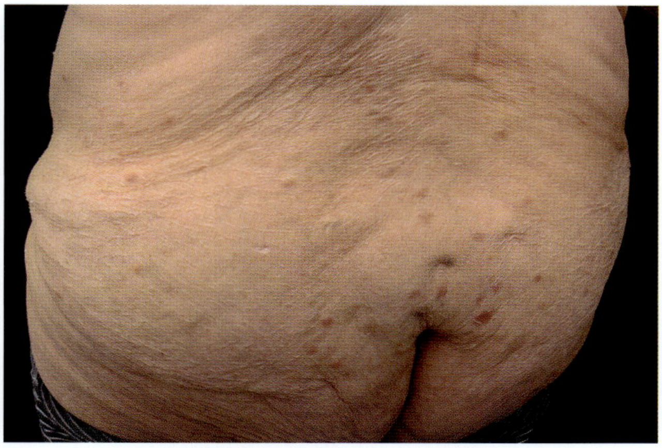

Figure 14.2 Cutaneous infiltrate of nodal T-follicular helper cell lymphoma, angioimmunoblastic type. Localized papules and small tumors on the lower back and buttocks.

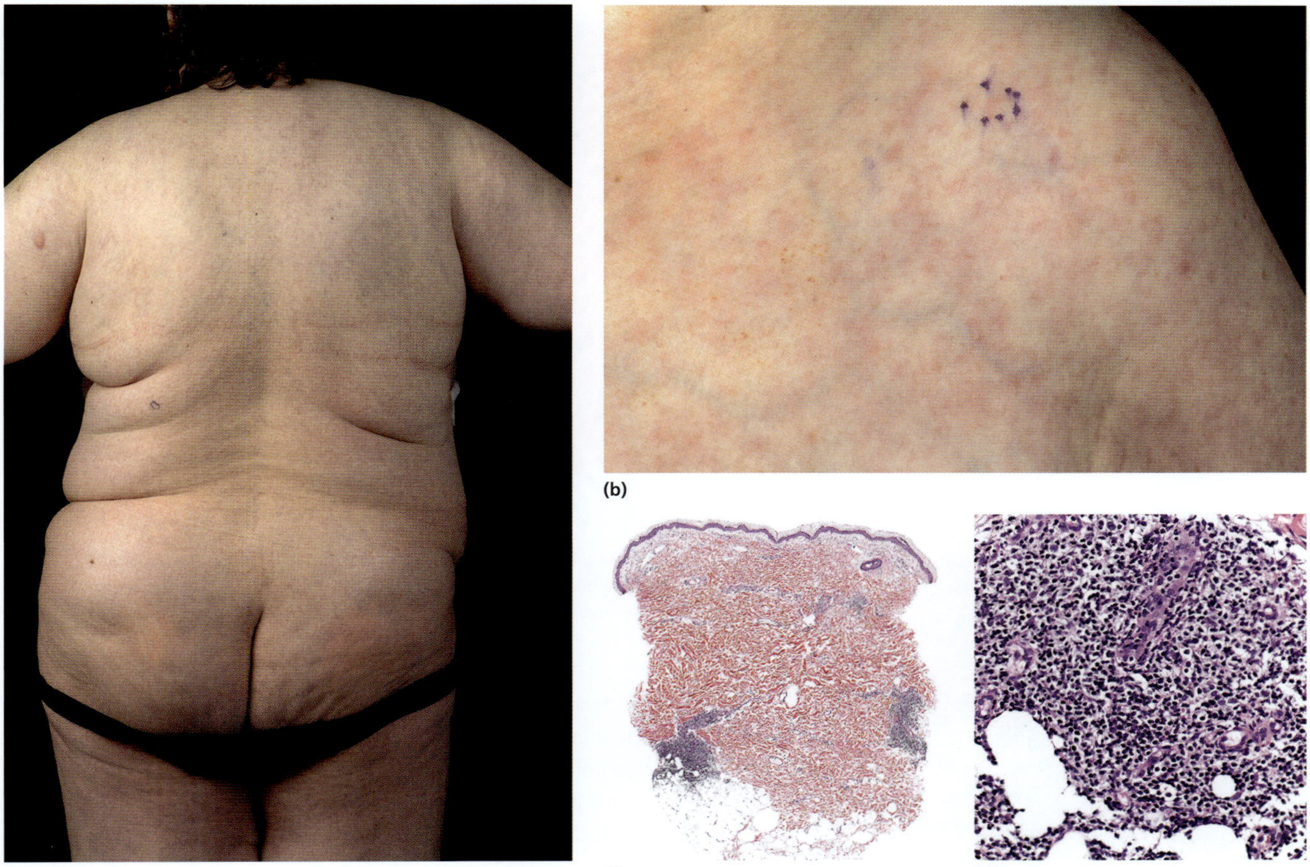

(a) (b) (c) (d)

Figure 14.3 Cutaneous infiltrate of nodal T-follicular helper cell lymphoma, angioimmunoblastic type. (a) Generalized skin "rash" mimicking an inflammatory condition; (b) detail of the skin lesions (the marked area corresponds to the biopsy site); (c, d) histology shows deep lymphoid infiltrates.

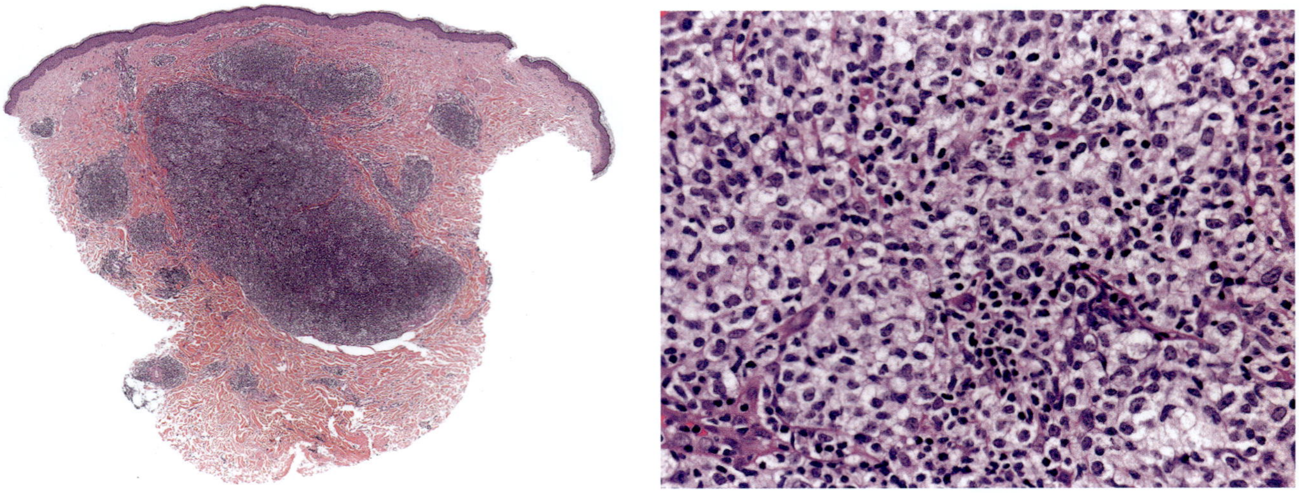

(a) (b)

**Figure 14.4** Cutaneous infiltrate of nodal T-follicular helper cell lymphoma, angioimmunoblastic type. (a) Dense dermal infiltrate with a biphasic pattern: the dark areas consist of small reactive lymphocytes, whereas the paler areas are composed of mid-sized and large neoplastic cells. (b) Detail of mid-sized and large pleomorphic cells admixed with small lymphocytes.

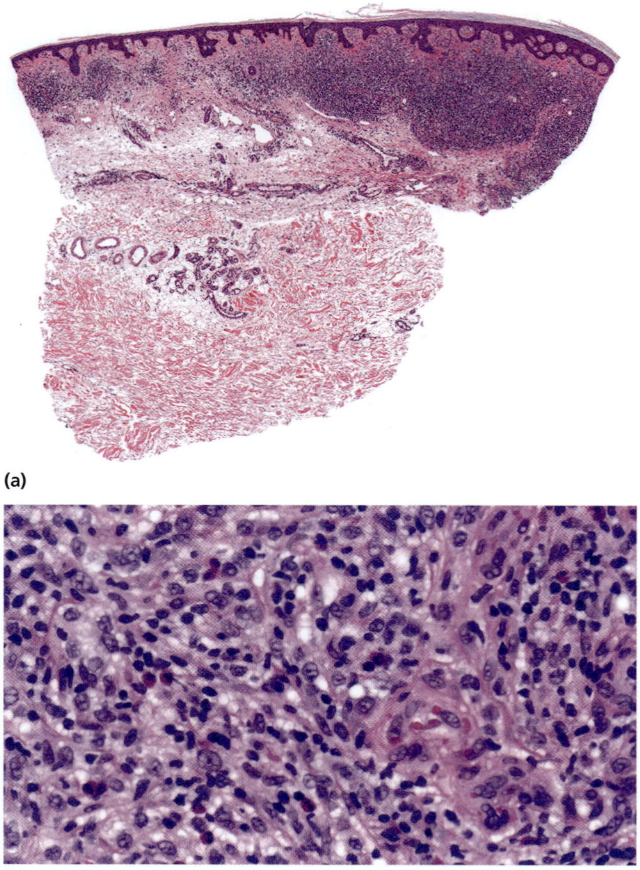

(a)

(b)

**Figure 14.5** Cutaneous infiltrate of nodal T-follicular helper cell lymphoma, angioimmunoblastic type. (a) Dense band-like infiltrate with only isolated intraepidermal cells. (b) Detail of mid-sized and large pleomorphic cells admixed with small lymphocytes and eosinophils.

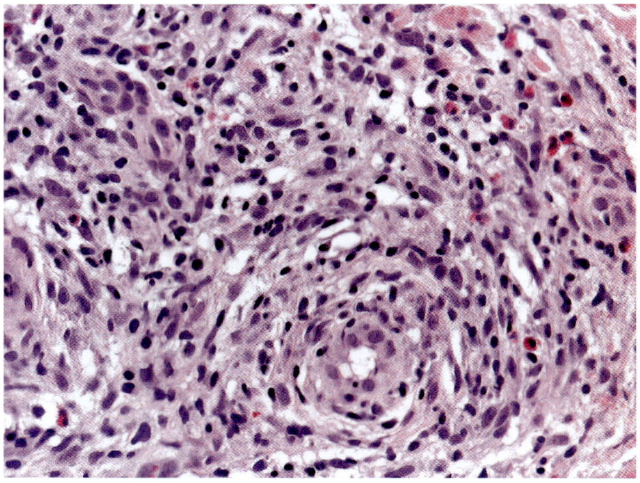

**Figure 14.6** Cutaneous infiltrate of nodal T-follicular helper cell lymphoma, angioimmunoblastic type. Pleomorphic cells admixed with several eosinophils. Note high endothelial venules.

with superficial, band-like infiltrates (Fig. 14.5). The number of neoplastic lymphocytes is often a minority; thus, the histopathologic features may be misinterpreted as those of a reactive infiltrate [8]. Increased numbers of venules with a prominent endothelial lining are typically found ("high endothelial venules") (Fig. 14.6) [9, 10]. A histopathologic presentation resembling an infectious process has also been reported [11], and some cases may mimic cutaneous B-cell lymphomas or cutaneous Hodgkin lymphoma [12]. Epidermotropism and folliculotropism may rarely be observed.

In some cases, cutaneous biopsies show only sparse perivascular and periadnexal infiltrates with mild atypia (Fig. 14.7), but the presence of monoclonal populations of T lymphocytes in the majority of these cases suggests that these lesions also represent specific manifestations of the disease (corresponding clinically to the "inflammatory dermatitis"-like presentation). In fact, the cases I have observed revealed the typical phenotype of nodal TFH cell lymphoma, angioimmunoblastic type (Fig. 14.7c to f).

Although in some cases, small, reactive lymphoid follicles may be observed, the three patterns described in nodal disease (pattern 1 mimicking reactive follicular hyperplasia, pattern 2 with a prominent perifollicular neoplastic T-cell infiltrate around lymphoid follicles partly effacing the normal nodal architecture, and pattern 3 characterized by complete effacement of the nodal architecture with no residual lymphoid follicles) are not applicable to skin manifestations of the disease.

## Immunophenotype

Neoplastic cells reveal a phenotype corresponding to TFH cells ($CD3^+$, $CD4^+$, $CD8^-$, $CD10^+$, Bcl-$6^+$, PD-$1^+$, $CXCL13^+$, and $ICOS^+$) (Figs. 14.7c to f and 14.8a to d). CXCL13 is a chemokine which is expressed by helper T lymphocytes involved in the normal maturation process of germinal center B lymphocytes within the lymph nodes. Several studies have shown that $CXCL13^+$ T lymphocytes can be identified in most cutaneous cases of nodal TFH cell lymphoma, angioimmunoblastic type, whereas the expression of CD10 can be found in a minority of cases only [13–19]. In this context, it must be underlined that evaluation of CD10 in skin biopsies is very difficult because of strong background and positivity of dermal dendritic cells, and evaluation of a Bcl-6 staining is usually more informative (Fig. 14.8d). Clusters of polyclonal B lymphocytes are commonly present. Irregular aggregates of $CD21^+$ follicular dendritic cells can be observed, especially around the high endothelial venules (Fig. 14.8e). EBV can be demonstrated by in situ hybridization within the B lymphocytes (Fig. 14.8f) [20], but the neoplastic T-cells are constantly negative. However, in my experience, EBV-encoded small RNAs ($EBER^+$) cells are lacking in many cases of specific cutaneous infiltrates, and negative cases have been reported by other authors as well [3a, 21]. In a study on 22 skin samples of cutaneous manifestations of angioimmunoblastic T-cell lymphoma, $EBER^+$ cells were found in of 45.5% of cases [22]. An increased number of $TdT^+$ cells has been observed in lymph nodes of patients with angioimmunoblastic T-cell lymphoma [23].

## Molecular genetics

Molecular genetics shows a monoclonal rearrangement of T-cell receptor (TCR) genes and usually a polyclonal pattern of immunoglobulin (Ig) genes (a monoclonal rearrangement of the Ig genes can be found in 20–30% of nodal cases, related to the expansion of the $EBV^+$ B-cell population). Next-generation sequencing of nodal TFH cell lymphoma, angioimmunoblastic type showed the presence of genetic mutations strongly associated with this type of lymphoma (*IDH2*), and of other mutations found also in other T-cell lymphomas with TFH phenotype (*TET2*, *DNMT3A*, and *RHOA*) [24–28]. Similar genetic alterations have been observed also in cutaneous manifestations of the disease [29].

Trisomy 3 and 5 and an additional X chromosome are frequent genetic aberrations in nodal cases. Gains of 22q, 19, and 11q13 and losses of 13q have been shown in some cases by comparative genomic hybridization. In a case with cutaneous involvement, DNA microarrays in the affected lymph nodes revealed the expression of an apoptosis-inhibitory protein and of secondary lymphoid tissue chemokines, including tumor necrosis factor-β [30].

## Treatment

Cutaneous involvement is always secondary to nodal disease; thus, patients should be managed in a hematological setting. The treatment may be difficult to administer due to frequent, potentially lethal infections. There are only limited data on treatment and prognosis of patients with specific skin involvement of nodal TFH cell lymphoma, angioimmunoblastic type. Systemic treatment options include chemotherapy with cyclophosphamide, adriamycin, vincristine, and prednisone (CHOP), often associated to immunomodulators including rituximab and bortezomib among others [31]. Romidepsin combined with oral azacytidine induced complete remission in three patients with relapsing/refractory nodal TFH cell lymphoma, angioimmunoblastic type [32]. A recent study revealed that *CCR7*, *MAP3K14*, *CD69*, *TGFB1*, *EOMES*, *CD63*, *CARD11*, and *CD34* were strongly overexpressed in patients not responding to standard treatment, whereas *SIGLEC5*, *EFH1*, *CPA3*, *NCAM1*, *MUC1*, and *ANGP1* were highly overexpressed in the group responding to treatment [33]. Stratification of data in this study suggested that patients not responding to standard CHOP therapy may benefit from treatment with an anti-PD1/CD3 antibody, or with a combination of pembrolizumab + romidepsin or brentuximab vedotin, or with a bispecific anti-CD30/CD16A antibody.

## Prognosis

The prognosis is generally poor. Onset of a second diffuse large B-cell lymphoma (usually, but not always, related to EBV) is a bad prognostic sign. Commencing therapy at an early stage of the disease may give better results in terms of survival. Skin involvement did not affect survival in one study [21].

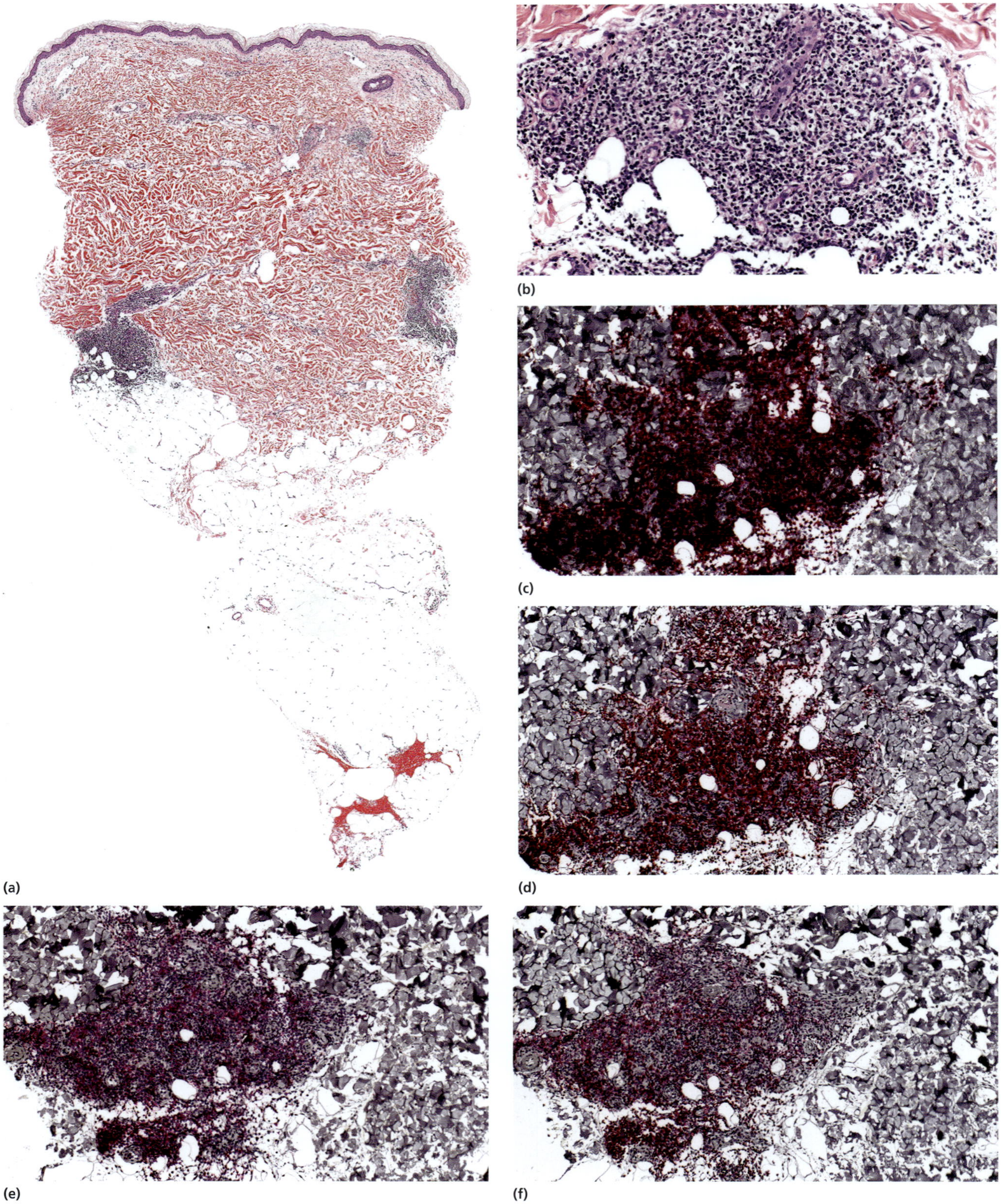

**Figure 14.7** Cutaneous infiltrate of nodal T-follicular helper cell lymphoma, angioimmunoblastic type. (a) Sparse, perivascular, and periadnexal dermal infiltrates reaching the superficial part of the subcutaneous fat. (b) Predominance of small and medium-sized cells. (c) Many lymphocytes are positive for CD3, and (d) other for CD20; stainings for (e) ICOS and (f) PD-1 highlights neoplastic T lymphocytes with a TFH phenotype.

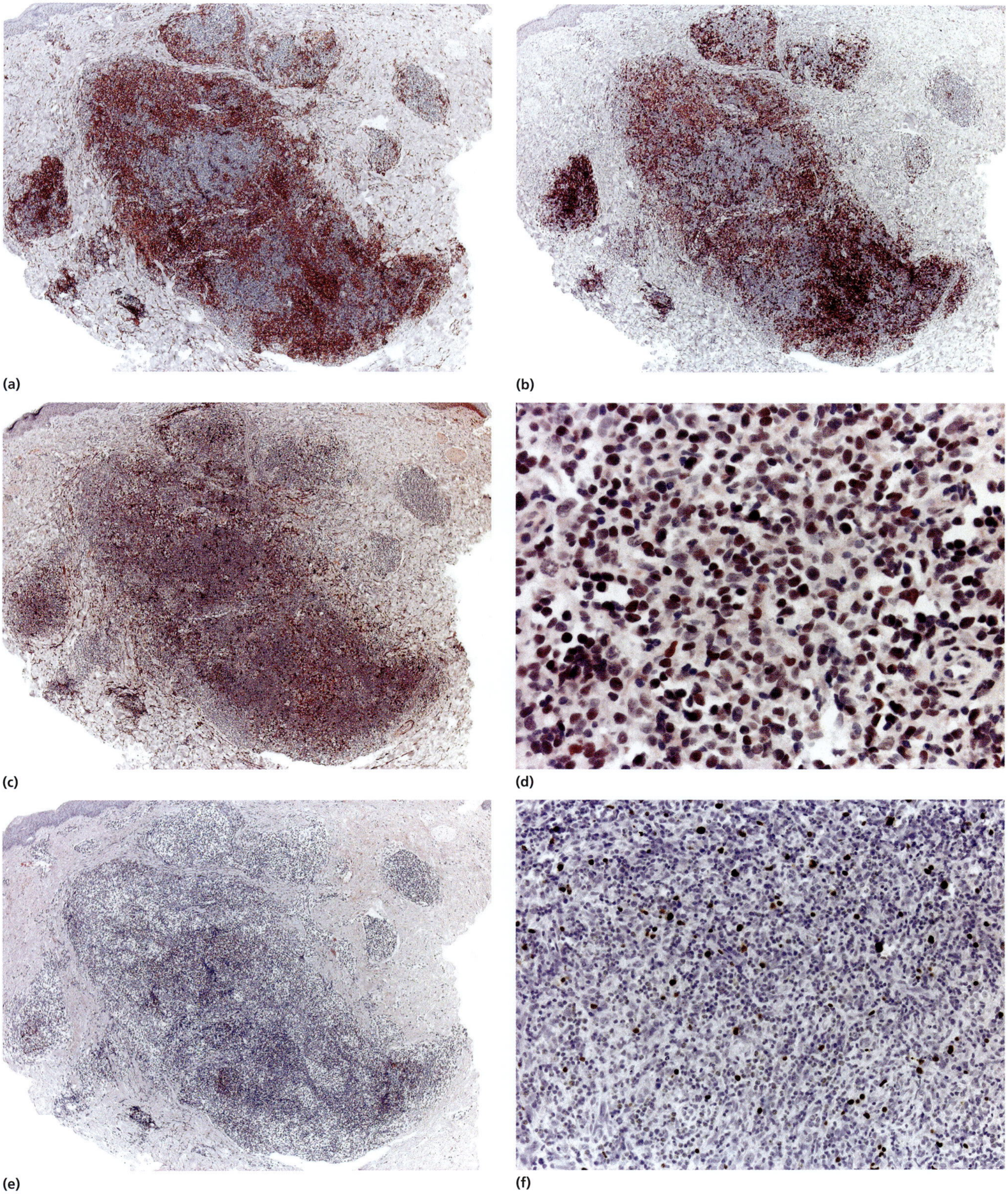

**Figure 14.8** Cutaneous infiltrate of nodal T-follicular helper cell lymphoma, angioimmunoblastic type. Positivity of most neoplastic cells for (a) CD4, (b) PD-1, (c) CXCL-13, and (d) Bcl-6. (e) Note faint, irregular clusters of CD21$^{+}$ cells. (f) Scattered B lymphocytes are positive for EBV (EBER-1).

## Résumé

**Specific cutaneous manifestations of nodal T-follicular helper cell lymphoma, angioimmunoblastic type**

| | | |
|---|---|---|
| **Clinical** | Elderly adults. Cutaneous lesions may be rarely the first manifestation of the disease, but primary cutaneous cases do not occur. | |
| **Morphology** | Small-, medium-, or large-sized pleomorphic lymphocytes intermingled with plasma cells, eosinophils, and histiocytes. High-endothelial venules. | |
| **Immunohistochemistry** | CD3, CD4, CD5 | + |
| | CXCL13, PD-1, ICOS, Bcl-6 | + |
| | CD10 | – (+) |
| | CD8 | – |
| | CD20 | + (–) (non-neoplastic B lymphocytes) |
| | EBER1 | – (+) (non-neoplastic B lymphocytes) |
| | CD21 | + (non-neoplastic follicular dendritic cells in clusters) |
| **Genetics** | Monoclonal rearrangement of the TCR genes (concomitant monoclonal rearrangement of the Ig genes in 20–30% of cases). Genetic mutations in *IDH2*, *TET2*, *DNMT3A*, and *RHOA*. | |
| **Treatment guidelines** | Management in a hematological setting. Chemotherapy with CHOP associated to other substances (risk of potentially lethal infections). | |

## References


1. Dogan A, Gaulard P, Lemonnier F, *et al*. Follicular helper T-cell lymphoma. In: Arber DA, Borowitz MJ, Cook JR, *et al*., eds. *The International Consensus Classification of Myeloid and Lymphoid Neoplasms*. Philadelphia (US): Wolters Kluver, 2025: 720–732.
2. Attygalle AD, Sekata-Yamagimoto M, Amador C, *et al*. Nodal T follicular helper cell lymphoma, angioimmunoblastic type. In: *WHO Classification of Tumours Editorial Board. Haematolymphoid Tumours*. 5th edition. Lyon (France): IARC, 2024: 744–751.
3. (a) Botros N, Cerroni L, Shawwa A, *et al*. Cutaneous manifestations of angioimmunoblastic T-cell lymphoma: clinical and pathological characteristics. *Am J Dermatopathol* 2015;**37**:274–283.(b) Díaz de la Pinta FJ, Cuevas MA, Manso R, *et al*. Clinical, pathologic, and molecular spectrum of angioinmmunoblastic T-cell lymphoma cutaneous lesions. clinical, pathologic, and molecular analysis. *Am J Surg Pathol* 2025;**49**:403–410.
4. Suárez AE, Artiga MJ, Santonja C, *et al*. Angioimmunoblastic T-cell lymphoma with a clonal plasma cell proliferation that underwent immunoglobulin isotype switch in the skin, coinciding with cutaneous disease progression. *J Cutan Pathol* 2016;**43**: 1203–1210.
5. Schotte U, Megahed M, Jansen T, *et al*. Angio-immunoblastische Lymphadenopathie mit kutanen Manifestationen bei einem 13 jährigen Mädchen. *Hautarzt* 1992;**43**:728–734.
6. Suarez-Vilela D, Izquierdo-Garcia FM. Angio-immunoblastic lymphadenopathy-like T-cell lymphoma: cutaneous clinical onset with prominent granulomatous reaction. *Am J Surg Pathol* 2003;**27**: 699–700.
7. Jacobson RK, Lee KC, Muglia JJ, *et al*. Cutaneous manifestations of angioimmunoblastic T-cell lymphoma. *J Am Acad Dermatol* 2013;**69**:e25–e26.
8. Oishi N, Sartori-Valinotti JC, Bennani NN, *et al*. Cutaneous lesions of angioimmunoblastic T-cell lymphoma: clinical, pathological, and immunophenotypic features. *J Cutan Pathol* 2019;**46**:637–644.
9. Martel P, Laroche L, Courville P, *et al*. Cutaneous involvement in patients with angio-immunoblastic lymphadenopathy with dysproteinemia. *Arch Dermatol* 2000;**136**:881–886.
10. Schmuth M, Ramaker J, Trautmann C, *et al*. Cutaneous involvement in prelymphomatous angio-immunoblastic lymphadenopathy. *J Am Acad Dermatol* 1997;**36**:290–295.
11. Jayaraman AG, Cassarino D, Advani R, *et al*. Cutaneous involvement by angio-immunoblastic T-cell lymphoma: a unique histologic presentation, mimicking an infectious etiology. *J Cutan Pathol* 2006;**33**(suppl. 2):6–11.
12. Szablewski V, Dereure O, René C, *et al*. Cutaneous localization of angioimmunoblastic T-cell lymphoma may masquerade as B-cell lymphoma or classical Hodgkin lymphoma: a histologic diagnostic pitfall. *J Cutan Pathol* 2019;**46**:102–110.
13. Attygalle A, Al-Jehani R, Diss TC, *et al*. Neoplastic T cells in angio-immunoblastic T-cell lymphoma express CD10. *Blood* 2002;**99**:627–633.
14. Grogg KL, Attygalle AD, Macon WR, *et al*. Angio-immunoblastic T-cell lymphoma: a neoplasm of germinal-center T-helper cells? *Blood* 2005;**106**:1501–1502.
15. Ortonne N, Dupuis J, Plonquet A, *et al*. Characterization of CXCL13+ neoplastic T cells in cutaneous lesions of angio-immunoblastic T-cell lymphoma (AITL). *Am J Surg Pathol* 2007;**31**:1068–1076.
16. de Leval L, Rickman DS, Thielen C, *et al*. The gene expression profile of nodal peripheral T-cell lymphoma demonstrates a molecular link between angioimmunoblastic T-cell lymphoma (AITL) and follicular helper T ($T_{FH}$) cells. *Blood* 2007;**109**:4952–4963.
17. Grogg KL, Attygale AD, Macon WR, *et al*. Expression of CXCL13, a chemokine highly upregulated in germinal center T-helper cells, distinguishes angioimmunoblastic T-cell lymphoma from peripheral T-cell lymphoma, unspecified. *Mod Pathol* 2006;**19**: 1101–1107.
18. Yu H, Shahsafaei A, Dorfman DM. Germinal-center T-helper-cell markers PD-1 and CXCL13 are both expressed by neoplastic cells

in angioimmunoblastic T-cell lymphoma. *Am J Clin Pathol* 2009;**131**:33–41.

19. Balaraman B, Conley JA, Sheinbein DM. Evaluation of cutaneous angioimmunoblastic T-cell lymphoma. *J Am Acad Dermatol* 2011;**65**:855–862.
20. Brown HA, Macon WR, Kurtin PJ, Gibson LE. Cutaneous involvement by angio-immunoblastic T-cell lymphoma with remarkable heterogeneous Epstein–Barr virus expression. *J Cutan Pathol* 2001;**28**: 432–438.
21. Lee WJ, Won KH, Choi JW, *et al.* Cutaneous angioimmunoblastic T-cell lymphoma: Epstein–Barr virus positivity and its effects on clinicopathologic features. *J Am Acad Dermatol* 2019;**81**:989–997.
22. Díaz de la Pinta FJ, Cuevas MAPG, Manso R, *et al.* Clinical, pathologic, and molecular spectrum of angioinmmunoblastic T-cell lymphoma cutaneous lesions: clinical, pathologic, and molecular analysis. *Am J Surg Pathol* 2025;**49**:403–410.
23. Ohgami RS, Zhao S, Ohgami JK, *et al.* TdT$^+$ T-lymphoblastic populations are increased in Castleman disease, in Castleman disease in association with follicular dendritic cell tumors, and in angioimmunoblastic T-cell lymphoma. *Am J Surg Pathol* 2012;**36**:1619–1628.
24. Odejide O, Weigert O, Lane AA, *et al.* A targeted mutational landscape of angioimmunoblastic T-cell lymphoma. *Blood* 2014;**123**:1293–1296.
25. Sakata-Yanagimoto M, Enami T, Yoshida K, *et al.* Somatic RHOA mutation in angioimmunoblastic T cell lymphoma. *Nature Gen* 2014;**46**:171–175.
26. Vallois D, Dobay MPD, Morin RD, *et al.* Activating mutations in genes related to TCR signaling in angioimmunoblastic and other follicular helper T-cell–derived lymphomas. *Blood* 2016;**128**: 1490–1502.
27. Palomero T, Couronné L, Khiabanian H, *et al.* Recurrent mutations in epigenetic regulators, RHOA and FYN kinase in peripheral T cell lymphomas. *Nat Genet* 2014;**46**:166–170.
28. Pileri SA. Follicular helper T-cell–related lymphomas. *Blood* 2015;**126**:1733–1734.
29. Leclaire Alirkilicarslan AL, Dupuy A, Pujals A, *et al.* Expression of TFH markers and detection of RHOA p.G17V and IDH2 p.R172K/S mutations in cutaneous localizations of angioimmunoblastic T-cell lymphomas. *Am J Surg Pathol* 2017;**41**:1581–1592.
30. Murakami T, Ohtsuki M, Nakagawa H. Angio-immunoblastic lymphadenopathy-type peripheral T-cell lymphoma with cutaneous infiltration: report of a case and its gene expression profile. *Br J Dermatol* 2001;**144**:878–884.
31. Zhang Q, Yin L, Lai Q, *et al.* Advances in the pathogenesis and therapeutic strategies of angioimmunoblastic T-cell lymphoma. *Clin Exp Med* 2023;**23**:4219–4235.
32. O'Connor OA, Falchi L, Lue JK, *et al.* Oral 5-azacytidine and romidepsin exhibit marked activity in patients with PTCL: a multicenter phase 1 study. *Blood* 2019;**134**:1395–1405.
33. Díaz-Alejo JF, Morillo-Giles D, Díaz de la Pinta FJ, *et al.* New therapies for angioimmunoblastic T-cell lymphoma: a comprehensive review and analysis. *Leuk Lymphoma* 2024;**65**:2056–2059.

CHAPTER 15

# Cutaneous manifestations in Epstein–Barr virus-positive T-cell and NK-cell lymphoid proliferations and lymphomas of childhood

Epstein–Barr virus (EBV)-related lymphoproliferative diseases in children and adolescents represent a peculiar group of disorders ranging from indolent to aggressive disease. Some of these entities are confined to or arise primarily in the skin. In the International Consensus Classification (ICC) *of Myeloid and Lymphoid Neoplasms* and in the new World Health Organization (WHO) *Classification of Haematolymphoid Tumours*, EBV$^+$ T-cell and NK-cell lymphoid proliferations and lymphomas of childhood are included as a distinct group of mature NK/T-cell neoplasms [1, 2]. The two entities within this group that are relevant for the skin and will be discussed in this chapter are severe mosquito bite allergy and hydroa vacciniforme lymphoproliferative disorder.

## Severe mosquito bite allergy

Severe mosquito bite allergy is characterized by high fever and severe local skin symptoms including bullae, ulcers, necrosis, and scarring following mosquito bites [3]. As for other EBV-positive T/NK-cell lymphoproliferative diseases of childhood, severe mosquito bite allergy is observed almost exclusively in specific countries (East Asia – Japan, Taiwan, China, and South Korea, and some American countries, particularly Mexico, but also other Central American and South American countries). The disease is included as a distinct entity in the ICC classification *of Myeloid and Lymphoid Neoplasms* and in the WHO *Classification of Haematolymphoid Tumors* [1, 4].

In the context of reactions to mosquito bites, "severe mosquito bite allergy" should not be mixed up with so-called Skeeter syndrome, an intense local reaction to mosquito bites that can also be accompanied by systemic symptoms such as fever and vomiting, but that is not associated to EBV. In addition, "exaggerated insect bite-like reactions" can be observed in different hematological malignancies and bear no relationship to the severe mosquito bite allergy discussed in this paragraph (see also Chapter 29). In short, the term "severe mosquito bite allergy" to define a potentially lethal hematological condition seems a bit unfortunate, as it may be misunderstood or used in the wrong context (a less confusing terminology may be "EBV-associated severe mosquito bite allergy").

### Clinical features

Severe mosquito bite allergy is characterized by an overreaction to insect bites (particularly, but not only, mosquitos) with hemorrhagic blisters, ulceration, and necrosis followed by scarring at the site of the bite, and with systemic symptoms such as fever, lymphadenopathy, and elevation of liver enzymes. Large granular lymphocytes are found in the peripheral blood, and there are high levels of IgE due to a strong T helper 2 shift in the immune response. Symptoms in severe mosquito bite allergy are transient, in contrast to systemic chronic active EBV disease.

Some patients with severe mosquito bite allergy may progress to overt hematological malignancies (particularly NK/T-cell lymphoma or aggressive NK-cell leukemia), and up to 50% die due to severe hemophagocytic syndrome or to the associated lymphoma/leukemia [5, 6].

### Histopathology

Histology of cutaneous lesions shows features similar to those of hydroa vacciniforme (intraepidermal vesiculation and bullae resulting in necrosis, and moderately dense, perivascular, and periadnexal dermal infiltrates of lymphocytes). Eosinophils are usually abundant, but differentiation from systemic hydroa vacciniforme lymphoproliferative disorder cannot be done upon this finding alone. The infiltrate is not as dense as that observed in systemic hydroa vacciniforme lymphoproliferative disorder, but it may reveal atypical cells and often shows angiocentricity.

### Immunophenotype

Immunohistology shows an NK-cell phenotype with positivity for CD3ε (surface CD3 is negative in true NK-cell cases) and CD56, expression of cytotoxic proteins (TIA-1, granzyme B, perforin), common positivity for CD30, and positive in situ-hybridization for EBV (EBER-1) in large, activated

*Skin Lymphoma: The Illustrated Guide*, Sixth Edition. Lorenzo Cerroni.

lymphocytes (LMP-1 is usually negative on tissue sections). CD56 may be rarely negative [7]. Rare cases may present with a T-cell phenotype.

### Molecular genetics

Somatic mutations in EBV-positive cells, including particularly mutations in the *DDX3X* gene, cause clonal evolution in multiple cell lineages [8].

### Treatment

In the absence of hemophagocytic syndrome or signs of progression to leukemia/lymphoma, the mosquito bites are treated symptomatically.

### Prognosis

Although the course is prolonged with remissions and relapses, as already mentioned patients with severe mosquito bite allergy are at high risk of developing a severe hemophagocytic syndrome or a concomitant lymphoma/leukemia [9], and approximately 50% die of causes related to these diseases [6]. The onset of the disease at age >9 and expression in the skin lesions of an EBV-encoded immediate-early gene transcript (BZLF1 mRNA) were associated with a worse prognosis in one study [5]. Severe mosquito bite allergy also seems to be a risk factor for disease progression in patients with hydroa vacciniforme lymphoproliferative disorder [10].

**Résumé**

| | | |
|---|---|---|
| **Severe mosquito bite allergy** | | |
| **Clinical** | Children from East Asia or Mexico. High fever and intense local skin symptoms including bullae, ulcers, necrosis, and scarring following mosquito bites. | |
| **Morphology** | Variably dense lymphoid infiltrates with atypical lymphocytes. Frequent angiocentricity. | |
| **Immunohistochemistry** | CD3ε | + (surface CD3 negative) (rare cases have a T-cell phenotype) |
| | CD16, CD56 | + |
| | EBER-1 | + |
| | LMP1 | – |
| | CD30 | +/– |
| **Genetics** | Monoclonal integration of EBV. | |
| **Treatment guidelines** | Symptomatic treatment after insect bite. Associated conditions (hemophagocytic syndrome, leukemia/lymphoma) treated accordingly. | |

## Hydroa-vacciniforme lymphoproliferative disorders

A rare, peculiar NK/T-cell lymphoma affecting mainly children and resembling hydroa vacciniforme clinically has been described in Latin America (particularly Mexico, Guatemala, and Peru) and some Asiatic countries (China, Japan, Korea, Nepal, and Taiwan) [11–22]. A putative case occurring in a white patient has also been reported [23]. In the last edition of the WHO *Classification of Haematolymphoid Tumours* and in the ICC classification *of Myeloid and Lymphoid Neoplasms*, the term hydroa vacciniforme lymphoproliferative disorder has been introduced to encompass cases of conventional hydroa vacciniforme (in the WHO classification referred to as "classic" hydroa vacciniforme lymphoproliferative disorder) as well as aggressive cases of "systemic" hydroa vacciniforme lymphoproliferative disorder [1, 24]. This last term has replaced the former one of "hydroa-like lymphoma." Other terms used in the past for this unusual lymphoproliferative disorder were hydroa vacciniforme-like lymphoma, hydroa vacciniforme-like T-cell lymphoma, atypical hydroa vacciniforme, angiocentric T-cell lymphoma of childhood, and edematous, scarring vasculitic panniculitis.

To my eyes, the relationship of systemic hydroa vacciniforme lymphoproliferative disorder to classic hydroa vacciniforme is unclear, although cases with intermediate features have been described ("borderline" hydroa vacciniforme/hydroa vacciniforme-like lymphoma) [25–28]. EBV is implicated in the etiology and pathogenesis of both the classic and the systemic forms, and the cutaneous clinical presentation shows overlapping features, suggesting that a spectrum of hydroa vacciniforme ranging from classic hydroa vacciniforme to systemic hydroa vacciniforme lymphoproliferative disorder likely exist. However, systemic hydroa vacciniforme lymphoproliferative disorder has never been observed in white patients (and almost never been observed at all) as a progression from classic hydroa vacciniforme, and systemic hydroa vacciniforme lymphoproliferative disorder occurs almost exclusively in specific ethnical backgrounds [29]. In fact, in white patients, the disease usually resolves by early adulthood. In addition, even in Asiatic populations, progression from classic hydroa vacciniforme to systemic hydroa vacciniforme lymphoproliferative disorder seems to be infrequent [5, 30]. In short, it seems that without the proper ethnical background the aggressive, systemic form of the disease does not occur, thus genetic susceptibility probably represents a crucial factor. Differences in the EBV-infected cells have also been detected between the two forms: patients with classic hydroa vacciniforme have an increased number of EBV-infected γδT-cells but no infected αβT-cells, whereas the systemic form can show an αβ or, less frequently, a γδ EBV-infected T-cell population [31].

## Classic hydroa vacciniforme

Classic hydroa vacciniforme (termed classic hydroa vacciniforme lymphoproliferative disorder in the WHO *Classification of Haematolymphoid Tumours* [24]) is a rare cutaneous disorder characterized by photosensitivity with the formation of bullae that heal with scars, located mainly on photoexposed areas [32]. The onset is during childhood and usually resolution happens in adolescence or early adulthood [32]. An association with EBV has been demonstrated. Progression from classic hydroa vacciniforme to systemic hydroa vacciniforme lymphoproliferative disorder has been documented, but almost exclusively in patients from Latin America and Japan [29, 33]. Although it seems likely that classic hydroa vacciniforme and systemic hydroa vacciniforme lymphoproliferative disorder exist in a spectrum, the last condition is restricted almost uniquely to particular ethnical backgrounds, and is observed in specific countries (particularly Mexico, Guatemala, Peru, China, Japan, Korea, Nepal, and Taiwan), in contrast to classic hydroa vacciniforme which is rare but recognized globally, including in the white population in the United States and Europe. In this context, referring to the inclusion of classic hydroa vacciniforme in a WHO scheme designed for lymphomas rather than for inflammatory disorders, Lim and Rosen in 2024 wrote: "However, inclusion of classic hydroa vacciniforme remains controversial" [32].

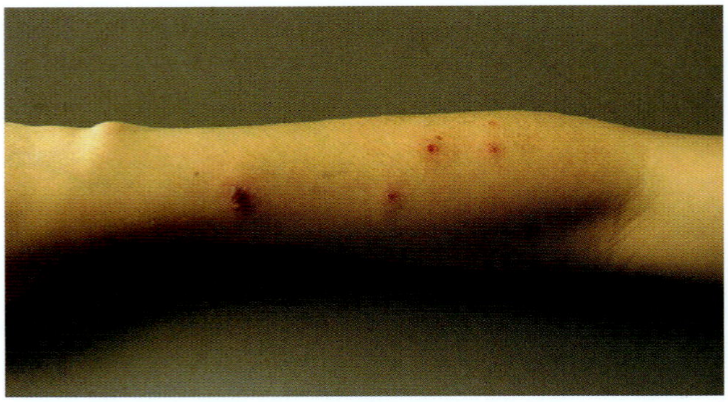

**Figure 15.1** Classic hydroa vacciniforme. Partly crusted lesions on the right arm. (*Courtesy of Prof. Fabio Facchetti, Brescia, Italy.*)

### Clinical features

Clinically, classic hydroa vacciniforme presents in childhood with pruritic or burning erythematous macules on photoexposed skin, especially the face and dorsal aspects of the hands (Fig. 15.1). The lesions arise within a few hours from sun exposure, then vesicles or bullae develop, followed by hemorrhagic crusts and varioliform scars. Similar lesions can be induced at the site of phototesting (Fig. 15.2).

### Histopathology

Histopathology reveals intraepidermal vesiculation resulting in necrosis (Fig. 15.3). In the dermis there are moderately dense, mainly perivascular, and periadnexal infiltrates of lymphocytes. Early lesions show subepidermal edema and dermal inflammatory infiltrates (Fig. 15.4a). Neutrophils and eosinophils may be present (Fig. 15.4b). In some cases, a wedge-shaped pattern with central ulceration may resemble a severe arthropod bite reaction (Fig. 15.5a). The infiltrate is usually not as dense as that observed in systemic hydroa vacciniforme lymphoproliferative disorder, but it may reveal focally atypical cells and some degree of angiocentricity (Fig. 15.5b).

### Immunophenotype

Analysis of data is hindered by the frequent inclusion of cases of severe hydroa vacciniforme (now referred to as systemic hydroa vacciniforme lymphoproliferative disorder) together with those of the classic variant of the disease. There is a predominance of T-lymphocytes (Fig. 15.6), often positive for CD8, and in several cases characterized by a γ/δ T-cell phenotype [9, 31]. Staining for Ki-67 demonstrates a low proliferation rate. In situ hybridization for EBV is positive (Fig. 15.3d).

### Molecular genetics

Analysis of TCR genes rearrangement reveals a polyclonal or monoclonal pattern. EBV is usually monoclonally integrated into the lymphocytes.

### Treatment

There is no effective treatment for hydroa vacciniforme. Photoprotection helps reducing the number and severity of the flares. PUVA has been used with variable results, but its efficacy is questionable. Antimalarials, azathioprine, thalidomide, and cyclosporine have been used in occasional cases.

### Prognosis

The prognosis of classic hydroa vacciniforme is excellent, and most patients experience resolution during adolescence or early adulthood. Cases with a prolonged course and persistence in adulthood have been reported [34].

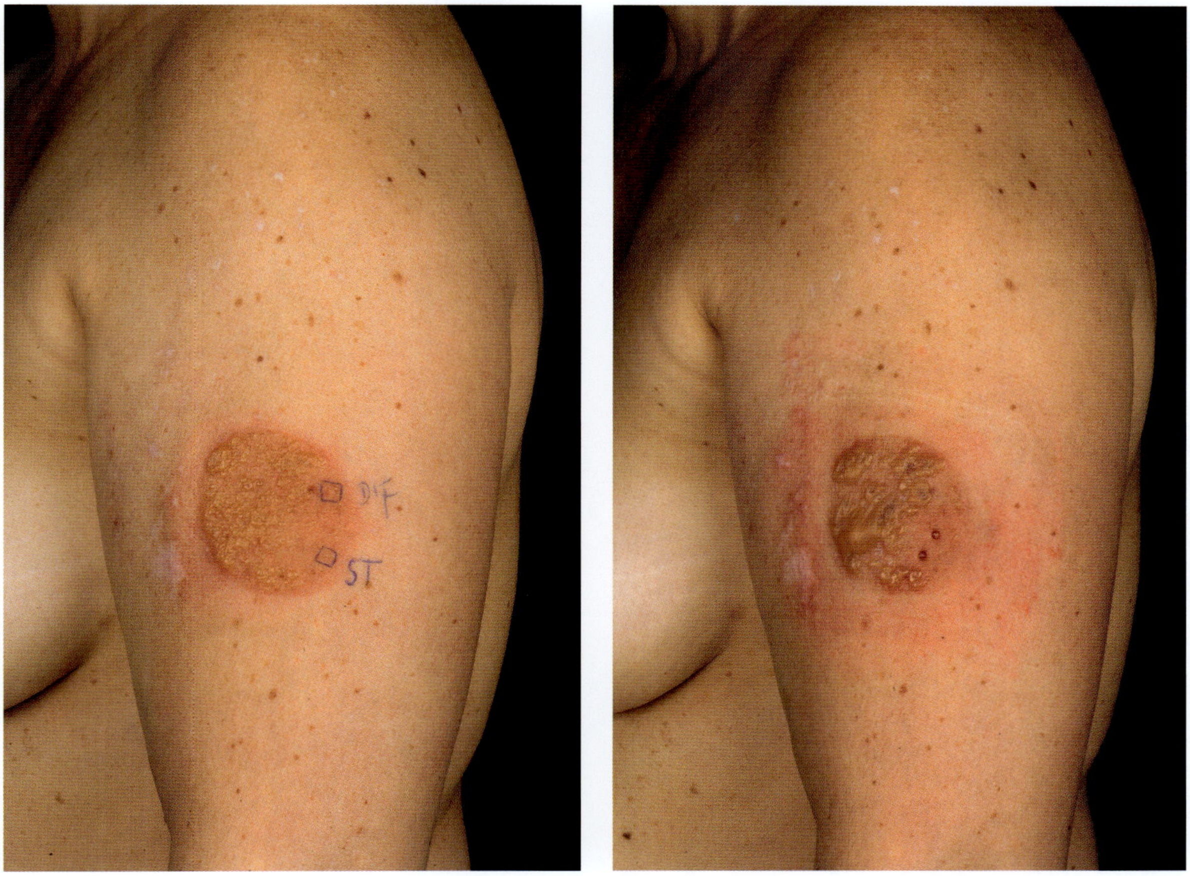


(a) (b)

**Figure 15.2** Classic hydroa vacciniforme. Clinical appearance of a UV-A phototest area in an adult patient. (a) One day after irradiation multiple, partly confluent vesicles are visible. The markings correspond to the sites of punch biopsies for routine histology (ST) and direct immunofluorescence studies (DIF); DIF was negative. (b) One day later confluence of the vesicles in large bullae.

## Résumé

| | | |
|---|---|---|
| **Classic hydroa vacciniforme** | | |
| **Clinical** | Children presenting a few hours after photoexposure with pruritic or burning erythematous macules on photoexposed skin, especially the face and dorsal aspects of the hands, followed by vesiculation, hemorrhagic crusts, and varioliform scars. | |
| **Morphology** | Intraepidermal vesiculation. Moderately dense, mainly perivascular and periadnexal dermal infiltrate of lymphocytes, often admixed with neutrophils and in some cases with eosinophils. | |
| **Immunohistochemistry** | CD3 | + |
| | CD8 | + |
| | EBER-1 | + |
| | TCRγ, TCRδ | + (–) |
| | TCRß | – (+) |
| | LMP1 | – |
| **Genetics** | Polyclonal or monoclonal TCR genes rearrangement pattern. Monoclonal integration of EBV. | |
| **Treatment guidelines** | Refractory to most treatment modalities. Photoprotection paramount in the management of patients. Efficacy of phototherapy questionable. Many cases resolve with early adulthood. | |

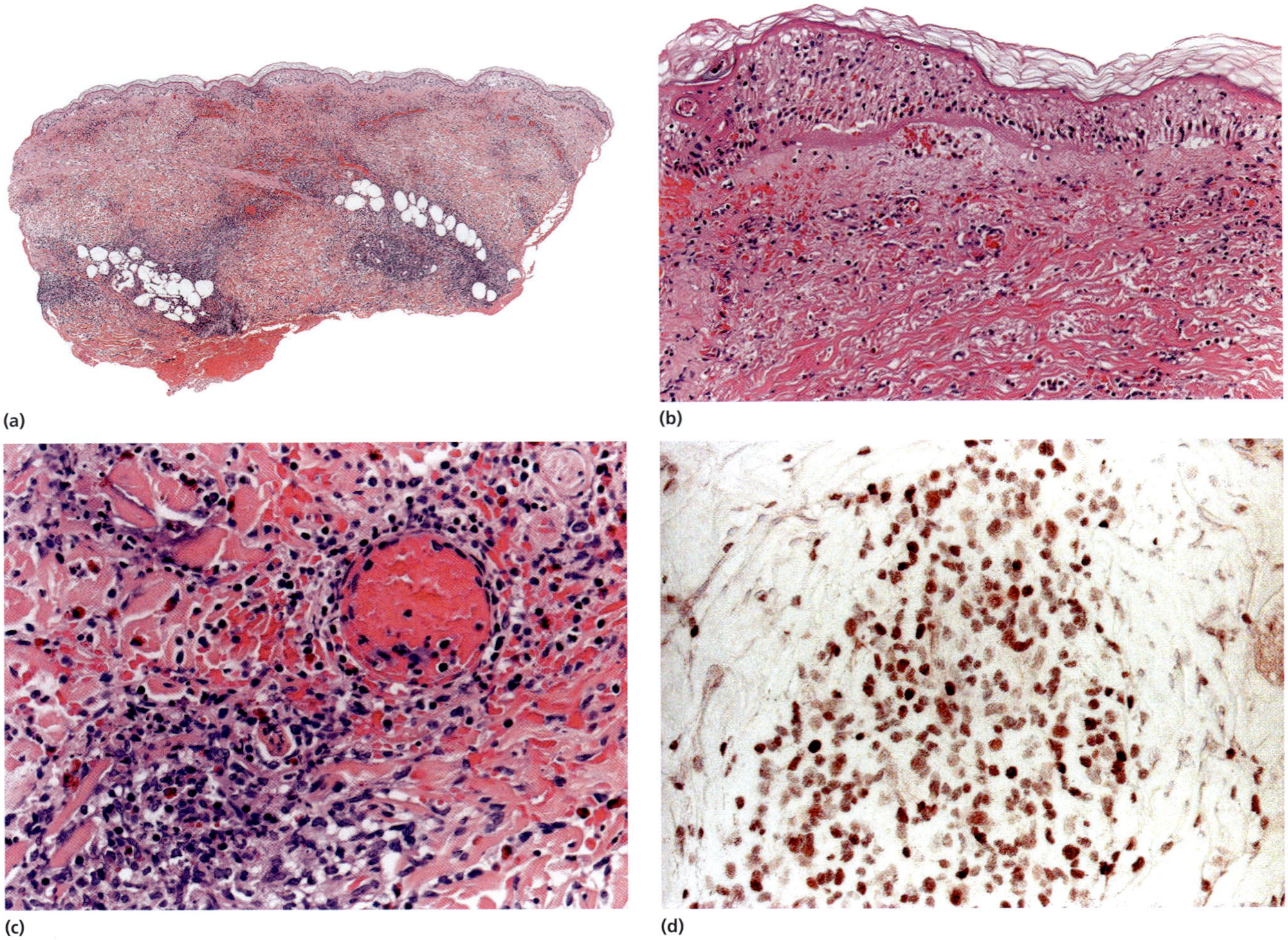

**Figure 15.3** Classic Hydroa vacciniforme. (a, b) Necrosis of the epidermis and of part of the dermis with hemorrhage and lymphoid infiltrates. (c) Detail of the infiltrate with several eosinophils; note a thrombosed vessel. (d) In situ hybridization for EBV (EBER-1) shows a positive signal in several lymphocytes.

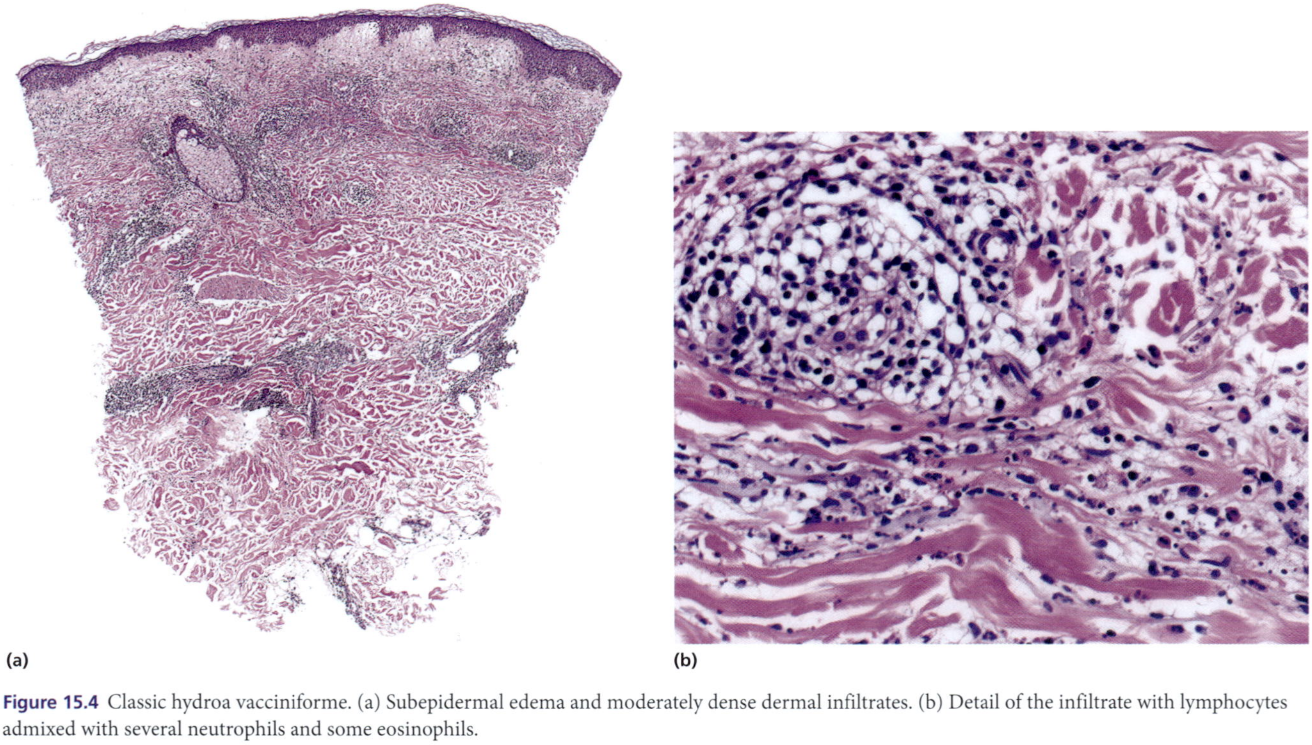

**Figure 15.4** Classic hydroa vacciniforme. (a) Subepidermal edema and moderately dense dermal infiltrates. (b) Detail of the infiltrate with lymphocytes admixed with several neutrophils and some eosinophils.

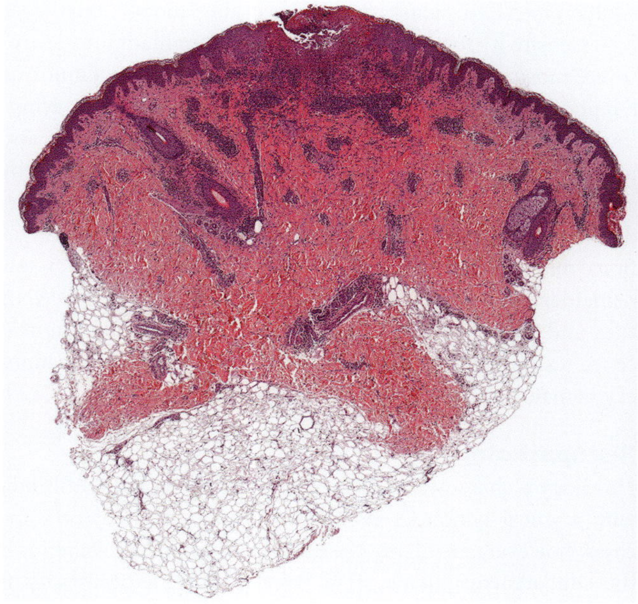

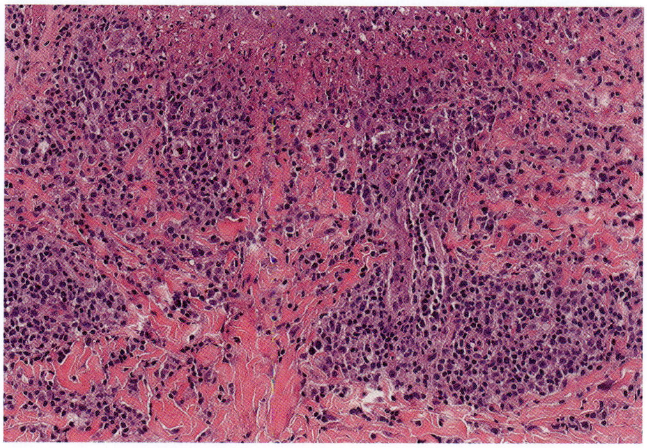

(a) (b)

**Figure 15.5** Classic hydroa vacciniforme. (a) Central ulceration and wedge-shaped dermal infiltrate. (b) Some of the lymphocytes are larger with hyperchromatic nuclei; a few eosinophils are present. Similar features may be misinterpreted as those of severe arthropod bite reactions.

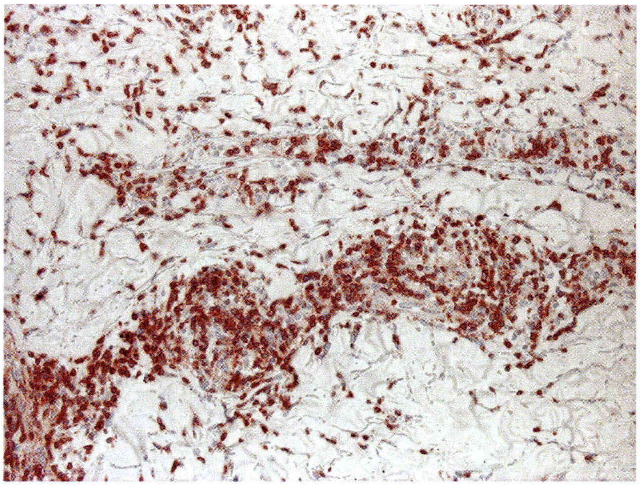

**Figure 15.6** Classic hydroa vacciniforme. Predominance of $CD3^+$ T-lymphocytes.

## Systemic hydroa vacciniforme lymphoproliferative disorder

### Clinical features

Most reported patients with systemic hydroa vacciniforme lymphoproliferative disorder are children, but rarely adults with a similar clinical presentation have been observed. Lesions arise especially on sun-exposed areas, particularly the face and ears, the lower parts of the arms, and the back of the hands, but other lesions are found on sun-covered skin, too. Clinically there are infiltrated plaques, often crusted and/or ulcerated, associated with blisters, edema, and varioliform scars (Fig. 15.7). Large tumors may be observed. Facial swelling is common (Fig. 15.8) [35] (this clinical presentation is similar to what can be observed in extranodal NK/T-cell lymphoma, nasal-type, another EBV-associated lymphoma). Blisters and severe facial swelling seem to be more common in children than in

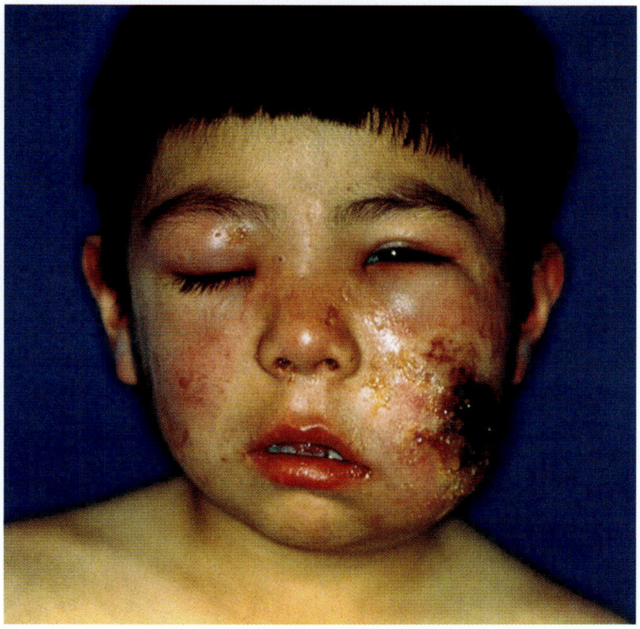

**Figure 15.7** Systemic hydroa vacciniforme lymphoproliferative disorder. Ulcerated, crusted lesions on the face with a large mass on the cheek and prominent swelling. (*Courtesy of Dr. Mario Magana, Mexico City, Mexico.*)

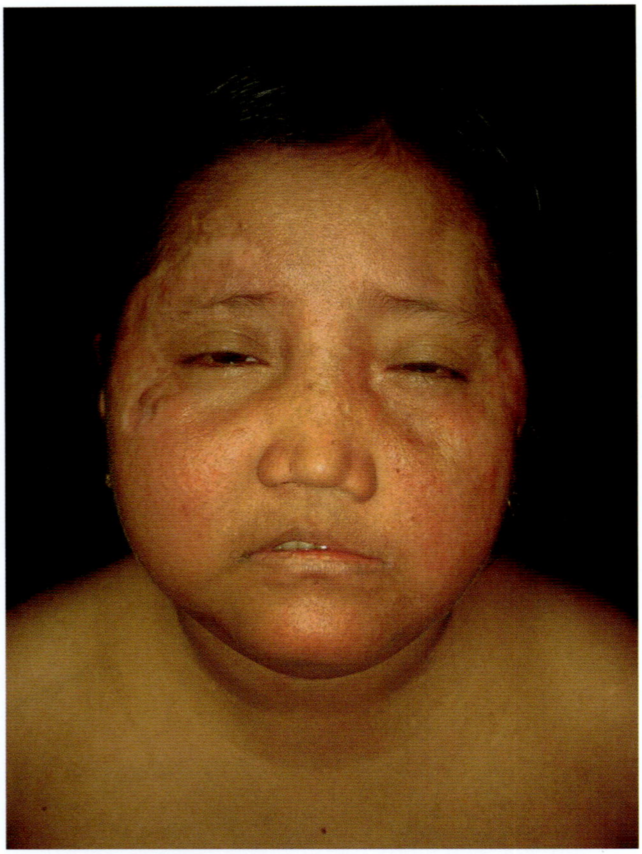

**Figure 15.8** Systemic hydroa vacciniforme lymphoproliferative disorder. Pronounced facial swelling and scarring. (*Courtesy of Dr. Schettini, Manau, Brazil.*)

adults [36]. Photosensitivity is invariably found, as well as hypersensitivity to mosquito bites (the concomitant presence of severe mosquito bite allergy and systemic hydroa vacciniforme lymphoproliferative disorder, however, is rare). Systemic symptoms are present in the vast majority of the patients and include malaise, fever, weight loss, and often lymphadenopathy and hepatosplenomegaly. A hemophagocytic syndrome may develop, particularly in advanced cases. Laboratory investigations may reveal decreased levels of hemoglobin and a low hematocrit level, in addition to other alterations. High ANA titer and granular IgM deposition on direct immunofluorescence testing led to an initial misdiagnosis of cutaneous lupus erythematosus in a case from South Korea [37].

## Histopathology

Histology is characterized by variably dense lymphoid infiltrates with atypical lymphocytes (atypia may be minimal in some cases, however), involving the entire dermis and in some cases the subcutaneous tissues (Fig. 15.9) [38]. Angiocentricity is frequently found (Fig. 15.10), as well as infiltration of adnexal structures. Neurotropism may be present as well (Fig. 15.11). The epidermis shows variable degrees of necrosis, spongiosis, and ulceration. Eosinophils may be found within the infiltrate, rendering differentiation from severe mosquito bite allergy difficult on histopathological grounds alone.

## Immunophenotype

Neoplastic cells are positive for CD2, CD3, and CD5 (Fig. 15.12a). Most cases express CD8 or are $CD4^-/CD8^-$, and are positive for cytotoxic proteins (TIA-1, granzyme B, perforin)

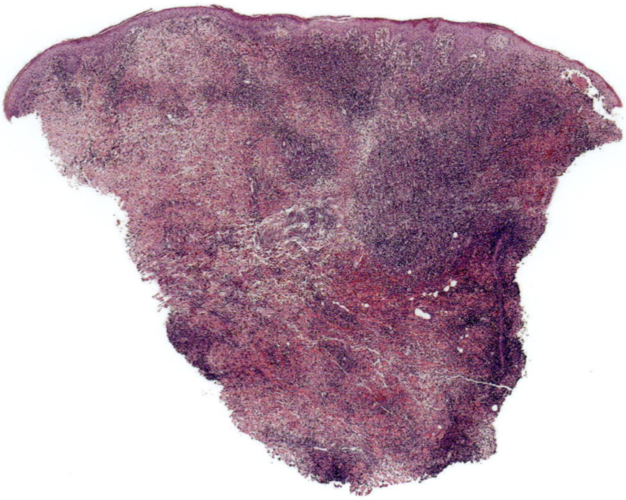

(a)

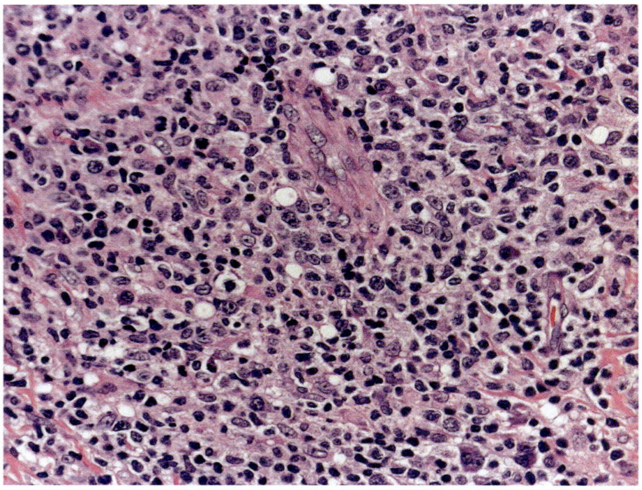

(b)

**Figure 15.9** Systemic hydroa vacciniforme lymphoproliferative disorder. (a) Dense lymphoid infiltrates in the entire dermis. (b) Small and medium-sized pleomorphic lymphocytes admixed with several large cells.

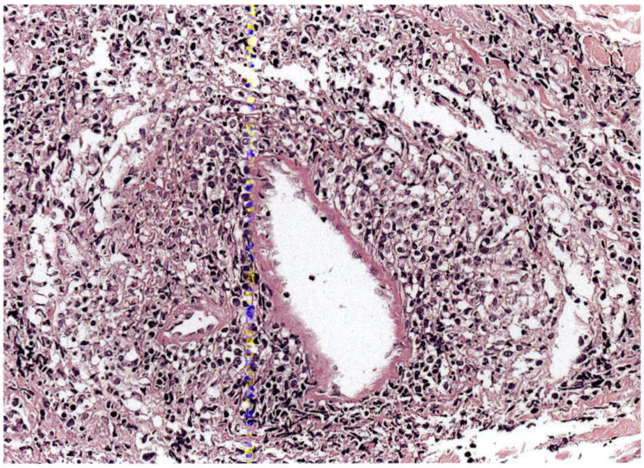

**Figure 15.10** Systemic hydroa vacciniforme lymphoproliferative disorder. Angiocentricity of neoplastic cells infiltrating a large vessel.

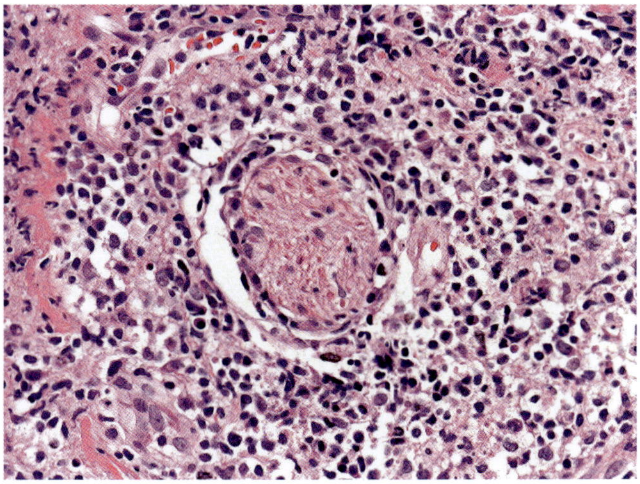

**Figure 15.11** Systemic hydroa vacciniforme lymphoproliferative disorder. Perineural infiltrate with some neurotropic lymphocytes.

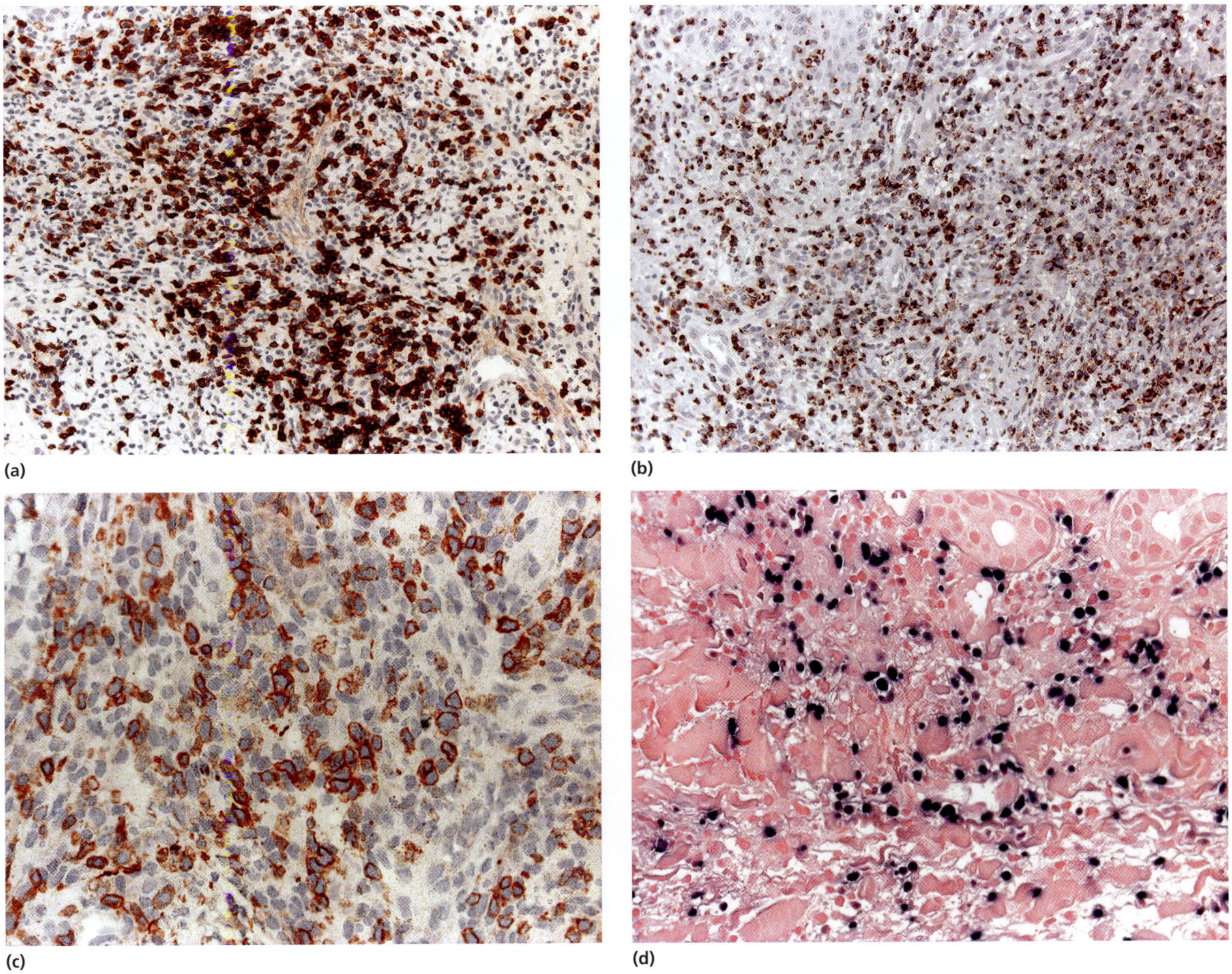

**Figure 15.12** Systemic hydroa vacciniforme lymphoproliferative disorder. (a) Neoplastic cells are positive for CD5, (b) TIA-1, and (c) CD56. (d) Several cells are positive for EBV (EBER-1).

(Fig. 15.12b). CD4$^+$ cases expressing cytotoxic proteins and CD4$^+$/CD8$^+$ cases seem to be more frequent in Chinese patients [39]. The α/β phenotype is much more common than the γ/δ or the true NK ones [40]. CD30 and CD56 expressions have been observed in a proportion of cases (Fig. 15.12c) [41, 42]. In situ hybridization for EBV (EBER-1) shows a positive signal in variable numbers of tumor cells in practically all tested specimens (Fig. 15.12d), but latent membrane protein (LMP1) is usually negative.

### Molecular genetics

A monoclonal rearrangement of the TCR genes can be detected in a proportion of cases (those with a T-cell phenotype) [23].

### Treatment

Due to the rarity of the disease management is not standardized, and large studies have not been performed. Photoprotection is paramount but not sufficient to avoid the progression of the disease. Patients with a diagnosis of systemic hydroa vacciniforme lymphoproliferative disorder have been managed, among others, by phototherapy (narrowband UV-B), systemic corticosteroids, polychemotherapy, and hematopoietic stem cell transplantation with variable rates of success [39, 43]. Some patients have been treated with interferon-α with good responses. Thalidomide has been used in a few cases [44].

### Prognosis

Systemic hydroa vacciniforme lymphoproliferative disorder has a prolonged course but a bad prognosis, intermediate between aggressive cutaneous cytotoxic NK/T-cell lymphomas and more indolent types of cutaneous T-cell lymphoma [19, 40]. Most cases published in the literature are either alive with specific manifestations of the disease or dead of systemic lymphoma. In a series of 19 Asiatic patients, EBV-DNA loads, elevated lactate dehydrogenase, cytopenia, and multiorgan destructive involvement were poor independent prognostic factors [39]. The course may be less aggressive in Asiatic patients than in those from Latin America [10, 43]. Concomitant severe mosquito bite allergy was found to be a risk factor for disease progression in Chinese patients [10].

### Résumé

**Systemic hydroa vacciniforme lymphoproliferative disorder**

| | | |
|---|---|---|
| **Clinical** | Mostly children. Infiltrated, ulcerated plaques, sometimes large tumors. Lesions may resemble hydroa vacciniforme clinically, and "borderline" cases exist. Photosensitivity; hypersensitivity to mosquito bites. | |
| **Morphology** | Variably dense lymphoid infiltrates with atypical lymphocytes. Frequent angiocentricity. | |
| **Immunohistochemistry** | CD2, CD3, CD5 | + |
| | CD4 | – |
| | CD8 | + |
| | CD56 | + (–) |
| | TCRβ | + (–) |
| | TCRγ, TCRδ | – (+) |
| | EBER-1 | + |
| | LMP1 | – |
| | CD30 | +/– |
| **Genetics** | Rearrangement of the TCR genes detected in a proportion of cases. | |
| **Treatment guidelines** | Probably systemic chemotherapy should be administered. Stem cell transplantation has been performed. Phototherapy, interferon-α, thalidomide used in some cases. | |

## References


1. Quinanilla-Martinez L, Barrionuevo C, Cohen JI, *et al.* Epstein–Barr virus-positive T- and natural killer-cell lymphoproliferative disorders of childhood. In: Arber DA, Borowitz MJ, Cook JR, *et al.*, eds. *The International Consensus Classification of Myeloid and Lymphoid Neoplasms.* Philadelphia (US): Wolters Kluver, 2025: 613–626.
2. Alaggio R, Amador C, Anagnostopoulos I, *et al.* The 5th edition of the World Health Organization classification of haematolymphoid tumours: lymphoid neoplasms. *Leukemia* 2022;**36**:1720–1748.
3. Tokura Y, Ishihara S, Ohshima K, *et al.* Severe mosquito bite hypersensitivity, natural killer cell leukaemia, latent or chronic active Epstein–Barr virus infection and hydroa vacciniforme-like eruption. *Br J Dermatol* 1998;**138**:905–906.
4. Kimura H, Arauio I, Kato S, Ng SB. Severe mosquito bite allergy. In: *WHO Classification of Tumours Editorial Board. Haematolymphoid Tumours.* 5th edition. Lyon (France): IARC, 2024: 772–773.
5. Miyake T, Yamamoto T, Hirai Y, *et al.* Survival rates and prognostic factors of Epstein–Barr virus-associated hydroa vacciniforme and hypersensitivity to mosquito bites. *Br J Dermatol* 2015;**172**:56–63.
6. Tokura Y, Ishihara S, Tagawa S, *et al.* Hypersensitivity to mosquito bites as the primary clinical manifestation of a juvenile type of Epstein–Barr virus-associated natural killer cell leukemia/lymphoma. *J Am Acad Dermatol* 2001;**45**:569–578.

7. Said J, Smart C. Severe mosquito bite allergy: an unusual EBV+ NK cell lymphoproliferative disorder. *Blood* 2019;**133**:999.
8. Okuno Y, Murata T, Sato Y, *et al.* Defective Epstein-Barr virus in chronic active infection and haematological malignancy. *Nat Microbiol* 2019;**4**:404–413.
9. Kimura H, Ito Y, Kawabe S, *et al.* EBV-associated T/NK-cell lymphoproliferative diseases in non-immunocompromised hosts: prospective analysis of 108 cases. *Blood* 2012;**119**:673–686.
10. Zhang Y, Liu Y, Xu J, *et al.* Hydroa vacciniforme lymphoproliferative disorder: a retrospective study of 42 paediatric cases. *Eur J Dermatol* 2024;**34**:144–149.
11. Ruiz-Maldonado R, Parrilla F, Orozco-Covarrubias M, *et al.* Edematous, scarring vasculitic panniculitis: a new multisystemic disease with malignant potential. *J Am Acad Dermatol* 1995;**32**:37–44.
12. Magana M, Sangueza P, Gil-Beristain J, *et al.* Angiocentric cutaneous T-cell lymphoma of childhood (hydroa-like lymphoma): a distinctive type of cutaneous T-cell lymphoma. *J Am Acad Dermatol* 1998;**38**:574–579.
13. Chen HH, Hsiao CH, Chiu HC. Hydroa vacciniforme-like primary cutaneous CD8-positive T-cell lymphoma. *Br J Dermatol* 2002; **147**:587–591.
14. Barrionuevo C, Anderson VM, Zevallos-Giampietri E, *et al.* Hydroa-like cutaneous T-cell lymphoma: a clinicopathologic and molecular genetic study of 16 pediatric cases from Peru. *Appl Immunohistochem Mol Morphol* 2002;**10**:7–14.
15. Cho KH, Kim CW, Heo DS, *et al.* Epstein–Barr virus-associated peripheral T-cell lymphoma in adults with hydroa vacciniforme-like lesions. *Clin Exp Dermatol* 2001;**26**:242–247.
16. Cho KH, Lee SH, Kim CW, *et al.* Epstein–Barr virus-associated lymphoproliferative lesions presenting as a hydroa vacciniforme-like eruption: an analysis of six cases. *Br J Dermatol* 2004;**151**:372–380.
17. Oono T, Arata J, Masuda T, *et al.* Coexistence of hydroa vacciniforme and malignant lymphoma. *Arch Dermatol* 1986;**122**:1306–1309.
18. Xu Z, Lian S. Epstein–Barr virus-associated hydroa vacciniforme-like cutaneous lymphoma in seven Chinese children. *Ped Dermatol* 2010;**27**:463–469.
19. Sangueza M, Plaza JA. Hydroa vacciniforme-like cutaneous T-cell lymphoma: clinicopathologic and immunohistochemical study of 12 cases. *J Am Acad Dermatol* 2013;**69**:112–119.
20. Rodriguez-Pinilla SM, Barrionuevo C, Garcia J, *et al.* EBV-associated cutaneous NK/T-cell lymphoma. Review of a series of 14 cases from Peru in children and young adults. *Am J Surg Pathol* 2010;**34**:1773–1782.
21. Santos M, Nogueira L, Talahri C, *et al.* Hydroa vacciniforme-like lymphoma in a patient from the Brazilian Amazon. *Int J Dermatol* 2013;**52**:641–643.
22. Zhang X, Wang T, Wang L. Hydroa vacciniforme-like lymphoma in Tibetan children: 2 cases and a literature review. *Am J Dermatopathol* 2018;**40**:358–361.
23. Steger GG, Dittrich C, Hönigsmann H, Moser K. Permanent cure of hydroa vacciniforme after chemotherapy for Hodgkin's disease. *Br J Dermatol* 1988;**119**:684–685.
24. Kimura H, Plaza JA, Araujo I, *et al.* Hydroa vacciniforme lymphoproliferative disorder. In: *WHO Classification of Tumours Editorial Board. Haematolymphoid Tumours.* 5th edition. Lyon (France): IARC, 2024: 774–776.
25. Wu YH, Chen HC, Hsiao PF, *et al.* Hydroa vacciniforme-like Epstein–Barr virus-associated monoclonal T-lymphoproliferative disorder in a child. *Int J Dermatol* 2007;**46**:1081–1086.
26. Iwatsuki K, Ohtsuka K, Harada JI, *et al.* Clinicopathologic manifestations of Epstein–Barr virus-associated cutaneous lymphoproliferative disorders. *Arch Dermatol* 1997;**133**:1081–1086.
27. Iwatsuki K, Xu Z, Takata M, *et al.* The association of latent Epstein–Barr virus infection with hydroa vacciniforme. *Br J Dermatol* 1999;**140**:715–721.
28. Iwatsuki K, Yamamoto T, Tsuji K, *et al.* A spectrum of clinical manifestations caused by host immune responses against Epstein–Barr virus infections. *Acta Med Okayama* 2004;**58**:169–180.
29. Cohen JI, Manoli I, Dowdell K, *et al.* Hydroa vacciniforme-like lymphoproliferative disorder: an EBV disease with a low risk of systemic illness in whites. *Blood* 2019;**133**:2753–2764.
30. Chen CC, Chang KC, Medeiros LJ, Lee JYY. Hydroa vacciniforme and hydroa vacciniforme-like T-cell lymphoma: an uncommon event for transformation. *J Cutan Pathol* 2016;**43**:1102–1111.
31. Iwatsuki K, Miyake T, Hirai Y, Yamamoto T. Hydroa vacciniforme: a distinctive form of Epstein–Barr virus-associated T-cell lymphoproliferative disorders. *Eur J Dermatol* 2019;**29**:21–28.
32. Lim HW, Rosen CF. Photodermatologic disorders. In: Bolognia JL, Schaffer JV, Cerroni L, eds. *Dermatology.* 5th edition. Elsevier: Philadelphia, 2024: 1564–1584.
33. Iwatsuki K, Satoh M, Yamamoto T, *et al.* Pathogenic link between hydroa vacciniforme and Epstein–Barr virus-associated hematologic disorders. *Arch Dermatol* 2006;**142**:587–595.
34. Gupta G, Man I, Kemmett D. Hydroa vacciniforme: a clinical and follow-up study of 17 cases. *J Am Acad Dermatol* 2000;**42**:208–213.
35. Plaza JA, Sangueza M. Hydroa vacciniforme–like lymphoma with primarily periorbital swelling: 7 cases of an atypical clinical manifestation of this rare cutaneous T-cell lymphoma. *Am J Dermatopathol* 2015;**37**:20–25.
36. Wen PF, Zhang M, Wang TT, *et al.* Comparative study of the clinical pathology, immunophenotype, Epstein–Barr virus infection status, and gene rearrangements in adult and child patients with hydroa vacciniforme-like lymphoproliferative disorder. *Am J Dermatopathol* 2019;**41**:7–15.
37. Kim TH, Lee JH, Kim YC, Lee SE. Hydroa vacciniforme-like lymphoma misdiagnosed as cutaneous lupus erythematosus. *J Cutan Pathol* 2015;**42**:229–231.
38. Magana M, Massone C, Magana P, Cerroni L. Clinicopathologic features of hydroa vacciniforme-like lymphoma. A series of 9 patients. *Am J Dermatopathol* 2016;**38**:20–25.
39. Guo N, Chen Y, Wang Y, *et al.* Clinicopathological categorization of hydroa vacciniforme-like lymphoproliferative disorder: an analysis of prognostic implications and treatment based on 19 cases. *Diagn Pathol* 2019;**14**:82.
40. Quintanilla-Martinez L, Ridaura C, Nagl F, *et al.* Hydroa vacciniforme-like lymphoma: a chronic EBV+ lymphoproliferative disorder with risk to develop a systemic lymphoma. *Blood* 2013;**122**:3101–3110.
41. Doeden K, Molina-Kirsch H, Perez E, *et al.* Hydroa-like lymphoma with CD56 expression. *J Cutan Pathol* 2008;**35**:488–494.
42. Feng S, Jin P, Zeng X. Hydroa vacciniforme-like primary cutaneous CD8-positive T-cell lymphoma. *Eur J Dermatol* 2008;**18**:364–365.
43. Liu Y, Ma C, Wang G, Wang L. Hydroa vacciniforme-like lymphoproliferative disorder: clinicopathologic study of 41 cases. *J Am Acad Dermatol* 2019;**81**:534–540.
44. Beltran BE, Maza I, Moises-Alfaro CB, *et al.* Thalidomide for the treatment of hydroa vacciniforme-like lymphoma: report of four pediatric cases from Peru. *Am J Hematol* 2014;**89**:1160–1161.

SECTION 2

# Cutaneous B-cell lymphomas and lymphoproliferative disorders

## CHAPTER 16

# Cutaneous follicle center lymphoma

Cutaneous follicle center lymphoma is defined as the neoplastic proliferation of germinal center cells confined to the skin. The pattern of growth can be purely follicular, purely diffuse, or mixed. This lymphoma is listed as a specific entity in the 2018 and 2024 updates of the classification of cutaneous lymphomas by the European Organization for Research and Treatment of Cancer (EORTC) World Health Organization (WHO), and is included as a specific entity in the International Consensus Classification (ICC) *of Myeloid and Lymphoid Neoplasms* [1–3]. In the 5th edition of the WHO *Classification of Haematolymphoid Tumours* cutaneous follicle center lymphoma is listed as a distinct entity within the group of "mature B-cell neoplasms" [4].

It must be underlined that primary cutaneous follicle center lymphoma with a diffuse pattern of growth is characterized by a predominance of large cells without follicular structures, which in the lymph nodes would be diagnostic of a large B-cell lymphoma. On the other hand, irrespective of the morphology of the infiltrate cases of primary cutaneous follicle center lymphoma have the same prognosis, and are managed in the same way. The concept of primary cutaneous follicle center lymphoma as a morphologic spectrum including also cases with diffuse patterns of growth has been acknowledged in general lymphoma classifications, and has been a major step in understanding the heterogeneity of lymphomas showing similar histopathological features, but arising at different body sites. It may be that other extranodal follicle center lymphomas besides the cutaneous ones have analogous biological and prognostic features, different from those observed in nodal cases. In fact, it has been suggested that the model of a follicle center lymphoma that includes the diffuse variant may be useful to describe some extranodal diffuse large B-cell lymphomas characterized by an indolent course and by phenotypic features similar to those of cutaneous follicle center lymphoma, and that the concept of cutaneous follicle center lymphoma should be expanded to encompass some large cell lymphomas at extranodal sites [5]. In the WHO classification, however, cutaneous follicle center lymphoma is the only recognized organ-specific, distinct entity of follicular lymphoma [4].

Complete staging investigations must be performed in all patients, as secondary cutaneous manifestations of nodal follicular lymphoma may present with exactly the same clinicopathologic features as primary cutaneous cases [6]. However, in otherwise asymptomatic patients upgrade of the stage upon complete investigations is rare [7]. Bone marrow biopsy is not performed routinely. In this context, it should also be underlined that positivity or negativity for Bcl-2 on neoplastic cells cannot be considered as a surrogate of complete staging investigations.

A tumor, node, metastasis (TNM) staging system for cutaneous lymphomas other than mycosis fungoides and Sézary syndrome has been proposed by the EORTC and International Society of Cutaneous Lymphomas (ISCL) (see Chapter 1, Table 1.3), and subsequently slightly modified in conjunction with the US Cutaneous Lymphoma Consortium (USCLC) [8, 9].

In the lymph nodes, rare cases of so-called "lineage plasticity" of follicle center lymphoma with transdifferentiation into Langerhans cell tumor have been observed (see also Chapter 1) [10]. Similar cases have not been reported in the skin.

## Clinical features

Patients are adults of both genders. Onset in children has been reported, but is exceptional [11, 12]. Cutaneous follicle center lymphoma presents with erythematous papules, plaques, and tumors, usually non-ulcerated, located mostly on the head and neck and the trunk (Fig. 16.1). A distinct clinical presentation with plaques and tumors on the back surrounded by erythematous macules and papules expanding centrifugally around the central tumors has been described in the past as "reticulohistiocytoma of the dorsum" or "Crosti lymphoma" (Fig. 16.2) [13]. In most instances, this particular presentation occurs on the back, but identical lesions may be observed anywhere on the trunk (Fig. 16.2b). In some cases, a wide perilesional erythema can extend on a large part of the trunk resembling a figurate erythema (Fig. 16.3). Early lesions of Crosti lymphoma show only small, circumscribed areas of erythema and/or small clustered papules and plaques, and may be very difficult to diagnose clinically (Fig. 16.4) [14]. These lesions grow at a variable rate but it is usually possible to appreciate the progression in sequential

*Skin Lymphoma: The Illustrated Guide*, Sixth Edition. Lorenzo Cerroni.

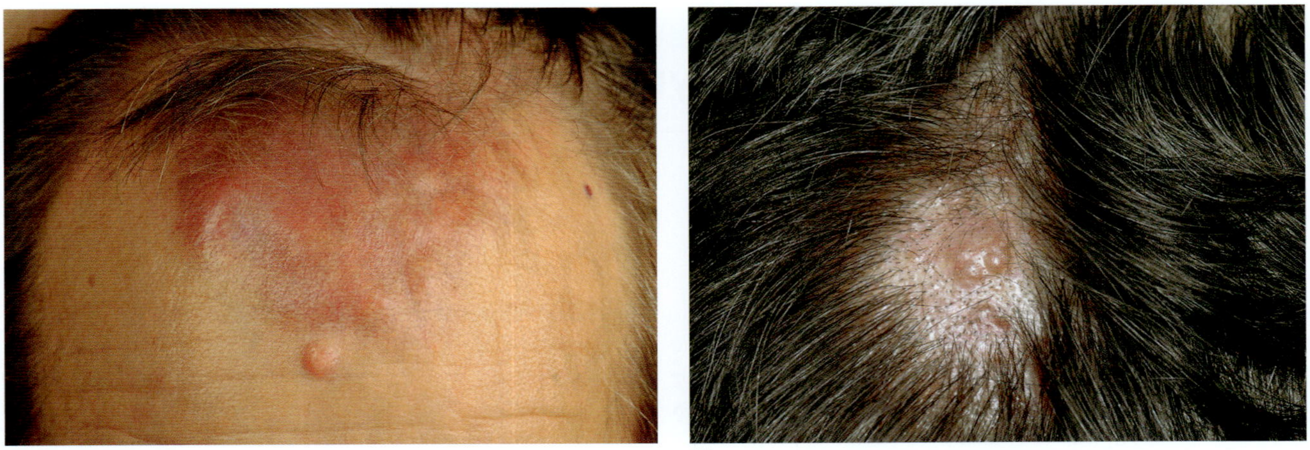

(a) (b)

Figure 16.1 Cutaneous follicle center lymphoma. (a) Large, flat erythematous tumor on the forehead. (b) Early lesion characterized by a small nodule with surrounding papules on the scalp.

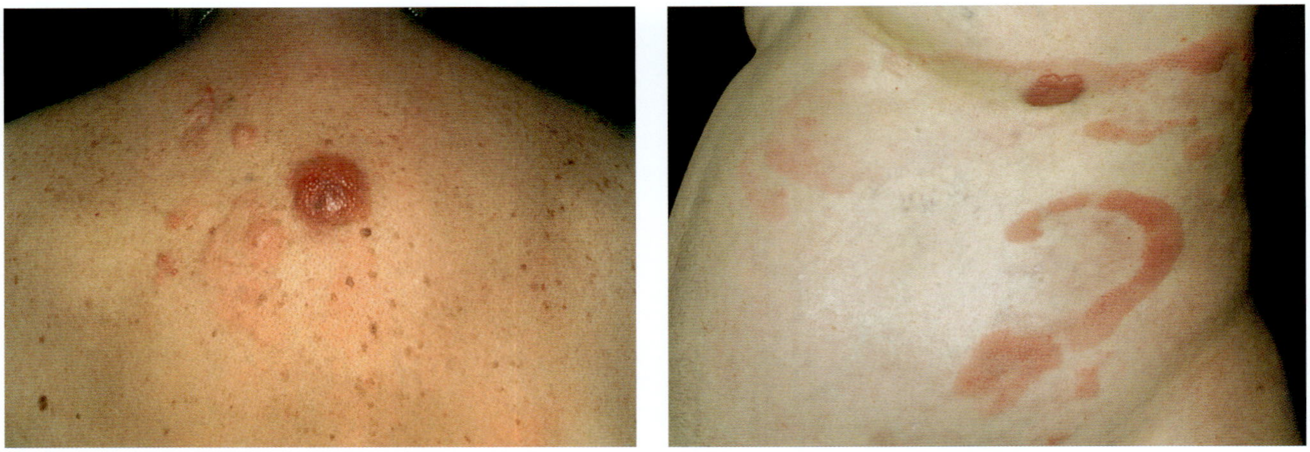

(a) (b)

Figure 16.2 Cutaneous follicle center lymphoma ("reticulohistiocytoma of the dorsum," "Crosti lymphoma"). (a) Large erythematous tumor surrounded by plaques, papules, and erythematous macules on the back. (b) Large, infiltrated lesions with annular morphology and erythematous tumor on the flank. (*Courtesy of Dr. Cornelia Müller, Homburg* [*Saar, Germany*].)

pictures (Fig. 16.5). In several patients with the clinical presentation of Crosti lymphoma, small erythematous papules located far from the main lesions can be observed (Fig. 16.6) [14]. These papules represent early manifestations of the disease and reveal histopathologically specific features of follicle center lymphoma (Fig. 16.7). The question arises as to whether local radiotherapy is the more appropriate treatment modality for these patients, and what the radiation field should be. The relatively high incidence of local recurrences observed in Crosti lymphoma treated by radiotherapy is very likely to be caused by the presence of early lesions far from the main tumor, which had not been identified clinically at the time of treatment planning and had not been included in the radiation field.

Follicle center lymphoma on the head may be clinically deceptive and present only with small papules, area of diffuse, slightly indurated erythema, or alopecia (Figs. 16.8–16.10) [15, 16]. Interestingly, alopecia may be observed also as a specific manifestation of extracutaneous follicular lymphoma (Fig. 16.11). Other cases show miliary and/or agminated papules, resembling rosacea or arthropod bite reactions (Fig. 16.12), irregular teleangectasia (Fig. 16.13) [17], or rarely rhinophyma-like lesions [18]. Miliary and agminated lesions, too, have been observed also in secondary cutaneous cases [19, 20], again underlining the fact that primary and secondary cutaneous follicle center lymphoma may show identical clinical features.

In a small proportion of patients, lesions of cutaneous follicle center lymphoma arise on the leg(s). Differentiation of these cases from those of diffuse large B-cell lymphoma, leg-type is crucial but may be difficult, as morphology may show a predominance of large cells in both entities (see also below the paragraph on differential diagnosis).

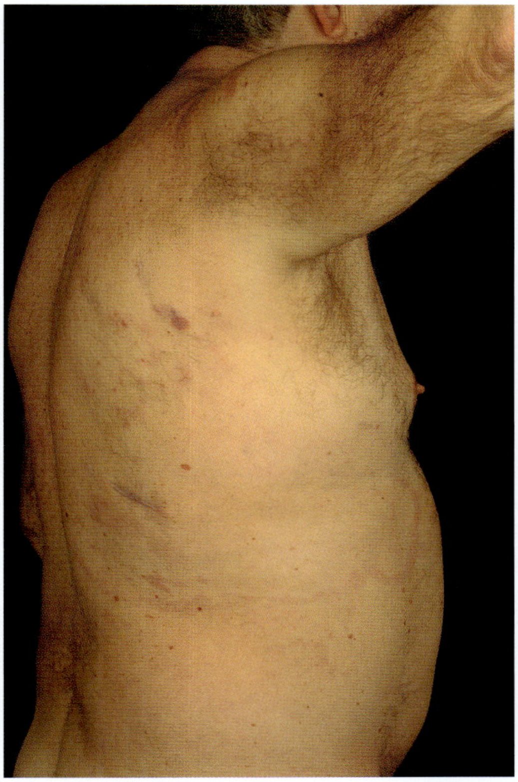

Figure 16.3 Cutaneous follicle center lymphoma ("reticulohistiocytoma of the dorsum," "Crosti lymphoma"). Papules and small erythematous plaque with a broad, figurate erythema-like arrangement on the distal part of the lesion, extending from the back to the abdomen. Note large scars from previous surgical excisions.

Although there are no clear-cut differences in clinical presentation between the diffuse and follicular variants of cutaneous follicle center lymphoma, cases with a follicular pattern have a predilection for the head and neck region, whereas tumors of Crosti lymphoma correspond in the majority of cases to a follicle center lymphoma with a diffuse pattern of growth (not only in the tumoral areas but also in the flat ones).

Some patients report that small papular lesions (particularly on the back) undergo spontaneous regression [14]. I have

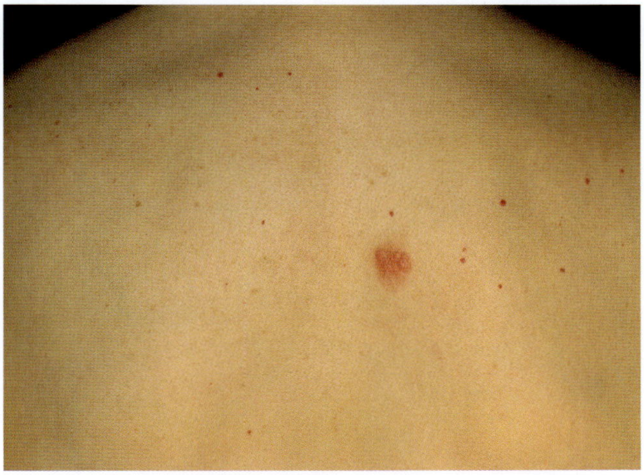

Figure 16.4 Cutaneous follicle center lymphoma ("reticulohistiocytoma of the dorsum," "Crosti lymphoma"), early lesion. Clustered papules on the back with a small erythematous halo.

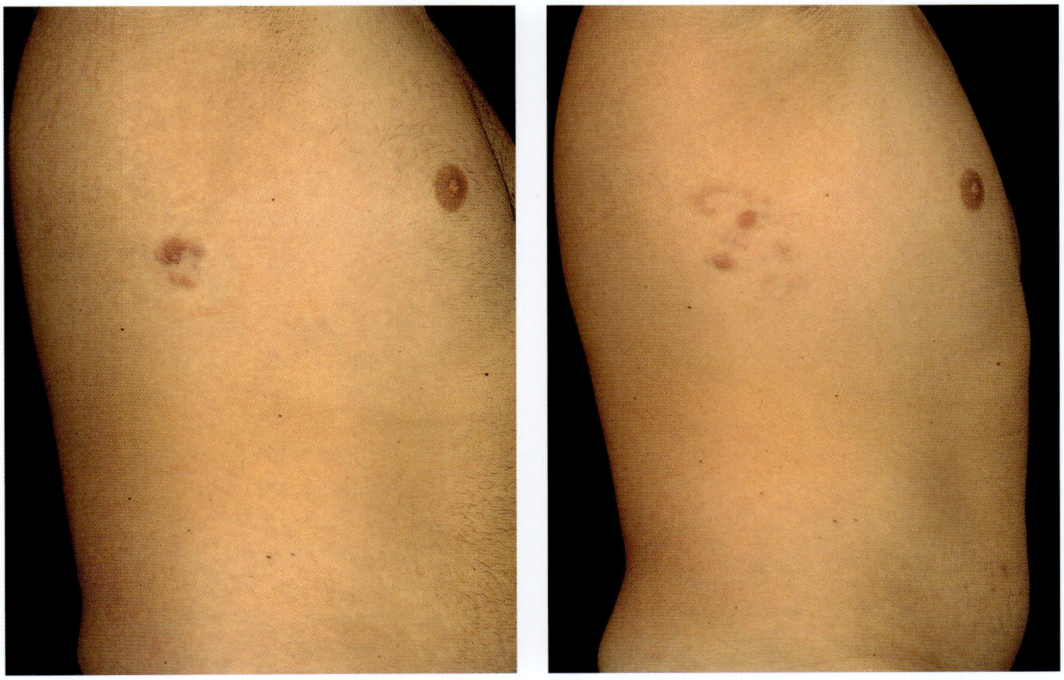

(a) (b)

Figure 16.5 Cutaneous follicle center lymphoma ("reticulohistiocytoma of the dorsum," "Crosti lymphoma"), early lesion. (a) Clustered papules and small areas of erythema on the flank at first presentation. (b) Fourteen months later the lesions have changed morphology and have spread centrifugally. Note a small scar of the previous diagnostic biopsy.

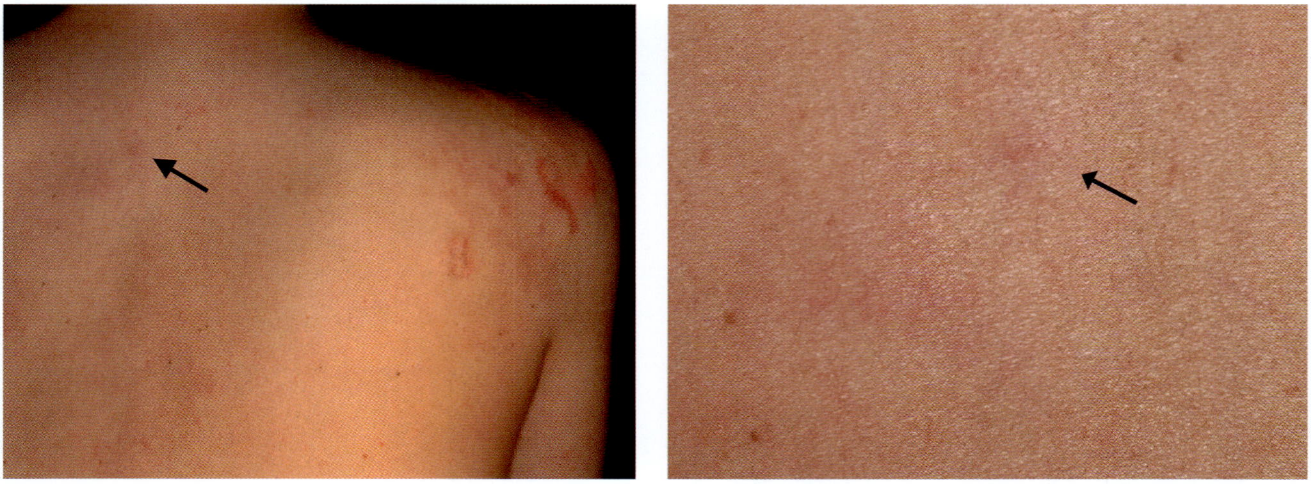

(a) (b)

**Figure 16.6** Cutaneous follicle center lymphoma. (a) Infiltrated plaques and several scars from previous surgical procedures on the right shoulder. Note a small erythematous papule on the paravertebral area (arrow). (b) Detail of the small papule (arrow). Biopsy revealed a specific infiltrate (see text).

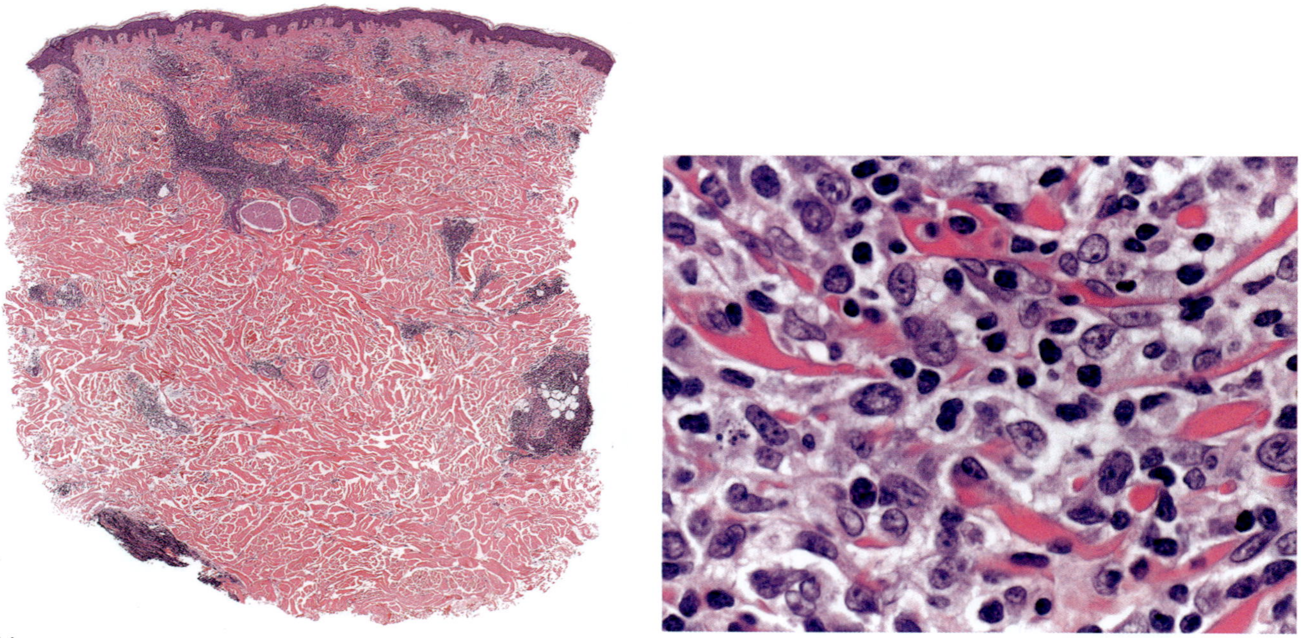

(a) (b)

**Figure 16.7** Cutaneous follicle center lymphoma, early lesion. (a) Histology reveals lymphoid infiltrates predominantly in the superficial and mid-dermis with involvement of the deep dermis. (b) Cytomorphology shows small lymphocytes admixed with many mid-sized and large centrocytes.

observed this phenomenon in several patients, and it is probably much more common than we currently realize. Spontaneous regression of specific manifestations of a cutaneous malignant tumor, on the other hand, is not rare and can be observed in several solid tumors as well.

Anetoderma has been observed rarely in cases of primary cutaneous follicle center lymphoma, and in some patients were associated with the presence of antiphospholipid antibodies [21]. In one patient, the lesions arose at the site of previous radiotherapy for breast cancer [22]. Association with infections such

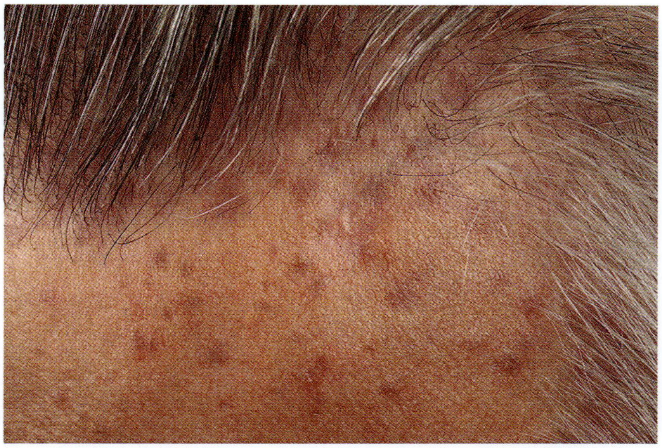

**Figure 16.8** Cutaneous follicle center lymphoma. Small livid papules on the scalp extending to the forehead.

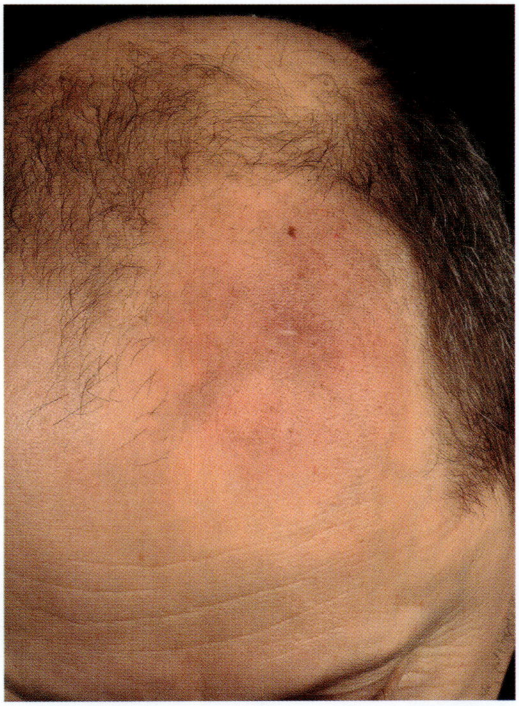

**Figure 16.9** Cutaneous follicle center lymphoma. Diffuse, infiltrated erythematous area on the scalp. Note the central scar of a diagnostic biopsy.

as *Borrelia burgdorferi*, hepatitis C, or human herpesvirus 8 has been described in sporadic patients, but does not seem to be an important etiologic factor for cutaneous follicle center lymphoma [23, 24]. In spite of the figurate erythema-like morphology reminiscent of erythema chronicum migrans, lesions of Crosti lymphoma are negative for *Borrelia*.

Cases of follicular lymphoma with features similar to those of cutaneous follicle center lymphoma have been described in the lower female genital tract, and it has been suggested that such cases may represent a variant of cutaneous follicle center lymphoma [25].

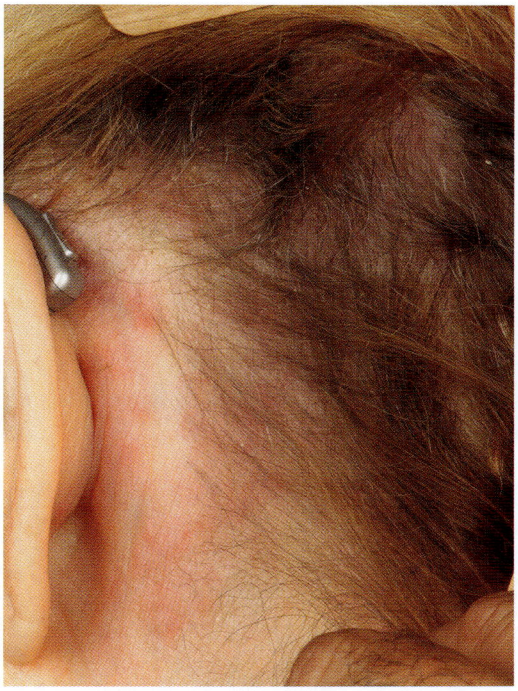

**Figure 16.10** Cutaneous follicle center lymphoma. Irregular, infiltrated erythema behind the ear and on the scalp.

## Histopathology, immunophenotype, and molecular genetics

### Histopathology

The histopathologic features of cases with a ***follicular pattern of growth*** consist of nodular infiltrates extending into the entire dermis, usually involving the subcutaneous tissues, characterized by a prominent follicular pattern (Fig. 16.14). The epidermis is spared as a rule. Neoplastic follicles in follicle center lymphoma show several morphologic abnormalities, such as a reduced or absent mantle zone, a reduced number or complete lack of tingible body macrophages, and a monomorphous appearance without a clear-cut distinction between dark and light areas (lack of "polarization") (Fig. 16.15). These features are readily observed at low power and provide valuable clues for the diagnosis. Cytomorphologically, neoplastic follicles consist of small and large centrocytes admixed with centroblasts, often intermingled with reactive small lymphocytes. Small clusters of neoplastic cells can be found in the interfollicular areas as well. It should be underlined that in some cases of cutaneous follicle center lymphoma neoplastic follicles may coexist with reactive ones, thus examination of partial biopsies (e.g., punch biopsies) may be misleading.

In some cases, cutaneous follicle center lymphoma with a follicular pattern of growth may show an "inversion" of the architecture of the lymphoid follicles, characterized by a pale area located at the periphery of the nodules (corresponding to neoplastic cells), surrounding a darker, and central area

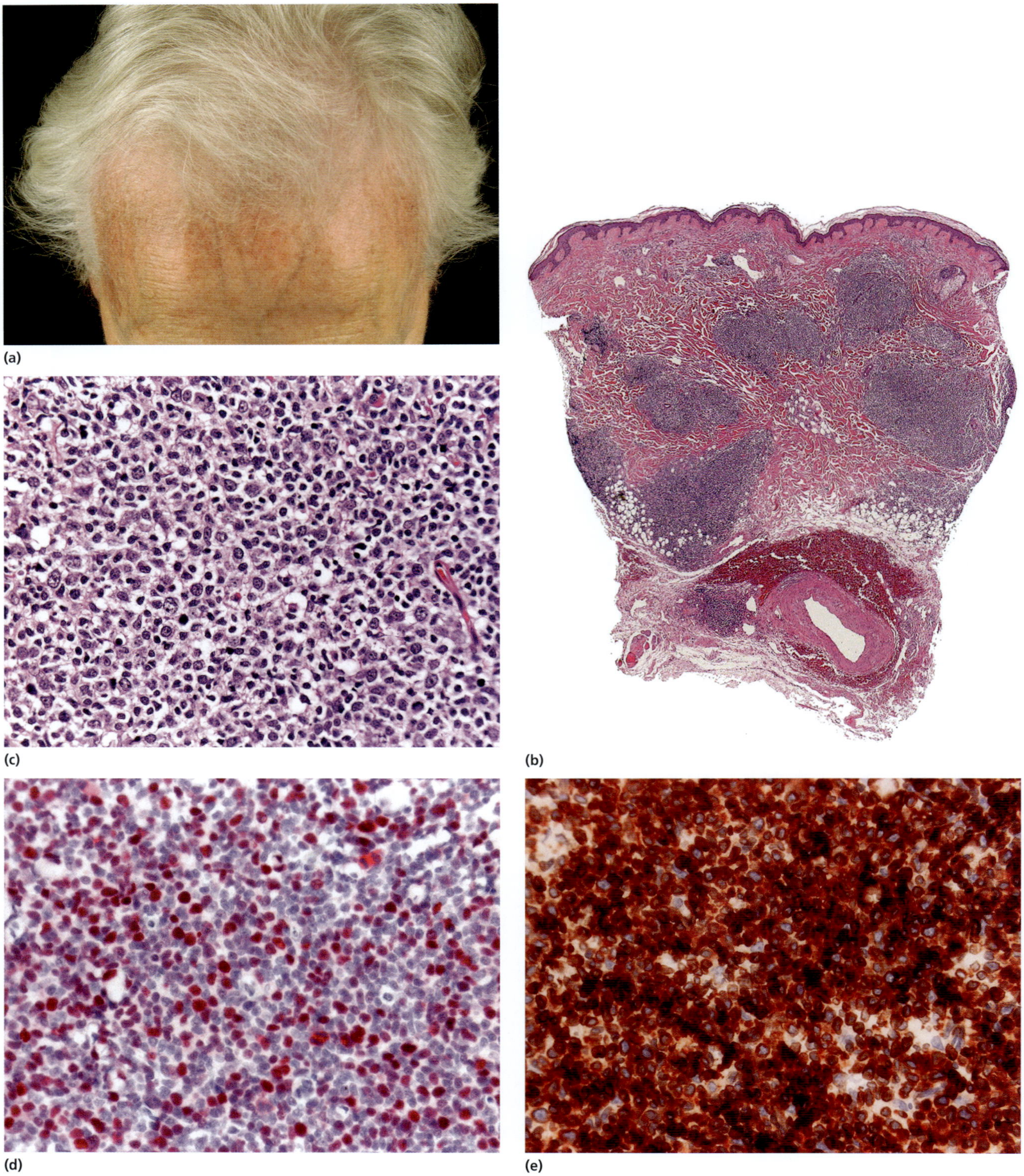

Figure 16.11 Secondary cutaneous manifestation of nodal follicular lymphoma. (a) Frontal "alopecia" with only very subtle erythema in a 71-year-old woman; (b) a biopsy showed dense lymphoid infiltrates with (c) irregular aggregates of follicular cells. (d) The follicular cells are positive for Bcl-6 and (e) Bcl-2. Staging investigations disclosed a follicular lymphoma in the abdominal lymph nodes.

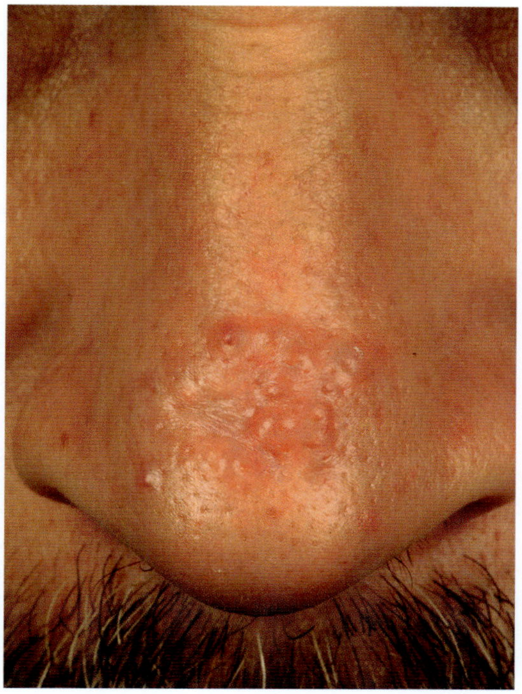

Figure 16.12 Cutaneous follicle center lymphoma. Agminated erythematous papules on the nose.

(corresponding to reactive lymphocytes) (Fig. 16.16). These features are never encountered in reactive follicular infiltrates and represent a clue to the diagnosis of lymphoma.

A morphologic variant of cutaneous follicle center lymphoma with a follicular pattern of growth showing nodules of medium–large centrocytes admixed with some centroblasts without a

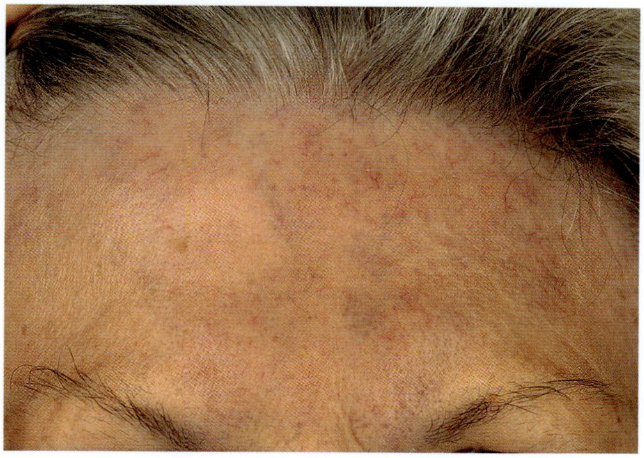

Figure 16.13 Cutaneous follicle center lymphoma. Widespread teleangectasia on the forehead and livid, infiltrated areas over the eyebrows.

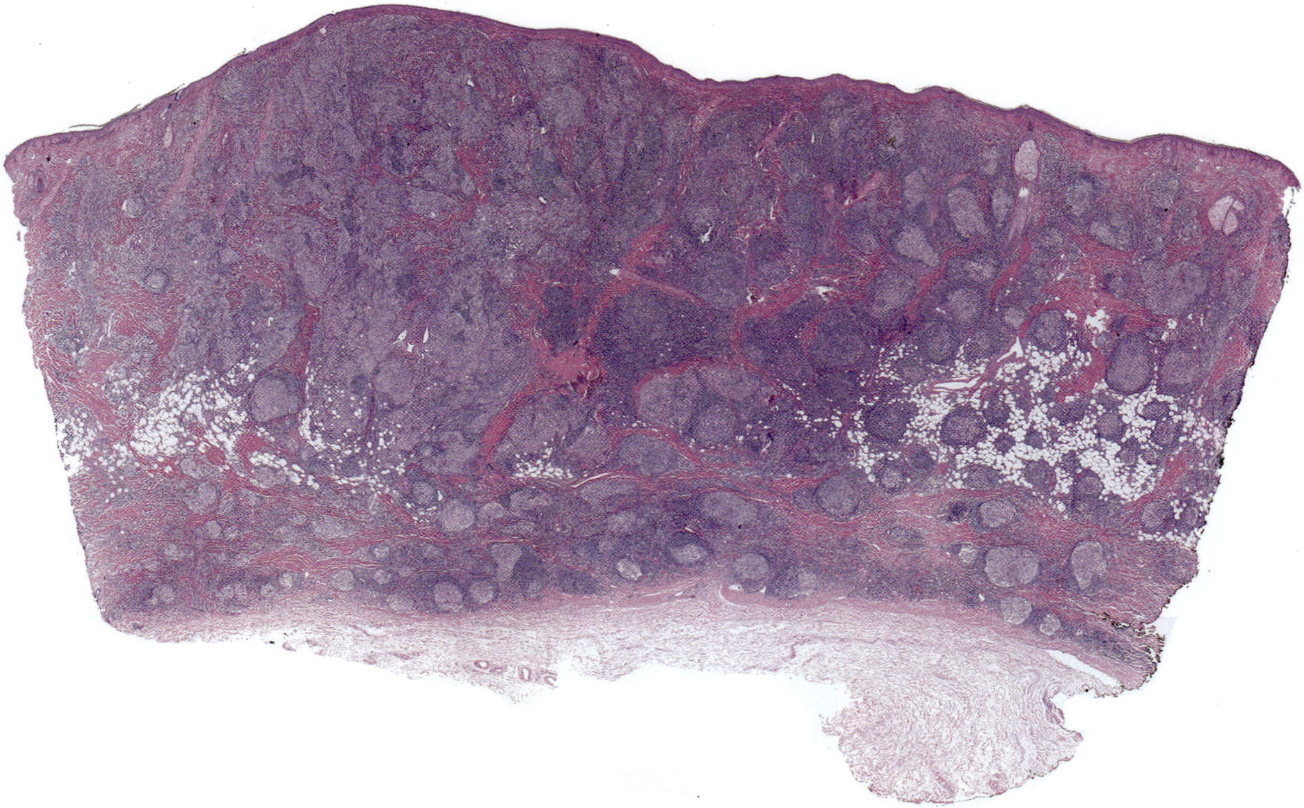

Figure 16.14 Cutaneous follicle center lymphoma, follicular type. Dense infiltrate within the entire dermis and subcutaneous fat. Note prominent lymphoid follicles with a reduced or absent mantle.

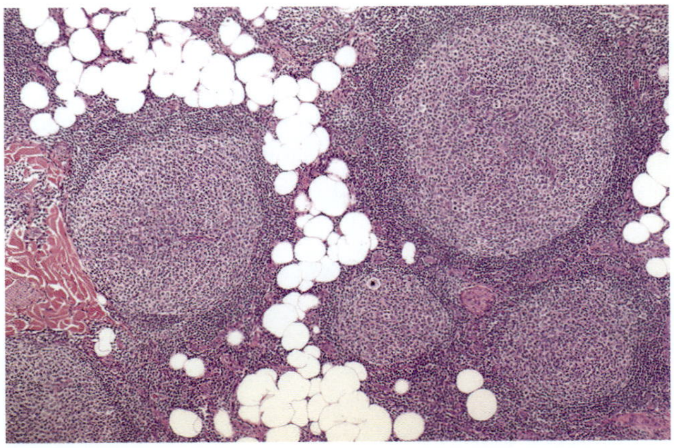

**Figure 16.15** Cutaneous follicle center lymphoma, follicular type. Lymphoid follicles reveal several atypical morphologic aspects: reduced mantle zone, lack of polarization (lack of dark and light areas), and the absence of tingible body macrophages.

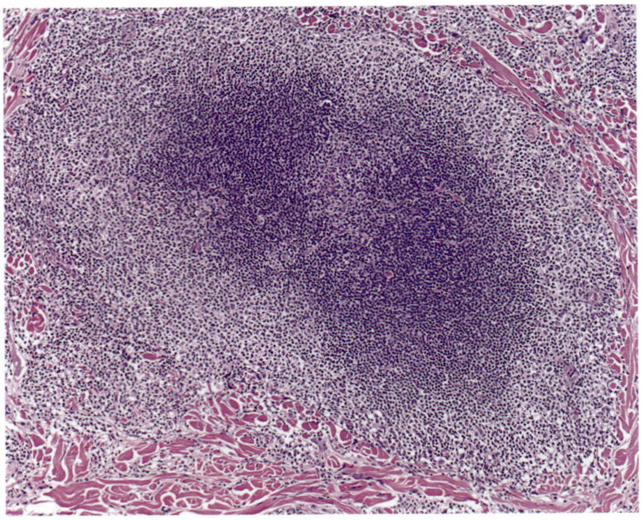

**Figure 16.16** Cutaneous follicle center lymphoma, follicular type. "Inverted" architecture of the lymphoid follicle, characterized by a pale area located at the periphery of the nodule (corresponding to neoplastic cells), surrounding a darker, central area (corresponding to reactive lymphocytes).

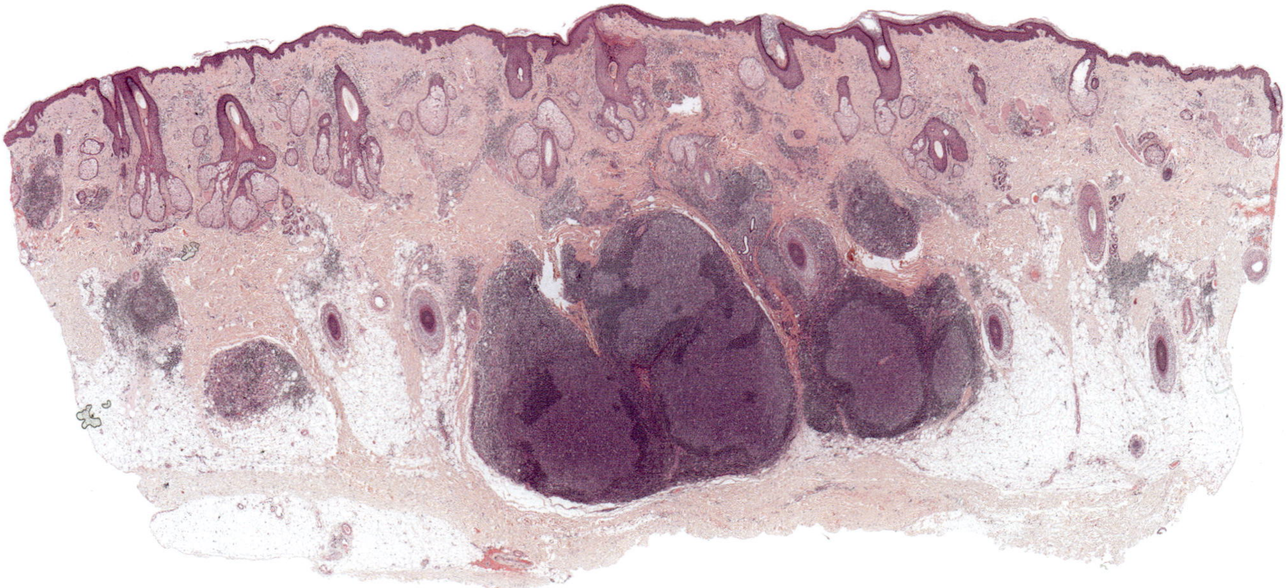

**Figure 16.17** Cutaneous follicle center lymphoma ("large cell lymphocytoma"). Nodular lymphoid infiltrate in the deep dermis and subcutaneous fat, composed almost exclusively of large lymphoid follicles with little mantle zone.

prominent interfollicular infiltrate has been termed in the past "large cell lymphocytoma" (Fig. 16.17) [26, 27]. This pattern reflects the almost exclusive presence of large, atypical lymphoid follicles devoid of a mantle but still retaining a recognizable nodular, rather than diffuse, architecture (and a network of $CD21^+$ follicular dendritic cells).

In the lymph nodes, cases of follicle center lymphoma may uncommonly show plasmacytic differentiation, posing differential diagnostic problems with marginal zone lymphoma (MALT-lymphomas) [28]. A clonal relationship between neoplastic lymphocytes and plasma cells has been demonstrated in some of these cases, confirming that they are morphologic variations of follicle center lymphoma [29]. I have observed similar cases in the skin, with clonal neoplastic plasma cells within a lesion of otherwise typical follicle center lymphoma, and rare cases have been published [30, 31]. These cases may be

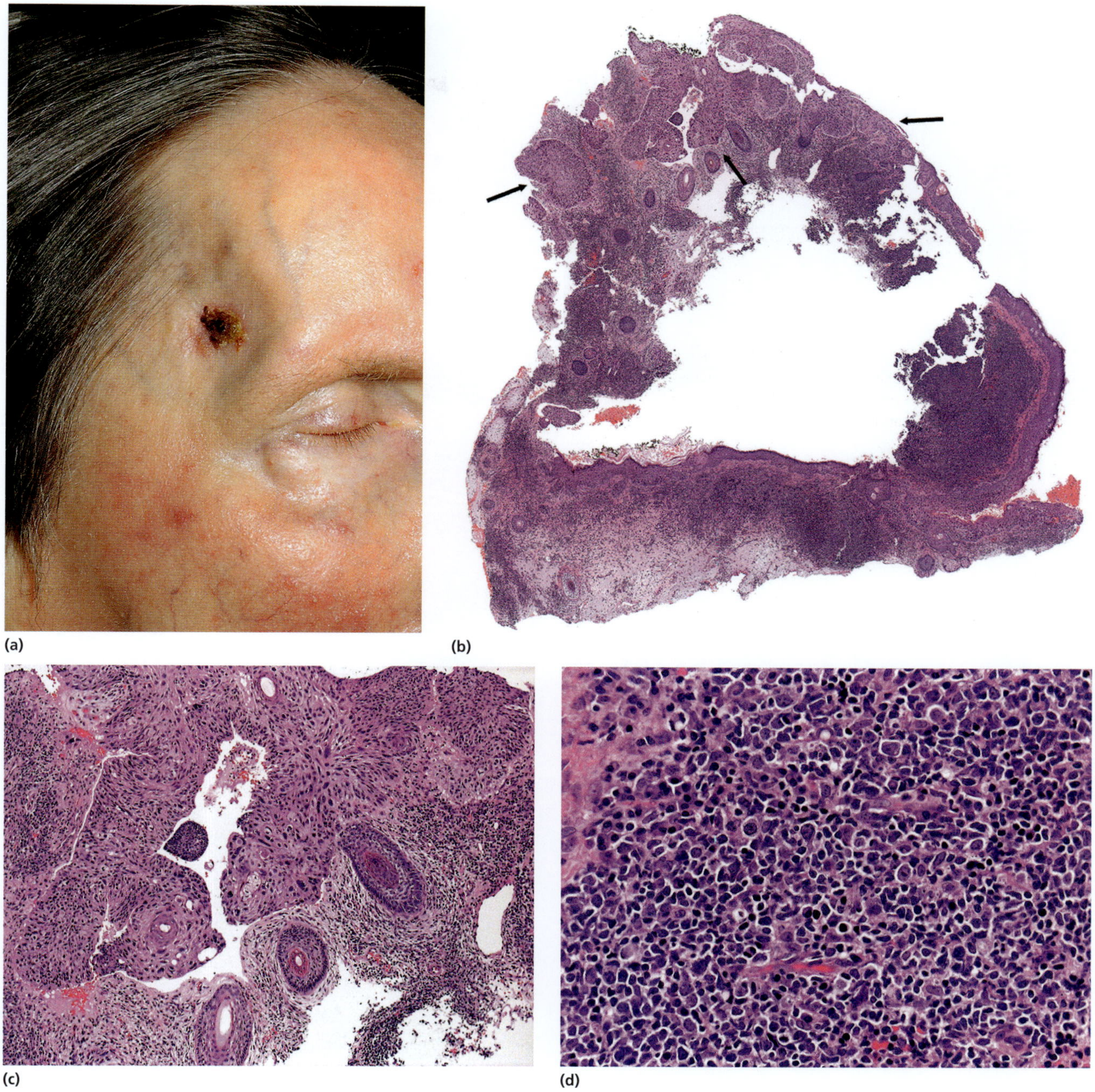

Figure 16.18 Cutaneous follicle center lymphoma at the site of squamous cell carcinoma. (a) Crusted plaque on the right temple in an elderly patient, clinically consistent with an epithelial tumor. (b) A shaving biopsy shows irregular complexes of a superficial squamous cell carcinoma (arrows) and a dense lymphoid infiltrate. (c) Detail of the squamous cell carcinoma. (d) The lymphoid infiltrate is characterized by many medium-sized and large cells with morphological features of centrocytes. (e) Staining for CD20 is positive in most lymphoid cells; (f) staining for CD21 shows focal remnants of a network of follicular dendritic cells; (g) neoplastic cells are positive for Bcl-6 and (h) negative for Bcl-2.

misinterpreted as cutaneous marginal zone lymphoproliferative disorder, and indeed in some patients overlapping features of the two conditions may be observed, and precise classification may be very difficult. Similar overlapping features may be encountered at extracutaneous sites as well [28].

I have observed rarely cutaneous follicle center lymphoma at the site of other cutaneous tumors in the head and neck area (Fig. 16.18). Similar cases may be misinterpreted as reactive inflammation. In fact, reactive germinal centers can be observed rarely at the sites of cutaneous basal or squamous cell carcinoma, and should be distinguished from atypical lymphoid follicles of genuine cutaneous follicle center lymphoma.

Well-developed lesions of cutaneous follicle center lymphoma with a ***diffuse pattern of growth*** involve the entire dermis, often extending into the subcutaneous fat (Fig. 16.19). They are characterized by a proliferation of medium and large

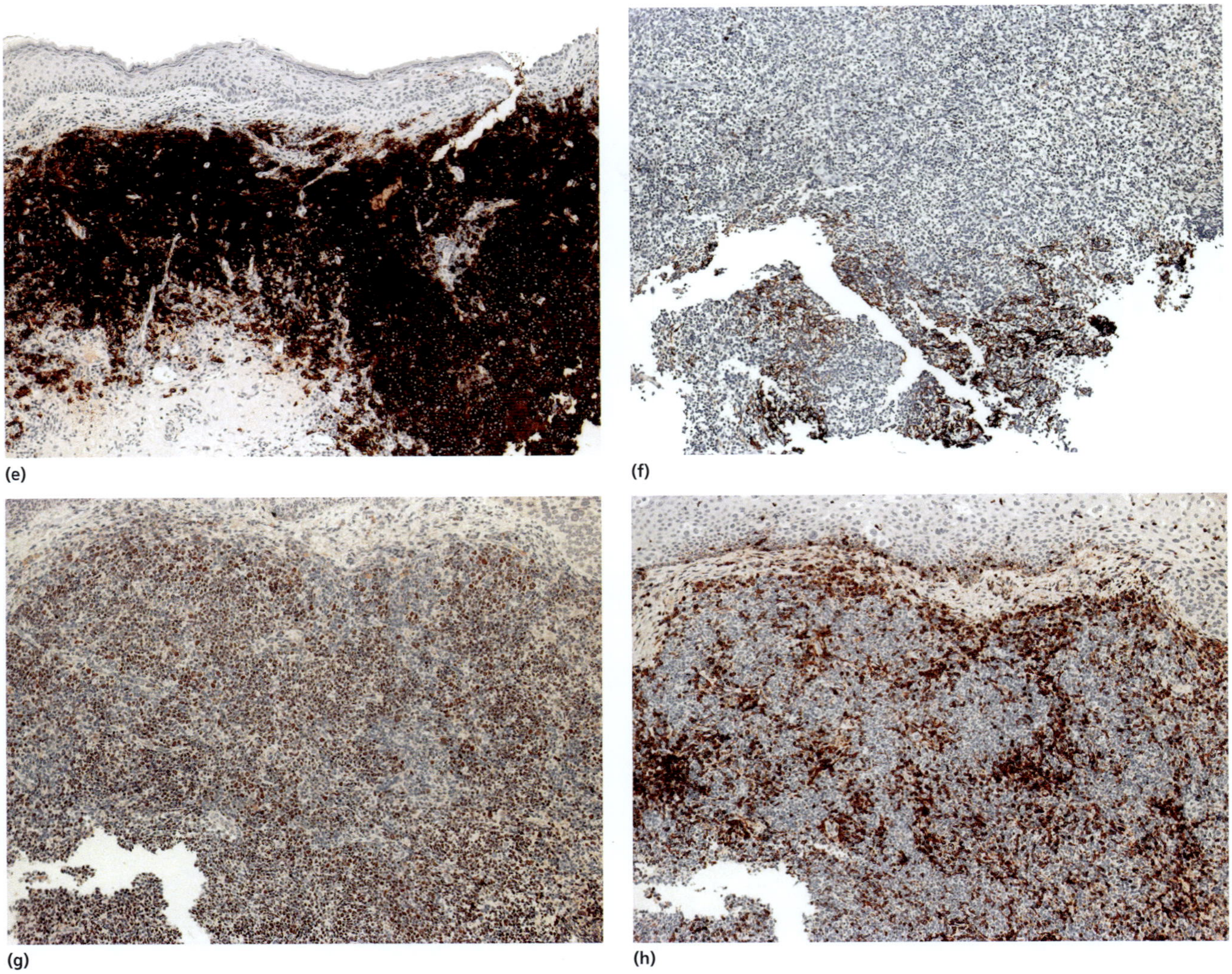


Figure 16.18 (Continued)

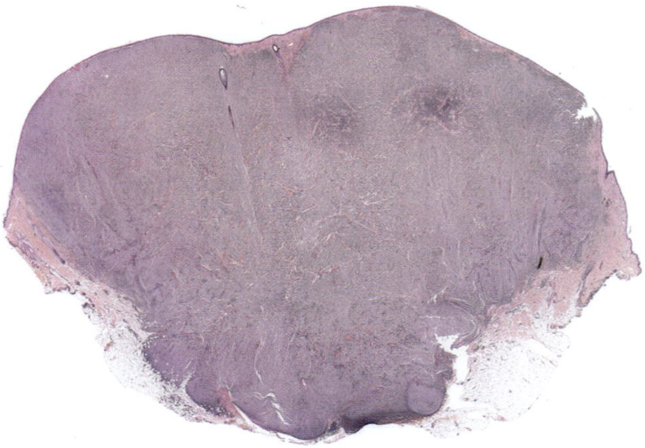

Figure 16.19 Cutaneous follicle center lymphoma, diffuse type. Dense nodular infiltrates within the entire dermis.

cleaved cells (centrocytes) admixed with a minority of rounded cells with large, vesicular nuclei and nucleoli located close to the nuclear membrane (centroblasts) (Fig. 16.20). It is crucial to underline that cases with a diffuse pattern of growth and predominance of centroblasts should be classified as diffuse large B-cell lymphoma, leg-type. Small reactive lymphocytes are almost invariably admixed with the tumor cells, mostly dispersed through the infiltrate. As already mentioned, follicular structures may be observed focally in some cases with a predominantly diffuse pattern of growth. In these cases, too, the follicles are usually irregular and display atypical features (Fig. 16.21). Sometimes both patterns of growth (diffuse and follicular) represent approximately equal parts of one and the same tumor (Fig. 16.22).

Early lesions of follicle center lymphoma, diffuse type, are composed of relatively small, dermal lymphoid aggregates.

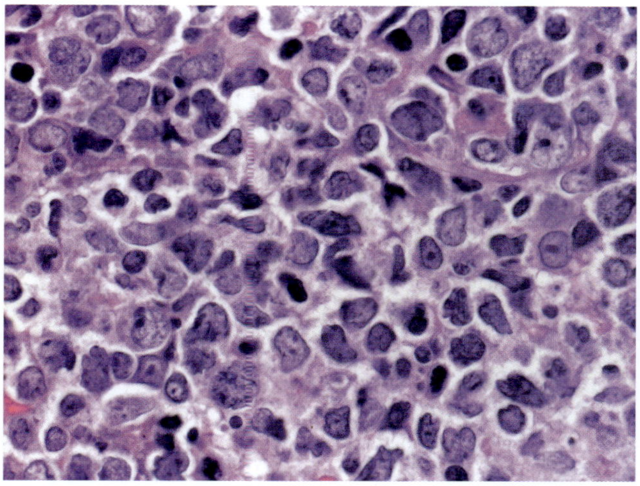

Figure 16.20 Cutaneous follicle center lymphoma, diffuse type. Medium-sized and large centrocytes predominate, admixed with some centroblasts.

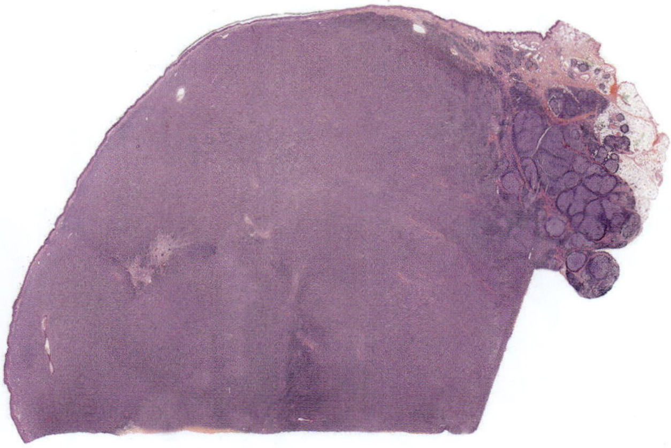

Figure 16.21 Cutaneous follicle center lymphoma, mainly diffuse type. The large, nodular area representing sheets of centrocytes admixed with some centroblasts, and a small area with neoplastic lymphoid follicles at the periphery of the lesion.

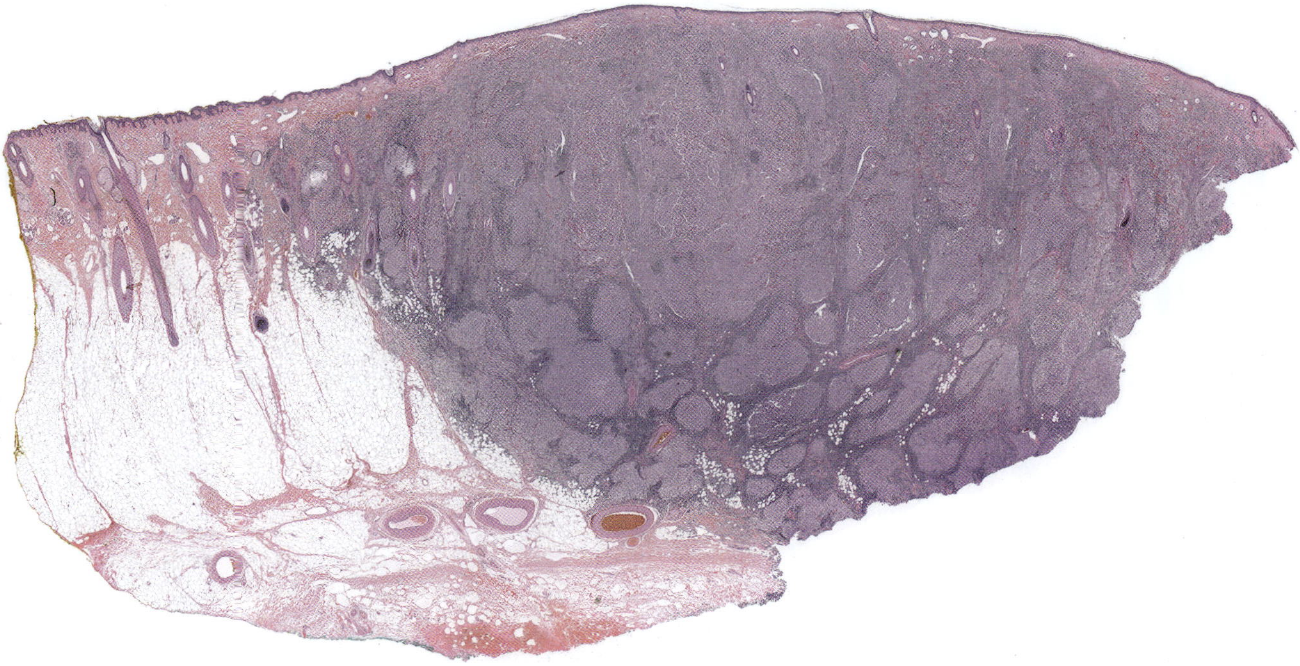

Figure 16.22 Cutaneous follicle center lymphoma, mixed follicular and diffuse type. Dense nodular infiltrates within the dermis and subcutaneous fat. Note large, irregular, confluent neoplastic follicles and a broad area with a diffuse pattern of growth.

There are variable numbers of medium and large cells, mostly showing morphologic features of centrocytes, admixed with many small reactive lymphocytes (Fig. 16.7) [14]. Clear-cut lymphoid follicles are not observed as a rule. This finding, together with the absence of follicular dendritic cells in about half of the specimens, suggests that at least some of the cases of early follicle center lymphoma, diffuse type, are characterized by a diffuse pattern of growth from the outset, never showing a clear-cut follicular arrangement [14].

A peculiar histopathologic variant of cutaneous follicle center lymphoma with a diffuse pattern of growth is characterized by diffuse infiltrates with predominance of spindle and bizarre

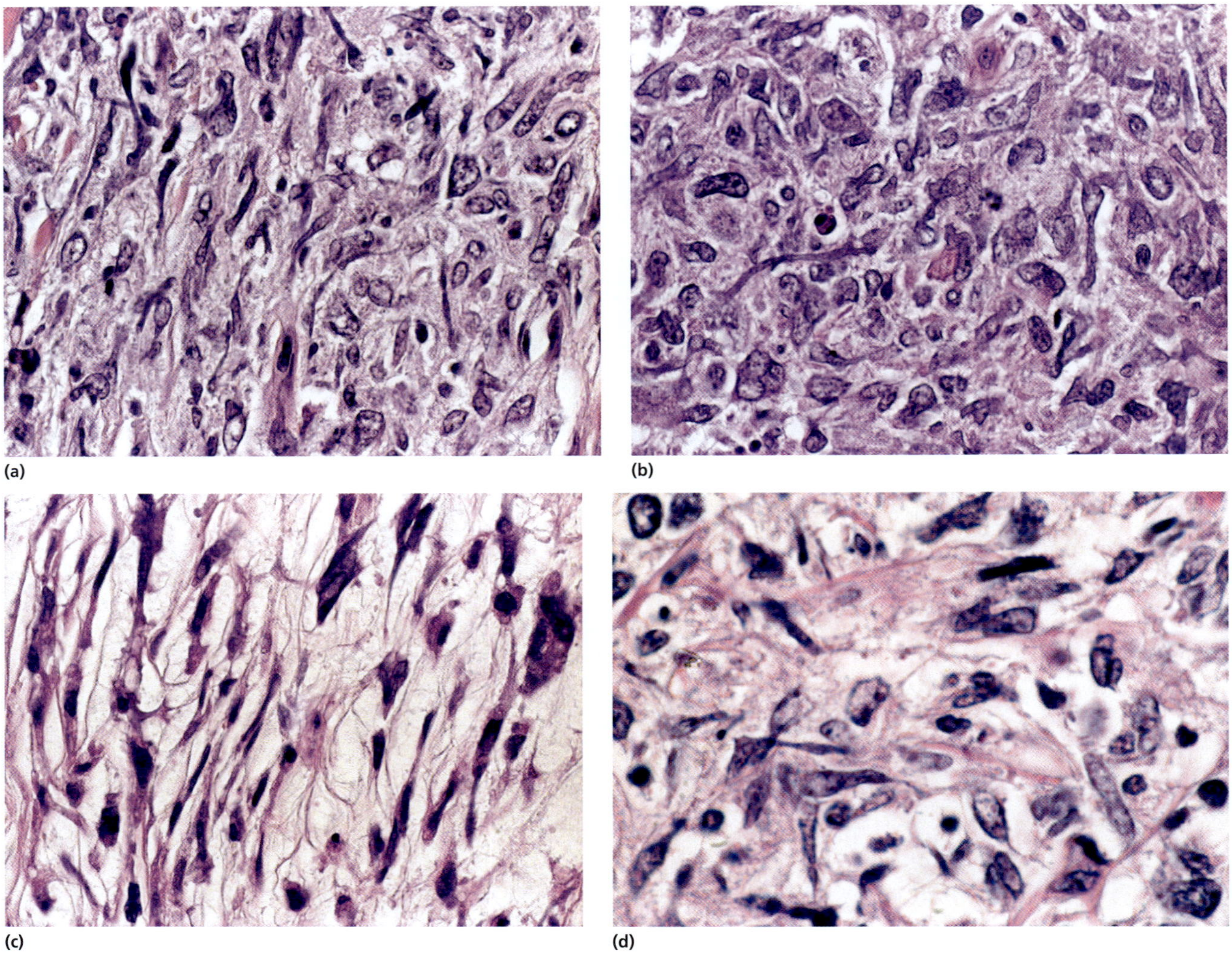

Figure 16.23 Cutaneous follicle center lymphoma, spindle cell variant. (a), (b), (c), and (d) show variations in the morphologic features of neoplastic cells, representing centrocytes with bizarre, elongated, partly spindled, twisted nuclei.

cells, and has been termed "***cutaneous spindle cell B-cell lymphoma***" or "cutaneous sarcomatoid B-cell lymphoma" (Fig. 16.23) [32–38]. The bizarre cells are centrocytes that show different sizes and shapes. The peculiar shapes of these cells are not due to drying or fixation artifacts (see Chapter 1), as they can be observed in otherwise impeccable specimens. Although these cases were previously interpreted as a variant of cutaneous diffuse large B-cell lymphoma, the vast majority of them represent examples of cutaneous follicle center lymphoma, diffuse type [34, 38], and have a gene signature of germinal center B-cells [39]. At extracutaneous sites, too, the spindle cell variant is characterized by genotypic and phenotypic markers of germinal center cell origin [40]. Sclerosis and myxoid areas may also be observed in cases of cutaneous follicle center lymphoma, particularly in the spindle cell variant of the disease (Figs. 16.24 and 16.25) [41]. Interestingly, variable numbers of spindle cells

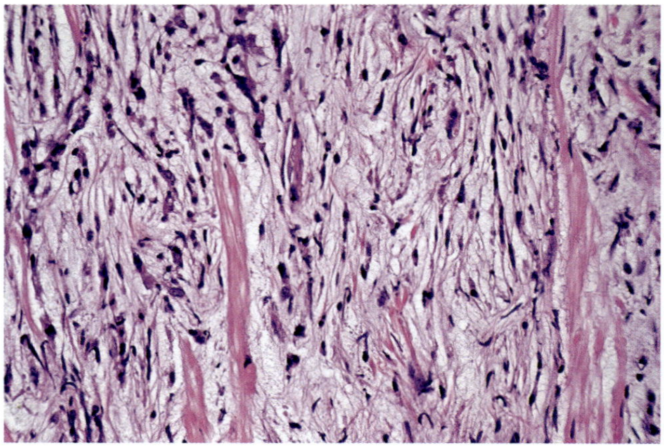

Figure 16.24 Cutaneous follicle center lymphoma, spindle cell variant. Proliferation of spindled lymphocytes within a myxoid stroma.

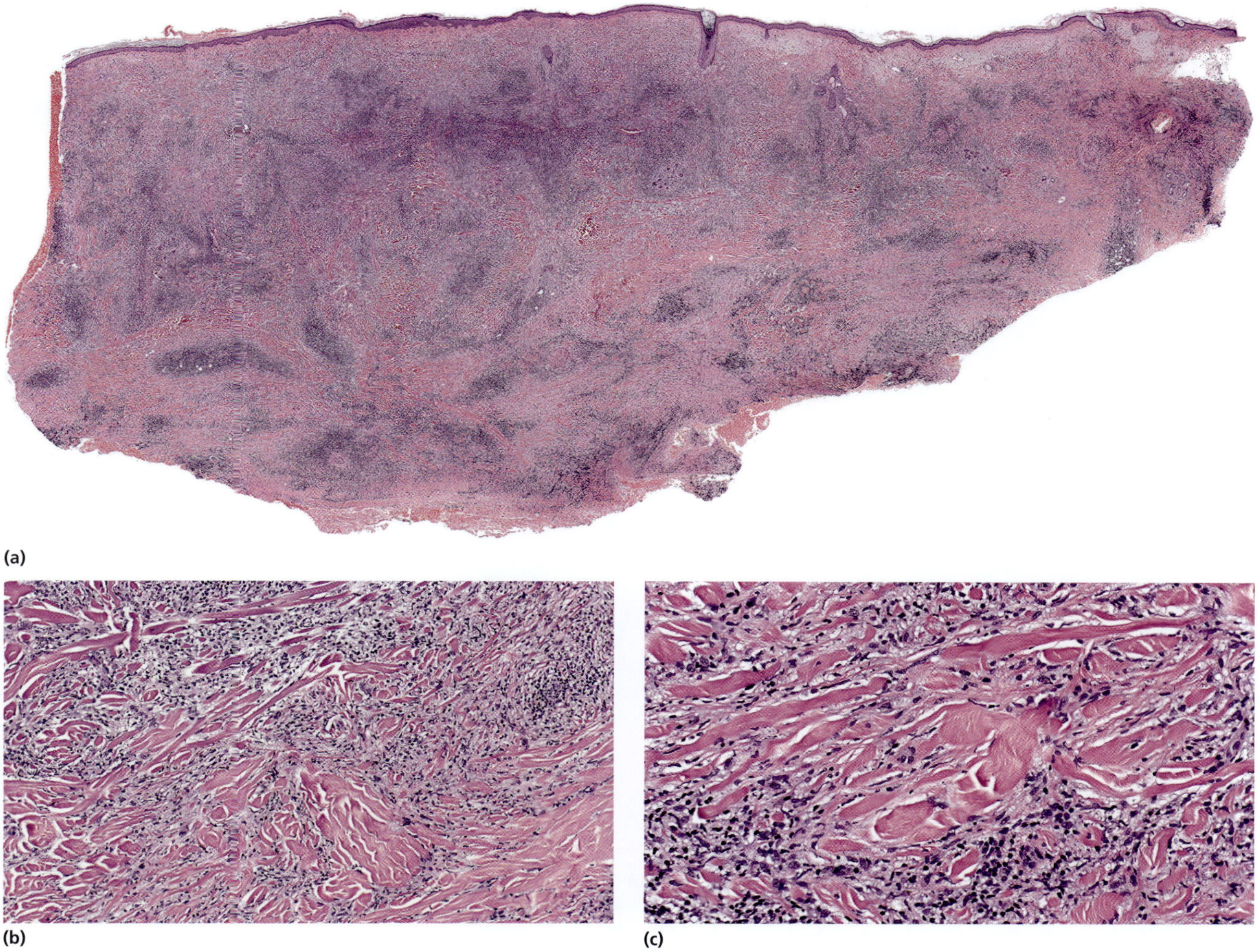


**Figure 16.25** Cutaneous follicle center lymphoma, spindle cell variant with sclerosis. (a) Diffuse infiltrate within the entire dermis with focal areas of sclerosis; (b, c) detail of spindled lymphocytes and sclerotic collagen bundles.

or cells with other bizarre morphology can be observed within neoplastic follicles of cutaneous follicle center lymphoma, follicular type as well, confirming that this shape represents a peculiar morphologic variation of the centrocytes (Fig. 16.26).

At sites other than the skin, cases of so-called ***T-cell/histiocyte-rich large B-cell lymphoma*** are classified as a specific entity of large B-cell lymphoma, but in my experience, cutaneous cases represent a variant of follicle center lymphoma (see Chapter 20). In this context, Hodgkin and Reed-Sternberg-like cells can be observed in cases of cutaneous follicle center lymphoma (Fig. 16.27) [42].

## Immunophenotype

In all variants of cutaneous follicle center lymphoma neoplastic cells are positive for B-cell markers, such as CD19, CD20, and CD79a, and for Bcl-6. There is no aberrant expression of CD5 or CD43 by the neoplastic B lymphocytes.

Follicular cells in cases with a ***follicular pattern of growth*** are positive for markers of germinal center cells such as CD10 and Bcl-6 (Fig. 16.28a and b) [43]. Staining for CD10 may be negative in some cases. The presence of small clusters of $CD10^+$ and/or $Bcl\text{-}6^+$ cells outside neoplastic follicles can be observed in a proportion of these cases. This phenomenon, caused by the active "migration" of neoplastic follicular cells from the follicle to the interfollicular area and back, has been described in nodal follicular lymphomas as well, and is not observed as a rule in reactive lymphoid infiltrates, thus being virtually diagnostic of follicle center lymphoma. A good diagnostic clue for cutaneous follicle center lymphoma with a follicular pattern is provided also by the staining for proliferating cells (Ki67/MIB-1). Reactive germinal centers show a high degree of proliferation (more than 90% of cells), whereas neoplastic follicles often show a proliferative fraction of less than 50% of the cells (Fig. 16.28c) [43]. A network of $CD21^+$ follicular dendritic cells is present in all cases

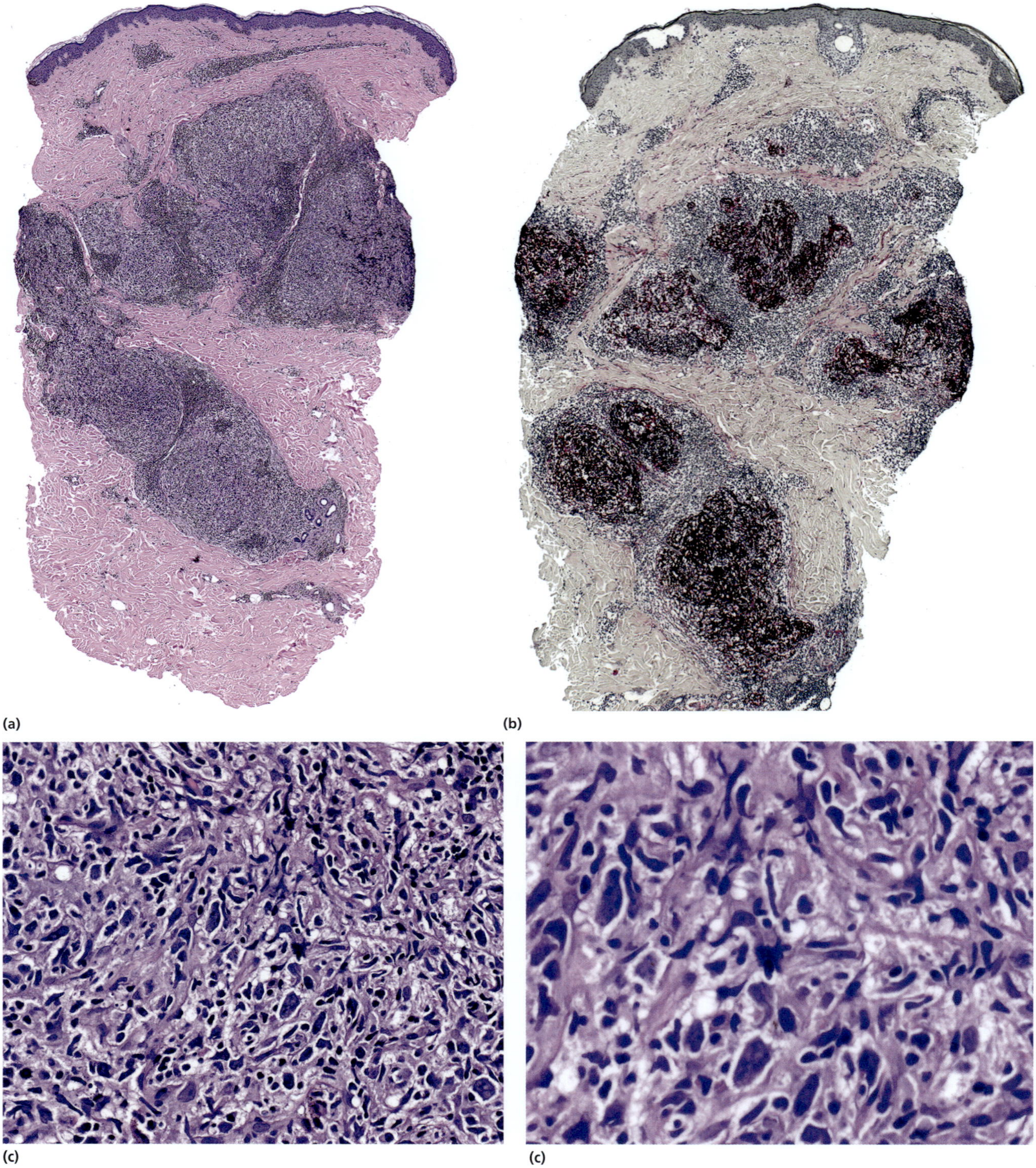


**Figure 16.26** Cutaneous follicle center lymphoma, a follicular variant with spindle cells. (a) Nodular infiltrate within the dermis with a follicular pattern. (b) Staining for CD21 confirms the presence of networks of follicular dendritic cells. (c, d) Detail of spindled and bizarre lymphocytes within the lymphoid follicles.

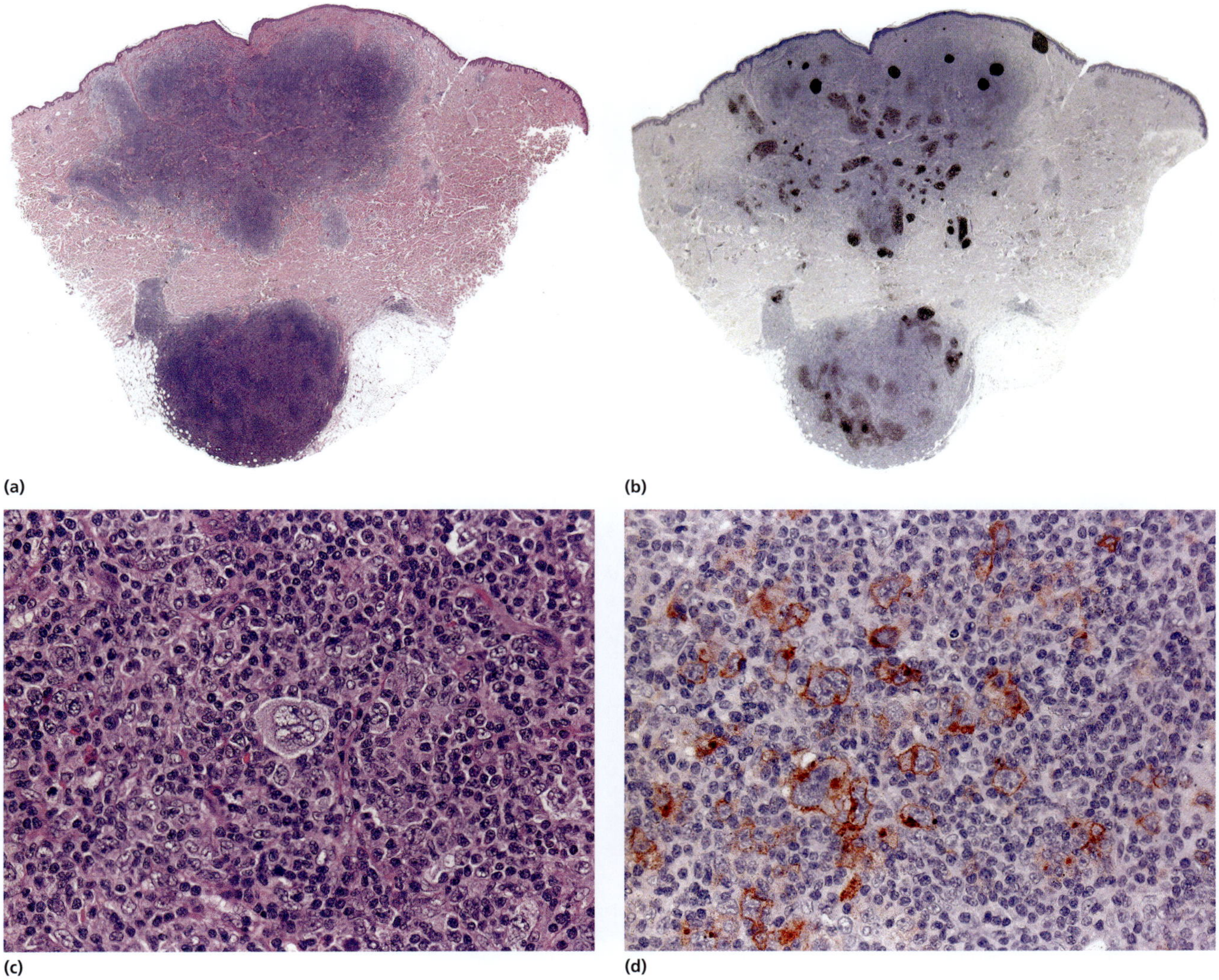


Figure 16.27 Cutaneous follicle center lymphoma, "Hodgkin type." (a) Nodular dermal lymphoid infiltrate extending to the subcutaneous fat in a 72-year-old man. (b) Lymphoid follicles outlined by the staining for CD21. (c) Some of the cells within the infiltrate had large, binucleated nuclei resembling Reed-Sternberg cells and (d) positive for CD30. In situ hybridization for EBV (EBER-1) was negative. Staging investigations were negative. This is an example of so-called "Hodgkin-like" cutaneous follicle center lymphoma. The presence of Reed-Sternberg-like and Hodgkin-like cells positive for CD30 may be misleading. Similar cases show overlapping histopathological features with cutaneous T-cell/histiocyte-rich large B-cell lymphoma, a type of lymphoma that in the skin in my opinion represents a variant of the follicle center lymphoma (see Chapter 20).

with follicular patterns. In lesions showing a mixed pattern (follicular and diffuse), $CD21^+$ follicular dendritic cells are usually located at the periphery of large areas with a diffuse pattern of growth (Fig. 16.29). CD23 and CD30 may be positive within neoplastic cells (Fig. 16.30, Fig. 16.31).

Although conflicting statements have been proposed, analysis of published reports shows that Bcl-2 expression can be found only in a minority of cases of primary cutaneous follicle center lymphoma [43–45]. The pattern of Bcl-2 negativity in cutaneous follicle center lymphoma is variable from negativity in virtually all neoplastic cells (Fig. 16.32a) to the presence of a minority of weakly positive cells (Fig. 16.32b). Only very rarely Bcl-2 is positive in the whole neoplastic population, akin to what is observed in nodal cases. On the other hand, when present Bcl-2 positivity in lymphoid follicles is virtually diagnostic of follicle center lymphoma and rules out a reactive process (Fig. 16.33). It should be underlined that the follicular mantle is always $Bcl\text{-}2^+$, and that only the expression within germinal center cells should be considered as evidence of malignancy. Positivity for Bcl-2 is not synonymous with cutaneous spread by nodal lymphoma, but positive cases should be staged very carefully. On the other hand, the intensity of Bcl-2

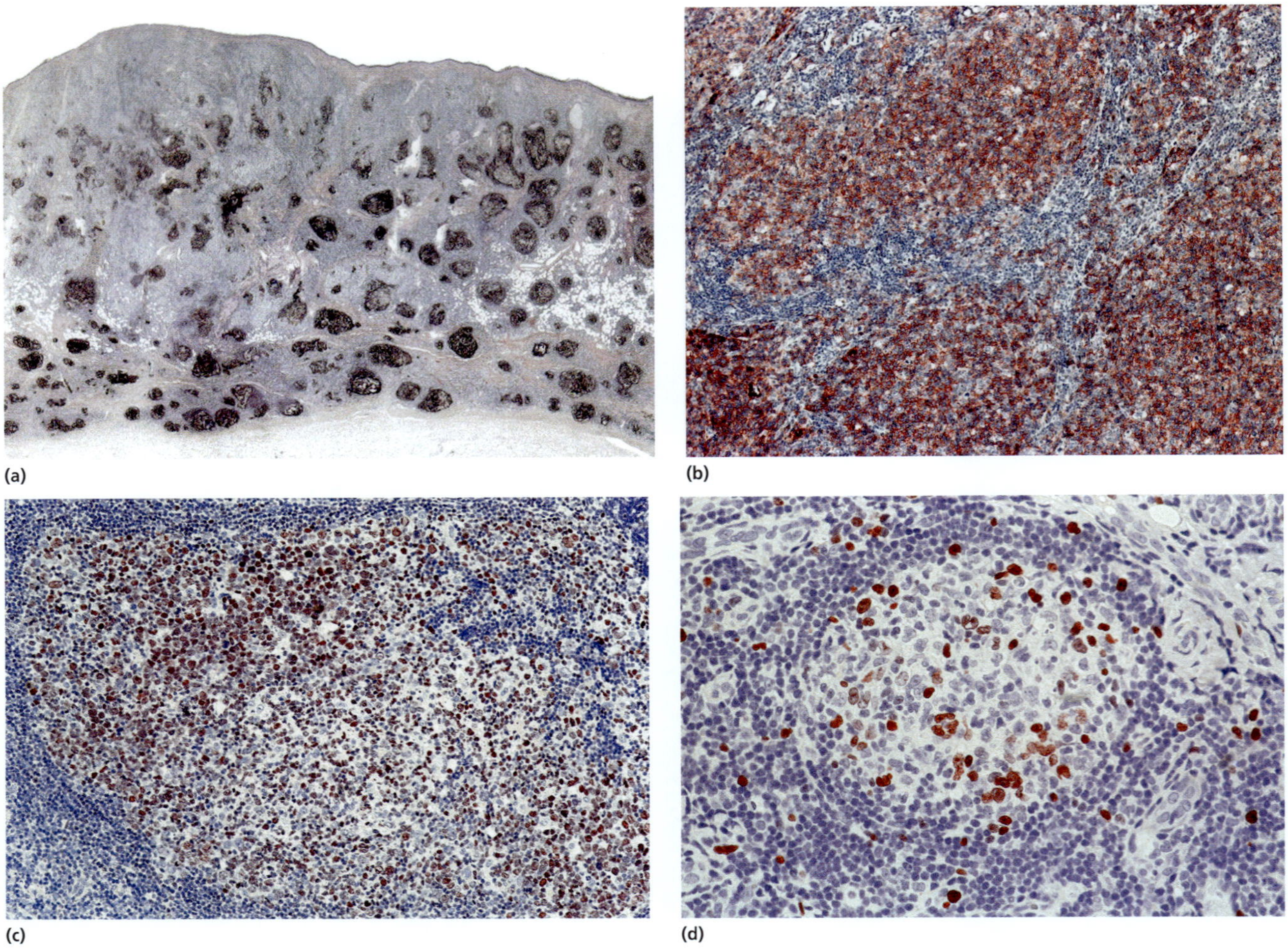


**Figure 16.28** Cutaneous follicle center lymphoma, follicular type. (a) Follicular pattern outlined by the CD21 staining. Neoplastic follicles stain for (b) CD10 and (c) Bcl-6; note CD10⁺ as well as Bcl-6⁺ cells extending beyond the follicles. (d) Markedly reduced proliferation rate within a neoplastic follicle detected by Ki-67 staining. In spite of the small size and regular shape of the follicle, this pattern of Ki-67 is inconsistent with a reactive germinal center and diagnostic of follicular lymphoma.

expression has been evaluated as the most useful single criterion for differentiating between primary cutaneous and secondary cutaneous follicle center lymphomas [46]. Cases of cutaneous follicle center lymphoma positive for Bcl-2 may harbor *BCL2* gene breaks and may present a 1p36 deletion [47].

Cases showing a ***diffuse pattern of growth*** are positive for Bcl-6, mostly negative for CD10, and consistently negative for Bcl-2. The multiple myeloma oncogene-1 (MUM-1) is positive only in a minority of cells (<30%) in cutaneous follicle center lymphoma (Fig. 16.34a) [48]. In rare cases, the percentage of positive cells may be higher (Fig. 16.34b), but the homogeneous positivity observed in diffuse large B-cell lymphoma, leg type, is never found. Negativity for Bcl-2 and MUM-1 represents the most important criterion for differentiation of cutaneous follicle center lymphoma, diffuse type, from cutaneous diffuse large B-cell lymphoma, leg type (see also the section on differential diagnosis of cutaneous follicle center lymphoma, diffuse type, from cutaneous diffuse large B-cell lymphoma, leg type, in this chapter). Forkhead box protein 1 (FOX-P1) and IgM are negative. Early lesions of follicle center lymphoma, diffuse type, are characterized by small, irregular clusters of cells positive for Bcl-6 and negative for Bcl-2 and MUM-1, often arranged at the periphery of the lymphoid infiltrates (Fig. 16.35). Although there are no recognizable follicles, irregular clusters of CD21⁺ cells can be found focally in about half of the cases. The presence of Bcl-6⁺ clusters without a recognizable follicular structure is strongly suggestive of cutaneous follicle center lymphoma, as they are never encountered in reactive infiltrates or in other types of low-grade cutaneous B-cell lymphoma. It should be underlined that scattered Bcl-6⁺ cells within an infiltrate (not

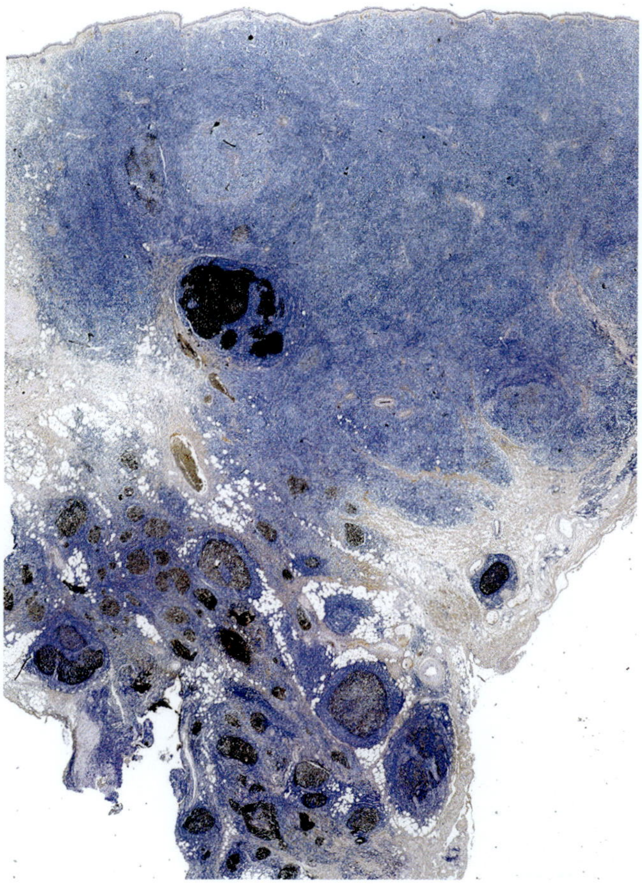

**Figure 16.29** Cutaneous follicle center lymphoma, mixed follicular and diffuse. Clusters of CD21⁺ follicular dendritic cells are arranged predominantly at the periphery of the lesion.

arranged in clusters) usually represent T follicular helper lymphocytes and should not be misinterpreted as follicular B cells.

Besides Bcl-6 and CD10, other markers can be used in order to confirm germinal center differentiation of neoplastic cells in all variants of cutaneous follicle center lymphoma. Paired box gene (PAX)-5 and interferon regulatory factor (IRF)8 are usually expressed, but other B cells are positive as well. Human germinal center-associated lymphoma (HGAL) and LIM-only transcription factor 2 – LMO2 have been reported as useful markers for the detection of the interfollicular and diffuse components [49]. In my experience, these markers do not offer information beyond that provided by Bcl-6, but may be helpful in cases with equivocal Bcl-6 staining.

The proliferation index (as detected by staining for Ki-67) is usually high in the diffuse type of cutaneous follicle center lymphoma. It has been suggested that a lower index may be a sign of a secondary cutaneous infiltration by nodal follicle center lymphoma [50], but this should be confirmed by additional data.

In cutaneous follicle center lymphoma, the detection of an immunoglobulin (Ig) light chain restriction is difficult in paraffin sections, but can be observed on snap-frozen tissue sections. As already mentioned, rarely a monoclonal population of plasma cells belonging to the same neoplastic clone as the follicular cells may be observed. Care should be taken to distinguish these cases from cutaneous marginal zone lymphoproliferative disorder, where monoclonal expression of Ig light chain kappa or lambda represents the most useful diagnostic criterion (see Chapter 17). Expression of 4 antigens (LMO2, HGAL, stathmin 1 – STMN1, and activation-induced cytidine deaminase – AID) has been suggested helpful in this differentiation (positive in cutaneous follicle center lymphoma

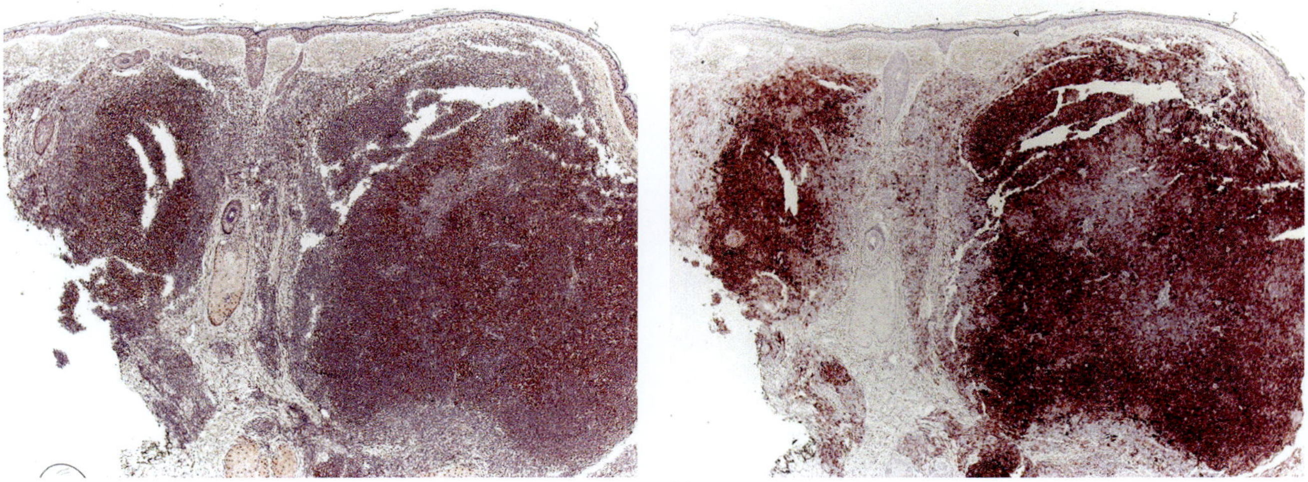

(a) (b)

**Figure 16.30** Cutaneous follicle center lymphoma, follicular type. Neoplastic cells are positive for (a) Bcl-6 and (b) CD23.

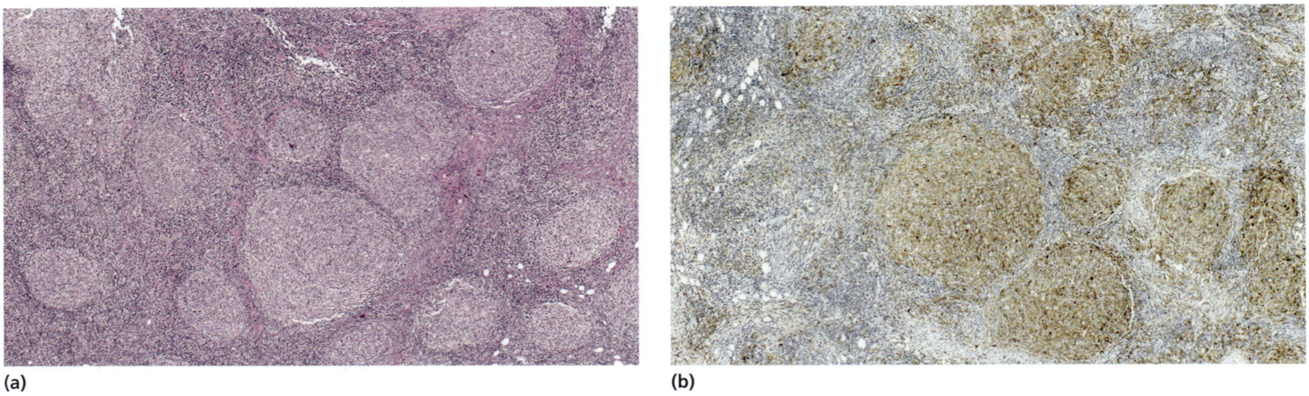

Figure 16.31 Cutaneous follicle center lymphoma, follicular type. (a) Atypical lymphoid follicles with lack of mantle zone, tingible body macrophages, and polarization; (b) Neoplastic cells are positive for CD30.

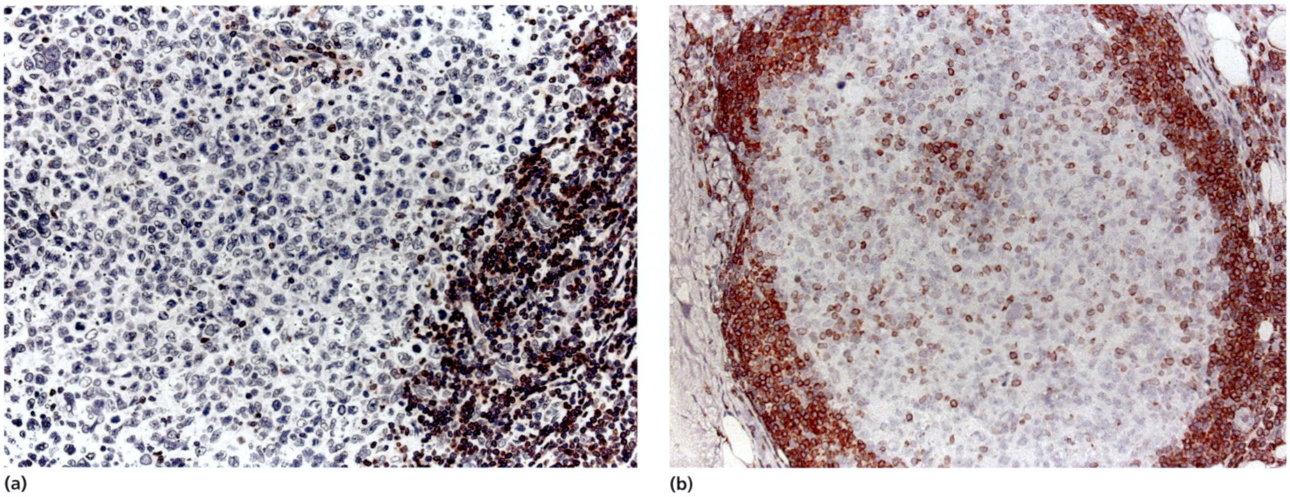

Figure 16.32 Cutaneous follicle center lymphoma, follicular type. (a) Neoplastic cells are completely negative for Bcl-2. Note positive small lymphocytes at the edge of the neoplastic aggregate representing positive internal controls. (b) Weak positivity of a few neoplastic lymphocytes (cells with strong positivity represent reactive lymphocytes).

and negative in cutaneous marginal zone lymphoproliferative disorder) [51]. In my experience, the distinction of cutaneous follicle center lymphoma from cutaneous marginal zone lymphoproliferative disorder is usually straightforward. However, I have seen cases classified initially as cutaneous marginal zone lymphoproliferative disorder and later reclassified as cutaneous follicle center lymphoma in biopsies of recurrent lesions. This is particularly true for cases classified based on small, partial biopsies (especially punch biopsies), in which only a small part of the entire infiltrate is visible on the biopsy specimen.

PD-1$^{+}$ reactive T lymphocytes have been observed in a proportion of cases of cutaneous follicle center lymphoma and less frequently in cutaneous marginal zone lymphoproliferative disorder (neoplastic cells are negative with this marker in both conditions) [52], but in my experience, this marker does not play a role in the differential diagnosis between the two diseases.

## Molecular genetics

Cutaneous follicle center lymphoma shows a monoclonal rearrangement of the Ig genes in the majority of cases. Analysis of the molecular clones in different biopsies taken from various skin sites of involvement or at the same cutaneous site at different time points showed that the same clone is present in most cases [48]. However, in a small percentage of patients different clones were detected in different specimens, suggesting the possibility that these cases represent multiple, unrelated primary cutaneous follicle center lymphomas [53]. Somatic hypermutations resulting in clonal evolution represent an alternative, more plausible explanation of this finding [54].

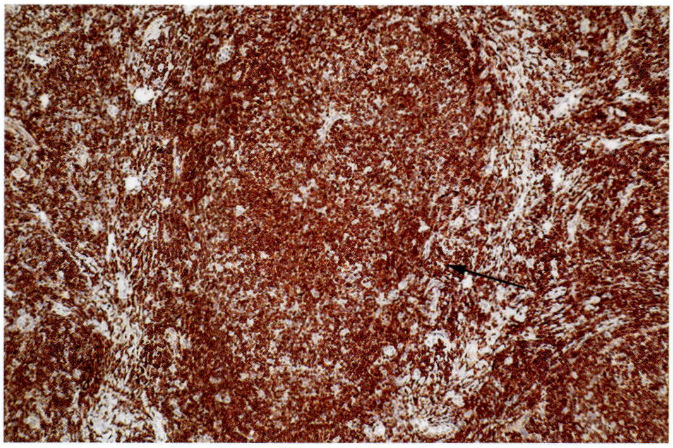

Figure 16.33 Cutaneous follicle center lymphoma, follicular type. A lymphoid follicle positive for Bcl-2 (arrow); note positivity of all reactive lymphocytes as well (mantle zone, perifollicular lymphocytes). Positivity of lymphocytes of a lymphoid follicle for Bcl-2 is diagnostic of follicular lymphoma and is found more frequently in secondary cutaneous involvement by nodal follicular lymphoma, but may be observed rarely in primary cutaneous cases as well.

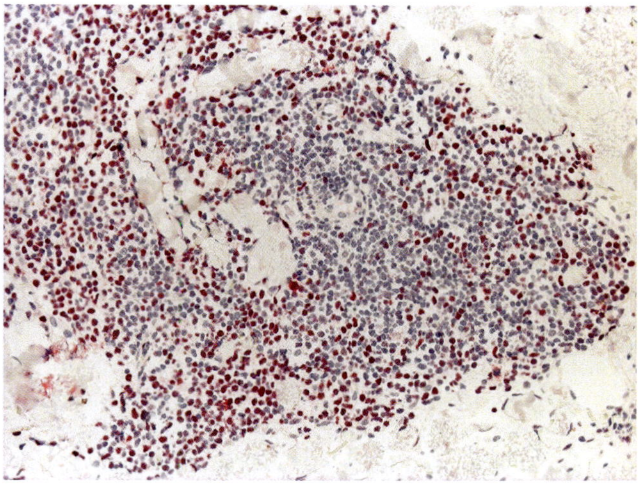

Figure 16.35 Cutaneous follicle center lymphoma, diffuse type. Early lesion showing clusters of Bcl-6⁺ cells without the background of a lymphoid follicle. This pattern is virtually diagnostic of cutaneous follicle center lymphoma.

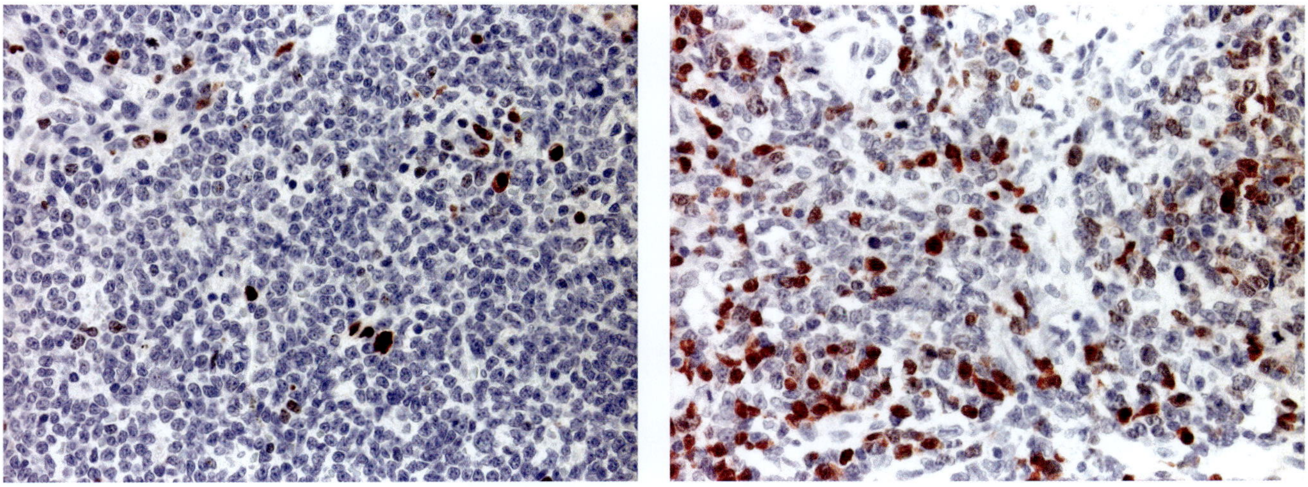

(a) (b)

Figure 16.34 Cutaneous follicle center lymphoma, diffuse type. (a) Staining for MUM-1 shows only a few positive cells. (b) In another case positivity for MUM-1 is found in a distinct proportion of the cells but not in the majority of them. Both staining patterns may be seen in cutaneous follicle center lymphoma, in contrast to the positivity of most cells found in cases of cutaneous diffuse large B-cell lymphoma, leg type.

Analysis of data from the literature clearly shows that the interchromosomal (14;18) translocation is extremely uncommon in primary cutaneous follicle center lymphoma, although the frequency varies in different studies (depending also on the method used for detection) [43, 44, 55]. It should be reminded that t(14;18)-negative cases of follicular lymphoma can be observed also in the lymph nodes, and may represent a distinct subgroup of nodal follicular lymphoma [56]. Analysis of nodal t(14;18)-negative cases revealed rearrangement of *BCL6* in about one-third of them [57], whereas this rearrangement is negative in cutaneous cases [58]. Interestingly, genetic studies on nodal t(14;18)-positive and negative cases revealed that t(14;18)-positive cases show the signature of germinal center B cells, whereas activated B-cell-like, NFκB, proliferation, and bystander cell signatures were increased in t(14;18)-negative cases [59]. These signatures are different from the germinal center cell one observed in cutaneous cases of follicle center lymphoma, again pointing at different genetic backgrounds between cutaneous and nodal diseases. In addition, some commonly mutated genes in nodal follicular lymphoma

(*KMT2D*, *CREBBP*, and *BCL2*) are significantly less commonly mutated in cutaneous follicle center cell lymphoma [58]. A t(12;21)(q13;q22) has been detected in one case of cutaneous follicle center lymphoma [60].

Gene expression studies using cDNA microarrays revealed that cases of cutaneous follicle center lymphoma have a germinal center cell signature and show hypermutated Ig variable genes with frequent use of the VH1-69 and VH4-59 segments and amplification of *REL* [61–63]. The genetic signature is similar in cases with different patterns of growth (follicular or diffuse).

Differential expression of a group of genes involved in the regulation of lymphopoiesis and malignant transformation (polycomb group) was found in cutaneous B-cell lymphomas arising on the head and trunk as opposed to those located on the legs, confirming that these lymphomas represent distinct entities [64].

## Differential diagnosis of cutaneous follicle center lymphoma, diffuse type, from cutaneous diffuse large B-cell lymphoma, leg type

Cutaneous follicle center lymphoma, diffuse type, and cutaneous diffuse large B-cell lymphoma, leg type, are both characterized by a predominant population of large B lymphocytes, thus creating problems in the precise classification. Morphologically, the diffuse type of cutaneous follicle center lymphoma shows predominance of large cleaved lymphocytes (centrocytes), in contrast to cutaneous diffuse large B-cell lymphoma, leg type, where large round cells (centroblasts and particularly immunoblasts) are the majority [48]. Immunohistology reveals negativity for Bcl-2, MUM-1, cytoplasmic IgM, MYC, and FOX-P1 in cutaneous follicle center lymphoma, as opposed to positivity for these markers in the vast majority of cases of cutaneous diffuse large B-cell lymphoma, leg type [48, 65a]. One study suggested that cytoplasmic positivity for IgM in otherwise conventional cutaneous follicle center lymphoma may be associated with more frequent extracutaneous dissemination [65b]. Markers of germinal center cells such as Bcl-6 and less frequently CD10 are positive in cutaneous follicle center lymphoma, but may also be positive in diffuse large B-cell lymphoma, leg type, thus not providing helpful clues for the differential diagnosis. Molecular studies showed that neoplastic cells in the two subgroups have different gene signatures (cutaneous follicle center lymphoma: germinal center cell signature; and cutaneous diffuse large B-cell lymphoma, leg type: activated B-lymphocyte signature) [62]. Expression of p63 has been proposed as another useful marker in differentiating between cutaneous follicle center lymphoma (rarely positive) and diffuse large B-cell lymphoma, leg-type (positive in the majority of cases) [66]. In contrast to diffuse large B-cell lymphoma, leg-type, cutaneous follicle center lymphoma does not show *MYD88*$^{L265P}$ gene mutations.

It should be noted that rare cases of cutaneous follicle center lymphoma, diffuse type, arising on the legs have a bad prognosis, similar to that of cutaneous diffuse large B-cell lymphoma, leg type [48, 67]. The reason for this peculiar behavior is currently unclear. It may be that, in spite of predominant large cleaved morphology and/or negativity for Bcl-2, MUM-1, and FOX-P1, these rare cases represent in fact morphologic and/or phenotypic variations of diffuse large B-cell lymphoma, leg type. Be that as it may, patients with cutaneous follicle center lymphoma arising on the legs should be managed with the greatest caution.

## Treatment

The best treatment for patients with cutaneous follicle center lymphoma is still a matter of debate. Most experts agree that aggressive strategies such as systemic chemotherapy should be reserved only for cases with extracutaneous involvement or with untreatable, generalized cutaneous disease (cases with generalized cutaneous disease, however, are very rare). A watchful waiting strategy may be considered, as the prognosis is excellent.

Local radiotherapy is still considered the first-line treatment [68–72], but some data question the validity of this approach, particularly for lesions located on the back (see the section on clinical features above in this chapter) [14]. Local radiotherapy is the best modality for solitary or clustered tumors, but relapses may occur even in this setting [73]. Surgical excision may also be considered for solitary lesions. Recommendations from the EORTC cutaneous lymphoma tumor group for radiation therapy have been published recently [74]. The anti-CD20 monoclonal antibody (rituximab) has been used both systemically and intralesionally with good results [75–77], but in my experience, recurrences are frequent when patients are treated with rituximab alone (recurrences in these cases may be CD20-negative). Rituximab can also be combined with systemic chemotherapy in patients with generalized skin or extracutaneous involvement and can be conjugated with radionuclides in order to provide selective irradiation of tumor cells. A short rituximab-lenalidomide regimen improved the complete remission rate and progression-free survival in untreated symptomatic follicular lymphomas of the lymph nodes [78].

Topical therapies such as corticosteroids, nitrogen mustard, imiquimod, or cryosurgery seem to be of limited value. Interferon-α (either systemically or intralesionally) has been used in the past for the treatment of patients with cutaneous follicle center lymphoma, sometimes associated with other treatment regimens [71], but is not considered an alternative option in actual guidelines.

It has been suggested that disrupting the crosstalk between malignant B cells and accessory cells may be a novel strategy for treating low-grade B-cell malignancies (irrespective of the site of origin) [79], but at present, there are no data on this approach for cutaneous follicle center lymphomas or other low-grade B-cell lymphomas of the skin.

## Prognosis

The prognosis of patients with primary cutaneous follicle center lymphoma is very good, regardless of the pattern of growth [1, 36, 58, 80–82]. In many cases, lesions grow slowly over years or decades and only seldom spread to extracutaneous sites (Fig. 16.36). Although local recurrences can be observed in a distinct proportion of patients, extracutaneous involvement is uncommon. Involvement of the central nervous system has been observed rarely [83]. Progression to extracutaneous disease seems to be more common in cases harboring a *BCL2* rearrangement [84], and expression of Bcl-2 protein is more common in cases showing cutaneous recurrences after treatment [85].

In exceptional cases, in spite of the absence of extracutaneous spread, local growth of tumors located on the scalp may cause infiltration of the underlying bone structures with osseous erosion and consequent meningeal exposure [86].

A prognostic index based on elevated LDH, number of lesions >2, and presence of nodular lesions has been suggested for indolent cutaneous B-cell lymphomas (cutaneous lymphomas prognostic index – CLIPi) [87]. However, in my experience the presence of more than two lesions and/or of nodular lesions does not have any impact on behavior; thus I do not think that this index adds any new information concerning the prognosis of indolent cutaneous B-cell lymphomas, including cutaneous follicle center lymphoma.

As already mentioned, it is important to underline the fact that rare cases of follicle center lymphoma presenting clinically with lesions located on the legs and histopathologically with a diffuse pattern of growth characterized by predominance of large centrocytes may have a worse prognosis, and should probably be managed as diffuse large B-cell lymphoma, leg type [48, 67].

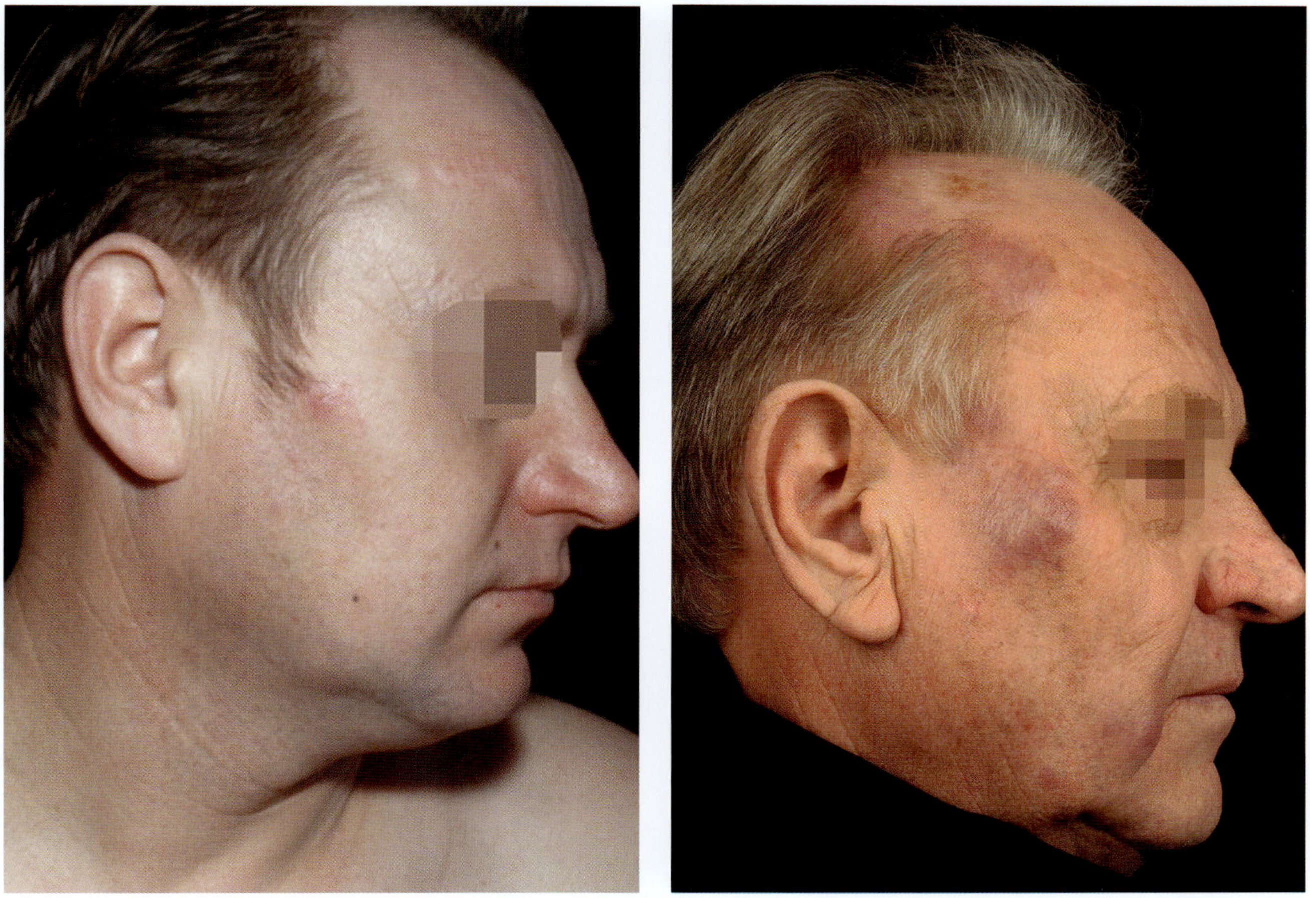

(a) (b)

Figure 16.36 Natural history of cutaneous follicle center lymphoma. (a) This patient presented for the first time in 1978 at the age of 38 with a preauricular infiltrated plaque; according to the patient the lesion was present for >10 years. The patient refused treatment. He presented again in 1985, 1999, and (b) 2009 with persistent disease (31 years after the first presentation and >40 years after the onset of the first lesion). Local radiotherapy in 1985 was the only treatment he had accepted.

## Résumé

**Cutaneous follicle center lymphoma**

| | | |
|---|---|---|
| **Clinical** | Adults. Solitary or grouped papules, plaques, and tumors, often surrounded by erythematous patches. Broad, indurated erythema or alopecia in some cases. Preferential locations: scalp, back (Crosti lymphoma). | |
| **Morphology** | Nodular or diffuse infiltrates characterized by predominance of centrocytes admixed with some centroblasts and with small lymphocytes. The pattern of growth can be follicular, diffuse, or mixed. Cases with a diffuse pattern of growth and predominance of centroblasts should be classified as diffuse large B-cell lymphoma. | |
| **Immunohistochemistry** | CD19, CD20, CD79a | + |
| | Bcl-6 | + |
| | CD10 | –(+) |
| | IgM, MYC, FOX-P1 | – |
| | Bcl-2 | –(+) |
| | CD5, CD43 | – |
| | MUM-1 | – (a minority of cells may be positive) |
| | Ki67 | Reduced proliferation of neoplastic follicles; high proliferation in the diffuse variant. |
| **Genetics** | Monoclonal rearrangement of the Ig genes detected in the majority of cases; t(14;18) absent in most cases. Germinal center cell signature of neoplastic cells. | |
| **Treatment guidelines** | Watchful waiting; surgical excision; local radiotherapy; rituximab. Systemic chemotherapy is reserved for generalized lesions and/or extracutaneous spread. | |

## References


1. Willemze R, Cerroni L, Kempf W, *et al.* The 2018 update of the WHO-EORTC classification for primary cutaneous lymphomas. *Blood* 2019;**133**:1703–1714.
2. Kempf W, Mitteldorf C, Cerroni L, *et al.* Classifications of cutaneous lymphomas and lymphoproliferative disorders: an update from the EORTC cutaneous lymphoma histopathology group. *J Eur Acad Dermatol Venereol* 2024;**38**:1491–1503.
3. Goodlad JR, Rosen ST. Primary cutaneous follicle center lymphoma. In: Arber DA, Borowitz MJ, Cook JR, *et al.*, eds. *The International Consensus Classification of Myeloid and Lymphoid Neoplasms.* Philadelphia (US): Wolters Kluver, 2025: 446–449.
4. Louissaint A Jr, Santucci M, Jansen PM, *et al.* Primary cutaneous follicle centre lymphoma. In: *WHO Classification of Tumours Editorial Board. Haematolymphoid Tumours.* 5th edition. Lyon (France): IARC, 2024: 440–442.
5. Aigner F, Korol D, Schmitt AM, *et al.* Extranodal diffuse large B cell lymphoma of cutaneous follicle centre lymphoma type: a study of 24 patients with non-cutaneous primary limited stage extranodal diffuse large B cell lymphoma in support of a new concept. *Histopathology* 2012;**60**:774–784.
6. Senff NJ, Kluin-Nelemans JC, Willemze R. Results of bone marrow examination in 275 patients with histological features that suggest an indolent type of cutaneous B-cell lymphoma. *Br J Haematol* 2008;**142**:52–56.
7. Vachhani P, Neppalli VT, Cancino CJ, *et al.* Radiological imaging and bone marrow biopsy in staging of cutaneous B-cell lymphoma. *Br J Haematol* 2019;**184**:674–676.
8. Olsen EA, Whittaker S, Willemze R, *et al.* Primary cutaneous lymphoma: recommendations for clinical trial design and staging update from the ISCL, USCLC, and EORTC. *Blood* 2022;**140**:419–437.
9. National Comprehensive Cancer Network. Primary Cutaneous Lymphomas (Version 3.2025). Accessed September 15, 2025. https://www.nccn.org/professionals/physician_gls/pdf/primary_cutaneous.pdf
10. West DS, Dogan A, Quint PS, *et al.* Clonally related follicular lymphomas and Langerhans cell neoplasms – expanding the spectrum of transdifferentiation. *Am J Surg Pathol* 2013;**37**:978–986.
11. Ghislanzoni M, Gambini D, Perrone T, *et al.* Primary cutaneous follicular center cell lymphoma of the nose with maxillary sinus involvement in a pediatric patient. *J Am Acad Dermatol* 2005;**52**:s73–s75.
12. Amitay-Laish I, Feinmesser M, Ben-Amitai D, *et al.* Juvenile onset of primary low-grade cutaneous B-cell lymphoma. *Br J Dermatol* 2009;**161**:140–147.
13. Berti E, Alessi E, Caputo R, *et al.* Reticulohistiocytoma of the dorsum. *J Am Acad Dermatol* 1988;**19**:259–272.
14. Gulia A, Saggini A, Wiesner T, *et al.* Clinicopathologic features of early lesions of primary cutaneous follicle center lymphoma, diffuse type: implications for early diagnosis and treatment. *J Am Acad Dermatol* 2011;**65**:991–1000.
15. Kliuk J, Charles-Holmes R, Carr RA. Primary cutaneous follicle centre cell lymphoma of the scalp presenting with scarring alopecia. *Br J Dermatol* 2011;**165**:205–207.
16. Massone C, Fink-Puches R, Cerroni L. Atypical clinical presentation of primary and secondary cutaneous follicle center lymphoma (FCL) on the head characterized by macular lesions. *J Am Acad Dermatol* 2016;**75**:1000–1006.
17. Massone C, Fink-Puches R, Laimer M, *et al.* Miliary and agminated-type primary cutaneous follicle center lymphoma: report of 18 cases. *J Am Acad Dermatol* 2011;**65**:749–755.
18. Barzilai A, Feuerman H, Quaglino P, *et al.* Cutaneous B-cell neoplasms mimicking granulomatous rosacea or rhinophyma. *Arch Dermatol* 2012;**148**:824–831.
19. Aventin DL, Garcia M, Pedro C, *et al.* Miliary and agminated papules as clinical presentation of a secondary cutaneous follicular lymphoma. *J Am Acad Dermatol* 2012;**67**:e195–e196.
20. Sahil M, Prins C, Kaya G, *et al.* Unusual clinical presentation of a follicular lymphoma. *Rev Med Suisse* 2014;**10**:744–748.

21. Hodak E, Feuerman H, Barzilai A, *et al.* Anetodermic primary cutaneous B-cell lymphoma: a unique clinicopathological presentation of lymphoma possibly associated with antiphospholipid antibodies. *Arch Dermatol* 2010;**146**:175–182.
22. Bachmeyer C, Khosrotehrani K, Moguelet P, Aractingi S. Primary cutaneous follicular B-cell lymphoma arising at the site of radiotherapy for breast cancer. *Br J Dermatol* 2006;**156**:198–199.
23. Cerroni L, Zöchling N, Pütz B, Kerl H. Infection by Borrelia burgdorferi and cutaneous B-cell lymphoma. *J Cutan Pathol* 1997;**24**:457–461.
24. Goodlad JR, Davidson MM, Hollowood K, *et al.* Primary cutaneous B-cell lymphoma and Borrelia burgdorferi infection in patients from the highlands of Scotland. *Am J Surg Pathol* 2000;**24**:1279–1285.
25. Saksena A, Jain A, Pack SD, *et al.* Follicle center lymphoma (FCL) of the lower female genital tract (LFGT): a novel variant of primary cutaneous follicle center lymphoma (PCFCL). *Am J Surg Pathol* 2023;**47**:409–419.
26. English JSC, Smith NP, Spaull J, *et al.* Large cell lymphocytoma: a clinicopathological study. *Clin Exp Dermatol* 1989;**14**:181–185.
27. Winkelmann RK, Dabski K. Large cell lymphocytoma: follow-up, immunopathology studies, and comparison to cutaneous follicular and Crosti lymphoma. *Arch Dermatol Res* 1987;**279**:S81–S87.
28. Chapman JR, Alvarez JP, White K, *et al.* Unusual variants of follicular lymphoma: case-based review. *Am J Surg Pathol* 2020;**44**:329–339.
29. Gradowski JF, Jaffe ES, Warnke RA, *et al.* Follicular lymphomas with plasmacytic differentiation include two subtypes. *Mod Pathol* 2010;**23**:71–79.
30. Kelley JT, Brown NA, Hristov AC, Bresler SC. Primary cutaneous follicle center lymphoma with extensive plasmacytic differentiation and t(14;18) in both the lymphoid and plasma cell components. *J Cutan Pathol* 2021;**48**:969–974.
31. Skala SL, Harms PW, Fullen DR, *et al.* Cutaneous follicle center lymphomas with plasmacytic differentiation. *J Cutan Pathol* 2021;**48**:632–636.
32. Cerroni L, El-Shabrawi-Caelen L, Fink-Puches R, *et al.* Cutaneous spindle-cell B-cell lymphoma: a morphologic variant of cutaneous large B-cell lymphoma. *Am J Dermatopathol* 2000;**22**:299–304.
33. Ferrara G, Bevilacqua M, Argenziano G. Cutaneous spindle B-cell lymphoma: a reappraisal. *Am J Dermatopathol* 2002;**24**:526–527.
34. Cerroni L. Reply to cutaneous spindle B-cell lymphoma: a reappraisal. *Am J Dermatopathol* 2002;**24**:527–528.
35. Goodlad JR. Spindle-cell B-cell lymphoma presenting in the skin. *Br J Dermatol* 2001;**145**:313–317.
36. Ries S, Barr R, LeBoit P, *et al.* Cutaneous sarcomatoid B-cell lymphoma. *Am J Dermatopathol* 2007;**29**:96–98.
37. Wang L, Lv Y, Wang X, *et al.* Giant primary cutaneous spindle cell B-cell lymphoma of follicle center cell origin. *Am J Dermatopathol* 2010;**32**:628–632.
38. Yann CJ, Cerroni L, LeBoit PE. Cutaneous spindle-cell B-cell lymphomas. Most are neoplasms of follicular center cell origin. *Am J Surg Pathol* 2015;**39**:737–743.
39. Oschlies I, Kohler CW, Szczepanowski M, *et al.* Spindle-cell variants of primary cutaneous follicle center B-cell lymphomas are germinal center B-cell lymphomas by gene expression profiling using a formalin-fixed paraffin-embedded specimen. *J Invest Dermatol* 2017;**137**:2450–2453.
40. Carbone A, Gloghini A, Libra M, *et al.* A spindle cell variant of diffuse large B-cell lymphoma possesses genotypic and phenotypic markers characteristic of a germinal center B-cell origin. *Mod Pathol* 2006;**19**:299–306.
41. Li L, Majerowski J, Sokumbi O. Cutaneous spindled follicle center cell lymphoma with abundant mucin: A diagnostic pitfall. *J Cutan Pathol* 2020;**47**:394–397.
42. Marie D, Houda B-R, Béatrice V, *et al.* Primary cutaneous follicle center lymphoma with Hodgkin and Reed-Sternberg-like cells: a new histopathologic variant. *J Cutan Pathol* 2014;**41**:797–801.
43. Cerroni L, Arzberger E, Pütz B, *et al.* Primary cutaneous follicle center cell lymphoma with follicular growth pattern. *Blood* 2000;**95**:3922–3928.
44. Cerroni L, Volkenandt M, Rieger E, *et al.* Bcl-2 protein expression and correlation with the interchromosomal 14;18 translocation in cutaneous lymphomas and pseudolymphomas. *J Invest Dermatol* 1994;**102**:231–235.
45. Goodlad JR, Krajewski AS, Batstone PJ, *et al.* Primary cutaneous follicular lymphoma: a clinicopathologic and molecular study of 16 cases in support of a distinct entity. *Am J Surg Pathol* 2002;**26**: 733–741.
46. Servitje O, Climent F, Colomo L, *et al.* Primary cutaneous vs secondary cutaneous follicular lymphomas: A comparative study focused on BCL2, CD10, and t(14;18) expression. *J Cutan Pathol* 2019;**46**:182–189.
47. Szablewski V, Ingen-Housz-Oro S, Baia M, *et al.* Primary cutaneous follicle center lymphomas expressing BCL2 protein frequently harbor BCL2 gene break and may present 1p36 deletion. A study of 20 cases. *Am J Surg Pathol* 2016;**40**:127–136.
48. Kodama K, Massone C, Chott A, *et al.* Primary cutaneous large B-cell lymphomas: clinicopathologic features, classification, and prognostic factors in a large series of patients. *Blood* 2005;**106**:2491–2497.
49. Younes SF, Beck AH, Lossos IS, *et al.* Immunoarchitectural patterns in follicular lymphoma: efficacy of HGAL and LMO2 in the detection of the interfollicular and diffuse components. *Am J Surg Pathol* 2010;**34**:1266–1276.
50. Zhou XA, Yang J, Ringbloom KG, *et al.* Genomic landscape of cutaneous follicular lymphomas reveals 2 subgroups with clinically predictive molecular features. *Blood Adv* 2021;**5**:649–661.
51. Verdanet E, Dereure O, Rene C, *et al.* Diagnostic value of STMN1, LMO2, HGAL, AID expression and 1p36 chromosomal abnormalities in primary cutaneous B cell lymphomas. *Histopathology* 2017;**71**:648–660.
52. Cetinözman F, Koens L, Jansen PM, Willemze R. Programmed death-1 expression in cutaneous B-cell lymphoma. *J Cutan Pathol* 2014;**41**:14–21.
53. Fujiwara M, Morales AV, Seo K, *et al.* Clonal identity and differences in primary cutaneous B-cell lymphoma occurring at different sites or time points in the same patient. *Am J Dermatopathol* 2013;**35**:11–18.
54. Golembowsky S, Gellrich S, von Zimmermann M, *et al.* Clonal evolution in a primary cutaneous follicle center B cell lymphoma revealed by single cell analysis in sequential biopsies. *Immunobiology* 2000;**201**:631–644.
55. Delia D, Borrello MG, Berti E, *et al.* Clonal immunoglobulin gene rearrangements and normal T-cell receptor, bcl-2, and c-myc genes in primary cutaneous B-cell lymphomas. *Cancer Res* 1989;**49**: 4901–4905.

56. Siddiqi IN, Friedman J, Barry-Holson KQ, *et al.* Characterization of a variant of t(14;18) negative nodal diffuse follicular lymphoma with CD23 expression, 1p36/TNFRSF14 abnormalities, and STAT6 mutations. *Mod Pathol* 2016;**29**:570–581.
57. Gu K, Fu K, Jain S, *et al.* t(14;18)-negative follicular lymphomas are associated with a high frequency of BCL6 rearrangement at the alternative breakpoint region. *Mod Pathol* 2009;**22**:1251–1257.
58. Barasch NJK, Liu YC, Ho J, *et al.* The molecular landscape and other distinctive features of primary cutaneous follicle center lymphoma. *Hum Pathol* 2020;**106**:93–105.
59. Leich E, Salaverria I, Bea S, *et al.* Follicular lymphomas with and without translocation t(14;18) differ in gene expression profiles and genetic alterations. *Blood* 2009;**114**:826–834.
60. Jetic TM, Berry PK, Jubetirer SJ, *et al.* Primary cutaneous follicle center lymphoma of the arm with a novel chromosomal translocation t(12;21)(q13;q22): a case report. *Am J Hematol* 2006;**81**:448–453.
61. Storz MN, van de Rijn M, Kim YH, *et al.* Gene expression profiles of cutaneous B cell lymphoma. *J Invest Dermatol* 2003;**120**:865–870.
62. Hoefnagel JJ, Dijkman R, Basso K, *et al.* Distinct types of primary cutaneous large B-cell lymphoma identified by gene expression profiling. *Blood* 2005;**105**:3671–3678.
63. Perez M, Pacchiarotti A, Frontani M, *et al.* Primary cutaneous B-cell lymphoma is associated with somatically hypermutated immunoglobulin variable genes and frequent use of VH1-69 and VH4-59 segments. *Br J Dermatol* 2010;**162**:611–618.
64. Raaphorst FM, Vermeer M, Fieret E, *et al.* Site-specific expression of polycomb-group genes encoding the HPC-HPH/PRC1 complex in clinically defined primary nodal and cutaneous large B-cell lymphomas. *Am J Pathol* 2004;**164**:533–542.
65. (a) Koens L, Vermeer MH, Willemze R, *et al.* IgM Expression on paraffin sections distinguishes primary cutaneous large B-cell lymphoma, leg type from primary cutaneous follicle center lymphoma. *Am J Surg Pathol* 2010;**34**:1043–1048.(b) Schrader AMR, de Groen RAL, Willemze R, *et al.* IgM immunohistochemical expression is a potential risk factor for extracutaneous dissemination in patients with primary cutaneous follicle center lymphoma. *Am J Surg Pathol* 2025;**49**:931–941.
66. Robson A, Shukur Z, Ally M, *et al.* Immunocytochemical p63 expression discriminates between primary cutaneous follicle centre cell and diffuse large B cell lymphoma-leg type, and is of the TAp63 isoform. *Histopathology* 2016;**69**:11–19.
67. Senff NJ, Hoefnagel JJ, Jansen PM, *et al.* Reclassification of 300 primary cutaneous B-cell lymphomas according to the new WHO–EORTC classification for cutaneous lymphomas: comparison with previous classifications and identification of prognostic markers. *J Clin Oncol* 2007;**25**:1581–1587.
68. Pimpinelli N, Santucci M, Bosi A, *et al.* Primary cutaneous follicular centre-cell lymphoma: a lymphoproliferative disease with favourable prognosis. *Clin Exp Dermatol* 1989;**14**:12–19.
69. Rijlaarsdam JU, Toonstra J, Meijer CJLM, *et al.* Treatment of primary cutaneous B-cell lymphomas of follicle center cell origin: a clinical follow-up study of 55 patients treated with radiotherapy or polychemotherapy. *J Clin Oncol* 1996;**14**:549–555.
70. Piccinno R, Caccialanza M, Berti E. Dermatologic radiotherapy of primary cutaneous follicle center cell lymphoma. *Eur J Dermatol* 2003;**13**:49–52.
71. Senff NJ, Noordijk EM, Kim YH, *et al.* European organization for research and treatment of cancer and international society for cutaneous lymphoma consensus recommendations for the management of cutaneous B-cell lymphomas. *Blood* 2008;**112**:1600–1609.
72. Willemze R, Hodak E, Zinzani PL, *et al.* Primary cutaneous lymphomas: ESMO Clinical Practice Guidelines for diagnosis, treatment and follow-up. *Ann Oncol* 2018;**29**(Suppl. 4):iv30–iv40. on behalf of the ESMO Guidelines Committee
73. Christensen L, Cooper K, Honda K, Mansur D. Relapse rates in patients with unilesional primary cutaneous B-cell lymphoma treated with radiation therapy: a single-institution experience. *Br J Dermatol* 2018;**179**:1172–1173.
74. Elsayad K, Guenova E, Assaf C, *et al.* Radiotherapy in cutaneous lymphomas: Recommendations from the EORTC cutaneous lymphoma tumour group. *Eur J Cancer* 2024;**212**:115064.
75. Fink-Puches R, Wolf IH, Zalaudek I, *et al.* Treatment of primary cutaneous B-cell lymphoma with rituximab. *J Am Acad Dermatol* 2005;**52**:847–853.
76. Heinzerling LM, Urbanek M, Funk JO, *et al.* Reduction of tumor burden and stabilization of disease by systemic therapy with anti-CD20 antibody (rituximab) in patients with primary cutaneous B-cell lymphoma. *Cancer* 2000;**89**:1835–1844.
77. Penate Y, Hernandez-Machin B, Perez-Mendez LI, *et al.* Intralesional rituximab in the treatment of indolent primary cutaneous B-cell lymphomas: an epidemiological observational multicentre study. The Spanish Working Group on Cutaneous Lymphoma. *Br J Dermatol* 2012;**167**:174–179.
78. Zucca E, Rondeau S, Vanazzi A, *et al.* Short regimen of rituximab plus lenalidomide in follicular lymphoma patients in need of first-line therapy. *Blood* 2019;**134**:353–362.
79. Burger JA, Ghia P, Rosenwald A, *et al.* The microenvironment in mature B-cell malignancies: a target for new treatment strategies. *Blood* 2009;**114**:3367–3375.
80. Fink-Puches R, Zenahlik P, Bäck B, *et al.* Primary cutaneous lymphomas: applicability of current classification schemes (European Organization for Research and Treatment of Cancer, World Health Organization) based on clinicopathologic features observed in a large group of patients. *Blood* 2002;**99**:800–805.
81. Zinzani PL, Quaglino P, Pimpinelli N, *et al.* Prognostic factors in primary cutaneous B-cell lymphoma: the Italian Study Group for Cutaneous Lymphomas. *J Clin Oncol* 2006;**24**:1376–1382.
82. Chan SA, Shah F, Chaganti S, *et al.* Primary cutaneous B-cell lymphoma: systemic spread is rare while cutaneous relapses and secondary malignancies are frequent. *Br J Dermatol* 2017;**177**:287–289.
83. Bekkenk MW, Postma TJ, Meijer CJLM, Willemze R. Frequency of central nervous system involvement in primary cutaneous B-cell lymphoma. *Cancer* 2000;**89**:913–919.
84. Pham-Ledard A, Cowppli-Bony A, Doussau A, *et al.* Diagnostic and prognostic value of BCL2 rearrangement in 53 patients with follicular lymphoma presenting as primary skin lesions. *Am J Clin Pathol* 2015;**143**:362–373.
85. Pileri A, Grandi V, Agostinelli C, *et al.* BCL-2 expression in primary cutaneous follicle center lymphoma is associated with a higher risk of cutaneous relapses: a study of 126 cases. *J Eur Acad Dermatol Venereol* 2022;**36**:e811–e813.
86. Fierro MT, Marenco F, Novelli M, *et al.* Long-term evolution of an untreated primary cutaneous follicle center lymphoma of the scalp. *Am J Dermatopathol* 2010;**32**:91–94.
87. Mian M, Marcheselli L, Luminari S, *et al.* CLIPI: a new prognostic index for indolent cutaneous B cell lymphoma proposed by the International Extranodal Lymphoma Study Group (IELSG 11). *Ann Hematol* 2011;**90**:401–408.

CHAPTER 17

# Primary cutaneous marginal zone lymphoproliferative disorder (primary cutaneous marginal zone lymphoma) and variants

Primary cutaneous marginal zone lymphoproliferative disorder is an indolent cutaneous B-cell lymphoproliferative disorder characterized by the proliferation of marginal zone cells, lymphoplasmacytoid cells, and plasma cells in the skin. In the 2018 and 2024 updates of the classification of cutaneous lymphomas by the European Organization for Research and Treatment of Cancer (EORTC)/World Health Organization (WHO), this entity is listed as primary cutaneous marginal zone lymphoma [1, 2]. In the 5th edition of the WHO *Classification of Haematolymphoid Tumours*, cutaneous marginal zone lymphoma has been included within the group of marginal zone lymphoma of the lymph nodes and other organs [3]. In the International Consensus Classification (ICC) *of Myeloid and Lymphoid Neoplasms*, the entity has been downgraded to a lymphoproliferative disorder rather than a lymphoma, as it is characterized by an indolent behavior and almost never spreads to extracutaneous sites [4]. This is the major difference among the two classification schemes for what concerns primary cutaneous lymphomas and lymphoproliferative disorders. However, the difference is more semantic than practical, as in the WHO classification, it is stated that "primary cutaneous marginal zone lymphoproliferative disorder" is an accepted related terminology [3]. Personally, as I wrote in previous editions of the book, I favor the terminology of cutaneous marginal zone lymphoproliferative disorder, and use it in routine practice. Thus, I will use this denomination in the rest of this Chapter (as well as in the entire book).

Marginal zone lymphomas in various organs and cutaneous marginal zone lymphoproliferative disorder are characterized by several common features, particularly the association with chronic inflammation due to autoimmune disorders or infections [5]. Many cases of extranodal marginal zone lymphoma of the mucosa-associated lymphoid tissue (MALT) are related to infection organisms, including *Helicobacter pylori* (involved in gastric cases) and *Chlamydia jejuni* and *Chlamydia psittaci* (involved in ocular cases); in the skin, some cases of marginal zone lymphoproliferative disorder are associated with infection by *Borrelia burgdorferi* (involved in cutaneous cases), suggesting that different microorganisms play a role in the etiology of this group of diseases [6]. The hepatitis C virus (HCV) has been detected in splenic marginal zone lymphoma [6]. In contrast to the Epstein–Barr virus (EBV)-related lymphoproliferative disorders, in all types of marginal zone lymphoma and lymphoproliferative disorder, the implicated microorganisms do not directly infect lymphoid cells, but rather induce chronic stimulation of the immune system, eventually leading to lymphoid transformation and in some organs to onset of lymphoma. I have seen cutaneous marginal zone lymphoproliferative disorder arising at the same time in two adult brothers, but they shared the same housing; thus, the association may be environmental rather than genetic. In one study, various gastrointestinal disorders (reflux, gastric ulcers, positive serology for *Helicobacter*, and irritable bowel disease) and autoimmune diseases of uncertain significance were observed at higher frequency in patients with cutaneous marginal zone lymphoproliferative disorder [7], but I have not observed a similar association in patients from my Hospital.

The relationship (if any) between the different types of marginal zone lymphoproliferative disorders arising in different settings (lymph nodes, spleen, MALT organs, skin, and pediatric patients) is unclear. A study showed that unbalanced genomic alterations differ between the splenic and the extranodal MALT-type groups, with nodal cases being intermediate between them [8]. However, this study lumped all MALT-type cases together; thus, any putative difference between cutaneous and extracutaneous lesions would not be detected. The *MYD88* L265P somatic mutation has been detected in a subset of splenic marginal zone lymphomas (as well as in a majority of cases of Waldenström macroglobulinemia/lymphoplasmacytic lymphoma) but not in cutaneous or nodal variants [9]. The frequency of specific molecular alterations differs among tumors arising in different organs. *BRAF* mutations have been identified in 16% of cases of nodal marginal zone lymphoma, but not in splenic, cutaneous, or MALT-related cases [10]. In fact, in the last edition of the WHO classification, splenic marginal zone lymphoma is included in the group of splenic B-cell lymphomas

*Skin Lymphoma: The Illustrated Guide*, Sixth Edition. Lorenzo Cerroni.

and leukemias rather than in the group of marginal zone lymphomas. The so-called lymphoepithelial lesions, a hallmark of marginal zone lymphoma arising at mucosal sites (conceptually comparable to the epidermotropism observed in cutaneous T-cell lymphomas), are not found in cutaneous marginal zone lymphoproliferative disorder. Finally, site-specific work-up for marginal zone lymphomas arising in different organs has been suggested [11]. Interestingly, the IgG4 expression by neoplastic cells has been observed in a distinct proportion of cutaneous cases with plasmacytic differentiation, but only in sporadic cases from other organs [12], thus suggesting that some organ-related differences may indeed exist. No significant clinical differences have been identified between IgG4 positive and negative cutaneous cases in one study [13], whereas a higher frequency of IgG4 positivity was observed in class-switched cases in another one [14]. In this context, it is also of interest that in one patient a metachronic occurrence of primary cutaneous marginal zone lymphoproliferative disorder and primary cutaneous Rosai-Dorfman disease (another cutaneous disorder that can be associated with $IgG4^+$ cells) has been described [15]. However, in my opinion, cutaneous marginal zone lymphoproliferative disorder is not related to the so-called IgG4-related sclerosing disorders, and detection of IgG4 does not play any relevant diagnostic role.

Cutaneous marginal zone lymphoproliferative disorder includes lesions that were formerly classified as primary cutaneous immunocytoma and primary cutaneous plasmacytoma [16–20]. Some cases reported previously as "cutaneous lymphoid hyperplasia" or as "cutaneous follicular lymphoid hyperplasia with monotypic plasma cells" also represent examples of marginal zone lymphoproliferative disorder of the skin [21, 22], again underlying the indolent nature of the disease. In my experience, there are five main histopathologic presentations of cutaneous marginal zone lymphoproliferative disorder:

1. Cutaneous marginal zone lymphoproliferative disorder, conventional variant (approximately 82% of cases of the Dermatopathology Unit of the Medical University of Graz, Austria).
2. Cutaneous marginal zone lymphoproliferative disorder, lymphoplasmacytic variant (formerly cutaneous immunocytoma) (approximately 13% of cases of the Dermatopathology Unit of the Medical University of Graz, Austria).
3. Cutaneous marginal zone lymphoproliferative disorder, plasmacytic variant (formerly cutaneous plasmacytoma) (approximately 3% of cases of the Dermatopathology Unit of the Medical University of Graz, Austria).
4. Cutaneous marginal zone lymphoproliferative disorder, blastoid variant (approximately 2% of cases of the Dermatopathology Unit of the Medical University of Graz, Austria). This type has been observed de novo, or in recurrent lesions in patients with a previous diagnosis of one of the other variants of cutaneous marginal zone lymphoproliferative disorder.
5. Cutaneous amyloidoma (this variant includes very rare cases characterized by prominent amyloid deposition).

Overlapping features exist, particularly between the conventional and the plasmacytic types, and some patients show lesions that are classified within a given group and subsequently recurrences that would be better classified within another one. A relationship between marginal zone lymphoma and extramedullary plasmacytoma has been postulated also at sites other than the skin [23], suggesting that these entities of low-grade B-cell lymphoma may be related. In addition, transformation to pure proliferations of plasma cells has been observed in six cases of extracutaneous marginal zone lymphoma treated with rituximab [24], showing that the transition between morphologic types can be observed also at sites other than the skin. However, I have never seen examples of the lymphoplasmacytic variant recurring with features of conventional or plasmacytic types. In my view, particularly between the conventional and the lymphoplasmacytic variants of cutaneous marginal zone lymphoproliferative disorder, there are differences that are worth mentioning, and that can be summarized as follows:

- The conventional variant of cutaneous marginal zone lymphoproliferative disorder is observed mostly in younger adults and adults, whereas the lymphoplasmacytic variant is seen more often in the elderly.
- The preferential location differs (trunk and upper extremities for the conventional variant, lower extremities for the lymphoplasmacytic variant).
- Association with *B. burgdorferi* infection is more common in the lymphoplasmacytic variant [25]. I have observed cases of the lymphoplasmacytic variant, but not of conventional marginal zone lymphoproliferative disorder arising on the background of acrodermatitis chronica atrophicans.
- The histopathologic pattern differs (see below); intranuclear inclusions (Dutcher bodies) are seen mostly in the lymphoplasmacytic variant. Parenthetically, although in the skin, Dutcher bodies are seen mostly in marginal zone lymphoproliferative disorder, they may be encountered rarely also in reactive conditions characterized by the presence of lymphoplasmacytoid cells (in this setting always as an isolated finding).

The analysis of the molecular clones in different biopsies of marginal zone lymphoproliferative disorder taken from various skin sites of involvement, or at the same cutaneous site at different time points, showed that the same clone is present in most cases [26]. However, in a small percentage of patients, different clones were detected in different specimens, suggesting the possibility that these cases represent multiple, unrelated primary cutaneous marginal zone lymphoproliferative disorders [26]. Somatic hypermutations resulting in clonal evolution may represent an alternative explanation. I have observed rarely an immunoglobulin (Ig) light chain expression "switch" in sequential biopsies of cutaneous marginal zone lymphoproliferative disorder (from kappa to lambda or vice versa), and even the presence of distinct populations of kappa and lambda monoclonal cells in one and the same specimen. Similar cases have been reported [27, 28], but whether they represent true different lymphoproliferative disorders or just clonal evolution has not been elucidated yet.

A rare presentation of cutaneous marginal zone lymphoproliferative disorder is represented by so-called "cutaneous amyloidoma" [29, 30]. These peculiar tumors are characterized by prominent amyloid deposition and comparatively few monoclonal plasma cells, and are not related to multiple myeloma (or other light chain producing low-grade B-cell lymphoproliferative disorders) or systemic amyloidosis. Although, in one study, a minority of patients with cutaneous marginal zone lymphoproliferative disorder showed a suspicious serum protein electrophoresis in terms of paraproteinemia, only in less than half of these patients the heavy and light chain restriction in tissue samples correlated with the serological findings [31], thus suggesting that in the majority of patients with both cutaneous marginal zone lymphoproliferative disorder and paraproteinemia, this last is not related to the cutaneous disease.

I have come across patients affected by both cutaneous marginal zone lymphoproliferative disorder and mycosis fungoides. Either disease could arise prior to the other one, and in rare instances, both would be detected at the same time in one and the same lesion (see also composite lymphomas in Chapter 28). This association is infrequent but not exceptional, yet I do not think that there is any etiologic or pathogenetic relationship between cutaneous marginal zone lymphoproliferative disorder and mycosis fungoides. In this context, one exceptional case of epidermotropic cutaneous marginal zone lymphoproliferative disorder has been described, [32] and care should be taken not to misdiagnose such cases as mycosis fungoides. Cutaneous marginal zone lymphoproliferative disorder has been described also following successful treatment of nodal Hodgkin lymphoma [33], and rarely in the setting of immunosuppression (particularly post-transplant) [34], and as a lymphoproliferative disorder of donor origin after allogeneic hematopoietic stem cell transplantation [35].

Over the years, I have seen a number of cases classified initially as cutaneous marginal zone lymphoproliferative disorder and later reclassified as cutaneous follicle center lymphoma on biopsy of recurrent lesions. Although the differential diagnosis between these two entities is usually easy, the rare presence in cases of cutaneous follicle center lymphoma of monoclonal plasma cells belonging to the neoplastic clone may be a source of mistakes. I must admit that, in rare instances, the differentiation between these two entities is difficult and subjective; in such cases, the working diagnosis of "atypical lymphoid proliferation with monotypic plasma cells, suspicious for low-grade cutaneous B-cell lymphoma" may be used, rather than providing a more precise but potentially wrong classification. Interestingly, overlapping features between these two B-cell lymphomas can be observed also at sites other than the skin. In addition, overlapping histopathological, immunophenotypic, and molecular features between cutaneous marginal zone lymphoproliferative disorder and cutaneous $CD4^+$ small/medium T-cell lymphoproliferative disorder have been described as well [36, 37]. However, in my experience, the differential diagnosis between these two conditions does not represent a problem, and cases can be distinguished easily based on clinicopathological features.

Finally, it should be underlined that, although in some classifications, cutaneous marginal zone lymphoproliferative disorder is currently classified as a lymphoma, and the prognosis is excellent. In fact, heavy-chain class-switched cases (representing the vast majority of cases; see below for details) present with frequent cutaneous recurrences but almost never with extracutaneous disease (Fig. 17.1); even before the ICC classification adopted a new nomenclature, it had been suggested that this condition may be better classified as a "lymphoproliferative disorder" rather than a true malignant lymphoma [38, 39]. A similar option has been adopted for the "cutaneous $CD4^+$ small–medium T-cell lymphoma," which has been reclassified as "cutaneous $CD4^+$ small–medium T-cell lymphoproliferative disorder" in all recent lymphoma classifications. Personally, I classify these cases as a lymphoproliferative disorder, according to the ICC classification. Interestingly, in a recent study on recurrent cutaneous marginal zone lymphoproliferative disorder, 0/19 (0%) distant recurrences and 23/42 (55%) local recurrences revealed the same clone at a molecular level [40], suggesting that in several cases, the "recurrent disease" represented a new lesion rather than a true recurrence. In addition, in the same study, polyclonality (rather than monoclonality) in both original and recurrent lesions was observed in 3/19 (16%) cases with distant recurrences, and 5/42 (12%) with local recurrences. These data support the concept that cutaneous marginal zone lymphoproliferative disorder is not a true lymphoma.

## Cutaneous marginal zone lymphoproliferative disorder, conventional variant

The conventional variant of primary cutaneous marginal zone lymphoproliferative disorder is by far the most frequent among the morphologic subtypes. The association with *B. burgdorferi* has been detected in some cases in areas with or without endemic infection [22, 41, 42]. However, this association may be regional, as other studies on cutaneous marginal zone lymphoproliferative disorder did not show evidence of infection by *B. burgdorferi* [43–46]. In addition, in my experience, the association with *B. burgdorferi* is more frequent in the lymphoplasmacytic type of cutaneous marginal zone lymphoproliferative disorder (see the corresponding section in this chapter). There is no link with other infectious agents including *H. pylori*, HCV, EBV, and human herpes viruses (HHV)-7 and 8. The knowledge that different examples of cutaneous marginal

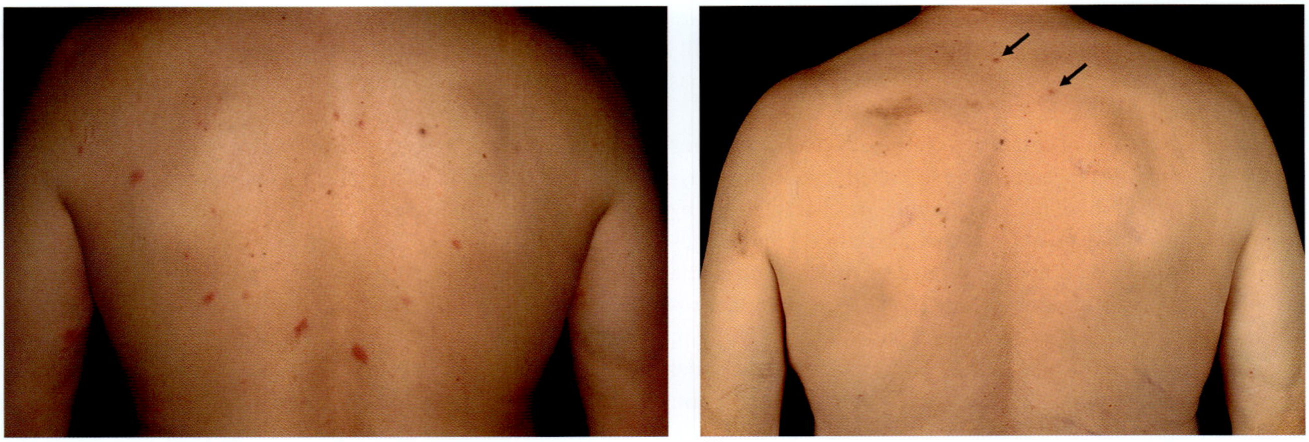

(a) (b)

Figure 17.1 "Natural history" of cutaneous marginal zone lymphoproliferative disorder (conventional variant). (a) This patient presented for the first time in 1995, at the age of 45, with multiple lesions of cutaneous marginal zone lymphoproliferative disorder on the back and upper extremities. He returned regularly over the years for excision of recurrent lesions (he only accepted surgical excision as a treatment option). (b) In 2019, 24 years after the first presentation, he still had recurrent lesions on the back (arrows), besides scars from >40 previous excisions. At last follow-up, the patient is alive with recurrent lesions 30 years after the first presentation.

zone lymphoproliferative disorder recognize similar antigens supports the hypothesis of an antigen-driven disorder [5, 47, 48], similar to what happens in other types of extracutaneous lymphoma. A similar mechanism related to chronic antigenic stimulation may be responsible for the onset of cutaneous marginal zone lymphoproliferative disorder after vaccination or in the context of fluoxetine (Prozac®) therapy [49, 50]. In this context, monoclonal populations of plasma cells have been observed at the injection site of talimogene laherparepvec (T-VEC), a genetically engineered herpes simplex virus type 1 used for treatment of cutaneous metastases of melanoma (see Chapter 31, Fig. 31.87) [51].

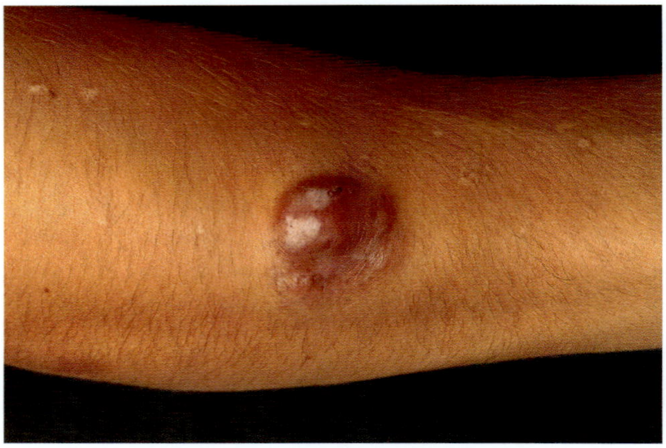

Figure 17.2 Cutaneous marginal zone lymphoproliferative disorder, conventional variant. Solitary, large erythematous tumor on the arm.

## Clinical features

Cutaneous marginal zone lymphoproliferative disorder, conventional variant, occurs typically in young adults with a male predominance [17, 52, 53]. Onset in childhood may be observed [54, 55]. Patients present with red to reddish brown papules, plaques, and nodules localized particularly to the upper extremities or the trunk. Lesions are commonly solitary but may be multiple (Figs. 17.2 and 17.3). The clinical picture of "Crosti's lymphoma," typical of cutaneous follicle center lymphoma, is not found in patients with cutaneous marginal zone lymphoproliferative disorder, but clustered lesions on the back may resemble the early manifestations of cutaneous follicle center lymphoma (Fig. 17.4). In some cases, the clinical picture resembles that of rosacea [56]. However, in my experience, this clinical presentation is observed more frequently in patients with cutaneous follicle center lymphoma (see Chapter 16). Cutaneous recurrences are frequent and often distant from the primary site of involvement (Fig. 17.5).

In one patient, cutaneous marginal zone lymphoproliferative disorder occurred on the background of erythema ab igne [57], and I have observed cases at sites of chronic antigen stimulation such as tattoo (Fig. 17.6).

The onset of anetoderma in some lesions of cutaneous marginal zone lymphoproliferative disorder has been reported [58, 59], and in some patients, it has been related to the presence of serum antiphospholipid antibodies [60].

In the absence of extracutaneous symptoms, the need for complete staging investigations in patients with conventional lesions of cutaneous marginal zone lymphoproliferative disorder is questionable [61], although they may be considered for unmutated cases ($IgM^+$). In a study, whole-body imaging allowed to detect the presence of extracutaneous lesions in only 3.6% of patients with cutaneous marginal zone lymphoproliferative disorder [62]. Bone marrow involvement has been

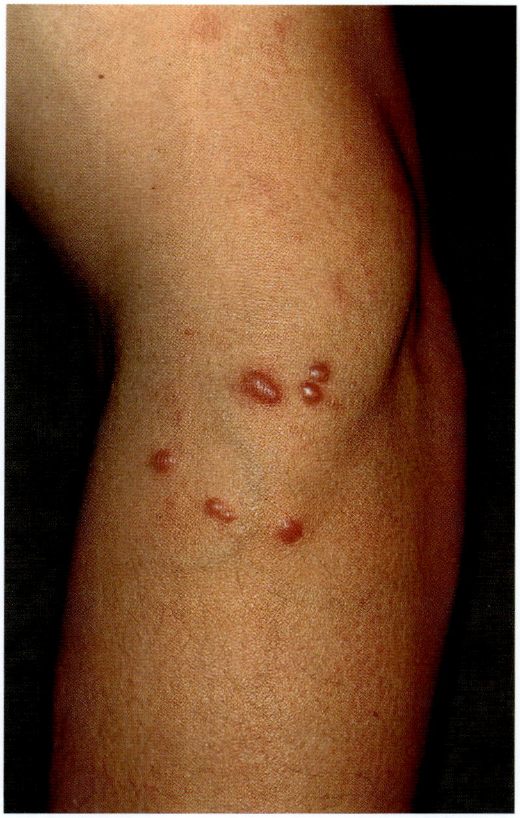

**Figure 17.3** Cutaneous marginal zone lymphoproliferative disorder, conventional variant. Cluster of papules and small erythematous nodules on the arm.

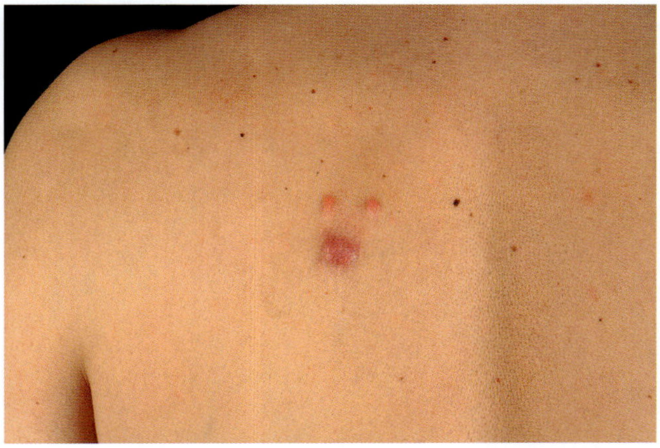

**Figure 17.4** Cutaneous marginal zone lymphoproliferative disorder, conventional variant. Clustered papules and small nodule on the left shoulder.

described only rarely in patients with cutaneous disease [63, 64] and in my experience, it is almost never present, thus questioning the need for bone marrow biopsy in these patients [65]. In this context, it should be remembered that extranodal marginal zone lymphoma of the MALT organs may present rarely with

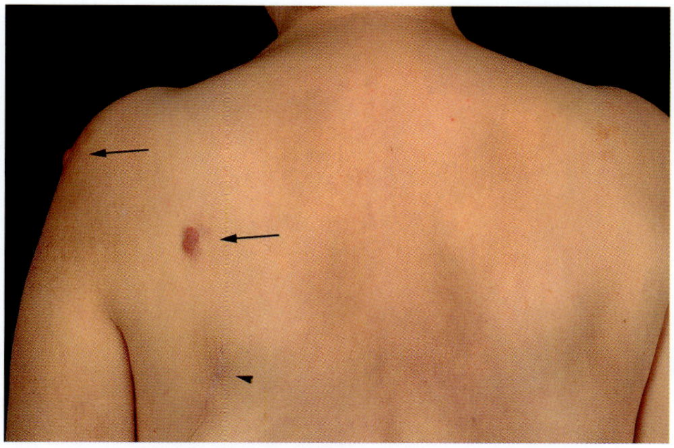

**Figure 17.5** Cutaneous marginal zone lymphoproliferative disorder, conventional variant. Two erythematous nodules on the left shoulder (arrows). Note a scar from a previous excision of a similar lesion (arrowhead).

secondary cutaneous manifestations, a possibility that should be kept in mind, particularly in patients with unusual clinical presentations [66].

## Histopathology, immunophenotype, and molecular genetics

### Histopathology

Histology shows patchy, nodular, or diffuse infiltrates within the dermis and sometimes the superficial part of the subcutaneous fat. The infiltrate may be top-heavy (Fig. 17.7) or bottom-heavy (Fig. 17.8). The epidermis is not involved (intraepidermal T lymphocytes may be observed in some cases, and exceptional cases may show also a few intraepidermal neoplastic B lymphocytes). A characteristic pattern can be observed at low magnification: nodular infiltrates with lymphoid follicles, often containing reactive germinal centers, are surrounded by a pale-staining peri- and interfollicular population of small- to medium-sized cells with indented nuclei, inconspicuous nucleoli, and abundant pale cytoplasm (marginal zone cells, centrocyte-like cells) (Fig. 17.9) [17]. In addition, plasma cells (at the margins of the infiltrate), lymphoplasmacytoid cells, small lymphocytes, and occasional large blasts are observed. It should be emphasized that in the conventional variant of cutaneous marginal zone lymphoproliferative disorder, neoplastic cells represent a minority of the infiltrate and are invariably admixed with large numbers of reactive lymphocytes (Fig. 17.10) and with other inflammatory cells (histiocytes, sometimes with the formation of small granulomas, and eosinophils). Reactive germinal centers are almost always present (Fig. 17.9). Large, $CD30^+$ cells, some resembling Hodgkin cells, have been described in cases of cutaneous marginal zone lymphoproliferative disorder [67, 68]. Periadnexal and perineural clusters of neoplastic cells can be observed rarely (Fig. 17.11). In some cases, the infiltrate is superficial with a band-like

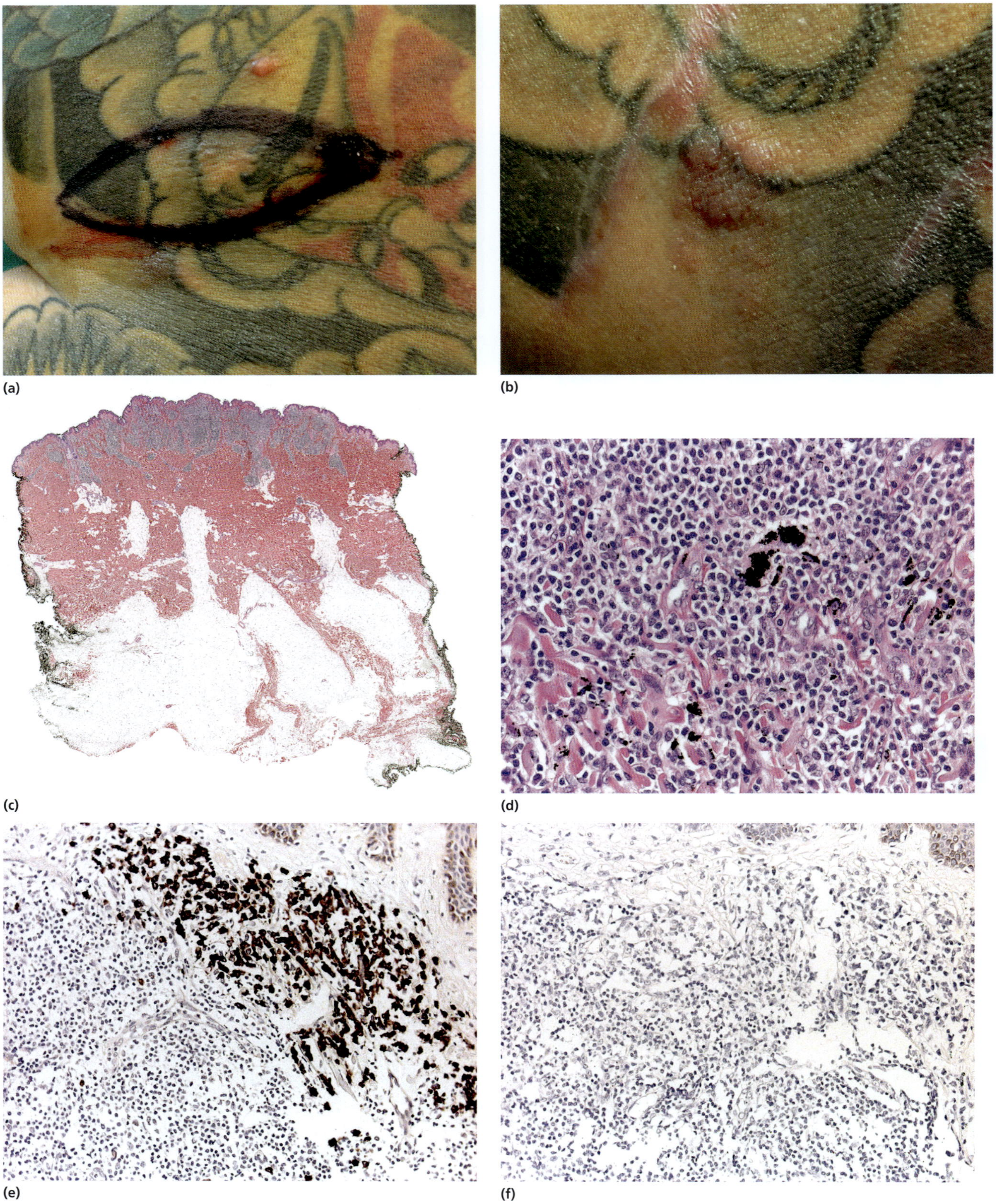

**Figure 17.6** Cutaneous marginal zone lymphoproliferative disorder, conventional variant, arising within a tattoo. (a, b) Multicoloured tattoo with irregular erythematous lesions (*Courtesy Dr. C. Massone, Genua*). (c) Dense dermal lymphoid infiltrate admixed (d) with plasma cells and plasmacytoid cells; note pigmented particles of the tattoo. In situ hybridization for the immunoglobulin light chains shows (e) positivity of the majority of plasma cells for kappa and (f) negativity for lambda.

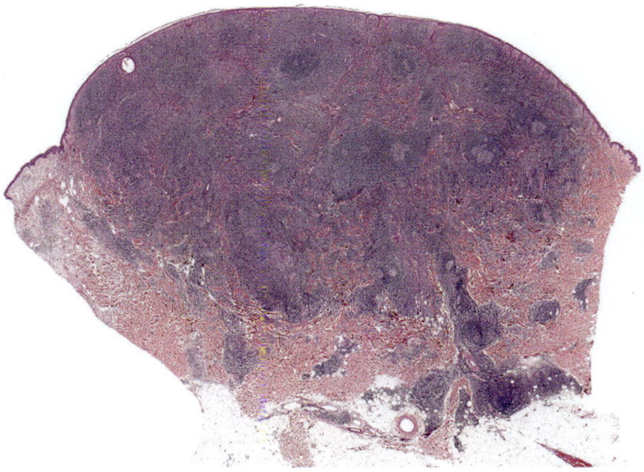

Figure 17.7 Cutaneous marginal zone lymphoproliferative disorder, conventional variant. "Top-heavy" infiltrate with dark and pale areas (see text).

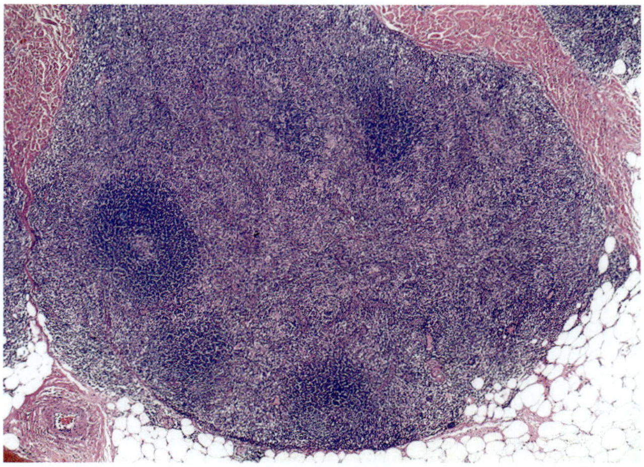

Figure 17.9 Cutaneous marginal zone lymphoproliferative disorder, conventional variant. Nodular infiltrate within the deep dermis and superficial subcutaneous fat. Note small nodules of reactive lymphocytes (dark area), one with a germinal center, surrounded by large numbers of neoplastic cells (pale area) (see text).

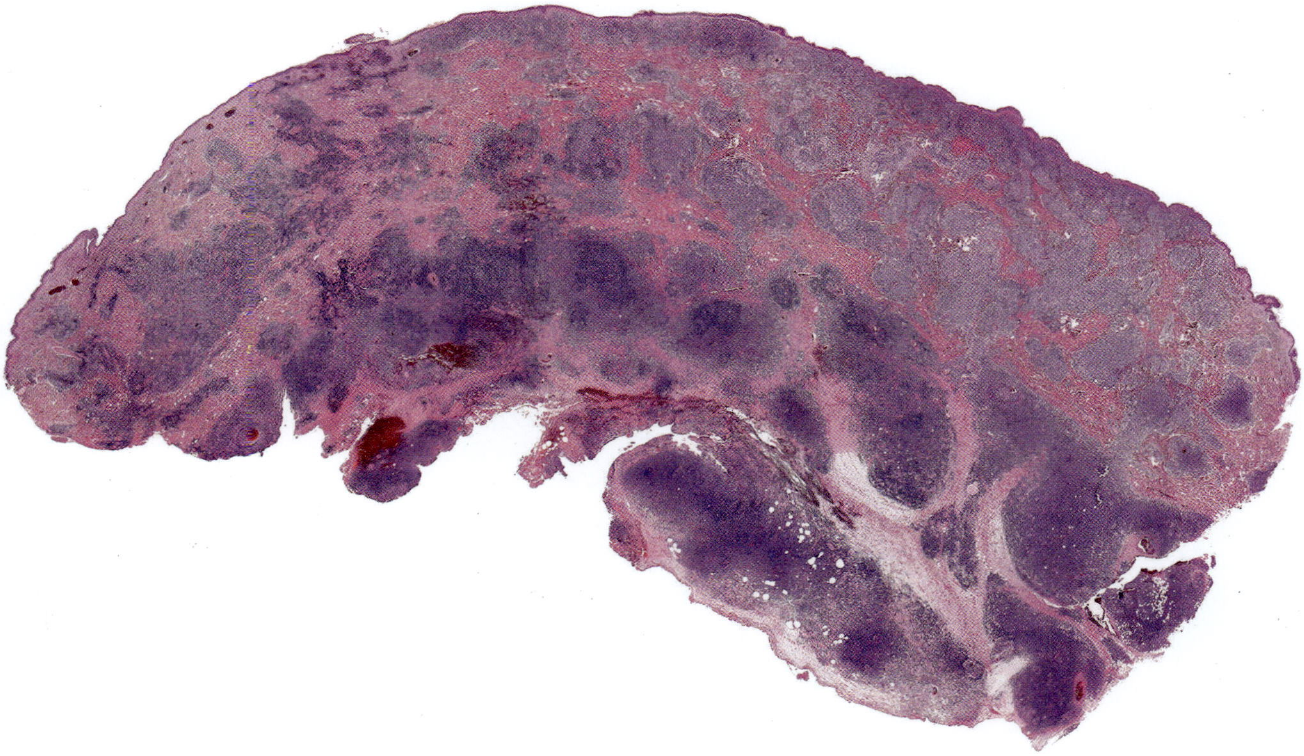

Figure 17.8 Cutaneous marginal zone lymphoproliferative disorder, conventional variant. Dense, "bottom-heavy" lymphoid infiltrates with reactive germinal centers.

arrangement (Fig. 17.12a and b); in these cases, too, monoclonal plasma cells are located mainly at the periphery of the infiltrate (Fig. 17.12b and c).

The neoplastic population in the conventional variant of cutaneous marginal zone lymphoproliferative disorder is composed of a combination of marginal zone cells, lymphoplasmacytoid lymphocytes, and plasma cells. Marginal zone cells represent usually only a proportion of the neoplastic lymphocytes (Fig. 17.13a), but they may predominate, at least focally, forming small sheets without plasma cell differentiation (Fig. 17.13b). In other lesions, neoplastic plasma cells and lymphoplasmacytoid cells represent the majority of tumoral cells

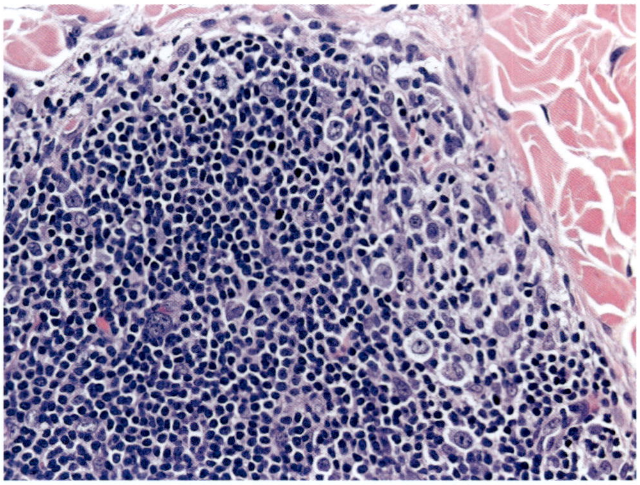

Figure 17.10 Cutaneous marginal zone lymphoproliferative disorder, conventional variant. Reactive lymphocytes predominate, admixed with some larger, paler cells (marginal zone cells) arranged at the periphery of the infiltrate.

(Fig. 17.13c). Cases where blastoid marginal zone cells, lymphoplasmacytoid cells, or plasma cells represent the majority of the entire infiltrate should be classified within the corresponding variant. There is no precise cut-off point: I use the definition "neoplastic cells representing >50% of the infiltrate," but that is as subjective a number as any other. Usually, however, the distinction is easy, as infiltrates in the blastoid, lymphoplasmacytoid, and plasma cell variants are much more monomorphous than those of the conventional variant. The predominance of marginal zone cells (>50% of the total infiltrate) may also be observed very rarely, but infiltrates in these cases are less monomorphous and resemble the conventional variant of cutaneous marginal zone lymphoproliferative disorder (Fig. 17.14). I classify these cases within the conventional variant, as they present neither with the histopathologic picture classified formerly as cutaneous immunocytoma or cutaneous plasmacytoma, nor with a predominance of blastoid cells.

## Immunophenotype

Phenotypic analyses reveal a mixed population composed of many reactive T- and B-lymphocytes admixed with variable numbers of neoplastic plasma cells ($CD20^-$, $CD38^+$, and $CD138^+$ with a monoclonal expression of the Ig light chain kappa or lambda), and marginal zone cells ($CD20^+$, $CD79a^+$, Bcl-$2^+$, $CD5^-$, $CD10^-$, Bcl-$6^-$, cyclin-$D1^-$, and monoclonal light chain) (Fig. 17.15). Bcl-6, and to a lesser extent, CD10 antibodies are particularly useful for differentiation of cutaneous marginal zone lymphoproliferative disorder (negative) from cutaneous follicle center lymphoma (positive), keeping in mind that follicular B lymphocytes in reactive germinal centers are Bcl-6-positive [69]. Myeloid cell nuclear differentiation antigen (MNDA) is positive in neoplastic cells in 60–70% of cases of marginal zone lymphoproliferative disorder, but negative in cells of follicle center lymphoma. The aberrant nuclear expression of Bcl-10 may be observed.

Extranodal marginal zone lymphomas arising in various MALT organs as well as cutaneous cases, but not other low-grade B-cell lymphomas, express Ig receptor translocation associated 1 (IRTA1), a molecule recognizing the equivalent of the marginal zone in human lymphoid tissues other than the spleen, providing a useful diagnostic criterion [70, 71].

The expression of four antigens (LIM-only transcription factor 2 – LMO2, human germinal center-associated lymphoma – HGAL, stathmin 1 – STMN1, and activation-induced cytidine deaminase – AID) has been suggested helpful in differentiating cutaneous marginal zone lymphoproliferative disorder (negative) from cutaneous follicle center lymphoma (positive) [72]. It should be underlined that reactive germinal

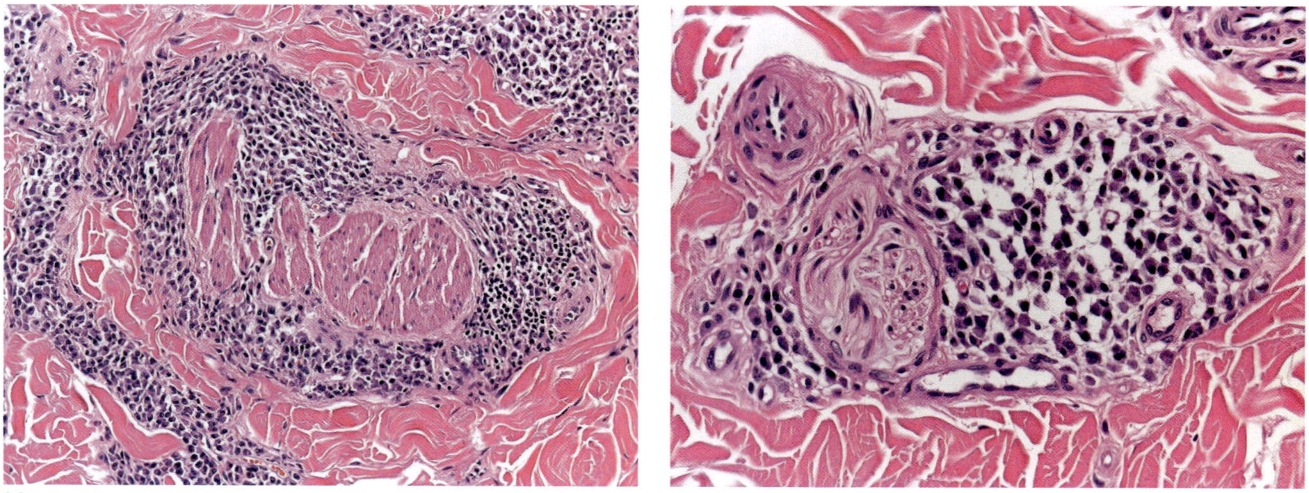

(a) (b)

Figure 17.11 Cutaneous marginal zone lymphoproliferative disorder, conventional variant. (a) Neoplastic plasma cells surrounding a smooth muscle and (b) a nerve.

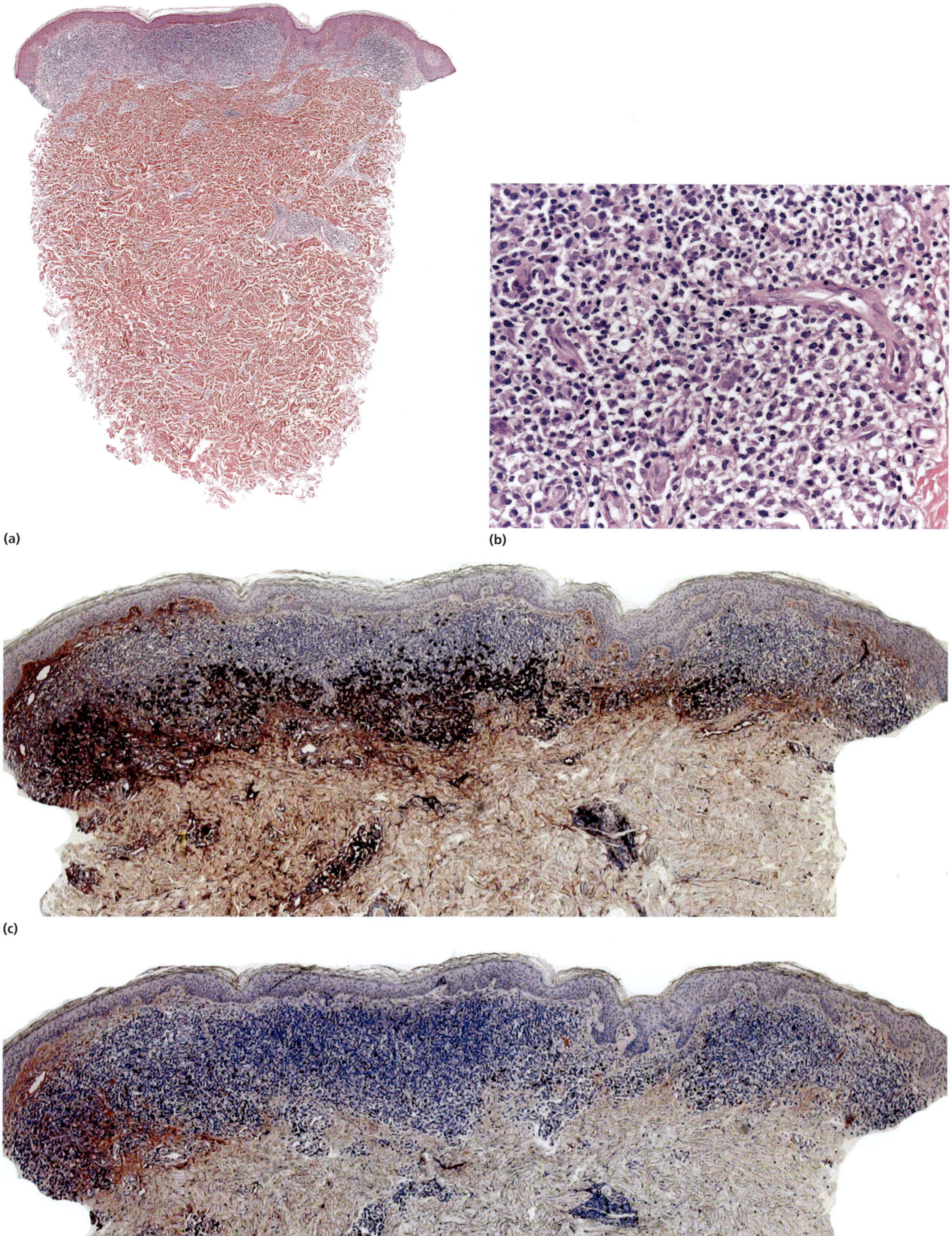


**Figure 17.12** Cutaneous marginal zone lymphoproliferative disorder. (a) Band-like infiltrate with (b) many plasmacytoid cells and plasma cells. Staining for immunoglobulin light chains shows (c) positivity for lambda and (d) negativity for kappa.

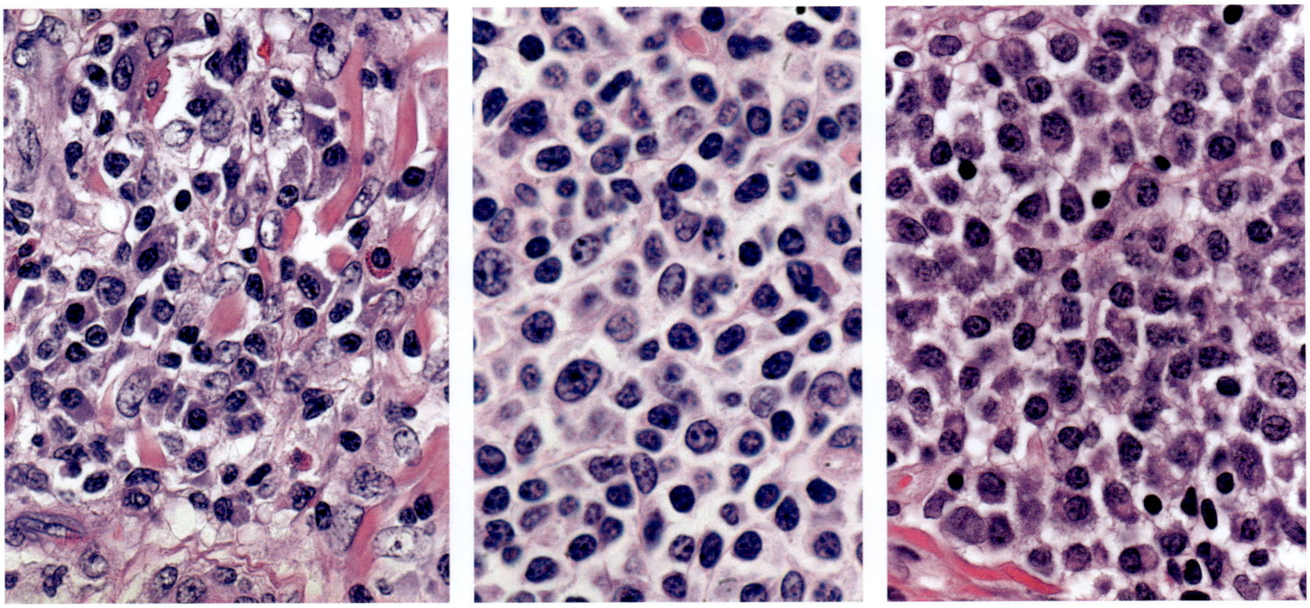

(a) (b) (c)

**Figure 17.13** Cutaneous marginal zone lymphoproliferative disorder. Morphologic variations of the conventional variant. (a) Marginal zone cells ("centrocyte-like") with abundant cytoplasm admixed with plasma cells, small lymphocytes, and eosinophils. (b) "Monocytoid" cells, some with blastoid morphology. (c) Lymphoplasmacytoid cells and plasma cells, admixed with some blastoid cells.

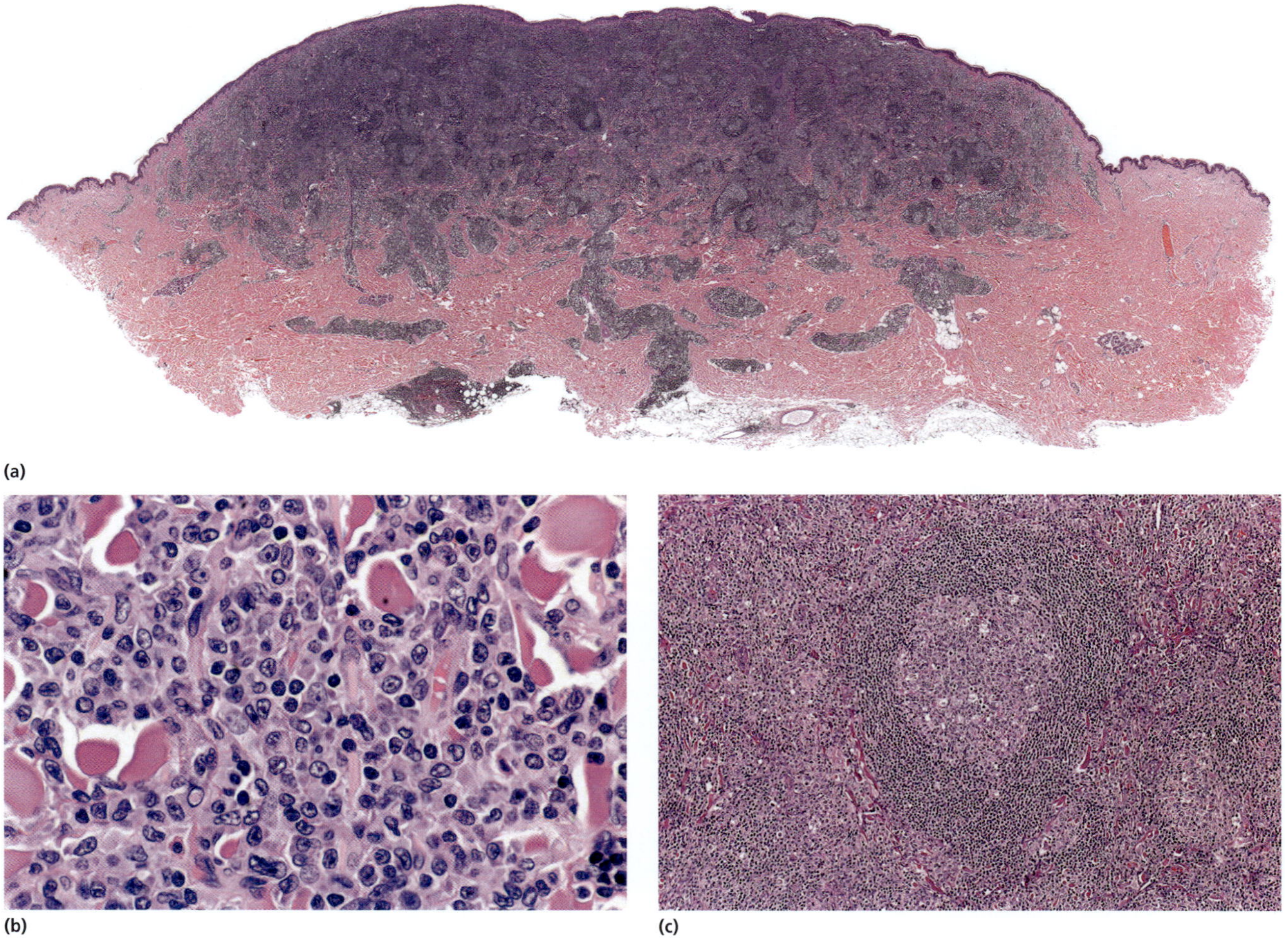

(a) (b) (c)

**Figure 17.14** Cutaneous marginal zone lymphoproliferative disorder, conventional variant. (a) "Top-heavy" infiltrate with the characteristic pale and dark areas typical of this variant of cutaneous marginal zone lymphoma. (b) The atypical population consists predominantly of marginal zone cells. (c) Reactive germinal centers are present in most cases of cutaneous marginal zone lymphoproliferative disease.

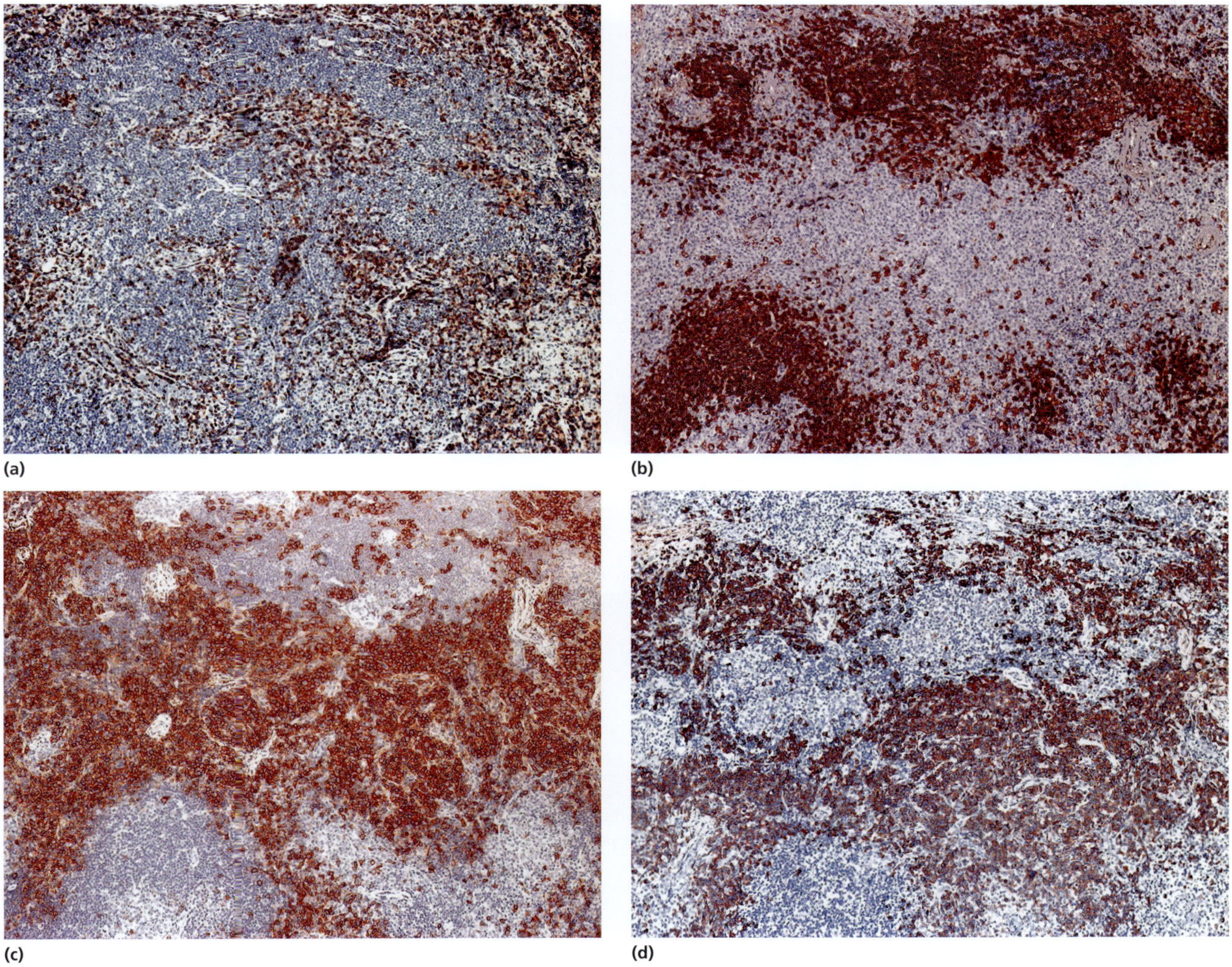


**Figure 17.15** Cutaneous marginal zone lymphoproliferative disorder, conventional variant. Staining for (a) CD3 and (b) CD20 shows many reactive lymphocytes, admixed with (c) CD138$^{+}$ neoplastic plasma cells showing (d) monoclonal expression of the immunoglobulin light chain kappa.

centers are present in the vast majority of cases of cutaneous marginal zone lymphoproliferative disorder, thus reactive follicular B lymphocytes are constantly present.

In practically all cases of cutaneous marginal zone lymphoproliferative disorder, the intracytoplasmic monotypic expression of Ig light chains can be observed, and is more prominent when the number of plasma cells is larger. The monoclonal expression of either kappa or lambda Ig light chain represents the most important immunohistochemical feature, and for practical purposes, a diagnosis of cutaneous marginal zone lymphoproliferative disorder should be seriously questioned if monoclonality cannot be demonstrated on the biopsy specimen. In this context, in situ hybridization for the Ig light chains is a more specific method than immunohistochemistry for the detection of clonality (Fig. 17.16), and automated RNA in situ hybridization for kappa and lambda mRNA has been shown to have a sensitivity comparable or superior to flow cytometry [73]. Double staining for kappa and lambda may be helpful in evaluating the ratio of positive cells (a κ:λ ratio of 10:1 is considered diagnostic of monoclonality, or 4:1 if λ:κ) (Fig. 17.17), but in the vast majority of cases, the staining pattern is clear-cut, and it is not necessary to compare counts of positive cells. The monotypic cells are arranged in variably large clusters, usually located at the periphery of the lymphoid aggregates. A typical distribution of monotypic plasma cells is that observed as a variably large band located in the subepidermal area. When reactive germinal centers are present, sometimes features of so-called "follicular colonization" may be observed, consisting of neoplastic plasma cells located within the germinal centers (Fig. 17.18). However, in my experience, this finding is not common in cutaneous cases.

Staining for Ki67 shows that the proliferating population of cells is characteristically disposed at the periphery of the lymphoid aggregates (Fig. 17.19).

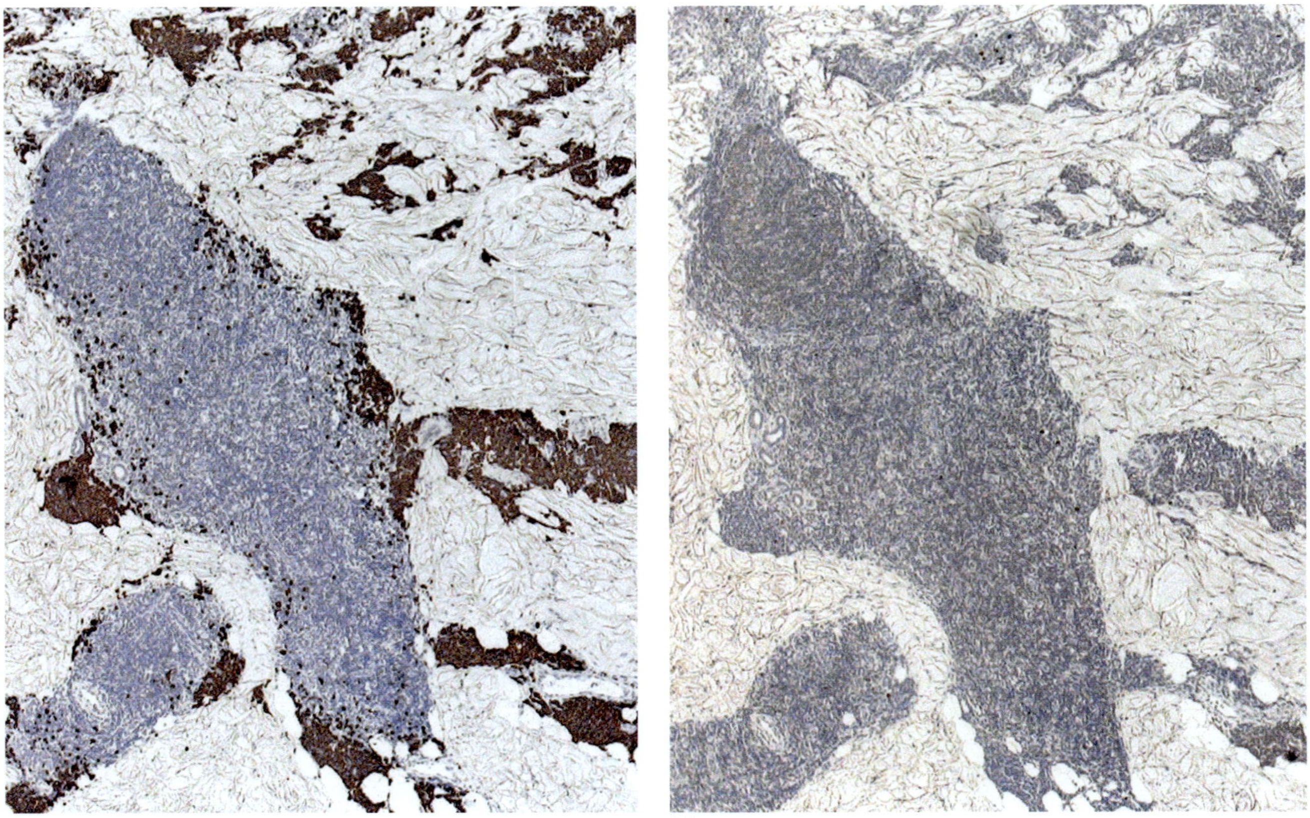

(a) (b)

**Figure 17.16** Cutaneous marginal zone lymphoproliferative disorder, conventional variant. In situ hybridization for the Ig light chains kappa and lambda. (a) Monoclonal population of plasma cells positive for lambda, located at the periphery of the nodular infiltrates and arranged in variably large clusters. (b) Negative in situ hybridization for kappa.

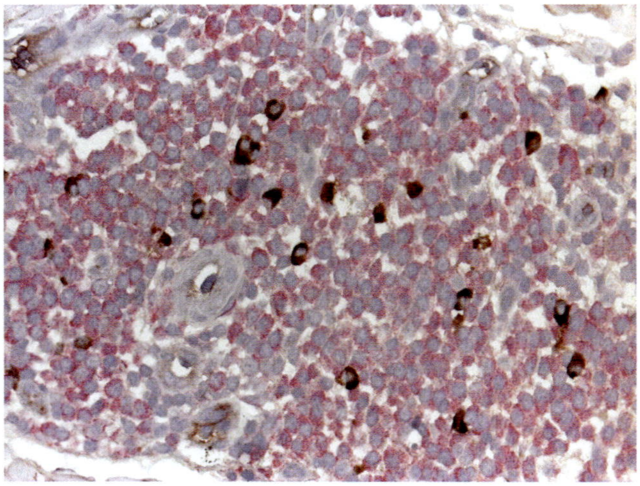

**Figure 17.17** Cutaneous marginal zone lymphoproliferative disorder, conventional variant. Double staining for kappa (red) and lambda (brown) allows a better comparison of the immunoglobulin light chain ratio. A ratio of 10:1 is considered diagnostic of monoclonality if kappa predominates (4:1 if lambda predominates).

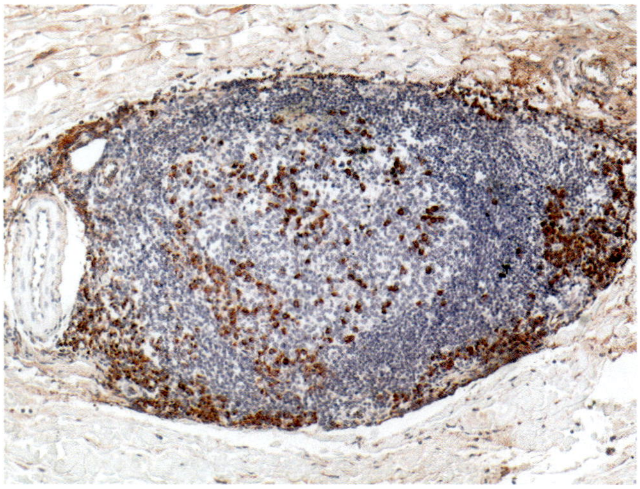

**Figure 17.18** Cutaneous marginal zone lymphoproliferative disorder, conventional variant. Monoclonal plasma cells expressing the immunoglobulin light chain lambda located at the periphery of the nodule and colonizing a reactive germinal center ("follicular colonization").

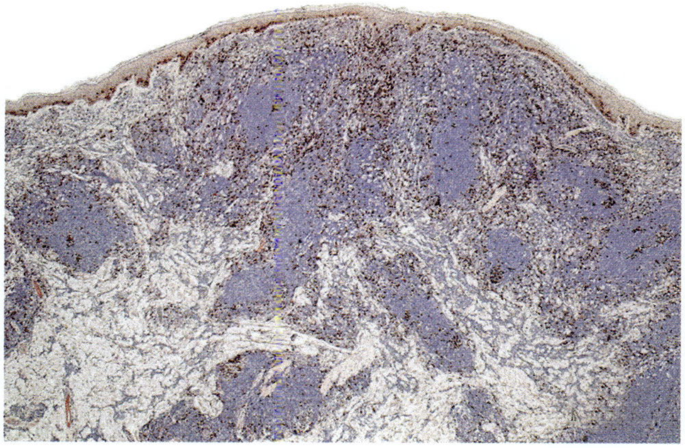

Figure 17.19 Cutaneous marginal zone lymphoproliferative disorder, conventional variant. Staining for Ki-67 highlights proliferating cells arranged at the periphery of the lymphoid aggregates.

The IgM expression can be observed in a small subset of cutaneous cases characterized by larger numbers of B-lymphocytes and more frequent extracutaneous dissemination (Fig. 17.20) [74]. These cases correspond to the ones without Ig class switch (see below), and present with a more monomorphous histopathological pattern rather than with the admixture of several cell types seen in most cases of cutaneous marginal zone lymphoproliferative disorder. It is possible that most of the nonclass-switched cases fall into the group of cutaneous marginal zone lymphoproliferative disorder with lymphoplasmacytic differentiation (the old "cutaneous immunocytoma"), but IgM-positivity is rare and there are no detailed data about its frequency in different morphological variants.

Clusters of CD123$^{+}$ plasmacytoid dendritic cells have been reported in some cases of cutaneous marginal zone lymphoproliferative disorder, and a pathogenetic role of these cells has

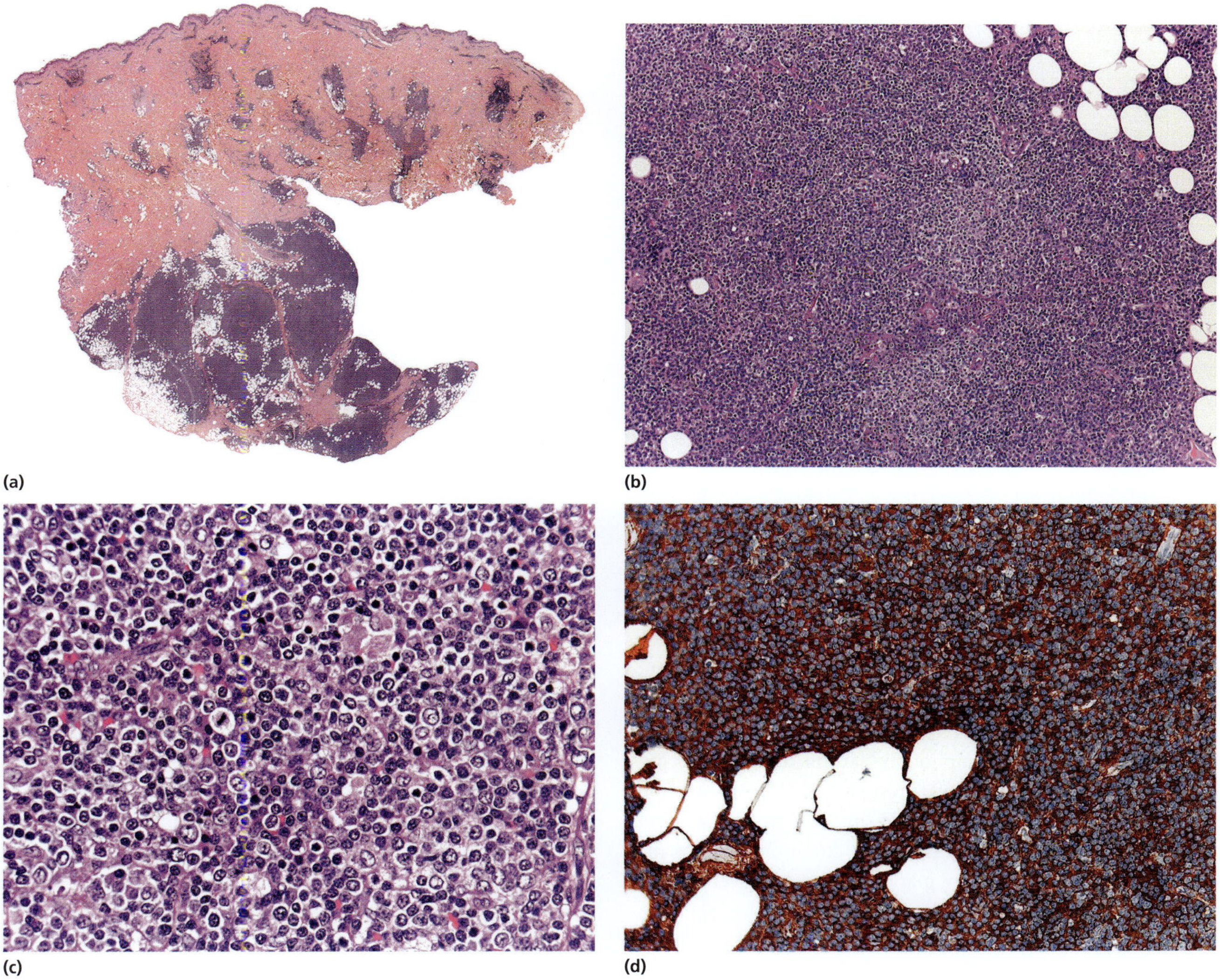


Figure 17.20 Cutaneous marginal zone lymphoproliferative disorder, conventional variant. (a) Bottom-heavy, (b) dense lymphoid infiltrated with (c) many marginal zone cells and plasmacytoid cells and (d) strong positivity for IgM.

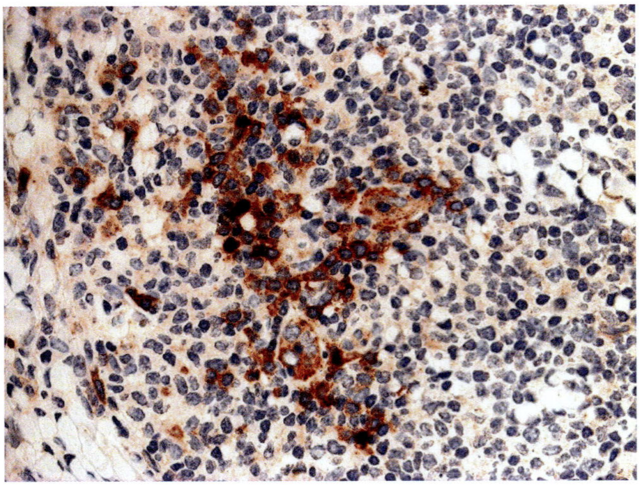

**Figure 17.21** Cutaneous marginal zone lymphoproliferative disorder, conventional variant. Staining for CD123 shows a small cluster of positive plasmacytoid dendritic cells.

been proposed [75]. In my experience and in that of others [74], these clusters are always small and are unrelated to the neoplastic cells (Fig. 17.21). In my opinion, plasmacytoid dendritic cells do not play any role in the disease. PD-1$^{+}$ reactive T lymphocytes have been observed more often in cutaneous follicle center lymphoma than in cutaneous marginal zone lymphoproliferative disorder (neoplastic cells are negative with this marker) [76], but in my experience, it does not play a role in the differential diagnosis between the two entities.

## Molecular genetics

A monoclonal rearrangement of the Ig genes can be observed in approximately 50–60% of cases. The t(11;18)(q21;q21), detected mostly in gastric and lung tumors, is almost never present in cutaneous cases [3, 4, 43, 77, 78]. A specific interchromosomal 14;18 translocation involving *IGH* and *MALT1* has been described in a subset of cutaneous marginal zone lymphoproliferative disorders as well as of marginal zone lymphomas of other organs including the liver, ocular adnexa, and salivary glands [78]. It seems that rare cases of cutaneous marginal zone lymphoproliferative disorder may harbor a conventional t(14;18) involving *IGH* and *BCL2* as well [79]. A t(3;14)(p14;q32) involving *IGH* and *FOXP1* has been detected in a subset of MALT lymphomas arising at different sites, including 2/20 cutaneous cases tested [80]. Cases showing a trisomy 3 may be characterized by the upregulation of *FOXP1* [80]. Trisomy 18 is relatively common in intestinal, ocular adnexal, and salivary glands tumors, but very rare in cutaneous cases.

A study on class-switched Igs revealed that cutaneous marginal zone lymphoproliferative disorder deviates from the general profile of extranodal marginal zone lymphoma of MALT [81]. IgM is expressed in most noncutaneous cases, whereas cutaneous marginal zone lymphoproliferative disorders express IgG, IgA, and IgE and do not show an obvious Ig repertoire bias. In addition, in contrast to other extranodal marginal zone lymphomas of MALT, the isotype-switched cutaneous marginal zone lymphoproliferative disorders lack the chemokine receptor CXCR3 and seem to arise in a different inflammatory environment [81].

Gene expression studies using cDNA microarrays revealed that cutaneous marginal zone lymphoproliferative disorder is characterized by a plasma cell signature [82], but selection of cases may have introduced a bias. As already mentioned, unbalanced genomic alterations differ between splenic and extranodal marginal zone lymphomas, with nodal cases being intermediate between the two groups [8]. Genetic aberrations found in adult and pediatric cases seem to be similar [83].

In one study, a majority of cases presented alterations in the *FAS* gene affecting the functionally relevant death domain of the apoptosis-regulating FAS/CD95 protein [84], suggesting that the cells may acquire a survival advantage by escaping apoptosis. This molecular mechanism could explain the very indolent behavior of this low-grade cutaneous lymphoproliferative disorder. Other aberrations include hypermethylation of p15 and/or p16 and expression of p15 and/or p16 protein observed in some patients with cutaneous marginal zone lymphoproliferative disorder [85]. Aberrant somatic hypermutations and frequent use of VH1-69 and VH4-59 segments can also be observed, suggesting that they could contribute to the pathogenesis of the disease by mutating regulatory and coding sequences of specific genes, including the proto-oncogenes *PAX5*, *RhoH/TTF*, *c-MYC*, and *MIM1* [86, 87]. *BRAF* mutations have been identified in a minority of cases of nodal marginal zone lymphoma (4/25, 16%), but not in four cutaneous cases analyzed [10]. Methylation of *DAPK1* and *CDKN2A* seems to be common [88], whereas *MYD88*$^{L265P}$ mutations are not observed.

A distinct percentage of disseminated marginal zone lymphoma of the MALT shows the emergence of different neoplastic clones over time; as already mentioned; however, extracutaneous spread is exceedingly rare in primary cutaneous marginal zone lymphoproliferative disorder, and studies on clone variability are not available.

## Treatment

Solitary lesions may be excised. Complete responses may be achieved after administration of intralesional or systemic steroids [89]. Many patients can be managed with a so-called "watchful waiting" strategy [90]. Patients with multiple lesions can be treated with anti-CD20 antibody (rituximab). The anti-CD20 antibody may be administered either intralesionally or systemically and is usually effective, but recurrences are frequent. Radiotherapy may be used, particularly for single tumors. However, recurrences are often at sites different from those treated initially, so this option is usually not suggested as first-line treatment, particularly for young patients. In this context, marginal zone lymphoma of the MALT probably represents a multifocal disease with neoplastic cells entering the blood and relocating to distant sites. Such a mechanism may explain the clinical behavior of cutaneous marginal zone lymphoproliferative disorder as well, and suggests some conceptual similarities with the most common form of indolent cutaneous lymphoma, namely, mycosis fungoides. Recommendations for radiation therapy from the EORTC cutaneous lymphoma tumor group have been published recently [91].

Complete responses after systemic antibiotics have been reported, and this should be the first-line therapy for patients with evidence of *B. burgdorferi* infection (see also the section on cutaneous marginal zone lymphoproliferative disorder, lymphoplasmacytic variant, in this chapter) [92, 93].

For patients presenting with multiple lesions requiring treatment, chlorambucil is often used in European centers (but less so in the United States), especially in older patients and for a maximum of 3 months [90]. Systemic multiagent chemotherapy should be reserved for those rare cases with extracutaneous dissemination.

## Prognosis

The prognosis of cutaneous marginal zone lymphoproliferative disorder, conventional variant, is excellent, and the estimated five-year survival is 98% [94–96]. A similar prognosis has been demonstrated for cases occurring in pediatric age [97]. Recurrences can be observed in 40–50% of patients after successful treatment but usually retain the low-grade features of the primary tumor [98, 99]. In my experience, there is no prognostic significance related to the main histopathologic subtypes (conventional, lymphoplasmacytic, and plasmacytic). Blastic transformation in recurrent lesions has been associated with a worse prognosis [100], but cases presenting with a blastoid morphology from the beginning do not seem to have a more aggressive course [101a]. It has been suggested that cases with Bcl-10 nuclear expression have a locally more aggressive behavior [43] and that IgM positive cases are more frequently complicated by extracutaneous spread [40, 84]. In a recent study from the French Study Group of Cutaneous Lymphoma, three out of three IgM positive cases exhibited large cell transformation and extracutaneous spread [101b], Detection of specific cells in the bone marrow does not have an impact on the prognosis of patients with cutaneous marginal zone lymphoproliferative disorder [63, 64].

Cutaneous cases have a better prognosis compared to that of lesions arising in the gastrointestinal tract or in the lungs [102], again pointing at possible differences among extranodal marginal zone lymphomas arising in different organs.

A prognostic index based on elevated LDH, number of lesions >2, and the presence of nodular lesions has been suggested for indolent cutaneous B-cell lymphomas (cutaneous lymphomas prognostic index – CLIPi) [103]. However, in my experience, LDH is never elevated in these patients and the presence of more than two lesions and/or of nodular lesions does not have any impact on prognosis. Thus, I do not believe that this index has any utility in assessing prognosis of indolent cutaneous B-cell lymphomas, including cutaneous marginal zone lymphoproliferative disorder.


**Résumé**

**Cutaneous marginal zone lymphoproliferative disorder, conventional variant**

| | | |
|---|---|---|
| **Clinical** | Young adults and adults; can occur in children. Solitary or grouped papules or small nodules. Preferential locations: upper extremities, trunk. | |
| **Morphology** | Patchy, nodular, or diffuse infiltrates. Characteristic pattern with central nodular dark area composed of small reactive lymphocytes with or without the formation of germinal centers, surrounded by a pale area where neoplastic marginal zone cells, lymphoplasmacytoid cells, and plasma cells predominate. | |
| **Immunohistochemistry** | CD20, CD79a | + |
| | Bcl-2 | + |
| | IRTA1 | + |
| | MNDA | –/+ |
| | CD5, CD10, Bcl-6, Cyclin-D1 | – |
| | cIg | + (monoclonal) |
| | IgM | positive cases may show a more aggressive course (cases without class-switch) |
| **Genetics** | Monoclonal rearrangement of the Ig genes detected in 50–60% of cases. t(14;18)(q32;q21) or trisomy 3 in a minority of cases. Class-switched immunoglobulins in the majority of cases. | |
| **Treatment guidelines** | Excision of solitary lesions; rituximab; local radiotherapy; "watchful waiting." Antibiotic treatment should be used as first-line treatment in cases with evidence of *Borrelia burgdorferi* infection. Systemic chemotherapy reserved for rare patients with extracutaneous spread. | |

## Cutaneous marginal zone lymphoproliferative disorder, lymphoplasmacytic variant

The lymphoplasmacytic variant of cutaneous marginal zone lymphoproliferative disorder is characterized by a monomorphous proliferation of small lymphocytes, lymphoplasmacytoid cells, and plasma cells showing monotypic intracytoplasmic Igs. Patients do not show the features of Waldenström macroglobulinemia and have an excellent prognosis and response to treatment. Rare reports on cutaneous lymphoplasmacytic lymphoma in patients with Waldenström macroglobulinemia probably represent secondary cutaneous involvement rather than primary cutaneous lymphoplasmacytic lymphoma (see also Chapter 20) [104]. Most of the cases described in the past as "primary cutaneous immunocytoma" would be classified today as "conventional" marginal zone lymphoproliferative disorders, but some showed the peculiar clinicopathologic features described in this section [105, 106].

There may be a strong link between this variant of marginal zone lymphoproliferative disorder and an infection by *B. burgdorferi*. Cases of "cutaneous immunocytoma" arising within skin lesions of acrodermatitis chronica atrophicans have been reported [107]. In a study using the polymerase chain reaction (PCR) technique, 75% of cases classified as "cutaneous immunocytoma" were positive for *Borrelia* DNA, as compared to 10% of cases of conventional marginal zone lymphoproliferative disorder [25].

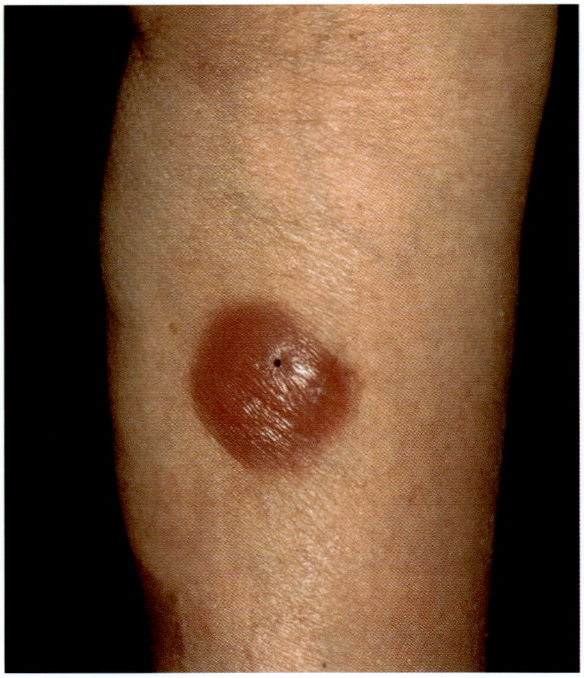

**Figure 17.22** Cutaneous marginal zone lymphoproliferative disorder, lymphoplasmacytic variant. Large dome-shaped tumor on the lower leg.

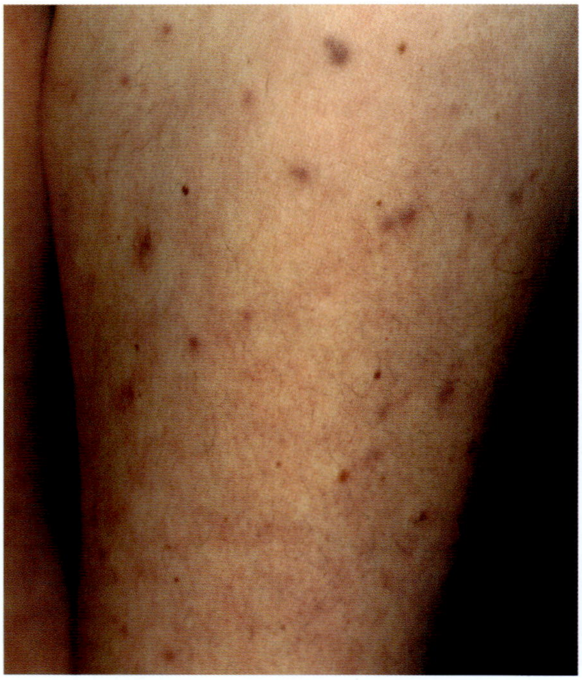

**Figure 17.23** Cutaneous marginal zone lymphoproliferative disorder, lymphoplasmacytic variant. Miliary, livid papules on the thigh.

## Clinical features

Patients are typically elderly, of either gender. Clinical examination reveals erythematous, reddish-brown plaques or dome-shaped tumors located especially on the lower extremities (Fig. 17.22). Ulceration is uncommon. Generalized tumors are never encountered. Rarely, patients present with miliary lesions restricted to an anatomic area (Fig. 17.23). Anetoderma may develop within skin lesions of the lymphoplasmacytic variant of cutaneous marginal zone lymphoma (Fig. 17.24).

## Histopathology, immunophenotype, and molecular genetics

### Histopathology

The architectural pattern is characterized by dense, monomorphous, nodular, or diffuse infiltrates with involvement of the dermis and subcutis (Fig. 17.25). The epidermis is usually spared. At scanning magnification, the biphasic pattern observed in conventional cases of cutaneous marginal zone lymphoma is not seen because the infiltrate is monomorphous. In addition, the neoplastic cells do not possess the abundant clear cytoplasm of marginal zone cells, conveying to the tumor a "darker" appearance compared to conventional cutaneous marginal zone lymphoproliferative disorder.

The predominating cell types are lymphoplasmacytoid cells (Fig. 17.26). In addition, plasma cells are usually present, often located at the periphery of the infiltrates. Periodic acid-Schiff

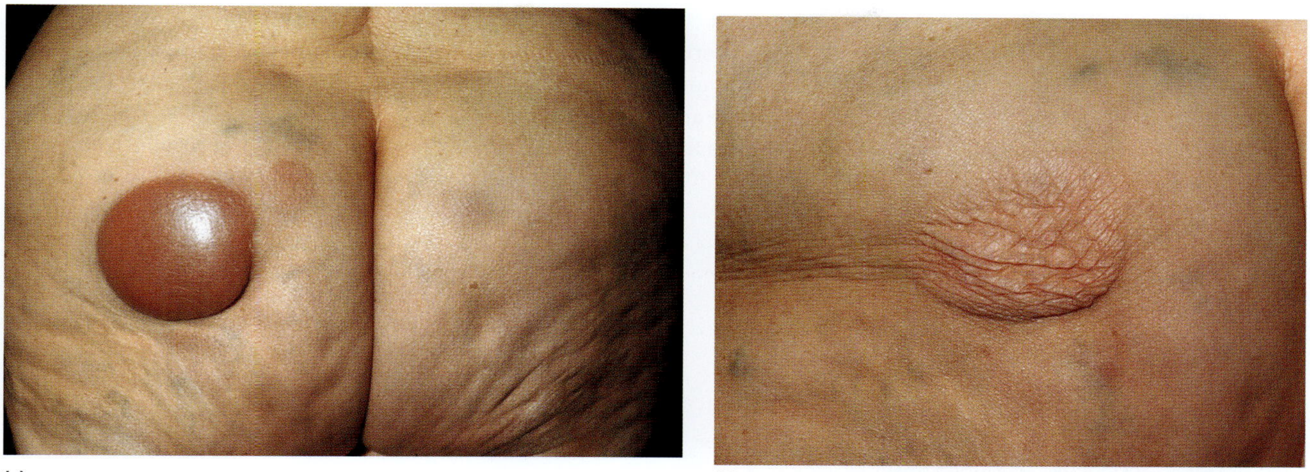

(a) (b)

Figure 17.24 Cutaneous marginal zone lymphoproliferative disorder, lymphoplasmacytic variant. (a) Large dome-shaped tumor on the buttocks. (b) Note resolution with anetoderma after radiotherapy.

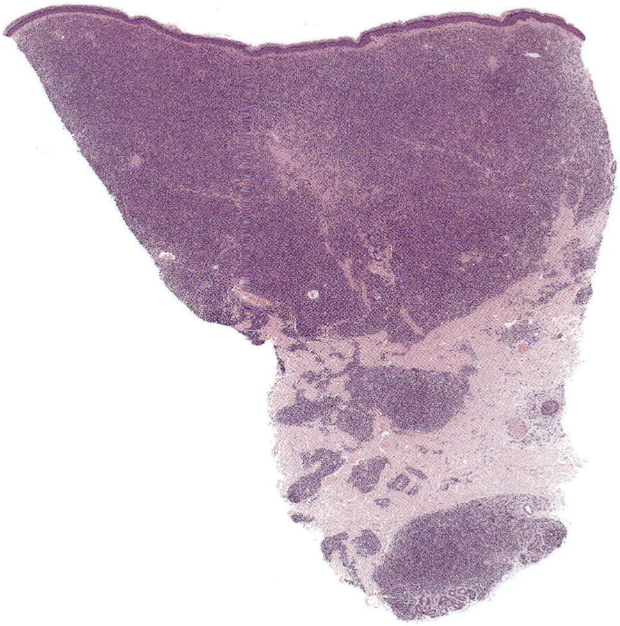

Figure 17.25 Cutaneous marginal zone lymphoproliferative disorder, lymphoplasmacytic variant. Dense, diffuse, monomorphous infiltrate within the entire dermis and the superficial part of the subcutaneous fat.

(PAS)-positive intranuclear inclusions (Dutcher bodies) are observed as a rule and represent a valuable diagnostic clue (Fig. 17.26 inset). Reactive lymphoid follicles and germinal centers are rare.

In contrast to the conventional variant of cutaneous marginal zone lymphoproliferative disorder, neoplastic cells in the lymphoplasmacytic variant represent the great majority of the infiltrate, and reactive T and B lymphocytes and histiocytes are only a minority. Eosinophils and a granulomatous reaction are usually absent.

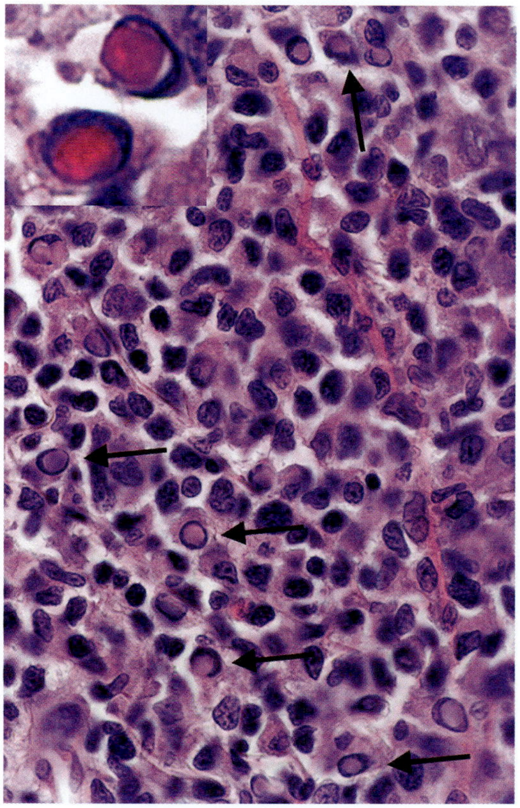

Figure 17.26 Cutaneous marginal zone lymphoproliferative disorder, lymphoplasmacytic variant. Lymphoplasmacytoid lymphocytes predominate. Note several eosinophilic intranuclear inclusions ("Dutcher bodies") (arrows). Intranuclear inclusions ("Dutcher bodies") stain bright purple–red with periodic acid-Schiff (PAS) (inset).

## Immunophenotype

The cells express B-cell markers and monoclonal cytoplasmic Igs, more often IgG (but nonclass-switched cases positive for IgM may be more common than in other variants of cutaneous marginal zone lymphoproliferative disorder). In contrast to the conventional variant, staining for CD20 shows a uniform positivity of the vast majority of the cells, which also show monoclonal light chain restriction (Fig. 17.27). The cells are positive for Bcl-2, and in some cases for CD43, and negative for CD5, CD10, Bcl-6, and cyclin D1.

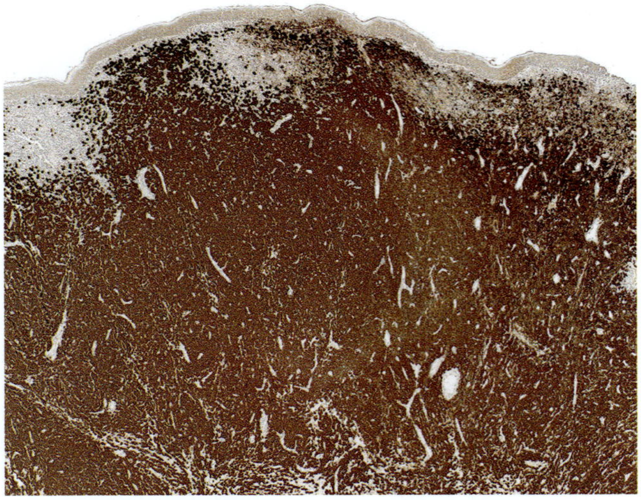

**Figure 17.27** Cutaneous marginal zone lymphoproliferative disorder, lymphoplasmacytic variant. In situ hybridization for the immunoglobulin light chain kappa shows positivity of nearly all cells.

## Molecular genetics

The molecular analysis reveals monoclonal rearrangement of the Ig genes in most cases. The evaluation of specific genetic abnormalities is difficult, as cases are lumped together with those of the conventional variant of marginal zone lymphoproliferative disorder.

## Treatment

Small solitary nodules can be excised surgically. Larger lesions can be treated by local radiotherapy. As for other types of low-grade lymphoma, a "watchful waiting" strategy may be appropriate in some patients. Systemic chemotherapy should be considered only for patients with extracutaneous spread.

Cases with proven association with *B. burgdorferi* infection should be managed with systemic antibiotics first. In areas endemic for *Borrelia* infection, systemic antibiotic treatment may be considered as a first-line treatment for patients with the lymphoplasmacytic variant of cutaneous marginal zone lymphoproliferative disorder regardless of the results of serologic investigations.

## Prognosis

The prognosis of the lymphoplasmacytic variant of cutaneous marginal zone lymphoproliferative disorder is excellent, with only a few patients experiencing a more aggressive course. Cutaneous recurrences can be observed after treatment (even after chemotherapy), usually at the same site of the original lesion(s).

### Résumé

**Cutaneous marginal zone lymphoproliferative disorder, lymphoplasmacytic variant**

| | | |
|---|---|---|
| **Clinical** | Adults and elderly. Solitary or grouped plaques or dome-shaped tumors. Preferential location: lower extremities. Frequent association with *Borrelia burgdorferi* infection. | |
| **Morphology** | Monomorphous, nodular, or diffuse infiltrates characterized by predominance of lymphoplasmacytoid lymphocytes (representing the majority) and plasma cells (often arranged at the periphery of the infiltrates). Intranuclear $PAS^+$ inclusions (Dutcher bodies) frequent. | |
| **Immunohistochemistry** | CD20, CD79a | + |
| | Bcl-2 | + |
| | CD5, CD10, Bcl-6 | – |
| | cIg | + (monoclonal) |
| | IgM | positive cases may show a more aggressive course (cases without class-switch) |
| **Genetics** | Monoclonal rearrangement of the Ig genes detected in the majority of cases. | |
| **Treatment guidelines** | Radiotherapy; surgical excision of small solitary lesions; "watchful waiting;" rituximab. Antibiotic treatment may be effective and may be used as a first-line treatment in countries with endemic *Borrelia burgdorferi* infection. | |

## Cutaneous marginal zone lymphoproliferative disorder, plasmacytic variant

The plasmacytic variant of cutaneous marginal zone lymphoproliferative disorder is characterized by an almost exclusive proliferation of neoplastic plasma cells, hence the former classification as "primary cutaneous plasmacytoma." In fact, most cases reported under this diagnosis probably represent examples of cutaneous marginal zone lymphoproliferative disorder with a prominent plasma cell differentiation. This variant of cutaneous marginal zone lymphoproliferative disorder is exceedingly rare and should be distinguished from secondary skin involvement by multiple myeloma (see Chapter 20) [108]. In this context, it must be underlined that plasma cells are present in all types of cutaneous marginal zone lymphoproliferative disorder, and only when they represent the majority of the entire infiltrate a case should be classified as plasmacytic variant. The literature, however, is confusing and cases reported as "plasmacytic variant" would be classified as conventional marginal zone lymphoproliferative disorder in other centers [109]. I have observed patients with "primary cutaneous plasmacytoma" who, after successful treatment, relapsed with skin lesions showing histopathologic and phenotypic features of conventional marginal zone lymphoproliferative disorder. In addition, in a Workshop on Cutaneous Plasmacytoma organized by the EORTC-Cutaneous Lymphomas Task Force in Bilbao in 2001, no clear-cut cases of primary cutaneous plasmacytoma could be identified. The literature on primary cutaneous plasmacytoma (even cases published more recently [110]) should be analyzed with a critical eye, keeping in mind that most of these cases should probably be classified as cutaneous marginal zone lymphoproliferative disorder, plasmacytic variant.

A study revealed that the expression of IgG4 by neoplastic cells can be observed in almost 40% of cases of cutaneous marginal zone lymphoproliferative disorder, plasmacytic type [12]. None of the $IgG4^{+}$ cases had other signs of systemic IgG4 disease, suggesting that IgG4 positivity may be considered as a chance finding. The real percentage of cases of cutaneous marginal zone lymphoproliferative disorder positive for IgG4 has not been confirmed by large studies.

## Clinical features

The clinical presentation is similar to that of the conventional variant of cutaneous marginal zone lymphoproliferative disorder, with papules and small nodules, often solitary, located mostly on the upper extremities and the trunk.

## Histopathology, immunophenotype, and molecular genetics

### Histopathology

Lesions consist of dense nodules and/or sheets of cells within the entire dermis and subcutis (Fig. 17.28), predominantly composed of mature plasma cells admixed with some blastoid cells (Fig. 17.29). In some cases, it may be difficult to distinguish the plasmacytic from the blastoid variant of marginal zone lymphoproliferative disorder. Dutcher bodies are found occasionally, whereas Russell bodies (intracytoplasmic Igs' inclusions) are more common and may rarely be predominant within the infiltrate (Fig. 17.30). Small reactive lymphocytes are usually few. Reactive germinal centers may be observed rarely.

Amyloid deposits are usually not found in cutaneous marginal zone lymphoproliferative disorder, plasmacytic variant (but cutaneous amyloidoma is characterized by prominent amyloid deposition – see below the specific section). Crystalloid intracytoplasmic inclusions within histiocytes and macrophages ("crystal storing histiocytosis") are a rare feature of secondary cutaneous involvement by multiple myeloma rather than of primary cutaneous marginal zone lymphoproliferative disorder, plasmacytic variant (see Chapter 29).

### Immunophenotype

Plasma cells show the monoclonal expression of one Ig light chain, which is usually easy to detect in routine specimens. Most B-cell-associated markers are negative, but cells can be stained by antibodies specific for CD38 or CD138, and in some cases for CD79a. The immunohistochemical expression of cytokeratins, HMB45 and CD30, can be observed within plasma cells, representing a source of diagnostic error.

### Molecular genetics

Molecular analyses usually reveal a monoclonal rearrangement of the Ig genes. As already mentioned for the lymphoplasmacytic variant, for the plasmacytic variant of cutaneous marginal zone lymphoproliferative disorder, the evaluation of specific genetic abnormalities is also difficult, as cases are lumped together with those of the conventional variant.

## Treatment and prognosis

The analysis of data on treatment of this variant of cutaneous marginal zone lymphoproliferative disorder is hindered by the fact that some cases reported in the past as cutaneous plasmacytoma may have represented in truth as examples of specific skin manifestations of multiple myeloma, thus being characterized by a worse prognosis. In my experience, the prognosis is excellent and the treatment of choice is the same as for the conventional variant of cutaneous marginal zone lymphoproliferative disorder.

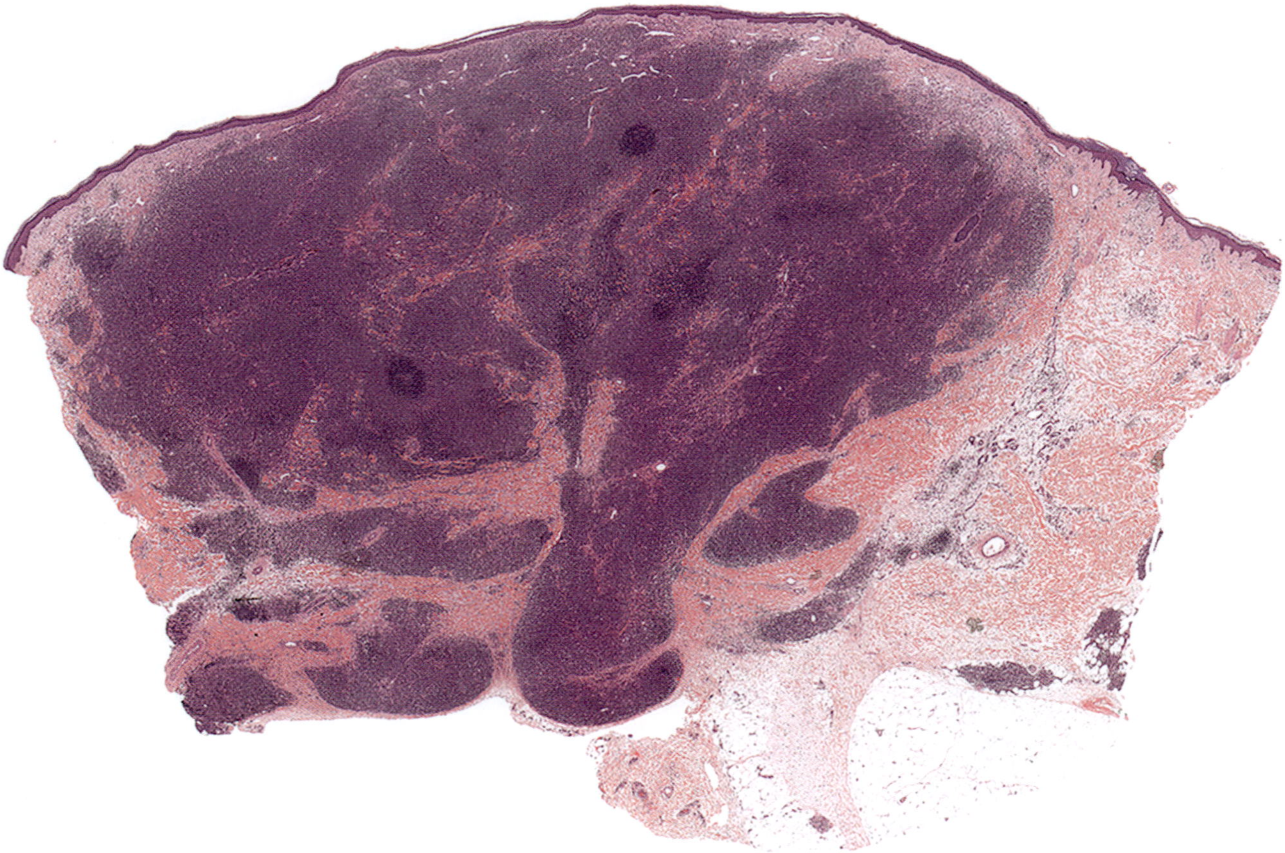

Figure 17.28 Cutaneous marginal zone lymphoproliferative disorder, plasmacytic variant. Dense infiltrates within the entire dermis. Note the predominance of pale areas representing sheets of neoplastic cells and only a few small, darker nodules (one with a germinal center) composed of reactive lymphocytes.

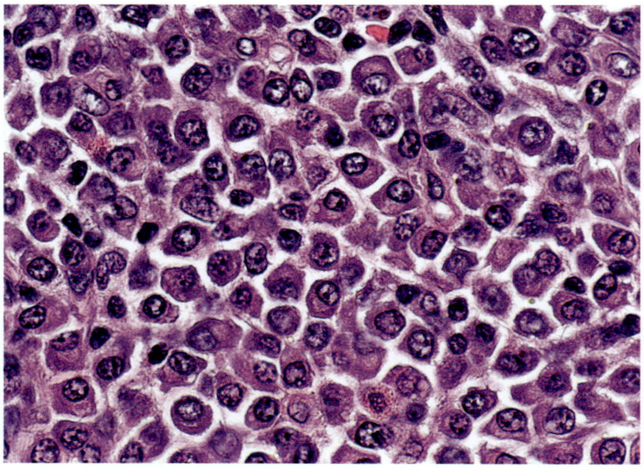

Figure 17.29 Cutaneous marginal zone lymphoproliferative disorder, plasmacytic variant. Predominance of atypical plasma cells admixed with some blastoid cells.

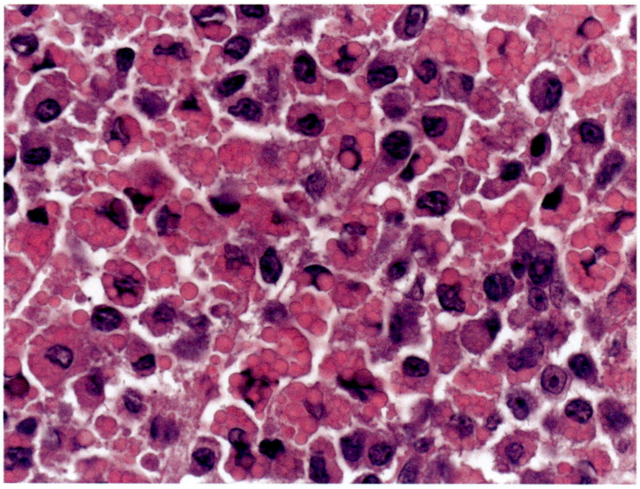

Figure 17.30 Cutaneous marginal zone lymphoproliferative disorder, plasmacytic variant. Note innumerable Russell bodies (intracytoplasmic immunoglobulins' inclusions) in this particular example.

## Résumé

**Cutaneous marginal zone lymphoproliferative disorder, plasmacytic variant**

| | | |
|---|---|---|
| **Clinical** | Same features as the conventional variant of cutaneous marginal zone lymphoproliferative disorder. | |
| **Morphology** | Nodular or diffuse infiltrates characterized by the predominance of plasma cells. Some of the plasma cells may have a blastic appearance. | |
| **Immunohistochemistry** | CD20 | – |
| | CD38, CD138 | + |
| | CD79a | +/– |
| | cIg | + (monoclonal) |
| **Genetics** | Monoclonal rearrangement of the Ig genes detected in the majority of cases. | |
| **Treatment guidelines** | Same as for the conventional variant of cutaneous marginal zone lymphoproliferative disorder. | |

## Cutaneous marginal zone lymphoproliferative disorder, blastoid variant

The blastoid variant of cutaneous marginal zone lymphoproliferative disorder is characterized by the predominance of large, blastoid cells, usually admixed with neoplastic plasma cells and with reactive cells. This variant may arise de novo or as transformation of a previous cutaneous marginal zone lymphoproliferative disorder [101a]. There may be overlapping histopathologic features with the plasmacytic variant in cases where several plasma cells display a blastoid morphology. Patients may have a more aggressive course, but fatal outcomes were not observed in a recent series [111].

## Clinical features

The clinical presentation is similar to that of the conventional variant of cutaneous marginal zone lymphoproliferative disorder. Patients present with papules and small nodules, often solitary, located mostly on the upper extremities and the trunk.

## Histopathology, immunophenotype, and molecular genetics

### Histopathology

Lesions consist of dense infiltrates within the entire dermis and subcutis, predominantly composed of mid-sized and large blastoid cells (Fig. 17.31). Mature plasma cells may be found

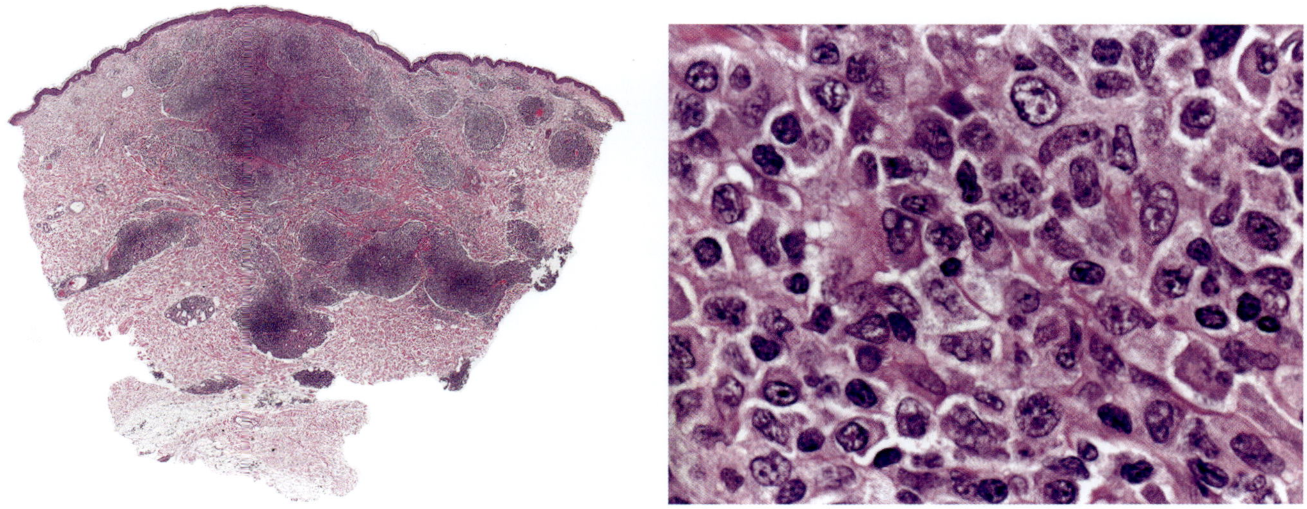

(a) (b)

**Figure 17.31** Cutaneous marginal zone lymphoproliferative disorder, blastoid variant. (a) Diffuse infiltrates involving the entire dermis. (b) Large cells with blastoid features, some resembling plasmablasts.

admixed with the blastoid cells and the differentiation from the plasmacytic variant may be difficult in some cases. Dutcher bodies and Russell bodies are absent. Small reactive lymphocytes and/or germinal centers are few, and the blastoid cells represent the majority of the infiltrate.

### Immunophenotype

The cells show the monoclonal expression of one Ig light chain. B-cell-associated markers are variably positive, as well as CD38 and CD138. The proliferation rate (Ki-67) is usually high (>50%). Bcl-6 and CD10 are negative, allowing distinction from cutaneous follicle center lymphoma, diffuse type. The cells are usually positive for MUM-1 and focal positivity for CD30 may be observed as well. CD5 and CD23 are positive in some of the cases [101a].

### Molecular genetics

Molecular analyses usually reveal a monoclonal rearrangement of the Ig genes. As already mentioned for other variants, for the blastoid variant of cutaneous marginal zone lymphoproliferative disorder, specific genetic data are also not available. Isolated cases revealed cytogenetic abnormalities suggesting a possible transformation into a diffuse large B cell lymphoma, but prognosis was not worse than in cases lacking these molecular features [111]. We studied one case that was negative for the t(14;18) and the t(11;18), and did not display a trisomy of chromosome 3.

## Treatment and prognosis

There are no data on the treatment of the blastoid variant of cutaneous marginal zone lymphoproliferative disorder, as cases have been lumped together with those of other variants. As already mentioned, blastic transformation in recurrent lesions has been associated with a worse prognosis [100], thus suggesting that these patients should probably be treated in a more aggressive fashion. Patients presenting with a blastoid morphology from the beginning seem to have a good prognosis, similar to that of other types of cutaneous marginal zone lymphoproliferative disorder [101a]. In fact, I have seen patients starting with blastoid cutaneous marginal zone lymphoproliferative disorder and relapsing with conventional lesions after treatment, without any sign of extracutaneous involvement.

The expression of CD5 and CD23 by neoplastic cells was observed in biopsies from patients with blastic transformation, thus suggesting a prognostic role for these two markers, but the number of cases was very small [101a].

**Résumé**

**Cutaneous marginal zone lymphoproliferative disorder, blastoid variant**

| | | |
|---|---|---|
| **Clinical** | Two main settings: arising de novo or in patients with a previous diagnosis of cutaneous lymphoproliferative disorder. | |
| **Morphology** | Dense infiltrates characterized by predominance of blastoid cells admixed with some plasma cells. | |
| **Immunohistochemistry** | CD20, CD79a, CD138 | +/– |
| | MUM-1 | + |
| | Bcl-6, CD10 | – |
| | CD5, CD23 | –/+ |
| | CD30 | +/– |
| | cIg | + (monoclonal) |
| **Genetics** | Monoclonal rearrangement of the Ig genes detected in the majority of cases. No genetic aberrations described specifically for this variant. | |
| **Treatment guidelines** | De novo cases: same as for the conventional variant of cutaneous marginal zone lymphoproliferative disorder. Cases with transformation should probably be treated in a more aggressive way, but specific data are not available. | |

## Cutaneous amyloidoma

In the vast majority of cases, cutaneous amyloidoma represents a lesion composed by few monoclonal plasma cells with prominent amyloid deposition (amyloid L) [29, 112]. Although the relationship with cutaneous marginal zone lymphoproliferative disorder has not been proved beyond doubt yet, the knowledge that some cases may harbor similar genetic alterations, and that recurrences of cutaneous amyloidoma may present with histopathological features of conventional cutaneous marginal zone lymphoproliferative disorder lends support to the hypothesis that the two disease exist in a spectrum [29]. In addition, I have observed rarely cases of "conventional" cutaneous marginal zone lymphoproliferative disorder showing focally areas of amyloid deposition (Fig. 17.32).

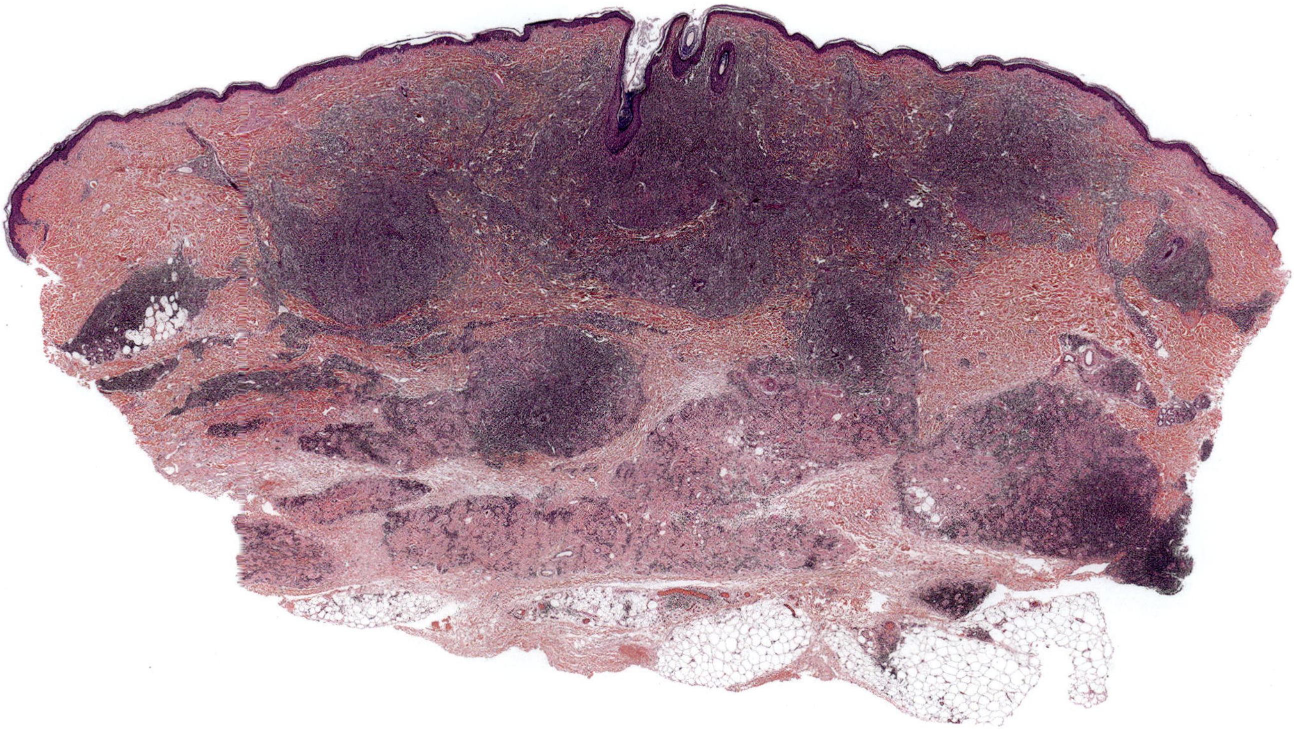

(a)

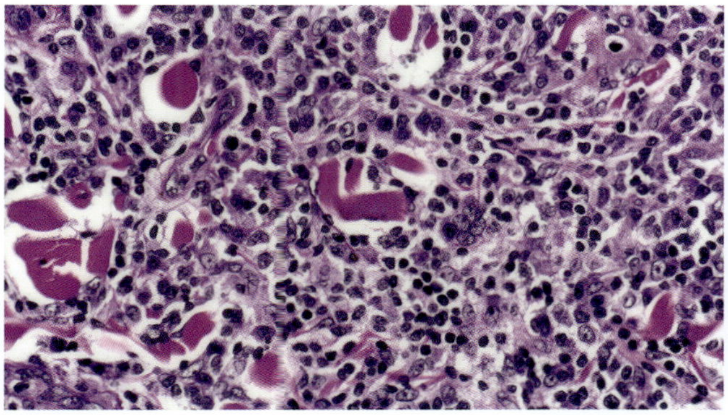

(b)

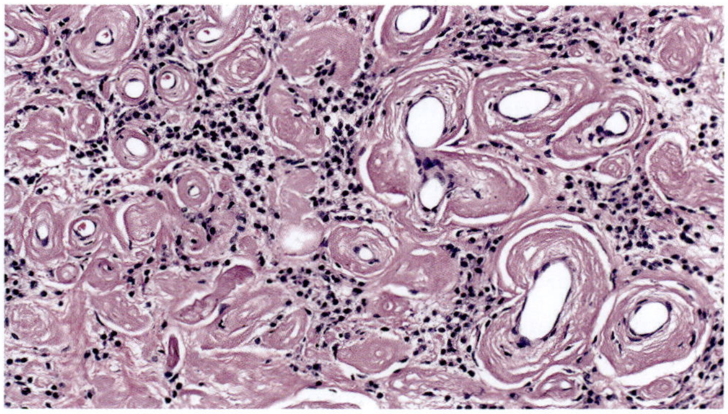

(c)

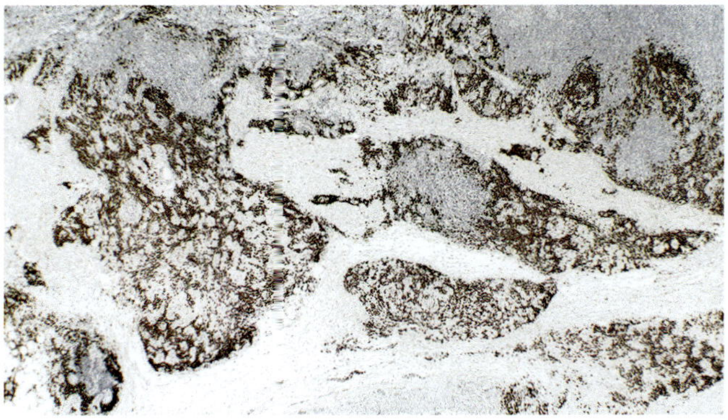

(d)

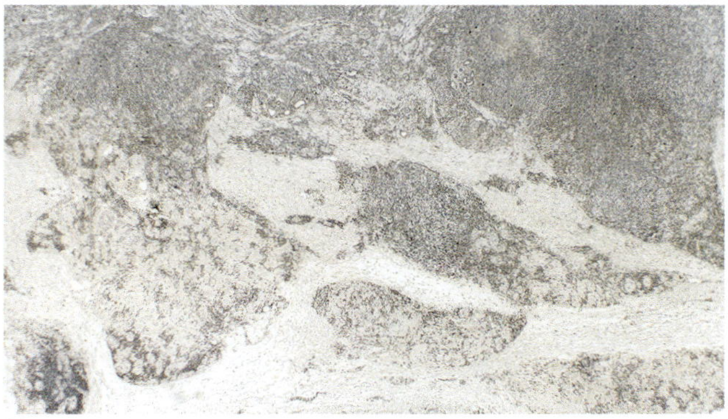

(e)

**Figure 17.32** Cutaneous marginal zone lymphoproliferative disorder with amyloid deposition. (a) Dense lymphoid infiltrate within the entire dermis. (b) Mononuclear cells with features of plasmacytoid cells and marginal zone cells admixed with numerous small lymphocytes. (c) Amyloid deposition around the vessels in the deeper part of the lesion. In situ hybridization for the immunoglobulin light chains shows (d) positivity of the majority of plasma cells for lambda and (e) negativity for kappa.

Interestingly, a condition analogous to cutaneous amyloidoma, termed "nodular pulmonary amyloidosis," may be detected in the lungs of patients with Sjögren syndrome [113]. Similar features can be observed also in other forms of AL-amyloidosis localized to single sites in different organs [114]. Nodular pulmonary amyloidosis is characterized by circumscribed deposits of AL-amyloid in the connective tissue of the lungs, associated with a sparse lymphoplasmacytic infiltrate characterized by monotypic light chain restriction [113]. Nodular pulmonary amyloidosis may be regarded as the pulmonary counterpart of cutaneous amyloidoma, and in fact, these patients may present with cutaneous lesions of marginal zone lymphoma at onset or recurrence [115]. In analogy to cutaneous amyloidoma, nodular pulmonary amyloidosis is considered as a localized low-grade B-cell neoplasm closely related to MALT lymphomas [115].

## Clinical features

Patients present with solitary, waxy small nodules, located mostly on the extremities (Fig. 17.33). In one patient presenting with two separate cutaneous lesions, the second one showed features of conventional cutaneous marginal zone lymphoproliferative disorder [29].

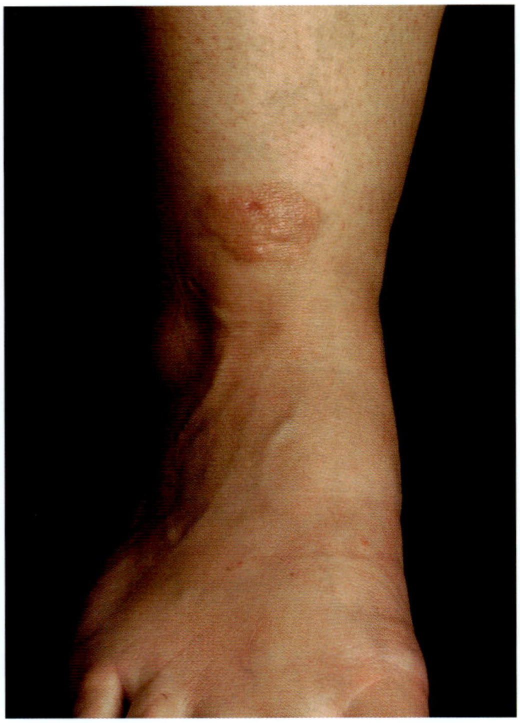

**Figure 17.33** Cutaneous amyloidoma. Waxy plaque on the distal part of the leg.

## Histopathology, immunophenotype, and molecular genetics

### Histopathology

Lesions show a prominent amyloid deposition in the dermis and subcutaneous fat, often with perivascular accentuation of the deposits (Fig. 17.34a and b). The infiltrate is usually sparse with predominance of plasma cells. As already mentioned, dense infiltrates with histopathological features of conventional cutaneous marginal zone lymphoproliferative disorder can be observed rarely in cases showing amyloid deposition (Fig. 17.32), supporting the inclusion of cutaneous amyloidoma in the group of cutaneous marginal zone lymphoproliferative disorder.

### Immunophenotype

The plasma cells show a monoclonal expression of one Ig light chain (Fig. 14.34c and d).

### Molecular genetics

In one case, a t(14;18)(q32;q21)/*IGH-MALT1* translocation has been described, underlining the relationship to conventional cutaneous marginal zone lymphoproliferative disorder [29].

## Treatment and prognosis

Cutaneous amyloidoma is characterized by an excellent prognosis, and association to systemic amyloidosis and/or multiple myeloma or other Ig-producing extracutaneous lymphoproliferative disorders have not been reported. The lesions are treated by surgical excision. Local recurrence of cutaneous amyloidoma or onset of conventional variants of cutaneous marginal zone lymphoproliferative disorder are observed in a distinct proportion of cases, but evolution into extracutaneous lymphoma or systemic amyloidosis has not been observed [29].

### Résumé

| | |
|---|---|
| **Cutaneous amyloidoma** | |
| **Clinical** | Solitary, waxy small nodules located mostly on the extremities. |
| **Morphology** | Prominent amyloid deposition; few perivascular plasma cells. Rare cases show dense infiltrates with histopathological features of conventional cutaneous marginal zone lymphoproliferative disorder. |
| **Immunology** | cIg + (monoclonal) |
| **Genetics** | In one case, a t(14;18)(q32;q21)/*IGH-MALT1* translocation has been described. |
| **Treatment guidelines** | Surgical excision. |

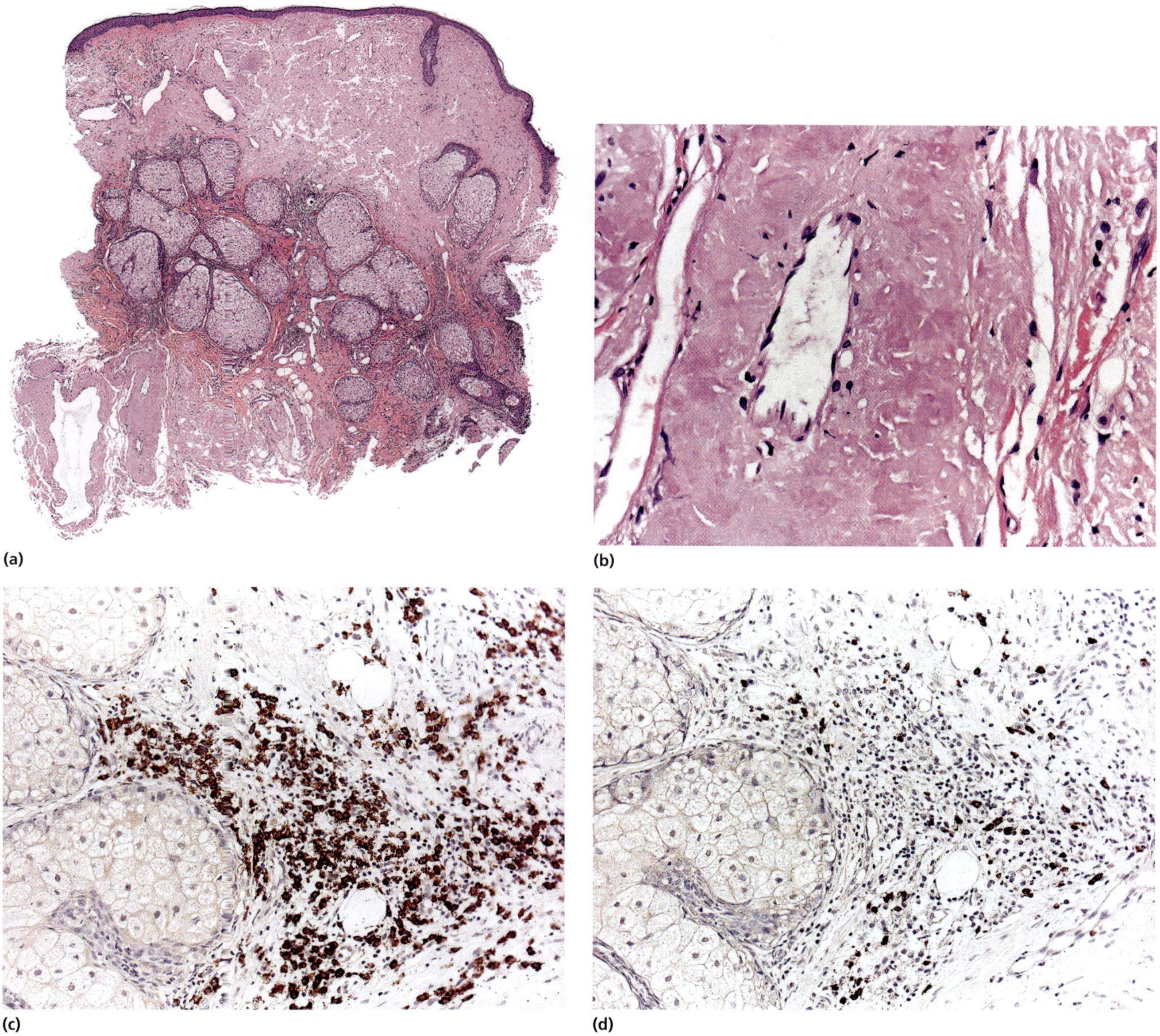


**Figure 17.34** Cutaneous amyloidoma. (a) Amyloid deposition within the entire dermis with only sparse infiltrates of lymphocytes and plasma cells. (b) Accentuation of amyloid deposition around the vessels. In situ hybridization for the immunoglobulin light chains shows (c) positivity of the majority of plasma cells for lambda and (d) of a few cells only for kappa.

## References

1. Willemze R, Cerroni L, Kempf W, *et al.* The 2018 update of the WHO-EORTC classification for primary cutaneous lymphomas. *Blood* 2019;**133**:1703–1714.
2. Kempf W, Mitteldorf C, Cerroni L, *et al.* Classifications of cutaneous lymphomas and lymphoproliferative disorders: an update from the EORTC cutaneous lymphoma histopathology group. *J Eur Acad Dermatol Venereol* 2024;**38**:1491–1503.
3. Geyer J, Willemze R. Primary cutaneous marginal zone lymphoma. In: *WHO Classification of Tumours Editorial Board. Haematolymphoid Tumours*. 5th editing edition. Lyon (France): IARC, 2024: 409–411.
4. Goodlad JR, Gibson SE, Rosen ST, Zamò A. Primary cutaneous marginal zone lymphoproliferative disorder. In: Arber DA, Borowitz MJ, Cook JR, *et al.*, eds. *The International Consensus Classification of Myeloid and Lymphoid Neoplasms*. Philadelphia (US): Wolters Kluver, 2025: 417–420.
5. Bende RJ, van Maldegem F, van Noesel CJM. Chronic inflammatory disease, lymphoid tissue neogenesis and extranodal marginal zone B-cell lymphomas. *Haematologica* 2009;**94**:1109–1123.
6. Suarez F, Lortholary O, Hermine O, Lecuit M. Infection-associated lymphomas derived from marginal zone B cells: a model of antigen-driven lymphoproliferation. *Blood* 2006;**107**:3034–3044.
7. Guitart J, Deonizio J, Bloom T, *et al.* High incidence of gastrointestinal tract disorders and autoimmunity in primary cutaneous marginal zone B-cell lymphomas. *JAMA Dermatol* 2014;**150**:412–418.

8. Rinaldi A, Mian M, Chigrinova E, *et al.* Genome-wide DNA profiling of marginal zone lymphomas identifies subtype-specific lesions with an impact on the clinical outcome. *Blood* 2011;**117**:1595–1604.
9. Martinez-Lopez A, Curiel-Olmo S, Mollejo M, *et al.* MYD88 (L265P) somatic mutation in marginal zone B-cell lymphoma. *Am J Surg Pathol* 2015;**39**:644–651.
10. Pillonel V, Juskevicius D, Ng CKY, *et al.* High-throughput sequencing of nodal marginal zone lymphomas identifies recurrent BRAF mutations. *Leukemia* 2018;**32**:2412–2426.
11. Zucca E, Bertoni F. The spectrum of MALT lymphoma at different sites: biological and therapeutic relevance. *Blood* 2016;**127**:2082–2092.
12. Brenner I, Roth S, Puppe B, *et al.* Primary cutaneous marginal zone lymphomas with plasmacytic differentiation show frequent IgG4 expression. *Mod Pathol* 2013;**26**:1568–1576.
13. De Souza A, Ferry JA, Burghart DR, *et al.* IgG4 expression in primary cutaneous marginal zone lymphoma: a multicenter study. *Appl Immunohistochem Mol Morphol* 2018;**26**:462–467.
14. Carlsen ED, Swerdlow SH, Cook JR, Gibson SE. Class-switched primary cutaneous marginal zone lymphomas are frequently IgG4-positive and have features distinct from IgM-positive cases. *Am J Surg Pathol* 2019;**43**:1403–1412.
15. Gonzalez-Quesada A, Bastida J, Rivero-Vera JC, *et al.* Image gallery: metachronic occurrence of primary cutaneous marginal zone B-cell lymphoma and primary cutaneous Rosai-Dorfman disease in the same patient. *Br J Dermatol* 2017;**177**:e355.
16. Bailey EM, Ferry JA, Harris NL, *et al.* Marginal zone lymphoma (low-grade B-cell lymphoma of mucosa-associated lymphoid tissue type) of skin and subcutaneous tissue: a study of 15 patients. *Am J Surg Pathol* 1996;**20**:1011–1023.
17. Cerroni L, Signoretti S, Höfler G, *et al.* Primary cutaneous marginal zone B-cell lymphoma: a recently described entity of low-grade malignant cutaneous B-cell lymphoma. *Am J Surg Pathol* 1997;**21**:1307–1315.
18. Duncan LN, LeBoit PE. Are primary cutaneous immunocytoma and marginal zone lymphoma the same disease? *Am J Surg Pathol* 1997;**21**:1368–1372.
19. Aberer E, Cerroni L, Kerl H. Cutaneous immunocytoma presenting with multiple infiltrated macules and papules. *J Am Acad Dermatol* 2001;**44**:324–329.
20. Servitje O, Gallardo F, Estrach T, *et al.* Primary cutaneous marginal zone B-cell lymphoma: a clinical, histopathological, immunophenotypic and molecular genetic study of 22 cases. *Br J Dermatol* 2002;**147**:1147–1158.
21. Schmid U, Eckert F, Griesser H, *et al.* Cutaneous follicular lymphoid hyperplasia with monotypic plasma cells: a clinicopathologic study of 18 patients. *Am J Surg Pathol* 1995;**19**:12–20.
22. Arai E, Shimizu M, Hirose T. A review of 55 cases of cutaneous lymphoid hyperplasia: reassessment of the histopathologic findings leading to reclassification of 4 lesions as cutaneous marginal zone lymphoma and 19 as pseudolymphomatous folliculitis. *Hum Pathol* 2005;**36**:505–511.
23. Hussong JW, Perkins SL, Schnitzer B, *et al.* Extramedullary plasmacytoma: a form of marginal zone cell lymphoma? *Am J Clin Pathol* 1999;**111**:111–116.
24. Dimosthenous K, Papanikolaou A, Athanasiadou I, *et al.* Transformation of marginal zone lymphomas to pure plasma cell histology following treatment with the anti-CD20 antibody rituximab. *J Haematopathol* 2008;**1**:170–171.
25. Cerroni L, Zöchling N, Pütz B, Kerl H. Infection by Borrelia burgdorferi and cutaneous B-cell lymphoma. *J Cutan Pathol* 1997;**24**:457–461.
26. Fujiwara M, Morales AV, Seo K, *et al.* Clonal identity and differences in primary cutaneous B-cell lymphoma occurring at different sites or time points in the same patient. *Am J Dermatopathol* 2013;**35**:11–18.
27. Edinger JT, Lorenzo CR, Breneman DL, *et al.* Primary cutaneous marginal zone lymphoma with subclinical cutaneous involvement and biclonality. *J Cutan Pathol* 2011;**38**:724–730.
28. Nicholson KM, Patel KP, Duvic M, *et al.* Bi-clonal, multifocal primary cutaneous marginal zone B-cell lymphoma: report of a case and review of the literature. *J Cutan Pathol* 2012;**39**:866–871.
29. Walsh NM, Lano IM, Green P, *et al.* AL amyloidoma of the skin/subcutis: cutaneous amyloidosis, plasma cell dyscrasia or a manifestation of primary cutaneous marginal zone lymphoma? *Am J Surg Pathol* 2017;**41**:1069–1076.
30. Dangien A, Beylot-Barry M, Battistella M, *et al.* Clinical presentation, therapeutic approach and outcome of primary cutaneous marginal zone B-cell lymphoma presenting as AL amyloidoma of the skin. *Br J Dermatol* 2019;**181**:607–609.
31. Frings VG, Röding K, Strate A, *et al.* Paraproteinaemia in primary cutaneous marginal zone lymphoma. *Acta Derm Venereol* 2018;**98**:956–962.
32. Lee BA, Jacobson M, Seidel G. Epidermotropic marginal zone lymphoma simulating mycosis fungoides. *J Cutan Pathol* 2013;**40**:569–572.
33. Servitje O, Marti RM, Estrach T, *et al.* Occurrence of Hodgkin's disease and cutaneous B cell lymphoma in the same patient: a report of two cases. *Eur J Dermatol* 2000;**10**:43–46.
34. Gong S, Crane GM, McCall CM, *et al.* Expanding the spectrum of EBV-positive marginal zone lymphomas: a lesion associated with diverse immunodeficiency settings. *Am J Surg Pathol* 2018;**42**:1306–1316.
35. Bejarano PL, Sayagués JM, Alcoceba M, *et al.* Primary cutaneous marginal zone lymphoproliferative disorder of donor origin after allogeneic hematopoietic stem cell transplantation. *Am J Dermatopathol* 2023;**45**:378–382.
36. Obiorah IE, Karrs J, Brown L, *et al.* Overlapping features of primary cutaneous marginal zone lymphoproliferative disorder and primary cutaneous CD4+ small/medium T-cell lymphoproliferative disorder: a diagnostic challenge examined by genomic analysis. *Am J Surg Pathol* 2023;**47**:344–353.
37. Palos K, Szakony J, Csomor J, *et al.* Primary cutaneous lymphoproliferations in the grey zone between marginal zone lymphoma and CD4+ small/medium T-cell lymphoproliferative disease. *J Cutan Pathol* 2024;**51**:868–875.
38. Swerdlow SH. Cutaneous marginal zone lymphomas. *Semin Diagn Pathol* 2017;**34**:76–84.
39. Guitart J. Rethinking primary cutaneous marginal zone lymphoma: shifting the focus to the cause of the infiltrate. *J Cutan Pathol* 2015;**42**:600–603.
40. Beltzung F, Beylot-Barry M, Battistella M. Recurrent primary cutaneous marginal zone lymphoma: a comparative study of initial tumours, recurrences, and outcomes in 61 patients. *Histopathology* 2025;**86**:704–714.

41. Goodlad JR, Davidson MM, Hollowood K, *et al.* Primary cutaneous B-cell lymphoma and Borrelia burgdorferi infection in patients from the highlands of Scotland. *Am J Surg Pathol* 2000;**24**:1279–1285.
42. de la Fouchardiére A, Vandenesch F, Berger F. Borrelia-associated primary cutaneous MALT lymphoma in a non-endemic region. *Am J Surg Pathol* 2003;**27**:702–703.
43. Li C, Inagaki H, Kuo TT, *et al.* Primary cutaneous marginal zone B-cell lymphoma: a molecular and clinicopathologic study of 24 Asian cases. *Am J Surg Pathol* 2003;**27**:1061–1069.
44. Wood GS, Kamath NV, Guitart J, *et al.* Absence of Borrelia burgdorferi DNA in cutaneous B-cell lymphomas from the United States. *J Cutan Pathol* 2001;**28**:502–507.
45. Goteri G, Ranaldi R, Simonetti O, *et al.* Clinicopathological features of primary cutaneous B-cell lymphomas from an academic regional hospital in central Italy: no evidence of Borrelia burgdorferi association. *Leukem Lymph* 2007;**48**:2184–2188.
46. Ponzoni M, Ferreri AJ, Mappa S, *et al.* Prevalence of Borrelia burgdorferi infection in a series of 98 primary cutaneous lymphomas. *Oncologist* 2011;**16**:1582–1588.
47. Bahler DW, Kim BK, Gao A, Swerdlow SH. Analysis of immunoglobulin VH genes suggests cutaneous marginal zone B-cell lymphomas recognise similar antigens. *Br J Haematol* 2006;**132**:571–575.
48. Lenze D, Berg E, Volkmer-Engert R, *et al.* Influence of antigen on the development of MALT lymphoma. *Blood* 2006;**107**:1141–1148.
49. May SA, Netto G, Domiati-Saad R, Kasper C. Cutaneous lymphoid hyperplasia and marginal zone B-cell lymphoma following vaccination. *J Am Acad Dermatol* 2005;**53**:512–516.
50. Breza TS Jr, Zheng P, Porcu P, Magro CM. Cutaneous marginal zone B-cell lymphoma in the setting of fluoxetine therapy: a hypothesis regarding pathogenesis based on in vitro suppression of T-cell-proliferative response. *J Cutan Pathol* 2006;**33**:522–528.
51. Richtig G, Cerroni L, Schmidt H, *et al.* Talimogene laherparepvec can initiate plasma cell invasion into infiltrated melanoma lesions – a case series. *J Eur Acad Dermatol Venereol* 2021;**35**:e209–e211.
52. Hoefnagel JJ, Vermeer MH, Jansen PM, *et al.* Primary cutaneous marginal zone B-cell lymphoma. Clinical and therapeutic features in 50 cases. *Arch Dermatol* 2005;**141**:1139–1145.
53. Taddesse-Heath L, Pittaluga S, Sorbara L, *et al.* Marginal zone B-cell lymphoma in children and young adults. *Am J Surg Pathol* 2003;**27**:522–531.
54. Fink-Puches R, Chott A, Ardigo M, *et al.* The spectrum of cutaneous lymphomas in patients less than 20 years of age. *Ped Dermatol* 2004;**21**:525–533.
55. Amitay-Laish I, Feinmesser M, Ben-Amitai D, *et al.* Juvenile onset of primary low-grade cutaneous B-cell lymphoma. *Br J Dermatol* 2009;**161**:140–147.
56. Barzilai A, Feuerman H, Quaglino P, *et al.* Cutaneous B-cell neoplasms mimicking granulomatous rosacea or rhinophyma. *Arch Dermatol* 2012;**148**:824–831.
57. Wharton J, Roffwarg D, Miller J, *et al.* Cutaneous marginal zone lymphoma arising in the setting of erythema ab igne. *J Am Acad Dermatol* 2010;**62**:1080–1081.
58. Kasper RC, Wood GS, Nihal M, LeBoit PE. Anetoderma arising in cutaneous B-cell lymphoproliferative disease. *Am J Dermatopathol* 2001;**23**:124–132.
59. Child FJ, Woollons A, Price ML, *et al.* Multiple cutaneous immunocytoma with secondary anetoderma: a report of two cases. *Br J Dermatol* 2000;**143**:165–170.
60. Hodak E, Feuerman H, Barzilai A, *et al.* Anetodermic primary cutaneous B-cell lymphoma: a unique clinicopathological presentation of lymphoma possibly associated with antiphospholipid antibodies. *Arch Dermatol* 2010;**146**:175–182.
61. Vachhani P, Neppalli VT, Cancino CJ, *et al.* Radiological imaging and bone marrow biopsy in staging of cutaneous B-cell lymphoma. *Br J Haematol* 2019;**184**:674–676.
62. Kheterpal MK, Dai J, Geller S, *et al.* Role of imaging in low-grade cutaneous B-cell lymphoma presenting in the skin. *J Am Acad Dermatol* 2019;**81**:970–976.
63. Senff NJ, Kluin-Nelemans JC, Willemze R. Results of bone marrow examination in 275 patients with histological features that suggest an indolent type of cutaneous B-cell lymphoma. *Br J Haematol* 2008;**142**:52–56.
64. Bathelier E, Thomas L, Balme B, *et al.* Asymptomatic bone marrow involvement in patients presenting with cutaneous marginal zone B-cell lymphoma. *Br J Dermatol* 2008;**159**:498–500.
65. Quereux G, Frot AS, Brocard A, *et al.* Routine bone marrow biopsy in the initial evaluation of primary cutaneous B-cell lymphoma does not appear justified. *Eur J Dermatol* 2009;**19**:216–220.
66. Gerami P, Wickless SC, Querfeld C, *et al.* Cutaneous involvement with marginal zone lymphoma. *J Am Acad Dermatol* 2010;**63**: 142–145.
67. Prieto-Torres L, Manso R, Cieza-Díaz DE, *et al.* Large cells with CD30 expression and hodgkin-like features in primary cutaneous marginal zone B-cell lymphoma: a study of 13 cases. *Am J Surg Pathol* 2019;**43**:1191–1202.
68. Di Napoli A, Rogges E, Noccioli N, *et al.* Deep sequencing of immunoglobulin genes identifies a very low percentage of monoclonal B cells in primary cutaneous marginal zone lymphomas with CD30-positive hodgkin/reed-sternberg-like cells. *Diagnostics* 2022;**12**:290.
69. de Leval L, Harris NL, Longtine J, *et al.* Cutaneous B-cell lymphomas of follicular and marginal zone types: use of Bcl-6, CD10, Bcl-2, and CD21 in differential diagnosis and classification. *Am J Surg Pathol* 2001;**25**:732–741.
70. Falini B, Agostinelli C, Bigerna B, *et al.* IRTA1 is selectively expressed in nodal and extranodal marginal zone lymphomas. *Histopathology* 2012;**61**:930–941.
71. Ikeda JI, Kohara M, Tsuruta Y, *et al.* Immunohistochemical analysis of the novel marginal zone B-cell marker IRTA1 in malignant lymphoma. *Hum Pathol* 2017;**59**:70–79.
72. Verdanet E, Dereure O, Rene C, *et al.* Diagnostic value of STMN1, LMO2, HGAL, AID expression and 1p36 chromosomal abnormalities in primary cutaneous B cell lymphomas. *Histopathology* 2017;**71**:648–660.
73. Guo L, Wang Z, Anderson CM, *et al.* Ultrasensitive automated RNA in situ hybridization for kappa and lambda light chain mRNA detects B-cell clonality in tissue biopsies with performance comparable or superior to flow cytometry. *Mod Pathol* 2018;**31**:385–394.
74. Edinger JT, Kant JA, Swerdlow SH. Cutaneous marginal zone lymphomas have distinctive features and include 2 subsets. *Am J Surg Pathol* 2010;**34**:1830–1841.
75. Kutzner H, Kerl H, Pfaltz M, *et al.* CD123-positive plasmacytoid dendritic cells in primary cutaneous marginal zone B-cell lymphoma. Diagnostic and pathogenetic implications. *Am J Surg Pathol* 2009;**33**:1307–1313.

76. Cetinözman F, Koens L, Jansen PM, Willemze R. Programmed death-1 expression in cutaneous B-cell lymphoma. *J Cutan Pathol* 2014;**41**:14–21.
77. Gallardo F, Bellosillo B, Espinet B, *et al.* Aberrant nuclear BCL10 expression and lack of t(11;18)(q21;q21) in primary cutaneous marginal zone B-cell lymphoma. *Hum Pathol* 2006;**37**:867–873.
78. Streubel B, Lamprecht A, Dierlamm J, *et al.* T(14;18)(q32;q21) involving IGH and MALT1 is a frequent chromosomal aberration in MALT lymphoma. *Blood* 2003;**101**:2335–2339.
79. Palmedo G, Hantschke M, Rütten A, *et al.* Primary cutaneous marginal zone B-cell lymphoma may exhibit both the t(14;18)(q32;q21) IGH/BCL2 and the t(14;18)(q;32;q21) IGH/MALT1 translocation: an indicator for clonal transformation towards higher-grade B-cell lymphoma? *Am J Dermatopathol* 2007;**29**:231–236.
80. Streubel B, Vinatzer U, Lamprecht A, *et al.* t(3;14)(p14.1;q32) involving IgH and FOXP1 is a novel recurrent chromosomal aberration in MALT lymphoma. *Leukemia* 2005;**19**:652–658.
81. van Maldegem F, van Dijk R, Wormhoudt TA, *et al.* The majority of cutaneous marginal zone B-cell lymphomas expresses class-switched immunoglobulins and develops in a T-helper type 2 inflammatory environment. *Blood* 2008;**112**:3355–3361.
82. Storz MN, van de Rijn M, Kim YH, *et al.* Gene expression profiles of cutaneous B cell lymphoma. *J Invest Dermatol* 2003;**120**:865–870.
83. Rizzo KA, Streubel B, Pittaluga S, *et al.* Marginal zone lymphomas in children and the young adult population; characterization of genetic aberrations by FISH and RT-PCR. *Mod Pathol* 2010;**23**:866–873.
84. Maurus K, Appenzeller S, Roth S, *et al.* Panel sequencing shows recurrent genetic FAS alterations in primary cutaneous marginal zone lymphoma. *J Invest Dermatol* 2018;**138**:1573–1581.
85. Child FJ, Scarisbrick JJ, Calonje E, *et al.* Inactivation of tumor suppressor genes $p15^{INK4b}$ and $p16^{INK4a}$ in primary cutaneous B cell lymphoma. *J Invest Dermatol* 2002;**118**:941–948.
86. Deutsch AJA, Frühwirth M, Aigelsreiter A, *et al.* Primary cutaneous marginal zone B-cell lymphomas are targeted by aberrant somatic hypermutation. *J Invest Dermatol* 2009;**129**:476–479.
87. Perez M, Pacchiarotti A, Frontani M, *et al.* Primary cutaneous B-cell lymphoma is associated with somatically hypermutated immunoglobulin variable genes and frequent use of VH1-69 and VH4-59 segments. *Br J Dermatol* 2010;**162**:611–618.
88. Takino H, Li C, Hu S, *et al.* Primary cutaneous marginal zone B-cell lymphoma: a molecular and clinicopathological study of cases from Asia, Germany, and the United States. *Mod Pathol* 2008;**21**:1517–1526.
89. Willemze R, Hodak E, Zinzani PL, *et al.* Primary cutaneous lymphomas: ESMO Clinical Practice Guidelines for diagnosis, treatment and follow-up. *Ann Oncol* 2018;**29**(Supplement 4):iv30–iv40.on behalf of the ESMO Guidelines Committee
90. Senff NJ, Noordijk EM, Kim YH, *et al.* European Organization for Research and Treatment of Cancer and International Society for Cutaneous Lymphoma consensus recommendations for the management of cutaneous B-cell lymphomas. *Blood* 2008;**112**:1600–1609.
91. Elsayad K, Guenova E, Assaf C, *et al.* Radiotherapy in cutaneous lymphomas: recommendations from the EORTC cutaneous lymphoma tumour group. *Eur J Cancer* 2024;**212**:115064.
92. Roggero E, Zucca E, Mainetti C, *et al.* Eradication of Borrelia burgdorferi infection in primary marginal zone B-cell lymphoma of the skin. *Hum Pathol* 2000;**31**:263–268.
93. Kütting B, Bonsmann G, Metze D, *et al.* Borrelia burgdorferi-associated primary cutaneous B cell lymphoma: complete clearing of skin lesions after antibiotic pulse therapy or intralesional injection of interferon-α2a. *J Am Acad Dermatol* 1997;**36**:311–314.
94. Fink-Puches R, Zenahlik P, Bäck B, *et al.* Primary cutaneous lymphomas: applicability of current classification schemes (European Organization for Research and Treatment of Cancer, World Health Organization) based on clinicopathologic features observed in a large group of patients. *Blood* 2002;**99**:800–805.
95. Bouaziz JD, Bastuji-Garin S, Poszepczynska-Guigne E, *et al.* Relative frequency and survival of patients with primary cutaneous lymphomas: data from a single-centre study of 203 patients. *Br J Dermatol* 2006;**154**:1206–1207.
96. Zinzani PL, Quaglino P, Pimpinelli N, *et al.* Prognostic factors in primary cutaneous B-cell lymphoma: The Italian Study Group for Cutaneous Lymphomas. *J Clin Oncol* 2006;**24**:1376–1382.
97. Amitay-Laish I, Tavallaee M, Kim J, *et al.* Paediatric primary cutaneous marginal zone B-cell lymphoma: does it differ from its adult counterpart? *Br J Dermatol* 2017;**176**:1010–1020.
98. Servitje O, Muniesa C, Benavente Y, *et al.* Primary cutaneous marginal zone B-cell lymphoma: response to treatment and disease-free survival in a series of 137 patients. *J Am Acad Dermatol* 2013;**69**:357–365.
99. Chan SA, Shah F, Chaganti S, *et al.* Primary cutaneous B-cell lymphoma: systemic spread is rare while cutaneous relapses and secondary malignancies are frequent. *Br J Dermatol* 2017;**177**:287–289.
100. Gronbaeck K, Moller PH, Nedergaard T, *et al.* Primary cutaneous B-cell lymphoma: a clinical, histological, phenotypic and genotypic study of 21 cases. *Br J Dermatol* 2000;**142**:913–923.
101. (a)Magro CM, Yang A, Fraga G. Blastic marginal zone lymphoma: a clinical and pathological study of 8 cases and review of the literature. *Am J Dermatopathol* 2013;**35**:319–326.(b) Beltzung F, Beylot-Barry M, Battistella M, *et al.* Recurrent primary cutaneous marginal zone lymphoma: a comparative study of initial tumours, recurrences, and outcomes in 61 patients. *Histopathol* 2025;**86**:704–714.
102. Oliszewski AJ, Castillo JJ. Survival of patients with marginal zone lymphoma. *Cancer* 2013;**119**:629–638.
103. Mian M, Marcheselli L, Luminari S, *et al.* CLIPI: a new prognostic index for indolent cutaneous B cell lymphoma proposed by the International Extranodal Lymphoma Study Group (IELSG 11). *Ann Hematol* 2011;**90**:401–408.
104. Lin P, Bueso-Ramos C, Wilson CS, *et al.* Waldenström macroglobulinemia involving extramedullary sites: morphologic and immunophenotypic findings in 44 patients. *Am J Surg Pathol* 2003;**27**:1104–1113.
105. LeBoit PE, McNutt NS, Reed JA, *et al.* Primary cutaneous immunocytoma: a B-cell lymphoma that can easily be mistaken for cutaneous lymphoid hyperplasia. *Am J Surg Pathol* 1994;**18**:969–978.
106. Rijlaarsdam JU, van der Putte SCJ, Berti E, *et al.* Cutaneous immunocytomas: a clinicopathologic study of 26 cases. *Histopathology* 1993;**23**:117–125.

107. Goos N. Acrodermatitis chronica atrophicans and malignant lymphoma. *Acta Derm Venereol (Stockh)* 1971;**51**:457–459.
108. Requena L, Kutzner H, Palmedo G, *et al.* Cutaneous involvement in multiple myeloma: a clinicopathologic, immunohistochemical, and cytogenetic study of 8 cases. *Arch Dermatol* 2003;**139**:475–486.
109. Turbiner Geyer J, Ferry JA, Longtine JA, *et al.* Characteristics of cutaneous marginal zone lymphomas with marked plasmacytic differentiation and a T cell-rich background. *Am J Clin Pathol* 2010;**133**:59–69.
110. Koletsa T, Patsatsi A, Kostopoulos I, *et al.* A case of primary cutaneous plasmacytoma presenting in adolescence. *Am J Dermatopathol* 2012;**34**:537–540.
111. Magro CM, Kalomeris T, Roberts A. Primary cutaneous blastic marginal zone lymphoma: a comprehensive clinical, light microscopic, phenotypic and cytogenetic appraisal. *Ann Diagn Pathol* 2023;**63**:152101.
112. Ueberdiek S, Kempf W, Kretschmer L, *et al.* AL-amyloidoma of the skin – A rare manifestation of primary cutaneous marginal zone lymphoma. *Am J Dermatopathol* 2019;**41**:518–521.
113. Hernandez-Molina G, Faz-Munoz D, Astudillo-Angel M, *et al.* Coexistance of amyloidosis and primary Sjögren's syndrome: an overview. *Curr Rheumatol Rev* 2018;**14**:231–238.
114. Mahmood S, Bridoux F, Venner CP, *et al.* Natural history and outcomes in localised immunoglobulin light-chain amyloidosis: a long-term observational study. *Lancet Haematol* 2015;**2**: e241–e250.
115. Grogg KL, Aubry MC, Vrana JA, *et al.* Nodular pulmonary amyloidosis is characterized by localized immunoglobulin deposition and is frequently associated with an indolent B-cell lymphoproliferative disorder. *Am J Surg Pathol* 2013;**37**: 406–412.

CHAPTER 18

# Cutaneous diffuse large B-cell lymphoma, leg type

Cutaneous diffuse large B-cell lymphoma, leg type, is a malignant lymphoma occurring mostly on the leg(s) in elderly patients [1–2]. The nomenclature of this entity has been the source of a long controversy, but the term cutaneous diffuse large B-cell lymphoma, leg type, is now established, and this lymphoma is listed as a specific entity in the 2018 and 2024 update of the classification of cutaneous lymphomas by the European Organization for Research and Treatment of Cancer (EORTC)/World Health Organization (WHO) [3, 4], in the International Consensus Classification (ICC) *of Myeloid and Lymphoid Neoplasms* and in the 5th edition of the WHO *Classification of Haematolymphoid Tumours* [5, 6]. On the other hand, it has been shown that primary cutaneous diffuse large B-cell lymphoma, leg type, and secondary cutaneous involvement by testicular B-cell lymphoma share identical clinicopathological and immunophenotypic features [7]. It is a matter of discussion whether cutaneous diffuse large B-cell lymphoma, leg type, is a specific entity *per se*, or does simply represent a primary cutaneous variant of diffuse large B-cell lymphoma, not otherwise specified (NOS). In fact, there are more similarities than differences between these two groups, and it has been suggested that cutaneous diffuse large B-cell lymphoma, leg type, should not be considered as a separate entity, but rather classified within the group of diffuse large B-cell lymphoma, NOS [8]. On the other hand, diffuse large B-cell lymphoma, NOS represents a heterogeneous group, whereas the new WHO classification recognizes 17 distinct subtypes of diffuse large B-cell lymphoma classified according to particular site of origin, genetic characteristics, or specific clinical context [9]. For what concerns the skin, particularly in the light of the problematic of the differentiation of primary cutaneous follicle center lymphoma, diffuse type from primary cutaneous diffuse large B-cell lymphoma, leg type, I believe that nomenclature should not be changed, and cutaneous diffuse large B-cell lymphoma, leg type should be listed as a separate entity.

Although cutaneous diffuse large B-cell lymphoma, leg type, and follicle center lymphoma, diffuse type, may present morphologically with overlapping features (both are comprised of a neoplastic population of large B lymphocytes), it is crucial to distinguish them, as the latter has an indolent course with excellent prognosis. A thorough discussion of differential diagnostic features is presented in Chapter 13.

Cutaneous diffuse large B-cell lymphoma, leg type, is the main entity of primary cutaneous large cell lymphoma and diagnosis is made according to relatively simple, conventional clinicopathological criteria. In this context, it must be underlined that diagnostic scores such as the Hans algorithm [10, 11] have been devised for diagnosis and classification of nodal, not cutaneous, diffuse large B-cell lymphomas, and in my opinion, and that of others [12], they do not have any value in cutaneous cases. In contrast to the lymph nodes, in fact, in the skin cases of large B-cell lymphoma with predominance of large centrocytes are classified in the group of follicle center lymphoma already by morphology. Although some authors advocate the use of a modified Hans algorithm for diagnosis of cutaneous diffuse large B-cell lymphoma, leg type [13], I think that there is no need whatsoever to use it in order to establish diagnosis and to properly classify cases of cutaneous B-cell lymphoma with predominance of large lymphocytes.

Several studies on extracutaneous diffuse large B-cell lymphoma pointed at the existence of molecular variants associated with a worse prognosis. These variants are characterized by a first rearrangement of *MYC*, associated to further rearrangements in the *BCL2* and/or *BCL6* genes ("double hit" or "triple hit" cases) [14, 15]. In the last revision of the WHO classification, cases with *MYC* and *BCL2* rearrangements are classified as a specific category of high-grade diffuse large B-cell lymphomas with an aggressive behaviour under the term "diffuse large B-cell lymphoma/high-grade B-cell lymphoma with *MYC* and *BCL2* rearrangements" (cases with *MYC* and *BCL6* rearrangements, on the other hand, are not classified within this group, but in the group of diffuse large B-cell lymphoma, NOS) [16]. The absence of the expression of LMO2 has been suggested as a surrogate evidence of the presence of *MYC* translocations [17], but LMO2-negativity is not accepted as a replacement of molecular studies. Data in the skin show that *MYC* rearrangements are more common than at extracutaneous sites, whereas double-hits are very rare and don't affect prognosis [18], or are not found at all [19]. In addition, double-hit cases are characterized by the rearrangement of *MYC* and *BCL6* rather than *BCL2* [20]. In the

*Skin Lymphoma: The Illustrated Guide*, Sixth Edition. Lorenzo Cerroni.

skin, although *MYC* rearrangements affect the disease-free survival, they do not seem to affect the overall survival of the patients [18]; other studies pointed at a possible prognostic value of double-hit cases [20]. Besides the presence or absence of specific rearrangements at the molecular level, the prognosis in extracutaneous cases is related also to the expression of the proteins detected by conventional immunohistology, and "double expression" or "triple expression" patterns can be identified [21–23]. In my experience, the expression of MYC, Bcl-2, and Bcl-6 is common in primary cutaneous cases, and data from other centers confirmed that the double expression of MYC and Bcl-2 is frequent [18]. MYC expression was associated with cutaneous relapses in one study [13]. However, data on the prognostic value of double expression in patients with primary cutaneous diffuse large B-cell lymphoma, leg type are contradictory, with some authors suggesting a worse prognosis [19], and others reporting no effect on prognosis [18]. In the literature, the cut-off point to establish immunohistochemical positivity of MYC and Bcl-2 lacks uniformity; at present, cut-off points considered valid are 50% of positive cells for Bcl-2, and 40% for MYC.

In the lymph nodes, different genetic subtypes of diffuse large B-cell lymphoma with different clinicopathological and prognostic features have been identified, characterized by the co-occurrence of *MYD88*$^{L265P}$ and *CD79B* mutations (MCD type), *BCL6* fusions and *NOTCH2* mutations (BN2 type), *NOTCH1* mutations (N1 type), and *EZH2* mutations and *BCL2* translocations (EZB type), respectively [24]. The majority of cutaneous cases shows highly recurrent mutations involving *MYD88* [25]. It must be underlined, however, that attempts to define genetic relevant subtypes of diffuse large B-cell lymphoma have resulted in the identification of different molecular groups [26], suggesting that further data are needed before more solid conclusions can be drawn, even at the nodal site. At present, besides the diffuse large B-cell lymphoma/high-grade B-cell lymphoma with *MYC* and *BCL2* rearrangements, genetically defined subtypes include ALK-positive large B-cell lymphoma, large B-cell lymphoma with *IRF4* rearrangement, and high-grade B-cell lymphoma with 11q aberration [9].

Cutaneous diffuse large B-cell lymphoma, leg type, can be seen in immunocompromised patients and has been observed in association with Kaposi sarcoma, but is not specifically linked to infection by human herpesvirus (HHV)-8 [27, 28]. The presence of specific sequences of *Borrelia burgdorferi* DNA has been demonstrated in rare cases from countries with endemic infection [29–31]. Cases with a positive nuclear signal for Epstein–Barr virus (EBV) detected by in situ hybridization have been rarely reported in the literature [32, 33], but probably should be better classified in the category of EBV$^{+}$ cutaneous diffuse large B-cell lymphoma, NOS (see Chapter 20). EBV$^{+}$ cases arising in the setting of immune suppression should be better classified among the immunosuppression-associated lymphomas [34]. Primary cutaneous diffuse type or diffuse large B-cell lymphoma, leg type should also be differentiated from rare examples of plasmablastic lymphoma that may arise primary in the skin (see Chapter 20), and from other cutaneous diffuse large cell lymphomas arising in the setting of immune deficiency.

An exceptional case of composite lymphoma consisting of a subcutaneous panniculitic-like T-cell lymphoma and a diffuse large B-cell lymphoma, leg type coexisting in the same lesion has been reported [35] (see also Chapter 28).

It must be remembered that a diagnosis of cutaneous diffuse large B-cell lymphoma, leg type, can be made only upon negative staging investigations, as any extracutaneous diffuse large B-cell lymphoma may involve the skin secondarily (keeping in mind that secondary cutaneous diffuse large B-cell lymphoma may be confined to the leg(s), thus being clinically and histopathologically indistinguishable from primary cutaneous diffuse large B-cell lymphoma, leg type). Radiological imaging positron emission tomography-computed tomography (PET-CT) and bone marrow biopsy modify the clinical stage in a distinct proportion of patients with cutaneous diffuse large B-cell lymphoma [36]. The term "leg-type" should be used only for cases without extracutaneous involvement at presentation. In nodal diffuse large B-cell lymphoma, PET-CT imaging is as specific and sensitive as a biopsy in identifying bone marrow involvement, suggesting that it can replace bone marrow biopsy as the method of choice [37].

## Clinical features

The disease predominantly affects the leg(s) of elderly patients (over 70 years of age), especially females. A wide spectrum of clinical presentations can be observed at onset: irregular, partly infiltrated patches and small, flat plaques (Fig. 18.1a), sometimes with superficial erosions and crusts (Fig. 18.1b); solitary or localized, sometimes ulcerated nodules (Fig. 18.1c, d); confluent plaques and tumors covering a large part of the leg (Fig. 18.1e); variably large ulcerations with infiltrated borders, which may lead to the misdiagnosis of chronic venous ulceration ("neoplastic ulcera") (Fig. 18.1f, g); and localized lesions involving both legs (Fig. 18.1h). Recurrent and/or lesions in advanced stages may display features similar to the primary ones or become more widespread, usually still retaining the peculiar tropism for the legs (Fig. 18.2).

Some patients may present clinically with patches similar to the lesions of early mycosis fungoides (Fig. 18.3a), or with solitary or multiple annular lesions that resemble erythema chronicum migrans or gyrate erythema (Fig. 18.3b and c) [38, 39]. In these cases, due to both the inconspicuous clinical presentation and the histopathologic features characterized by relatively sparse perivascular aggregates of cells, the correct diagnosis may be missed. Although I believed previously that these lesions may represent early phases of the disease, today

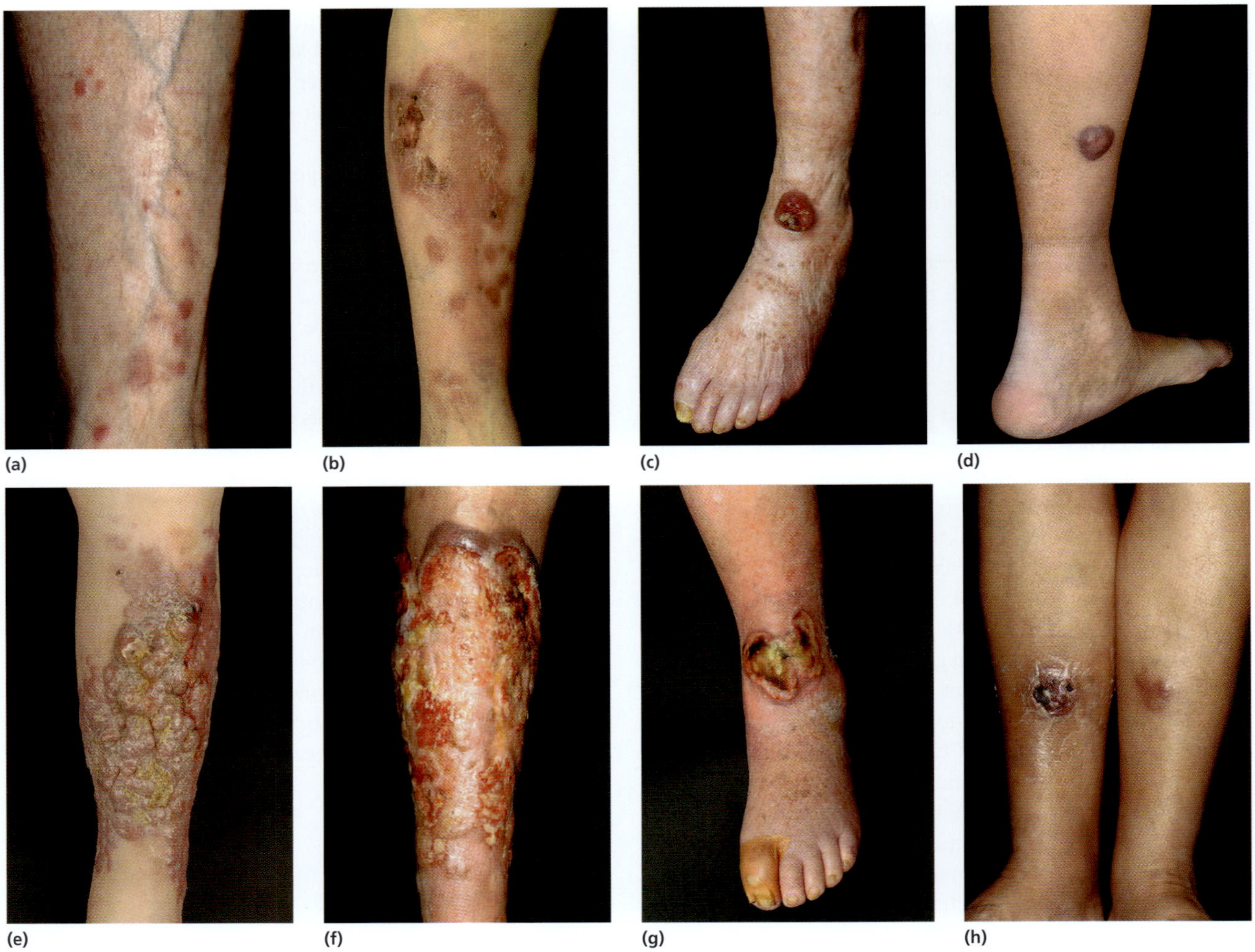

Figure 18.1 Clinical spectrum of cutaneous diffuse large B-cell lymphoma, leg type. (a) Erythematous papules and small plaques on the lower part of one leg. (b) Large, partly erosive patches and plaques on the lower leg. (c) Solitary, ulcerated tumor on the ankle. (d) Solitary, nonulcerated tumor on the lower leg. (e) Confluent plaques and tumors on the left lower leg. (f) Large ulcerated lesion with infiltrated margins involving the entire lower leg ("neoplastic ulcera"). (g) Ulceration with raised, infiltrated borders on the distal portion of the left leg. (h) Tumors in the pretibial region of both legs.

I am convinced that this is a peculiar presentation which is independent of the length of the clinical manifestations, and in some patients, I have observed identical lesions as a manifestation of recurrence after treatment. In this context, one unusual case, annular lesions present for 20 years were eventually proved by biopsy to be a diffuse large B-cell lymphoma, leg type [40].

It is important to underline that lesions with similar clinical, histopathologic, and phenotypical features can arise at cutaneous sites other than the legs (diffuse large B-cell lymphoma, leg type, occurs in approximately 80–85% of cases on the leg(s) only) [41]. Onset at body sites other than the legs is usually characterized by solitary or localized tumors (Fig. 18.4).

Cutaneous diffuse large B-cell lymphoma, leg type, has been observed on the background of chronic lymphedema [42], but the association is most likely fortuitous (I have also seen cases arising on the background of chronic stasis dermatitis without lymphedema – Fig. 18.5). Spontaneous regression after biopsy has been reported in exceptional cases [43].

## Histopathology, immunophenotype, and molecular genetics

### Histopathology

There are dense, diffuse lymphoid infiltrates within the entire dermis and subcutaneous fat (Fig. 18.6), consisting predominantly of large cells with round nuclei (immunoblasts and centroblasts) (Fig. 18.7). Involvement of the epidermis by large neoplastic cells may be observed rarely, sometimes indistinguishable from Darier nests (Fig. 18.8). Rare cases may even show band-like infiltrates in the superficial and mid-dermis, simulating the histopathologic pattern of mycosis fungoides

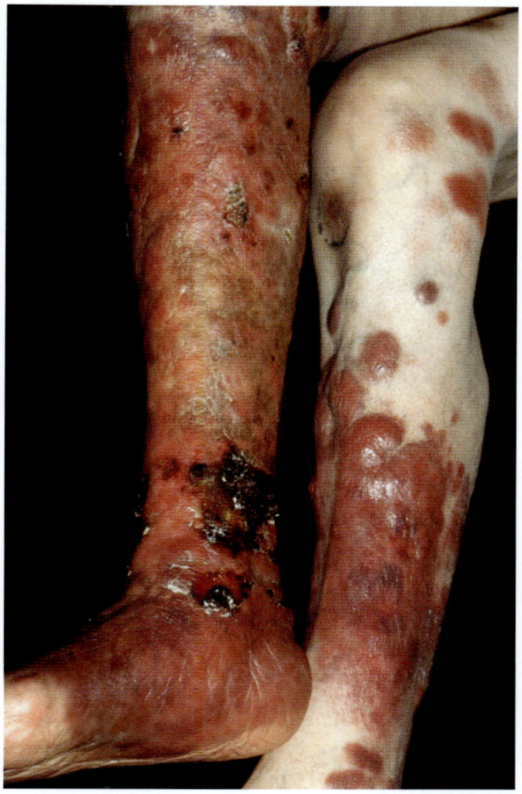

Figure 18.2 Cutaneous diffuse large B-cell lymphoma, leg type. Confluent tumors involving almost the entire surface of both legs and feet.

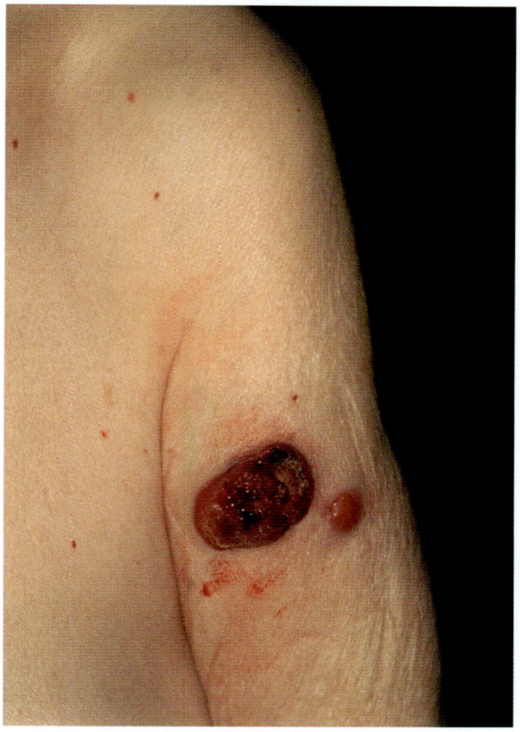

Figure 18.4 Cutaneous diffuse large B-cell lymphoma, leg type. Two contiguous tumors, one of which ulcerated, located on the upper arm.

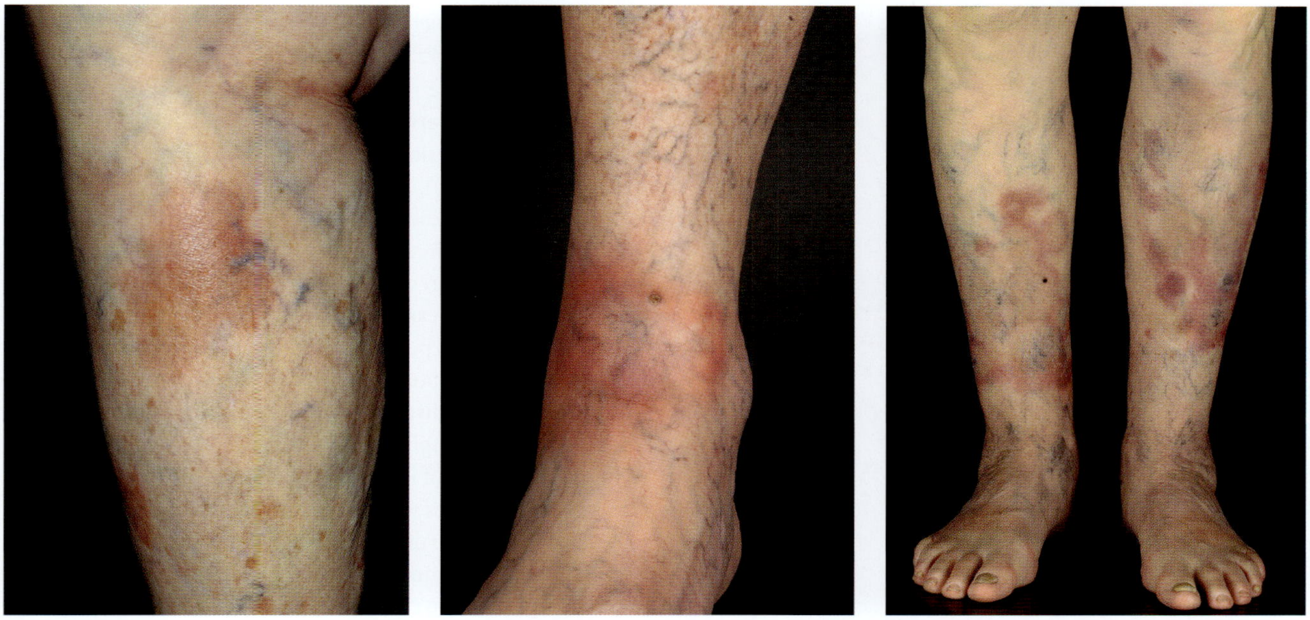

(a) (b) (c)

Figure 18.3 Cutaneous diffuse large B-cell lymphoma, leg type presenting with infiltrated patches or with annular lesions. (a) Infiltrated patches on the left lower leg. (b) Solitary annular lesion on the distal part of one leg. (c) Confluent, annular lesions on both lower legs.

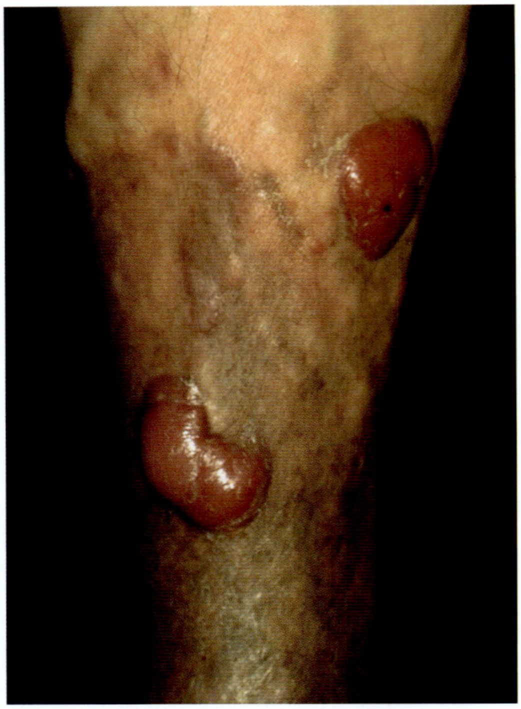

Figure 18.5 Cutaneous diffuse large B-cell lymphoma, leg type. Two large tumors arising on the background of hyperpigmentation due to chronic stasis dermatitis, but without evidence of chronic lymphedema.

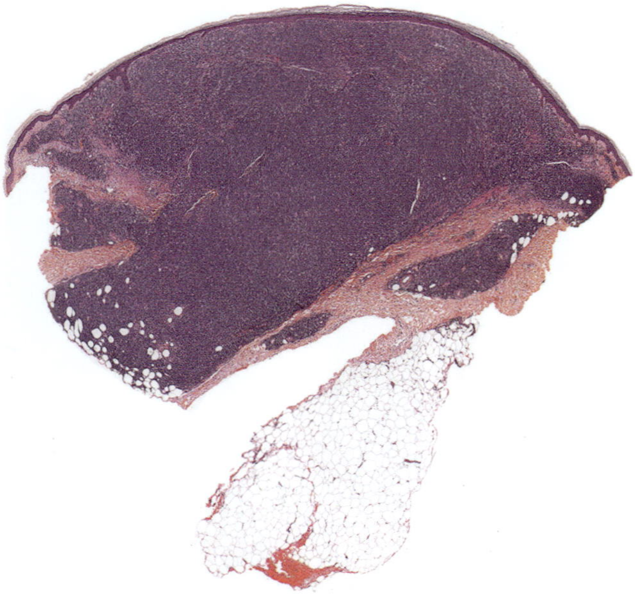

Figure 18.6 Cutaneous diffuse large B-cell lymphoma, leg type. Dense, nodular-diffuse lymphoid infiltrates involving the entire dermis and superficial part of the subcutaneous fat.

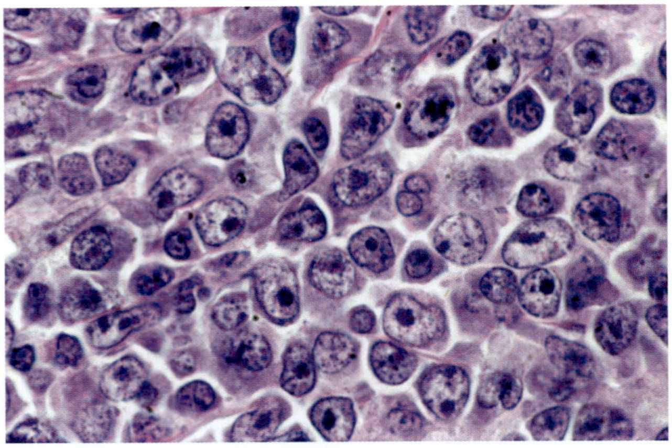

Figure 18.7 Cutaneous diffuse large B-cell lymphoma, leg type. Immunoblasts predominate.

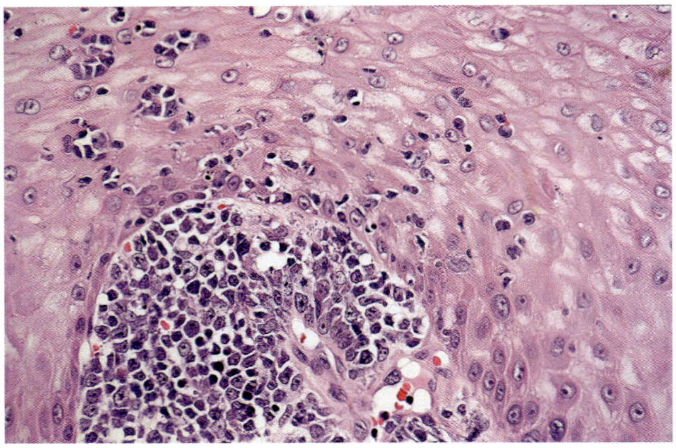

Figure 18.8 Cutaneous diffuse large B-cell lymphoma, leg type. Epidermotropism of neoplastic B lymphocytes forming intraepidermal collections indistinguishable from Darier nests.

(Fig. 18.9). Sparse perivascular collections of large cells may be observed in early lesions and may be the source of diagnostic problems (Fig. 18.10). Angiocentricity is an uncommon finding (Fig. 18.11) [22]. Reactive small lymphocytes are usually only sparse. Mitoses are frequent.

Although the predominance of spindle cells has been described in some cases [44], in my experience, most of the lesions showing this peculiar morphology represent a variant of cutaneous follicle center lymphoma, diffuse type (see Chapter 16 for a more detailed discussion). In rare instances, cutaneous diffuse large B-cell lymphoma, leg type, may relapse with clinicopathologic features of intravascular large B-cell lymphoma [45]. I have observed cases with bulky tumors and focal intravascular complexes at the site of the main tumor (Fig. 18.12); these cases represent an uncommon variant of cutaneous diffuse large B-cell lymphoma, leg type, and should not be classified as intravascular large B-cell lymphoma (extravascular neoplastic cells are not observed as a rule in intravascular large B-cell lymphoma, allowing an easy differentiation between the two entities).

A rare histopathologic variant of cutaneous diffuse large B-cell lymphoma, leg type, shows a starry sky and/or mosaic stone-like pattern with "squared" lymphocytes (Fig. 18.13). This histopathologic presentation is similar to what is observed in cutaneous Burkitt lymphoma or in cutaneous lymphoblastic lymphomas. Cases with this peculiar morphology have the same phenotype and behavior of diffuse large B-cell lymphoma, leg type.

## Immunophenotype

Neoplastic cells express B-cell markers (CD19, CD20 and CD79a), but there can be (partial) loss of antigen expression. Bcl-2 protein is usually strongly positive and is evaluated exclusively on neoplastic cells, with small reactive lymphocytes serving as normal positive controls (Fig. 18.14) [46]. Other markers positive in the great majority of cases are multiple

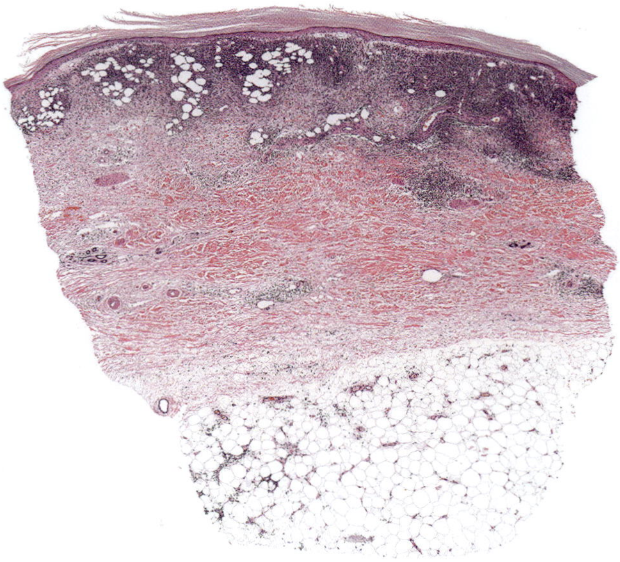

Figure 18.9 Cutaneous diffuse large B-cell lymphoma, leg type characterized by dense, band-like lymphoid infiltrates in the upper and mid-dermis.

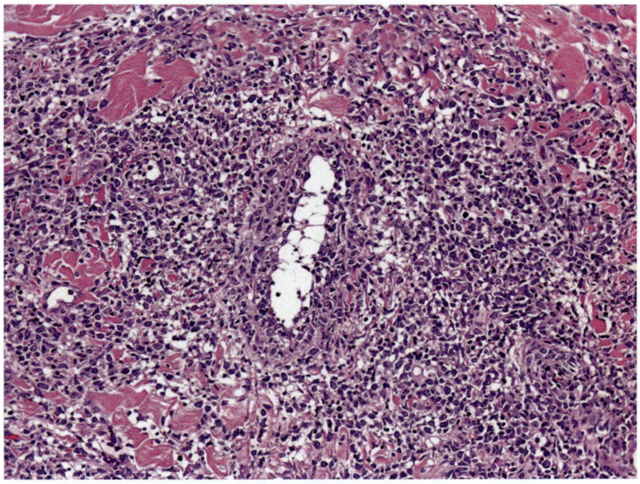

Figure 18.11 Cutaneous diffuse large B-cell lymphoma, leg type. Angiocentric infiltrates with angiotropism.

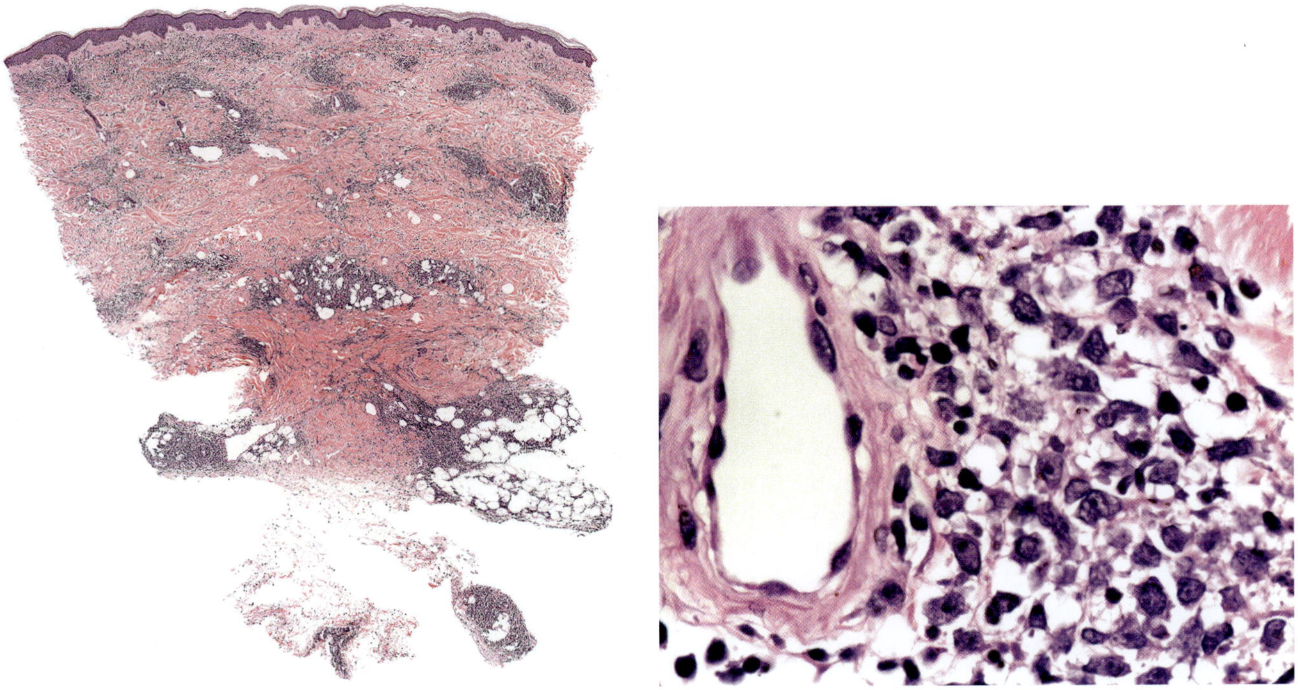

(a) (b)

Figure 18.10 Cutaneous diffuse large B-cell lymphoma, leg type presenting clinically with annular lesions. (a) Early lesion showing mild perivascular lymphoid infiltrates. (b) Detail of neoplastic cells.

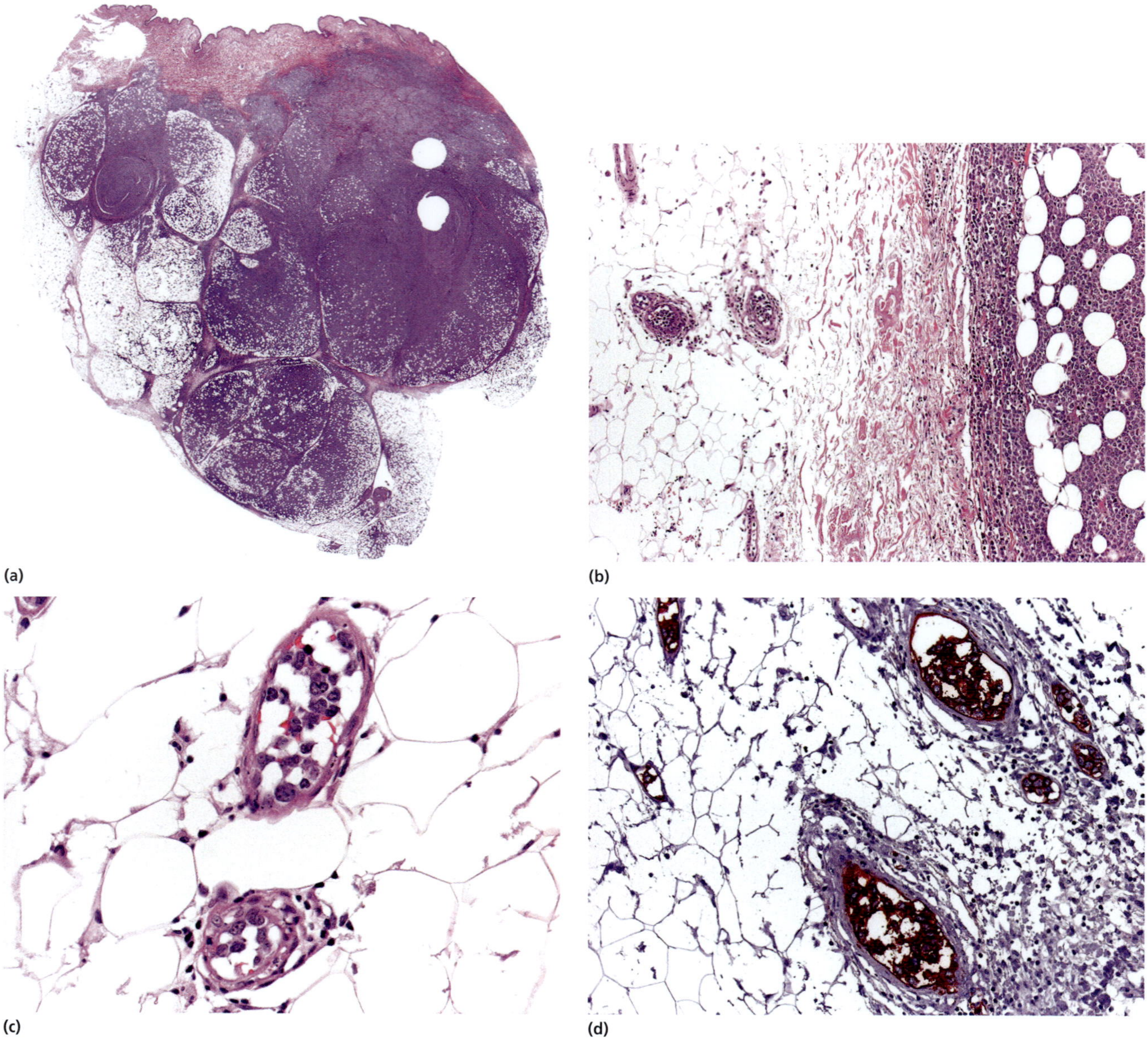


**Figure 18.12** Cutaneous diffuse large B-cell lymphoma, leg type. (a) Bulky tumor mass in the deep dermis and subcutaneous tissue; within the subcutaneous fat at the side of the main tumor there are (b, c) intravascular complexes of neoplastic cells (d) positive for CD20.

myeloma oncogene-1 (MUM-1) and forkhead box protein 1 (FOX-P1) (Fig. 18.15a and b) [47–49]. In the majority of cases, neoplastic cells express Bcl-6 and only rarely CD10, demonstrating a derivation from germinal center cells (Fig. 18.15c) [50], but CD21, a marker of follicular dendritic cells, is negative. IgM is strongly positive (sometimes with the coexpression of IgD), in contrast to negativity observed in follicle center lymphoma, diffuse type (Fig. 18.15d) [51]. Early lesions with sparse infiltrates display the same phenotype as advanced tumors. A useful marker in this setting is Ki-67, which allows both detection of a high proliferation index inconsistent with inflammatory dermatoses and, due to nuclear staining, also a better evaluation of the size of the nuclei (Fig. 18.16).

Rare Bcl-2-negative cases that otherwise fit into this group should not be classified as cutaneous follicle center lymphoma or as cutaneous diffuse large B-cell lymphoma, other. Expression of MYC can be evaluated at the protein level by immunohistology, and may be important for characterization of the prognosis (data on cutaneous cases are still partly contradictory, though). Evaluation and scoring of the staining may be difficult and subjective, particularly in case with heterogeneous staining pattern. The cut-off value to define positivity of neoplastic cells is 40% (50% for Bcl-2). It has been suggested that digital image analysis may be more reliable than conventional observation for assessing the degree of positivity [52]. Evaluation of positivity for Bcl-2 may also be affected by the choice of the monoclonal antibody [53].

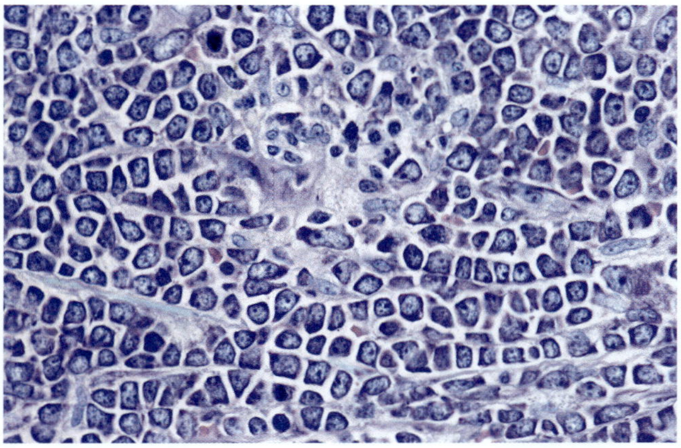

**Figure 18.13** Cutaneous diffuse large B-cell lymphoma, leg type. "Mosaic stone"-like arrangement of "squared" neoplastic cells resembling the histopathological features of Burkitt lymphoma or of lymphoblastic lymphoma (Giemsa staining).

Markers of plasma cell differentiation (CD138) are negative as a rule, allowing a distinction to be made from plasmablastic lymphoma (see Chapter 20). Some cases of cutaneous diffuse large B-cell lymphoma, leg type, show an anaplastic morphology histopathologically, and expression of CD30 phenotypically [54]. A better behavior has been reported for nodal cases positive for CD30 [55], but prognostic data on cutaneous cases are not available.

PD-1 and PD-L1 are expressed in variable amounts in neoplastic cells and inflammatory cells in extracutaneous diffuse large B-cell lymphoma [56, 57]. Tissue PD-L1$^+$ expression and T-cell-derived PD-1$^+$ expression seem to have significant adverse impact in nodal diffuse large B-cell lymphoma, but only in patients with high numbers of reactive T-cells (not in those with low numbers of CD3$^+$ infiltrating lymphocytes) [58]. In the skin, a study suggested that PD-L1$^+$ tumor cells and PD-L1$^+$ myeloid-derived suppressor cells may shield the tumor against the activity of PD-1$^+$ tumor-infiltrating lymphocytes, suggesting that targeting these cells by specific antibodies may be a novel therapeutic strategy for cutaneous diffuse large B-cell lymphoma, leg type [59].

Follicular dendritic cells are usually absent in primary cutaneous diffuse large B-cell lymphoma, leg type (yet it may be observed in secondary cutaneous diffuse large B-cell

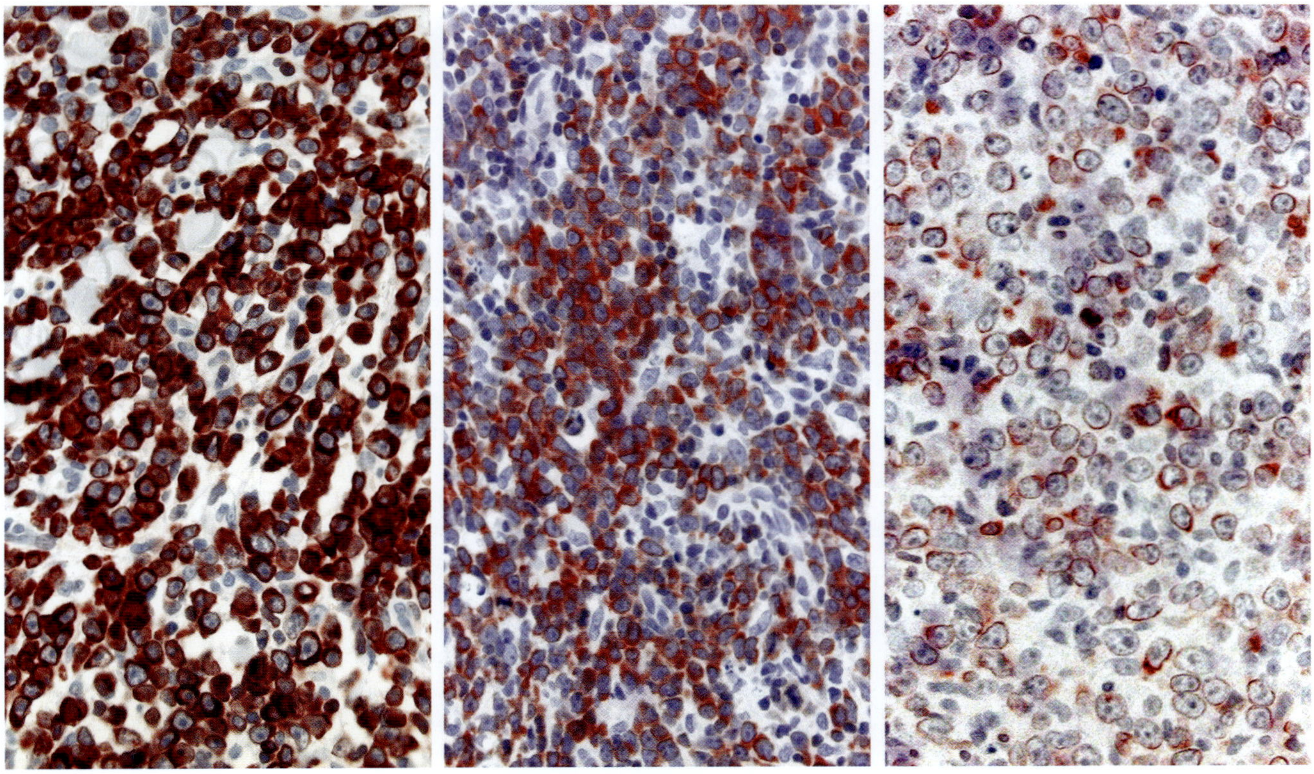

**Figure 18.14** Patterns of positivity for Bcl-2 in cutaneous diffuse large B-cell lymphoma, leg type. Strong positivity in virtually all neoplastic cells (left); variable positivity in the majority of neoplastic cells (middle); weak positivity in the majority of neoplastic cells (right). Positivity is defined as any staining pattern in ≥50% of neoplastic cells.

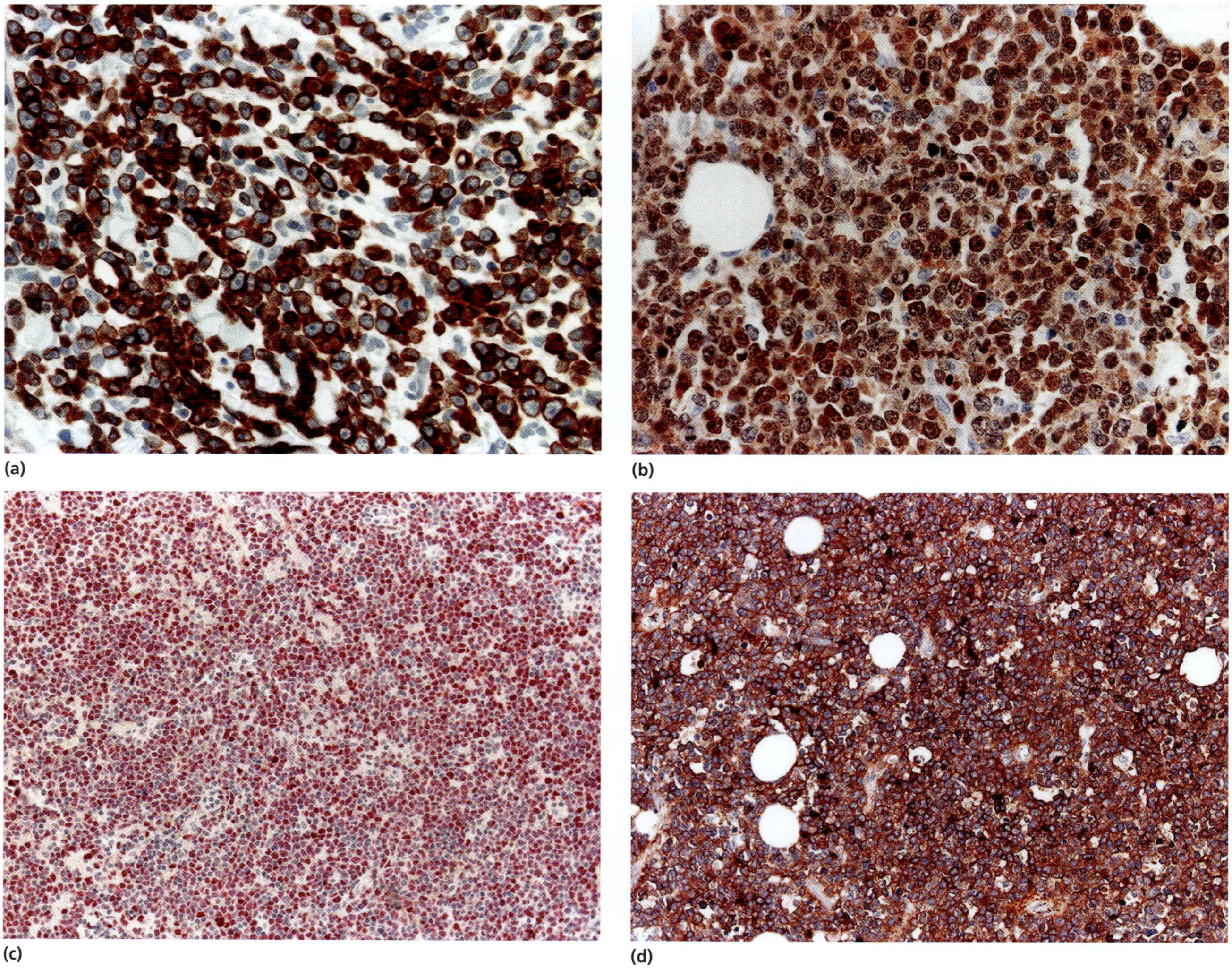


Figure 18.15 Cutaneous diffuse large B-cell lymphoma, leg type. Positive staining for (a) Bcl-2, (b) MUM-1, (c) Bcl-6, and (d) IgM.

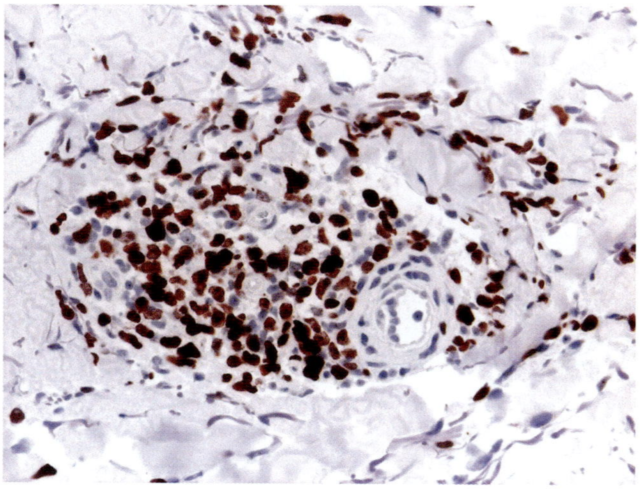

Figure 18.16 Cutaneous diffuse large B-cell lymphoma, leg type. Ki-67 staining in an early lesion demonstrates high proliferation rate of neoplastic cells, providing a helpful diagnostic clue.

lymphoma), and the presence of $CD21^+$ clusters of cells may suggest a diagnosis of cutaneous follicle center lymphoma, diffuse type. However, in rare cases clusters of $CD21^+$ cells can be observed on the background of otherwise typical features of cutaneous diffuse large B-cell lymphoma, leg type (Fig. 18.17), thus complete phenotypic analyses are always necessary, and interpretation of any given finding must be done in the context of all histopathological and phenotypic data. In my experience, clinicopathological evaluation is sufficient for diagnosis in the vast majority of cases, and molecular features are almost never needed for purpose of differential diagnosis from cutaneous follicle center lymphoma, diffuse type.

## Molecular genetics

A monoclonal rearrangement of the immunoglobulin (Ig) genes is found in most cases. The analysis of single cells by micromanipulation and polymerase chain reaction (PCR) showed that cutaneous diffuse large B-cell lymphoma, leg type, is characterized by

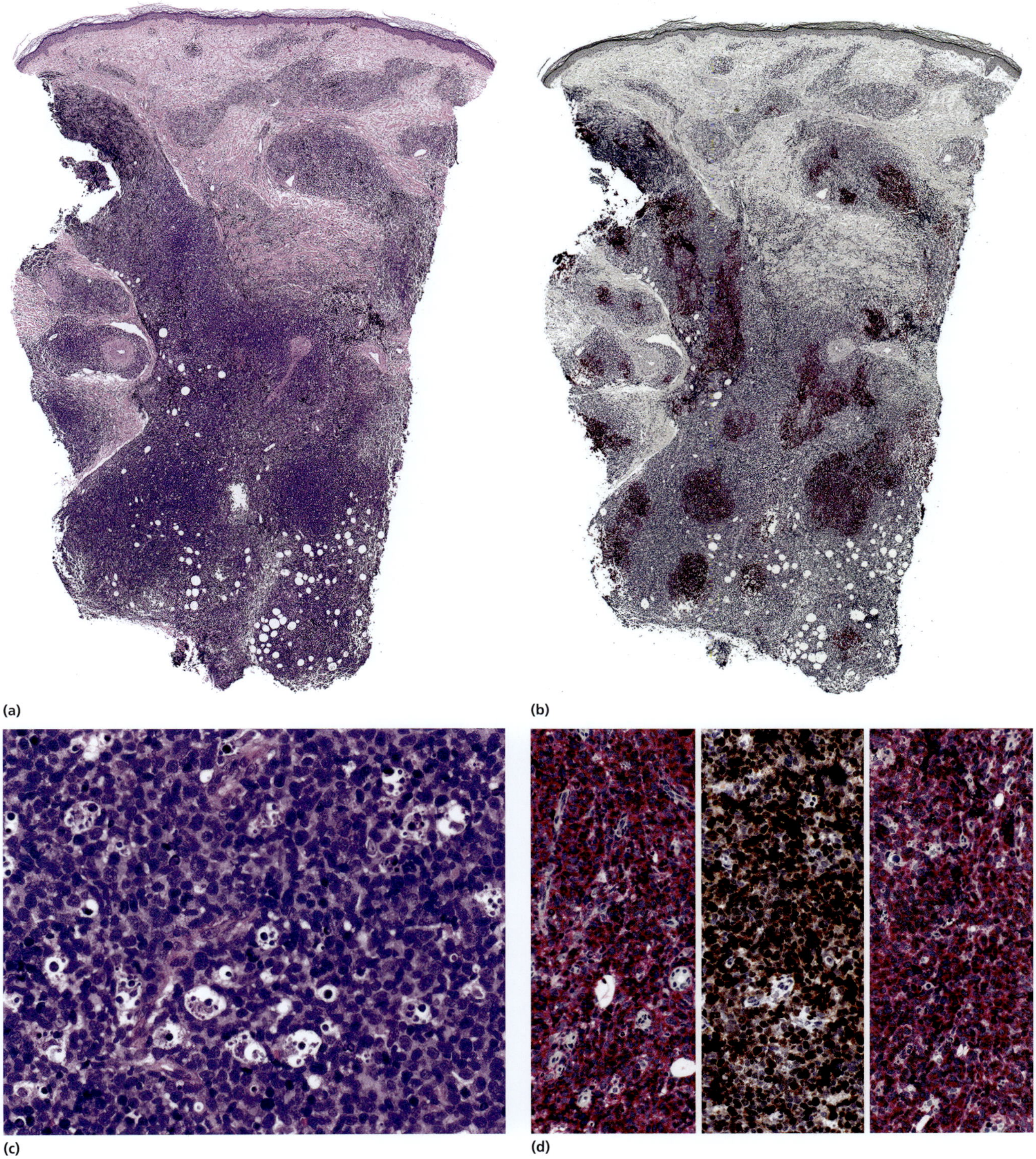


**Figure 18.17** Cutaneous diffuse large B-cell lymphoma, leg type. (a) Dense, diffuse infiltrates involving the entire dermis and visible subcutaneous fat in an 82-year-old woman with a tumor on the lower leg. (b) Irregular networks of CD21⁺ follicular dendritic cells. (c) Predominance of large lymphocytes with focally a "starry sky" pattern. Immunohistology showed positivity of neoplastic cells for CD20 (d, left), MUM-1 (d, middle), and Bcl-2 (d, right), as well as for Bcl-6, IgM, and CD10. Approximately half of the cells were positive for C-MYC. The proliferation rate (Ki-67) was >80%. The in situ hybridization for EBV (EBER-1) was negative. The presence of CD21⁺ follicular dendritic cells is usually a feature of secondary cutaneous involvement by nodal diffuse large B-cell lymphoma with a germinal center cell origin rather than of primary cutaneous diffuse large B-cell lymphoma, leg type.

a proliferation of postgerminal center cells [60]. The expression profile is that of activated B-cells with a strong expression of the transcription factor MUM-1/IRF4 and constitutive activation of the NF-κB pathway [61]. Hypermethylation of p15 and/or p16 has been observed in some patients with cutaneous diffuse large B-cell lymphoma, leg type, [62]; 9p21 deletions, possibly resulting in the inactivation of p16, have been detected in several cases, and may have a prognostic significance [63–65].

Mutations in the *MYD88*$^{L265P}$ gene, coding for a universal adaptor protein involved in the activation of signal pathways including the NF-κB one, are found in the majority of cutaneous diffuse large B-cell lymphoma, leg type, but not in cutaneous follicle center lymphoma [66–68]. Other mutations affecting the B-cell receptor signaling pathway involve the *TNFAIP3*, *CD79B*, and *CARD11* genes [8, 66, 69], again suggesting constitutional activation of the NF-κB pathway. As already mentioned, molecular variants characterized by double hit (rearrangements of *MYC* and *BCL6*) have been described in a minority of primary cutaneous cases [20] (see above in this Chapter). Besides *MYC*, other genetic alterations include the overexpression of genes associated with cell proliferation, of the protooncogenes *PIM1* and *PIM2*, and of the transcription factor Oct-2 [61]. The overexpression of FOX-P1 is not related to *FOXP1* translocations [49].

A considerable body of evidence shows that cutaneous diffuse large B-cell lymphoma, leg type, has a molecular profile different from that of cutaneous follicle center lymphoma, diffuse type, thus supporting the classification of these lymphomas into separate categories [61, 64, 70]. Cutaneous diffuse large B-cell lymphoma, leg type, has the gene signature of activated B lymphocytes, whereas follicle center lymphoma displays the signature of germinal center cells [61, 71]. A site-specific expression pattern of some polycomb-group genes, which are involved in the regulation of lymphopoiesis and malignant transformation, has been observed in cases of cutaneous B-cell lymphomas with large cell morphology arising on the head and neck or on the trunk as opposed to those located on the leg, again confirming that these tumors represent distinct types of cutaneous B-cell lymphoma [72].

The t(14;18) involving the *BCL-2* und *IGH* genes is not present in cutaneous diffuse large B-cell lymphoma, leg type. Amplifications of 18q21.31–21.33, including the *MALT1* and *BCL2* loci, have been detected in several cases, providing a possible explanation for the Bcl-2 expression in spite of the absence of the t(14;18) translocation [70]. A t(14,18)(q32;q21) involving the *IGH* and *MALT1* genes has been detected in one patient, but this case may have represented in truth a secondary cutaneous spread from an extracutaneous B-cell lymphoma [73].

## Treatment

The therapy of choice is anthracycline-containing systemic chemotherapy combined with anti-CD20 antibody (rituximab) [74–78]. However, this treatment can be difficult to administer because of the advanced age of most patients (often over 80 years), particularly in relapsing cases. Age-adapted schemes have been proposed [74]. Rituximab may be used alone, but recurrences are the rule. Lenalidomide, an analog of thalidomide, induced response in some patients and may be considered in relapses or in refractory cases [79]. The absence of the *MYD88*$^{L265P}$ mutation was associated with a higher overall response to lenalidomide [79]. Ibrutinib, a molecule that binds permanently to Bruton's tyrosine kinase, has been used successfully in some cases.

If chemotherapy cannot be given, solitary lesions may be treated by radiotherapy. Recommendations from the EORTC cutaneous lymphoma tumour group for radiation therapy have been published recently [80]. Intralesional interferon-α and antibiotic therapy have also been administered in the past, but nonaggressive options should not be considered if more appropriate modalities can be used.

Anti-CD19–directed autologous chimeric antigen receptor–modified T cells (CAR-T) are being used for relapsed or refractory large B-cell lymphomas [81], but there are no data concerning cutaneous cases. Molecular analyses may improve monitoring of patients with well-defined molecular aberrations [82].

## Prognosis

Cutaneous diffuse large B-cell lymphoma, leg type, has an aggressive behavior, and the estimated disease-specific five-year survival is 40–50% [77, 83]. A major improvement in survival has been observed using systemic polychemotherapy associated to rituximab [84]. Relapse after treatment is common and extracutaneous spread often occurs a few years after onset of the disease. Involvement of the central nervous system can be observed in some cases. Chemoresistance may be linked to mutations in the B-cell receptor signaling genes [85].

The analysis of prognostic factors is hindered by the fact that in the past cases of cutaneous B-cell lymphoma with large cell morphology belonging to different diagnostic groups (diffuse large B-cell lymphoma, leg type, and follicle center lymphoma, diffuse type) were lumped together. In this context, reports on a better prognosis of cases with a predominance of cleaved cells over those with a predominance of round cells were due to the inclusion of examples of both lymphoma types in the same category. In a similar way, the prognostic value of the Bcl-2 expression observed in the past was due to the fact that Bcl-2 is expressed by most cases of cutaneous diffuse large B-cell lymphoma, leg type, but usually not by those of cutaneous follicle center lymphoma, diffuse type. Other markers discriminating between the two types of lymphoma (e.g., MUM-1) do not have an independent prognostic value [86]. Thus, all of these parameters have no prognostic meaning if cases are classified correctly.

The presence of an *MYC* rearrangement is associated with a worse prognosis [18]. As already mentioned, nodal diffuse large

B-cell lymphoma with a double expression of Bcl-2 and MYC proteins is characterized by a worse prognosis [21–23]. Double expression of MYC and Bcl-2 seems to be frequent in cutaneous cases [18], but the prognostic value in patients with primary cutaneous diffuse large B-cell lymphoma, leg type is unclear, with one study suggesting a worse prognosis [19], and another one reporting no effect on prognosis [18]. P53 expression has been reported to augment the negative prognostic effect of *MYC* rearrangement, expression, or concurrent MYC/BCL2 expression in diffuse large B-cell lymphoma, even in the absence of *BCL2* and *BCL6* rearrangements, but data on cutaneous cases are lacking [87, 88]. The reduced expression of CD37, a B-cell surface antigen widely expressed on mature B cells, has been linked to a statistically significant worse prognosis and resistance to R-CHOP therapy (independent of other parameters) in patients with nodal diffuse large B-cell lymphoma [89]. Data on cutaneous cases are not available.

The number of lesions at presentation may be related to prognosis in cases of cutaneous diffuse large B-cell lymphoma, leg type [41]. As already mentioned, cases with deletion of 9p21 seem to be characterized by a more aggressive course [63]. High numbers of reactive, FOX-P3$^+$ regulatory T-cells were related to a better prognosis in one study [90], but this data has not been confirmed by further analyses. In nodal diffuse large B-cell lymphoma, unspecified positivity for CD30 is associated with a better prognosis [55], but data on cutaneous cases are not available.

Finally, the prognosis of cases presenting with figurate lesions is unclear. As already mentioned, one case with long-standing lesions over 20 years has been reported [40], and the few cases that I have seen seem to have a more indolent behavior. However, at the present state of knowledge, no conclusions can be drawn, and these patients should be managed in the same way as those with more conventional clinico-pathologic presentation.

**Résumé**

| **Cutaneous diffuse large B-cell lymphoma, leg type** | | |
|---|---|---|
| **Clinical** | Elderly; female to male ratio 3:1. Broad spectrum of presentations; usually solitary or clustered tumors, often ulcerated. Location on the leg(s) in >80% of cases. | |
| **Morphology** | Dense diffuse infiltrates characterized by predominance of large cells with round nuclei (centroblasts, immunoblasts). Occasionally shows epidermotropism or angiotropism. | |
| **Immunohistochemistry** | CD20, CD79a, PAX-5 | + |
| | cytoplasmic IgM | + (+/– coexpression of IgD) |
| | Bcl-2 | + |
| | MUM-1 | + |
| | FOX-P1 | + |
| | MYC | +/– |
| | Bcl-6 | +(–) |
| | CD10 | –(+) |
| | CD21 | – |
| **Genetics** | Monoclonal rearrangement of the Ig genes detected in the majority of cases. Loss of *CDKN2A* and *CDKN2B* on 9p21 bears a worse prognosis. Gene signature of activated B lymphocytes. $MYD88^{L265P}$ and other gene mutations suggest constitutional activation of the NF-κB pathway. Double-hit rearrangement of *MYC* and *BCL6* in a proportion of cases. | |
| **Treatment guidelines** | Anthracycline-containing systemic chemotherapy with rituximab. Solitary lesions may be treated by radiotherapy if chemotherapy is not possible. | |

## Primary cutaneous diffuse large B-cell lymphoma, NOS

The existence of a further category of primary cutaneous diffuse large B-cell lymphoma, other (or "NOS") has been proposed for cases of cutaneous lymphoma with predominance of large B cells that do not fit into the most common categories (cutaneous follicle center lymphoma, diffuse type and cutaneous diffuse large B-cell lymphoma, leg type) [91, 92]. The 2018 and 2024 updates WHO/EORTC classification of cutaneous lymphomas do not include a "NOS" category for cutaneous diffuse large B-cell lymphoma [3, 4]. In my experience, the inclusion of a given case in such a category is very subjective, and in routine practice, only exceptional cases cannot be classified confidently within one of the two established categories of cutaneous follicle center lymphoma, diffuse type or diffuse large B-cell lymphoma, leg type. The high percentage of "NOS" cases detected in one study (25% of cutaneous B-cell lymphomas other than marginal

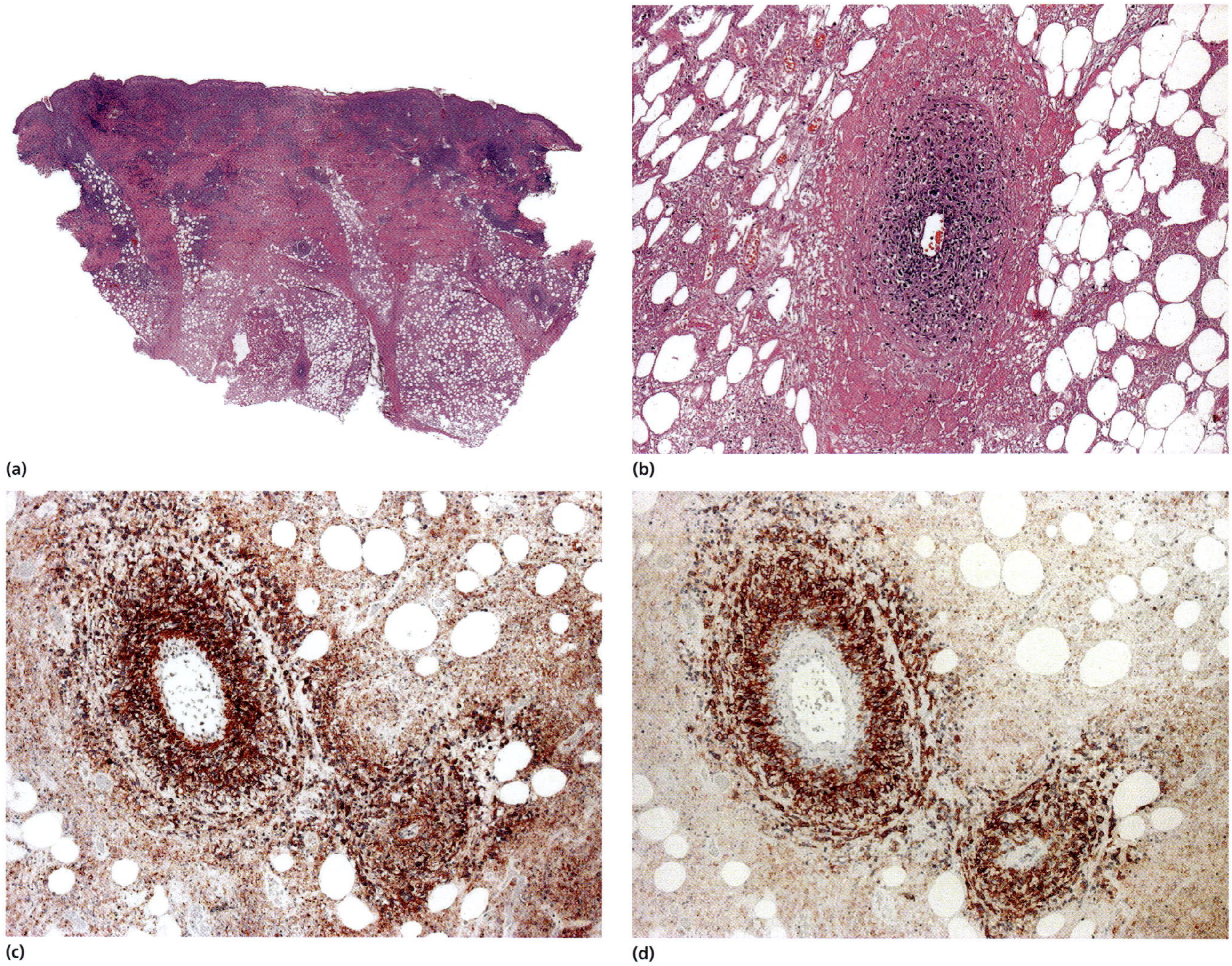

Figure 18.18 Cutaneous diffuse large B-cell lymphoma with prominent angiocentricity and necrosis. (a) Dense lymphoid infiltrates with marked necrosis within the entire dermis and subcutaneous fat. (b) Prominent angiocentricity/angiodestruction with surrounding necrosis. Neoplastic cells are positive for (c) CD79a and (d) CD30 (this case was negative for EBV).

zone lymphoma) [92] and in a second one (44% of cases of primary cutaneous diffuse large B-cell lymphoma) [93] does not reflect my personal experience. Negativity for Bcl-2, used as diagnostic criterion for the category "diffuse large B-cell lymphoma, other" in another study [91], is not sufficient to classify differently cases that show otherwise typical histopathological and phenotypic features of diffuse large B-cell lymphoma, leg type. In cases of cutaneous lymphoma characterized by a predominance of large cells and arising primary in the skin, the presence of a network of follicular dendritic cells, and a negative staining for BCL2, MUM1, MYC, and cytoplasmic IgM, support a diagnosis of primary cutaneous follicle center lymphoma. Cases that do not meet the diagnostic criteria of either primary cutaneous diffuse large B-cell lymphoma, leg type, or primary cutaneous follicle center lymphoma are very rare and may be referred to as primary cutaneous diffuse large B-cell lymphoma, NOS. I have encountered only exceptional cases of primary cutaneous diffuse large B-cell lymphoma that could not be classified into existing categories; some of these cases reveal very peculiar features like angiocentricity and angiodestruction, similar to lymphomatoid granulomatosis but without association to EBV (Fig. 18.18).

Rare cases of primary cutaneous $ALK^+$ diffuse large B-cell lymphoma have also been reported [94]. Although in the lymph nodes these cases are considered to represent a distinct entity and are included as such in the WHO *Classification of Haematolymphoid Tumours* [95], it is unclear whether cases arising primary in the skin should be considered as phenotypic and molecular variants of cutaneous diffuse large B-cell lymphoma, leg type, or represent a distinct entity comparable to the nodal one.

Finally, as already mentioned, it should be reminded that cases classified as follicle center lymphoma, diffuse type, according to the criteria of the WHO classification, but arising on the legs, have a bad prognosis, similar to that of cutaneous diffuse large B-cell lymphoma, leg type (see Chapter 16) [41, 96]. Thus, patients with follicle center lymphoma arising on the legs should be managed with the greatest caution, as the behavior may be more aggressive than that of the conventional variant arising on the head and neck area or on the trunk.

## References


1. Vermeer MH, Geelen FAMJ, van Haselen CW, *et al.* Primary cutaneous large B-cell lymphomas of the legs: a distinct type of cutaneous B-cell lymphoma with an intermediate prognosis. *Arch Dermatol* 1996;**132**:1304–1308.
2. Paulli M, Viglio A, Vivenza D, *et al.* Primary cutaneous large B-cell lymphoma of the leg: histogenetic analysis of a controversial entity. *Hum Pathol* 2002;**33**:937–943.
3. Willemze R, Cerroni L, Kempf W, *et al.* The 2018 update of the WHO-EORTC classification for primary cutaneous lymphomas. *Blood* 2019;**133**:1703–1714.
4. Kempf W, Mitteldorf C, Cerroni L, *et al.* Classifications of cutaneous lymphomas and lymphoproliferative disorders: an update from the EORTC cutaneous lymphoma histopathology group. *J Eur Acad Dermatol Venereol* 2024;**38**:1491–1503.
5. Goodlad JR, Rosen ST, Schrader AR. Primary cutaneous diffuse large B-cell lymphoma, leg type. In: Arber DA, Borowitz MJ, Cook JR, *et al.*, eds. *The International Consensus Classification of myeloid and Lymphoid Neoplasms*. Philadelphia (US): Wolters Kluver, 2025: 502–504.
6. Oschlies I, Parrens M, Battistella M, *et al.* Primary cutaneous diffuse large B-cell lymphoma, leg-type. In: *WHO Classification of Tumours Editorial Board. Haematolymphoid Tumours*. 5th edition. Lyon (France): IARC, 2024: 517–519.
7. Muniesa C, Pujol RM, Estrach T, *et al.* Primary cutaneous diffuse large B-cell lymphoma, leg type and secondary cutaneous involvement by testicular B-cell lymphoma share identical clinicopathological and immunophenotypic features. *J Am Acad Dermatol* 2012;**66**:650–654.
8. Pham-Ledard A, Prochazkova-Carlotti M, Andrique L, *et al.* Multiple genetic alterations in primary cutaneous large B-cell lymphoma, leg type support a common lymphomagenesis with activated B-cell-like diffuse large B-cell lymphoma. *Mod Pathol* 2014;**27**:402–411.
9. Ott G, Alaggio R, Dave SS, *et al.* Diffuse large B-cell lymphomas: introduction. In: *WHO Classification of Tumours Editorial Board. Haematolymphoid Tumours*. 5th edition. Lyon (France): IARC, 2024: 461–462.
10. Choi WW, Weisenburger DD, Greiner TC, *et al.* A new immunostain algorithm classifies diffuse large B-cell lymphoma into molecular subtypes with high accuracy. *Clin Cancer Res* 2009;**15**:5494–5502.
11. Hans CP, Weisenburger DD, Greiner TC, *et al.* Confirmation of the molecular classification of diffuse large B-cell lymphoma by immunohistochemistry using a tissue microarray. *Blood* 2004;**103**:275–282.
12. Schrader AMR, de Groen RAL, Willemze R, *et al.* Cell-of-origin classification using the Hans and Lymph2Cx algorithms in primary cutaneous large B-cell lymphomas. *Virchows Arch* 2022;**480**:667–675.
13. Menguy S, Beylot-Barry M, Parrens M, *et al.* Primary cutaneous large B-cell lymphomas: relevance of the 2017 World Health Organization classification: clinicopathological and molecular analyses of 64 cases. *Histopathology* 2019;**74**:1067–1080.
14. Sesques P, Johnson NA. Approach to the diagnosis and treatment of high-grade B-cell lymphomas with MYC and BCL2 and/or BCL6 rearrangements. *Blood* 2017;**129**:280–288.
15. Huang W, Medeiros LJ, Lin P, *et al.* MYC/BCL2/BCL6 triple hit lymphoma: a study of 40 patients with a comparison to MYC/BCL2 and MYC/BCL6 double hit lymphomas. *Mod Pathol* 2018;**31**:1470–1478.
16. Rosenwald A, Gujral S, Barrans SL, *et al.* Diffuse large B-cell lymphoma NOS. In: *WHO Classification of Tumours Editorial Board. Haematolymphoid Tumours*. 5th edition. Lyon (France): IARC, 2024: 463–472.
17. Colomo L, Vazquez I, Papaleo N, *et al.* LMO2-negative expression predicts the presence of MYC translocations in aggressive B-cell lymphomas. *Am J Surg Pathol* 2017;**41**:877–886.
18. Schrader AMR, Jansen PM, Vermeer MH, *et al.* High incidence and clinical significance of MYC rearrangements in primary cutaneous diffuse large B-cell lymphoma, leg type. *Am J Surg Pathol* 2018;**42**:1488–1494.
19. Menguy S, Frison E, Prochazkova-Carlotti M, *et al.* Double-hit or dual expression of MYC and BCL2 in primary cutaneous large B-cell lymphomas. *Mod Pathol* 2018;**31**:1332–1342.
20. Lucioni M, Pescia C, Bonometti A, *et al.* Double expressor and double/triple hit status among primary cutaneous diffuse large B-cell lymphoma: a comparison between leg type and not otherwise specified subtypes. *Hum Pathol* 2021;**111**:1–9.
21. Kluk MJ, Chapuy B, Sinha P, *et al.* Immunohistochemical detection of MYC-driven diffuse large B-cell lymphomas. *PLoS One* 2012;**7**:e33813.
22. Hu S, Xu-Monette ZY, Tzankov A, *et al.* MYC/BCL2 protein coexpression contributes to the inferior survival of activated B-cell subtype of diffuse large B-cell lymphoma and demonstrates high-risk gene expression signatures: a report from The International DLBCL Rituximab–CHOP Consortium Program. *Blood* 2013;**121**:4021–4031.
23. Green TM, Young KH, Visco C, *et al.* Immunohistochemical double-hit score is a strong predictor of outcome in patients with diffuse large B-cell lymphoma treated with rituximab plus cyclophosphamide, doxorubicin, vincristine, and prednisone. *J Clin Oncol* 2012;**30**:3460–3467.
24. Schmitz R, Wright GW, Huang DW, *et al.* Genetics and pathogenesis of diffuse large B-cell lymphoma. *N Engl J Med* 2018;**378**:1396–1407.
25. Mareschal S, Pham-Ledard A, Julien Viailly P, *et al.* Identification of somatic mutations in primary cutaneous diffuse large B-cell lymphoma, leg type by massive parallel sequencing. *J Invest Dermatol* 2017;**137**:1984–1994.
26. Chapuy B, Stewart C, Dunford AJ, *et al.* Molecular subtypes of diffuse large B cell lymphoma are associated with distinct pathogenic mechanisms and outcomes. *Nat Med* 2018;**24**:679–690.
27. Berti E, Marzano AV, Decleva I, *et al.* Simultaneous onset of primary cutaneous B-cell lymphoma and human herpes virus 8-associated Kaposi's sarcoma. *Br J Dermatol* 1997;**136**:924–949.

28. Zöchling N, Pütz B, Wolf P, *et al.* Human herpes virus 8-specific DNA sequences in primary cutaneous B-cell lymphomas. *Arch Dermatol* 1998;**134**:246–247.
29. Cerroni L, Zöchling N, Pütz B, Kerl H. Infection by Borrelia burgdorferi and cutaneous B-cell lymphoma. *J Cutan Pathol* 1997;**24**:457–461.
30. Goodlad JR, Davidson MM, Hollowood K, *et al.* Primary cutaneous B-cell lymphoma and Borrelia burgdorferi infection in patients from the Highlands of Scotland. *Am J Surg Pathol* 2000;**24**:1279–1285.
31. Ponzoni M, Ferreri AJ, Mappa S, *et al.* Prevalence of Borrelia burgdorferi infection in a series of 98 primary cutaneous lymphomas. *Oncologist* 2011;**16**:1582–1588.
32. Tokuda Y, Fukushima M, Nakazawa K, *et al.* A case of primary Epstein–Barr virus associated cutaneous diffuse large B-cell lymphoma unassociated with iatrogenic or endogenous immune dysregulation. *J Cutan Pathol* 2008;**35**:666–671.
33. Gaitonde S, Kavuri S, Alagiozian-Angelova V, *et al.* EBV positivity in primary cutaneous large B-cell lymphoma with immunophenotypic features of leg type: an isolated incidence or something more significant? *Acta Oncol* 2008;**47**:461–464.
34. Chan BCY, Stefanato CM, Moonim MT, *et al.* Diffuse large B-cell lymphoma developing in erythrodermic cutaneous T-cell lymphoma: a case series. *Br J Dermatol* 2017;**177**:e138–e140.
35. Szablewski V, Costes-Martineau V, René C, *et al.* Composite cutaneous lymphoma of diffuse large B-cell lymphoma-leg type and subcutaneous panniculitis-like T-cell lymphoma. *J Cutan Pathol* 2018;**45**:716–720.
36. Vachhani P, Neppalli VT, Cancino CJ, *et al.* Radiological imaging and bone marrow biopsy in staging of cutaneous B-cell lymphoma. *Br J Haematol* 2019;**184**:674–676.
37. Khan AB, Barrington SF, Mikhaeel NG, *et al.* PET-CT staging of DLBCL accurately identifies and provides new insight into the clinical significance of bone marrow involvement. *Blood* 2013;**122**:61–67.
38. Ekmekci TR, Koslu A, Sakiz D, Barutcuoglu B. Primary cutaneous large B-cell lymphoma, leg type, presented with a migratory lesion. *J Eur Acad Dermatol Venereol* 2007;**21**:1000–1001.
39. Massone C, Fink-Puches R, Wolf I, *et al.* Atypical clinicopathologic presentation of primary cutaneous diffuse large B-cell lymphoma, leg type. *J Am Acad Dermatol* 2015;**72**:1016–1020.
40. Lin CP, Mulvaney PM, Lian CG, Clarissa Yang FS. Figurate erythema for 20 years. *JAAD Case Rep* 2019;**5**:475–477.
41. Kodama K, Massone C, Chott A, *et al.* Primary cutaneous large B-cell lymphomas: clinicopathologic features, classification, and prognostic factors in a large series of patients. *Blood* 2005;**106**:2491–2497.
42. Torres-Paoli D, Sanchez JL. Primary cutaneous B-cell lymphoma of the leg in a chronic lymphoedematous extremity. *Am J Dermatopathol* 2000;**22**:257–260.
43. Marrero-Aleman G, Montenegro-Damaso T, Penate Y. Primary cutaneous diffuse large B-cell lymphoma, leg type, with spontaneous regression after biopsy. *Am J Dermatopathol* 2017; **39**:785–787.
44. Plaza JA, Kacerovska D, Stockman DL, *et al.* The histomorphologic spectrum of primary cutaneous diffuse large B-cell lymphoma: a study of 79 cases. *Am J Dermatopathol* 2011;**33**:649–658.
45. Kamath NV, Gilliam AC, Nihal M, *et al.* Primary cutaneous large B-cell lymphoma of the leg relapsing as cutaneous intravascular large B-cell lymphoma. *Arch Dermatol* 2001;**137**:1637–1638.
46. Tsuyama N, Sakata S, Baba S, *et al.* BCL2 expression in DLBCL: reappraisal of immunohistochemistry with new criteria for therapeutic biomarker evaluation. *Blood* 2017;**130**:489–500.
47. Geelen FAMJ, Vermeer MH, Meijer CJLM, *et al.* Bcl-2 protein expression in primary cutaneous large B-cell lymphoma is site-related. *J Clin Oncol* 1998;**16**:2080–2085.
48. Gronbaeck K, Moller PH, Nedergaard T, *et al.* Primary cutaneous B-cell lymphoma: a clinical, histological, phenotypic and genotypic study of 21 cases. *Br J Dermatol* 2000;**142**:913–923.
49. Espinet B, Garcia-Herrera A, Gallardo F, *et al.* FOXP1 molecular cytogenetics and protein expression analyses in primary cutaneous large B cell lymphoma, leg-type. *Histol Histopathol* 2011;**26**:213–221.
50. Hoefnagel JJ, Vermeer MH, Jansen PM, *et al.* Bcl-2, Bcl-6 and CD10 expression in cutaneous B-cell lymphoma: further support for a follicle centre cell origin and differential diagnostic significance. *Br J Dermatol* 2003;**149**:1183–1191.
51. Koens L, Vermeer MH, Willemze R, *et al.* IgM expression on paraffin sections distinguishes primary cutaneous large B-cell lymphoma, leg type from primary cutaneous follicle center lymphoma. *Am J Surg Pathol* 2010;**34**:1043–1048.
52. Hupp M, Williams S, Dunnette B, *et al.* Comparison of evaluation techniques, including digital image analysis, for MYC protein expression by immunohistochemical stain in aggressive B-cell lymphomas. *Hum Pathol* 2019;**83**:124–132.
53. Kendrick SL, Redd L, Muranyi A, *et al.* BCL2 antibodies targeted at different epitopes detect varying levels of protein expression and correlate with frequent gene amplification in diffuse large B cell lymphoma. *Hum Pathol* 2014;**45**:2144–2153.
54. Herrera E, Gallardo M, Bosch R, *et al.* Primary cutaneous CD30 (Ki-1)-positive non-anaplastic B-cell lymphoma. *J Cutan Pathol* 2002;**29**:181–184.
55. Hu S, Xu-Monette ZY, Balasubramanyam A, *et al.* CD30 expression defines a novel subgroup of diffuse large B-cell lymphoma with favorable prognosis and distinct gene expression signature: a report from the International DLBCL Rituximab-CHOP Consortium Program Study. *Blood* 2013;**121**:2715–2724.
56. Kwon D, Kim S, Kim PJ, *et al.* Clinicopathological analysis of programmed cell death 1 and programmed cell death ligand 1 expression in the tumour microenvironments of diffuse large B cell lymphomas. *Histopathology* 2016;**68**:1079–1089.
57. Menguy S, Prochazkova-Carlotti M, Beylot-Barry M, *et al.* PD-L1 and PD-L2 are differentially expressed by macrophages or tumor cells in primary cutaneous diffuse large B-cell lymphoma, leg type. *Am J Surg Pathol* 2018;**42**:326–334.
58. Li L, Sun R, Miao Y, *et al.* PD-1/PD-L1 expression and interaction by automated quantitative immunofluorescent analysis show adverse prognostic impact in patients with diffuse large B-cell lymphoma having T-cell infiltration: a study from the International DLBCL Consortium Program. *Mod Pathol* 2019;**32**:741–754.
59. Mitteldorf C, Berisha A, Pfaltz MC, *et al.* Tumor microenvironment and checkpoint molecules in primary cutaneous diffuse large B-cell lymphoma-new therapeutic targets. *Am J Surg Pathol* 2017;**41**:998–1004.
60. Gellrich S, Rutz S, Golembowski S, *et al.* Primary cutaneous follicle center cell lymphomas and large B cell lymphomas of the leg descend from germinal center cells: a single cell polymerase chain reaction analysis. *J Invest Dermatol* 2001;**117**:1512–1520.

61. Hoefnagel JJ, Dijkman R, Basso K, *et al.* Distinct types of primary cutaneous large B-cell lymphoma identified by gene expression profiling. *Blood* 2005;**105**:3671–3678.
62. Child FJ, Scarisbrick JJ, Calonje E, *et al.* Inactivation of tumor suppressor genes $p15^{INK4b}$ and $p16^{INK4a}$ in primary cutaneous B cell lymphoma. *J Invest Dermatol* 2002;**118**:941–948.
63. Senff NJ, Zoutman WH, Vermeer MH, *et al.* Fine-mapping chromosomal loss at 9p21: correlation with prognosis in primary cutaneous diffuse large B-cell lymphoma, leg type. *J Invest Dermatol* 2009;**129**:1149–1155.
64. Wiesner T, Obenauf AC, Geigl JB, *et al.* 9p21 deletion in primary cutaneous large B-cell lymphoma, leg type, may escape detection by standard FISH assays. *J Invest Dermatol* 2009;**129**:238–240.
65. Kaune KM, Neumann C, Hallermann C, *et al.* Simultaneous aberrations of single CDKN2A network components and a high Rb phosphorylation status can differentiate subgroups of primary cutaneous B-cell lymphomas. *Exp Dermatol* 2011;**20**:331–335.
66. Pham-Ledard A, Cappellen D, Martinez F, *et al.* MYD88 somatic mutation is a genetic feature of primary cutaneous diffuse large B-cell lymphoma, leg type. *J Invest Dermatol* 2012;**132**: 2118–2120.
67. Menguy S, Gros A, Pham-Ledard A, *et al.* MYD88 somatic mutation is a diagnostic criterion in primary cutaneous large B-cell lymphoma. *J Invest Dermatol* 2016;**136**:1741–1744.
68. Zhou XA, Louissaint A Jr, Wenzel A, *et al.* Genomic analyses identify recurrent alterations in immune evasion genes in diffuse large B-cell lymphoma, leg type. *J Invest Dermatol* 2018;**138**:2365–2376.
69. Koens L, Zoutman WH, Ngarmlertsirichai P, *et al.* Nuclear factor-κB pathway-activating gene aberrancies in primary cutaneous large B-cell lymphoma, leg type. *J Invest Dermatol* 2014;**134**:290–292.
70. Dijkman R, Tensen CP, Jordanova ES, *et al.* Array-based comparative genomic hybridization analysis reveals recurrent chromosomal alterations and prognostic parameters in primary cutaneous large B-cell lymphoma. *J Clin Oncol* 2006;**24**:296–305.
71. Storz MN, van de Rijn M, Kim YH, *et al.* Gene expression profiles of cutaneous B cell lymphoma. *J Invest Dermatol* 2003;**120**: 865–870.
72. Raaphorst FM, Vermeer M, Fieret E, *et al.* Site-specific expression of polycomb-group genes encoding the HPC–HPH/PRC1 complex in clinically defined primary nodal and cutaneous large B-cell lymphomas. *Am J Pathol* 2004;**164**:533–542.
73. Cook JR, Sherer M, Craig FE, *et al.* t(14;18)(q32;q21) involving MALT1 and IGH genes in an extranodal diffuse large B-cell lymphoma. *Hum Pathol* 2003;**34**:1212–1215.
74. Grange F, Maubec E, Bagot M, *et al.* Treatment of cutaneous B-cell lymphoma, leg type, with age-adapted combinations of chemotherapies and rituximab. *Arch Dermatol* 2009;**145**:329–330.
75. Guyot A, Ortonne N, Valeyrie-Allenore L, *et al.* Combined treatment with rituximab and anthracycline-containing chemotherapy for primary cutaneous large B-cell lymphomas, leg-type, in elderly patients. *Arch Dermatol* 2010;**146**:89–91.
76. Senff NJ, Noordijk EM, Kim YH, *et al.* European Organization for Research and Treatment of Cancer and International Society for Cutaneous Lymphoma consensus recommendations for the management of cutaneous B-cell lymphomas. *Blood* 2008;**112**: 1600–1609.
77. Grange F, Beylot-Barry M, Courville P, *et al.* Primary cutaneous diffuse large B-cell lymphoma, leg type. Clinicopathologic features and prognostic analysis in 60 cases. *Arch Dermatol* 2007;**143**: 1144–1150.
78. Willemze R, Hodak E, Zinzani PL, *et al.* Primary cutaneous lymphomas: ESMO Clinical Practice Guidelines for diagnosis, treatment and follow-up. *Ann Oncol* 2018;**29**(Suppl. 4):iv30–iv40. on behalf of the ESMO Guidelines Committee
79. Beylot-Barry M, Mermin D, Maillard A, *et al.* A single-arm phase II trial of lenalidomide in relapsing or refractory primary cutaneous large B-cell lymphoma, leg type. *J Invest Dermatol* 2018;**138**: 1982–1989.
80. Elsayad K, Guenova E, Assaf C, *et al.* Radiotherapy in cutaneous lymphomas: recommendations from the EORTC cutaneous lymphoma tumour group. *Eur J Cancer* 2024;**212**:115064.
81. Ghobadi A, Munoz J, Westin JR, *et al.* Outcomes of subsequent anti-lymphoma therapies after second-line axicabtagene ciloleucel or standard of care in ZUMA-7. *Blood Adv* 2024;**8**:2982–2990.
82. Schrader AMR, de Groen RAL, Willemze R, *et al.* Genetic stability of driver alterations in primary cutaneous diffuse large B-cell lymphoma, leg type and their relapses: a rationale for the use of molecular-based methods for more effective disease monitoring. *Cancer* 2022;**14**:5152.
83. Fink-Puches R, Zenahlik P, Bäck B, *et al.* Primary cutaneous lymphomas: applicability of current classification schemes (European Organization for Research and Treatment of Cancer, World Health Organization) based on clinicopathologic features observed in a large group of patients. *Blood* 2002;**99**:800–805.
84. Grange F, Joly P, Barbe C, *et al.* Improvement of survival in patients with primary cutaneous diffuse large B-cell lymphoma, leg type, in France. *JAMA Dermatol* 2014;**150**:535–541.
85. Ducharme O, Beylot-Barry M, Pham-Ledard A, *et al.* Mutations of the B-cell receptor pathway confer chemoresistance in primary cutaneous diffuse large B-cell lymphoma leg type. *J Invest Dermatol* 2019;**139**:2334–2342.
86. Hallermann C, Niermann C, Fischer RJ, Schulze HJ. New prognostic relevant factors in primary cutaneous diffuse large B-cell lymphomas. *J Am Acad Dermatol* 2007;**56**:588–597.
87. Wang XJ, Medeiros LJ, Bueso-Ramos CE, *et al.* P53 expression correlates with poorer survival and augments the negative prognostic effect of MYC rearrangement, expression or concurrent MYC/BCL2 expression in diffuse large B-cell lymphoma. *Mod Pathol* 2017;**30**:194–203.
88. Li S, Weiss VL, Wang XJ, *et al.* High-grade B-cell lymphoma with MYC rearrangement and without BCL2 and BCL6 rearrangements is associated with high P53 expression and a poor prognosis. *Am J Surg Pathol* 2016;**40**:253–261.
89. Xu-Monette ZY, Li L, Byrd JC, *et al.* Assessment of CD37 B-cell antigen and cell of origin significantly improves risk prediction in diffuse large B-cell lymphoma. *Blood* 2016;**128**:3083–3100.
90. Felcht M, Heck M, Weiss C, *et al.* Expression of the T-cell regulatory marker FOXP3 in primary cutaneous large B-cell lymphoma tumour cells. *Br J Dermatol* 2012;**167**:348–358.
91. Felcht M, Klemke CD, Nicolay JP, *et al.* Primary cutaneous diffuse large B-cell lymphoma, NOS and leg type: clinical, morphologic and prognostic differences. *J Dtsch Dermatol Ges* 2019;**17**:275–285.
92. Lucioni M, Berti E, Arcaini L, *et al.* Primary cutaneous B-cell lymphoma other than marginal zone: clinicopathologic analysis of 161 cases: comparison with current classification and definition of prognostic markers. *Cancer Med* 2016;**5**:2740–2755.

93. Uccella S, Goteri G, Maiorana A, *et al.* Clinicopathological, cytogenetic, and molecular profiles of primary cutaneous diffuse large B-cell lymphomas. *Hum Pathol* 2023;**136**:44–55.
94. Kempf W, Torricelli R, Zettl A, *et al.* Primary cutaneous anaplastic lymphoma kinase–positive large B-cell lymphoma. *Am J Dermatopathol* 2019;**41**:602–605.
95. Medeiros JL, Sengar M, Delabie J, *et al.* ALK-positive large B-cell lymphoma. In: *WHO Classification of Tumours Editorial Board. Haematolymphoid Tumours.* 5th edition. Lyon (France): IARC, 2024: 481–483.
96. Senff NJ, Hoefnagel JJ, Jansen PM, *et al.* Reclassification of 300 primary cutaneous B-cell lymphomas according to the new WHO–EORTC classification for cutaneous lymphomas: comparison with previous classifications and identification of prognostic markers. *J Clin Oncol* 2007;**25**:1581–1587.

## CHAPTER 19

# Intravascular large cell lymphomas

It is yet unclear whether the two phenotypic variants of intravascular large cell lymphoma, namely, the more frequent B-cell type and the exceedingly rare natural killer (NK)/T-cell type, represent different phenotypes of one category of lymphoma or completely different entities. In addition, it has been clearly demonstrated that CD30$^{+}$ "intravascular" anaplastic large T-cell lymphoma is unrelated to conventional intravascular large cell lymphomas, as they present with neoplastic cells located within the lymphatic rather than the blood vessels, and are characterized by an indolent course (see Chapter 5). In this edition of the book, intravascular large cell lymphomas have been included in the section on cutaneous B cell lymphomas, as in most instances, they represent indeed a peculiar type of large B-cell lymphoma. The NK/T-cell variant is included in this chapter as a separate entity, because the intravascular location of the cells is a least common denominator with the B-cell type, and because intravascular NK/T-cell lymphoma is not included in current lymphoma classifications.

Intravascular large B-cell lymphoma is considered as a distinct entity in the International Consensus Classification (ICC) *of Myeloid and Lymphoid Neoplasms* and in the 5th edition of the World Health Organization (WHO) *Classification of Haematolymphoid Tumours* [1, 2]. By contrast, the NK/T-cell variant is probably the only lymphoma type that is not covered by any classification. The 4th update of the WHO classification mentioned it only with the following words: "An increasing number of intravascular NK/T-cell lymphomas with EBV-positive tumor cells and rarely intralymphatic anaplastic large cell lymphomas, ALK-negative, have been reported, but they should be considered different entities." [3]; further details were not provided, and there is no mention of the entity neither in the 5th edition of the WHO classification nor in the ICC classification. In addition, in that sentence, the aggressive intravascular NK/T-cell lymphoma was lumped together with the indolent intralymphatic anaplastic large cell lymphoma: it should be clearly understood, however, that the second group represents a variant of anaplastic large cell lymphoma and that it has no relationship whatsoever with intravascular large NK/T-cell lymphoma (intralymphatic anaplastic large cell lymphoma is covered in detail in Chapter 5). In my opinion, intravascular large NK/T-cell lymphoma represents a specific entity of non-Hodgkin lymphoma, clearly separated from intravascular large B-cell lymphoma: the first is commonly associated with EBV and is treated with T-cell directed therapy, whereas the second shows no association with EBV and is managed like a diffuse large B-cell lymphoma.

The skin may be the only affected site in intravascular large cell lymphomas, but more frequently, the disease presents with generalized lesions and common neurologic symptoms due to involvement of the central nervous system. Random skin biopsy has been suggested in order to confirm the diagnosis in patients with neurological symptoms and suspect diagnosis of intravascular large B-cell lymphoma [4–7]. In fact, in a large study on 42 patients, diagnosis was achieved by "random" skin biopsy in 69% of cases, although according to the authors, only 14% of cases presented with skin changes [8]. A similar study on Western patients revealed a sensitivity of 50% [9]. In order to achieve diagnosis, an incisional biopsy should be performed rather than a punch biopsy [10]. On the other hand, the issue on "skin changes" as reported in published series may be difficult to judge, as cutaneous signs are often characterized only by unusual telangiectasias and/or inconspicuous erythema or purpura ("panniculitis-like"), and may be overlooked or considered nonspecific.

Intravascular large cell lymphoma is characterized by the presence of neoplastic cells confined almost exclusively to the lumina of vessels, and it was formerly misinterpreted as a vascular neoplasm (malignant angioendotheliomatosis) [11]. Cases classified in the past as large B-cell lymphoma recurring as intravascular lymphoma [12, 13] or as "mixed" intravascular and diffuse large B-cell lymphoma [14] should not be included in this category but rather classified as diffuse large B-cell lymphoma with intravascular component (see Chapter 18 and Fig. 18.12) [15].

The reason(s) why neoplastic cells in intravascular large cell lymphoma are confined within the vessels is unclear. The absence of molecules crucial for adhesion of lymphocytes to endothelial cells and migration out of the vessels (CD29 and CD54) has been observed in some cases with the B-cell phenotype, leading to the hypothesis that neoplastic lymphocytes in intravascular large

*Skin Lymphoma: The Illustrated Guide*, Sixth Edition. Lorenzo Cerroni.

B-cell lymphoma are unable to escape outside the vessel walls [16]. Molecular studies in cases with B-cell phenotype demonstrated the expression of angiogenic factors *VEGFA*, *VEGFC*, *FIGF*, and *SPP1* by neoplastic cells in one case of cutaneous intravascular large B-cell lymphoma [17]. In one patient, CXCR3 was expressed by tumor lymphocytes, and its ligand CXCL9 was detected in blood vessels, thus providing a further possible explanation for intraluminal location of neoplastic cells [18]. These findings are mostly anecdotal and observed only in a limited number of cases, though seem to point at a pathogenetic mechanism characterized by neoplastic cells expressing molecules that make them capable of adhesion to the endothelium, but unlike diffuse large B-cell lymphoma lacking molecules involved in extravasation from the blood vessels.

It should be remembered that in a distinct proportion of the reported cases, particularly in the NK/T-cell variant of the disease, the diagnosis of intravascular large cell lymphoma was a retrospective one made first at autopsy. In a large French-Canadian study, almost 25% of patients received a post-mortem diagnosis [19].

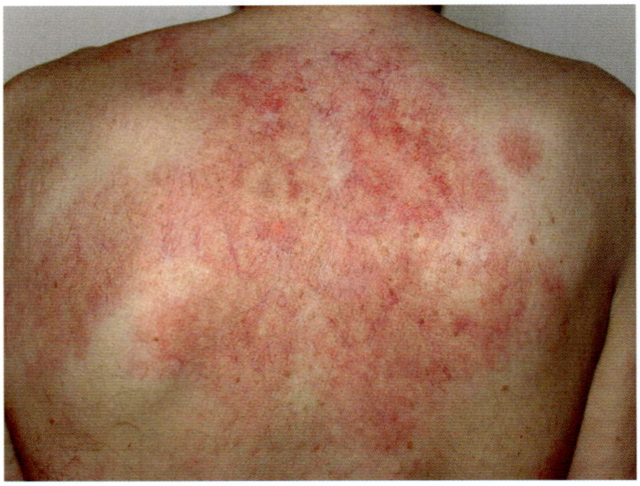

**Figure 19.1** Intravascular large B-cell lymphoma. Ill-defined, erythematous, infiltrated lesions with telangiectasia on the back. *(Courtesy of Dr. Fritz Breier, Vienna, Austria).*

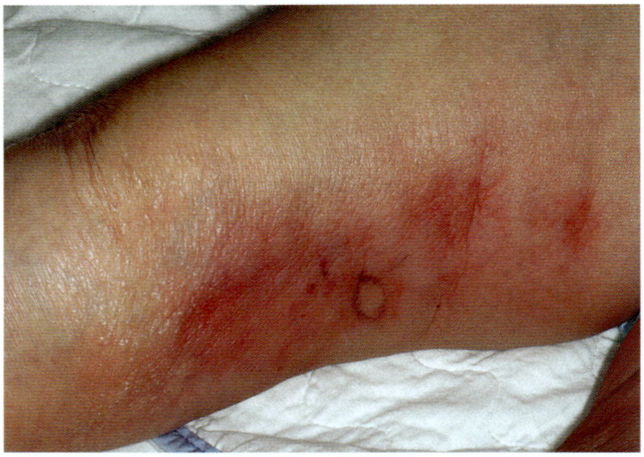

**Figure 19.2** Intravascular large B-cell lymphoma. Panniculitis-like lesion on the thigh. *(Courtesy of Prof. Robert Müllegger, Wiener Neustadt, Austria).*

## Intravascular large B-cell lymphoma

Intravascular large B-cell lymphoma is a malignant proliferation of large B lymphocytes confined within blood vessels. In rare cases, the skin may be the only affected site, though more often the lymphoma is disseminated with common involvement of the central nervous system. As already mentioned, cases of intravascular large B-cell lymphoma have been reported in patients with pre-existing cutaneous or, more often, nodal large B-cell lymphoma, representing recurrence of the original disease rather than a genuine intravascular large B-cell lymphoma [12, 13].

Intravascular large B-cell lymphoma should be distinguished from intralymphatic anaplastic large cell lymphoma (see Chapter 5). The differential diagnosis includes also reactive angioendotheliomatosis, a benign disorder due to an intravascular proliferation of endothelial cells, intralymphatic histiocytosis, a reactive condition characterized by presence of clusters of intralymphatic histiocytes [20], and the so-called benign intralymphatic proliferation of T-cell lymphoid blasts, a condition described rarely as an incidental finding in various skin diseases (see Chapter 31). Differential diagnosis among these entities is easily achieved by morphology and immunohistological stainings. Differentiation from intravascular large NK/T-cell lymphoma, too, is easily achieved by immunohistochemistry.

### Clinical features

Patients present with indurated, erythematous or violaceous, ill-defined patches and plaques, preferentially located on the trunk and thighs (Fig. 19.1). The clinical appearance is not typical of lymphoma and may sometimes suggest a diagnosis of panniculitis or purpura (Fig. 19.2) [21-25]. Telangiectasia is frequently found in affected areas (Fig. 19.3) [26], and generalized telangiectasia has been observed in one patient [27]. Neurologic symptoms as a sign of involvement of the central nervous system are commonly present [28a]. Other organs that are frequently involved are the liver and kidney.

A case of donor transmission of an intravascular large B-cell lymphoma to two recipients of kidney transplantation has been reported [28b], underlining the need for accurate pre-transplant screening.

Hemophagocytosis was reported in the majority of Asian patients [29, 30], but not in European ones [31-33]. It has been suggested that hemophagocytosis-associated cases represent a distinct variant of the disease with significantly different clinical features ("Asian" variant of intravascular large B-cell lymphoma), characterized by higher frequency of systemic symptoms (fever and fatigue) and hepatic, splenic, and bone marrow involvement, and lower frequency of neurologic and cutaneous involvement [31]. B symptoms, anemia, thrombocytopenia, hepatosplenomegaly, and bone marrow involvement are frequently observed in patients with associated hemophagocytic syndrome.

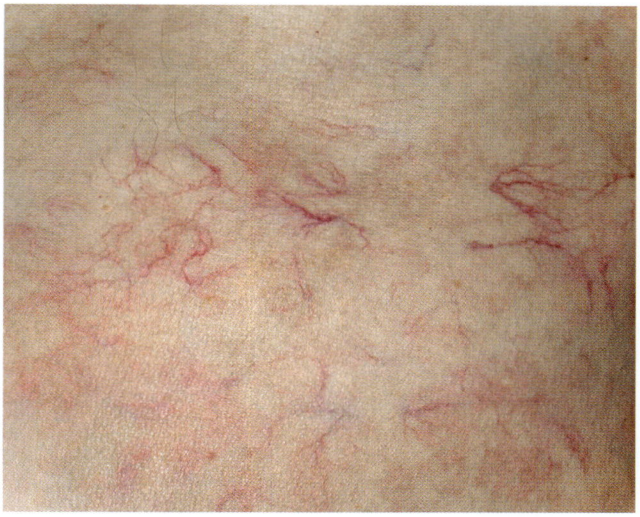

**Figure 19.3** Intravascular large B-cell lymphoma. Prominent, irregular telangiectatic vessels. *(Courtesy of Dr. Fritz Breier, Vienna, Austria).*

## Histopathology

Histology reveals a proliferation of large lymphocytes filling dilated blood vessels within the dermis and subcutaneous tissues, conveying at low power the impression of increased numbers of "thick" vessels within the dermis and sometimes the subcutaneous fat (Fig. 19.4a). A perivascular infiltrate of large atypical cells is not present as a rule (rare cases may present with isolated extravascular cells), and even perivascular reactive infiltrates are sparse or sometimes missing altogether. The malignant cells are large with scant cytoplasm and often with prominent nucleoli (immunoblasts) (Fig. 19.4b). In some cases, only a few neoplastic cells can be found within the vessels, representing a potential pitfall in the histopathological diagnosis (Fig. 19.5).

## Immunophenotype

Neoplastic cells are positive for B-cell-associated markers (CD19, CD20 and CD79a) (Fig. 19.6a), and in a subset of cases show the aberrant CD5 expression [34]. Positivity for Bcl-2 and multiple myeloma oncogene 1 (MUM-1) is observed in the vast majority of cases, highlighting the phenotypic similarities with other diffuse large B-cell lymphomas (Figs. 19.6b and c). Bcl-6 and CD10 are positive only in a small minority of cases, whereas cyclin D1 is consistently negative. The monoclonal expression of either κ or λ light chain can be demonstrated in the majority of cases on frozen sections of tissue, but detection is usually not possible on the routinely fixed material. Positivity for prostatic acid phosphatase has been reported in a small series [35]. MYC can be positive at the protein level. PD-L1 expression has been detected

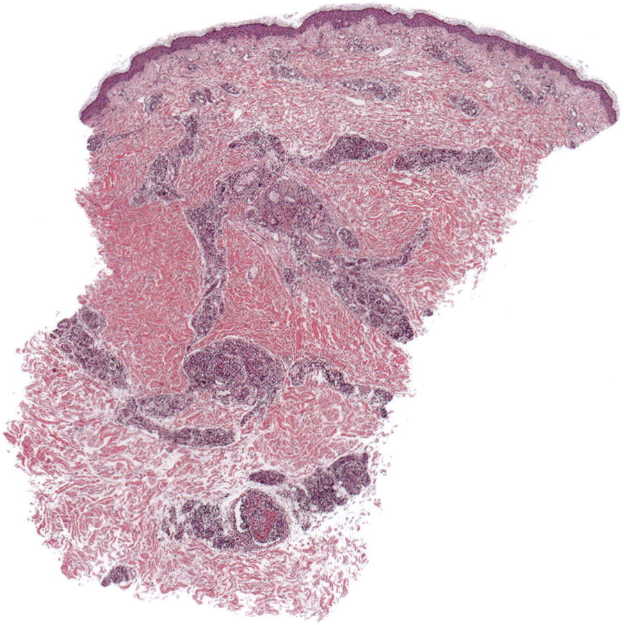

(a)

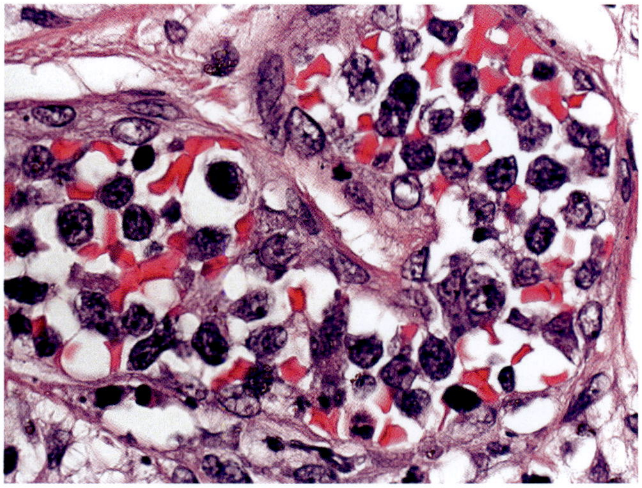

(b)

**Figure 19.4** Intravascular large B-cell lymphoma. (a) At low-power magnification, there is an increase in small vessels in the dermis with sparse perivascular reactive infiltrates. (b) Detail of large atypical cells within the vessels.

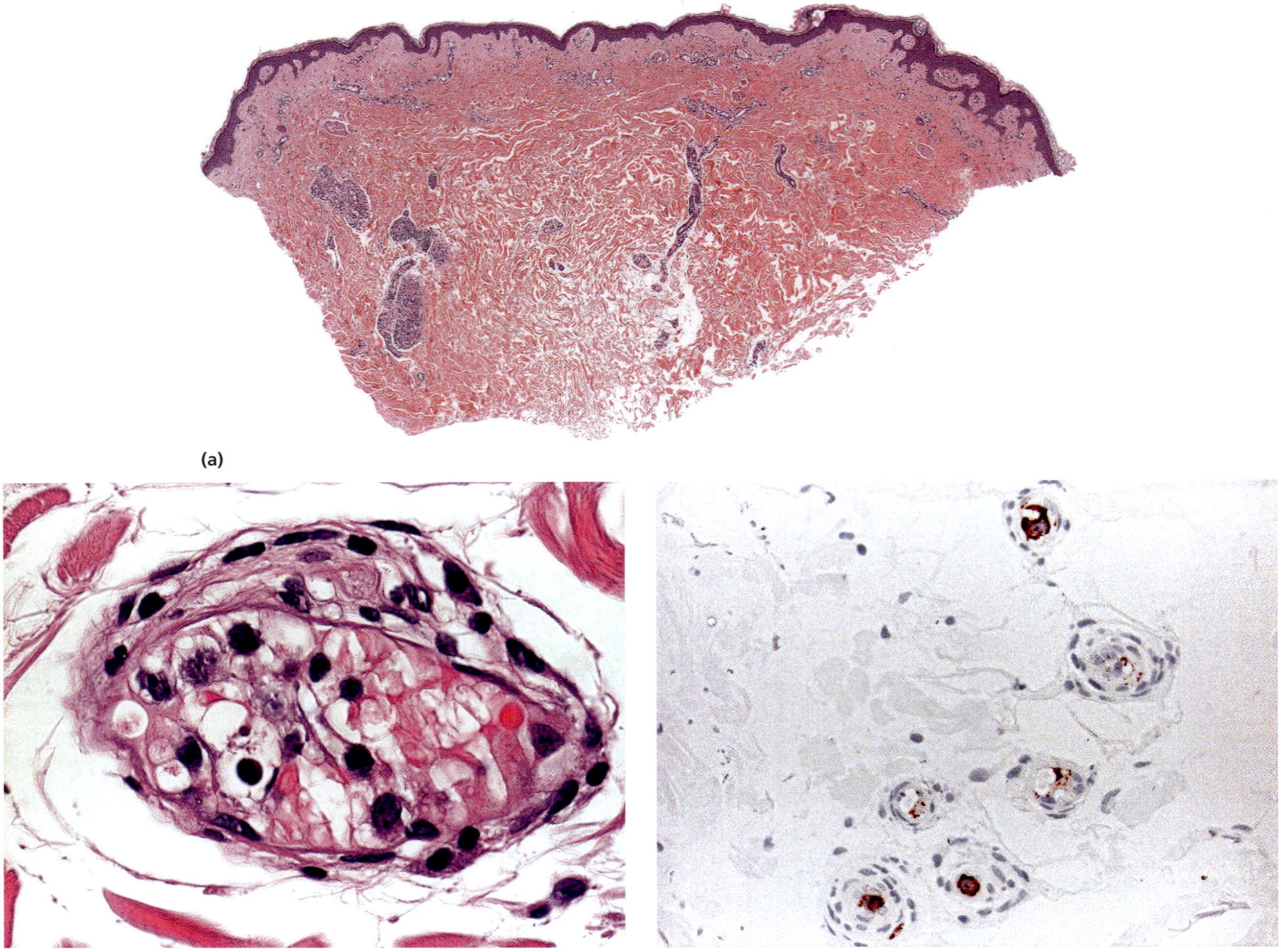

(a) (b) (c)

**Figure 19.5** Intravascular large B-cell lymphoma with minimal neoplastic infiltrate. (a) At low-power magnification, the pathological process is very difficult to identify. (b) Detail of few large atypical cells within the vessels. (c) Staining for CD20 shows that some of the vessels contain only isolated neoplastic cells.

in neoplastic cells in almost half of the cases, both in the "conventional" variant and in the variant associated with hemophagocytic syndrome, and was unrelated to CD5 positivity [36].

Staining with endothelial cell-related antibodies (i.e., CD31 and CD34) highlights the characteristic intravascular location of the cells (Fig. 19.6d), which are located in blood vessels (podoplanin-positive lymphatic vessels do not harbor neoplastic cells).

In situ hybridization for Epstein–Barr virus (EBV) was negative in a large study [29], but rare positive cases may be observed.

## Molecular genetics

The molecular analysis shows monoclonal rearrangement of the immunoglobulin genes. The high prevalence of *MYD88* and *CD79B* mutations are observed in intravascular large B-cell lymphoma [37], showing similarities to diffuse large B-cell lymphomas of nongerminal center cell origin [38]. Molecular studies revealed complex karyotypes abnormalities in cases of intravascular large B-cell lymphoma [39], involving particularly chromosome 1 (>70%) with almost one-third showing rearrangements of 1p13 or 1q21 [39, 40]. Aberrations in chromosomes 1 and 6 and trisomy of 18 have been reported in some patients [41]. A t(14;18) was observed in one case [42], but this translocation is usually not present in intravascular large B-cell lymphoma. The molecular features of intravascular large B-cell lymphoma suggest that constitutive NF-κB activation and immune evasion play a crucial role in the pathogenesis of the disease [43].

## Intravascular large B-cell lymphoma colonizing hemangiomas

Colonization of capillaries of cutaneous hemangiomas by neoplastic cells of intravascular large B-cell lymphoma has been observed in more cases than pure chance would justify, suggesting

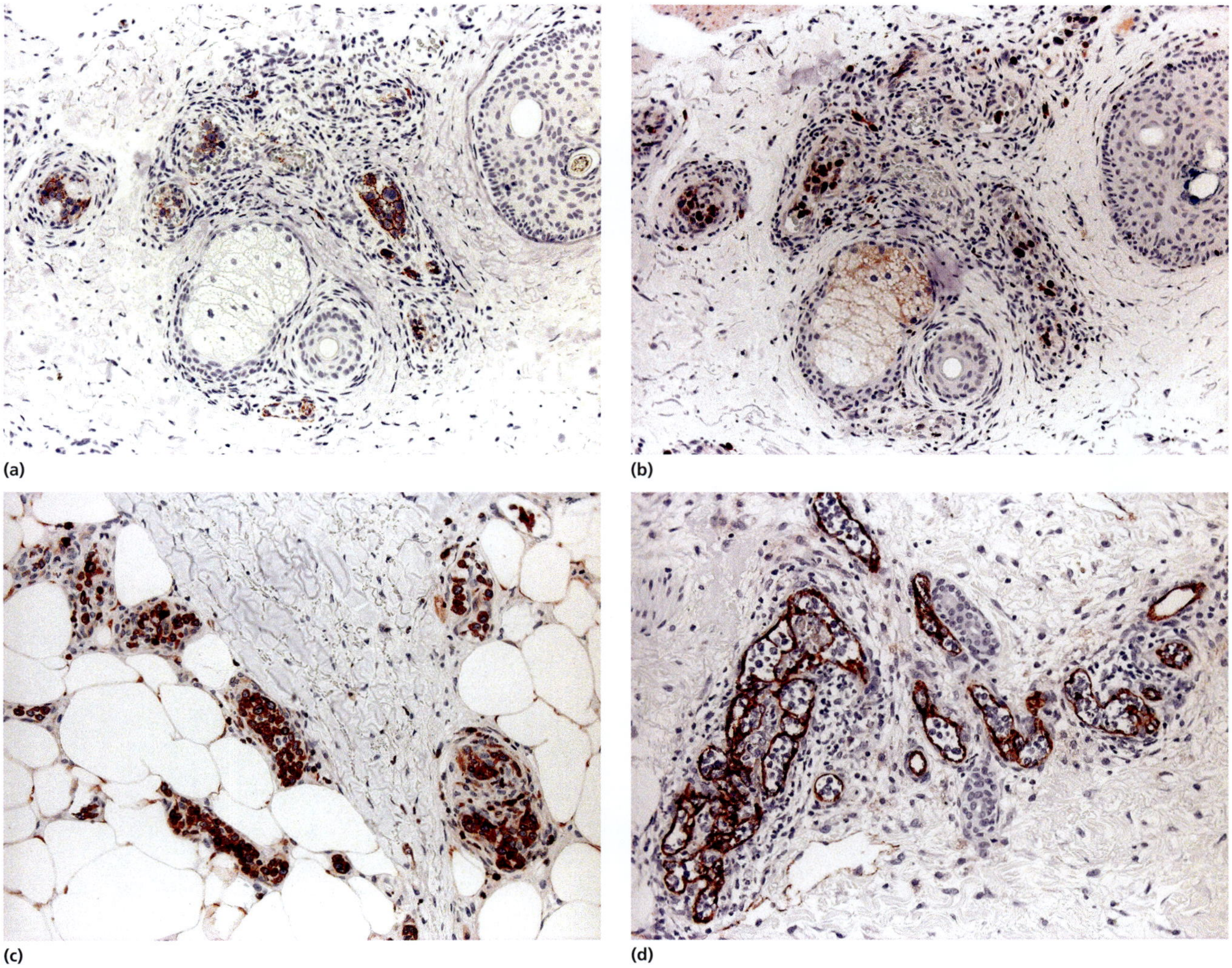

Figure 19.6 Intravascular large B-cell lymphoma. Neoplastic cells are positive for (a) CD20, (b) MUM-1, and (c) Bcl-2. (d) The intravascular arrangement of neoplastic cells is highlighted by the staining for CD31.

that these cells have a special tropism for neoplastic blood vessels [44-54]. Sometimes, this is the only manifestation of the lymphoma, and no other sites are involved [48-50], and biopsy of senile hemangiomas has been proposed as a better way to diagnose the disease than random skin biopsy [55-57]. We have observed a woman with intravascular large B-cell lymphoma confined to three out of six capillary hemangiomas that had been surgically removed, and with no other manifestations of the disease (Fig. 19.7) [49]. The three hemangiomas were located at different body sites, and several angiolipomas excised at the same time were completely negative. In a similar fashion, neoplastic cells have been detected in the vessels of Kaposi sarcoma and of other solid tumors [58]. This is probably one of the most intriguing features of this rare lymphoma, and investigation of such cases may provide some clues concerning the disease.

## Treatment

The treatment of choice of intravascular large B-cell lymphoma is anthracycline-based systemic chemotherapy associated with rituximab (R-CHOP) [30, 59-61]. It has also been suggested to add drugs with a higher bioavailability in the central nervous system, such as high-dose methotrexate or cytarabine [15, 62]. Autologous peripheral blood stem cell transplantation has been used in occasional patients with encouraging results [63], but data on large numbers of patients are lacking. Cases positive for PD-L1 expression might benefit from targeted immunotherapy.

Anti-CD19–directed autologous chimeric antigen receptor-modified T cells (CAR-T) are being used for relapsed or refractory large B-cell lymphomas [64], but there are no relevant data concerning intravascular large B-cell lymphoma.

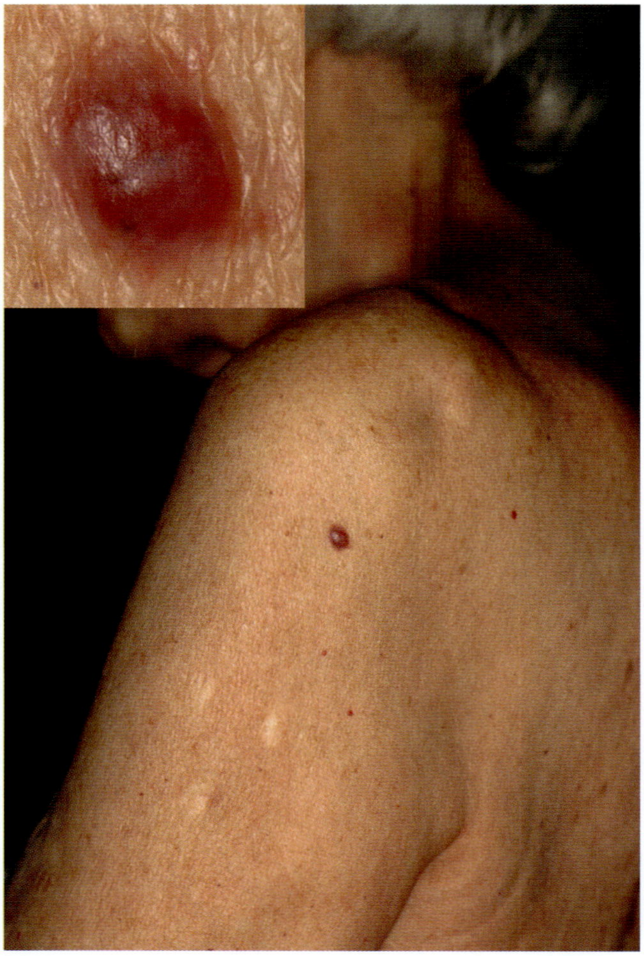

(a)

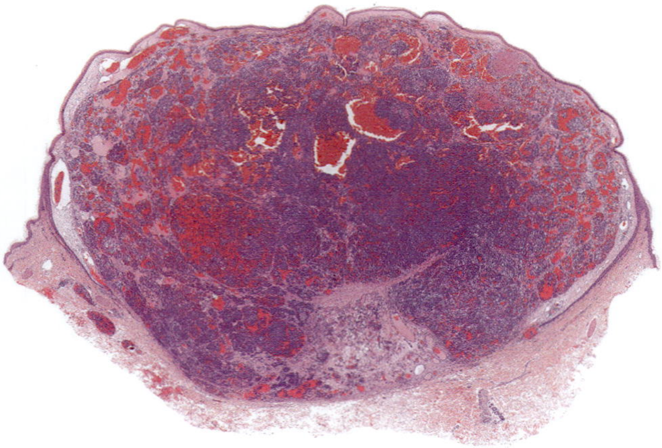

(b)

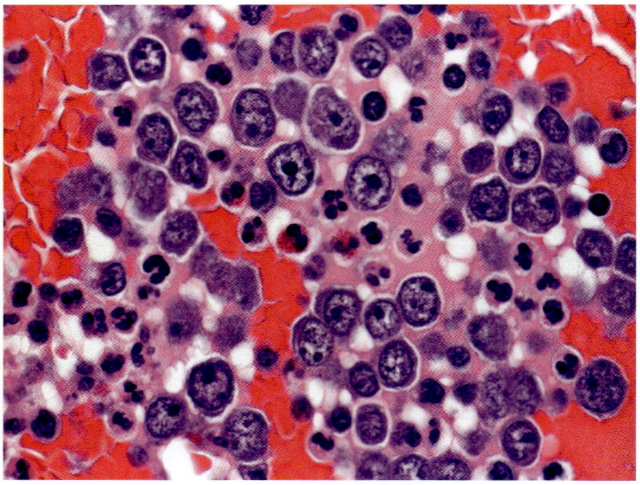

(c)

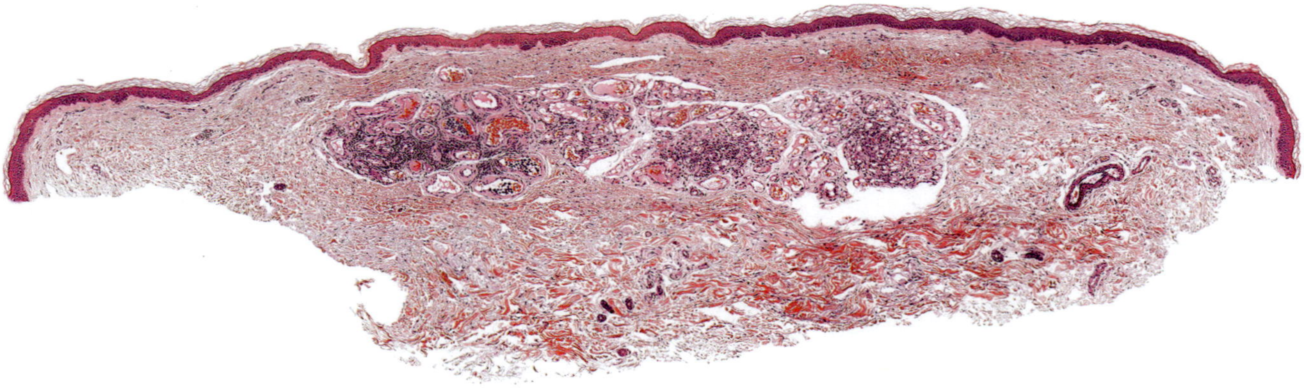

(d)

Figure 19.7 Intravascular large B-cell lymphoma colonizing the vessels of a cherry hemangioma. (a) Cherry hemangioma without distinctive clinical features on the left shoulder (detail of the lesion in the inset). (b) Histology shows, at low-power magnification, the features of a cherry hemangioma with vessels dilated by large clusters of neoplastic cells; (c) detail of large atypical cells admixed with neutrophils, some eosinophils, and erythrocytes; (d) low-power magnification of a second cherry hemangioma removed from the same patient, with less conspicuous involvement by intravascular large B-cell lymphoma; (e) high-power magnification shows large, atypical cells within some of the vessels. (f) Neoplastic cells in all affected hemangiomas were positive for CD20.

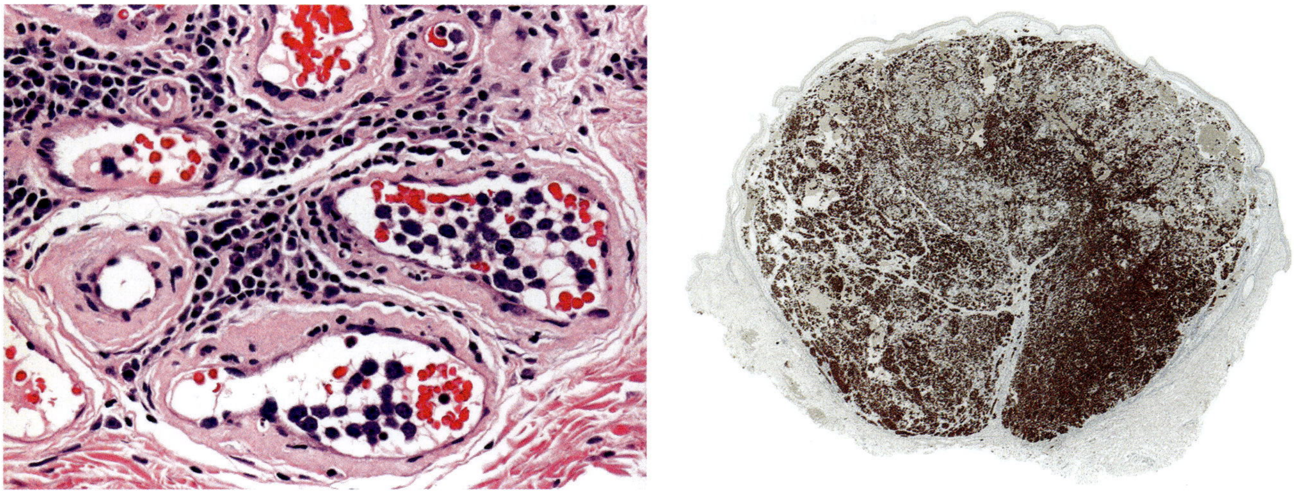

(e) (f)

**Figure 19.7** (Continued)

## Prognosis

The prognosis of cases limited to the skin seems to be better than that of the generalized (multisystem) disease [61, 65, 66]. The majority of deaths are directly due to the lymphoma; other most relevant causes of death are infections, cardiovascular disease, neurologic disease, and chronic obstructive pulmonary disease [67]. Unfavorable prognostic factors are lack of anthracycline-based chemotherapy, age older than 60 years, and thrombocytopenia <100 $\times 10^9$/L [29]. Positivity for CD5 does not influence the prognosis. The PD-L1 expression in neoplastic cells has been associated with a poorer prognosis in one study [68].

### Résumé

**Intravascular large B-cell lymphoma**

| | | |
|---|---|---|
| **Clinical** | Adults. Solitary or multiple indurated patches and plaques, sometimes resembling panniculitis or telangiectatic erythema. Preferential locations: trunk, thighs. Colonization of cherry hemangiomas reported in several patients. | |
| **Morphology** | Intravascular (blood vessels) proliferation of large atypical lymphoid cells. | |
| **Immunohistochemistry** | CD19, CD20, CD79a | + |
| | CD5 | +/– |
| | Bcl-2, MUM-1 | + |
| | Bcl-6, CD10 | –(+) |
| | CD29, CD54 | – |
| | PD-L1 | +/– |
| | $CD31^+$, $D2\text{-}40^-$ | (involved vessels) |
| **Genetics** | Monoclonal rearrangement of the Ig genes. High prevalence of *MYD88* and *CD79B* mutations. | |
| **Treatment guidelines** | Anthracycline-based systemic chemotherapy associated with rituximab (R-CHOP). High-dose methotrexate. | |

## Intravascular large NK/T-cell lymphoma

Rarely, cases of cutaneous intravascular large cell lymphoma may show a T-cell or NK-cell phenotype [69-87]. This is probably the rarest form of lymphoma (not only cutaneous), as few cases have been reported in the literature, and only in some of them have sufficient immunophenotypic studies been performed. Besides the phenotype, the most striking difference between intravascular large NK/T-cell lymphoma and intravascular large B-cell lymphoma seems to be the much more common association with EBV infection in the NK/T-cell variant [69, 70]. Intravascular large NK/T-cell lymphoma is not covered in the ICC *of Myeloid and Lymphoid Neoplasms* and in the WHO *Classification of Haematolymphoid Tumours*, (see the beginning of this chapter).

In the past, cases of intralymphatic CD30$^+$ anaplastic large cell lymphoma were included in this group, but there is sufficient evidence that they represent a completely different entity (see Chapter 5). In this context, however, it should be reminded that cases of genuine intravascular large NK/T-cell lymphoma may be rarely positive for CD30, thus representing a potential pitfall in the diagnosis. The two diseases can be easily distinguished by a simple staining for podoplanin: neoplastic cells in intralymphatic CD30$^+$ anaplastic large cell lymphoma are confined to podoplanin-positive lymphatic vessels, whereas cells of intravascular large NK/T-cell lymphoma are found within the podoplanin-negative blood vessels.

Patients are usually elderly adults though a congenital case (detected at autopsy and without skin involvement) has been reported [71]. The clinical presentation and histopathologic features are similar to those seen in the more common B-cell variant, but livid lesions are more common than telangiectasia (Fig. 19.8a). One case mimicked a panniculitis clinically [88]. Similarly to the B-cell variant, neoplastic cells of intravascular NK/T-cell lymphoma have been found in normal-looking skin [89]. Histopathologically, intravascular large NK/T-cell lymphoma is indistinguishable from the B-cell variant of the disease (Figs. 19.8b, c).

Neoplastic cells in intravascular large NK/T-cell lymphoma express CD2 and CD3, but are commonly negative for CD5 (Fig. 19.9a). Several studies demonstrated that the vast majority of cases have a cytotoxic NK/T phenotype (Fig. 19.9b) and are

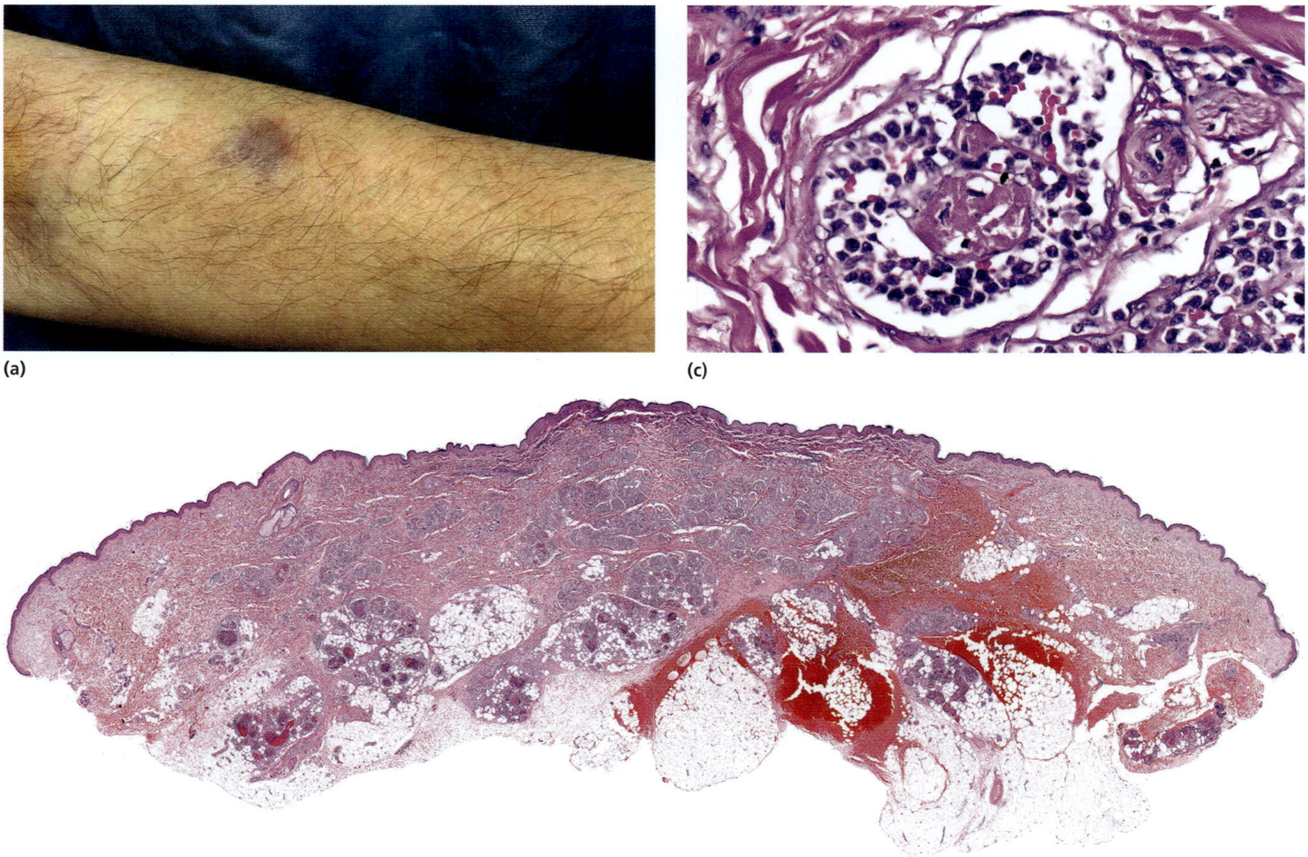

(a) (c) (b)

**Figure 19.8** Intravascular large NK/T-cell lymphoma. (a) Livid plaque on the lower arm *(Courtesy of Dr. Babak Itzlinger-Monshi, Vienna)*. (b) At scanning magnification there is a marked increase in small vessels in the dermis and subcutaneous fat. (c) Neoplastic lymphocytes fill the vessel; note a small fibrin thrombus.

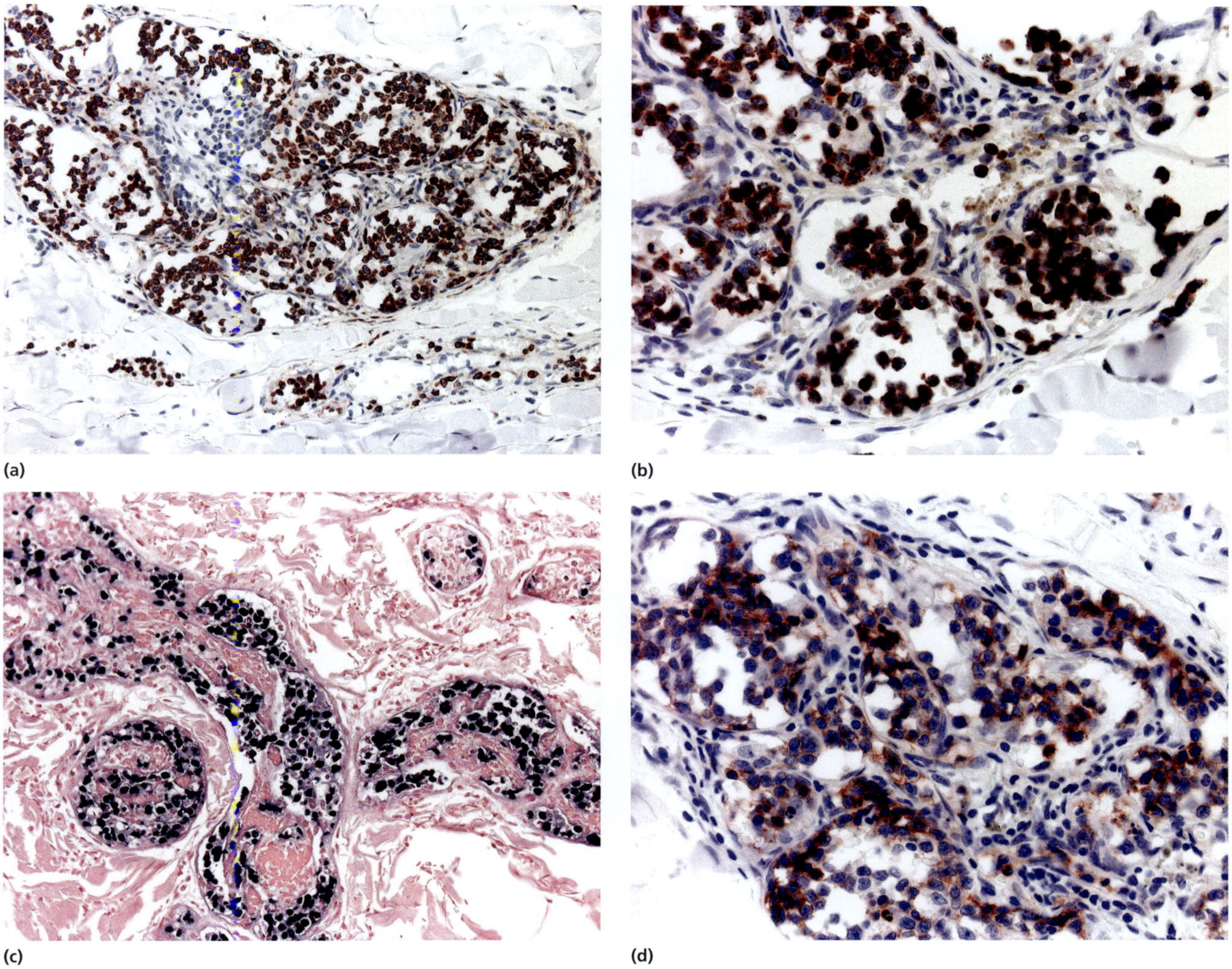

Figure 19.9 Intravascular large NK/T-cell lymphoma. Intravascular large lymphocytes are positive for (a) CD3 and (b) TIA-1. (c) Neoplastic cells also reveal a positive signal upon in situ hybridization for EBV (EBER-1) and (d) are positive for CD56.

associated with EBV (Fig. 19.9c), thus showing some similarities to extranodal NK/T-cell lymphoma, nasal type [69, 72, 73]. However, rarely cases are characterized by a T-helper or a CD30⁺ phenotype and EBV-negative cases are well documented; thus, it seems that intravascular large NK/T-cell lymphoma represents a relatively heterogeneous phenotypic entity [69, 90]. CD56 is expressed by neoplastic cells in the majority of cases (Fig. 19.9d), whereas βF1, a marker of α/β T lymphocytes, was negative in all cases tested [69, 72]. One case showed positivity for TCR-gamma [91], and one was negative for both βF1 and TCR-gamma [92]. In one case, intravascular large NK/T-cell lymphoma was associated with a specific infiltrate of B-CLL present in the same tissue sections as well as in the bone marrow (which was not colonized by cells of the intravascular NK/T-cell lymphoma) [69], representing a type of cutaneous composite lymphoma (see Chapter 28).

The molecular analysis of the T-cell receptor (TCR) genes rearrangement was conducted only in a few instances, revealing monoclonality in approximately one-third of cases (the negative cases possibly representing those with a genuine NK cell phenotype). Somatic mutations in some epigenetic regulators have been described in two cases [93].

Prognosis and treatment of intravascular large NK/T-cell lymphoma do not seem to differ from those of the B-cell type, but of course anti-CD20 antibodies do not have efficacy in the NK/T-cell variant. Data on treatment are available only for a handful of patients, and there are no clear-cut guidelines. The course is very aggressive. The prognosis seems to be better for patients with disease limited to one organ only, as compared to those with disease detected in two or more organs.

## Résumé

**Intravascular large NK/T-cell lymphoma**

| | | |
|---|---|---|
| **Clinical** | Very rare variant of intravascular large cell lymphoma. Adults. Solitary or multiple indurated patches and plaques; sometimes telangiectasia. | |
| **Morphology** | Intravascular proliferation of large atypical lymphoid cells. | |
| **Immunohistochemistry** | CD2, CD3 | + |
| | CD5 | − |
| | βF1 | − |
| | CD20, CD79a | − |
| | CD56 | +(−) |
| | TIA-1, granzyme B | + |
| | CD30 | −(+) (most positive cases represent examples of intralymphatic anaplastic large cell lymphoma) |
| | EBER-1 | +(−) |
| | $CD31^{+}$, $D2\text{-}40^{-}$ | (involved vessels) |
| **Genetics** | Monoclonal rearrangement of the TCR genes in approximately one-third of cases. | |
| **Treatment guidelines** | Systemic chemotherapy (value of anthracycline-based systemic chemotherapy not tested in cases with NK/T-cell phenotype). | |

## References


1. Nakamura S, Venkataraman G. Intravascular large B-cell lymphoma. In: Arber DA, Borowitz MJ, Cook JR, *et al*., eds. *The International Consensus Classification of Myeloid and Lymphoid Neoplasms*. Philadelphia, PA: Wolters Kluwer, 2025: 505–507.
2. De Jong D, Nagane M, Batchelor T, *et al*. Intravascular large B-cell lymphoma. In: *WHO Classification of Tumours Editorial Board. Haematolymphoid Tumours*. 5th edition. Lyon: IARC, 2024: 520–522.
3. Nakamura S, Ponzoni M, Campo E. Intravascular large B-cell lymphoma. In: Swerdlow SH, Campo E, Harris NL, *et al*., eds. *WHO Classification of Tumours of Haematopoietic and Lymphoid Tissues*. Revised 4th edition. Lyon, Cedex: IARC, 2017: 317–318.
4. Matsue K, Abe Y, Kitsdate A, *et al*. Sensitivity and specificity of incisional random skin biopsy for diagnosis of intravascular large B-cell lymphoma. *Blood* 2019;**133**:1257–1259.
5. Takigawa M, Yamasaki O, Nomura H, *et al*. Probability scoring system of intravascular large B-cell lymphoma for the application of random skin biopsy: a retrospective cohort study. *JAAD Int* 2022;**9**:146–152.
6. Enzan N, Kitadate A, Kono M. Optimizing random skin biopsies: a review of techniques and indications for intravascular large B-cell lymphoma. *Int J Hematol* 2024;**119**:619–625.
7. Obinwanne V, Falcone LM, Tung JK, James AJ. A diagnostic dilemma: the role of random skin biopsies to diagnose intravascular large B-cell lymphoma. *Int J Dermatol* 2024;**63**:1267–1268.
8. Matsue K, Abe Y, Narita K, *et al*. Diagnosis of intravascular large B-cell lymphoma: novel insights into clinicopathological features from 42 patients at a single institution over 20 years. *Br J Haematol* 2019;**187**:328–336.
9. Rozenbaum D, Tung J, Xue Y, Kroshinsky D. Skin biopsy in the diagnosis of intravascular lymphoma: a retrospective diagnostic accuracy study. *J Am Acad Dermatol* 2021;**85**:665–670.
10. Enzan N, Kitadate A, Tanaka A, Matsue K. Incisional random skin biopsy, not punch biopsy, is an appropriate method for diagnosis of intravascular large B-cell lymphoma: a clinicopathological study of 25 patients. *Br J Dermatol* 2019;**181**:200–201.
11. Sheibani K, Battifora H, Winberg CD, *et al*. Further evidence that "malignant angioendotheliomatosis" is an angiotropic large-cell lymphoma. *N Engl J Med* 1986;**314**:943–948.
12. Asagoe K, Fujimoto W, Yoshino T, *et al*. Intravascular lymphomatosis of the skin as a manifestation of recurrent B-cell lymphoma. *J Am Acad Dermatol* 2003;**48**:S1–S4.
13. Kamath NV, Gilliam AC, Nihal M, *et al*. Primary cutaneous large B-cell lymphoma of the leg relapsing as cutaneous intravascular large B-cell lymphoma. *Arch Dermatol* 2001; **137**:1637–1638.
14. Sukpanichnant S, Visuthisakchai S. Intravascular lymphomatosis: a study of 20 cases in Thailand and a review of the literature. *Clin Lymphoma Myeloma* 2006;**6**:319–328.
15. Ponzoni M, Ferreri AJM, Campo E, *et al*. Definition, diagnosis, and management of intravascular large B-cell lymphoma: proposals and perspectives from an international consensus meeting. *J Clin Oncol* 2007;**25**:3168–3173.
16. Ponzoni M, Arrigoni G, Gould VE, *et al*. Lack of CD29 (beta1 integrin) and CD54 (ICAM-1) adhesion molecules in intravascular lymphomatosis. *Hum Pathol* 2000;**31**:220–226.
17. Saurel CA, Personett DA, Edenfield BH, *et al*. Molecular analysis of intravascular large B-cell lymphoma with neoangiogenesis. *Br J Haematol* 2010;**152**:234–244.
18. Kato M, Ohshima K, Mizuno M, *et al*. Analysis of CXCL9 and CXCR3 expression in a case of intravascular large B-cell lymphoma. *J Am Acad Dermatol* 2009;**61**:889–891.
19. Brunet V, Marouan S, Routy JP, *et al*. Retrospective study of intravascular large B-cell lymphoma cases diagnosed in Quebec A retrospective study of 29 case reports. *Medicine* 2017;**96**(5):e5985.

20. Wick MR, Rocamora A. Reactive and malignant "angioendotheliomatosis:" a discriminant clinicopathological study. *J Cutan Pathol* 1988;**15**:260–271.
21. Chang A, Zic JA, Boyd AS. Intravascular large cell lymphoma: a patient with asymptomatic purpuric patches and a chronic clinical course. *J Am Acad Dermatol* 1998;**39**:318–321.
22. Di Giuseppe JA, Nelson WG, Seifter EJ, *et al.* Intravascular lymphomatosis: a clinicopathologic study of 10 cases and assessment of response to chemotherapy. *J Clin Oncol* 1994;**12**:2573–2579.
23. Kiyohara T, Kumakiri M, Kobayashi H, *et al.* A case of intravascular large B-cell lymphoma mimicking erythema nodosum: the importance of multiple skin biopsies. *J Cutan Pathol* 2000;**27**:413–418.
24. Stroup RM, Sheibani K, Moncada A, *et al.* Angiotropic (intravascular) lymphoma: a clinicopathologic study of seven cases with unique clinical presentations. *Cancer* 1990;**66**:1781–1788.
25. Yegappan S, Coupland R, Arber DA, *et al.* Angiotropic lymphoma: an immunophenotypically and clinically heterogeneous lymphoma. *Mod Pathol* 2001;**14**:1147–1156.
26. Feldmann R, Schierl M, Sittenthaler M, *et al.* Intravascular large B-cell lymphoma of the skin: typical clinical manifestations and a favourable response to rituximab-containing therapy. *Dermatology* 2009;**219**:344–346.
27. Özgüroglu E, Büyülbabani N, Ögzüroglu M, Baykal C. Generalized telangiectasia as the major manifestation of angiotropic (intravascular) lymphoma. *Br J Dermatol* 1997;**137**:422–425.
28. (a)Glass J, Hochberg FH, Miller DC. Intravascular lymphomatosis: a systemic disease with neurologic manifestations. *Cancer* 1993; **71**:3156–3164.(b) Fernandes BP, Pimenta AC, Henriques A, *et al.* Donor transmission of an intravascular large B-Cell lymphoma in multiorgan transplantation: A case report from a rare pitfall in the predonation screening for donor disease. *Transplant Proc* 2025.
29. Murase T, Yamaguchi M, Suzuki R, *et al.* Intravascular large B-cell lymphoma (IVLBCL): a clinicopathologic study of 96 cases with special reference to the immunophenotypic heterogeneity of CD5. *Blood* 2007;**109**:478–485.
30. Shimada K, Kinoshita T, Nace T, *et al.* Presentation and management of intravascular large B-cell lymphoma. *Lancet Oncol* 2009;**10**:895–902.
31. Ferreri AJM, Dognini GP, Campo E, *et al.* Variations in clinical presentation, frequency of hemophagocytosis and clinical behavior of intravascular lymphoma diagnosed in different geographical regions. *Haematologica* 2007;**92**:486–492.
32. Nakamura S, Murase T, Kinoshita T. Intravascular large B-cell lymphoma: the heterogeneous clinical manifestations of its classical and hemophagocytosis-related forms. *Haematologica* 2007;**92**:434–436.
33. Terrier B, Aouba A, Vasiliu V, *et al.* Intravascular lymphoma associated with haemophagocytic syndrome: a very rare entity in Western countries. *Eur J Haematol* 2005;**75**:341–345.
34. Khalidi HS, Brynes RK, Browne P, *et al.* Intravascular large B-cell lymphoma: the CD5 antigen is expressed by a subset of cases. *Mod Pathol* 1998;**11**:983–988.
35. Seki K, Miyakoshi S, Lee GH, *et al.* Prostatic acid phosphatase is a possible tumor marker for intravascular large B-cell lymphoma. *Am J Surg Pathol* 2004;**28**:1384–1388.
36. Gupta GK, Jaffe ES, Pittaluga S. A study of PD-L1 expression in intravascular large B cell lymphoma: correlation with clinical and pathological features. *Histopathology* 2019;**75**:282–286.
37. Schrader AMR, Jansen PM, Willemze R, *et al.* High prevalence of MYD88 and CD79B mutations in intravascular large B-cell lymphoma. *Blood* 2018;**131**:2086–2089.
38. Bauer WM, Aichelburg MC, Griss J, *et al.* Molecular classification of tumour cells in a patient with intravascular large B-cell lymphoma. *Br J Dermatol* 2018;**178**:215–221.
39. Khoury H, Lestou VS, Gascoyne RD, *et al.* Multicolor karyotyping and clinicopathologic analysis of three intravascular lymphoma cases. *Mod Pathol* 2003;**16**:716–724.
40. Klairmont MM, Cheng J, Martin MG, *et al.* Recurrent cytogenetic abnormalities in intravascular large B-cell lymphoma. *Am J Clin Pathol* 2018;**150**:18–26.
41. Tsukadaira A, Okubo Y, Ogasawara H, *et al.* Chromosomal aberrations in intravascular lymphomatosis. *Am J Clin Oncol* 2002;**25**:178–181.
42. Vieites B, Fraga M, Lopez-Presas E, *et al.* Detection of t(14;18) translocation in a case of intravascular large B-cell lymphoma: a germinal centre cell origin in a subset of these lymphomas? *Histopathology* 2005;**46**:466–468.
43. Gonzalez-Farre B, Ramis-Zaldivar JE, Castrejón de Anta N, *et al.* Intravascular large B-cell lymphoma genomic profile is characterized by alterations in genes regulating NF-κB and immune checkpoints. *Am J Surg Pathol* 2023;**47**:202–211.
44. Kobayashi T, Munakata S, Sugiura H, *et al.* Angiotropic lymphoma: proliferation of B cells in the capillaries of cutaneous angiomas. *Br J Dermatol* 2000;**143**:162–164.
45. Rubin MA, Cossman J, Freter CE, Azumi N. Intravascular large cell lymphoma coexisting within hemangiomas of the skin. *Am J Surg Pathol* 1997;**21**:860–864.
46. Nixon BK, Kussick SJ, Carlon MJ, Rubin BP. Intravascular large B-cell lymphoma involving hemangiomas: an unusual presentation of a rare neoplasm. *Mod Pathol* 2005;**18**:1121–1126.
47. Ishida M, Hotta M, Hodohara K, *et al.* A case of intravascular large B-cell lymphoma colonizing in senile hemangioma. *J Cutan Pathol* 2011;**38**:251–253.
48. Satoh S, Yamazaki M, Yahikozawa H, *et al.* Intravascular large B cell lymphoma diagnosed by senile angioma biopsy. *Intern Med* 2003;**42**:117–120.
49. Cerroni L, Zalaudek I, Kerl H. Intravascular large B-cell lymphoma colonizing cutaneous hemangiomas. *Dermatology* 2004;**209**:132–134.
50. Cerroni L. Hemangiomas with (bad) surprise. *Dermatology* 2004;**209**:79–80.
51. Krokowski M, Sellmann L, Feller AC. Intravascular large B-cell lymphoma within a subcutaneous cavernous haemangioma. *Br J Haematol* 2010;**151**:2.
52. Nakamura Y, Nakamagoe K, Kawachi Y, *et al.* Intravascular large B cell lymphoma with neurological symptoms diagnosed on the basis of a senile angioma-like eruption. *BMJ Case Rep* 2009;**2009**. doi: 10.1136/bcr.11.2008.1297.
53. Weingarten M, Weingarten M, Sidhu H, Sidhu JS. A poisoned cherry: migratory cutaneous intravascular large B-cell lymphoma with subsequent systemic nodal lymphoma. *JAAD Case Rep* 2020;**6**:1336–1338.
54. García de Sola-Llamas C, Pérez-Pérez M, Morrillo M, Ríos-Martín JJ. Intravascular large B-cell lymphoma with exclusively cutaneous involvement, colonizing pre-existing hemangiomas: a rare case with aberrant HMB45 expression. *Am J Dermatopathol* 2025; **47**:e43–e46.

55. Sakurai T, Wakida K, Takahashi T, *et al*. Usefulness of senile hemangioma biopsy for diagnosis of intravascular large B-cell lymphoma: a report of two cases and a literature review. *J Neurol Sci* 2017;**373**:52–54.
56. Ishida M, Hodohara K, Yoshida T, *et al*. Intravascular large B-cell lymphoma colonizing in senile hemangioma: a case report and proposal of possible diagnostic strategy for intravascular lymphoma. *Pathol Int* 2011;**61**:555–557.
57. Adachi Y, Kosami K, Mizuta N, *et al*. Benefits of skin biopsy of senile hemangioma in intravascular large B-cell lymphoma: a case report and review of the literature. *Oncol Lett* 2014;**7**:2003–2006.
58. Ashman D, Pantanowitz L. Kaposi sarcoma with coexisting intravascular lymphoma. *Int J Surg Pathol* 2019;**27**:62–63.
59. Ferreri AJM, Dognini GP, Bairey O, *et al*. The addition of rituximab to anthracycline-based chemotherapy significantly improves outcome in "Western" patients with intravascular large B-cell lymphoma. *Br J Haematol* 2008;**143**:253–257.
60. Fonkem E, Lok E, Robison D, *et al*. The natural history of intravascular lymphomatosis. *Cancer Med* 2014;**3**:1010–1024.
61. Ponzoni M, Campo E, Nakamura S. Intravascular large B-cell lymphoma: a chameleon with multiple faces and many masks. *Blood* 2018;**132**:1561–1567.
62. Kebir S, Kuchelmeister K, Niehusmann P, *et al*. Intravascular CNS lymphoma: successful therapy using high-dose methotrexate-based polychemotherapy. *Exp Hematol Oncol* 2012;**1**:37.
63. Koizumi M, Nishimura M, Yokota A, *et al*. Successful treatment of intravascular malignant lymphomatosis with high-dose chemotherapy and autologous peripheral blood stem cell transplantation. *Bone Marrow Transplant* 2001;**27**:1101–1103.
64. Ghobadi A, Munoz J, Westin JR, *et al*. Outcomes of subsequent anti-lymphoma therapies after second-line axicabtagene ciloleucel or standard of care in ZUMA-7. *Blood Adv* 2024;**8**:2982–2990.
65. Ferreri AJM, Campo E, Seymour JF, *et al*. Intravascular lymphoma: clinical presentation, natural history, management and prognostic factors in a series of 38 cases, with special emphasis on the 'cutaneous variant'. *Br J Haematol* 2004;**127**:173–183.
66. Kong YY, Dai B, Sheng WQ, *et al*. Intravascular large B-cell lymphoma with cutaneous manifestations: a clinicopathologic, immunophenotypic and molecular study of three cases. *J Cutan Pathol* 2009;**36**:865–870.
67. Goyal A, Goyal K, Bohjanen K. Mortality in intravascular large B-cell lymphoma: a SEER analysis. *J Am Acad Dermatol* 2018;**79**:1163–1165.
68. Suzuki Y, Kohno K, Matsue K, *et al*. PD-L1 (SP142) expression in neoplastic cells predicts a poor prognosis for patients with intravascular large B-cell lymphoma treated with rituximab-based multi-agent chemotherapy. *Cancer Med* 2020;**9**:4768–4776.
69. Cerroni L, Massone C, Kutzner H, *et al*. Intravascular large T-cell or NK-cell lymphoma. A rare variant of intravascular large cell lymphoma with frequent cytotoxic phenotype and association with Epstein–Barr virus infection. *Am J Surg Pathol* 2008;**32**:891–898.
70. Nakamichi N, Fukuhara S, Aozasa K, Morii E. NK-cell intravascular lymphomatosis–a mini-review. *Eur J Haematol* 2008;**81**:1–7.
71. Tateyama H, Eimoto T, Tada T, *et al*. Congenital angiotropic lymphoma (intravascular lymphomatosis) of the T-cell type. *Cancer* 1991;**67**:2131–2136.
72. Au WY, Shek WH, Nicholls J, *et al*. T-cell intravascular lymphomatosis (angiotropic large cell lymphoma): association with Epstein–Barr viral infection. *Histopathology* 1997;**31**:563–567.
73. Gleason BC, Brinster NK, Granter SR, *et al*. Intravascular cytotoxic T-cell lymphoma: a case report and review of the literature. *J Am Acad Dermatol* 2008;**58**:290–294.
74. Santucci M, Pimpinelli N, Massi D, *et al*. Cytotoxic/natural killer cell cutaneous lymphomas. Report of the EORTC Cutaneous Lymphoma Task Force Workshop. *Cancer* 2003;**97**:610–627.
75. Kaluza V, Rao DS, Said JW, *et al*. Primary extranodal nasal-type natural killer/T-cell lymphoma of the brain: a case report. *Hum Pathol* 2006;**37**:769–772.
76. Kuo TT, Chen MJ, Kuo M. Cutaneous intravascular NK-cell lymphoma: report of a rare variant associated with Epstein–Barr virus. *Am J Surg Pathol* 2006;**30**:1197–1201.
77. Merchant SH, Viswanatha DS, Zumwalt RE, *et al*. Epstein–Barr virus-associated intravascular large T-cell lymphoma presenting as acute renal failure in a patient with acquired immune deficiency syndrome. *Hum Pathol* 2003;**34**:950–954.
78. Song DE, Lee MW, Ryu MH, *et al*. Intravascular large cell lymphoma of the natural killer cell type. *J Clin Oncol* 2007;**25**: 1279–1282.
79. Takahashi E, Kajimoto K, Fukatsu T, *et al*. Intravascular large T-cell lymphoma: a case report of CD30-positive and ALK-negative anaplastic type with cytotoxic molecule expression. *Virchows Arch* 2005;**447**:1000–1006.
80. Wu H, Said JW, Ames ED, *et al*. First reported cases of intravascular large cell lymphoma of the NK cell type. Clinical, histologic, immunophenotypic, and molecular features. *Am J Clin Pathol* 2005;**123**:603–611.
81. Liu Y, Zhang W, An J, *et al*. Cutaneous intravascular natural killer-cell lymphoma: a case report and review of the literature. *Am J Clin Pathol* 2014;**142**:243–247.
82. Sharma TL, Yeaney GA, Soltanzadeh P, *et al*. Intravascular T-cell lymphoma: a rare, poorly characterized entity with cytotoxic phenotype. *Neuropathology* 2017;**37**:365–370.
83. Okonkwo L, Jaffe ES. Intravascular large cell lymphoma of NK/T-cell type, EBV positive. *Blood* 2017;**130**:837.
84. Wang L, Chen S, Ma H, *et al*. Intravascular NK/T-cell lymphoma: a report of five cases with cutaneous manifestation from China. *J Cutan Pathol* 2015;**42**:610–617.
85. Bi Y, Huo Z, liang Z, *et al*. Intravascular NK-cell lymphoma: a case report and review of the literature. *Diagn Pathol* 2015;**10**:84.
86. Jang YH, Lee SJ, Choi YH, *et al*. Intravascular cytotoxic T-cell lymphoma in a young immunocompetent woman. *Ann Dermatol* 2014;**26**:496–500.
87. Zanelli M, Mengoli MC, Del Sordo R, *et al*. Intravascular NK/T-cell lymphoma, Epstein–Barr virus positive with multiorgan involvement: a clinical dilemma. *BMC Cancer* 2018;**18**:1115.
88. Alhumidi A. Cutaneous Intravascular NK/T-cell lymphoma mimic panniculitis clinically, case report and literature brief review. *Diagn Pathol* 2015;**10**:107.
89. Obara K, Amoh Y. Case of extranodal natural killer/T-cell lymphoma, nasal type, presenting with intravascular localization of tumor cells in skin biopsies from both plaque and normal-appearing

skin: a case report and literature review. *Am J Dermatopathol* 2020;**42**:196–203.
90. Melchers RC, Willemze R, Jansen PM, *et al.* A rare case of cutaneous Epstein–Barr virus-negative intravascular cytotoxic T-cell lymphoma. *JAAD Case Rep* 2019;**5**:548–551.
91. Martinez-Escala ME, Guggina LM, Cotliar J, *et al.* Cutaneous involvement in a case of intravascular T-cell lymphoma with a gamma/delta phenotype. *Am J Dermatopathol* 2016;**38**:e27–e29.
92. Alegría-Landa V, Manzarbeitia F, Salvatierra Calderón MG, *et al.* Cutaneous intravascular natural killer/T cell lymphoma with peculiar immunophenotype. *Histopathology* 2017;**71**:994–1002.
93. Fujikura K, Yamashita D, Sakamoto R, *et al.* Intravascular NK/T-cell lymphoma: clinicopathological and integrated molecular analysis of two cases provides a clue to disease pathogenesis. *J Clin Pathol* 2019;**72**:642–646.

CHAPTER 20

# Other cutaneous B-cell lymphomas

Besides the lymphoma entities discussed in previous chapters, there are a few reports on other types of B-cell lymphoma arising primary in the skin. In addition, most malignant B-cell lymphomas observed at extracutaneous sites may secondarily involve the skin, especially in the advanced stages. It has been suggested that cases of extracutaneous B-cell lymphoma that spread to the skin within 6 months from first diagnosis have a worse prognosis than those showing cutaneous involvement six or more months after the first diagnosis [1]. In some cases, histopathological features may be deceptive, and epidermotropism may be observed [2].

The clinicopathologic features of skin manifestations of the most important B-cell lymphomas, other than those discussed in the previous Chapters, are summarized in the following sections.

## Cutaneous manifestations of Epstein–Barr virus (EBV)-positive diffuse large B-cell lymphoma

$EBV^+$ diffuse large B-cell lymphoma (formerly referred to as $EBV^+$ diffuse large B-cell lymphoma of the elderly) is a distinct entity in the World Health Organization (WHO) *Classification of Haematolymphoid Tumours* [3] and is included as $EBV^+$ diffuse large B-cell lymphoma, not otherwise specified (NOS), in the International Consensus Classification (ICC) [4]. This entity is defined as an EBV-associated diffuse large B-cell lymphoma occurring in patients without any known immunodeficiency and without features of other $EBV^+$ lymphoproliferative disorders or lymphomas [3–6]. In fact, in immunocompetent patients the diagnosis of $EBV^+$ diffuse large B-cell lymphoma in the lymph nodes can be accepted only if specific categories of $EBV^+$ diffuse large B-cell lymphoma, including lymphomatoid granulomatosis and diffuse large B-cell lymphoma arising in the setting of chronic inflammation, have been ruled out. Although originally described in elderly patients, all ages can be affected, and younger patients seem to have a better prognosis [7, 8]. The disease seems to be more common in Asian countries and in Mexico and is relatively rare in Western populations [9–13]. The number of neoplastic cells positive on in situ hybridization for EBV (EBER-1) necessary to make a diagnosis of $EBV^+$ diffuse large B-cell lymphoma varied from ≥20% to nearly all cells in different publications, with the most recent version of the WHO classification mentioning among essential criteria positivity of "the majority" of neoplastic cells (to my eyes a definition that leaves room for arbitrary decisions as well, as variable numbers of non-neoplastic lymphocytes are admixed with the neoplastic ones) [3]. The International Consensus Classification includes a minimal percentage of 80% $EBV^+$ neoplastic cells as a requisite for the diagnosis [4]. As several reactive cells are usually present within the infiltrate, though, particularly in the skin, it may be difficult to decide whether the positivity reaches the diagnostic mark.

In the context of the discussion concerning $EBV^+$ diffuse large B-cell lymphoma, it should be remembered that several lymphoproliferative disorders are associated with EBV infection, including benign and malignant proliferations with natural killer (NK)-, T-, or B-cell phenotypes such as classical Hodgkin lymphoma, lymphomatoid granulomatosis, primary effusion lymphoma, plasmablastic lymphoma, Burkitt lymphoma, some types of NK/T-cell lymphoma, EBV-positive mucocutaneous ulcers, hydroa vacciniforme lymphoproliferative disorders, and post-transplant lymphoproliferative disorders, among others. Distinction among these groups may be very difficult, and some of the $EBV^+$ entities represent a spectrum from reactive hyperplasia to lymphoma. These cases can be classified properly only when the presence of EBV is considered within the general context. For example, hydroa vacciniforme-like lymphoma ("systemic hydroa vacciniforme lymphoproliferative disorder") may show overlapping histopathologic and phenotypic features with other cytotoxic NK/T-cell lymphomas, but the constellation of clinical findings, the racial background, and the peculiar clinical aspects allow a precise categorization. In the same way, cutaneous B-cell infiltrates associated with EBV may be classified precisely only upon correlation with the clinical features and with data concerning the presence or absence of immune suppression.

$EBV^+$ diffuse large B-cell lymphoma is probably linked in most cases to aging and decreased competence of the immune system ("immunosenescence"). In this context, there are arguments for its inclusion among the lymphoproliferative disorders

*Skin Lymphoma: The Illustrated Guide*, Sixth Edition. Lorenzo Cerroni.

and lymphomas arising in the setting of immune deficiency and dysregulation (see Chapter 21), but it is still considered as a specific entity in actual classification schemes. It represents a post-germinal center B-cell neoplasm characterized by activation of the JAK/STAT and NF-κB pathways [3, 14].

## Clinical features

EBV⁺ diffuse large B-cell lymphoma mostly arises in the lymph nodes, but the skin may be affected, usually showing localized or generalized infiltrated plaques and tumors [15]. Lesions are usually not ulcerated. Cutaneous involvement is observed more commonly in Asian patients than in Western patients [11, 16]. Some patients may present with a solitary tumor on the leg, prompting the differential diagnosis with diffuse large B-cell lymphoma, leg type [17, 18].

## Histopathology, immunophenotype, and molecular genetics

The histopathologic pattern may be polymorphous or monomorphic. Polymorphic cases show a mixed infiltrate with the presence of large cells resembling Hodgkin and Reed–Sternberg cells as well as centroblasts, immunoblasts, and plasmablasts, admixed with a variable number of reactive cells including small lymphocytes, plasma cells, and histiocytes. Monomorphic cases are characterized by a predominance of large, rounded B-cells (immunoblasts), sometimes showing features of plasmablasts, revealing the picture of a diffuse large B-cell lymphoma (Fig. 20.1) [15, 16]. Both variants are positive for EBV. Necrosis is common in affected lymph nodes, but less so in skin lesions.

In contrast to conventional diffuse large B-cell lymphoma, leg-type, cases of EBV⁺ diffuse large B-cell lymphoma may show loss of CD20 expression, but retain CD79a and PAX-5 positivity (Figs. 20.2a and b). CD30 is positive on neoplastic cells in the majority of cases, as well as multiple myeloma oncogene-1 (MUM-1), PD-1, and PD-L1 (Figs. 20.3a and b). Detection of EBV by in situ hybridization is a prerequisite for the diagnosis (Fig. 20.4). As already mentioned, positivity of 80% of neoplastic cells is required for the diagnosis ("the majority" in the WHO classification).

EBV⁺ diffuse large B-cell lymphoma is characterized by prominent activation of the JAK/STAT and NF-κB pathways [3, 14]. Immunoglobulin (Ig) genes are usually monoclonally rearranged. Cytogenetic complexity is low, and it has been suggested that for lymphomagenesis, the EBV oncogenic properties are sufficient in the context of immunosenescence [14]. Although both EBV⁺ diffuse large B-cell lymphoma and diffuse large B-cell lymphoma have the signature of activated B lymphocytes, some genes are differentially expressed in EBV⁺ diffuse large B-cell lymphoma [13], and relatively frequent mutations in *ARID1A*, *KMT2A/KMT2D*, *ANKRD11*, or *NOTCH2* distinguish nodal EBV⁺ diffuse large B-cell lymphoma from EBV-negative diffuse large B-cell lymphomas [19].

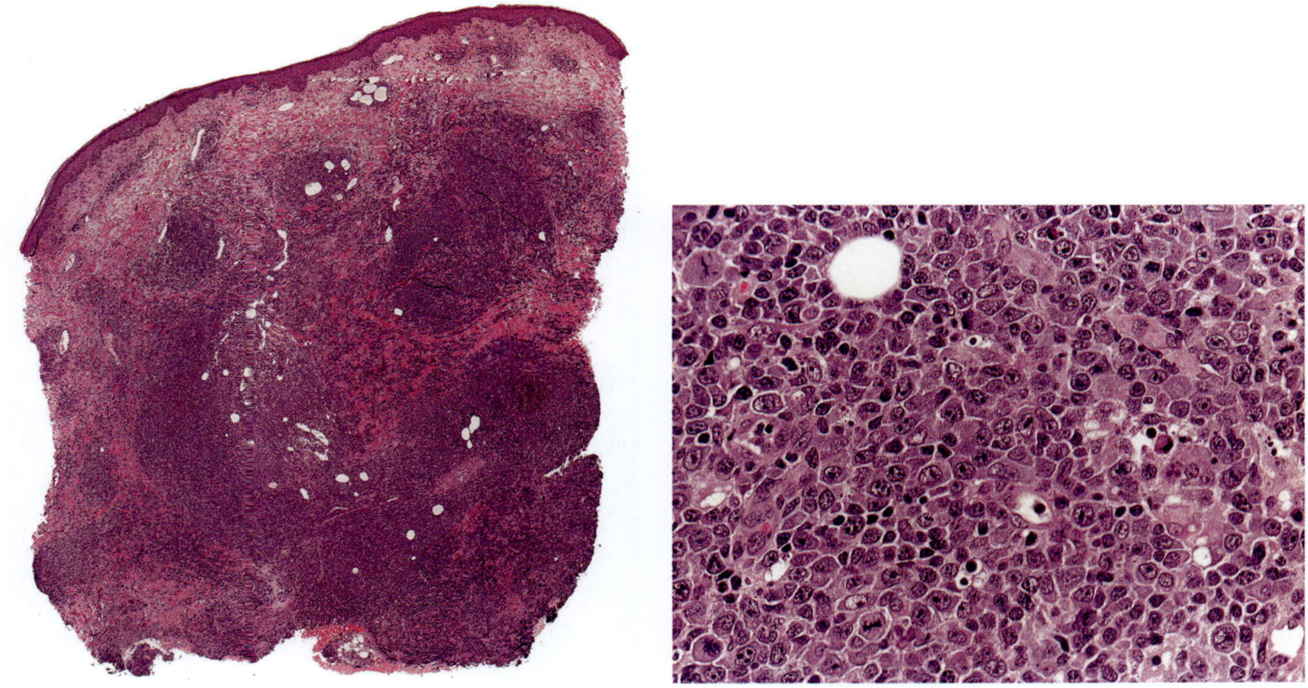

(a) (b)

**Figure 20.1** Cutaneous manifestations of EBV⁺ diffuse large B-cell lymphoma. (a) Diffuse infiltrate within the entire dermis with (b) sheets of large atypical cells.

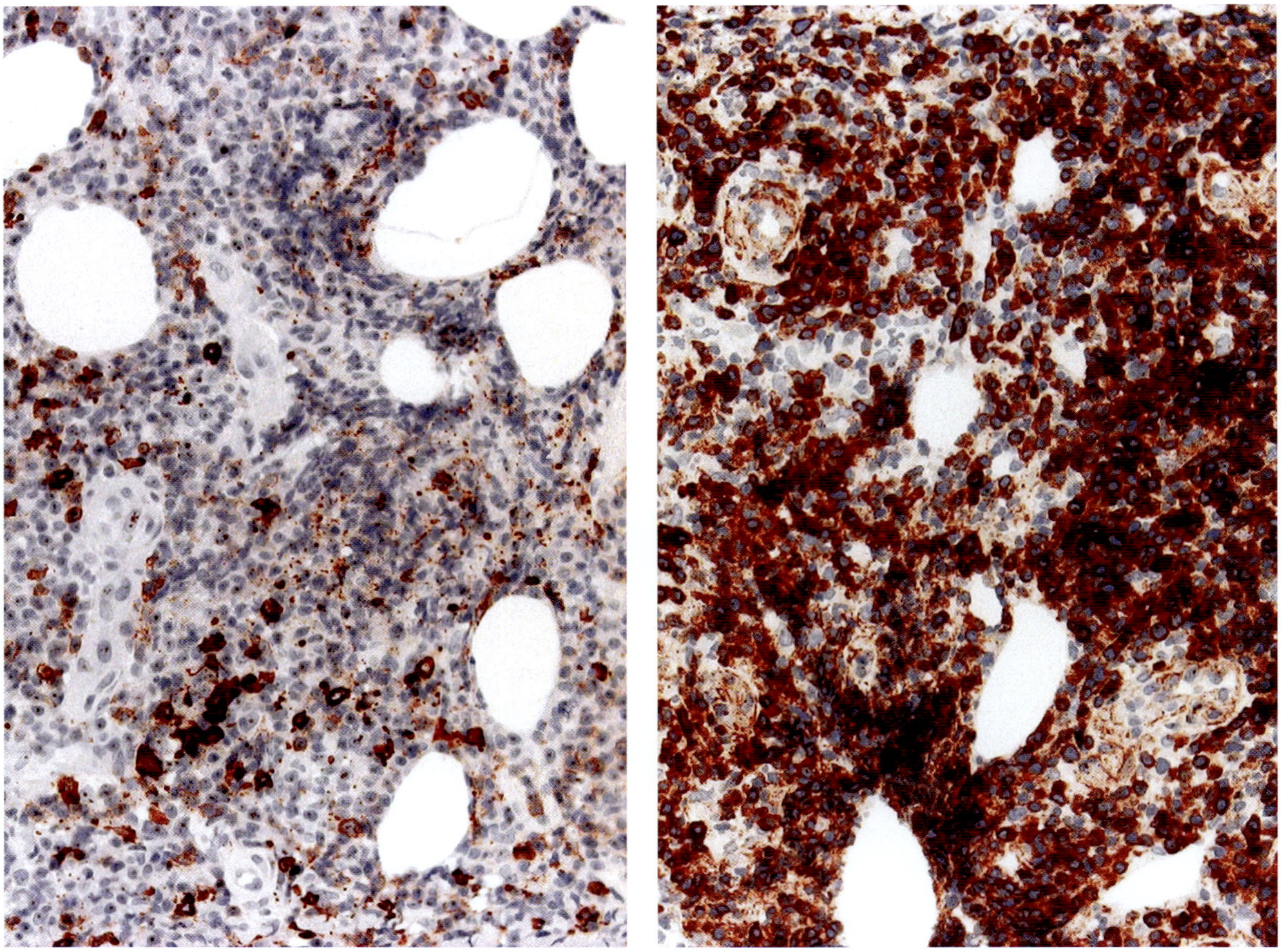

(a) (b)

**Figure 20.2** Cutaneous manifestations of EBV+ diffuse large B-cell lymphoma. Neoplastic cells are (a) negative for CD20 and (b) positive for CD79a.

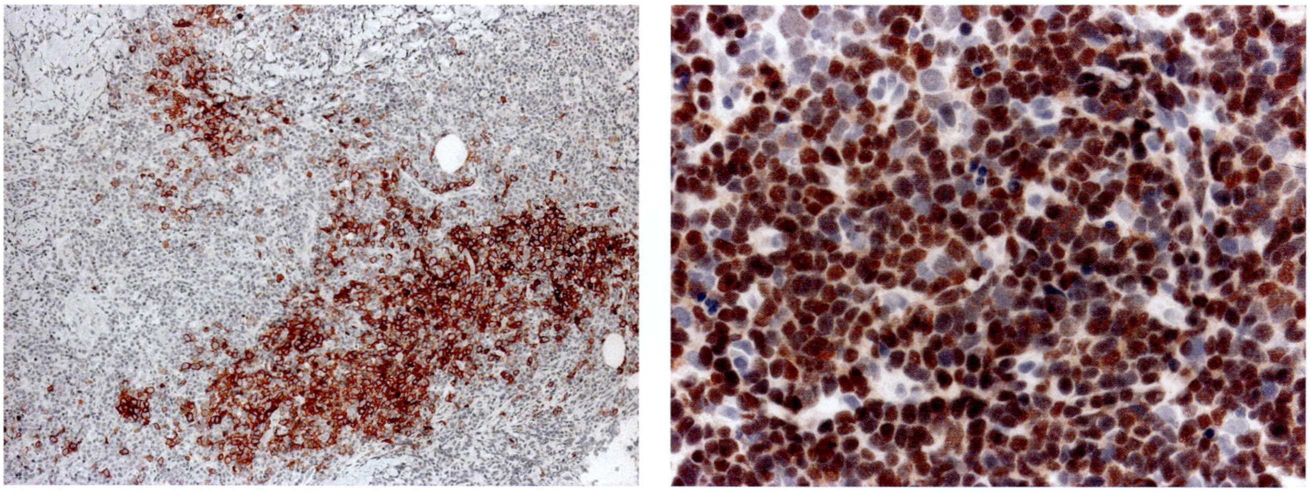

(a) (b)

**Figure 20.3** Cutaneous manifestations of EBV+ diffuse large B-cell lymphoma. Neoplastic cells are (a) focally positive for CD30 and (b) strongly positive for MUM-1.

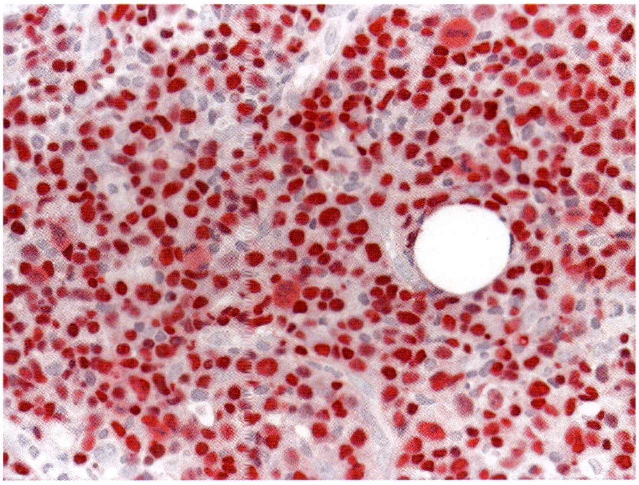

**Figure 20.4** Cutaneous manifestations of EBV+ diffuse large B-cell lymphoma. Strong positive signal in >80% of the cells upon in situ hybridization for EBV (EBER-1).

### Treatment and prognosis

EBV+ diffuse large B-cell lymphoma is a very aggressive lymphoma with a median survival of about 2 years in elderly patients, but the prognosis of the rare cases arising in younger patients seems to be much better. The treatment is often complicated by the advanced age of patients. The histopathologic pattern (polymorphic or monomorphic) does not have any prognostic meaning.

Different therapeutic approaches based on tumor biology and association with EBV infection have been suggested. Systemic chemotherapy, as well as anti-CD20 antibody (rituximab) and anti-CD30 antibody (brentuximab vedotin), may be used to target tumor cells. EBV-specific adoptive immunotherapy, miRNA-targeted therapy, and EBV lytic phase induction followed by anti-herpes virus drugs have been proposed as possible treatment strategies [13], but there is a lack of comprehensive studies, and reports of cutaneous cases are only anecdotal. The use of bortezomib or other inhibitors of the NF-κB pathway may be another alternative approach, based on the prominent NF-κB activation in tumor cells [13].

**Résumé**

**Cutaneous manifestations of EBV+ diffuse large B-cell lymphoma**

| | | |
|---|---|---|
| **Clinical** | Elderly patients. Skin is a relatively common site of presentation. | |
| **Morphology** | Polymorphous or monomorphic picture. Monomorphic infiltrates show features of diffuse large B-cell lymphoma. | |
| **Immunohistochemistry** | CD19, CD20 | + (−) |
| | CD79a, PAX-5 | + |
| | MUM-1, PD-1, PD-L1 | + |
| | Bcl-2, CD30 | + (−) |
| | Bcl-6 | − (+) |
| | CD3, CD5 | − |
| | EBER-1 | + (majority of neoplastic cells) |
| **Genetics** | Monoclonal rearrangement of the Ig genes. Activation of the JAK/STAT and NF-κB pathways. Signature of activated B lymphocytes. Relatively frequent mutations in *ARID1A*, *KMT2A/KMT2D*, *ANKRD11*, or *NOTCH2*. | |
| **Treatment guidelines** | Systemic chemotherapy + rituximab. Treatment of cutaneous cases is not standardized (only anecdotal cases). | |

## Cutaneous manifestations of mantle cell lymphoma

Mantle cell lymphoma is a rare B-cell lymphoma deriving from the inner mantle zone of lymphoid follicles [20, 21]. Cutaneous involvement is uncommon, but in rare cases, specific skin lesions may be the first manifestation of the disease [22–26]. Cutaneous involvement correlates with relapse or progression of nodal disease and a poor prognosis [27]. A few cases of mantle cell lymphoma arising primary in the skin have been reported [28], but the uniformly good prognosis observed in these patients casts doubt on the classification of these cases. Personally, I have never come across convincing cases of primary cutaneous mantle cell lymphoma and would consider such a diagnosis as the result of either a wrong classification of the case or an insufficient staging of the patient.

### Clinical features

Patients are middle-aged or older individuals, with a predominance of males. Clinically, the lesions are characterized by solitary or, more commonly, multiple reddish tumors. I have observed one patient with a solitary tumor on the navel, presenting clinically with the picture of so-called Sister Mary

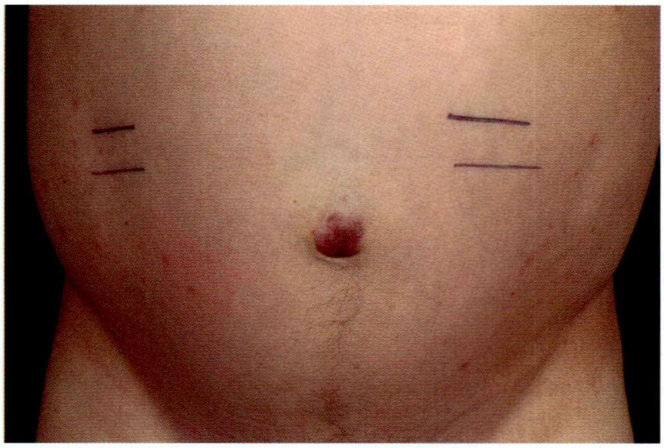

**Figure 20.5** Cutaneous manifestations of mantle cell lymphoma. Specific manifestation presenting with a solitary nodule in the navel ("Sister Mary Joseph's nodule"). Note also prominent ascites due to diffuse involvement of the peritoneum.

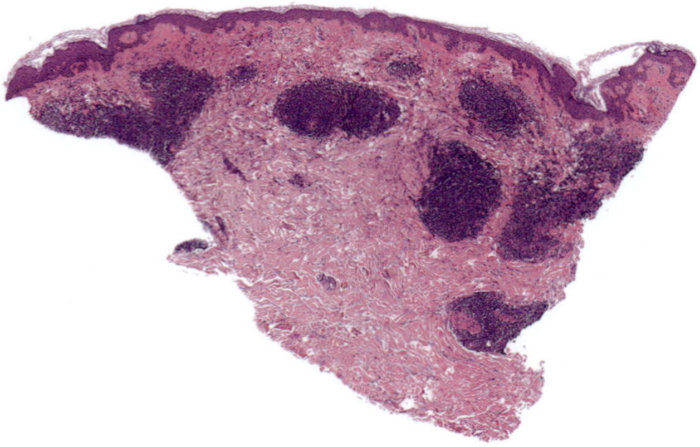

(a)

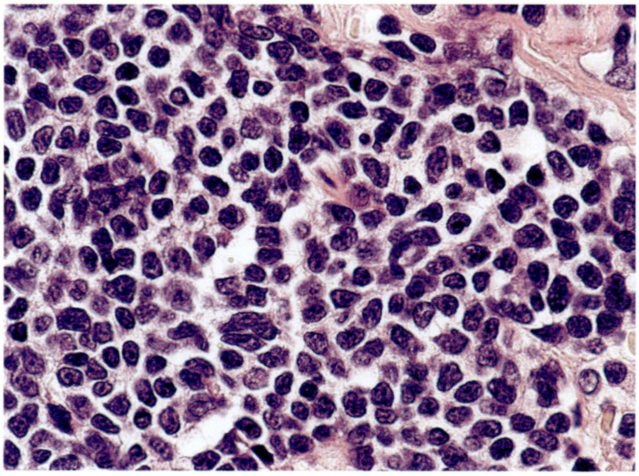

(b)

**Figure 20.6** Cutaneous manifestations of mantle cell lymphoma. (a) Dense nodular infiltrates in the dermis, composed of (b) monomorphous medium-sized cells with irregular nuclei.

Joseph's nodule as a recurrence of mantle cell lymphoma with diffuse peritoneal involvement and ascites (Fig. 20.5).

## Histopathology, immunophenotype, and molecular genetics

Histology shows nodular or diffuse, monomorphous infiltrates throughout the entire dermis and sometimes subcutis, composed of small- to medium-sized lymphocytes with irregular nuclei (Fig. 20.6). In one case prominent involvement of the subcutaneous fat resembled subcutaneous panniculitis-like T-cell lymphoma [29]. The blastoid variant, with either lymphoblast-like or large, cleaved cells, is frequently observed in cutaneous infiltrates, probably reflecting an increased propensity to skin involvement by tumors that undergo progression (Fig. 20.7), and should be differentiated from cutaneous diffuse large B-cell lymphoma, leg-type [30]. In one exceptional case, a specific skin infiltrate of mantle cell lymphoma has been observed at the cutaneous site of metastatic melanoma [31].

Immunohistology is characterized by positivity for CD19, CD20, and CD5 (Figs. 20.8a and b) and negativity for other T-cell markers. In contrast to cases of B-cell chronic lymphocytic leukemia (B-CLL), CD23 and CD200 are negative or only weakly expressed in neoplastic cells of mantle cell lymphoma, but cases positive for CD23 have been reported [32]. Nuclear staining for cyclin-D1 is a helpful tool for the differentiation of cutaneous mantle cell lymphoma from other malignant B-cell lymphomas, especially B-CLL and B-lymphoblastic lymphoma (Fig. 20.8c) [33]. According to the cyclin-D1 pattern, nodal cases are classified into two subtypes (cyclin-D1-positive, about 95% of cases, and cyclin-D1-negative, about 5% of cases). Cutaneous cases negative for cyclin-D1 are usually positive for SOX-11, which represents a useful antibody to avoid diagnostic pitfalls (cyclin-D2 and cyclin-D3 are also positive in extracutaneous cases, but there are no data on cutaneous ones) (Fig. 20.9). Negativity for SOX-11 has been reported in the less common, less aggressive variant of mantle cell lymphoma denominated leukemic non-nodal mantle cell lymphoma [34], but data on cases involving the skin are lacking. Aberrant expression of CD10 and Bcl-6 has been reported [35].

Molecular analyses reveal a monoclonal rearrangement of the Ig genes in the majority of cases. The typical t(11;14)(q13;q32), juxtaposing *CCND1* to *IGH*, can be demonstrated by different cytogenetic and molecular methods. The rare negative cases show rearrangements of *CCND2* or *CCND3* as alternative mechanisms of cell-cycle dysregulation.

## Treatment and prognosis

The treatment of choice is systemic chemotherapy, often followed by stem cell transplantation. Ibrutinib, as well as other

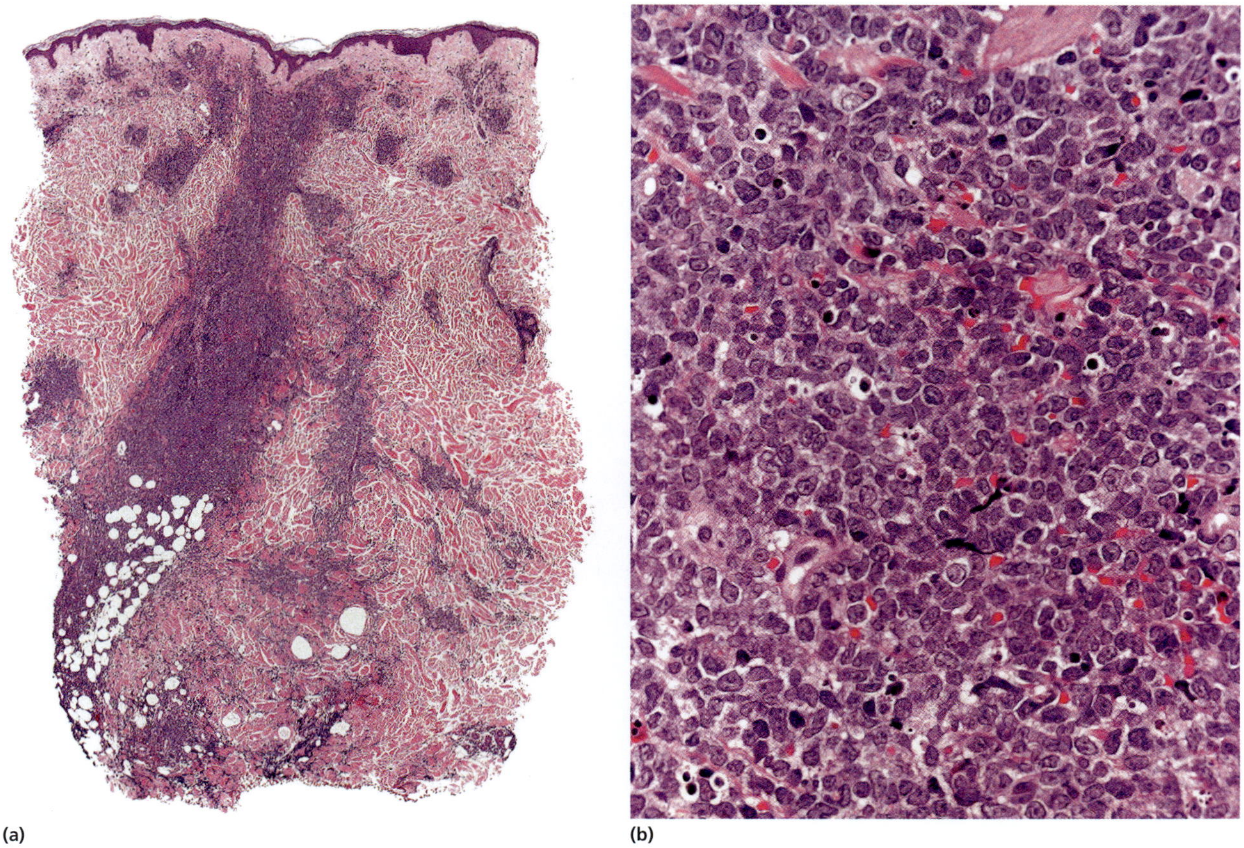



**Figure 20.7** Cutaneous manifestations of mantle cell lymphoma, blastoid variant. (a) Nodular and diffuse infiltrates within the dermis and visible subcutaneous fat, composed of (b) monomorphous, large, atypical cells resembling diffuse large B-cell lymphoma.

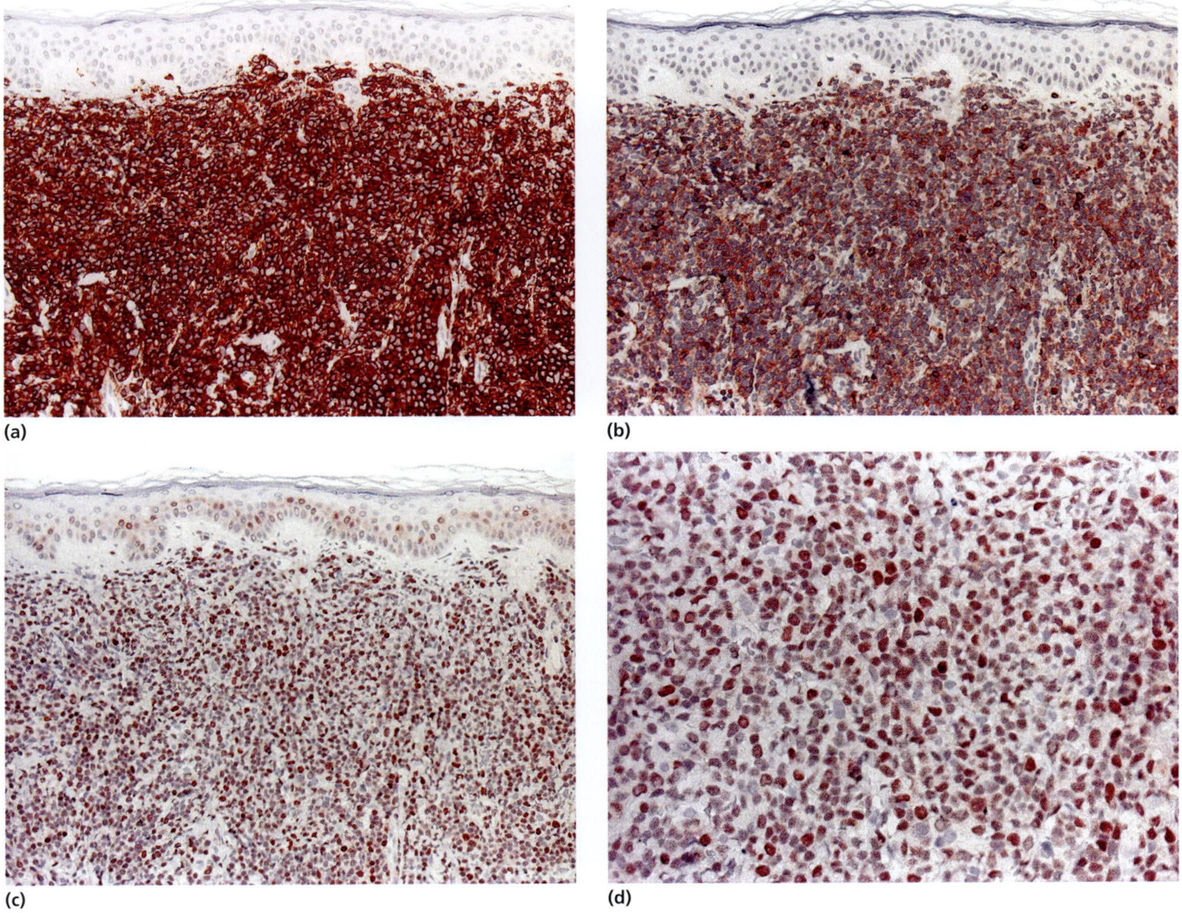



**Figure 20.8** Cutaneous manifestations of mantle cell lymphoma. Neoplastic cells positive for (a) CD20, (b) CD5, and (c, d) cyclin D1.

covalent Bruton tyrosine kinase inhibitors such as acalabrutinib and Zanubrutinib, has been increasingly used in relapsed cases. Chimeric antigen receptor (CAR) T-cell treatment can also be considered in appropriate settings [36]. As cutaneous cases are invariably due to secondary spread, management of these patients should be done in a hematological setting. The prognosis is poor, but new treatment modalities have dramatically increased survival rates. As already mentioned, nodal cases negative for SOX-11 have a better prognosis. Ki-67 and p53 expression in >30% and in ≥50% of neoplastic cells, respectively, are associated with a worse overall survival [37].

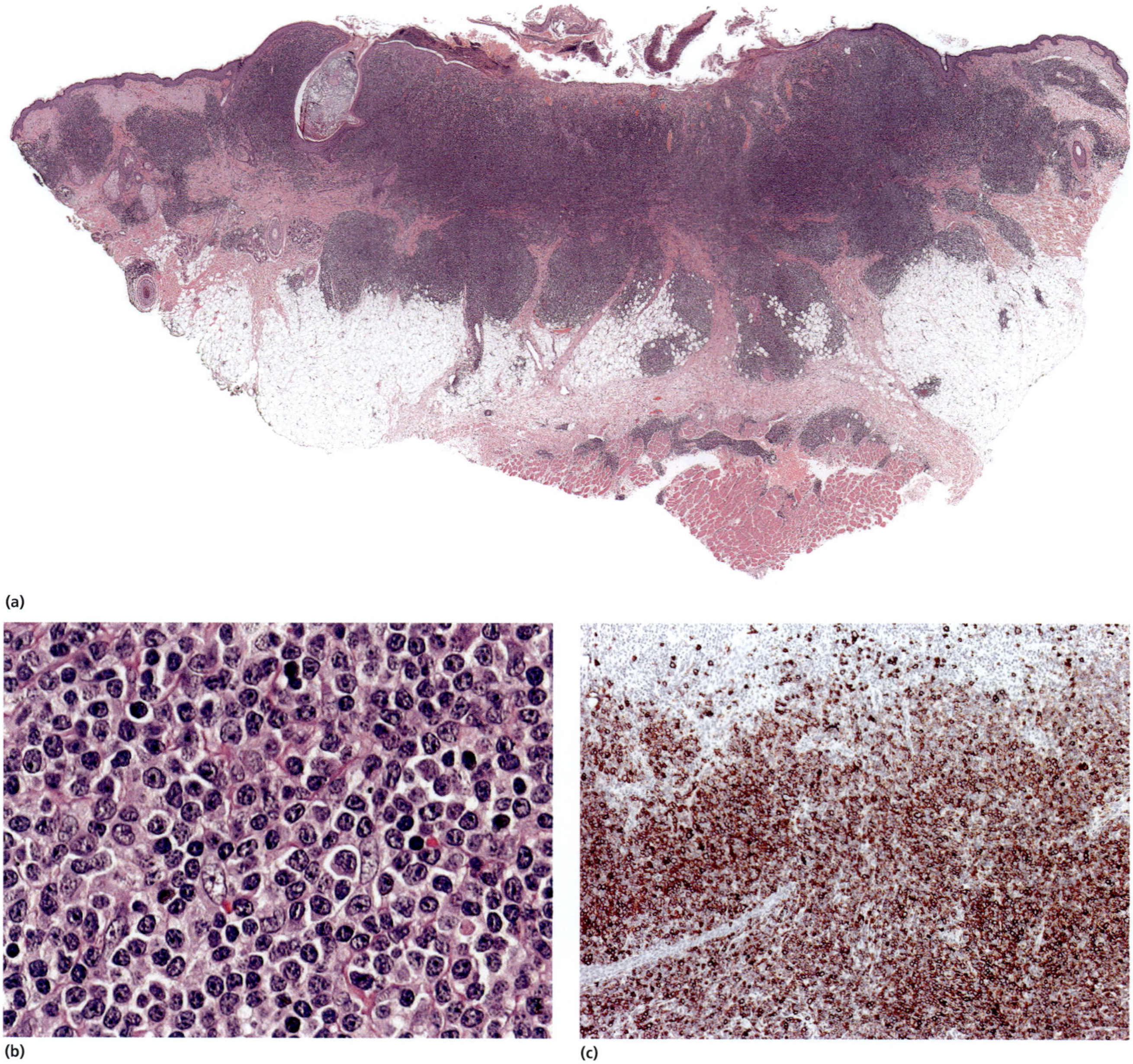


**Figure 20.9** Cutaneous manifestations of mantle cell lymphoma. (a) Dense lymphoid infiltrates within the entire dermis, characterized by (b) predominance of medium-sized and large, partly blastoid lymphocytes. Immunohistology revealed (c) positivity for CD20, (d) negativity for cyclin-D1, and positivity for (e) cyclin-D2, (f) SOX-11, and (g) MUM1.

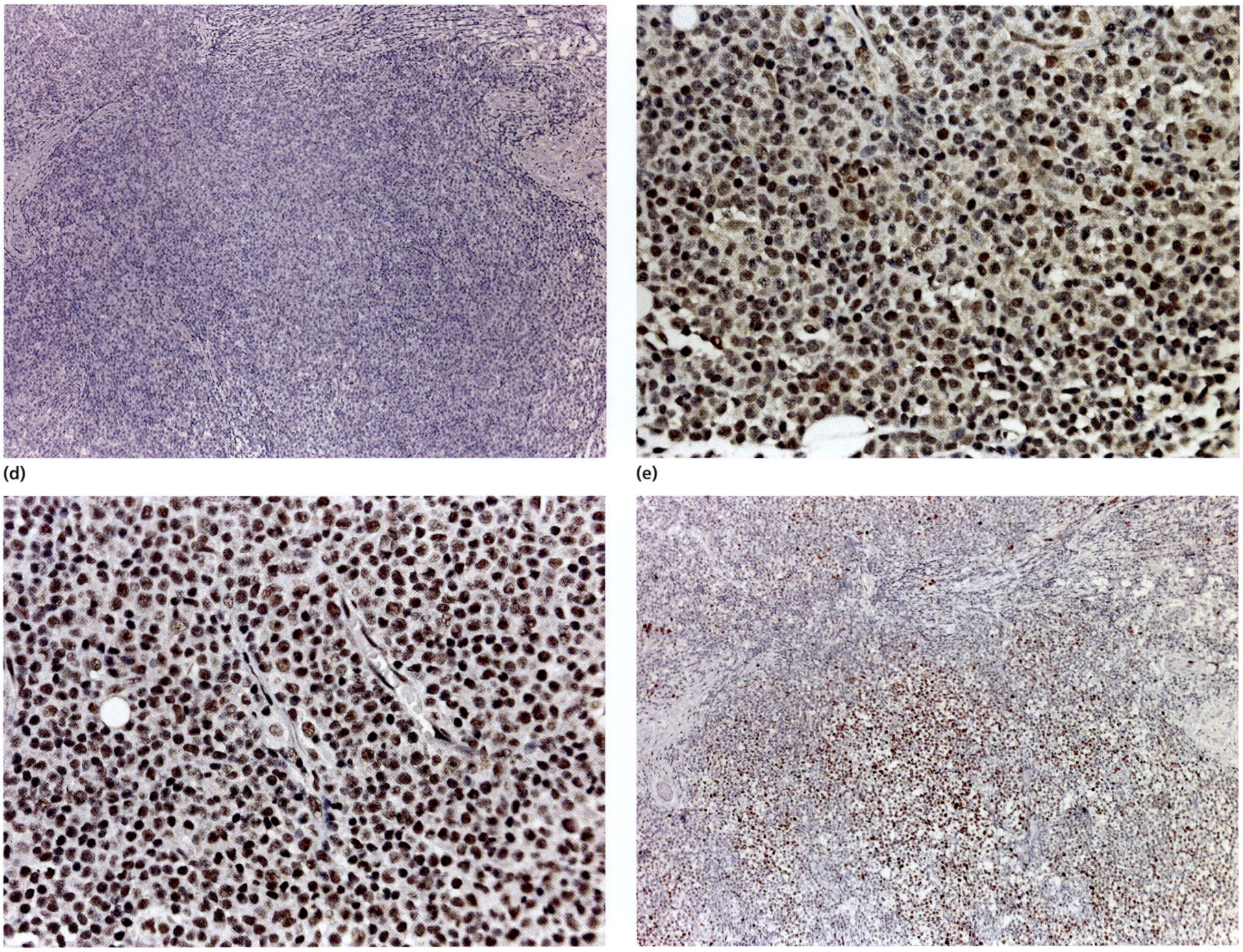

(d) (e) (f) (g)

Figure 20.9 (Continued)

## Résumé

**Cutaneous manifestations of mantle cell lymphoma**

| | | |
|---|---|---|
| **Clinical** | Adults. Usually, multiple tumors as secondary skin involvement. The existence of true primary cutaneous cases is questionable. | |
| **Morphology** | Monomorphous proliferation of small- to medium-sized lymphocytes with irregular nuclei. Lymphoblast-like cells in blastoid variant. | |
| **Immunohistochemistry** | CD19, CD20 | + |
| | CD5 | + (−) |
| | CD23, CD10 | − (+) |
| | Cyclin-D1 | + (−) |
| | SOX-11 | + (−) |
| **Genetics** | Monoclonal rearrangement of the Ig genes. Common t(11;14)(q13;q32). | |
| **Treatment guidelines** | Systemic chemotherapy; stem cell transplantation. Ibrutinib or other covalent Bruton tyrosine kinase inhibitors. Chimeric antigen receptor (CAR) T-cell treatment. | |

## Cutaneous manifestations of extracavitary primary effusion lymphoma

Primary effusion lymphoma is a large B-cell lymphoma presenting in serous effusions and associated with human herpes virus-8 (HHV-8) [38], usually arising in individuals infected with the human immunodeficiency virus (HIV). It is included in a section on "human herpesvirus 8-associated lymphoproliferative disorders" in the International Consensus Classification [39]. Tumors presenting as solid masses rather than serous effusions are classified as extracavitary effusion lymphoma [38, 40]. Cutaneous involvement may be seen in these cases as a secondary lymphoma manifestation, but primary cutaneous involvement has not been observed. It should be underlined that, at sites other than the skin, HHV-8-associated lymphoid proliferations represent a spectrum including reactive and neoplastic disorders [41], but there are no data on the existence of a primary cutaneous reactive HHV-8 lymphoid hyperplasia.

Earlier reports of HHV-8$^+$ plasmablastic lymphoma represent, in truth, examples of primary effusion lymphoma (see below the section on plasmablastic lymphoma). In rare patients, HHV-8-associated lymphoma has been observed concomitantly with Kaposi sarcoma and multicentric Castleman disease, showing that the entire repertoire of virus-associated malignancies may be observed in given patients [42].

### Clinical features

Extracavitary effusion lymphoma usually arises in HIV$^+$ young or middle-aged adults. Cutaneous involvement presents with nondescript, localized, or generalized cutaneous or subcutaneous nodules (Fig. 20.10) [43].

It should be underlined that a diagnosis of cutaneous involvement by extracavitary effusion lymphoma should be confirmed by the presence of a primary tumor at extracutaneous sites.

### Histopathology, immunophenotype, and molecular genetics

Histology shows cutaneous or subcutaneous infiltrates comprised of sheets of large cells with abundant eosinophilic cytoplasm and with anaplastic or plasmablastic appearance (Fig. 20.11). CD20 and CD79a are usually negative, but markers of plasma cell differentiation (CD38, CD138) are positive (Fig. 20.12). HHV-8 and EBV are expressed in virtually all neoplastic cells (Fig. 20.13). Aberrant expression of T-cell markers may be observed, representing a pitfall in the diagnosis (Fig. 20.14c). In some cases, cutaneous extracavitary effusion lymphoma may mimic histopathologically anaplastic large cell lymphoma and show expression of CD30, thus representing a diagnostic pitfall [44]. A rare case with intravascular distribution of tumor cells has been observed [45], and in other rare cases the skin infiltrate may be restricted to the subcutaneous fat tissue, mimicking the histopathological picture of subcutaneous panniculitis-like T-cell lymphoma (Fig. 20.14) [46].

The Ig genes are clonally rearranged. Only limited molecular data are available. Gains in chromosomes 7 and 12 have been reported.

### Treatment and prognosis

Patients are treated with systemic chemotherapy and anti-HIV drugs, but the prognosis is very poor, with a median survival of <6 months.

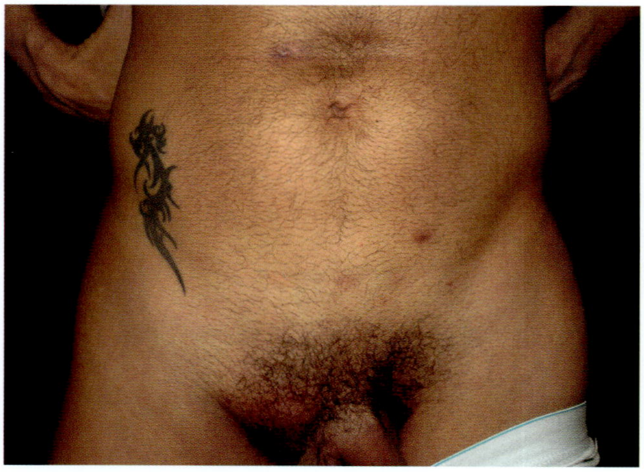

**Figure 20.10** Cutaneous manifestations of extracavitary primary effusion lymphoma. Several cutaneous–subcutaneous nodules on the abdomen and inguinal region. *(Courtesy of Prof. Luis Requena, Madrid, Spain.)*

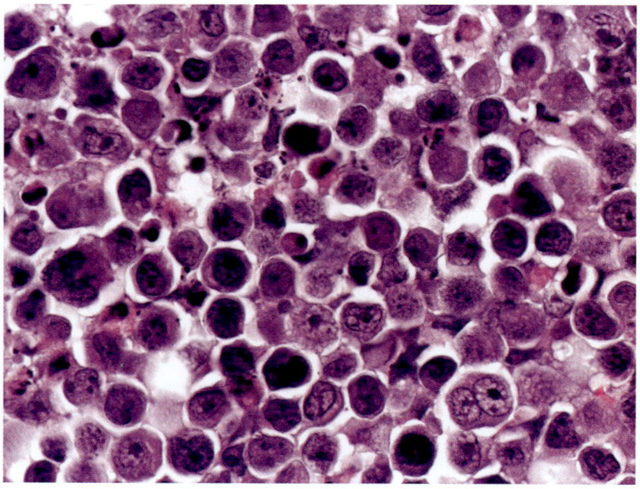

**Figure 20.11** Cutaneous manifestations of extracavitary primary effusion lymphoma. Large, atypical cells with anaplastic and plasmablastic morphology.

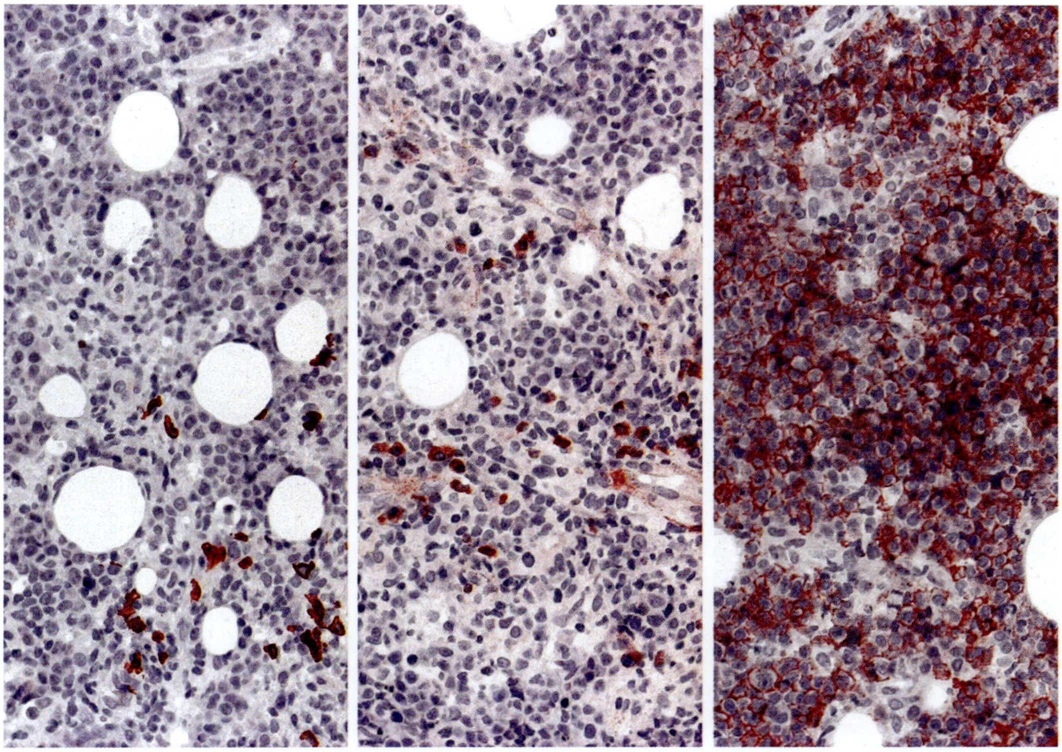

Figure 20.12 Cutaneous manifestations of extracavitary primary effusion lymphoma. Neoplastic cells are negative for CD20 (left) and CD79a (middle), and positive for CD138 (right).

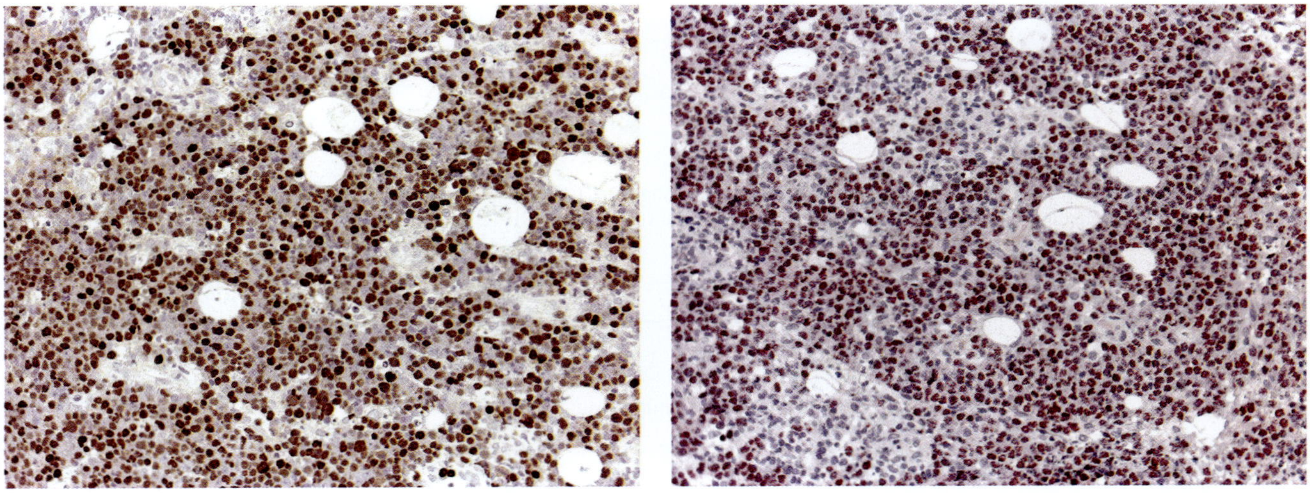

(a) (b)

Figure 20.13 Cutaneous manifestations of extracavitary primary effusion lymphoma. (a) Neoplastic cells reveal a positive signal upon in situ hybridization for EBV (EBER-1) and (b) are positive for HHV-8.

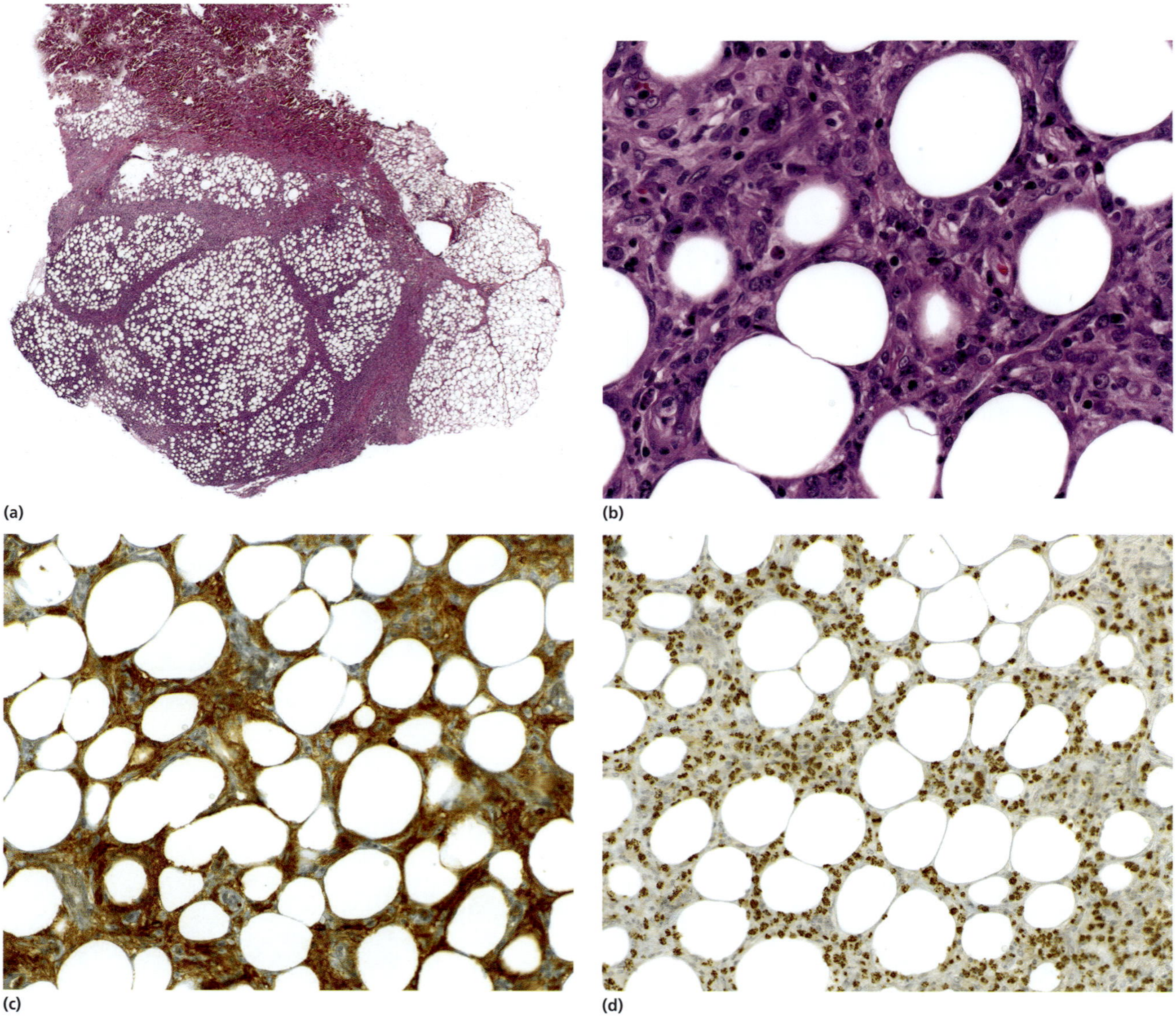

**Figure 20.14** Cutaneous manifestations of extracavitary primary effusion lymphoma. (a) Neoplastic cells restricted to the subcutaneous fat tissue with a "lobular panniculitis"-like pattern showing (b) rimming of adipocytes and positivity for (c) CD4 and (d) HHV-8 *(Case courtesy of Dr. Lucia Anemona and Dr. Andrea Saggini, Rome, Italy.)*

## Résumé

**Cutaneous manifestations of extracavitary primary effusion lymphoma**

| | | |
|---|---|---|
| **Clinical** | Mostly in HIV$^+$ adults. Usually multiple tumors as secondary skin involvement. | |
| **Morphology** | Sheets of large cells with abundant eosinophilic cytoplasm (anaplastic or plasmablastic appearance). | |
| **Immunohistochemistry** | CD19, CD20, CD79a | – |
| | CD38, CD138 | + |
| | HHV-8 | + |
| | EBER-1 | + |
| | CD30 | (+) |
| **Genetics** | Monoclonal rearrangement of the Ig genes. | |
| **Treatment guidelines** | Systemic chemotherapy. | |

## Cutaneous manifestations of multiple myeloma

Several cases of primary cutaneous plasmacytoma have been reported in the past, but in the WHO–European Organization for Research and Treatment of Cancer (EORTC) classification of cutaneous lymphomas, these cases have been reclassified as variants of marginal zone lymphoproliferative disorder with predominant plasmacytic differentiation (see Chapter 17) [47]. In this context, the existence of genuine primary cutaneous plasmacytoma seems unlikely, and cases of true plasmacytoma arising in the skin represent almost invariably secondary manifestations of multiple myeloma [48, 49]. Specific cutaneous involvement, however, seems to be rare: in a series from South Korea, cutaneous involvement in patients with multiple myeloma was found in approximately 1% of cases and was associated with a worse prognosis [50].

### Clinical features

Patients present clinically with solitary, clustered, or generalized cutaneous or subcutaneous plaques or tumors. The lesions often have a characteristic brown or purpuric color (Fig. 20.15). Similarly to what is observed in other hematological malignancies such as myeloid leukemia or B-cell chronic lymphocytic leukemia, neoplastic cells of multiple myeloma have been observed at the site of cutaneous injuries [51].

### Histopathology, immunophenotype, and molecular genetics

Cutaneous manifestations of multiple myeloma (cutaneous plasmacytoma) consist of dense nodules and/or sheets of cells within the entire dermis and subcutis. Mature and immature plasma cells with varying degrees of atypia predominate (Fig. 20.16). Dutcher bodies and Russell bodies are found occasionally. Small reactive lymphocytes are few or absent. Amyloid deposits may be observed within and/or surrounding the neoplastic infiltrates, particularly around blood vessels (Fig. 20.16c). Neoplastic cells may have a pleomorphic morphology and be difficult to identify as atypical plasma cells without phenotypic analyses (Fig. 20.17). As neoplastic plasma cells may express aberrant T-cell markers (see below), complete phenotypic analyses are always necessary in order to properly classify such cases. In some cases, cutaneous involvement may present with histopathological features of plasmablastic myeloma (Fig. 20.18) [52]. In contrast to plasmablastic lymphoma, which is often associated with EBV infection, plasmablastic myeloma

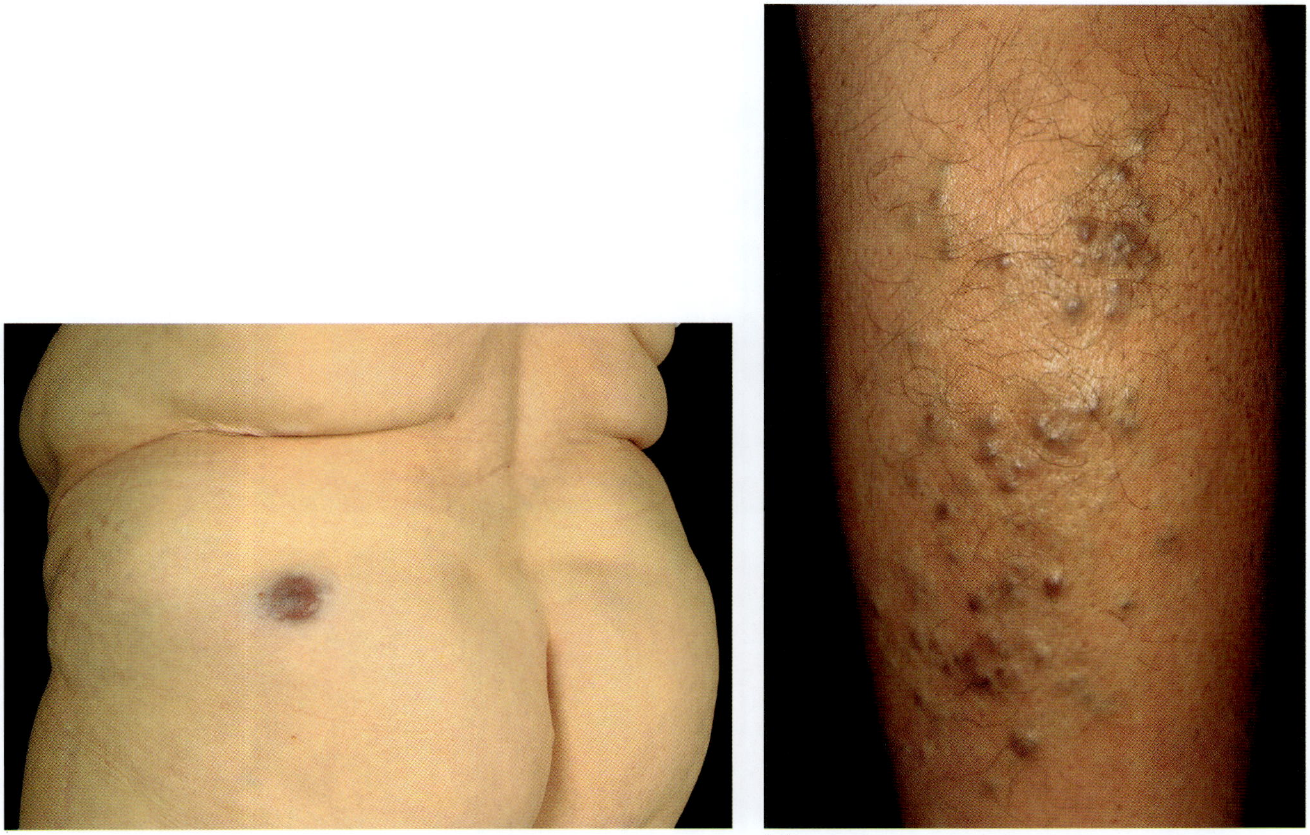

(a) (b)

**Figure 20.15** Specific cutaneous manifestations of multiple myeloma. (a) Solitary, large, livid nodule on the buttocks. (b) Miliary, livid papules and small nodules on the leg.

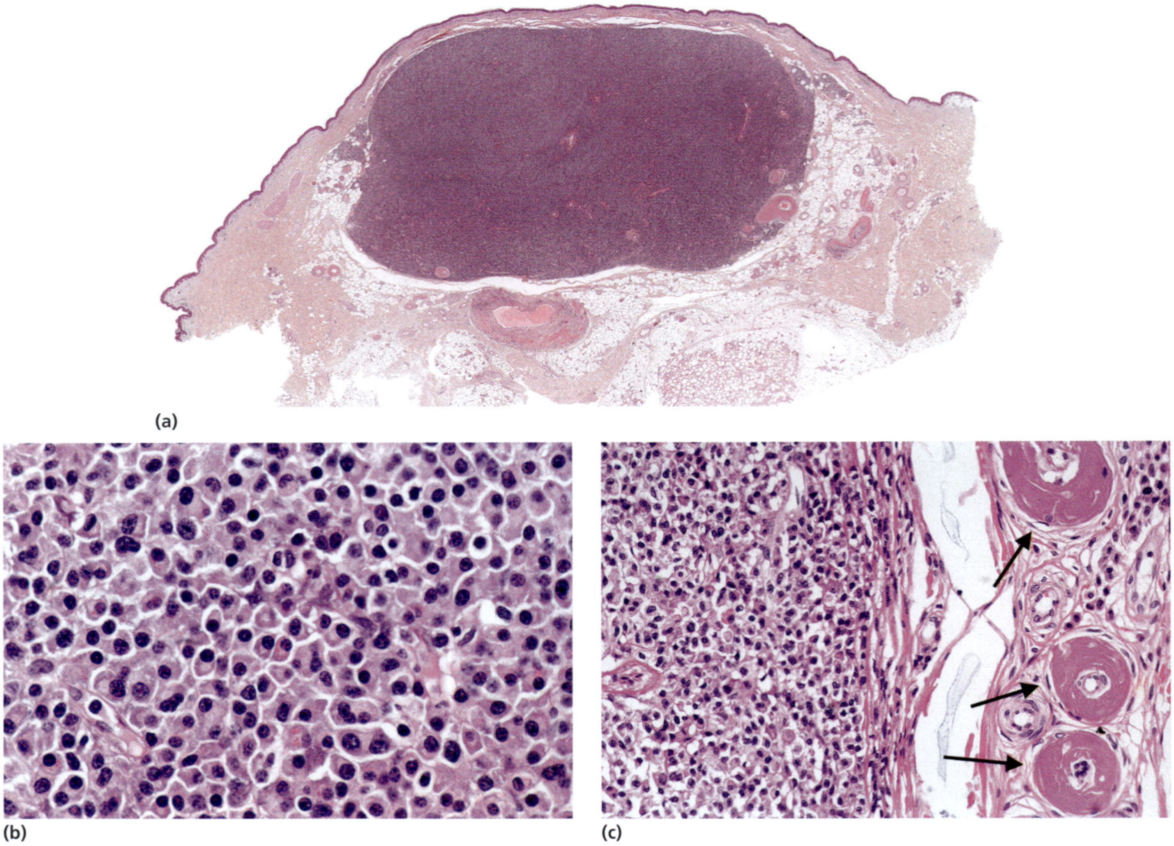

**Figure 20.16** Specific cutaneous manifestations of multiple myeloma. (a) Large nodule within the dermis and subcutis. (b) The nodule is composed of atypical plasma cells. (c) Note prominent amyloid deposits within the walls of three vessels (arrows).

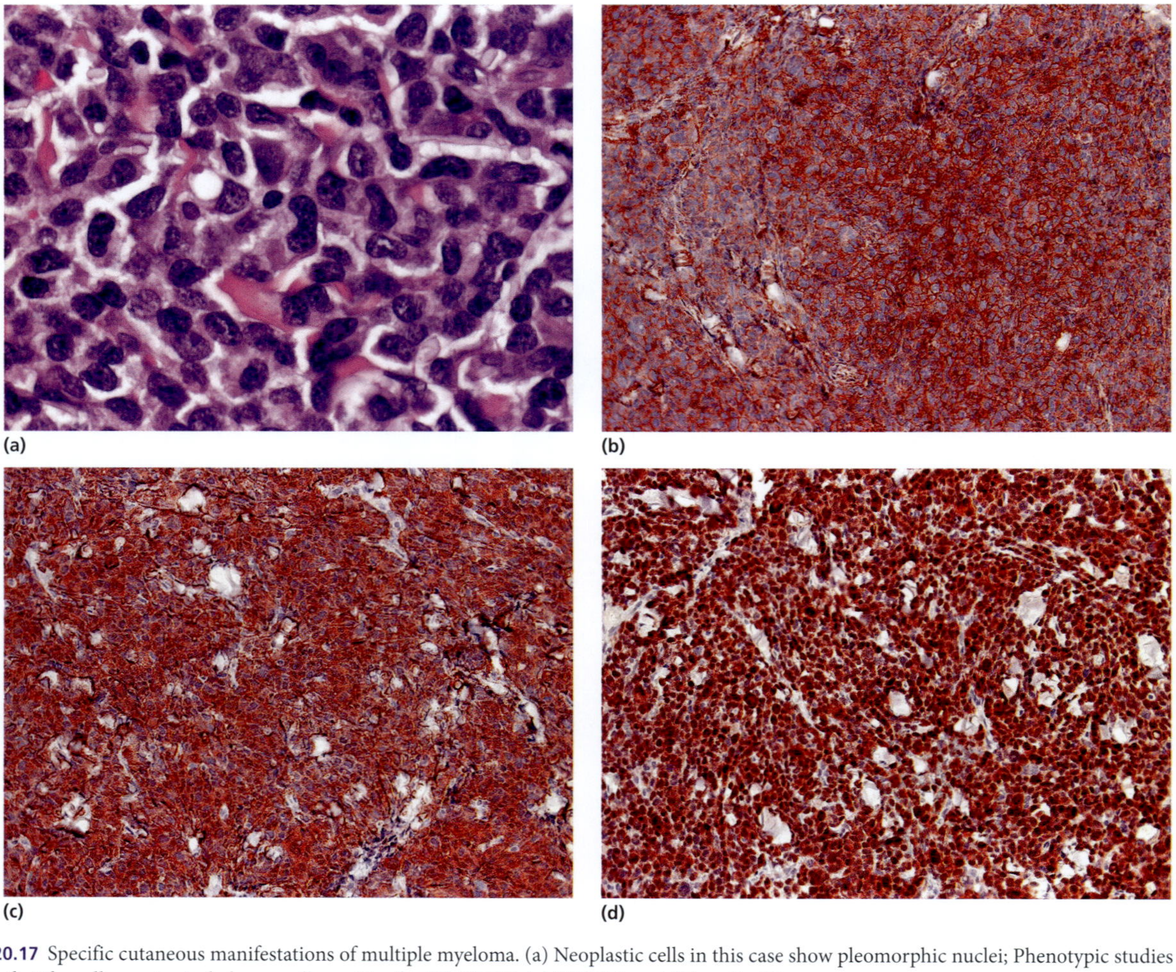

**Figure 20.17** Specific cutaneous manifestations of multiple myeloma. (a) Neoplastic cells in this case show pleomorphic nuclei; Phenotypic studies confirm that the cells are atypical plasma cells positive for (b) CD138, (c) MUM-1, and (d) cyclin D1.

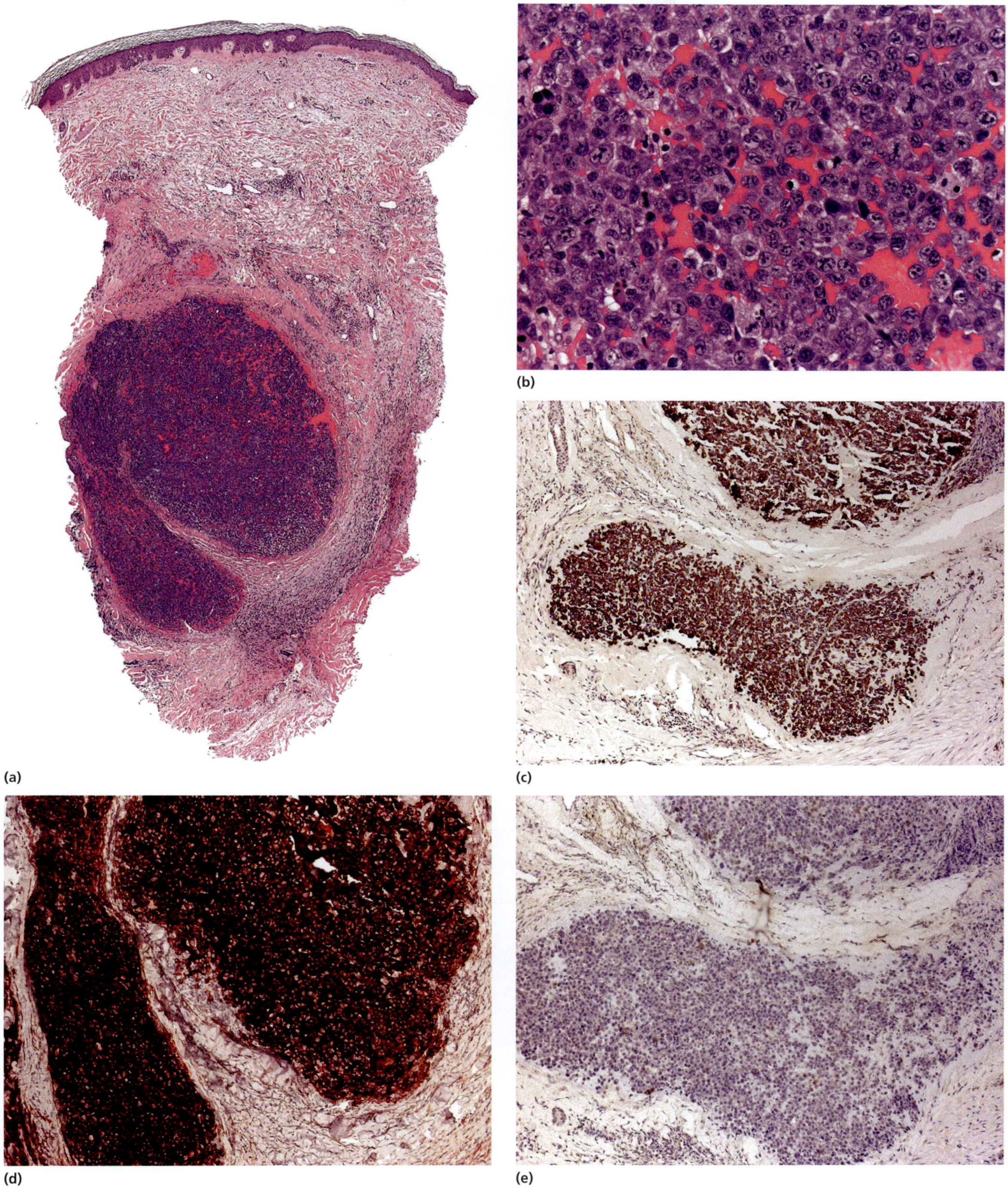

Figure 20.18 Specific cutaneous manifestations of plasmablastic multiple myeloma. (a) Nodular infiltrate within the deep dermis and subcutaneous fat, composed of (b) large plasmablasts positive for (c) the immunoglobulin light chain kappa, (d) negative for EBV (EBER-1), and (e) positive for CD138.

not arising in the setting of immune suppression is only rarely positive for EBV.

Neoplastic plasma cells contain cytoplasmic immunoglobulins (usually IgA) and show monoclonal expression of one immunoglobulin light chain. Biphenotypic plasma cell myeloma, characterized by secretion of paraprotein with two distinct heavy or light chain components, has been rarely described outside of the skin [53]. Leukocyte common antigen (CD45) and most B-cell-associated markers are negative, but cells can be stained by CD38, CD138, or MUM-1 in most cases and by CD56 and CD79a in some cases (Figs. 20.17b and c). Increased expression of MYC may be detected on immunohistochemistry. Positivity of neoplastic cells for CD117 has been advocated as a useful clue to differentiate plasma cell myeloma (positive) from plasmablastic lymphoma (negative) [54]. Cyclin-D1 may be positive in some cases (Fig. 20.17d). Immunohistochemical expression of cytokeratins, HMB45, and CD30 can be observed within neoplastic plasma cells, representing a potential source of diagnostic error. Rarely, an aberrant phenotype with expression of T-cell markers (CD3, CD4) can also be observed [52], representing a further pitfall in immunohistochemical characterization of neoplastic cells.

Molecular analysis usually reveals a monoclonal rearrangement of the Ig genes. Molecular alterations present already in early phases of the disease include trisomies of the odd-numbered chromosomes and chromosomal translocations involving the IGH locus, resulting in overexpression of several oncogenes, including *CCND1*, *CCND2*, *CCND3*, *NSD2*, *MAF*, *MAFA*, and *MAFB*.

### Treatment and prognosis

The treatment is tailored on the systemic manifestations. Radiotherapy may be administered for solitary cutaneous tumors.

The prognosis of cutaneous manifestations of multiple myeloma is poor. Analysis of data concerning cases of cutaneous plasmacytoma published in the literature, however, is hindered by the inclusion of cases with indolent behavior that today would be classified as cutaneous marginal zone lymphoproliferative disorder, plasmacytic variant.


**Résumé**

| | | |
|---|---|---|
| **Cutaneous manifestations of multiple myeloma** | | |
| **Clinical** | Solitary, grouped, or generalized (sub)cutaneous plaques and tumors. | |
| **Morphology** | Nodular or diffuse infiltrates are characterized by the predominance of mature and immature plasma cells. | |
| **Immunohistochemistry** | CD45 (LCA), CD19, CD20 | – |
| | CD38, CD138, MUM-1 | + |
| | CD56, CD79a | +/– |
| | Cyclin D1 | –/+ |
| | cIg | + (monoclonal) |
| **Genetics** | Monoclonal rearrangement of the Ig genes detected in the majority of cases. | |
| **Treatment guidelines** | Treatment is tailored on the systemic manifestations of the disease. Radiotherapy of solitary cutaneous tumors. | |


## Cutaneous manifestations of Burkitt lymphoma

Three variants of Burkitt lymphoma are recognized: (i) endemic (arising mostly in equatorial African and Papua New Guinean children and always associated with EBV); (ii) sporadic (arising mostly in children and young adults without racial predilection and associated with EBV in 20–30% of cases); and (iii) immunodeficiency-associated (arising mostly in immunocompromised HIV$^{+}$ patients and associated with EBV in 25–40% of cases) [55, 56]. Interestingly, the endemic variant is linked to malaria in addition to EBV, representing one of the examples of diseases with "polymicrobial" pathogenesis. Particular herpes viruses (HHV-5, HHV-8) are also found in the majority of cases of endemic Burkitt lymphoma, supporting again the polymicrobial etiology of this lymphoma. Skin involvement represents almost invariably a secondary manifestation of the disease [57, 58]. In rare cases of primary cutaneous diffuse large B-cell lymphoma, leg type, a Burkitt-like morphology may be observed, and these cases should be separated from genuine Burkitt lymphoma (see Chapter 18).

Burkitt lymphoma is characterized by a translocation involving *MYC* on chromosome 8, usually an *MYC/IGH* t(8;14)(q24;q32); strong expression of MYC (>80% of neoplastic cells); and/or demonstration of *MYC* translocation represent essential diagnostic criteria [55]. Some display a t(2;8)(p12;q24) (*IGK/MYC*), and others a t(8;22)(q24;q11) (*MYC/IGL*).

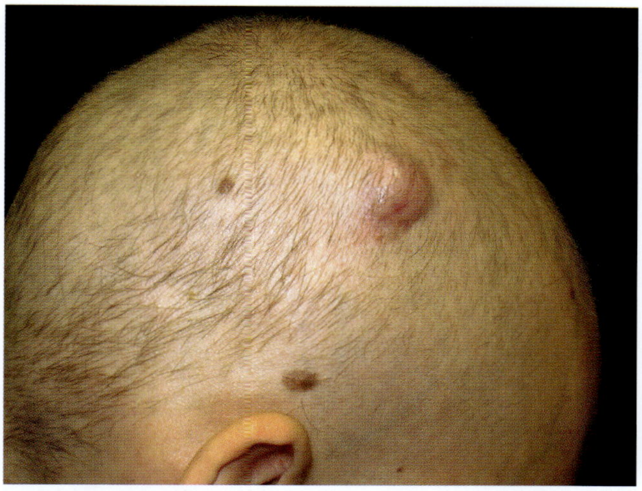

Figure 20.19 Specific cutaneous manifestations of Burkitt lymphoma. Large, solitary nodule on the scalp. *(Courtesy of Prof. Luis Requena, Madrid, Spain.)*

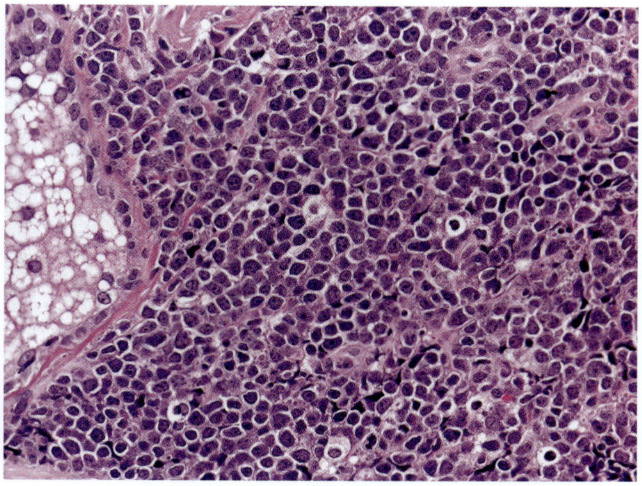

Figure 20.20 Specific cutaneous manifestations of Burkitt lymphoma. Diffuse proliferation of medium-sized and large blastoid cells. Note some hints of a "starry sky" pattern.

## Clinical features

Although Burkitt lymphoma is frequent in children and adolescents, most reports on skin involvement by the disease concern adult patients, with rare cases observed in children [59]. Cutaneous manifestations are characterized by solitary, localized, or generalized cutaneous or subcutaneous, rapidly expanding tumors (Fig. 20.19).

## Histopathology, immunophenotype, and molecular genetics

Histology shows diffuse infiltrates within the dermis and subcutaneous fat. A "starry sky" pattern may be observed. Cytomorphology reveals cohesive sheets of monomorphous, medium-sized or large, blastoid cells (Fig. 20.20). Tumor cells may acquire a polygonal shape with "squared" margins and show focally a "mosaic stone" and/or "Indian-filing" arrangement (Fig. 20.21).

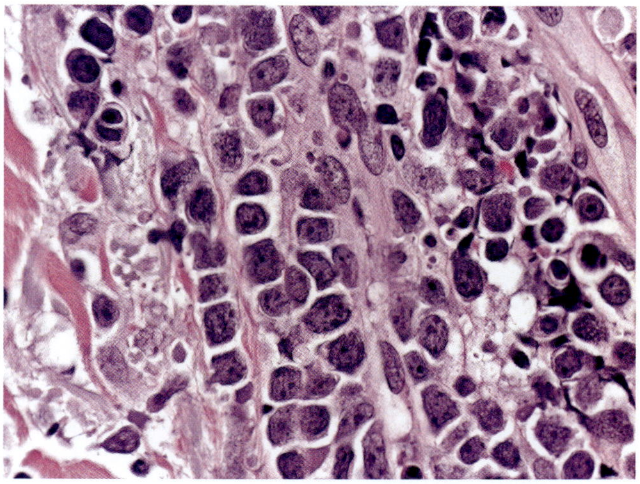

Figure 20.21 Specific cutaneous manifestations of Burkitt lymphoma. Note "Indian filing" and squared cells ("mosaic stone-like").

Tumor cells express B-cell-associated antigens and IgM with light chain restriction. Bcl-6 and CD10 are positive, whereas TdT is uniformly negative, allowing distinction from B-lymphoblastic lymphoma. Bcl-2 is usually negative or rarely weakly positive; alternative diagnoses should be considered in Bcl-2$^+$ cases. Ki-67 is positive in nearly all cells, representing a typical feature of Burkitt lymphoma (Fig. 20.22). In fact, for practical purposes, the diagnosis should not be considered if the proliferation rate is not nearly 100%. Neoplastic cells of Burkitt lymphoma are characterized by alterations in lipid metabolism, and immunohistochemical staining for adipophilin demonstrates characteristic intracytoplasmic positive vacuoles.

The typical *MYC* translocations t(8;14) (q24;q32) of Burkitt lymphoma can be detected by FISH using break-apart probes for *MYC* (Fig. 20.23) and result in protein expression at the immunohistochemical level. *MYC* translocations, however, are not specific for Burkitt lymphoma and have been observed also in primary cutaneous diffuse large B-cell lymphomas [60]. The gene expression signature is different from that observed in diffuse large B-cell lymphoma, but cases with overlapping features exist. Activation of the B-cell receptor signaling pathway has been demonstrated by next-generation sequencing studies. In non-endemic Burkitt lymphoma, there is an inverse correlation between association with EBV and number of mutations, suggesting that mutations in non-EBV-associated cases may serve for the activation of the B-cell receptor signaling.

*FOXO1* mutations have been detected in sporadic (about 1/3 of cases) and endemic (about half of the cases) pediatric Burkitt lymphoma cases [61]. *FOXO1* has an oncogenic role resulting in increased cell proliferation and may be targeted by specific therapy.

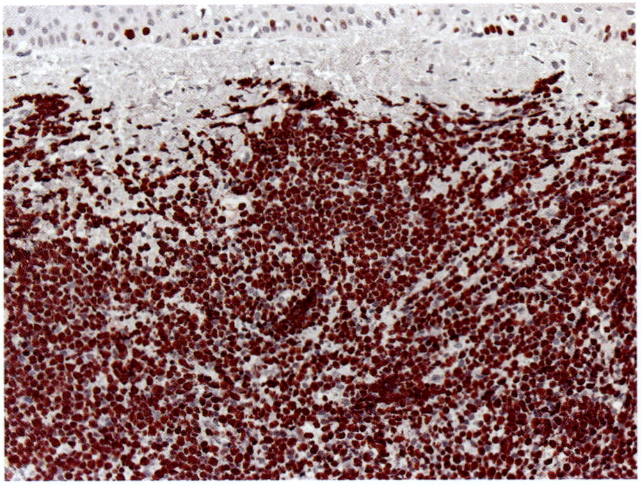

**Figure 20.22** Specific cutaneous manifestations of Burkitt lymphoma. Staining for Ki-67 reveals positivity of 100% of neoplastic cells.

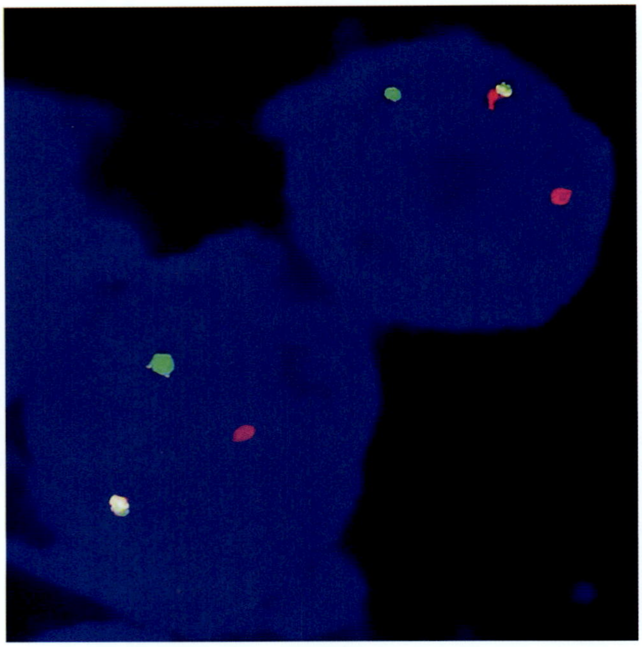

**Figure 20.23** Specific cutaneous manifestations of Burkitt lymphoma. FISH analysis with a dual-color break-apart probe flanking the MYC gene on chromosome 8 shows one split signal and one normal signal in two cells, indicating the presence of a MYC rearrangement. *(Courtesy of Prof. Fabio Facchetti, Brescia, Italy.)*

### Treatment and prognosis

Burkitt lymphoma is a highly aggressive but potentially curable neoplasm. Patients with sustained remission one year following initial treatment are considered cured. High-intensity chemotherapy regimens with the addition of rituximab are the treatment of choice. Children have a better prognosis than adults, and in general, prognosis is related to the staging results. Cases arising in the setting of immune suppression may have a worse prognosis [62].

**Résumé**

| **Cutaneous manifestations of Burkitt lymphoma** | | |
|---|---|---|
| **Clinical** | Solitary, localized, or generalized cutaneous or subcutaneous, rapidly expanding tumors. | |
| **Morphology** | Diffuse infiltrates, sometimes with a "starry sky" pattern. Cohesive sheets of monomorphous, medium-sized or large blastoid cells. | |
| **Immunohistochemistry** | CD19, CD20 | + |
| | MYC | + (>80% of cells) |
| | IgM, Bcl-6, CD10 | + |
| | TdT | – |
| | Ki-67 | + (nearly 100% of cells) |
| | Bcl-2 | – (or weakly +) |
| **Genetics** | Monoclonal rearrangement of the *MYC* gene: t(8;14)(q24;q32), t(2;8)(p12;q24), or t(8;22)(q24;q11). | |
| **Treatment guidelines** | High-intensity chemotherapy regimens with the addition of rituximab. | |

## Cutaneous lymphomatoid granulomatosis

Lymphomatoid granulomatosis is a B-cell lymphoproliferative disorder associated with EBV infection. The disease has a spectrum of presentations and may progress to an overt diffuse large B-cell lymphoma. Lymphomatoid granulomatosis was described first by Liebow *et al.* in 1972 as an angiocentric and angiodestructive lymphoproliferative process in the lungs [63]. The disease is rare and more common in individuals with predisposing conditions (HIV infection, iatrogenic immune suppression after allogeneic organ transplantation, Wiskott–Aldrich syndrome, and X-linked lymphoproliferative syndrome). It is divided into three grades according to the proportion of large cells and of $EBV^+$ B lymphocytes in relation to the reactive infiltrate [64, 65]. Cases characterized by a diffuse proliferation of large B lymphocytes should not be classified as lymphomatoid granulomatosis but rather as EBV-associated diffuse large B-cell lymphoma [64], but the distinction between grade 3 lesions and overt lymphoma may be subjective. Uniform diagnostic criteria are still a matter of debate [66]. Although patients are usually not immunosuppressed, the disease may be related to defective immune surveillance [67].

## Clinical features

The most common site affected is the lungs, followed by the skin and central nervous system [68–72]. Patients are usually adults, but skin lesions have been observed in children [73]. The clinical presentation is characterized by multiple erythematous papules, plaques, or tumors, commonly ulcerated (Fig. 20.24). Sites of predilection are the trunk and extremities. Pulmonary and/or constitutional symptoms are almost invariably present, and bilateral lung nodules can be demonstrated radiologically. Cutaneous lesions are present at the time of diagnosis in about one-third of patients and may precede the development of lung lesions in 10–15% of cases [74], but true primary cutaneous cases have not been observed. In this context it is still a controversial issue whether lymphomatoid granulomatosis should be diagnosed in the skin in the absence of lung involvement. Great caution should be exercised in these cases, and the diagnosis should be made only if the histopathologic and phenotypic features are completely convincing. In fact, cutaneous lymphomatoid granulomatosis may reveal overlapping clinicopathologic features with other EBV-associated entities.

## Histopathology, immunophenotype, and molecular genetics

The histopathologic features of cutaneous manifestations of lymphomatoid granulomatosis depend on the grade of disease and type of lesions. In some cases, only a nonspecific perivascular and periadnexal infiltrate of small- to medium-sized cells can be seen. Cutaneous tumors of lymphomatoid granulomatosis are characterized by the presence of an angiocentric/angiodestructive infiltrate with variable numbers of large B lymphocytes (Figs. 20.25a and b). Granulomatous features are often present.

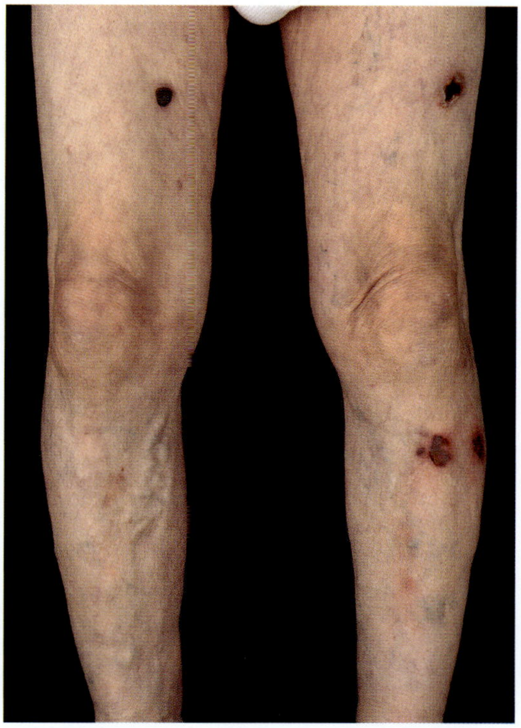

**Figure 20.24** Lymphomatoid granulomatosis. Ulcerated lesions on the legs.

The three histopathologic grades of lymphomatoid granulomatosis are defined as follows:

*Grade 1* lesions are characterized by a polymorphous lymphoid infiltrate without cytological atypia. Large cells are infrequent. EBER-1$^+$ cells, as detected by in situ hybridization techniques, are few or may even be absent in rare cases.

*Grade 2* lesions are characterized by a polymorphous inflammatory background with scattered large cells, sometimes organized in small clusters. EBER-1$^+$ cells are more numerous than in grade 1 lesions but do not form sheets.

In *grade 3* lesions, the polymorphous, inflammatory background is still detectable, but sheets of large B lymphocytes are present as well. As already mentioned, cases characterized by a diffuse proliferation of large B lymphocytes should not be classified as lymphomatoid granulomatosis but rather as EBV-associated diffuse large B-cell lymphoma, but the distinction may be subjective in given cases. In fact, it has been suggested that in the lung, lymphomatoid granulomatosis grades 2 and 3 cannot be clearly distinguished from diffuse large B-cell lymphoma [64].

The large B lymphocytes may show prominent pleomorphism and/or Hodgkin-like morphology. EBER-1$^+$ in situ hybridization shows many positive cells. The amount of necrosis increases in the three grades from absent or focal in grade 1 to prominent in grade 3 [72].

The large cells have a B-cell phenotype (Fig. 20.25c). It is important to remember that reactive small- to medium-sized lymphocytes with a T-helper phenotype are the predominant cells within the infiltrate, particularly in grades 1 and 2. As discussed before, most neoplastic B lymphocytes show a positive in situ hybridization signal for EBV (Fig. 20.25d). Molecular analyses reveal, in some cases, a monoclonal rearrangement of the Ig genes.

In the absence of a previous or concomitant diagnosis of lymphomatoid granulomatosis in the respiratory tract, a diagnosis of cutaneous lymphomatoid granulomatosis should be made only when all of the features described above are present.

## Treatment and prognosis

Different treatment modalities have been used for patients with cutaneous lesions of lymphomatoid granulomatosis, depending mainly on the grade of lesions at extracutaneous sites (e.g., interferon-α for grade 1 and 2 lesions, systemic chemotherapy and rituximab for grade 3) [67]. Successful treatment has been reported in isolated cases with autologous stem cell transplantation. The prognosis also depends on the grade and extent of extracutaneous involvement and is usually poor in advanced cases if aggressive treatment is not administered.

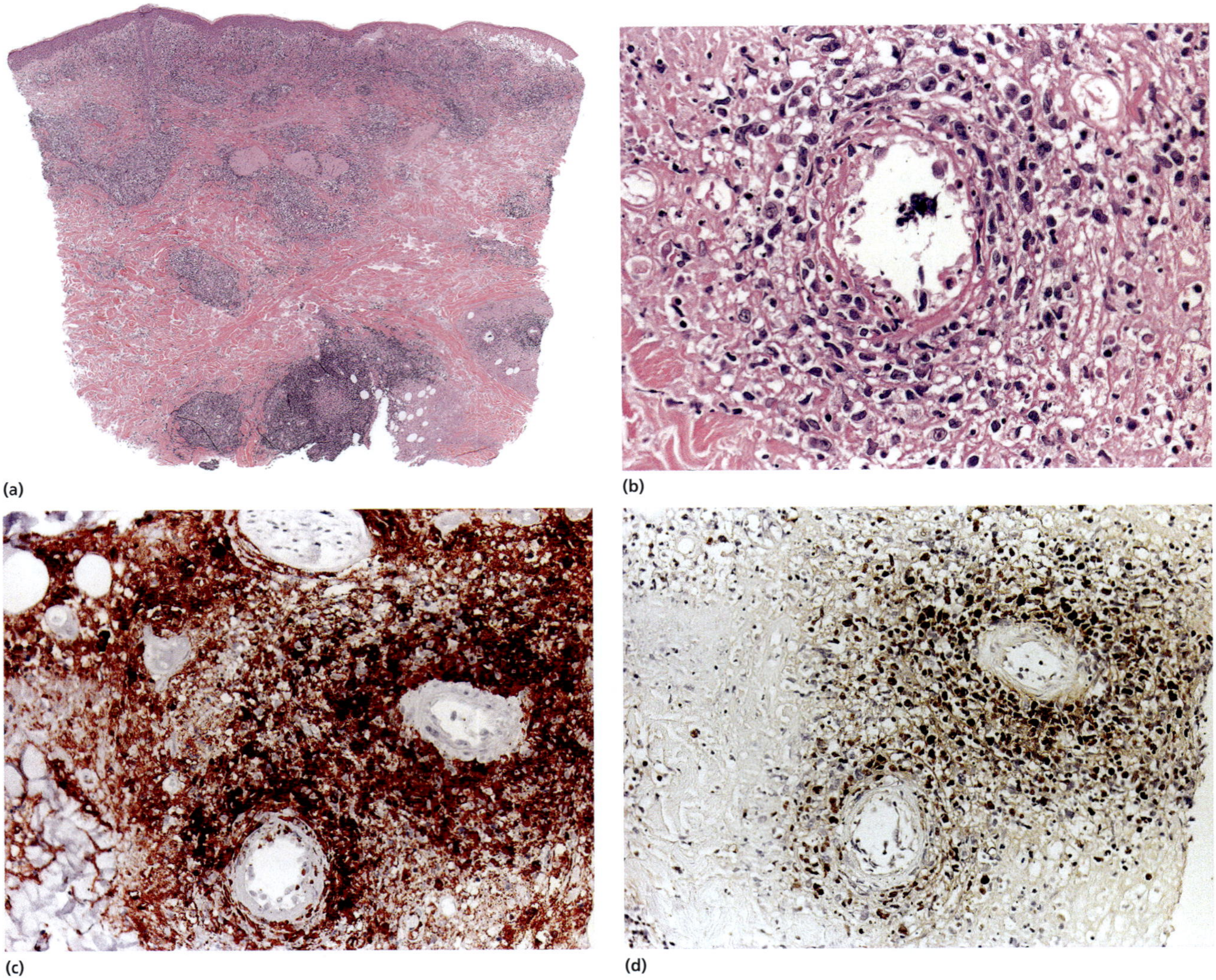


**Figure 20.25** Lymphomatoid granulomatosis. (a) Dense, partly angiocentric infiltrates within the entire dermis. (b) Detail of angiocentric architecture with large, atypical cells. (c) Expression of CD20 by perivascular large lymphocytes. (d) The large B lymphocytes reveal a positive signal upon in situ hybridization for EBV (EBER-1).

## Résumé

| **Cutaneous lymphomatoid granulomatosis** | | |
|---|---|---|
| **Clinical** | Adults (rarely children). Usually, multiple tumors. Lungs are almost invariably involved. | |
| **Morphology** | Depending on histopathologic grade, grade 2 and 3 lesions show angiocentric/angiodestructive infiltrates with the presence of variably large sheets of large B lymphocytes. Reactive T lymphocytes may predominate. | |
| **Immunohistochemistry** | CD19, CD20 | + (large B lymphocytes) |
| | CD3, CD4 | + (reactive small lymphocytes) |
| | EBER-1 | + (large B lymphocytes) |
| **Genetics** | Monoclonal rearrangement of the Ig genes. | |
| **Treatment guidelines** | Precise guidelines are not available for cutaneous cases. Systemic chemotherapy and rituximab are used for grade 3; interferon-α (grades 1 and 2). | |

## Cutaneous plasmablastic lymphoma

The entity of plasmablastic lymphoma of the oral cavity has been reported mainly (but not exclusively) in HIV+ individuals [75–78]. Cases have been observed less frequently also in other types of immunosuppression (including a post-transplant setting) or rarely in elderly immunocompetent individuals [79–83]. However, it seems that in HIV-endemic areas, virtually all cases are associated with HIV infection [84]. Although earlier reports suggested an association of plasmablastic lymphoma with HHV-8 infection [85], it has been demonstrated that most plasmablastic lymphomas are HHV-8-negative [86, 87]. Cases associated with HHV-8 represent a solid variant of primary effusion lymphoma rather than genuine plasmablastic lymphomas (see above in this Chapter) [87].

### Clinical features

Plasmablastic lymphoma presents mostly in adults with nodules and tumors arising in the oral mucosa (or at other mucosal sites). Cutaneous cases have been reported rarely [88–90].

### Histopathology, immunophenotype, and molecular genetics

Plasmablastic lymphoma shows a spectrum of morphologic presentations ranging from undifferentiated plasmablasts (large cells with immunoblast-like nuclei and only focally plasma cell-like cytoplasmic features) (Fig. 20.26) to plasmablasts with clear plasma cell differentiation (Fig. 20.27) and to more mature-looking plasma cells. An "Indian filing" arrangement of neoplastic cells may be observed (Fig. 20.28). The neoplastic cells are

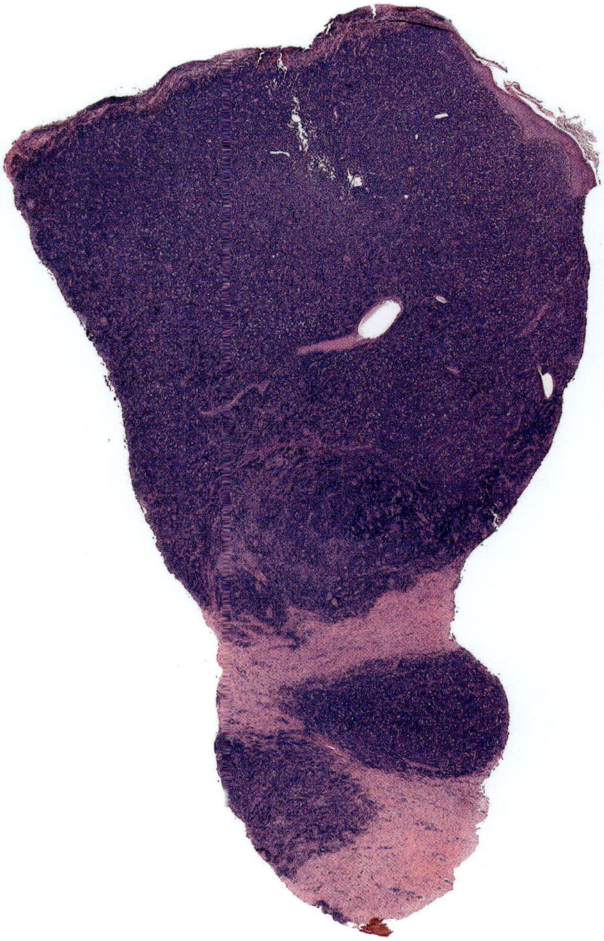

(a)

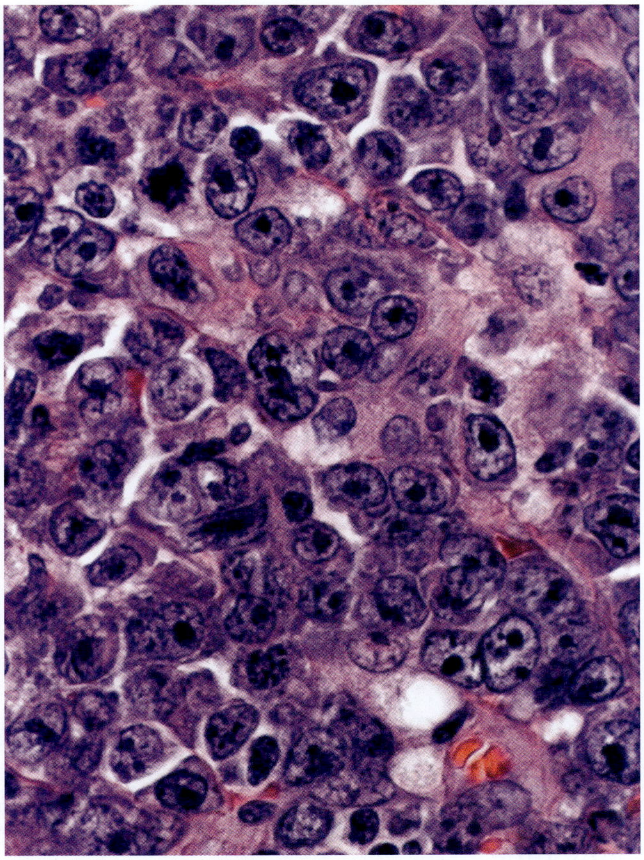

(b)

Figure 20.26 Cutaneous plasmablastic lymphoma. (a) Dense, monomorphous infiltrate within the entire dermis. (b) Plasmablasts with immunoblast-like nuclei, some of which are located eccentrically within a basophilic cytoplasm.

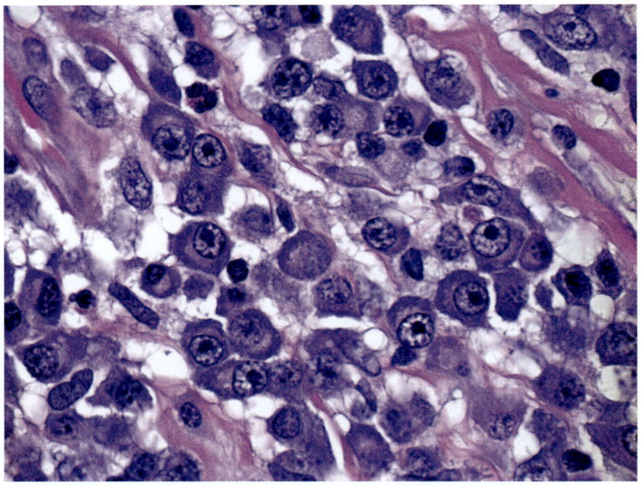

**Figure 20.27** Cutaneous plasmablastic lymphoma. More differentiated plasmablasts with plasma cell-like morphology and immunoblast-like nuclei.

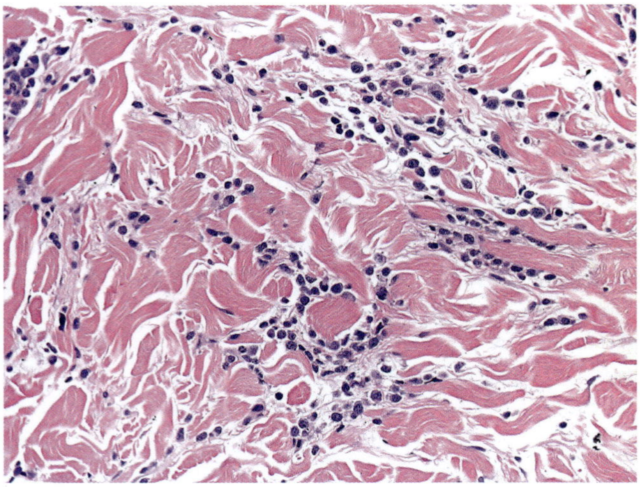

**Figure 20.28** Cutaneous plasmablastic lymphoma. Plasmablasts dissecting the collagen fibers with an “Indian filing” pattern.

usually negative for CD20, CD45, Bcl-6, Bcl-2, and PAX-5, but strongly positive for CD38, CD138, and MUM-1 and express monoclonal immunoglobulins in the majority of cases. CD56 and CD30 may be positive, and some cases may show aberrant expression of CD3 (Fig. 20.29) [91]. Two different phenotypic variants have been described, the first carrying a full plasmablastic phenotype and the second showing a defective phenotype [92]. ALK and HHV-8 stainings should be performed, and positive cases should be classified as ALK$^+$ diffuse large B-cell lymphoma or extracavitary primary effusion lymphoma, respectively.

In situ hybridization for EBV is positive in the majority of the cases, and in nearly all cases arising within the oral cavity (Fig. 20.30). Monoclonal rearrangement of the Ig genes is usually demonstrable. *MYC* translocations, associated with MYC protein expression, can be observed in the majority of the cases (more often in EBV$^+$ cases) [93].

### Treatment and prognosis

Plasmablastic lymphoma is extremely aggressive, and survival is usually very short (<1 year). Better management of the underlying disease may improve the prognosis in cases associated with HIV. The presence of *MYC* translocations may be associated with a worse prognosis.

### Résumé

**Cutaneous plasmablastic lymphoma**

| | | |
|---|---|---|
| **Clinical** | Adults. Cases arising within the oral cavity are related to HIV infection. Cutaneous cases have also been observed in other types of immune suppression and rarely in immune competent individuals. | |
| **Morphology** | Plasmablasts (large cells with mixed features of immunoblasts and plasma cells). | |
| **Immunohistochemistry** | CD19, CD20, CD45, PAX5, Bcl-2, Bcl-6 | – |
| | CD38, CD138 | + |
| | MUM-1 | + |
| | MYC | + (–) |
| | ALK | – |
| | Ig light chains | monoclonal expression |
| **Genetics** | Monoclonal rearrangement of the Ig genes. *MYC* translocations are found in the majority of cases. | |
| **Treatment guidelines** | Systemic chemotherapy: treatment of the background disease in HIV-associated cases. | |

## Cutaneous T-cell/histiocyte-rich large B-cell lymphoma

T-cell/histiocyte-rich large B-cell lymphoma is characterized by the malignant proliferation of B lymphocytes, admixed with a predominant population of reactive histiocytes and/or T lymphocytes. For a diagnosis of T-cell/histiocyte-rich large B-cell lymphoma, neoplastic large B-cells should not exceed 10% of the infiltrate and should be scattered without forming nodules or sheets. Nodal T-cell/histiocyte-rich B-cell lymphoma is considered to be a variant of the diffuse large B-cell lymphomas and is included as such in the ICC

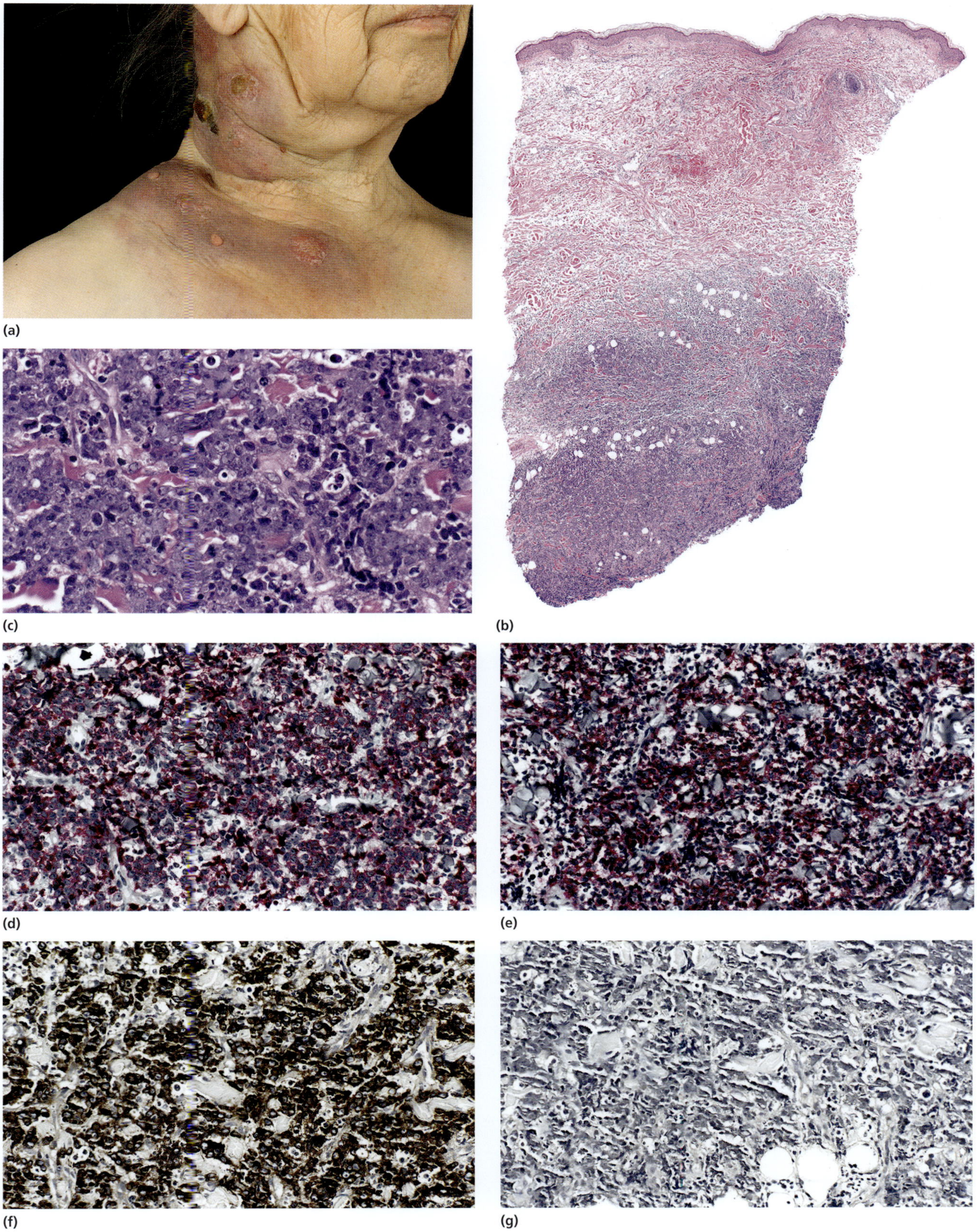

**Figure 20.29** Cutaneous plasmablastic lymphoma. (a) Infiltrated, confluent tumors on the lateral side of the neck. (b) Nodular infiltrate at the base of the biopsy, characterized by (c) large, blastoid cells, some with features of immunoblasts. Positivity of neoplastic cells for (d) CD3, (e) CD138 and (f) kappa light chain; (g) positivity for lambda. Positivity for CD3 and negativity for CD20 in this case was the reason for an initial misdiagnosis of T-cell lymphoma.

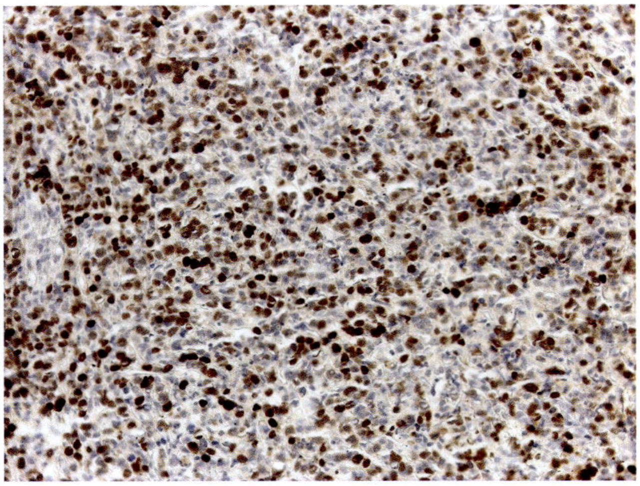

Figure 20.30 Cutaneous plasmablastic lymphoma. Most cells reveal a positive signal upon in situ hybridization for EBV (EBER-1).

Lymphoma Classification and the WHO *Classification of Haematolymphoid Tumours* [94, 95]. Cutaneous involvement seems to be extremely uncommon, but rare cases arising primary in the skin have been published [96–100]. In the past, this lymphoma was described under the term "T-cell-rich B-cell lymphoma".

Personally, I have never encountered convincing examples of primary cutaneous T-cell/histiocyte-rich large B-cell lymphoma as defined in the ICC or WHO classifications. On the other hand, I have observed rare cases of cutaneous follicle center lymphoma, diffuse type, that in one of the biopsies or, more frequently, in part of a biopsy showed histopathologic features similar to those of T-cell/histiocyte-rich large B-cell lymphoma. In this context, I believe that in the skin, this morphologic presentation represents a variation of the follicle center lymphoma, diffuse type.

## Clinical features

Patients with T-cell/histiocyte-rich large B-cell lymphoma are adults of either gender. Clinically, they present with erythematous papules, plaques, or nodules, usually on the face and trunk. As mentioned before, cases presenting primary in the skin probably represent variations of follicle center lymphoma, diffuse type.

## Histopathology, immunophenotype, and molecular genetics

Histology shows large blasts admixed with a predominant population of small lymphocytes (Figs. 20.31a and b). In a few patients, a biphasic pattern has been observed, suggesting that cutaneous T-cell/histiocyte-rich B-cell lymphoma represents a morphologic variation of a pre-existing low-grade (follicle center) B-cell lymphoma of the skin. Angiocentricity may be observed rarely [101].

Immunohistology reveals the B-cell phenotype of the large cells (CD20$^+$, CD30$^-$), often with positivity for markers of germinal center lineage such as Bcl-6 (Fig. 20.31c). The small reactive lymphocytes express a T-helper phenotype (CD3$^+$, CD4$^+$, CD8$^-$). Staining for Ki-67 highlights the proliferating large cells on the background of small reactive lymphocytes (Fig. 20.31d). EBV is not detected.

Molecular genetics shows a polyclonal pattern of T-cell receptor (TCR) genes, and in most cases, a monoclonal rearrangement of the Ig genes. In lesions showing no evidence of monoclonal rearrangement of the Ig genes, the negativity is probably due to the small number of neoplastic cells admixed with high numbers of reactive lymphocytes. PCR analysis after microdissection of large cells may be a useful tool for confirmation of monoclonality in such cases.

## Treatment and prognosis

As in other cases of primary cutaneous follicle center lymphoma, management of patients with disease confined to the skin should not be aggressive (surgical excision and/or local radiotherapy), at least as a first-line treatment strategy. An indolent behavior has been described in a small number of cases arising primary in the skin, confirming that they belong to the group of low-grade cutaneous B-cell lymphomas [97, 99].

### Résumé

**Cutaneous T-cell/histiocyte-rich large B-cell lymphoma**

| | | |
|---|---|---|
| **Clinical** | Adults. Erythematous papules, plaques, and nodules. Preferential locations: face, trunk. Primary cutaneous cases probably represent a variant of the cutaneous follicle center lymphoma, diffuse type. | |
| **Morphology** | <10% of large B cells, not forming nodules or sheets, are scattered in the background of a predominant population of T lymphocytes and histiocytes. | |
| **Immunohistochemistry** | CD19, CD20, CD79a | + |
| | Bcl-6 | + |
| | CD3, CD4 | + (reactive lymphocytes) |
| | CD30 | – |
| | EBER-1 | – |
| **Genetics** | Monoclonal rearrangement of the Ig genes (may be undetectable due to small numbers of neoplastic lymphocytes admixed with many reactive cells). | |
| **Treatment guidelines** | Primary cutaneous cases should be treated in the same manner as cutaneous follicle center lymphoma. | |

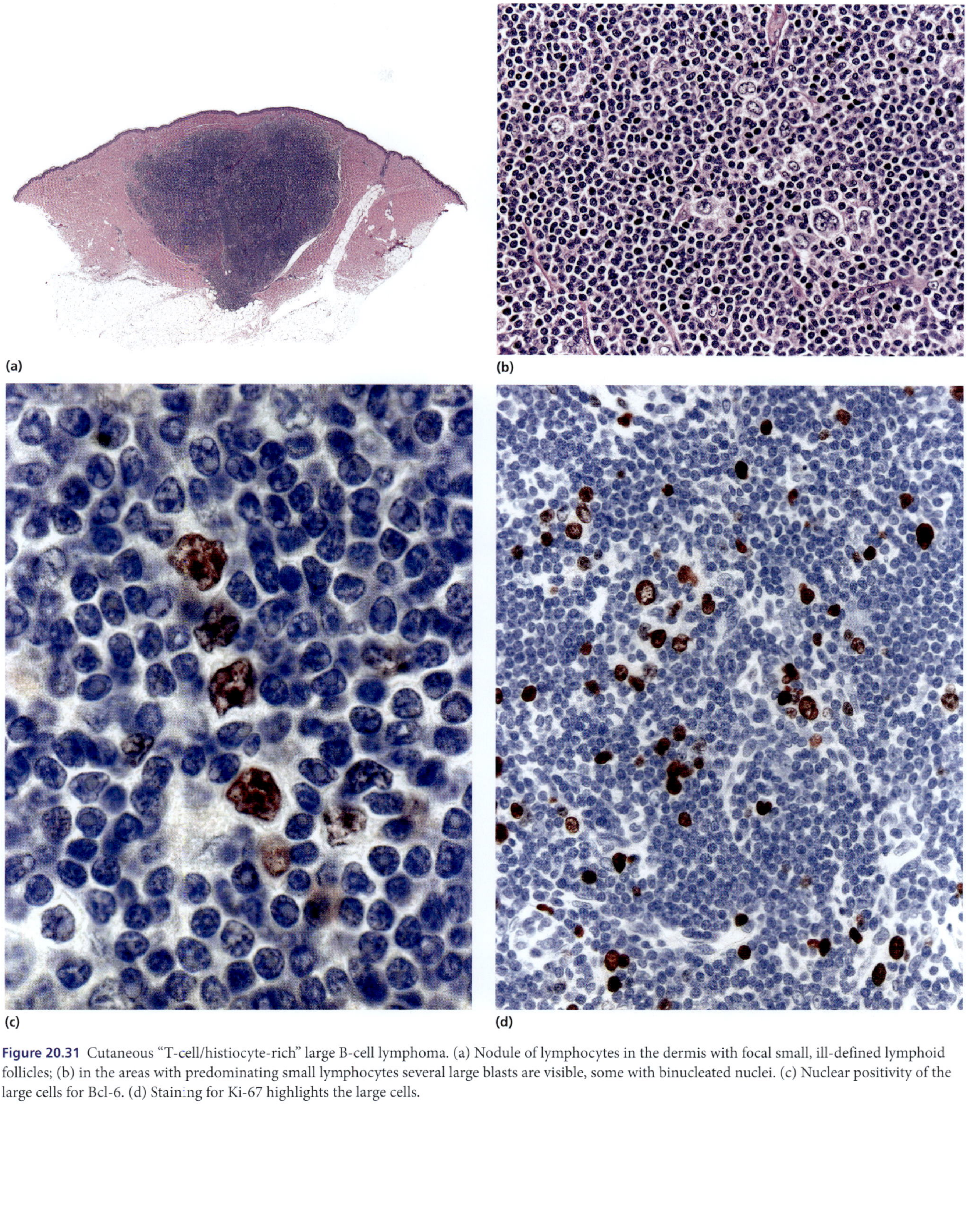

(a) (b) (c) (d)

Figure 20.31 Cutaneous "T-cell/histiocyte-rich" large B-cell lymphoma. (a) Nodule of lymphocytes in the dermis with focal small, ill-defined lymphoid follicles; (b) in the areas with predominating small lymphocytes several large blasts are visible, some with binucleated nuclei. (c) Nuclear positivity of the large cells for Bcl-6. (d) Staining for Ki-67 highlights the large cells.

## Cutaneous manifestations of Waldenström macroglobulinemia

Waldenström macroglobulinemia is characterized by the presence of a monoclonal IgM paraprotein in patients with lymphoplasmacytic lymphoma involving the bone marrow. In lymphoma classifications, it is considered as an IgM variant of lymphoplasmacytic lymphoma [102, 103]. Specific cutaneous involvement by neoplastic cells is rare but has been reported [104], whereas cutaneous manifestations related to the monoclonal paraprotein are less rare (including monoclonal cryoglobulinemia, bullous dermatoses, storage papules, crystal-storing histiocytosis, and cutaneous amyloidosis—see Chapter 29).

### Clinical features

Patients with specific (neoplastic) skin manifestations present with non-descript papules, infiltrated plaques, or tumors (Fig. 20.32). Paraproteinemia was present in all reported cases, with proteinuria detected in a minority of them (reviewed in [104]).

### Histopathology, immunophenotype, and molecular genetics

Most reported cases presented with dense, diffuse dermal infiltrates of lymphoplasmacytoid cells, often extending to the subcutis. In some cases, the infiltrate may be sparse, and neoplastic cells may also be identified within the blood vessels (Fig. 20.33). In one patient with known Waldenström macroglobulinemia, I have observed a specific manifestation of the disease at the site of a basal cell carcinoma on the ear (Fig. 20.34).

Immunohistochemical studies are fragmentary, but IgM heavy chain and kappa light chains were expressed in several reported cases. Molecular genetics shows a monoclonal rearrangement of the immunoglobulin genes. In one case involving the skin, the typical *MYD88* L265P mutation of lymphoplasmacytic lymphoma has been detected, representing a helpful clue to confirm the diagnosis [104].

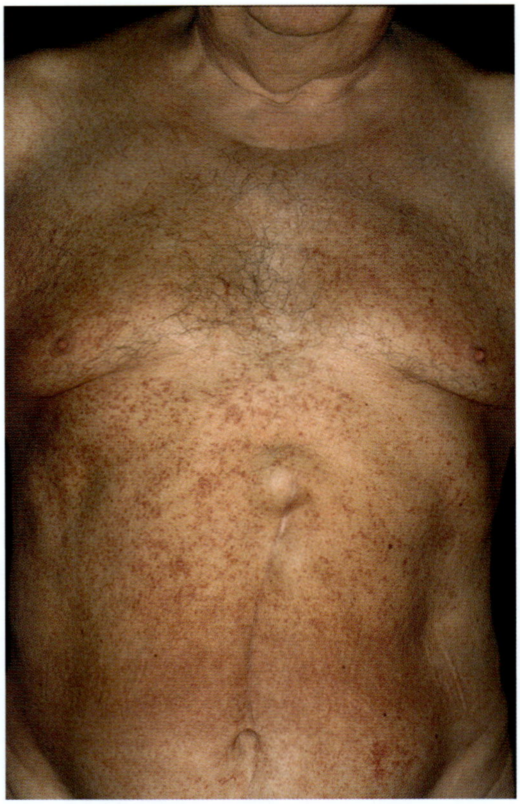

**Figure 20.32** Cutaneous manifestations of Waldenström macroglobulinemia. Generalized erythematous papules.

### Treatment and prognosis

Waldenström macroglobulinemia has an indolent course, but rare cases with large cell transformation have a worse prognosis [105]. Chlorambucil, fludarabine-based regimens, rituximab, and ibrutinib are used among other options, but the management of cutaneous cases should be done in a hematological setting. One cutaneous case presenting the typical *MYD88* L265P mutation has been successfully treated with ibrutinib [104].

### Résumé

**Cutaneous manifestations in Waldenström macroglobulinemia**

| | | |
|---|---|---|
| **Clinical** | Non-descript infiltrated papules or tumors (for skin manifestations related to paraproteinemia, see Chapter 29). | |
| **Morphology** | Histology shows a variably dense proliferation of lymphoplasmacytoid cells. | |
| **Immunohistochemistry** | CD20, CD79a | + |
| | IgM | + |
| | Ig light chains | + (mostly kappa) |
| **Genetics** | Monoclonal rearrangement of the immunoglobulin genes. The typical *MYD88* L265P mutation found in extracutaneous cases has also been reported in one case involving the skin. | |
| **Treatment guidelines** | Chlorambucil; fludarabine-based regimens; rituximab; ibrutinib. | |

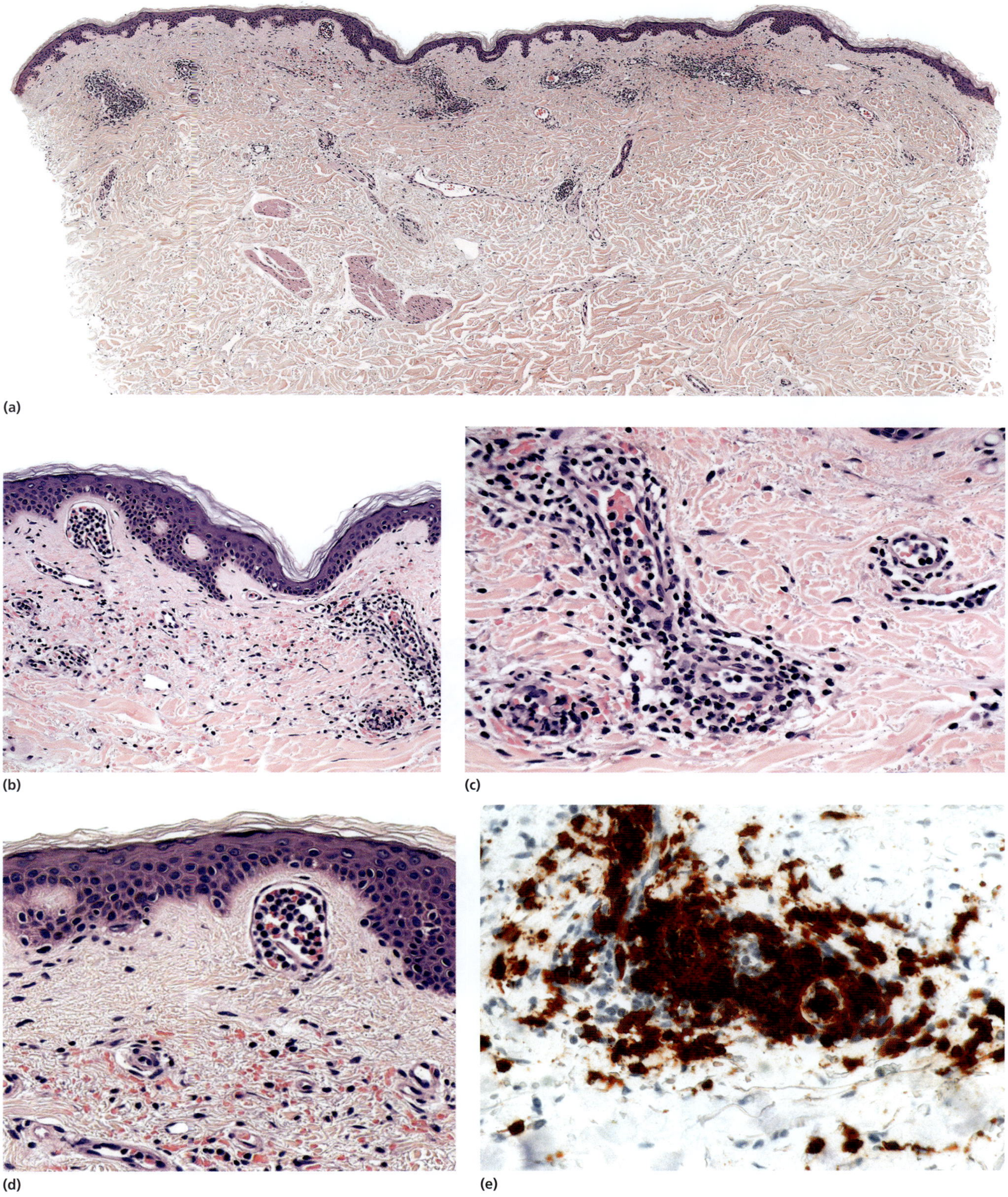


**Figure 20.33** Cutaneous manifestations of Waldenström macroglobulinemia. (a, b, c) Sparse, superficial dermal infiltrate composed of lymphoplasmacytoid cells with (d) intravascular complexes of cells. (e) All cells are positive for CD20.

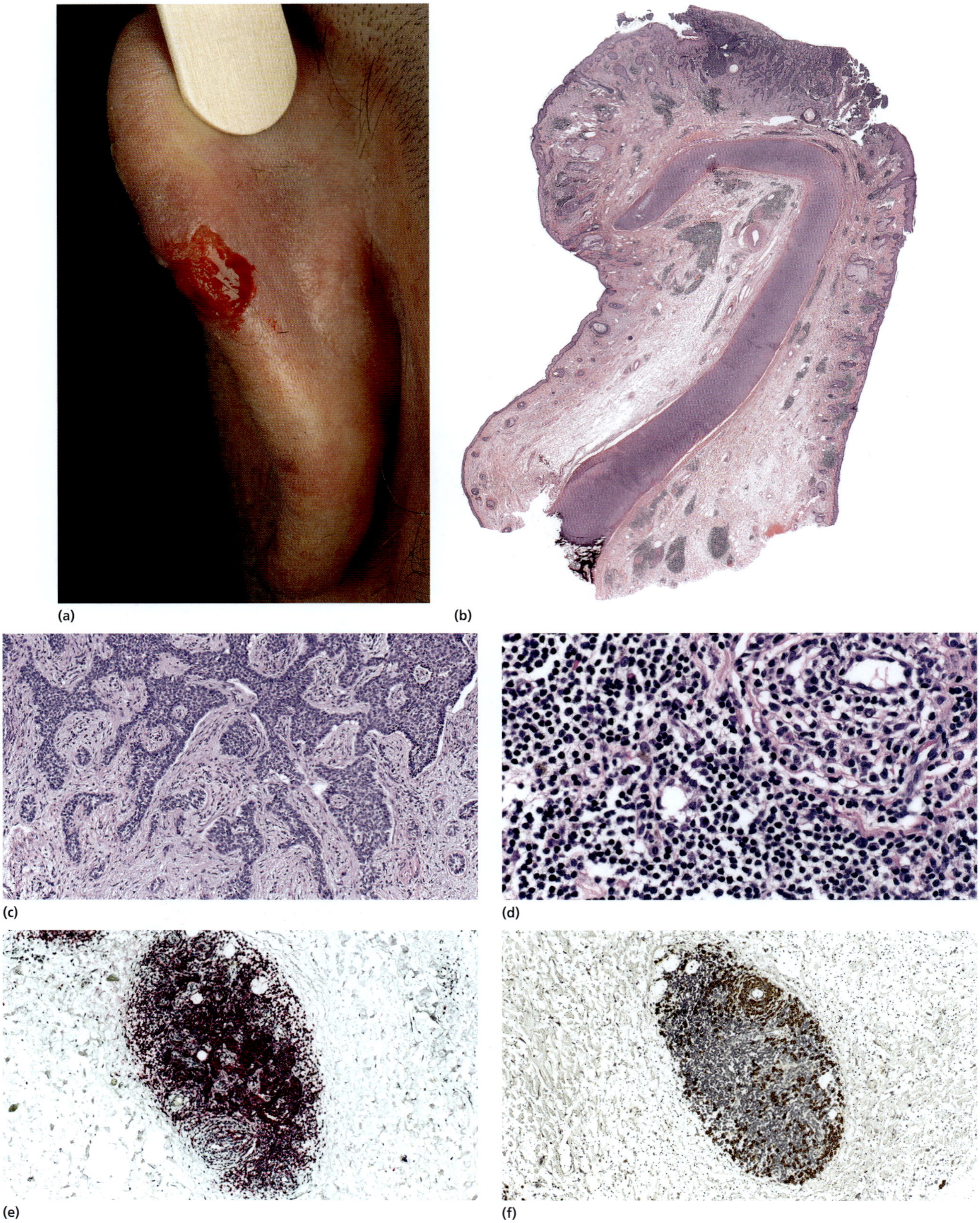

Figure 20.34 Cutaneous manifestations of Waldenström macroglobulinemia at the site of a basal cell carcinoma. (a) Ulcerated lesion on the left ear. (b) Histology shows an ulcerated basaloid tumor with (c) features of fibrosing basal cell carcinoma. (d) Dense perivascular lymphoid infiltrates admixed with several plasmacytoid cells and plasma cells. (e) Most lymphocytes are positive for CD20; (f) in situ-hybridization reveals monoclonal expression of kappa light chain.

## References


1. Lee WJ, Won KH, Won CH, *et al.* Secondary cutaneous lymphoma: comparative clinical features and survival outcome analysis of 106 cases according to lymphoma cell lineage. *Br J Dermatol* 2015;**173**:134–145.
2. Hedayat AA, Carter JB, Lansigan F, *et al.* Epidermotropic presentation by splenic B-cell lymphoma: the importance of clinical-pathologic correlation. *J Cutan Pathol* 2018;**45**:299–304.
3. Anagnostopoulos I, Lenz G, Asano N, *et al.* EBV-positive diffuse large B-cell lymphoma. In: *WHO Classification of Tumours Editorial Board. Haematolymphoid Tumours*. 5th edition. Lyon (France): IARC, 2024: 493–496.
4. Jaffe ES, Pittaluga S, Wilson WH. Epstein-Barr virus-positive diffuse large B-cell lymphoma, not otherwise specified. In: Arber DA, Borowitz MJ, Cook JR, *et al.*, eds. *The International Consensus Classification of Myeloid and Lymphoid Neoplasms*. Philadelphia (US): Wolters Kluver, 2025: 514–517.
5. Oyama T, Ichimura K, Suzuki R, *et al.* Senile EBV+ B-cell lymphoproliferative disorders A clinicopathologic study of 22 patients. *Am J Surg Pathol* 2003;**27**:16–26.
6. Wong HH, Wang J. Epstein–Barr virus positive diffuse large B-cell lymphoma of the elderly. *Leuk Lymphoma* 2009;**50**:335–340.
7. Nicolae A, Pittaluga S, Abdullah S, *et al.* EBV-positive large B-cell lymphomas in young patients: a nodal lymphoma with evidence for a tolerogenic immune environment. *Blood* 2015;**126**:863–872.
8. Hong JY, Yoon DH, Suh C, *et al.* EBVpositive diffuse large B-cell lymphoma in young adults: is this a distinct disease entity? *Ann Oncol* 2015;**26**:548–555.
9. Oyama T, Yamamoto K, Asano N, *et al.* Age-related EBV-associated B-cell lymphoproliferative disorders constitute a distinct clinicopathologic group: a study of 96 patients. *Clin Cancer Res* 2007;**13**: 5124–5132.
10. Dojcinov SD, Venkataraman G, Pittaluga S, *et al.* Age-related EBV-associated lymphoproliferative disorders in the Western population: a spectrum of reactive lymphoid hyperplasia and lymphoma. *Blood* 2011;**117**:4726–4735.
11. Hoeller S, Tzankov A, Pileri SA, *et al.* Epstein–Barr virus-positive diffuse large B-cell lymphoma in elderly patients is rare in Western populations. *Hum Pathol* 2010;**41**:352–357.
12. Hofscheier A, Ponciano A, Bonzheim I, *et al.* Geographic variation in the prevalence of Epstein–Barr virus-positive diffuse large B-cell lymphoma of the elderly: a comparative analysis of a Mexican and a German population. *Mod Pathol* 2011;**24**:1046–1054.
13. Ok CY, Papathomas TG, Medeiros LJ, Young KH. EBV-positive diffuse large B-cell lymphoma of the elderly. *Blood* 2013;**122**:328–340.
14. Montes-Moreno S, Odqvist L, Diaz-Perez JA, *et al.* EBV-positive diffuse large B-cell lymphoma of the elderly is an aggressive post-germinal center B-cell neoplasm characterized by prominent nuclear factor-kB activation. *Mod Pathol* 2012;**25**:968–982.
15. Lee LY, Namuduri R, Chan MMF, *et al.* Epstein-Barr virus positive diffuse large B-cell lymphoma presenting with vaginal sloughing and ulcerated skin nodule. *J Cutan Pathol* 2018;**45**:162–166.
16. Gibson SE, Hsi ED. Epstein–Barr virus-positive B-cell lymphoma of the elderly at a United States tertiary medical center: an uncommon aggressive lymphoma with a nongerminal center B-cell phenotype. *Hum Pathol* 2009;**40**:653–661.
17. Martin B, Whittaker S, Morris S, *et al.* A case of primary cutaneous senile EBV-related diffuse large B-cell lymphoma. *Am J Dermatopathol* 2010;**32**:190–193.
18. Gaitonde S, Kavuri S, Alagiozian-Angelova V, *et al.* EBV positivity in primary cutaneous large B-cell lymphoma with immunophenotypic features of leg type: an isolated incidence or something more significant? *Acta Oncol* 2008;**47**:461–464.
19. Gebauer N, Künstner A, Ketzer J, *et al.* Genomic insights into the pathogenesis of Epstein-Barr virus-associated diffuse large B-cell lymphoma by whole-genome and targeted amplicon sequencing. *Blood Cancer J* 2021;**11**:102.
20. Klapper W, Medeiros JL, Ferry JA, *et al.* Mantle cell lymphoma. In: *WHO Classification of Tumours Editorial Board. Haematolymphoid Tumours*. 5th edition. Lyon (France): IARC, 2024: 446–452.
21. Campo E, Dreyling M, Sander B, Zelenetz AD. Mantle cell lymphoma: conventional and leukemic nonmodal subtypes. In: Arber DA, Borowitz MJ, Cook JR, *et al.*, eds. *The International Consensus Classification of Myeloid and Lymphoid Neoplasms*. Philadelphia (US): Wolters Kluver, 2025: 462–471.
22. Sen F, Medeiros LJ, Lu D, *et al.* Mantle cell lymphoma involving skin: cutaneous lesions may be the first manifestation of disease and tumors often have blastoid cytologic features. *Am J Surg Pathol* 2002;**26**:1312–1318.
23. Dubus P, Young P, Beylot-Barry M, *et al.* Value of interphase FISH for the diagnosis of t(11,14)(q13;q32) on skin lesions of mantle cell lymphoma. *Am J Clin Pathol* 2002;**118**:832–841.
24. Marti RM, Campo E, Bosch F, *et al.* Cutaneous lymphocyte-associated antigen (CLA) expression in a lymphoblastoid mantle cell lymphoma presenting with skin lesions: comparison with other clinicopathologic presentations of mantle cell lymphoma. *J Cutan Pathol* 2001;**28**:256–264.
25. Geerts ML, Busschots AM. Mantle-cell lymphomas of the skin. *Dermatol Clin* 1994;**12**:409–417.
26. Gru AA, Hurley MY, Salavaggione AL, *et al.* Cutaneous mantle cell lymphoma: a clinicopathologic review of 10 cases. *J Cutan Pathol* 2016;**43**:1112–1120.
27. Kim DH, Medeiros LJ, Aung PP, *et al.* Mantle cell lymphoma involving skin: a clinicopathologic study of 37 cases. *Am J Surg Pathol* 2019;**43**:1421–1428.
28. Bertero M, Novelli M, Fierro MT, Bernengo MG. Mantle zone lymphoma: an immunohistologic study of skin lesions. *J Am Acad Dermatol* 1994;**30**:23–30.
29. Laggis C, Miles R, Stephens DM, *et al.* Cutaneous mantle cell lymphoma histomorphologically mimicking subcutaneous panniculitis-like T-cell lymphoma: case report. *J Cutan Pathol* 2019; **46**:538–541.
30. Wehkamp U, Pott C, Unterhalt M, *et al.* Skin involvement of mantle cell lymphoma may mimic primary cutaneous diffuse large B-cell lymphoma, leg type. *Am J Surg Pathol* 2015;**39**:1093–1101.
31. Panse G, Cowper S, Ko CJ, Subtil A. Cutaneous involvement by mantle cell lymphoma: expanding the spectrum of histopathologic findings in a Series of 9 Cases. *Am J Dermatopathol* 2020;**42**: 848–853.
32. Schlette E, Fu K, Medeiros LJ. CD23 expression in mantle cell lymphoma: clinicopathologic features of 18 cases. *Am J Clin Pathol* 2003;**120**:760–766.

33. Moody BR, Bartlett NL, George DW, *et al.* Cyclin D1 as an aid in the diagnosis of mantle cell lymphoma in skin biopsies: a case report. *Am J Dermatopathol* 2001;**23**:470–476.
34. Clot G, Jares P, Giné E, *et al.* A gene signature that distinguishes conventional and leukemic non-nodal mantle cell lymphoma helps predict outcome. *Blood* 2018;**132**:413–422.
35. Pizzi M, Agostinelli C, Righi S, *et al.* Aberrant expression of CD10 and BCL6 in mantle cell lymphoma. *Histopathology* 2017;**71**: 769–777.
36. Grainger BT, Cheah CY. "The End of the Golden Weather": therapeutic strategies for mantle cell lymphoma relapsed or refractory to covalent BTK inhibitors. *Haematologica* 2025;**110**: 576–587.
37. Hoster E, Rosenwald A, Berger F, *et al.* Prognostic value of Ki-67 index, cytology, and growth pattern in mantle-cell lymphoma: results from randomized trials of the European mantle cell lymphoma network. *J Clin Oncol* 2016;**34**:1386–1394.
38. Said JW, Chadburn A, Bacon CM, *et al.* Primary effusion lymphoma. In: *WHO Classification of Tumours Editorial Board. Haematolymphoid Tumours*. 5th edition. Lyon (France): IARC, 2024: 541–544.
39. Piris MA, Campo E, Carbone A. Human herpesvirus 8-associated lymphoproliferative disorders. In: Arber DA, Borowitz MJ, Cook JR, *et al.*, eds. *The International Consensus Classification of Myeloid and Lymphoid Neoplasms*. Philadelphia (US): Wolters Kluver, 2025: 538–545.
40. Pan ZG, Zhang QY, Lu ZB, *et al.* Extracavitary KSHV-associated large B-cell lymphoma – a distinct entity or a subtype of primary effusion lymphoma? Study of 9 cases and review of an additional 43 cases. *Am J Surg Pathol* 2012;**36**:1129–1140.
41. Gonzalez-Farre B, Martinez D, Lopez-Guerra M, *et al.* HHV8-related lymphoid proliferations: a broad spectrum of lesions from reactive lymphoid hyperplasia to overt lymphoma. *Mod Pathol* 2017;**30**:745–760.
42. Liu W, Lacouture ME, Jiang J, *et al.* KSHV/HHV8-associated primary cutaneous plasmablastic lymphoma in a patient with Castleman's disease and Kaposi's sarcoma. *J Cutan Pathol* 2006;**33**(suppl. 2):46–51.
43. Pielasinski U, Santonja C, Rodríguez-Pinilla SM, Requena L. Extracavitary primary effusion lymphoma presenting as a cutaneous tumor: a case report and literature review. *J Cutan Pathol* 2014;**41**:745–753.
44. Li MF, Hsiao CH, Chen YL, *et al.* Human herpesvirus 8-associated lymphoma mimicking cutaneous anaplastic large T-cell lymphoma in a patient with human immunodeficiency virus infection. *J Cutan Pathol* 2012;**39**:274–278.
45. Crane GM, Ambinder RF, Shirley CM, *et al.* HHV-8-positive and EBV-positive intravascular lymphoma. An unusual presentation of extracavitary primary effusion lymphoma. *Am J Surg Pathol* 2014;**38**:426–432.
46. Saggini A, Di Prete M, Facchetti S, *et al.* Panniculitis-like presentation of extracavitary primary effusion lymphoma. *Am J Dermatopathol* 2020;**42**:446–451.
47. Willemze R, Cerroni L, Kempf W, *et al.* The 2018 update of the WHO-EORTC classification for primary cutaneous lymphomas. *Blood* 2019;**133**:1703–1714.
48. Requena L, Kutzner H, Palmedo G, *et al.* Cutaneous involvement in multiple myeloma: a clinicopathologic, immunohistochemical, and cytogenetic study of 8 cases. *Arch Dermatol* 2003;**139**:475–486.
49. Hussong JW, Perkins SL, Schnitzer B, *et al.* Extramedullary plasmacytoma: a form of marginal zone cell lymphoma? *Am J Clin Pathol* 1999;**111**:111–116.
50. Woo YR, Kim JS, Lim JH, *et al.* Prevalence and clinicopathologic characteristics of multiple myeloma with cutaneous involvement: a case series from Korea. *J Am Acad Dermatol* 2018;**78**:471–478.
51. Boyle S, Hourigan M. Cutaneous seeding of neoplastic plasma cells to a site of bruising in a patient with relapsed myeloma. *Br J Haematol* 2018;**181**:723.
52. Varricchio S, Pagliuca F, Travaglino A, *et al.* Cutaneous localization of plasmablastic multiple myeloma with heterotopic expression of CD3 and CD4: skin involvement revealing systemic disease. *J Cutan Pathol* 2019;**46**:619–622.
53. Jiwani S, Bornhost J, Alapat D. Biphenotypic plasma cell myeloma: two cases of plasma cell neoplasm with a coexpression of kappa and lambda light chains. *Int J Clin Exp Pathol* 2015;**8**:8536–8544.
54. Marks E, Shi Y, Wang Y. CD117 (KIT) is a useful marker in the diagnosis of plasmablastic plasma cell myeloma. *Histopathology* 2017;**71**:81–88.
55. Sayed S, Leoncini L, Cheuk W, *et al.* Burkitt lymphoma. In: *WHO Classification of Tumours Editorial Board. Haematolymphoid Tumours*. 5th edition. Lyon (France): IARC, 2024: 532–538.
56. His ED, Friedberg JW, Link M, Perry AM. Burkitt lamphoma. In: Arber DA, Borowitz MJ, Cook JR, *et al.*, eds. *The International Consensus Classification of Myeloid and Lymphoid Neoplasms*. Philadelphia (US): Wolters Kluver, 2025: 546–551.
57. Fuhrmann TL, Ignatovich YV, Pentland A. Cutaneous metastatic disease: Burkitt lymphoma. *J Am Acad Dermatol* 2011;**64**:1196–1197.
58. Pettey AA, Walsh JS. Cutaneous involvement with Burkitt-like lymphoma. *Am J Dermatopathol* 2007;**29**:184–186.
59. Thakkar D, Lipi L, Misra R, Yadav SP. Skin involvement in Burkitt's lymphoma. *Hematol Oncol Stem Cell Ther* 2018;**11**:251–252.
60. Testo N, Olson LC, Subramaniyam S, *et al.* Primary cutaneous diffuse large B-cell lymphoma with a MYC-IGH rearrangement and gain of BCL2: expanding the spectrum of MYC/BCL2 double-hit lymphomas. *Am J Dermatopathol* 2016;**38**:769–774.
61. Zhou P, Blain AE, Newman AM, *et al.* Sporadic and endemic Burkitt lymphoma have frequent FOXO1 mutations but distinct hotspots in the AKT recognition motif. *Blood Adv* 2019;**3**: 2118–2127.
62. De Masson A, Velter C, Galicier L, *et al.* Disseminated skin involvement in HIV-associated Burkitt lymphoma: a rare clinical feature with poor prognosis. *Br J Dermatol* 2016;**174**:184–186.
63. Liebow AA, Carrington CR, Friedman PJ. Lymphomatoid granulomatosis. *Hum Pathol* 1972;**3**:457–558.
64. Anagnostopoulos I, Deckert M, Nicholson AG, Siebert R. Lymphomatoid granulomatosis. In: *WHO Classification of Tumours Editorial Board. Haematolymphoid Tumours*. 5th edition. Lyon (France): IARC, 2024: 489–492.
65. Jaffe ES, Melani C, Pittaluga S. Lymphomatoid granulomatosis. In: Arber DA, Borowitz MJ, Cook JR, *et al.*, eds. *The International Consensus Classification of Myeloid and Lymphoid Neoplasms*. Philadelphia (US): Wolters Kluver, 2025: 523–526.

66. Katzenstein ALA, Doxtader E, Narendra S. Lymphomatoid granulomatosis. Insights gained over 4 decades. *Am J Surg Pathol* 2010;**34**:e35–e48.
67. Melani C, Jaffe ES, Wilson WH. Pathobiology and treatment of lymphomatoid granulomatosis, a rare EBV-driven disorder. *Blood* 2020;**135**:1344–1352.
68. Katzenstein ALA, Carrington CB, Liebow AA. Lymphomatoid granulomatosis: a clinicopathologic study of 152 cases. *Cancer* 1979;**43**:360–373.
69. Beaty MW, Toro J, Sorbara L, *et al.* Cutaneous lymphomatoid granulomatosis: correlation of clinical and biologic features. *Am J Surg Pathol* 2001;**25**:1111–1120.
70. Carlson KC, Gibson LE. Cutaneous signs of lymphomatoid granulomatosis. *Arch Dermatol* 1991;**127**:1693–1698.
71. McNiff JM, Cooper D, Howe G, *et al.* Lymphomatoid granulomatosis of the skin and lung: an angiocentric T-cell-rich B-cell lymphoproliferative disorder. *Arch Dermatol* 1996;**132**:1464–1470.
72. Song JY, Pittaluga S, Dunleavy K, *et al.* Lymphomatoid granulomatosis—a single institute experience pathologic findings and clinical correlations. *Am J Surg Pathol* 2015;**39**:141–156.
73. LeSueur BW, Ellsworth L, Bangert JL, Hansen RC. Lymphomatoid granulomatosis in a 4-year-old boy. *Pediatr Dermatol* 2000;**17**:369–372.
74. Rysgaard CD, Stone MS. Lymphomatoid granulomatosis presenting with cutaneous involvement: a case report and review of the literature. *J Cutan Pathol* 2015;**42**:188–193.
75. Delecluse HJ, Anagnostopoulos I, Dallenbach F, *et al.* Plasmablastic lymphomas of the oral cavity: a new entity associated with the human immunodeficiency virus infection. *Blood* 1997;**89**:1413–1420.
76. Carbone A, Gloghini A, Gaidano G. Is plasmablastic lymphoma of the oral cavity an HHV8 associated disease? *Am J Surg Pathol* 2004;**28**:1251–1252.
77. Castillo J, Pantanowitz L, Dezube BJ. HIV-associated plasmablastic lymphoma: lessons learned from 112 published cases. *Am J Hematol* 2008;**83**:804–809.
78. Cota C, Lora V, Cerroni L. Primary cutaneous plasmablastic lymphoma as first sign of human immunodeficiency virus infection. *Pathol Case Rev* 2014;**19**:204–207.
79. Colomo L, Loong F, Rives S, *et al.* Diffuse large B-cell lymphomas with plasmablastic differentiation represent a heterogeneous group of disease entities. *Am J Surg Pathol* 2004;**28**:736–747.
80. Verma S, Nuovo GJ, Porcu P, *et al.* Epstein–Barr virus- and human herpesvirus 8-associated primary cutaneous plasmablastic lymphoma in the setting of renal transplantation. *J Cutan Pathol* 2005;**32**:35–39.
81. Montes-Moreno S, Leoncini L, Louissaint A Jr, *et al.* Plasmablastic lymphoma. In: *WHO Classification of Tumours Editorial Board. Haematolymphoid Tumours.* 5th edition. Lyon (France): IARC, 2024: 506–508.
82. Morscio J, Dierickx D, Nijs J, *et al.* Clinicopathologic comparison of plasmablastic lymphoma in HIV-positive, immunocompetent, and posttransplant patients: single-center series of 25 cases and meta-analysis of 277 reported cases. *Am J Surg Pathol* 2014;**38**:875–886.
83. Laurent C, Dirnhofer S, Lenz G. Plasmablastic lymphoma. In: Arber DA, Borowitz MJ, Cook JR, *et al.*, eds. *The International Consensus Classification of Myeloid and Lymphoid Neoplasms.* Philadelphia (US): Wolters Kluver, 2025: 535–537.
84. Meer S, Perner Y, McAlpine E, Willem P. Extra-oral plasmablastic lymphomas in a high HIV endemic area. *Histopathology* 2020; **76**:212–221.
85. Cioc AM, Allen C, Kalmar JR, *et al.* Oral plasmablastic lymphomas in AIDS patients are associated with human herpesvirus 8. *Am J Surg Pathol* 2004;**28**:41–46.
86. Goedhals J, Beukes CA, Hardie D. HHV8 in plasmablastic lymphoma. *Am J Surg Pathol* 2008;**32**:172.
87. Carbone A, Gloghini A, Gaidano G. KSHV/HHV8 doesn't play a significant role in the development of plasmablastic lymphoma of the oral cavity. *Am J Surg Pathol* 2008;**32**:172–174.
88. Jordan LB, Lessells AM, Goodlad JR. Plasmablastic lymphoma arising at a cutaneous site. *Histopathology* 2005;**46**:113–115.
89. Nicol I, Boye T, Carsuzaa F, *et al.* Post-transplant plasmablastic lymphoma of the skin. *Br J Dermatol* 2003;**149**:889–891.
90. Hernandez C, Cetner AS, Wiley EL. Cutaneous presentation of plasmablastic post-transplant lymphoproliferative disorder in a 14-month-old. *Pediatr Dermatol* 2009;**26**:713–716.
91. Pan Z, Chen M, Zhang Q, *et al.* CD3-positive plasmablastic B-cell neoplasms: a diagnostic pitfall. *Mod Pathol* 2018;**31**:718–731.
92. Montes-Moreno S, Gonzalez-Medina AR, Rodriguez-Pinilla SM, *et al.* Is there an immunophenotype for plasmablastic lymphoma? Immunohistochemical evaluation of the phenotype with new specific markers against XBP1, Blimp1, GCET1 and KLHL6. *J Haematopathol* 2008;**1**:208–209.
93. Frontzek F, Staiger AM, Zapukhlyak M, *et al.* Molecular and functional profiling identifies therapeutically targetable vulnerabilities in plasmablastic lymphoma. *Nat Commun* 2021;**12**:5183.
94. Hartmann S, Fromm JR, Medeiros JL, *et al.* T-cell/histiocyte-rich large B-cell lymphoma. In: *WHO Classification of Tumours Editorial Board. Haematolymphoid Tumours.* 5th edition. Lyon (France): IARC, 2024: 473–475.
95. Pileri SA, Advani RH, Shipp MA, Smith LB. T-cell/histiocyte-rich large B-cell lymphoma. In: Arber DA, Borowitz MJ, Cook JR, *et al.*, eds. *The International Consensus Classification of Myeloid and Lymphoid Neoplasms.* Philadelphia (US): Wolters Kluver, 2025: 490–493.
96. Arai E, Sakurai M, Nakayama H, *et al.* Primary cutaneous T-cell-rich B-cell lymphoma. *Br J Dermatol* 1993;**129**:196–200.
97. Dommann SN, Dommann-Scherrer CC, Zimmerman D, *et al.* Primary cutaneous T-cell-rich B-cell lymphoma: a case report with a 13-year follow-up. *Am J Dermatopathol* 1995;**17**:618–624.
98. Dunphy CH, Nahass GT. Primary cutaneous T-cell-rich B-cell lymphomas with flow cytometric immunophenotypic findings: report of 3 cases and review of the literature. *Arch Pathol Lab Med* 1999;**123**:1236–1240.
99. Li S, Griffin CA, Mann RB, Borowitz MJ. Primary cutaneous T-cell-rich B-cell lymphoma: clinically distinct from its nodal counterpart? *Mod Pathol* 2001;**14**:10–13.
100. Sander CA, Kaudewitz P, Kutzner H, *et al.* T-cell-rich B-cell lymphoma presenting in skin: a clinicopathologic analysis of six cases. *J Cutan Pathol* 1996;**23**:101–108.
101. Gogstetter D, Brown M, Seab J, Scott G. Angiocentric primary cutaneous T-cell-rich B-cell lymphoma: a case report and review of the literature. *J Cutan Pathol* 2000;**27**:516–525.

102. Montes-Moreno S, Manuyama D, Gaddie WR, *et al.* Lymphoplasmacytic lymphoma. In: *WHO Classification of Tumours Editorial Board. Haematolymphoid Tumours.* 5th edition. Lyon (France): IARC, 2024: 394–398.
103. Cook JR, Lin P, Treon S. Lymphoplasmacytic lymphoma. In: Arber DA, Borowitz MJ, Cook JR, *et al.*, eds. *The International Consensus Classification of Myeloid and Lymphoid Neoplasms.* Philadelphia (US): Wolters Kluver, 2025: 367–372.
104. Alegría-Landa V, Prieto-Torres L, Santonja C, *et al.* MYD88 L265P mutation in cutaneous involvement by Waldenström macroglobulinemia. *J Cutan Pathol* 2017;**44**:625–631.
105. Durot E, Tomowiak C, Michallet AS, *et al.* Transformed Waldenstrom macroglobulinaemia: clinical presentation and outcome. A multi-institutional retrospective study of 77 cases from the French Innovative Leukemia Organization (FILO). *Br J Haematol* 2017;**179**:439–448.

SECTION 3

# Cutaneous lymphomas and lymphoproliferative disorders in the setting of immune deficiency / dysregulation

CHAPTER 21

# Cutaneous lymphoproliferative disorders and lymphomas in the setting of immune deficiency/dysregulation

Individuals who are immunosuppressed, either due to a congenital immunodeficiency disorder ("inborn error of immunity") or as a consequence of disease (e.g., human immunodeficiency virus [HIV] infection), or of specific immunosuppressive treatment, are at higher risk of cutaneous and extracutaneous malignancies, including lymphomas. In the past, these disorders were classified into four groups: (i) lymphoproliferative diseases associated with primary immune disorders, (ii) lymphomas associated with HIV infection, (iii) post-transplant lymphoproliferative disorders, and (iv) other iatrogenic immunodeficiency-associated lymphoproliferative disorders. In the last years, growing evidence has shown that many overlapping features among different "entities" in different settings of immunodeficiency exist, and it has been suggested that a new nomenclature may be more appropriate for classification, including the name of the lesion, the associated virus, and the specific immunodeficiency setting [1]. In the International Consensus Classification (ICC) of lymphomas these disorders are included in a section on "Immunodeficiency-associated lymphoproliferative disorders", retaining in part the old classification schemes, and including a total of nine entities (posttransplant lymphoproliferative disorders, nondestructive posttransplant lymphoproliferative disorders, plasmacytic hyperplasia posttransplant lymphoproliferative disorder, infectious mononucleosis posttransplant lymphoproliferative disorder, florid follicular hyperplasia posttransplant lymphoproliferative disorder, polymorphic posttransplant lymphoproliferative disorder, monomorphic posttransplant lymphoproliferative disorder (B-cell and T-cell/natural killer [NK]-cell types), classic Hodgkin lymphoma posttransplant lymphoproliferative disorder, and other iatrogenic immunodeficiency-associated lymphoproliferative disorders) [2]. In the last World Health Organization (WHO) *Classification of Haematolymphoid Tumours,* these disorders are discussed in one section dedicated to "lymphoid proliferations and lymphomas associated with immune deficiency and dysregulation," including five subgroups (hyperplasias arising in immune deficiency/dysregulation, polymorphic lymphoproliferative disorders arising in immune deficiency/dysregulation, Epstein–Barr virus (EBV)-positive mucocutaneous ulcer, lymphomas arising in immune deficiency/dysregulation, and inborn error of immunity-associated lymphoid proliferations and lymphomas [3].

Although lymphoproliferative disorders associated with immune deficiency/dysregulation may arise primary in the skin, these conditions are not covered in the WHO-European Organization for Research and Treatment of Cancer (EORTC) classification of cutaneous lymphomas and in its new update [4, 5].

Cutaneous lymphoproliferative disorders and lymphomas in immunocompromised patients have peculiar aspects that warrant discussion in one specific section of this book. It should be underlined, however, that these disorders may present overlapping clinicopathological features with "conventional" variants of cutaneous lymphoproliferative disorders and lymphomas, and that in some cases, separation may be artificial. Sometimes the diagnosis may be one of exclusion, as clinicopathological features may not be clearly diagnostic of a specific entity (Fig. 21.1).

Similar to the situation in immune competent patients, in organs other than the skin, B-cell lymphomas clearly predominate also in immunocompromised patients. In the skin, on the other hand, T-cell lymphomas represent the majority of the cutaneous lymphomas arising in the setting of immune deficiency/dysregulation [6]. Besides several types of non-Hodgkin lymphoma, patients with solid organ transplantation have an increased risk of developing other cutaneous tumors such as squamous cell carcinoma, Merkel cell carcinoma, and Kaposi sarcoma, among others (melanoma representing a notable exception) [7]. Sometimes, cutaneous lymphomas arising in patients with immune deficiency/dysregulation may show unusual histopathological features similar to those observed in reactive (pseudolymphomatous) conditions arising in the same setting, such as predominance of $CD8^+$ lymphocytes and presence of a granulomatous reaction (see also Chapter 31) [8].

Although some lymphoproliferative diseases are typical of certain types of immune suppression, such as polymorphic B-cell posttransplant lymphoproliferative disorder, they can also arise in other types of immune deficiency/dysregulation.

*Skin Lymphoma: The Illustrated Guide*, Sixth Edition. Lorenzo Cerroni.

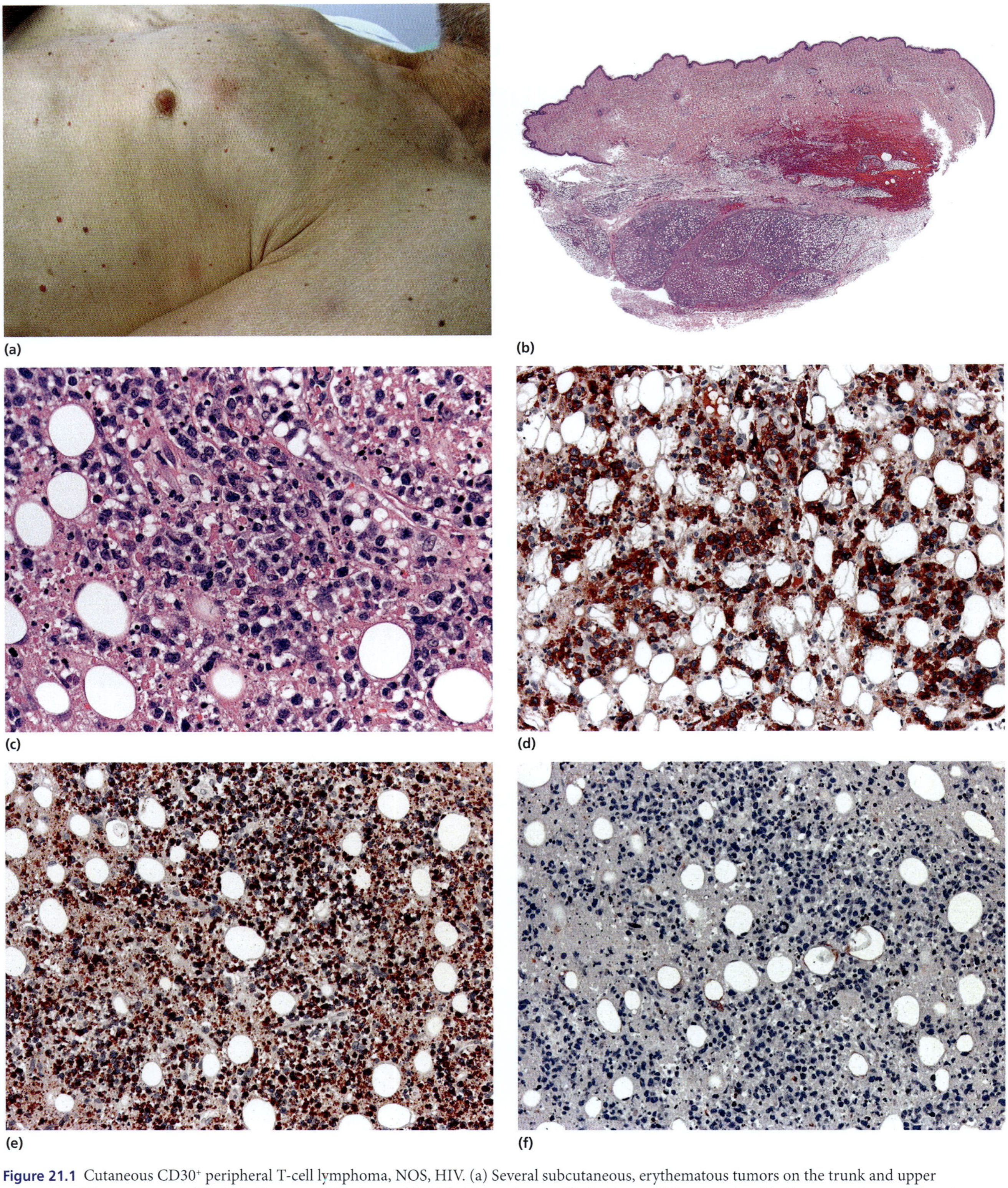

**Figure 21.1** Cutaneous CD30⁺ peripheral T-cell lymphoma, NOS, HIV. (a) Several subcutaneous, erythematous tumors on the trunk and upper extremities (*Photo courtesy of Dr. Isabel Viana and Dr. Esmeralda Vale, Lisbon, Portugal.*) (b) Dense, diffuse lymphoid infiltrates confined to the subcutaneous tissues, composed of (c) medium-sized and large pleomorphic lymphocytes. Immunohistology showed positivity of neoplastic cells for CD3, (d) CD30, (e) TIA-1, granzyme B, and focally for CD56, and negativity for CD2, (f) CD4, CD5, (g) CD8, (h) βF1, and TCR-δ. In situ hybridization for EBV (EBER-1) and staining for HHV-8 were negative. The diagnosis is one of exclusion: subcutaneous panniculitis-like T-cell lymphoma can be ruled out by negativity for CD8 and βF1. Negativity for TCR-δ and EBV rules out cutaneous γ/δ T-cell lymphoma and extranodal NK/T-cell lymphoma, nasal-type, respectively. Finally, the clinicopathologic features are not typical of cutaneous anaplastic large cell lymphoma, and the phenotype is not diagnostic of it as well.

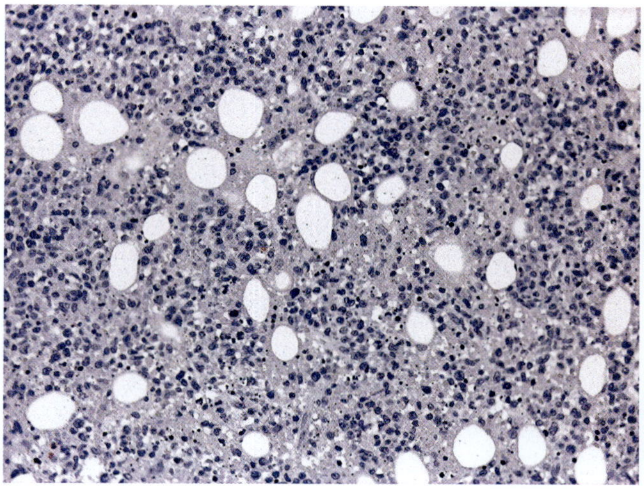

(g)

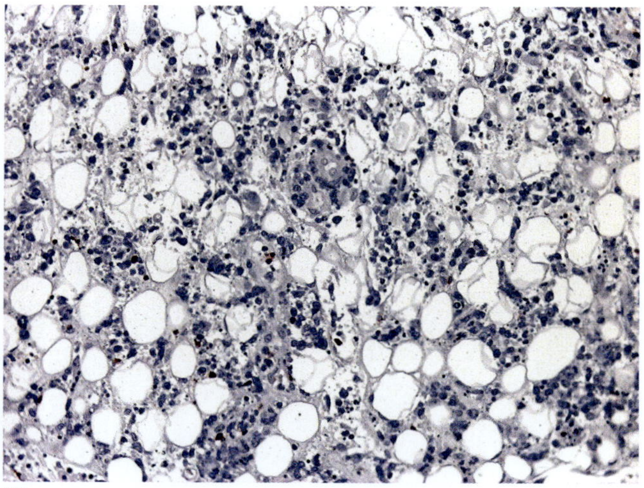

(h)

Figure 21.1 (Continued)

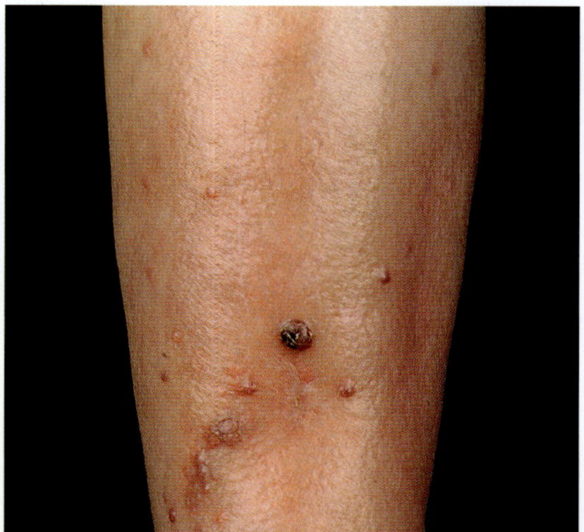

Figure 21.2 Cutaneous plasmablastic lymphoma, EBV⁺, posttransplant. Several papules and small nodules on the leg.

On the other hand, many conventional types of lymphoma may arise in individuals with immunodeficiency as well, such as mycosis fungoides and cutaneous anaplastic large cell lymphoma, for example. The occurrence of NK/T-cell lymphomas in patients with immune deficiency/dysregulation, and particularly of cutaneous anaplastic large cell lymphoma, seems to be more frequent in the skin than in other organs [6, 9]. As already mentioned, mycosis fungoides is the most frequent cutaneous lymphoma in the immune deficiency/dysregulation setting [6,10], and one case has been observed also in a pediatric patient as part of a post-transplant cutaneous composite lymphoma [11]. In immune deficiency/dysregulation-associated lymphomas arising at extracutaneous sites, the histopathologic picture is more frequently that of a B-cell lymphoma (diffuse large B-cell lymphoma, Burkitt lymphoma, plasma cell myeloma, or extramedullary plasmacytoma). Immune deficiency/dysregulation-associated B-cell lymphomas involving the skin often present with the features of diffuse large B-cell lymphoma or plasmablastic lymphoma (Figs. 21.2 and 21.3) [12, 13]. Cases of EBV⁺ cutaneous marginal zone lymphoproliferative disease and one case resembling lymphomatoid granulomatosis have also been observed [14, 15]. Rare cases are morphologically indistinguishable from plasmacytoma, with immunoglobulin light chain restriction and MUM-1 expression (Fig. 21.4) [16–19]. Immune deficiency/dysregulation-associated plasmacytomas are not always associated with EBV, usually arise several years after transplantation, and seem to have a better prognosis when compared to other immune deficiency/dysregulation-associated lymphomas [17]. As already mentioned, in the skin, the occurrence of immune deficiency/dysregulation-associated lymphoproliferative T-cell disorders, particularly mycosis fungoides and cutaneous anaplastic large cell lymphoma, is more common than at extracutaneous sites (Fig. 21.5) [6, 9, 20–25]. These cases represent approximately half of all cutaneous immune deficiency/dysregulation-associated lymphomas, again showing the higher frequency of T-cell lymphomas in the skin, as opposed to the lymph nodes. A case of subcutaneous panniculitis-like T-cell lymphoma has been observed in a cardiac allograft recipient [26]. Although cutaneous T-cell lymphomas in immunocompromised patients are usually not associated with EBV infection, EBV⁺ cases can be observed rarely [27].

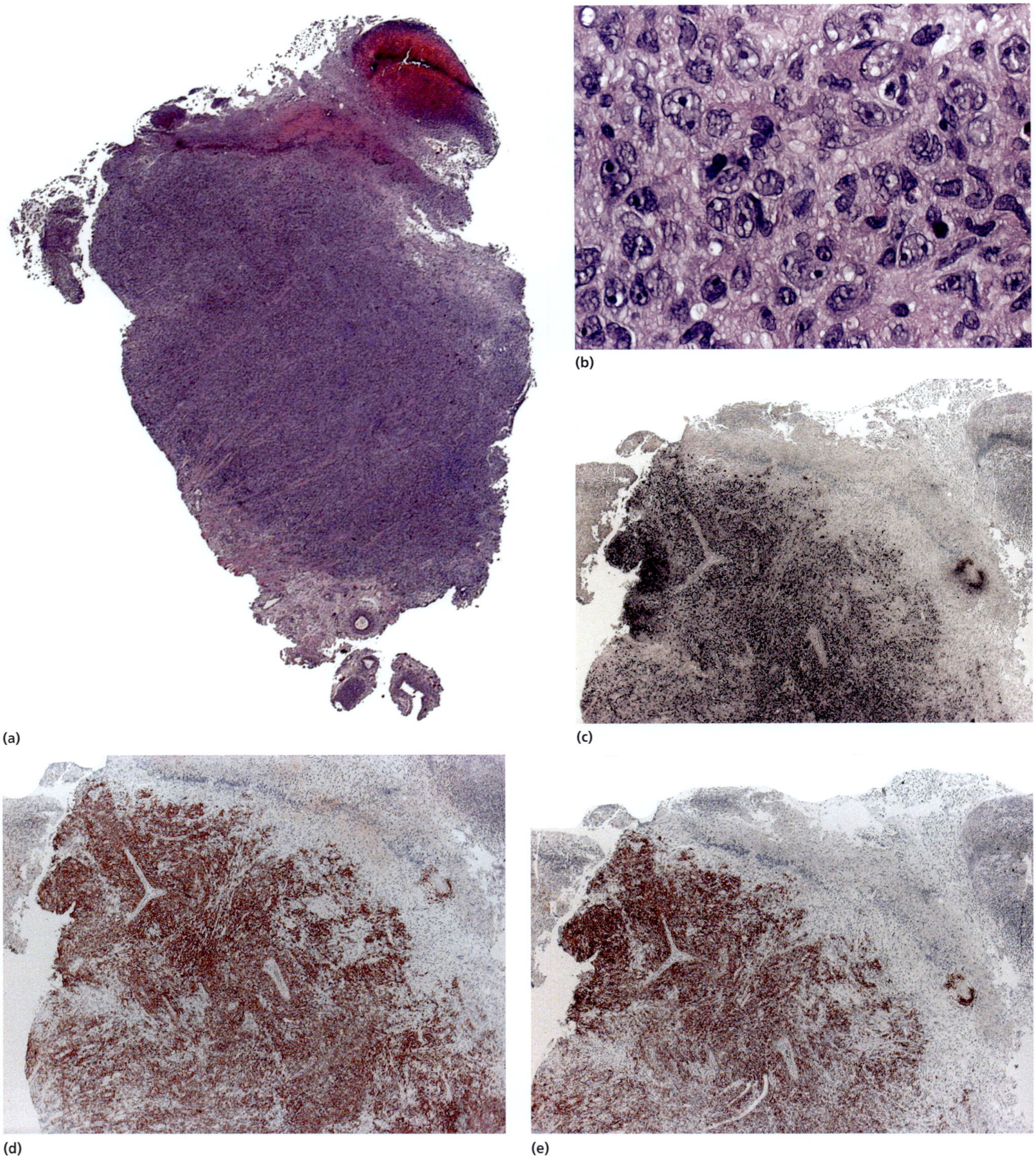

**Figure 21.3** Cutaneous diffuse large B-cell lymphoma, EBV$^{+}$, posttransplant. (a) Ulcerated tumor composed of (b) large, atypical cells that are positive for (c) EBV (EBER-1), (d) CD30, and (e) CD20.

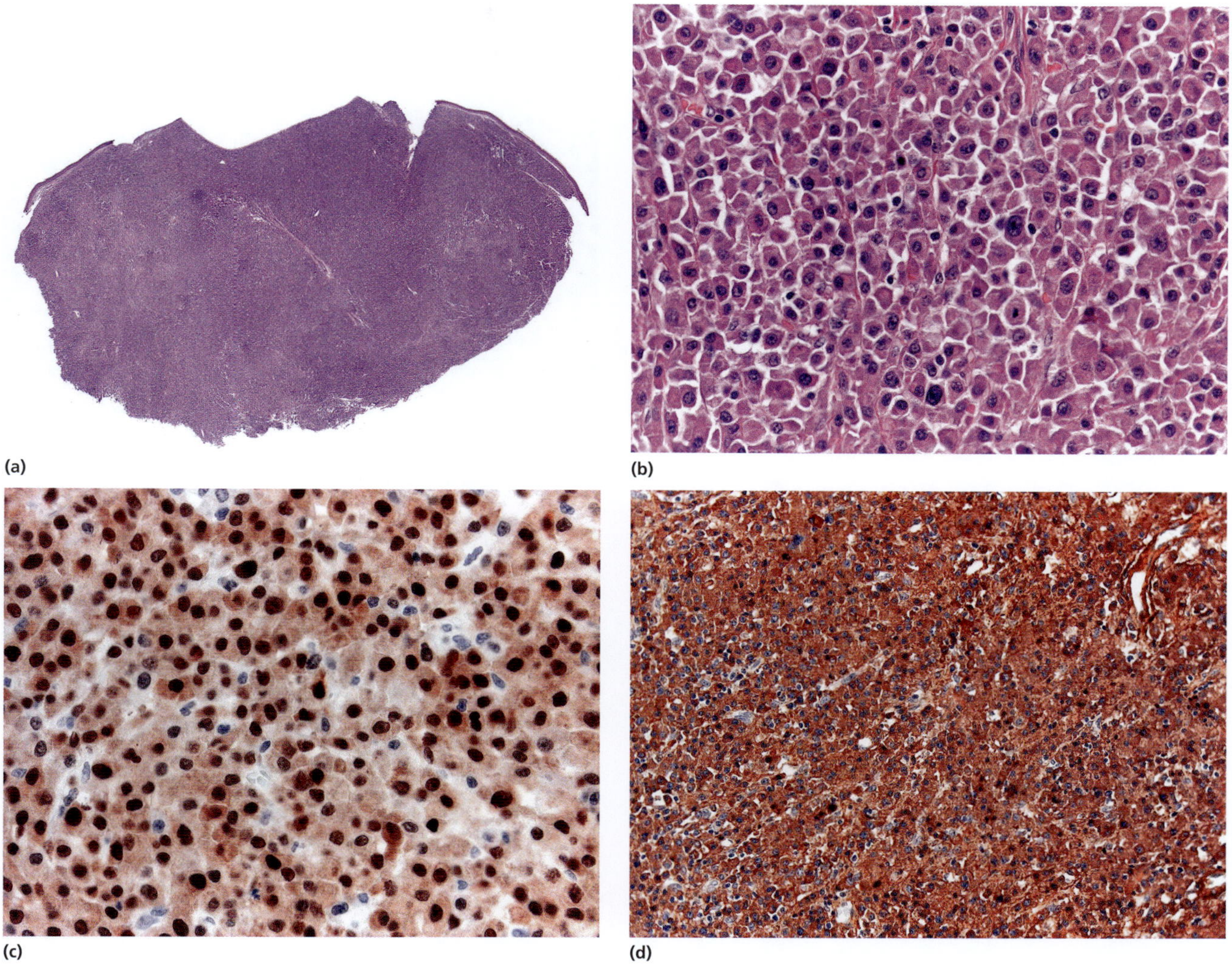

Figure 21.4 Cutaneous plasmacytoma, EBV$^+$, posttransplant. (a) Diffuse infiltrate replacing the entire dermis; (b) predominance of atypical plasma cells; (c) positivity for MUM-1; and (d) lambda immunoglobulin light chain.

In the context of lymphoproliferative disorders associated with immune deficiency/dysregulation, a few considerations should be borne in mind:

- One of the main differences between lymphomas in immunocompetent and immunosuppressed individuals is represented by the more frequent association with infectious agents in immunosuppressed patients, particularly with EBV and human herpes virus-8 (HHV-8), but also with other viruses. On the other hand, it should be reminded that in immunosuppressed patients, infectious agents may also be associated with atypical but benign cutaneous lymphoid infiltrates (for example, pseudolymphomatous syphilis in HIV infection).
- The same infectious agent may be associated with different types of lymphoma. Thus, demonstration of a particular microorganism should be interpreted only in the setting of complete clinical, morphologic, phenotypic, and molecular information and cannot be considered specific for a particular type of lymphoma.
- Although some types of lymphoma are frequently associated with particular forms of immune deficiency (e.g., plasmablastic lymphoma in HIV-infected patients), lymphomas with the same morphologic and phenotypic features may be observed in other types of immune deficiency/dysregulation, or even in immunocompetent individuals [28, 29].
- There are many overlaps among lymphoproliferative entities associated with different types of immune deficiency/dysregulation, and it is artificial to separate them according to the cause of immune suppression (e.g., posttransplant, HIV, iatrogenic). In fact, a new nomenclature including the histopathological name of the lesion, the associated virus, and the specific immunodeficiency setting has been proposed for classification of these cases (for example, "polymorphic

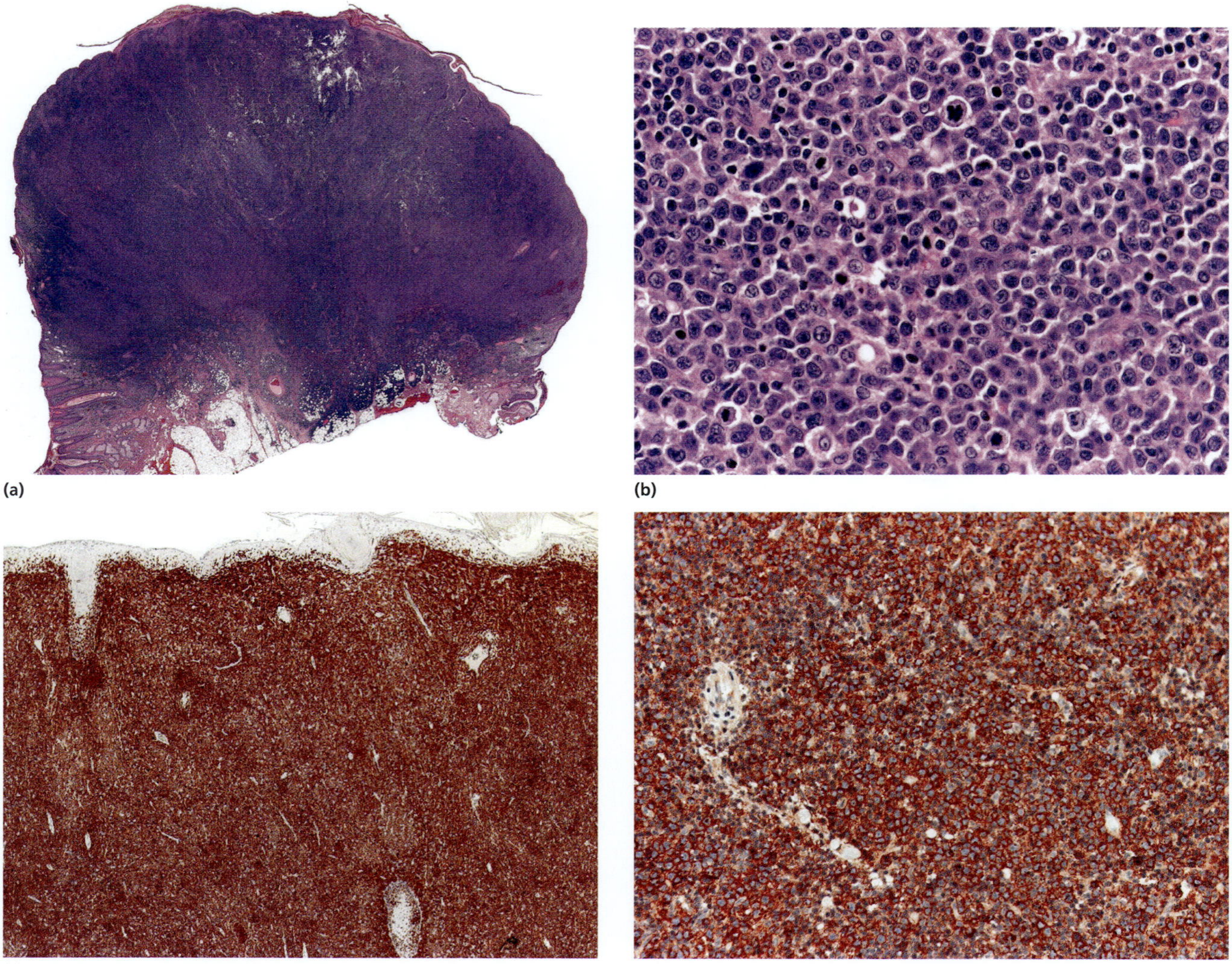


Figure 21.5 Cutaneous anaplastic large cell lymphoma, post-transplant. (a) Nodular infiltrate within the entire dermis and superficial part of the subcutaneous fat; (b) predominance of large, anaplastic lymphocytes; (c) positivity for CD3; and (d) CD30.

B-cell lymphoproliferative disorder, EBV1, iatrogenic (methotrexate)," or "diffuse large B-cell lymphoma, EBV2, HIV infection") [1].

- A single patient may present with lesions corresponding to different types of immunodeficiency/dysregulation-associated lymphoproliferative disorders at one site or at different sites. In fact, sometimes even "composite lymphomas" may be observed in this setting [11].

A last consideration concerns therapy. In some cases, reduction of the immune suppression, eventually combined with antiviral treatment, results in remission of the lymphoproliferative disorder or lymphoma, and conventional therapeutic options are usually left for more aggressive cases or for patients who are not responding to this approach. On the other hand, it should be reminded that "conventional" cutaneous lymphomas (e.g., mycosis fungoides, anaplastic large cell lymphoma) may behave differently (more aggressively) when they arise in the setting of immune deficiency/dysregulation.

In what follows, clinicopathological features of cutaneous lymphoproliferative disorders and lymphomas that are restricted to immune deficiency/dysregulation will be summarized, and the different settings of immune deficiency/dysregulation will be briefly reviewed; there will be no detailed discussion of specific entities that show overlapping clinicopathological features with the same conditions when observed in immune competent patients.

## Posttransplant immunodeficiency/dysregulation

Lymphoproliferative disorders are among the most common neoplasms in recipients of solid organ and bone marrow transplantation, developing in a small minority of patients. In a review of >14,400 transplantation recipients, the incidence was 0.8% for extracutaneous and 0.07% for cutaneous lymphoproliferative disorders [30]. For the most part, they represent examples of EBV-associated lymphoproliferative disorders. Although cutaneous manifestations are rare, some patients may present with disease localized solely to the skin [31–37]. Many cases arise within the first year after organ or bone marrow transplantation, but the time interval between transplantation and the onset of a posttransplant lymphoproliferative disorder may be much longer. The vast majority of cases of posttransplant lymphoproliferative disorders in solid organ recipients are of host origin, with only a small minority of donor origin (these last observed particularly in recipients of liver and lung allografts). On the other hand, most cases arising in recipients of allogeneic stem cell transplantation are of donor origin, as after successful engraftment, the immune system of the host has been replaced by that of the donor.

In general, posttransplant lymphoproliferative disorders occur more often in recipients of heart–lung allografts and less commonly in those who receive renal allografts. However, in a large European study on cutaneous cases, the majority of patients had a renal transplant [6]. Other risk factors include primary infection with EBV following transplantation, infection with cytomegalovirus, T-cell-specific immunosuppression, and younger age [38]. At extracutaneous sites, there is a higher risk of developing hepatosplenic T-cell lymphoma, Burkitt's lymphoma, NK/T-cell lymphoma, diffuse large B-cell lymphoma, and anaplastic large-cell lymphoma [39]. In the skin, on the other hand, about half of the cases are represented by mycosis fungoides [6]. Interestingly, in B-cell posttransplant lymphoproliferative disorders, clonal populations of T lymphocytes can also be detected, suggesting that a lack of immune surveillance may affect T as well as B cells [40]. Besides conventional posttransplant lymphoproliferative disorders, the onset of adult T-cell lymphoma/leukemia (ATLL) has been documented in three patients who received organs from a patient infected with human T lymphotropic virus 1 (HTLV-1) [41].

In the skin, besides cases showing clinicopathological features of different variants of cutaneous lymphomas, the most frequent entities are plasmacytic hyperplasia and polymorphic B-cell lymphoproliferative disorder (see the specific Sections in this Chapter).

Genetic analyses showed that gains of chromosomes 5p and 11p and deletions of chromosome 12p were common in the diffuse large B-cell lymphoma variant of post-transplant lymphoproliferative disorders and that some overlapping features between diffuse large B-cell lymphomas in immunocompetent and immunosuppressed individuals could be observed [42]. High levels of hypermethylation of the tumor suppressor gene *p16* have been demonstrated in one EBV-associated cutaneous case, supporting the evidence for a carcinogenic role of EBV in positive cases [43].

Reduction of immunosuppression, often associated with antiviral therapy, is the main strategy for treatment of posttransplant lymphoproliferative disorders [44–46]. Regression of the lesions may take place over a period of a few weeks up to a few months. Reduction of immune suppression, together with rituximab, may also be considered for cases with a B-cell phenotype [47]. Lesions that do not respond to these measures may be treated by more conventional modalities, including radiotherapy, interferon-α, and systemic chemotherapy, or with other strategies used for similar lymphomas arising in immune competent patients. For post-transplant lymphomas associated with EBV, gene therapy with genetically modified EBV-specific cytotoxic T cells may represent a further treatment option [48].

Plasmacytic hyperplasia and probably also plasmacytoma-like tumors almost always respond completely to the reduction of immunosuppression [17]. Although some cases of post-transplant cutaneous anaplastic large cell lymphoma had a favorable behavior [23, 49], in general, mycosis fungoides and cutaneous anaplastic large cell lymphoma in immunosuppressed individuals do not share the same favorable prognosis as in immunocompetent hosts [6, 9, 10, 50].

## Human immunodeficiency virus (HIV)-related immune deficiency/dysregulation

Patients infected with HIV may develop benign and malignant lymphoproliferative disorders [7, 51, 52]. It has been estimated that $HIV^+$ patients have a risk of developing a malignant lymphoma up to 200-fold higher than normal individuals. The onset of lymphoproliferative disorders has been observed particularly in individuals with overt acquired immunodeficiency syndrome (AIDS) [53–55]. There are overlapping features between the lymphomas arising in $HIV^+$ patients and those observed after solid organ or bone marrow transplantation, but also some aspects peculiar to $HIV^+$ individuals [2]. Most lymphoproliferative disorders that arise in $HIV^+$ patients occur at sites other than the skin, but primary cutaneous cases or secondary cutaneous involvement from extracutaneous lymphomas may be observed. Two types of lymphoma frequent in $HIV^+$ individuals, namely, primary effusion lymphoma and plasmablastic lymphoma, are only rarely observed in the skin (these two lymphomas are discussed in Chapter 20). However, cutaneous plasmablastic lymphoma may represent the first sign of AIDS in HIV-infected patients, and extracavitary primary effusion lymphoma may present in the skin as well [56, 57].

Cutaneous Burkitt lymphoma, too, has been observed in the setting of HIV infection [58, 59], as well as a case of primary cutaneous aggressive epidermotropic $CD8^+$ T-cell lymphoma [60]. In patients with HIV infection, mycosis fungoides should be distinguished from benign CD8+ cutaneous infiltrates, which may reveal similar clinicopathologic features (summarized in Chapter 31).

Most cutaneous lymphomas in $HIV^+$ patients represent examples of "conventional" skin lymphomas such as mycosis fungoides, anaplastic large cell lymphoma, or diffuse large B-cell lymphoma, leg type, similar to what can be observed in cutaneous lymphomas arising in post-transplant setting. In contrast to cutaneous lymphomas in the general population, however, mycosis fungoides represents a minority of the cases arising in $HIV^+$ patients, and B-cell lymphomas are more common. HIV-related cutaneous anaplastic large cell lymphoma presents with histopathologic and immunophenotypic features similar to those observed in the non-HIV-related type. Different morphologic subtypes may be observed [61, 62]. ALK-1 is not expressed by neoplastic cells. EBV and HHV-8 are usually negative, but may be detected in a minority of cases. Rarely, plasmacytic hyperplasia or polymorphic B-cell lymphoproliferative disorder may be observed in $HIV^+$ individuals [63].

Association with EBV has been documented in most cases of plasmablastic lymphoma and in other cutaneous B-cell lymphomas in $HIV^+$ individuals, and rarely also in cases of cutaneous anaplastic large cell lymphoma associated with HIV. Cases of HIV-related cutaneous anaplastic large cell lymphoma positive for HHV-8 have been documented as well [64], and infection with human T-lymphotropic virus 2 (HTLV-2) has been detected in one $HIV^+$ patient with a $CD8^+$ cutaneous T-cell lymphoma [65].

Patients are adults who are infected with HIV and have a very low CD4 count, but rarely children can also be affected as well [53, 66]. The onset of a cutaneous lymphoma may represent the first AIDS-defining illness in some of these patients. Cutaneous lesions are variable, depending on the type of lymphoma, and are not different from those observed in the corresponding lymphoma types arising in non-HIV-infected individuals. Accurate staging investigations should be performed in order to evaluate the extent (if any) of extracutaneous involvement. Of note, B-cell lymphomas associated with HHV-8 in $HIV^+$ patients may show an anaplastic morphology similar to that of anaplastic large cell lymphoma and express CD30 as well, thus representing a further potential pitfall [67, 68].

As these lymphomas arise in patients who are profoundly immunocompromised, death often ensues, resulting from complications of AIDS rather than from direct lymphoma spread. Therapy should be directed at both the HIV disease and the lymphoma [51]. Conservative treatment strategies have been advocated for cutaneous lymphomas [54]. In this context, it has been shown that after the introduction of antiretroviral treatment (ART, also known as highly active antiretroviral treatment – HAART) the frequency of the more aggressive types of HIV-associated lymphomas decreased, and the outcome has improved [69].

Mycosis fungoides in $HIV^+$ patients should be managed according to standard protocols (see Chapter 3) [53, 70]. Solitary or localized lesions of other lymphomas may be treated with local radiotherapy. If not already introduced, ART should be started. HIV-associated cutaneous anaplastic large cell lymphoma seems to have a worse prognosis than the non-HIV-related variant [71]; thus, conservative strategies may fail in this particular setting. Prognostic features for HIV-associated T-cell lymphomas have been studied for non-cutaneous cases [72], but representative data on primary cutaneous cases are lacking. Use of ART and the patient's performance status were associated with overall survival in multivariate analysis [72].

## Immune deficiency/dysregulation due to other iatrogenic and non-iatrogenic factors

Besides the post-transplant and HIV infection settings, cutaneous lymphoproliferative disorders may occur in any other iatrogenic or non-iatrogenic immunodeficiency, including inborn errors of immunity (also known as congenital immune deficiencies) and iatrogenic immune deficiencies related to the use of methotrexate or other immunosuppressive or immunomodulatory drugs. Lymphomas arising in inborn errors of immunity occur mostly in the lungs, gastrointestinal tract, and central nervous system and only rarely affect the skin [27]. On the other hand, it should be reminded that some distinct types of cutaneous pseudolymphoma may be observed in patients with inborn errors of immunity (discussed in Chapter 31).

The development of lymphomas in patients under methotrexate therapy is well known [73–76]. Lymphomatoid granulomatosis, a type of lymphoproliferative disease arising in this setting, may involve the skin in addition to the lungs (for a detailed discussion of lymphomatoid granulomatosis, see Chapter 20). An angiocentric pattern with angiodestruction and prominent necrosis, suggestive of lymphomatoid granulomatosis, has been observed in two cases of methotrexate-related cutaneous diffuse large B-cell lymphoma [77, 78]. Both cases were positive for CD30, and EBV was detected within tumor cells in one of the two cases only. The onset of cutaneous or extracutaneous lymphomas has also been described in patients undergoing treatment with immunosuppressive or immunomodulatory drugs ("biologics") [79–84]. In some of these cases, a wrong diagnosis of atopic dermatitis or psoriasis had been made, and treatment with one of the many immunologic agents had been started, resulting in rapid progression of an undiagnosed mycosis fungoides (see also Chapter 3) [81–83]. These particular cases have been termed "monoclonal antibody immunomodulator-related lymphoid proliferations" [84]. The lymphomas occurring in these settings have clinicopathologic features similar to corresponding entities observed in patients who do not take the drug, the main difference being represented by a higher rate of association with EBV infection. In some cases, rapid histopathologic progression from early changes to fully developed lesions has been documented [85]. As in other cutaneous lymphomas associated with immune deficiency/dysregulation, in some cases, precise classification may be difficult, and overlapping features of different lymphoma types may be present [86]. Besides conventional entities of cutaneous lymphoma, some patients show lesions of reactive plasmacytic hyperplasia or polymorphic B-cell lymphoproliferative disorder [87].

A case of cutaneous B-cell lymphoma associated with mycosis fungoides in a patient receiving methotrexate for a psoriasiform dermatitis has been reported, showing distinct cutaneous lesions relative to the two lymphoma types, one associated with EBV (B-cell lymphoma) and one not (mycosis fungoides) [88]. Interestingly, in this case, withdrawal of methotrexate resulted in complete regression of the EBV-associated cutaneous B-cell lymphoma but not of the mycosis fungoides, underlying the complexity of immune deficiency/dysregulation-related cutaneous lymphomas. On the other hand, it may be that the "psoriasiform dermatitis" treated by methotrexate in this patient was, in truth, an undiagnosed mycosis fungoides, thus providing a possible explanation for the different response to treatment.

A study of diffuse large B-cell lymphomas arising in the setting of methotrexate treatment showed a genetic profile closer to nongerminal center B-cell diffuse large B-cell lymphoma, but with characteristic 3q, 12q, and 20p gains and lower 9p losses, with no relevant differences between EBV$^+$ and EBV− cases (EBV$^+$ cases also had 4p focal gains) [89].

It should be remembered that knowledge of treatment with methotrexate or other immunosuppressive agents is an exclusion criterion for EBV$^+$ cutaneous diffuse large B-cell lymphoma, which represents a frequent differential diagnosis of EBV$^+$ cases with a B-cell phenotype (see Chapter 20).

In over half of the cases of methotrexate-associated cutaneous lymphoma, the lesions regress upon withdrawal of methotrexate [75]. Regression upon discontinuation of treatment may also be observed in cases associated with the use of cyclosporine and systemic steroids [44]. In patients with inborn errors of immunity, the treatment must be aimed at both the background condition and the lymphoma, depending also on the lymphoma type.

Similar to what was described in HIV-related cases, an aggressive course has been observed in cutaneous anaplastic large cell lymphoma related to other types of immune deficiency/dysregulation as well [50], suggesting that in immunosuppressed individuals, this lymphoma may have a worse prognosis irrespective of the cause of the immune deficiency. Brentuximab vedotin may be an option for refractory or relapsing CD30$^+$ cases [90].

## Cutaneous plasmacytic hyperplasia associated with immune deficiency/dysregulation

In the lymph nodes, immune deficiency/dysregulation-associated lymphoid hyperplasia includes follicular hyperplasia, infectious mononucleosis-like hyperplasia, plasmacytic hyperplasia, and HHV8-positive multicentric Castleman disease, but in the skin, only plasmacytic hyperplasia is observed. Patients are adults or children with different types of immunodeficiency/dysregulation, in my experience, mostly associated with HIV or in a post-transplant setting. Cutaneous lesions are variable, including mostly localized, non-descript macules and small plaques.

Histopathologic features are characterized by an inflammatory infiltrate comprising variable numbers of polyclonal plasma cells (Fig. 21.6). Staining for infectious organisms, especially syphilis, is crucial in such cases, as particularly in HIV$^+$ patients, cutaneous infections are common and may present with atypical lymphoid infiltrates resembling lymphoma (see Chapter 28).

Data on cutaneous cases are insufficient to draw conclusions regarding the best treatment options. Reduction of immune suppression is usually sufficient to achieve remission in extracutaneous cases; ART should be started in HIV-positive patients.

### Résumé

**Cutaneous plasmacytic hyperplasia associated with immune deficiency/dysregulation**

| | | |
|---|---|---|
| **Clinical** | Children and adults, mostly with immune deficiency/dysregulation associated with HIV or in a post-transplant setting. | |
| **Morphology** | Lymphoid infiltrates comprising variable numbers of plasma cells. | |
| **Immunohistochemistry** | CD3, CD20 | +/− (accompanying infiltrate) |
| | EBER-1 | + (−) |
| | Kappa, Lambda | Polyclonal pattern |
| **Genetics** | Not relevant. | |
| **Treatment guidelines** | Reduction of immunosuppression. | |

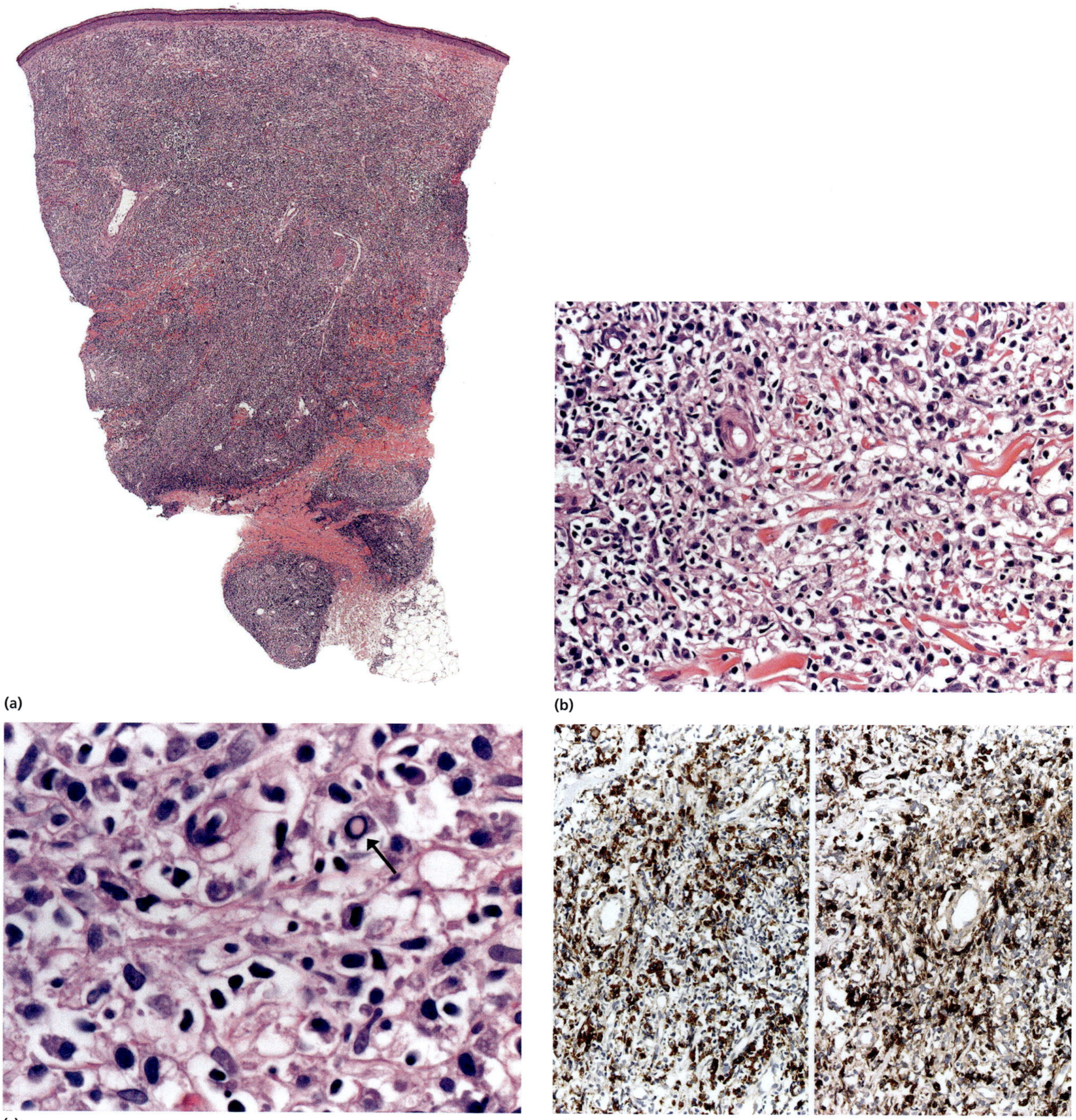

(a) (b) (c) (d)

Figure 21.6 Cutaneous plasmacytic hyperplasia, HIV. (a) Diffuse infiltrate involving the entire dermis showing (b) mixed cellularity with several mature plasma cells admixed with lymphocytes, some with medium-sized morphology. (c) Note a Dutcher body (arrow). (d) In situ hybridization for lambda (left) and kappa (right) reveals a polyclonal pattern of immunoglobulin light chain expression.

## Cutaneous polymorphic B-cell lymphoproliferative disorder associated with immune deficiency/dysregulation

Polymorphic B-cell lymphoproliferative disorder associated with immune deficiency/dysregulation has been observed particularly in post-transplant settings, but can also arise in other types of immunodeficiency/dysregulation, such as methotrexate treatment, and uncommonly in patients with HIV infection.

Patients are adults or children. Cutaneous lesions are variable, including erythematous plaques, nodules, and tumors, sometimes ulcerated (Figs. 21.7 and 21.8). They can be solitary, localized to a single anatomic region, or generalized. Staging investigations should be performed in order to evaluate the extent of involvement before planning the treatment.

Histopathologic features are characterized by a monoclonal infiltrate of B lymphocytes (admixed with reactive T cells), comprising the whole spectrum of maturation and including plasma cells, immunoblasts, and intermediate-sized lymphoid cells (Figs. 21.9 and 21.10). In-situ hybridization for EBV (EBER-1) is positive in most cases.

The management of patients depends on the type of immunodeficiency/dysregulation, but data on cutaneous cases are insufficient to draw conclusions regarding the best treatment options. Reduction of immune suppression is usually considered in a post-transplant setting, and ART should be started in HIV-positive patients. More aggressive options may be considered for patients with refractory disease and/or extracutaneous involvement.

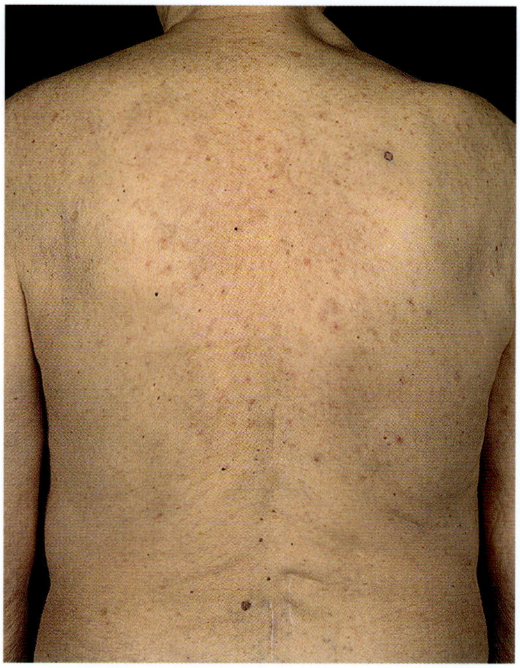

**Figure 21.8** Cutaneous polymorphic B-cell lymphoproliferative disorder, posttransplant. Generalized, small erythematous papules.

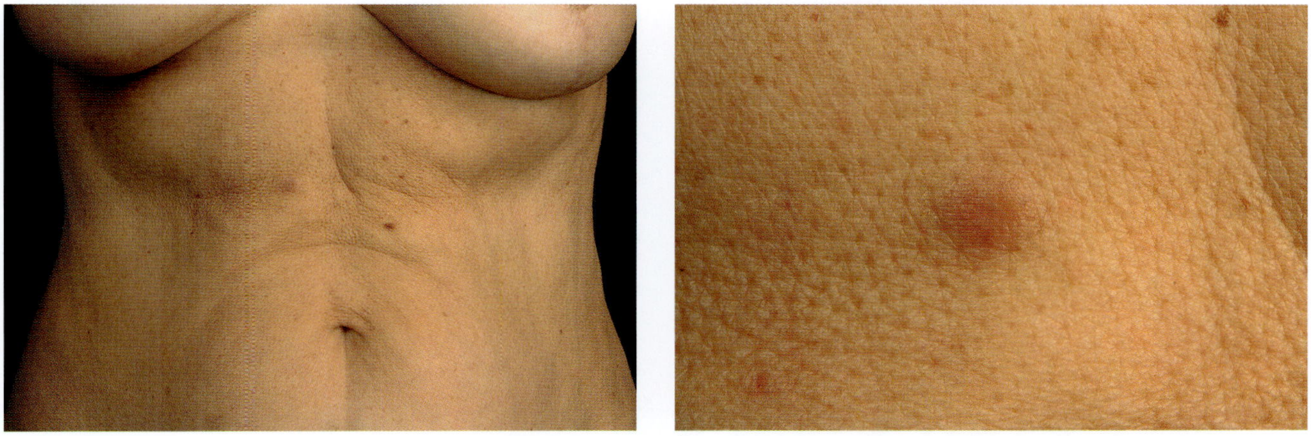

(a) (b)

**Figure 21.7** Cutaneous polymorphic B-cell lymphoproliferative disorder, posttransplant. (a) Small erythematous plaque on the abdomen; (b) detail of the plaque.

## Résumé

**Cutaneous polymorphic B-cell lymphoproliferative disorder associated with immune deficiency/dysregulation**

| | | |
|---|---|---|
| **Clinical** | Adults or children with different types of immunodeficiency/dysregulation; solitary, localized, or generalized erythematous plaques, nodules, and small tumors. | |
| **Morphology** | B and T lymphocytes (B lymphocytes comprising the whole spectrum of maturation and including plasma cells, immunoblasts, and intermediate-sized lymphoid cells). | |
| **Immunohistochemistry** | CD19, CD20, CD79a | + |
| | CD3, CD5 | + (reactive cells) |
| | CD30 | −/+ |
| | LMP-1, EBER-1 | + (B-cells) |
| **Genetics** | Monoclonal rearrangement of the Ig genes. | |
| **Treatment guidelines** | Reduction of immunosuppression. ART in patients positive for HIV. Radiotherapy (solitary or localized lesions); more aggressive treatments may be considered for non-responding cases with extracutaneous involvement. | |

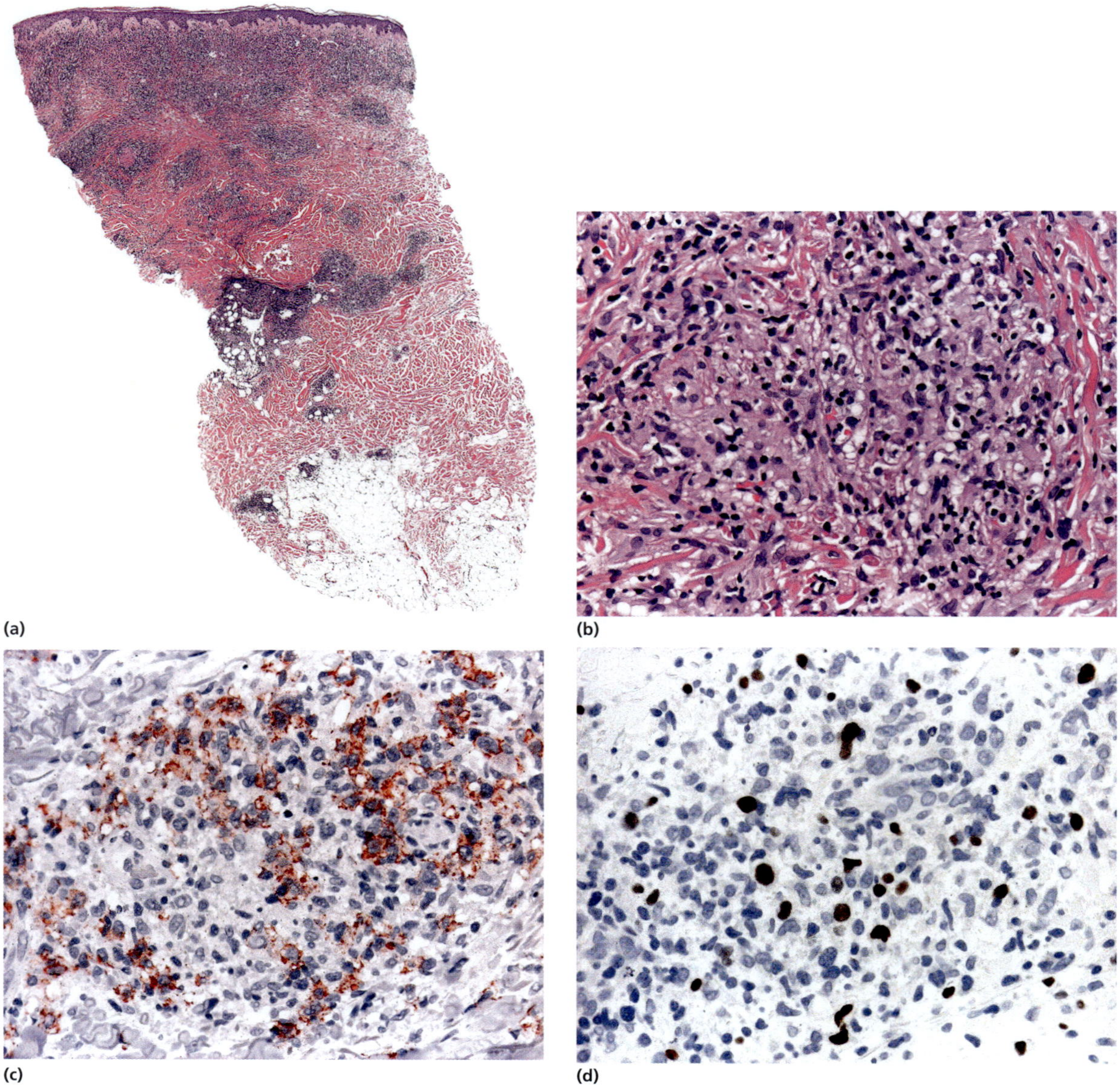

(a) (b) (c) (d)

**Figure 21.9** Cutaneous polymorphic B-cell lymphoproliferative disorder, posttransplant. (a) Dense infiltrate within the dermis; (b) mixed-cell infiltrate with small, medium-sized, and some large lymphocytes admixed with reactive cells; (c) staining for CD20 shows several large B-lymphocytes; (d) in situ hybridization for EBV (EBER-1) shows scattered positive lymphocytes.

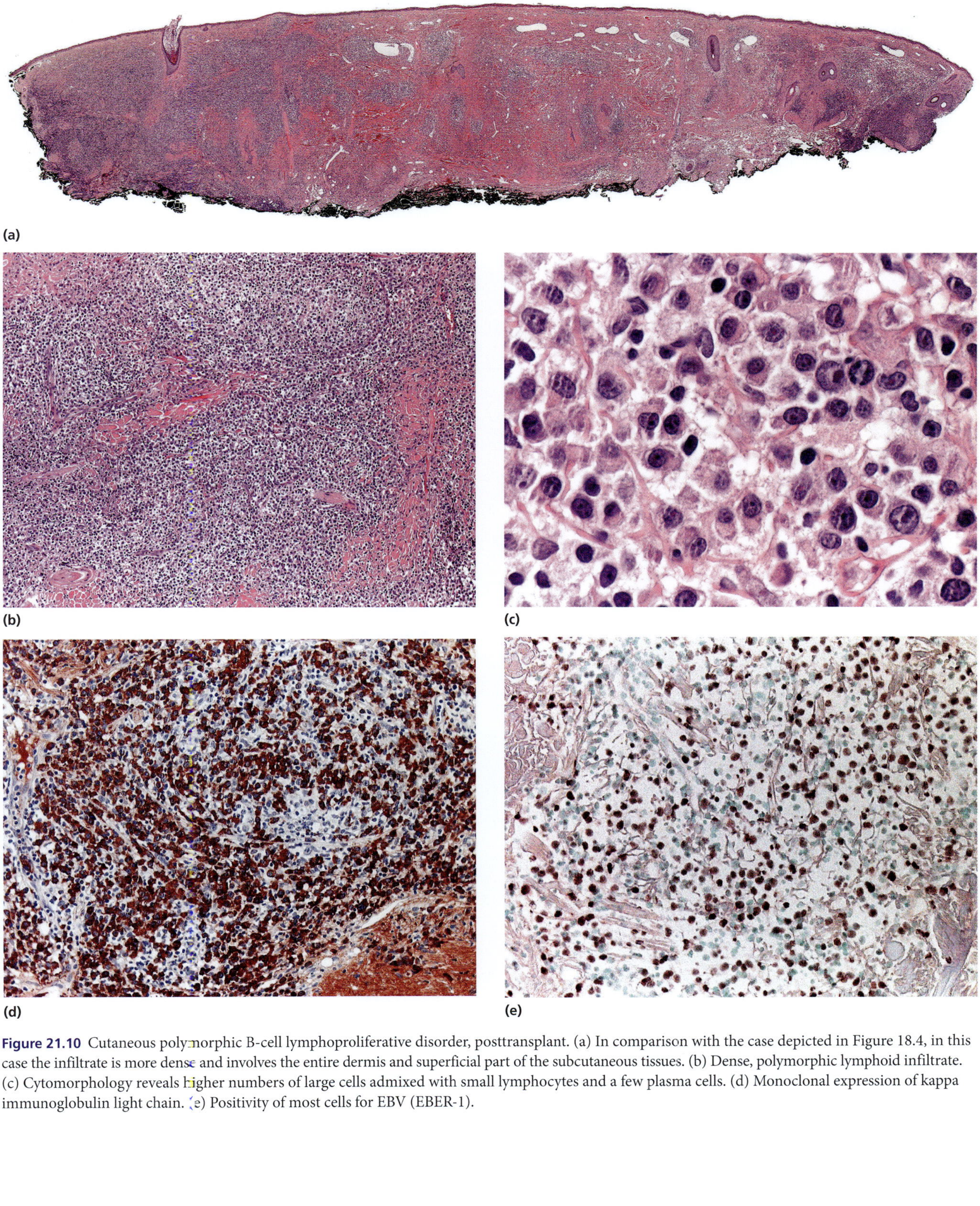

(a)

(b)

(c)

(d)

(e)

Figure 21.10 Cutaneous polymorphic B-cell lymphoproliferative disorder, posttransplant. (a) In comparison with the case depicted in Figure 18.4, in this case the infiltrate is more dense and involves the entire dermis and superficial part of the subcutaneous tissues. (b) Dense, polymorphic lymphoid infiltrate. (c) Cytomorphology reveals higher numbers of large cells admixed with small lymphocytes and a few plasma cells. (d) Monoclonal expression of kappa immunoglobulin light chain. (e) Positivity of most cells for EBV (EBER-1).

## Epstein–Barr virus (EBV)-associated mucocutaneous ulcers

A condition characterized by oropharyngeal and/or cutaneous ulcerative lesions associated with EBV infection and dense lymphoid infiltrates was described in the setting of immune suppression from a variety of origins [91]. This condition has been included as a distinct variant of B-cell lymphoproliferative disorder in the ICC classification and in the most recent edition of the WHO-EORTC classification of cutaneous lymphomas [2, 4, 5]. In the 5th update of the WHO *Classification of Haematolymphoid Tumours* and in the ICC *of Myeloid and Lymphoid Neoplasms,* EBV-associated mucocutaneous ulcer is included as a specific entity in the group of lymphoid proliferations and lymphomas associated with immune deficiency [92, 93].

Although in this edition of the book EBV-associated mucocutaneous ulcer is discussed in this Chapter, the rationale for the inclusion of this entity among the lymphomas is debatable, as the authors originally describing the condition had considered it as a form of pseudolymphoma [94]. Only one case originating in the colon has been described in association with Hodgkin lymphoma [95], and the prognosis of cutaneous cases is usually benign. EBV-associated mucocutaneous ulcers may result from a minimal and localized lapse in immunosurveillance over EBV [91]. In this context, EBV-associated mucocutaneous ulcer may be discussed in the Chapter on lymphoproliferative disorders associated with immune deficiency/dysregulation, or in the one on pseudolymphomas as well.

One major problem in the diagnosis of EBV-associated mucocutaneous ulcers is the presence of overlapping clinicopathological features with other EBV-associated conditions, particularly lymphomatoid granulomatosis and immunosuppression-related cutaneous lymphoproliferative diseases. In fact, besides cases arising in the setting of so-called immune senescence, EBV-associated mucocutaneous ulcers have been reported in patients with iatrogenic or HIV-related immune suppression. A case reported as "lymphomatoid granulomatosis" showed features that could have been interpreted also as those of EBV-associated mucocutaneous ulcer with an angiocentric pattern [96]. Precise classification of given cases into the four categories of (i) EBV-positive diffuse large B-cell lymphoma; (ii) lymphomatoid granulomatosis; (iii) EBV-associated lymphoproliferative disorders in immune suppressed patients; and (iv) EBV-associated mucocutaneous ulcer requires careful clinicopathological correlation and integration with other data. In the proper clinicopathological context, it has been suggested that the term "$EBV^+$ B-cell polymorphic lymphoproliferative disorder" or other specific type of $EBV^+$ lymphoma or lymphoproliferative disorder may be more appropriate for classification when patients present with two or more lesions [2].

### Clinical features

Patients with EBV-associated mucocutaneous ulcers are often elderly with so-called immune senescence. Other conditions determining immune suppression in these patients include immune suppressive treatment for solid organ allogeneic stem-cell transplantation, treatment with methotrexate, azathioprine, cyclosporine, or tumor necrosis factor inhibitors for autoimmune diseases, and HIV infection. Some intestinal cases are associated with Crohn's disease.

Clinically, variably large ulcerations are observed most commonly in the oral mucosa. Multiple lesions in one anatomical region may be observed [97], but alternative diagnoses should be considered in cases with multiple lesions.

### Histopathology, immunophenotype, and molecular genetics

Histology reveals dense lymphoid infiltrates with highly atypical, sometimes Reed–Sternberg-like cells within a polymorphous background, mimicking the features observed in Hodgkin lymphoma (Fig. 21.11). Angiocentricity may be observed in some cases; care should be taken to rule out lymphomatoid granulomatosis in such cases.

The atypical cells are positive for CD30 and PAX-5, with variable positivity for CD15 and reduced expression of CD20, thus simulating Reed–Sternberg cells phenotypically as well (Fig. 21.12a). OCT-2 and MUM-1 are positive, BOB1 is positive in a proportion of cases, and CD10 and Bcl-6 are negative. PD-L1 was expressed by neoplastic cells in all tested cases in one study (PD1 was positive only within the reactive infiltrate) [97].

EBV can be detected within the atypical cells in all cases, but positivity is also observed in small and mid-sized lymphocytes, representing a clue for differentiation from true Hodgkin lymphoma (where EBV-positivity is limited to large, atypical cells) (Fig. 21.12b). In addition, the large blasts are positive for CD45, unlike true Reed–Sternberg cells.

A monoclonal rearrangement of the immunoglobulin genes can be observed in less than half of the cases. There are no data on specific molecular alterations.

### Treatment and prognosis

In most patients, the clinical course was indolent without progression to disseminated disease, and spontaneous remission was observed in several cases following reduction of immune suppression, suggesting that conservative management is adequate [91, 94]. Local radiotherapy or rituximab may be used when the reduction of immune suppression is not possible. Spontaneous resolution has been observed in a distinct percentage of cases [97]. Systemic polychemotherapy is necessary only in exceptional cases [97].

## Résumé

**Epstein–Barr virus (EBV)-associated mucocutaneous ulcers**

| | | |
|---|---|---|
| **Clinical** | Onset in immune senescence or in immune suppressed patients. Variable large ulceration occurring mostly in the oral mucosa. Consider alternative diagnoses for patients with ≥2 lesions. | |
| **Morphology** | Dense lymphoid infiltrates with highly atypical, sometimes Reed–Sternberg-like cells within a polymorphous background. May show angiocentricity. | |
| **Immunohistochemistry** | CD20, CD79a | +/– (may be variable in a single case) |
| | OCT2, MUM1, PD-L1 | + |
| | CD30, PAX5 | + |
| | Bcl-6, CD10 | – |
| | EBER-1 | + (large cells and many small lymphocytes) |
| **Genetics** | Monoclonal rearrangement of the Ig genes in less than half of the cases. | |
| **Treatment guidelines** | Conservative treatment. Nearly all cases respond to the reduction of immune suppression if feasible. Local radiotherapy and rituximab may be used when reduction of immune suppression is not possible. | |

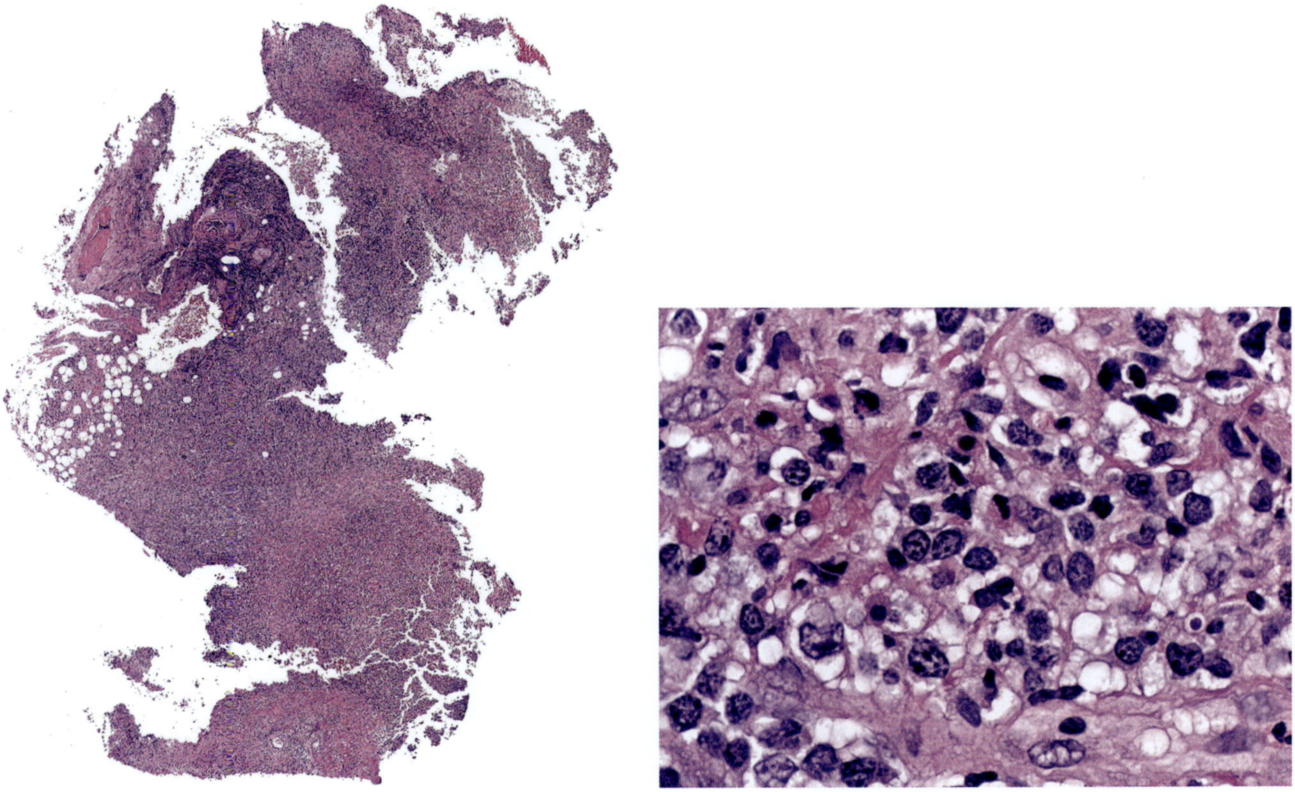

(a) (b)

**Figure 21.11** EBV⁺ mucocutaneous ulcer. (a) Ulcerated, dense lymphoid infiltrate in a lesion from the oral mucosa with (b) several large, atypical cells. *(Courtesy of Prof. Luis Requena, Madrid, Spain.)*

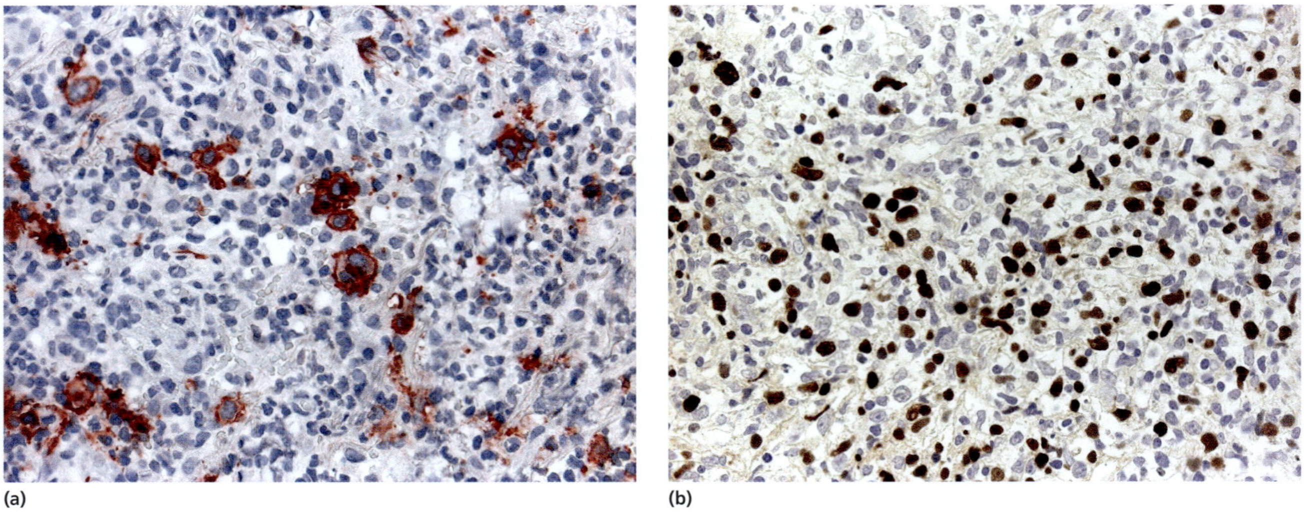

Figure 21.12 EBV+ mucocutaneous ulcer. (a) Positivity of large, atypical cells for CD30. (b) In-situ hybridization for EBV shows positivity of the atypical cells but also of several reactive cells in the background, unlike what is observed in Hodgkin lymphoma. *(Courtesy of Prof. Luis Requena, Madrid, Spain.)*

## Cutaneous manifestations of multicentric Castleman disease

Castleman disease is a peculiar, rare disorder of the lymph nodes (formerly known as angiofollicular or giant lymph node hyperplasia) that may present as unicentric or multicentric disease; in this last instance rarely involving the skin. A role of IL-6 in the pathogenesis of the disorder has been elucidated, and the multicentric disease is commonly associated with HHV-8 infection. Although the disease is not always associated with immunodeficiency/dysregulation, the majority of patients are positive for HIV, and other cases may be related to immune senescence. In previous editions of this book, Castleman disease was included among the pseudolymphomas, but due to the potentially aggressive course and association with immunodeficiency/dysregulation, it has been moved to this Chapter in this edition.

Several forms of Castleman disease are recognized in the lymph nodes: (i) the hyaline vascular variant, characterized by abnormal follicles with regressed germinal centers surrounded by widened mantle zones composed of small lymphocytes with a characteristic onion ring-like arrangement; (ii) the plasma cell variant, characterized by hyperplastic germinal centers and large accumulations of polyclonal plasma cells in the interfollicular region; and (iii) the plasmablastic variant, associated with HIV infection. Castleman disease is a benign, monotypic but polyclonal disorder, but may progress to diffuse large B-cell lymphoma or plasmablastic lymphoma, particularly in the setting of the multicentric variant associated with HIV infection.

Patients with multicentric Castleman disease have systemic symptoms such as fever, night sweats, weakness, fatigue, and weight loss. Virtually all patients have multifocal lymphadenopathy, and the majority of them have hepatosplenomegaly. Anemia and thrombocytopenia are frequent, as well as elevated serum IL-6 levels. Cutaneous lesions are observed mostly in the plasma cell variant and only exceptionally in the hyaline vascular type of Castleman disease. Skin lesions may be nonspecific (such as purpura or vasculitis, among others) or may show specific infiltrates histopathologically, retaining the features of the nodal disease. Multiple reddish-brownish plaques, reminiscent of Kaposi's sarcoma or of cutaneous plasmacytosis, are the most common clinical presentation of specific lesions. Genuine lesions of cutaneous Kaposi sarcoma may be coexistent with nodal multicentric Castleman disease, particularly in HIV+ patients. Histopathologically, variably large lymphoid follicles are surrounded by sheets of polyclonal plasma cells admixed with small lymphocytes (Fig. 21.13). Some of the cells may show features of plasmablasts. Staining for HHV-8 is usually positive. In one reported case, the plasma cells were positive for IgG4 [98]. The skin may also be involved by lymphomas arising on the background of nodal Castleman disease.

Lesions of cutaneous Castleman disease should be distinguished from other plasma cell-rich cutaneous infiltrates, particularly cutaneous marginal zone lymphoproliferative disorder and cutaneous and systemic plasmacytosis (both negative for HHV-8). A relationship between Castleman disease and cutaneous and systemic plasmacytosis has been postulated several times in the past, but differences in the IL-6 pattern, association with HHV-8, and the prognosis point at distinct disorders [99–101]. However, it cannot be excluded that the two diseases represent ends of a spectrum (see also the specific section on cutaneous and systemic plasmacytosis in Chapter 31).

Multicentric Castleman disease, with or without cutaneous involvement, is characterized by a potentially aggressive course. Solitary skin lesions may be excised surgically or

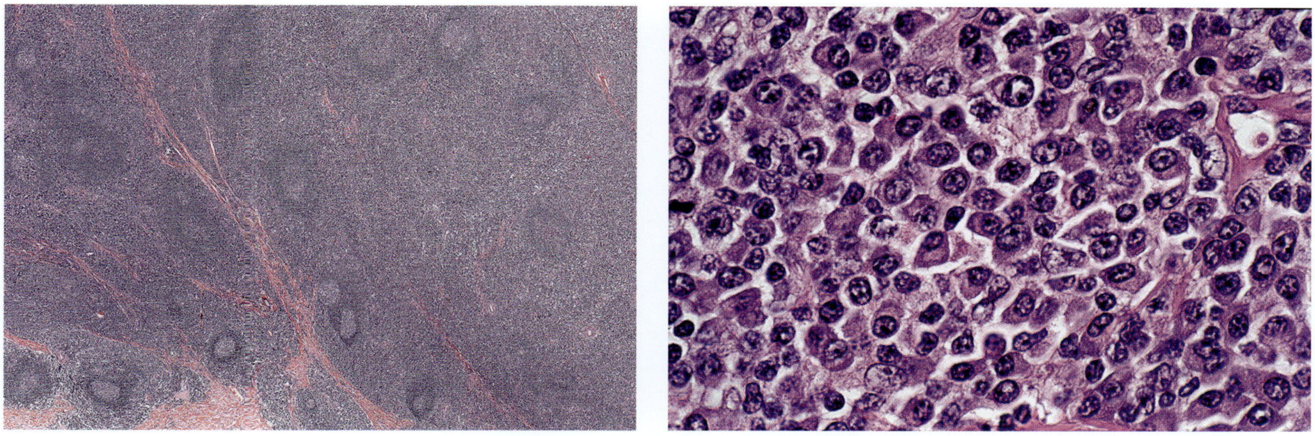

**(a)** **(b)**

**Figure 21.13** Cutaneous Castleman disease, plasma cell variant. (a) Germinal centers are surrounded by sheets of plasma cells. (b) Detail of the plasma cells, some with features of plasmablasts.

treated by local radiotherapy (options also used for unicentric Castleman disease of the lymph nodes). Several treatments have been used for multicentric Castleman disease, including systemic chemotherapy, siltuximab (anti-IL-6 chimeric antibody), interferon-α, and systemic steroids, among others, with rituximab (anti-CD20 antibody) now being considered a treatment of choice. The disease may relapse when treatment is discontinued. Anti-HHV-8 agents (e.g., cidofovir, foscarnet, ganciclovir, or valganciclovir) and liposomal doxorubicin may be used in patients with high viral load and/or concomitant Kaposi sarcoma. ART is used in patients positive for HIV.

### Résumé

| Cutaneous manifestations of multicentric Castleman disease | | |
|---|---|---|
| **Clinical** | Multiple reddish-brownish plaques. Fever, night sweats, weakness, fatigue, and weight loss. Multifocal lymphadenopathy, hepatosplenomegaly. Elevated serum IL-6 levels. | |
| **Morphology** | Variably large lymphoid follicles surrounded by sheets of polyclonal plasma cells admixed with small lymphocytes. Plasmablasts may be present. | |
| **Immunohistochemistry** | CD3, CD20 | +/– |
| | Kappa, Lambda | Polyclonal pattern |
| | HHV-8 | + |
| **Genetics** | Not relevant. | |
| **Treatment guidelines** | Solitary skin lesions may be excised surgically or treated by local radiotherapy. Rituximab. Management of nodal disorder in a hematological setting. | |

## References


1. Natkunam Y, Gratzinger D, Chadburn A, *et al.* Immunodeficiency-associated lymphoproliferative disorders: time for reappraisal? *Blood* 2018;**132**:1871–1878.
2. Campo E, Jaffe ES, Cook JR, *et al.* The International Consensus Classification of Mature Lymphoid Neoplasms: a report from the Clinical Advisory Committee. *Blood* 2022;**140**:1229–1253.
3. De Jong D, Chan JKC, Coupland SE, *et al.* Lymphoid proliferations and lymphomas associated with immune deficiency and dysregulation: Introduction. In: *WHO Classification of Tumours Editorial Board. Haematolymphoid Tumours.* 5th edition. Lyon (France): IARC, 2024: 549–554.
4. Willemze R, Cerroni L, Kempf W, *et al.* The 2018 update of the WHO-EORTC classification for primary cutaneous lymphomas. *Blood* 2019;**133**:1703–1714.

5. Kempf W, Mitteldorf C, Cerroni L, *et al.* Classifications of cutaneous lymphomas and lymphoproliferative disorders: an update from the EORTC cutaneous lymphoma histopathology group. *J Eur Acad Dermatol Venereol* 2024;**38**:1491–1503.
6. Seckin D, Barete S, Euvrard S, *et al.* Primary cutaneous post-transplant lymphoproliferative disorders in solid organ transplant recipients: a multicenter European case series. *Am J Transplant* 2013;**13**:2146–2153.
7. Lanoy E, Costagliola D, Engels EA. Skin cancers associated with HIV infection and solid-organ transplantation among elderly adults. *Int J Cancer* 2010;**126**:1724–1731.
8. Gammon B, Robson A, Deonizio J, *et al.* CD8(+) granulomatous cutaneous T-cell lymphoma: a potential association with immunodeficiency. *J Am Acad Dermatol* 2014;**71**:555–560.
9. Lok C, Viseux V, Denoeux JP, Bagot M. Post-transplant cutaneous T-cell lymphomas. *Crit Rev Oncol Hematol* 2005;**56**:137–145.
10. Pomerantz RG, Campbell LS, Jukic DM, *et al.* Posttransplant cutaneous T-cell lymphoma case reports and review of the Association of Calcineurin Inhibitor Use with Posttransplant Lymphoproliferative Disease Risk. *Arch Dermatol* 2010;**146**:513–516.
11. Mills KC, Sangüeza OP, Beaty MW, *et al.* Composite B-cell and T-cell lineage post-transplant lymphoproliferative disorder of the lung with unusual cutaneous manifestations of mycosis fungoides. *Am J Dermatopathol* 2012;**34**:220–225.
12. Nicol I, Boye T, Carsuzaa F, *et al.* Post-transplant plasmablastic lymphoma of the skin. *Br J Dermatol* 2003;**149**:889–891.
13. Samolitis NJ, Bharadwaj JS, Weis JR, Harris RM. Post-transplant lymphoproliferative disorder limited to the skin. *J Cutan Pathol* 2004;**31**:453–457.
14. Gong S, Crane GM, McCall CM, *et al.* Expanding the spectrum of EBV-positive Marginal Zone Lymphomas: a lesion associated with diverse immunodeficiency settings. *Am J Surg Pathol* 2018;**42**:1306–1316.
15. Kwon EJ, Katz KA, Draft KS, *et al.* Posttransplantation lymphoproliferative disease with features of lymphomatoid granulomatosis in a lung transplant patient. *J Am Acad Dermatol* 2006;**54**:657–663.
16. Molina-Ruiz AM, Pulpillo A, Lasanta B, *et al.* A rare case of primary cutaneous plasmacytoma-like lymphoproliferative disorder following renal transplantation. *J Cutan Pathol* 2012;**39**:685–689.
17. Richendollar BC, Hsi ED, Cook JR. Extramedullary plasmacytoma-like posttransplantation lymphoproliferative disorders clinical and pathologic features. *Am J Clin Pathol* 2009;**132**:581–588.
18. Salama S, Todd S, Cina DP, *et al.* Cutaneous presentation of post-renal transplant lymphoproliferative disorder: a series of four cases. *J Cutan Pathol* 2010;**37**:641–653.
19. Wang E, Stoecker M. Primary cutaneous giant cell plasmacytoma in an organ transplant patient: a rare presentation of a post-transplant lymphoproliferative disorder. *Am J Dermatopathol* 2010;**32**:479–485.
20. Ravat FE, Spittle MF, Russel-Jones R. Primary cutaneous T-cell lymphoma occurring after organ transplantation. *J Am Acad Dermatol* 2006;**54**:668–675.
21. Magro CM, Weinerman DJ, Porcu PL, Morrison CD. Posttransplant EBV-negative anaplastic large-cell lymphoma with dual rearrangement: a propos of two cases and review of the literature. *J Cutan Pathol* 2007;**34**(suppl. 1):1–8.
22. Coyne JD, Banerjee SS, Bromley M, *et al.* Post-transplant T-cell lymphoproliferative disorder/T-cell lymphoma: a report of three cases of T-anaplastic large-cell lymphoma with cutaneous presentation and a review of the literature. *Histopathology* 2004;**44**:387–393.
23. Belloni Fortina A, Montesco MC, Piaserico S, *et al.* Primary cutaneous CD30+ anaplastic large cell lymphoma in a heart transplant patient: case report and literature review. *Acta Derm Venereol (Stockh)* 2009;**89**:74–77.
24. Amin A, Burkhart C, Groben P, *et al.* Primary cutaneous T-cell lymphoma following organ transplantation in a 16-year-old boy. *Pediatr Dermatol* 2009;**26**:112–113.
25. Rogers TS, McGevna L, Cook DL. Pediatric cutaneous T-cell post-transplant lymphoproliferative disorder: case report and review of the literature. *J Cutan Pathol* 2018;**45**:858–863.
26. Bragman SG, Yeaney GA, Greig BW, *et al.* Subcutaneous panniculitic T-cell lymphoma in a cardiac allograft recipient. *J Cutan Pathol* 2005;**32**:366–370.
27. Wallet-Faber N, Bodemer C, Blanche S, *et al.* Primary cutaneous Epstein–Barr virus-related lymphoproliferative disorders in 4 immunosuppressed children. *J Am Acad Dermatol* 2008;**58**:74–80.
28. Colomo L, Loong F, Rives S, *et al.* Diffuse large B-cell lymphomas with plasmablastic differentiation represent a heterogeneous group of disease entities. *Am J Surg Pathol* 2004;**28**:736–747.
29. Morscio J, Dierickx D, Nijs J, *et al.* Clinicopathologic comparison of plasmablastic lymphoma in HIV-positive, immunocompetent, and posttransplant patients single-center series of 25 cases and meta-analysis of 277 reported cases. *Am J Surg Pathol* 2014;**38**:875–886.
30. Paik SH, Kim YJ, Won CH, *et al.* Cutaneous post-transplantation lymphoma: Clinical features and survival outcomes. *J Am Acad Dermatol* 2019;**81**:600–602.
31. Pacheco TR, Hinthner L, Fitzpatrick J. Extramedullary plasmacytoma in cardiac transplant recipients. *J Am Acad Dermatol* 2003;**49**:255–258.
32. Seckin D, Demirhan B, Gülec TO, *et al.* Posttransplantation primary cutaneous CD30 (Ki1)-positive large-cell lymphoma. *J Am Acad Dermatol* 2001;**45**:S197–S199.
33. Ward HA, Russo GG, McBurney E, *et al.* Posttransplant primary cutaneous T-cell lymphoma. *J Am Acad Dermatol* 2001;**44**:675–680.
34. Schumann KW, Oriba HA, Bergfeld WF, *et al.* Cutaneous presentation of post-transplant lymphoproliferative disorder. *J Am Acad Dermatol* 2000;**42**:923–926.
35. Chai C, White WL, Shea CR, Prieto VG. Epstein–Barr virus associated lymphoproliferative – disorders primarily involving the skin. *J Cutan Pathol* 1999;**26**:242–247.
36. Gonthier DM, Hartman G, Holley JL. Post-transplant lymphoproliferative disorder presenting as an isolated skin lesion. *Am J Kidney Dis* 1992;**19**:600–603.
37. McGregor JM, Yu CCW, Lu QL, *et al.* Post-transplant cutaneous lymphoma. *J Am Acad Dermatol* 1993;**29**:549–554.
38. Harris NL, Swerdlow SH. Post-transplant lymphoproliferative disorders: summary of Society for Hematopathology Workshop. *Semin Diagn Pathol* 1997;**14**:8–14.
39. Clarke CA, Morton LM, Lynch C, *et al.* Risk of lymphoma subtypes after solid organ transplantation in the United States. *Br J Cancer* 2013;**109**:280–288.
40. Ibrahim HAH, Menasce LP, Pomplun S, *et al.* Presence of monoclonal T-cell populations in B-cell post-transplant lymphoproliferative disorders. *Mod Pathol* 2011;**24**:232–240.

41. Glowacka I, Korn K, Potthoff SA, *et al.* Delayed seroconversion and rapid onset of lymphoproliferative disease after transmission of HTLV-1 from a multi organ donor. *Clin Infect Dis* 2013;**57**:1417–1424.
42. Rinaldi A, Kwee I, Poretti G, *et al.* Comparative genome-wide profiling of post-transplant lymphoproliferative disorders and diffuse large B-cell lymphomas. *Br J Haematol* 2006;**134**:27–36.
43. Arbiser JL, Mann KP, Losken EM, *et al.* Presence of p16 hypermethylation and Epstein–Barr virus infection in transplant-associated hematolymphoid neoplasms of the skin. *J Am Acad Dermatol* 2006;**55**:794–798.
44. Starzl TE, Nalesnik MA, Porter KA, *et al.* Reversibility of lymphomas and lymphoproliferative lesions developing under cyclosporin–steroid therapy. *Lancet* 1984;**8377**:583–587.
45. Green M. Management of Epstein–Barr virus-induced posttransplant lymphoproliferative disease in recipients of solid organ transplantation. *Am J Transplant* 2001;**1**:103–108.
46. Blokx WAM, Andriessen MPM, van Hamersvelt HW, van Krieken JHJM. Initial spontaneous remission of post-transplantation Epstein–Barr virus-related B-cell lymphoproliferative disorder of the skin in a renal transplant recipient: case report and review of the literature on cutaneous B-cell post-transplantation lymphoproliferative disease. *Am J Dermatopathol* 2002;**24**:414–422.
47. Ferguson NN, Thomas CP, Hohl RJ, *et al.* Primary Cutaneous Polymorphic EBV-Associated Posttransplant Lymphoproliferative Disorder After a Renal Transplant and Review of the Literature. *Am J Dermatopathol* 2015;**37**:790–794.
48. Ricciardelli I, Blundell MP, Brewin J, *et al.* Towards gene therapy for EBV-associated posttransplant lymphoma with genetically modified EBV-specific cytotoxic T cells. *Blood* 2014;**124**: 2514–2522.
49. Chiu LS, Choi PCL, Luk NM, *et al.* Spontaneous regression of primary cutaneous Epstein–Barr virus-positive, CD30-positive anaplastic large T-cell lymphoma in a heart-transplant recipient. *Clin Exp Dermatol* 2009;**34**:e21–e24.
50. Barete S, Frances C, Charlotte F, *et al.* Fatal outcome of deep-penetrating lower limb primary cutaneous anaplastic large cell lymphomas in two immunocompromised patients. *Acta Derm Venereol* 2009;**89**:627–630.
51. Carbone A, Cesarman E, Spina M, *et al.* HIV-associated lymphomas and gamma-herpesviruses. *Blood* 2009;**113**:1213–1224.
52. Chadburn A, Abdul-Nabi AM, Teruya BS, Lo AA. Lymphoid proliferations associated with human immunodeficiency virus infection. *Arch Pathol Lab Med* 2013;**137**:360–370.
53. Beylot-Barry M, Vergier B, Masquelier B, *et al.* The spectrum of cutaneous lymphomas in HIV infection: a study of 21 cases. *Am J Surg Pathol* 1999;**23**:1208–1216.
54. Kerschmann RL, Berger TG, Weiss LM, *et al.* Cutaneous presentations of lymphoma in human immunodeficiency virus disease: predominance of T-cell lineage. *Arch Dermatol* 1995;**131**:1281–1288.
55. Ribera JM, Navarro JT. Human immunodeficiency virus-related non-Hodgkin's lymphoma. *Haematologica* 2008;**93**:1129–1132.
56. Cota C, Lora V, Cerroni L. Primary cutaneous plasmablastic lymphoma as first sign of human immunodeficiency virus infection. *Pathol Case Rev* 2014;**19**:204–207.
57. Pielasinski U, Santonja C, Rodríguez-Pinilla SM, Requena L. Extracavitary primary effusion lymphoma presenting as a cutaneous tumor: a case report and literature review. *J Cutan Pathol* 2014;**41**:745–753.
58. De Masson A, Velter C, Galicier L, *et al.* Disseminated skin involvement in HIV-associated Burkitt lymphoma: a rare clinical feature with poor prognosis. *Br J Dermatol* 2016;**174**:184–186.
59. Corti M, De Carolis L, Solari R, *et al.* Non-Hodgkin's lymphoma with cutaneous involvement in AIDS patients. Report of five cases and review of the literature. *Braz J Infect Dis* 2010;**14**: 81–85.
60. Karkouche R, Ingen-Housz-Oro S, Le Gouvello S, *et al.* Primary cutaneous aggressive epidermotropic CD8+ T-cell lymphoma with KIR3DL2 and NKp46 expression in a human immunodeficiency virus carrier. *J Cutan Pathol* 2015;**42**:199–205.
61. Chadburn A, Cesarman E, Jagirdar J, *et al.* CD30 (Ki-1) positive anaplastic large cell lymphomas in individuals infected with the human immunodeficiency virus. *Cancer* 1993;**72**:3078–3090.
62. Jhala DN, Medeiros LJ, Lopez-Terrada D, *et al.* Neutrophil-rich anaplastic large cell lymphoma of T-cell lineage. A report of two cases arising in HIV-positive patients. *Am J Clin Pathol* 2000; **114**:478–482.
63. Nador RG, Chadburn A, Gundappa G, *et al.* Human immunodeficiency virus (HIV)-associated polymorphic lymphoproliferative disorders. *Am J Surg Pathol* 2003;**27**:293–302.
64. Fardet L, Blanche S, Brousse N, *et al.* Cutaneous EBV-related lymphoproliferative disorder in a 15-year-old boy with AIDS: an unusual clinical presentation. *J Pediatr Hematol Oncol* 2002;**24**:666–669.
65. Poiesz B, Dube D, Dube S, *et al.* HTLV-II-associated cutaneous T-cell lymphoma in a patient with HIV-1 infection. *N Engl J Med* 2000;**342**:930–936.
66. Gandemer V, Verkarre V, Quartier P, *et al.* Lymphomes chez l'enfant infecte par le HIV-1. *Arch Pediatr* 2000;**7**:738–744.
67. Katano H, Suda T, Morishita Y, *et al.* Human herpesvirus 8-associated solid lymphomas that occur in AIDS patients take anaplastic large cell morphology. *Mod Pathol* 2000;**13**:77–85.
68. Nakamura K, Katano H, Hoshino Y, *et al.* Human herpesvirus type 8 and Epstein–Barr virus-associated cutaneous lymphoma taking anaplastic large cell morphology in a man with HIV infection. *Br J Dermatol* 1999;**141**:141–145.
69. Liapis K, Clear A, Owen A, *et al.* The microenvironment of AIDS-related diffuse large B-cell lymphoma provides insight into the pathophysiology and indicates possible therapeutic strategies. *Blood* 2013;**122**:424–433.
70. Paech V, Lorenzen T, Stoehr A, *et al.* Remission of cutaneous mycosis fungoides in a patient with advanced HIV-infection. *Eur J Med Res* 2002;**7**:477–479.
71. Saggini A, Anemona L, Chimenti S, *et al.* HIV-associated primary cutaneous anaplastic large cell lymphoma: a clinicopathological subset with more aggressive behavior? Case report and review of the literature. *J Cutan Pathol* 2012;**39**:1100–1109.
72. Castillo JJ, Beltran BE, Bibas M, *et al.* Prognostic factors in patients with HIV-associated peripheral T-cell lymphoma: a multicenter study. *Am J Hematol* 2011;**86**:256–261.
73. Salloum E, Cooper DL, Howe G, *et al.* Spontaneous regression of lymphoproliferative disorders in patients treated with methotrexate for rheumatoid arthritis and other rheumatic diseases. *J Clin Oncol* 1996;**14**:1943–1949.
74. Feng WH, Cohen JI, Fischer S, *et al.* Reactivation of latent Epstein–Barr virus by methotrexate: a potential contributor to methotrexate-associated lymphomas. *J Natl Cancer Inst* 2004;**96**:1691–1702.

75. Koens L, Senff NJ, Vermeer MH, *et al.* Methotrexate-associated B-cell Lymphoproliferative Disorders Presenting in the Skin. A Clinicopathologic and Immunophenotypical Study of 10 Cases. *Am J Surg Pathol* 2014;**38**:999–1006.
76. Shimizu S, Inokuma D, Murata J, *et al.* Cutaneous manifestations of methotrexate-associated lymphoproliferative disorders: report of two cases and a review of the literature. *Acta Derm Venereol* 2015;**95**:366–367.
77. Pfistershammer K, Petzelbauer P, Stingl G, *et al.* Methotrexate-induced primary cutaneous diffuse large B-cell lymphoma with an "angiocentric" histological morphology. *Clin Exp Dermatol* 2010;**35**:59–62.
78. Shimura C, Satoh T, Takayama K, *et al.* Methotrexate-related lymphoproliferative disorder with extensive vascular involvement in a patient with rheumatoid arthritis. *J Am Acad Dermatol* 2009;**61**:126–129.
79. Corazza M, Zampino MR, Montanari A, *et al.* Primary cutaneous CD30+ large T-cell lymphoma in a patient with psoriasis treated with cyclosporine. *Dermatology* 2003;**206**:330–333.
80. Kirby B, Owen CM, Blewitt RW, Yates VM. Cutaneous T-cell lymphoma developing in a patient on cyclosporin therapy. *J Am Acad Dermatol* 2002;**47**:s165–s167.
81. Hernandez C, Worobec SM, Gaitonde S, *et al.* Progression of undiagnosed cutaneous T-cell lymphoma during efalizumab therapy. *Arch Dermatol* 2009;**145**:92–94.
82. Lafaille P, Bouffard D, Provost N. Exacerbation of undiagnosed mycosis fungoides during treatment with etanercept. *Arch Dermatol* 2009;**145**:94–95.
83. Chuang GS, Wasserman DI, Byers HR, Demierre MF. Hypopigmented T-cell dyscrasia evolving to hypopigmented mycosis fungoides during etanercept therapy. *J Am Acad Dermatol* 2008;**59**:s121–s122.
84. O'Malley DP, Chen S, Perkins SL, *et al.* Monoclonal antibody immunomodulator-related lymphoid proliferations. *J Haematopathol* 2008;**1**:228–229.
85. Clarke LE, Junkins-Hopkins JM, Seykora JT, *et al.* Methotrexate-associated lymphoproliferative disorder in a patient with rheumatoid arthritis presenting in the skin. *J Am Acad Dermatol* 2007;**56**:686–690.
86. Rausch T, Cairoli A, Benhattar J, *et al.* EBV+ cutaneous B-cell lymphoproliferation of the leg in an elderly patient with mycosis fungoides and methotrexate treatment. *APMIS* 2013;**121**:79–84.
87. Kurita D, Miyoshi H, Ichikawa A, *et al.* Methotrexate-associated Lymphoproliferative Disorders in Patients With Rheumatoid Arthritis: Clinicopathologic Features and Prognostic Factors. *Am J Surg Pathol* 2019;**43**:869–884.
88. Maderal AD, Malone JC, Callen JP. Methotrexate-Associated B-Cell Lymphoproliferative Disease in a Patient With Cutaneous T-Cell Lymphoma. *JAMA Dermatol* 2018;**154**:490–492.
89. Carreras J, Yukie KY, Miyaoka M, *et al.* Genomic Profile and Pathologic Features of Diffuse Large B-Cell Lymphoma Subtype of Methotrexate-associated Lymphoproliferative Disorder in Rheumatoid Arthritis Patients. *Am J Surg Pathol* 2018;**42**:936–950.
90. Claudino WM, Gibson B, Tse W, *et al.* Methotrexate-associated primary cutaneous CD30-positive cutaneous T-cell lymphoproliferative disorder: a case illustration and a brief review. *Am J Blood Res* 2016;**6**:1–5.
91. Dojcinov SD, Venkataraman G, Raffeld M, *et al.* EBV positive mucocutaneous ulcer- – a study of 26 cases associated with various sources of immunosuppression. *Am J Surg Pathol* 2010;**34**:405–417.
92. Natkunam Y, Gratzinger D, Bhagat G, *et al.* EBV-positive mucocutaneous ulcer. In: *WHO Classification of Tumours Editorial Board. Haematolymphoid Tumours.* 5th edition. Lyon (France): IARC, 2024: 565–567.
93. Dojcinov S, Cohen JI, Jaffe ES. Epstein-Barr virus-positive mucocutaneous ulcer. In: Arber DA, Borowitz MJ, Cook JR, *et al.*, eds. *The International Consensus Classification of Myeloid and Lymphoid Neoplasms.* Philadelphia (US): Wolters Kluver, 2025: 510–513.
94. Dojcinov SD, Venkataraman G, Pittaluga S, *et al.* Age-related EBV-associated lymphoproliferative disorders in the Western population: a spectrum of reactive lymphoid hyperplasia and lymphoma. *Blood* 2011;**117**:4726–4735.
95. Moran NR, Webster B, Lee KM, *et al.* Epstein Barr virus-positive mucocutaneous ulcer of the colon associated Hodgkin lymphoma in Crohn's disease. *World J Gastroenterol* 2015;**2015**(21): 6072–6076.
96. Nishida H, Oyama Y, Kusaba T, *et al.* A case of methotrexate-associated lymphoproliferative disorder (Lymphomatoid Granulomatosis) of the skin. *Am J Dermatopathol* 2019;**41**: 448–452.
97. Prieto-Torres L, Eraña I, Gil-Redondo R, *et al.* The spectrum of EBV-positive mucocutaneous ulcer: a study of 9 cases. *Am J Surg Pathol* 2019;**43**:201–210.
98. Takeuchi M, Sato Y, Takata K, *et al.* Cutaneous multicentric Castleman's disease mimicking IgG4-related disease. *Pathol Res Pract* 2012;**208**:746–749.
99. Honda R, Cerroni L, Tanikawa A, *et al.* Cutaneous plasmacytosis: report of 6 cases with or without systemic involvement. *J Am Acad Dermatol* 2013;**68**:978–985.
100. Haque M, Hou JS, Hisamichi K, *et al.* Cutaneous and systemic plasmacytosis vs. cutaneous plasmacytic Castleman disease: review and speculations about pathogenesis. *Clin Lymphoma Myeloma Leuk* 2011;**11**:453–461.
101. Shimizu S, Tanaka M, Shimizu H, Hanyaku H. Is cutaneous plasmacytosis a distinct clinical entity? *J Am Acad Dermatol* 1997;**36**:876–880.

SECTION 4

# Specific cutaneous manifestations of leukemias and of precursor hematologic neoplasms

## CHAPTER 22

# Cutaneous manifestations of B-cell chronic lymphocytic leukemia

B-cell chronic lymphocytic leukemia (B-CLL) (listed as "chronic lymphocytic leukaemia/small lymphocytic lymphoma") in the 5th edition of the World Health Organization (WHO) *Classification of Haematolymphoid Tumors* represents the most frequent type of adults' leukemia in Western countries [1]. In the International Consensus Classification (ICC) *of Myeloid and Lymphoid Neoplasms*, B-CLL is discussed in a chapter that includes also monoclonal B-cell lymphocytosis [2]. In patients affected by B-CLL, cutaneous lesions are common, representing in most instances nonspecific manifestations related to the impaired immune competence or to the administration of drugs. In some cases, however, neoplastic B lymphocytes are found within the skin [3]. Such lesions are referred to as specific cutaneous manifestations of B-CLL or as "leukemia cutis." It must be remembered that under the same term of "leukemia cutis," specific cutaneous manifestations of other types of leukemia, particularly myelogenous leukemia, have also been described. In contrast to cutaneous involvement by myeloid leukemia, which sometimes is observed before the diagnosis of leukemia is established in the bone marrow and/or blood ("aleukemic" leukemia cutis – see Chapter 23), specific cutaneous manifestations of B-CLL are usually concomitant to the first diagnosis or more commonly arise during the course of the disease, and only very rarely predate the diagnosis [4, 5].

Specific infiltrates of B-CLL have been frequently observed at the site of cutaneous inflammation due to different causes, showing that neoplastic cells retain at least in part the capability to answer chemotactic stimuli and to migrate to tissues where an immune response is being mounted [6–10]. This peculiar specific "inflammatory-like" response of B-CLL in the skin can be observed in various, unrelated conditions including benign and malignant cutaneous neoplasms (e.g., squamous cell carcinoma, seborrheic keratosis, and melanoma), cutaneous infections (e.g., herpes simplex and herpes zoster, and *Borrelia*), and inflammatory disorders (e.g., rosacea and xanthomas). Intravascular neoplastic cells have been documented also in a case of Kaposi sarcoma [11].

The skin may be involved in progression of B-CLL to a large cell lymphoma (Richter syndrome), and prognosis of Richter syndrome occurring in the skin may be better than when occurring at extracutaneous sites [12, 13].

## Clinical features

Clinically, patients with specific cutaneous manifestations of B-CLL present with localized or generalized erythematous papules, plaques, or tumors [3, 14–16]. Ulceration is uncommon. Multiple plaque and tumors on the face may result in the clinical picture of so-called "facies leonina" (Fig. 22.1).

Specific skin lesions of B-CLL at the sites of previous herpes simplex or herpes zoster eruptions are characterized by confluent papules arising a few days or weeks at the site of a healed herpes infection (Fig. 22.2) [6]. These lesions were often classified in the past as pseudolymphoma, but in most patients affected by B-CLL represent in fact specific cutaneous manifestations of the disease triggered by the immune response to the viruses [6]. It should be underlined that post-herpetic lymphoid infiltrates are not restricted to patients with B-CLL but may arise also in healthy individuals (in such cases representing a type of cutaneous pseudolymphoma – see Chapter 31).

In patients with B-CLL, cutaneous tumors arising at typical sites of *Borrelia burgdorferi*-associated lymphocytoma cutis (nipple, scrotum, and earlobe) represent specific manifestations of the disease caused by infection with *B. burgdorferi* (Fig. 22.3) [7]. Lesions arising on the nipple were well known in the past and were termed "leukemia lymphatica mammillae" in older textbooks, but of course relationship to *Borrelia* infection was not known at that time. Similar lesions can be observed also at other sites of the body, and respond slowly to antibiotic treatment (doxycycline of ceftriaxone for 3 weeks) (Fig. 22.4). Besides specific manifestations at sites typical of *Borrelia*-induced lymphocytoma, in one case, neoplastic infiltrates of B-CLL have also been observed at the site of *Borrelia*-associated erythema migrans [8], and I have rarely observed similar cases (Fig. 22.5).

*Skin Lymphoma: The Illustrated Guide*, Sixth Edition. Lorenzo Cerroni.

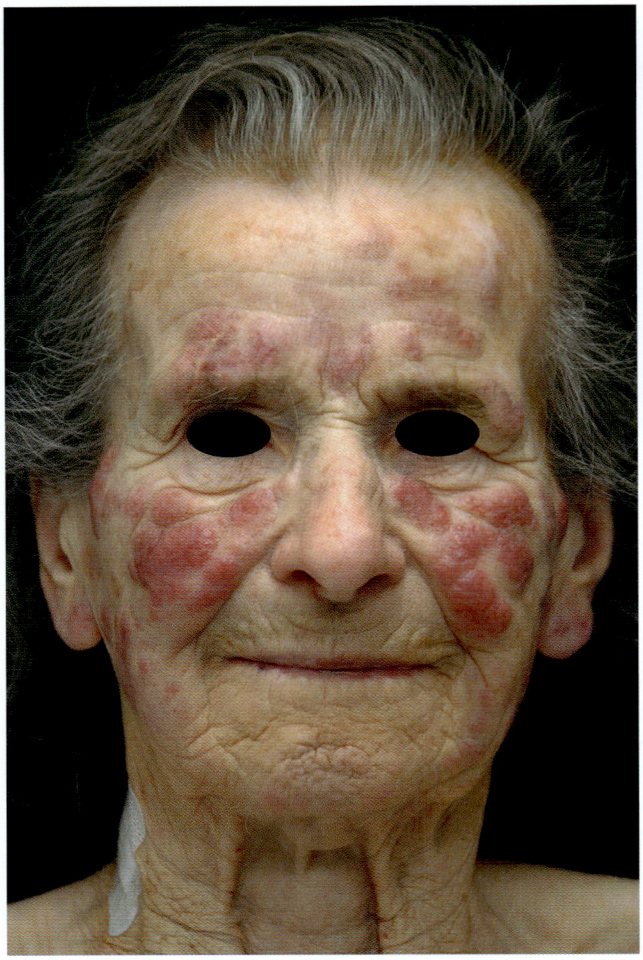

**Figure 22.1** Cutaneous B-CLL. Plaques and nodules on the face ("facies leonina").

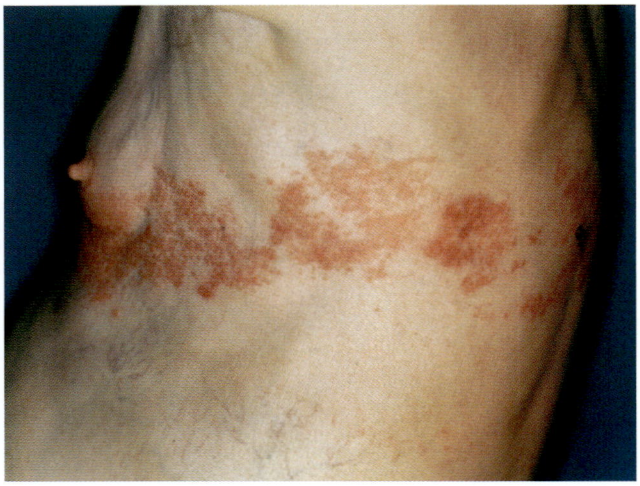

**Figure 22.2** Cutaneous B-CLL. Specific skin manifestations at the site of a previous herpes zoster eruption.

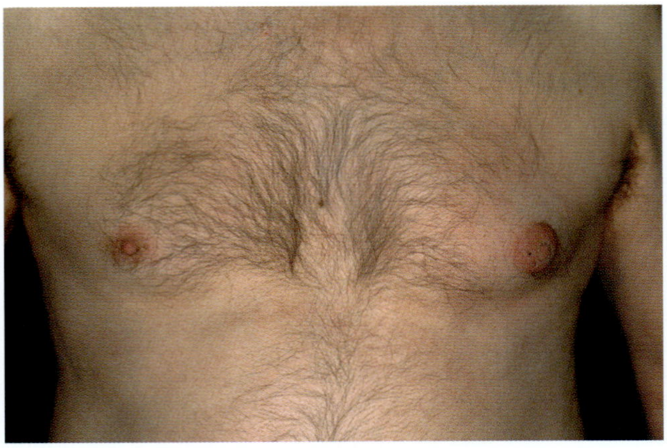

**Figure 22.3** Cutaneous B-CLL. Specific skin manifestation on the left nipple, at the site of a *Borrelia burgdorferi* infection (so-called "leukemia lymphatica mammillae").

Neoplastic cells of B-CLL can be observed also in several other "inflammatory" settings or in the context of cutaneous benign and malignant tumors. I have seen patients with rosacea or eruptive xanthomas associated with specific manifestations of B-CLL (Fig. 22.6). In these cases, lesions of rosacea appear more infiltrated than in conventional cases (Fig. 22.7). As for herpes and *Borrelia*-associated B-CLL, the lesions of the inflammatory dermatosis may be more resistant to conventional treatment. Cutaneous nonlymphoid tumors (e.g., squamous cell carcinoma and basal cell carcinoma) harboring neoplastic cells of B-CLL do not present any peculiar clinical aspect that may suggest the presence of these lymphocytes, and only upon histological examination it is possible to identify them.

Finally, a peculiar cutaneous hypersensitivity reaction has been observed in patients with B-CLL (and other types of non-Hodgkin lymphoma). This condition was previously referred to as "exaggerated insect bite-like reaction," but in many cases, it is not related to arthropod bites, and the term "eosinophilic dermatitis of haematological malignancies" has been proposed (see Chapter 29 for a more detailed discussion) [17–19]. When these lesions arise in the context of a B-CLL, neoplastic cells are sometimes found within the biopsy specimen admixed with large numbers of eosinophils and with reactive T lymphocytes [18]. The lesions are unrelated to laboratory findings, disease course, therapy, or prognosis, and usually resolve within a few weeks.

## Histopathology, immunophenotype, and molecular genetics

### Histopathology

Histology of specific manifestations of B-CLL may show either patchy, perivascular, and periadnexal lymphoid clusters or the presence of dense, monomorphous, nodular, or diffuse infiltrates of lymphocytes (Fig. 22.8) [6]. The subcutaneous fat is

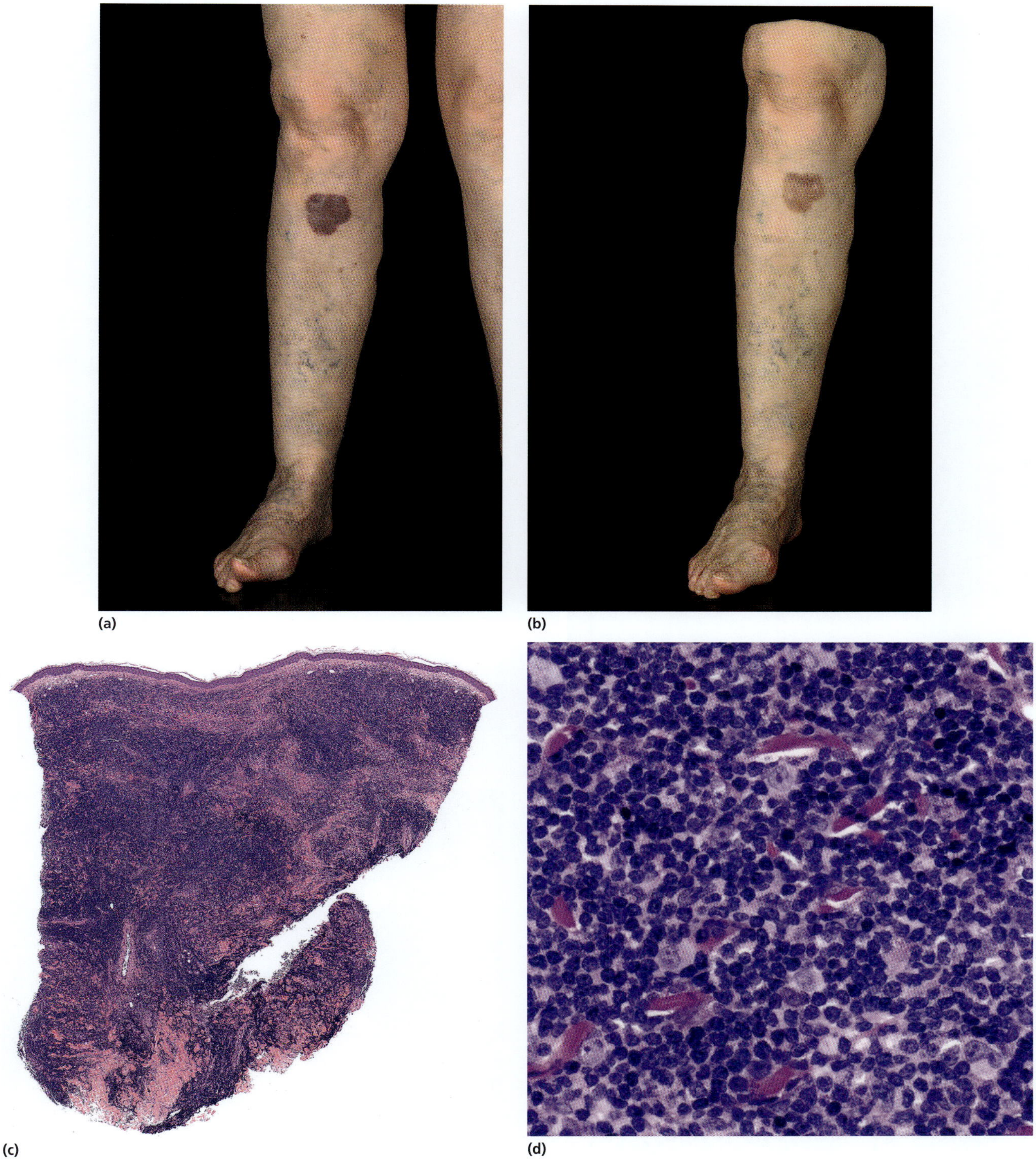

Figure 22.4 Cutaneous B-CLL. Specific skin manifestation on the right lower leg, at the site of a *Borrelia burgdorferi* infection. (a) Clinical picture at presentation; (b) complete resolution with post-inflammatory hyperpigmentation 10 months later (the antibiotic treatment was given for 3 weeks); (c) dense, diffuse infiltrate within the entire dermis; and (d) predominantly composed of small, monomorphous lymphocytes.

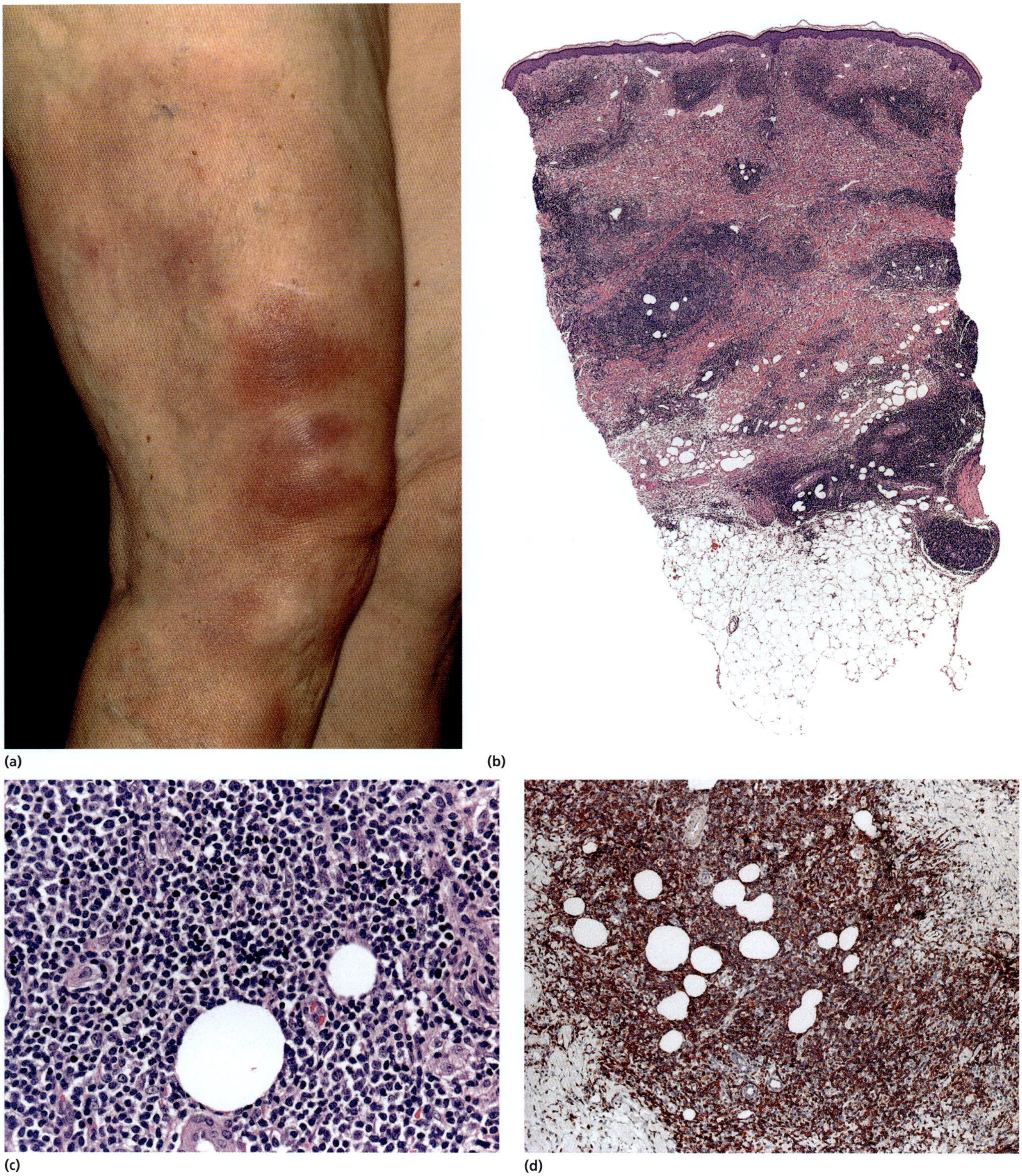


**Figure 22.5** Cutaneous B-CLL at the site of *Borrelia*-associated erythema migrans. (a) Partly annular, partly infiltrated, broad erythema extending from the middle of the right thigh to the area below the right knee of a 69-year-old woman with known B-CLL. (b) Dense lymphoid infiltrates within the entire dermis and involving the superficial part of the subcutaneous fat, (c) composed predominantly of small, hyperchromatic lymphocytes. Immunohistology revealed positivity for CD5 (d) and CD20 (e), as well as for CD23 and CD43. A PCR investigation for *Borrelia* DNA revealed the presence of a specific band. The lesions responded very slowly to antibiotic treatment and the patient was free of *Borrelia*-related skin lesions 7 months after observation.

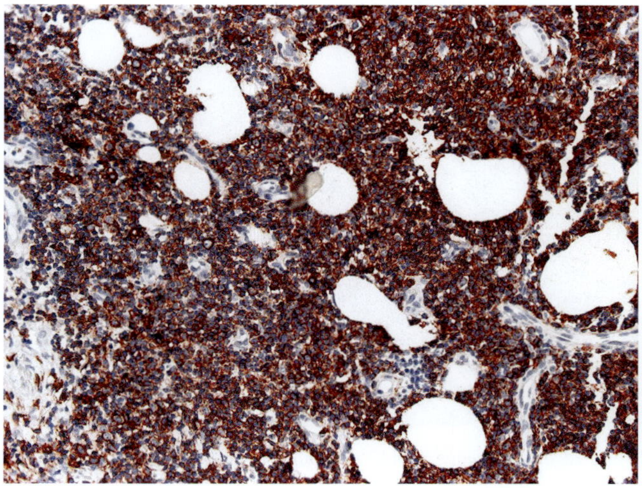

(e)

Figure 22.5 (Continued)

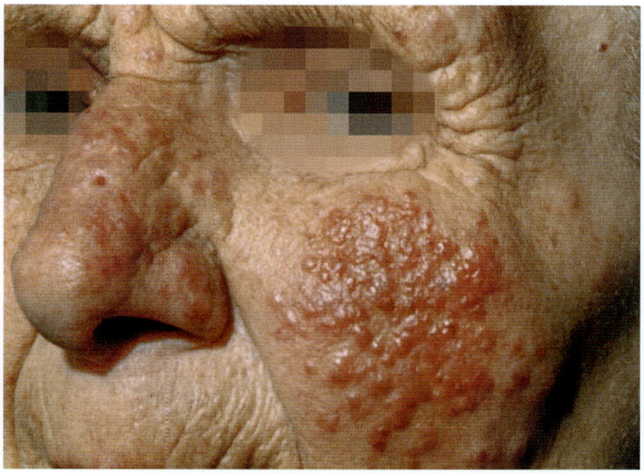

Figure 22.7 Cutaneous B-CLL in a patient with rosacea. The papules appear more infiltrated than in conventional papular rosacea.

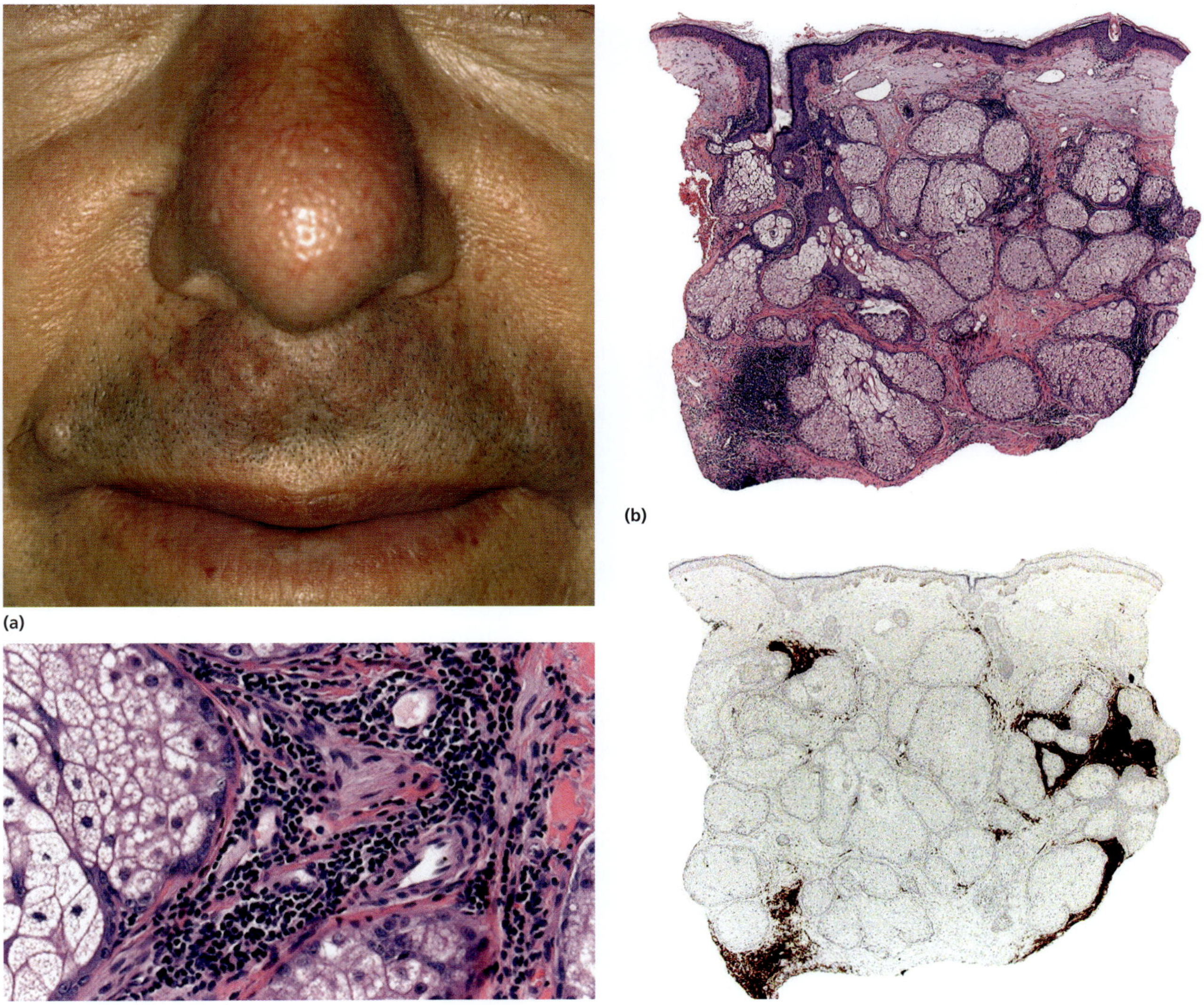

(a) (b) (c) (d)

Figure 22.6 Cutaneous B-CLL at the site of beginning rhinophyma. (a) Swelling of the distal part of the nose with telangiectatic vessels. (b, c) Hyperplasia of sebaceous glands with patchy lymphoid infiltrates, which are (d) positive for CD20.

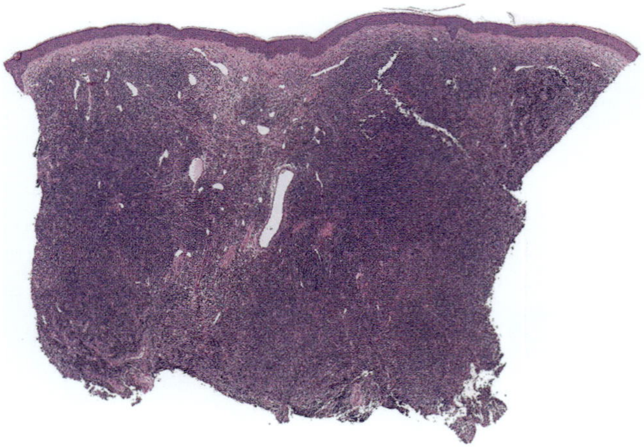

**Figure 22.8** Cutaneous B-CLL. Dense, diffuse lymphoid infiltrates within the entire dermis.

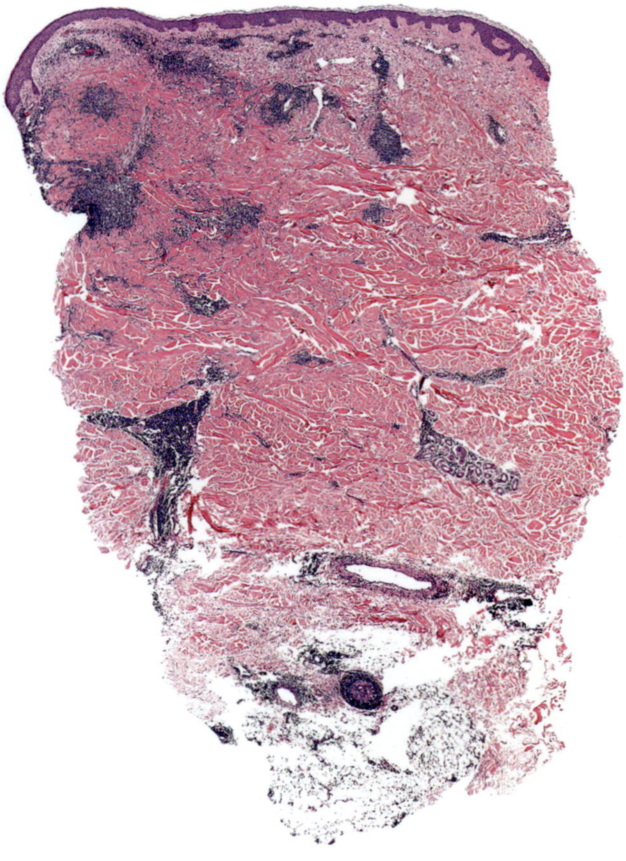

**Figure 22.9** Cutaneous B-CLL. Patchy, nodular lymphoid infiltrates in the dermis and subcutaneous fat.

almost invariably involved, even in cases in which the infiltrate is not very dense (Fig. 22.9). The infiltrate is composed predominantly of small hyperchromatic lymphocytes without prominent atypical features (Fig. 22.10). Small nodular areas with larger, paler cells showing features of prolymphocytes or

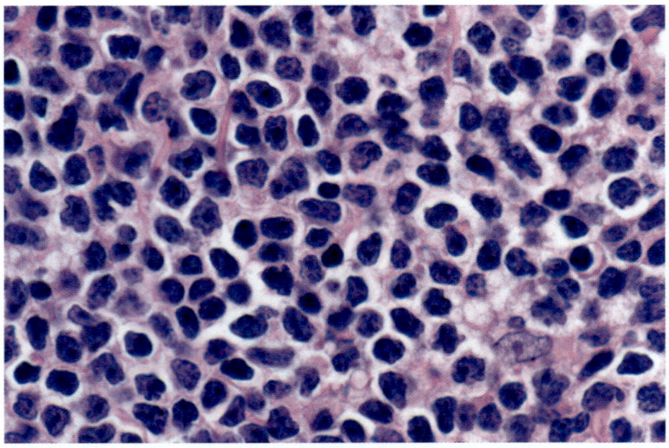

**Figure 22.10** Cutaneous B-CLL. Monomorphous infiltrate of small, hyperchromatic lymphocytes.

paraimmunoblasts (so-called "proliferation centers") can be observed occasionally (Fig. 22.11), and should not be misinterpreted as large cell transformation [6]. In some cases, other cells such as eosinophils and epithelioid histiocytes can be found.

In patients with B-CLL, neoplastic B-lymphocytes may be observed in biopsy specimens of different cutaneous conditions, representing specific manifestations of the disease at sites of skin inflammation (Fig. 22.12) [6–9]. In these cases, the neoplastic lymphocytes of the B-CLL are admixed with variable numbers of reactive cells (T lymphocytes, plasma cells, and histiocytes – sometimes with the formation of small granulomas, eosinophils, and neutrophils). In contrast to conventional *Borrelia*-associated "pseudolymphomas" arising in healthy patients, florid germinal centers are never observed in skin manifestations of B-CLL triggered by *Borrelia* infection, and the infiltrate shows a proliferation of mostly small, monomorphous lymphocytes (Figs. 22.4d, 22.5c). In patients with high numbers of lymphocytes in the blood, neoplastic cells can be observed mixed with erythrocytes at the site of surgical-related haemorrhage for biopsies performed for different reasons. In rare instances, small lymph nodes with infiltration of small lymphocytic lymphoma may be observed in skin biopsies below the subcutaneous fat (Fig. 22.13). The main clues for the identification of specific skin infiltrates of B-CLL in elderly patients on the background of a neoplastic or inflammatory skin conditions are listed in Table 22.1 (Figs. 22.14–22.17). If a B-CLL is not already known, these patients should be checked for the presence of it. As already mentioned, some cases of eosinophilic dermatitis of hematological malignancies in B-CLL patients are characterized by the presence of neoplastic cells besides T-lymphocytes, histiocytes, and large numbers of eosinophils.

Cases of cutaneous "composite" lymphoma with features of both mycosis fungoides and B-CLL have been observed [20], possibly representing a further example of migration of neoplastic B-lymphocytes at sites of various skin disorders

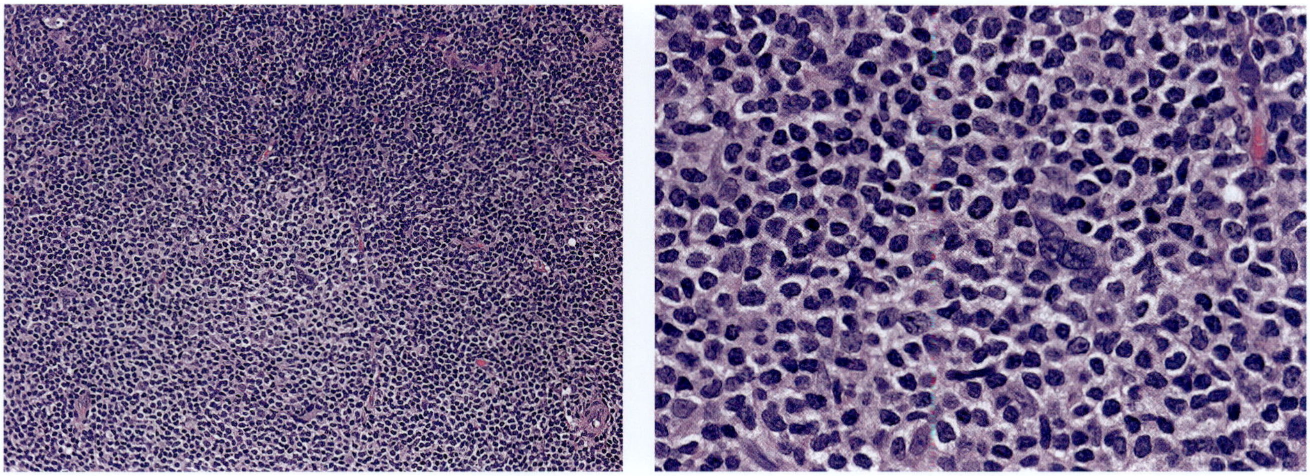

(a) (b)

**Figure 22.11** Cutaneous B-CLL. (a) Small lymphocytes admixed with a vaguely nodular, paler area with (b) several larger cells (prolymphocytes, paraimmunoblasts) representing a proliferation center.

(see also Chapter 28). I have also had the opportunity to observe a case of cutaneous intravascular large T-cell lymphoma arising in a patient with B-CLL (courtesy of Dr. Heinz Kutzner, Friedrichshafen, Germany), characterized by dermal vessels filled with neoplastic large T cells of the intravascular lymphoma and surrounded by perivascular infiltrates of CD20$^+$/CD5$^+$ small lymphocytes of the B-CLL (Fig. 28.2 in Chapter 28).

### Immunophenotype and molecular genetics

Immunohistology reveals the presence of B lymphocytes characterized by an aberrant immunophenotype (CD20$^+$, CD5$^+$, CD23$^+$, and CD43$^+$) (Fig. 22.12e) [3]. CD200, an OX-2 membrane glycoprotein, is expressed in nearly all cases of B-CLL, whereas CD5 may be negative in some cutaneous lesions. A cytoplasmic monoclonal expression of immunoglobulin (Ig) light chains may be detectable in rare examples. In contrast to mantle cell lymphoma, cyclin-D1 and SOX-11 are negative in B-CLL (cyclin-D1 may be positive in some of the cells of proliferation centres). The lymphoid enhancer-binding factor 1 (LEF1) is positive with a nuclear expression in cases of B-CLL but negative in marginal zone lymphoma and mantle cell lymphoma. A variable population of reactive T lymphocytes may be present.

The zeta-chain-associated protein kinase 70 (ZAP-70), a protein that is part of the T-cell receptor, correlates with the mutation status of B-CLL and is expressed in a subset of cases with a worse prognosis (both nuclear or cytoplasmic staining can be observed) (Fig. 22.18) [21, 22].

Molecular genetics shows in most cases a monoclonal rearrangement of the Ig genes. There is evidence that two relevant prognostic subgroups of B-CLL can be defined according to the presence or absence of somatic hypermutations in the neoplastic cells [1, 2, 22]. Reports of cutaneous involvement in patients with B-CLL did not mention the mutation status of the original leukemia, so data on the frequency of specific skin manifestations in the two subtypes are lacking.

At extracutaneous sites, B-CLL is characterized by various driver mutations found in different proportions during the course of the disease, such as mutations of *NOTCH1* (neurogenic locus notch homolog protein 1), *SF3B1* (splicing factor 3B subunit 1), *BIRC3* (baculoviral IAP repeat-containing protein 3), *TP53* (tumor protein 53), *ATM* (ataxia telangiectasia mutated), and *MYD88* (myeloid differentiation primary response gene 88) [23]. The disease is characterized by a peculiar clonal heterogeneity modulated over time, explaining in part the different features found in various organs and at different time during the course of the disease [24].

## Treatment and prognosis

Prognosis seems not to be affected by skin involvement [3, 10, 25]. The treatment must be planned according to the hematologic findings and the mutational status.

The management of cutaneous manifestations can often be carried out in a dermatological setting. Small solitary or clustered skin lesions may be removed surgically or by $CO_2$ laser vaporization. Larger lesions may be treated by radiotherapy. Positive responses to UV-B therapy, cladribine, and alemtuzumab have been reported [26, 27]. Rarely, skin manifestations may regress slowly without any specific treatment [28].

Chemotherapy should be used only if the hematological background requires it. Ibrutinib (a molecule that blocks B-cell receptor signaling) is considered as a first-line treatment if patients require therapy. Other drugs targeting molecular

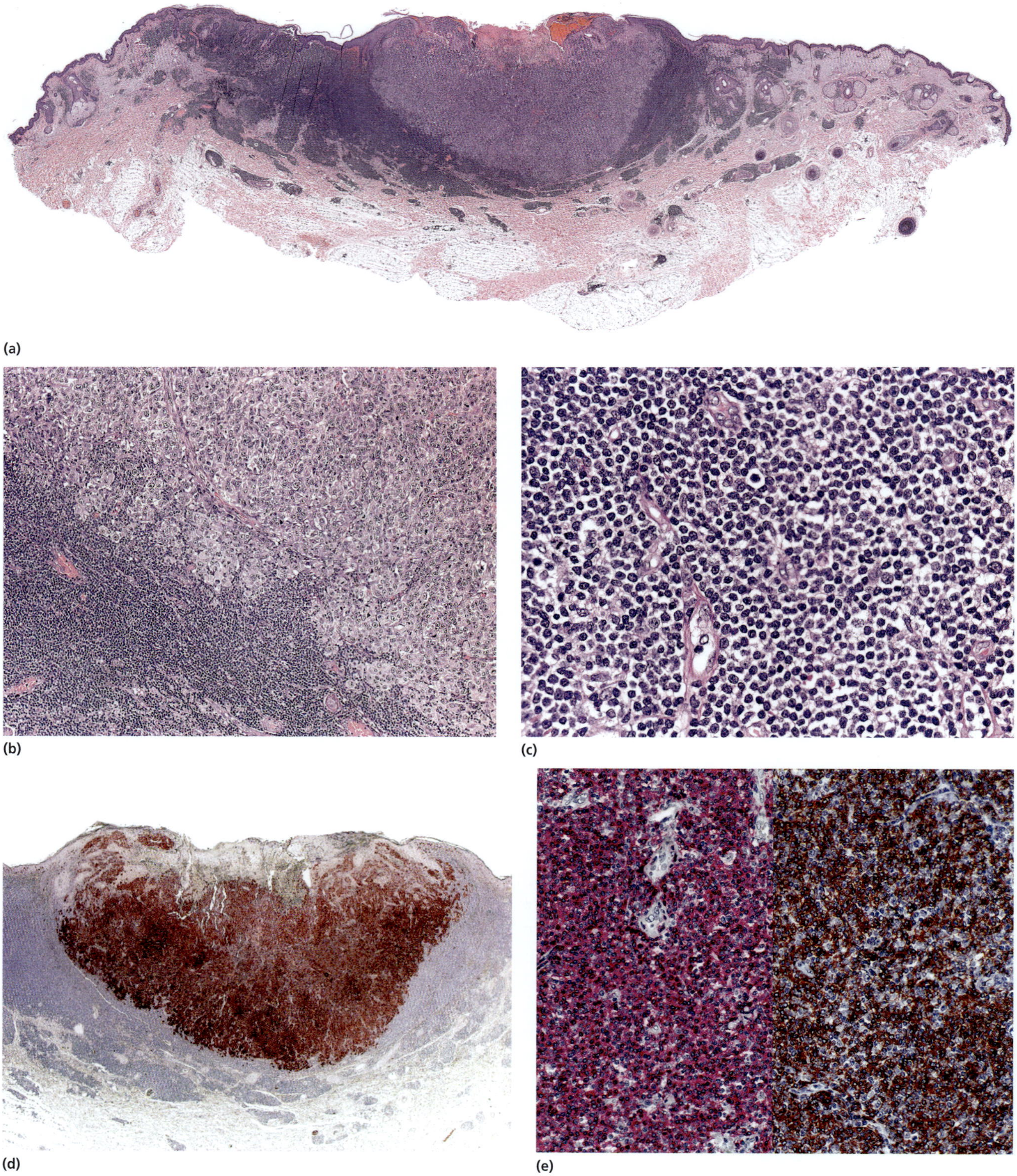


Figure 22.12 Cutaneous B-CLL at the site of a melanoma. (a) Large tumor surrounded by heavy lymphoid infiltrates; (b) epithelioid cells of melanoma and small, monomorphous, hyperchromatic lymphocytes of B-CLL; (c) detail of neoplastic lymphocytes of the B-CLL; (d) S100-positivity of melanoma cells; and (e) the lymphocytes are positive for CD20 (left) and CD23 (right).

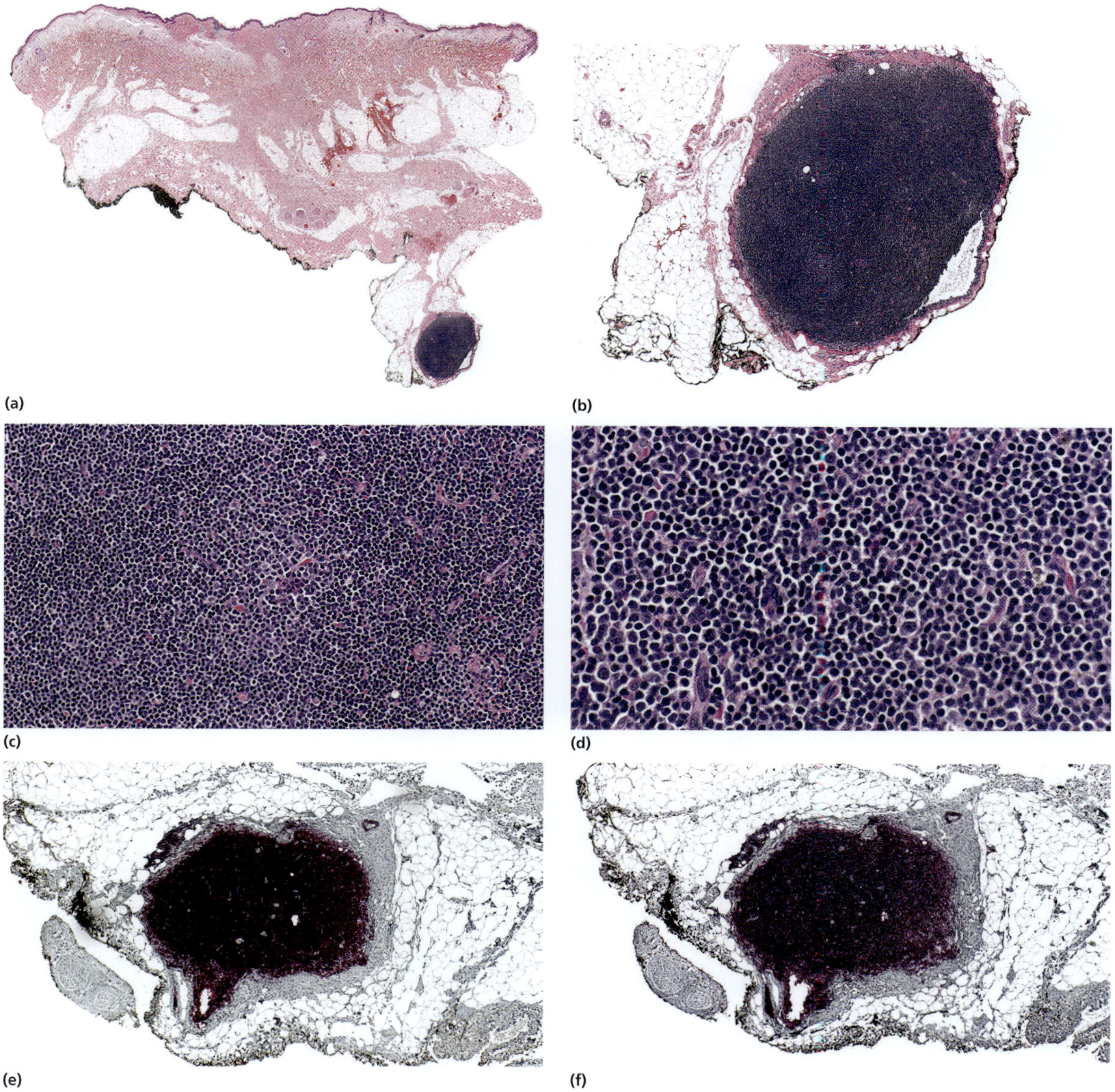


**Figure 22.13** B-CLL/small lymphocytic lymphoma within a lymph node in a biopsy specimen of re-excision of a previous squamous cell carcinoma. (a) Small lymph node at the base of the biopsy with (b) altered architecture; (c, d) predominance of small, hyperchromatic lymphocytes admixed with some larger cells. Most neoplastic cells are positive for CD20 (e) and CD23 (f).

**Table 22.1** Main clues for the identification of specific infiltrates of B-CLL in skin biopsies taken from elderly patients for other reasons (e.g., removal of a skin tumor)

| |
|---|
| Dense, monomorphous infiltrates composed mostly of small lymphocytes located in the immediate vicinity of a skin tumor (epithelial, melanocytic, or others) (Figs. 22.12 and 22.15). |
| Small, perivascular aggregates of small lymphocytes within the subcutaneous fat, distant from the main pathological substrate (Fig. 22.16). |
| Presence of lymphocytes within the hemorrhage associated with the surgical procedure (Fig. 22.14). |
| Presence of lymphocytes within the veins in the subcutaneous fat (Fig. 22.17). |

pathways that are used alone or in combination are venetoclax (a BH3-mimetic that blocks the antiapoptotic Bcl-2 protein), rituximab and obinutuzumab (anti-CD20 antibodies), and alemtuzumab (anti-CD52 antibody). Different chemotherapeutics including bendamustine, fludarabine, cyclophosphamide, and pentostatin are also used in combination with monoclonal antibodies (bendamustine and rituximab; FCR scheme: fludarabine, cyclophosphamide, and rituximab; PCR scheme: pentostatin, cyclophosphamide, and rituximab).

Patients with somatic hypermutations (mutated B-CLL) have a better prognosis than those without mutations (unmutated B-CLL), especially in earlier stages of the disease.

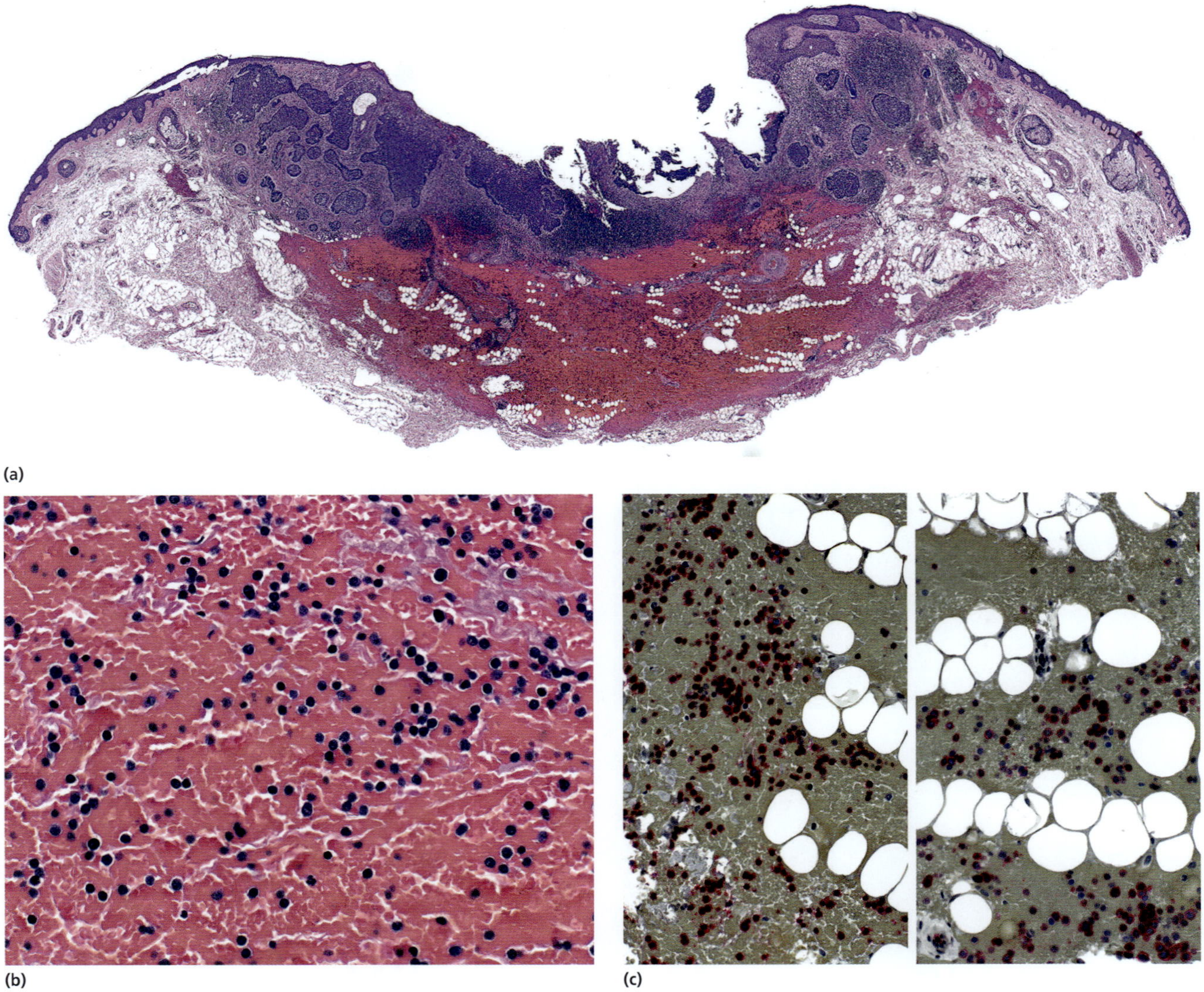

Figure 22.14 B-CLL cells within the hemorrhage. (a) Ulcerated basal cell carcinoma with large areas of hemorrhage; (b) numerous lymphocytes within the hemorrhage; and (c) positive for CD20 (left) and CD5 (right).

## Progression to diffuse large B-cell lymphoma (Richter syndrome)

Large cell transformation of B-CLL (Richter syndrome) has been reported occasionally in the skin [3, 29–34]. A role for Epstein–Barr virus has been postulated in transformation of B-CLL, but the exact etiology remains unclear. Patients present clinically with solitary or multiple, large cutaneous/subcutaneous tumors (Figs. 22.19a and b). As for manifestations of "conventional" B-CLL, skin lesions may be localized at the site of previous herpes zoster eruption (Fig. 22.20). Histology reveals features of a diffuse large B-cell lymphoma with many centroblasts and immunoblasts (Fig. 22.21). Immunohistology shows positivity for B-cell markers, often with an aberrant profile similar to that described above ($CD20^+$, $CD5^+$, $CD23^+$, and $CD43^+$), sometimes with the monoclonal expression of Ig light chains. Positivity for PD-1 has been observed in lesions of Richter syndrome and in prolymphocytes/paraimmunoblasts of the preceding B-CLL (but not in B-CLL-unrelated diffuse large B-cell lymphomas), suggesting that PD-1 expression by neoplastic cells may be used as a surrogate marker to determine clonal relationship between B-CLL and diffuse large B-cell infiltrates of Richter syndrome [35].

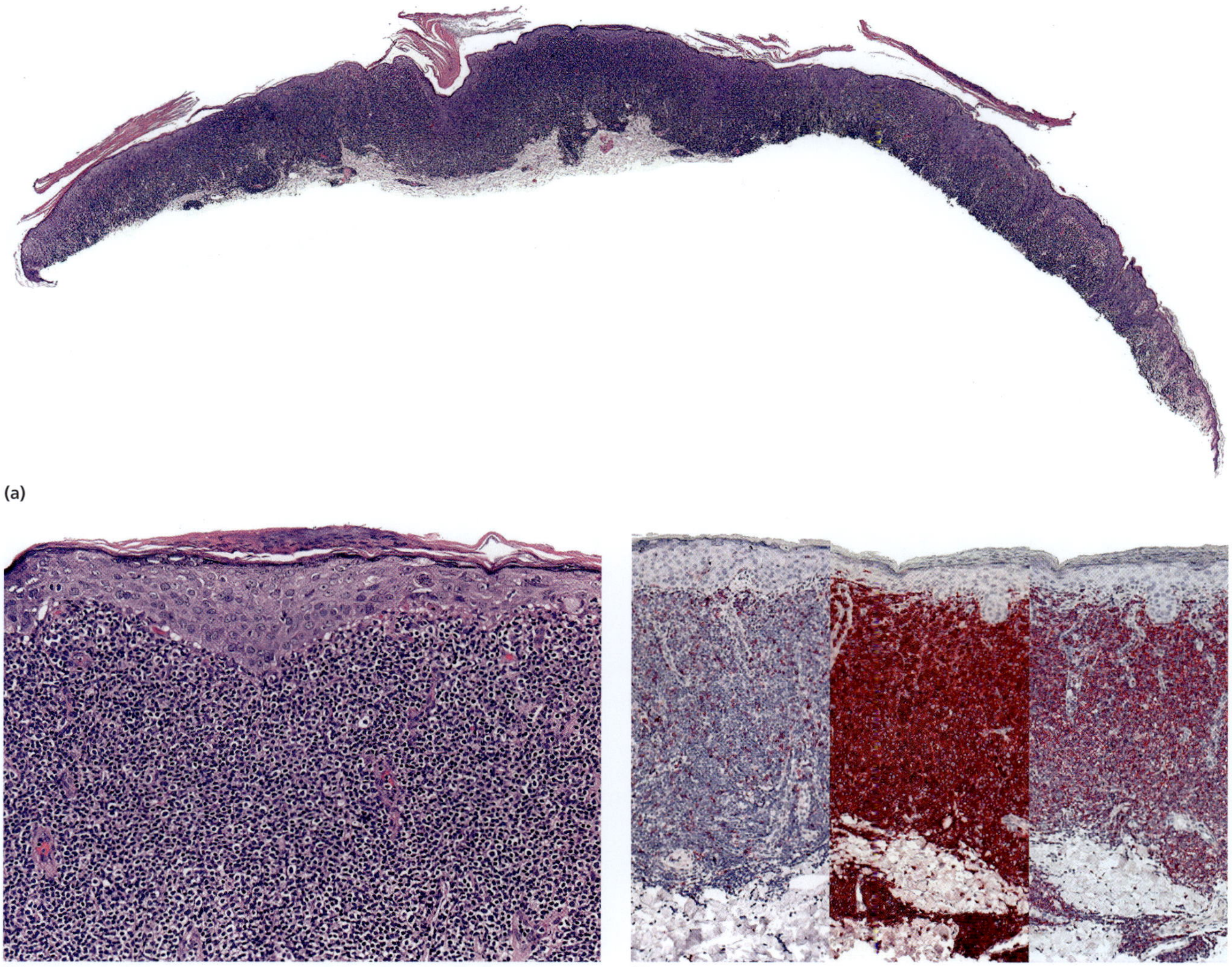

(a)

(b)

(c)

**Figure 22.15** Cutaneous B-CLL at the site of a carcinoma in situ. (a, b) Dense, monomorphous infiltrates of small lymphocytes in the immediate proximity of a squamous cell carcinoma in situ (Bowen disease) (c) The cells are negative for CD3 (left), and positive for CD5 (middle) and CD20 (right).

Molecular genetics reveals the presence of a monoclonal rearrangement of the Ig genes. The clone in most cases is the same as that observed in the lymphocytes of the preceding B-CLL, but in some cases, Richter syndrome represents the occurrence of a high-grade lymphoma unrelated to the previous B-CLL (so-called "second lymphoma") [29]. Richter syndrome in unmutated B-CLL is usually clonally related to the original neoplasm, whereas in mutated B-CLL, it represents more often a second lymphoma. The prognosis of patients with cutaneous Richter syndrome (and with Richter syndrome in general) is usually poor and treatment is ineffective [3, 32]. Rare cases with exclusive cutaneous involvement and prolonged survival have been reported [33, 34].

True skin lesions of Richter syndrome should be distinguished from the rare onset of a primary cutaneous B-cell lymphoma in patients with B-CLL, as the prognosis and management are completely different [31].

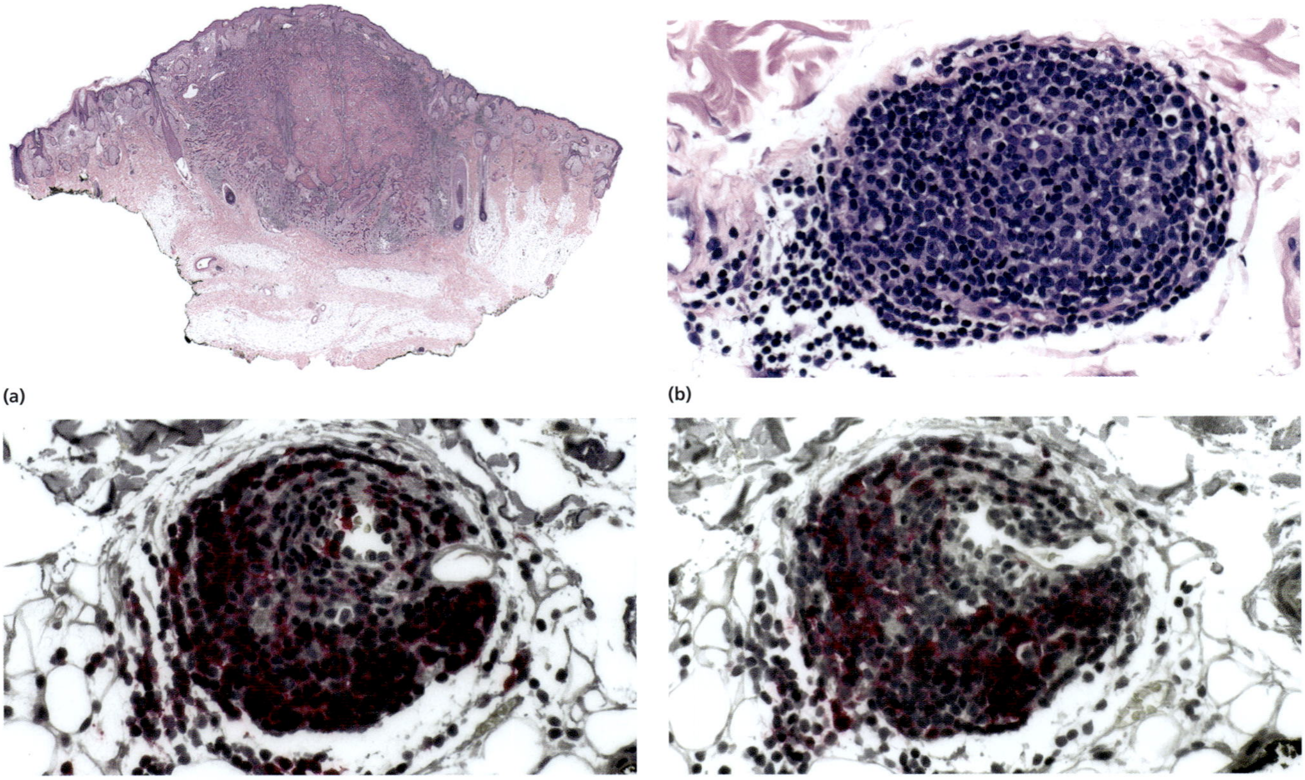

(a) (b) (c) (d)

**Figure 22.16** Cutaneous B-CLL in a biopsy of squamous cell carcinoma. (a, b) Small perivascular aggregate of lymphocytes within the subcutaneous fat, distant from the main tumor; the cells are positive for CD20 (c) and CD23 (d).

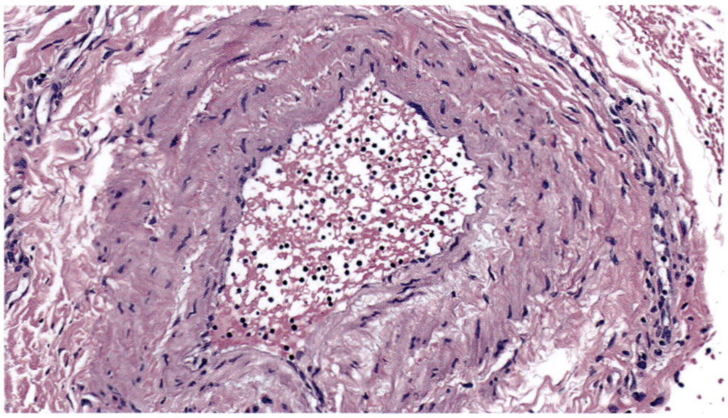

**Figure 22.17** B-CLL cells within a vein. Several lymphocytes are visible within a vein; lymphocytes are not observed within the veins in nonleukemic patients.

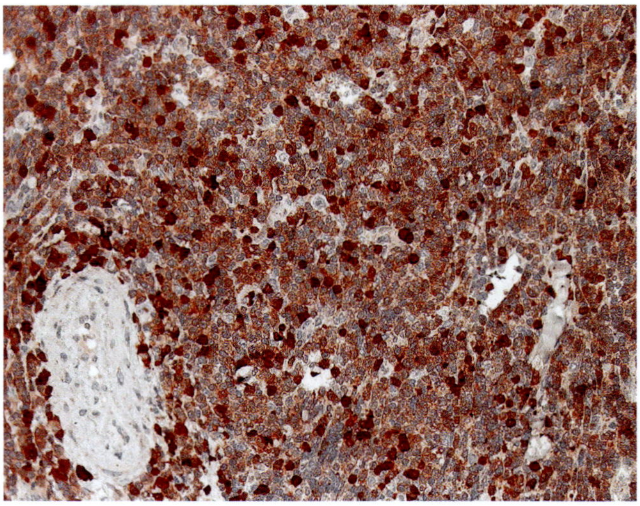

**Figure 22.18** Cutaneous B-CLL. Positivity of several neoplastic lymphocytes for ZAP70, typical of unmutated cases with a worse prognosis.

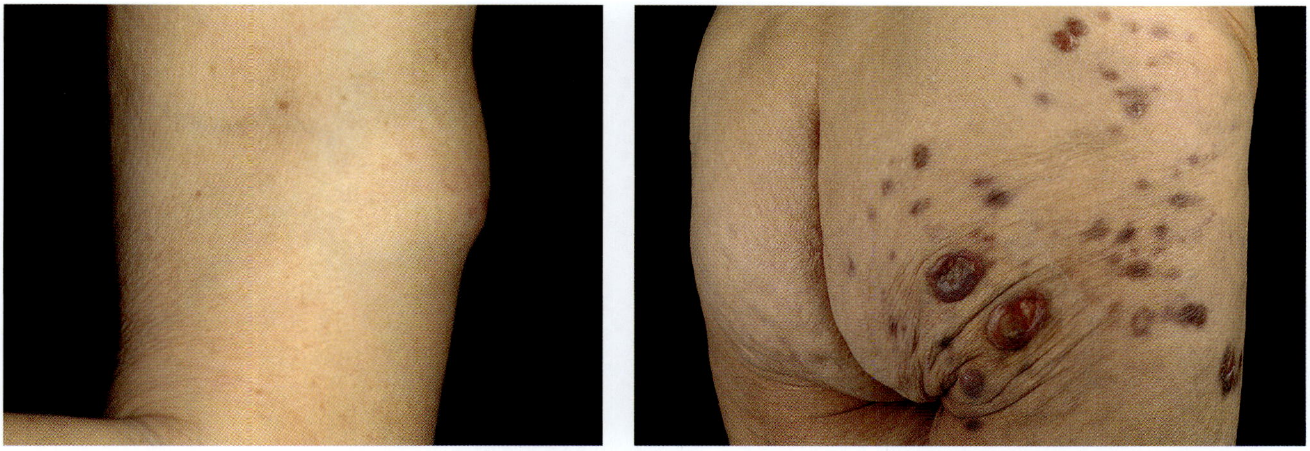

(a) (b)

**Figure 22.19** Cutaneous B-CLL with large cell transformation (Richter syndrome). (a) Large, solitary subcutaneous tumor on the arm. (b) Multiple, partly ulcerated plaques and tumors on the buttocks.

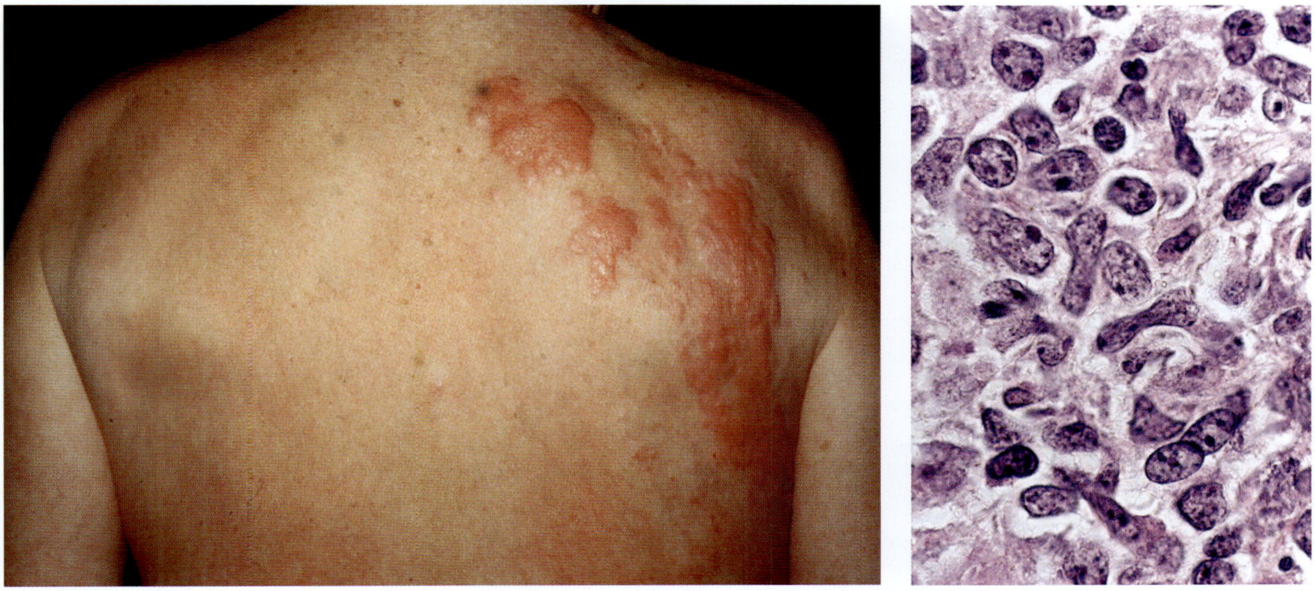

(a) (b)

**Figure 22.20** Cutaneous B-CLL with large cell transformation (Richter syndrome) at the site of previous Herpes zoster (a); (b) large cells predominate within the infiltrate.

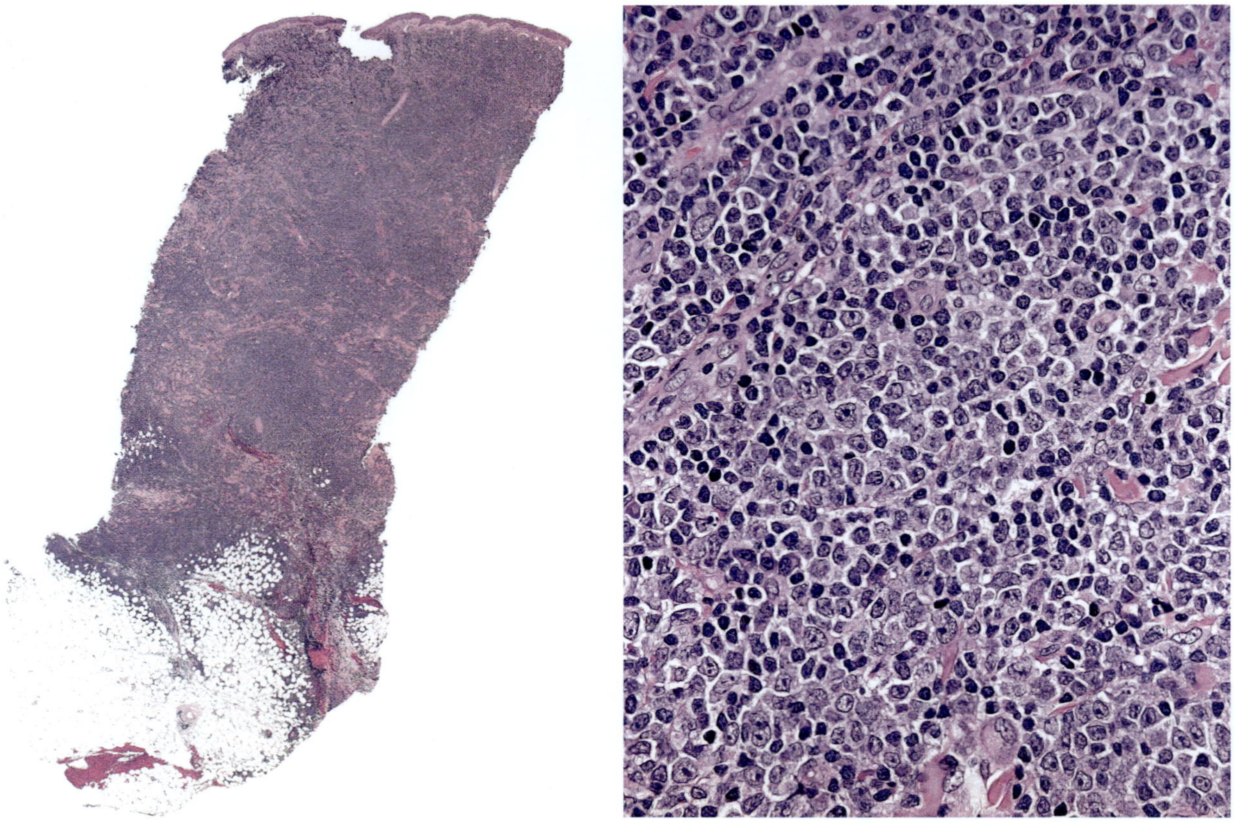

(a) (b)

**Figure 22.21** Cutaneous B-CLL with large cell transformation (Richter syndrome). (a) Dense, diffuse lymphoid infiltrates within the entire dermis involving the superficial subcutaneous fat; (b) predominance of large lymphocytes.

## Résumé

**Cutaneous manifestations of B-cell chronic lymphocytic leukemia**

| | | |
|---|---|---|
| **Clinical** | Elderly. Solitary, grouped, or generalized cutaneous papules, plaques, and tumors. Possible onset at sites of previous inflammation (e.g., rosacea, herpes simplex or herpes zoster infection, and infection by *Borrelia burgdorferi*) or at sites of cutaneous tumors. | |
| **Morphology** | Patchy or nodular infiltrates characterized by predominance of small, hyperchromatic, monomorphous lymphocytes. "Non-specific" cutaneous involvement in skin biopsies taken for other reasons. Predominance of large cells in Richter syndrome. | |
| **Immunohistochemistry** | CD19, CD20 | + |
| | CD5 | +(−) |
| | CD23 | + (usually negative in Richter syndrome) |
| | CD43 | + |
| | LEF1 | + |
| | CD200 | + |
| | Cyclin-D1, SOX11 | − |
| | ZAP-70 | + (unmutated cases, worse prognosis), − (mutated cases) |
| **Genetics** | Monoclonal rearrangement of the Ig genes detected in the majority of cases. Somatic hypermutations detected in 50–60% of cases. Mutated cases have better prognosis than unmutated cases. Richter syndrome may occur in the skin, and may be either clonally related to the B-CLL (usually in unmutated cases), or unrelated (second lymphoma, usually in mutated cases). | |
| **Treatment guidelines (skin manifestations)** | Radiotherapy; excision of solitary lesions. Systemic management, if needed, should be evaluated in a hematological setting (most cases of cutaneous infiltrates of B-CLL do not require a change in management due only to the skin lesions). Richter syndrome should be managed aggressively in a hematologic setting. | |

## References


1. Naresh, K.N., Rawstron, A.C., Akinola, N.O. et al. (2024). Chronic lymphocytic leukaemia/lymphoma. In: *WHO Classification of Tumours Editorial Board. Haematolymphoid Tumours*, 5the, 368–377. Lyon (France): IARC.
2. Sander, B., Bea, S., Gribben, J.G. et al. (2025). Chronic lymphocytic leukemia/small lymphocytic lymphoma and monoclonal B-cell lymphocytosis. In: *The International Consensus Classification of Myeloid and Lymphoid Neoplasms* (ed. D.A. Arber, M.J. Borowitz, J.R. Cook, et al.), 340–347. Philadelphia (US): Wolters Kluver.
3. Cerroni, L., Zenahlik, P., Höfler, G. et al. (1996). Specific cutaneous infiltrates of B-cell chronic lymphocytic leukemia. A clinicopathologic and prognostic study of 42 patients. *Am J Surg Pathol* **20**: 1000–1010.
4. Tapia, G., Mate, J.L., Fuente, M.J. et al. (2013). Cutaneous presentation of chronic lymphocytic leukemia as unique extramedullar involvement in a patient with normal peripheral blood lymphocyte count (monoclonal B-cell lymphocytosis). *J Cutan Pathol* **40**: 740–744.
5. Fulton, E., Alapat, D., Mabry, A. et al. (2016). CLL/SLL with initial presentation as a longstanding cutaneous plaque: a rare case. *J Cutan Pathol* **43**: 717–721.
6. Cerroni, L., Zenahlik, P., and Kerl, H. (1995). Specific infiltrates of B-cell chronic lymphocytic leukemia (B-CLL) arising at sites of herpes simplex and herpes zoster scars. *Cancer* **76**: 26–31.
7. Cerroni, L., Höfler, G., Bäck, B. et al. (2002). Specific cutaneous infiltrates of B-cell chronic lymphocytic leukemia (B-CLL) at sites typical for Borrelia burgdorferi infection. *J Cutan Pathol* **29**: 142–147.
8. Kash, N., Fink-Puches, R., and Cerroni, L. (2011). Cutaneous manifestations of B-cell chronic lymphocytic leukemia associated with Borrelia burgdorferi infection showing a marginal zone B-cell lymphoma-like infiltrate. *Am J Dermatopathol* **33**: 712–715.
9. Smoller, B.R. and Warnke, R.A. (1998). Cutaneous infiltrate of chronic lymphocytic leukemia and relationship to primary cutaneous epithelial neoplasms. *J Cutan Pathol* **25**: 160–164.
10. Thiesen, I., Wehkamp, U., Brüggemann, M. et al. (2019). Skin involvement by chronic lymphocytic leukaemia is frequently associated with unrelated neoplastic or inflammatory cutaneous disease and is not indicative of general disease progression. *Br J Dermatol* **180**: 227–228.
11. Saggini, A., Del Poeta, G., Santinelli, E. et al. (2019). Intravascular Colonization of Kaposi Sarcoma: Expanding the Spectrum of Specific Infiltrates of B-Cell Chronic Lymphocytic Leukemia. *Am J Dermatopathol* **41**: 940–944.
12. Kluk, J., Moonim, M., Duran, A. et al. (2015). Cutaneous Richter syndrome: a better place to transform? *Br J Dermatol* **172**: 513–521.
13. Reda, G., Cassin, R., Fabris, S. et al. (2017). Biological and molecular characterization of a rare case of cutaneous Richter syndrome. *Hematol Oncol* **35**: 869–874.
14. Paydas, S. and Zorludemir, S. (2000). Leukaemia cutis and leukaemic vasculitis. *Br J Dermatol* **143**: 773–779.
15. Schmid-Wendtner, M.H., Sander, C., Volkenandt, M., and Wendtner, C.M. (1999). Chronic lymphocytic leukemia presenting with cutaneous lesions. *J Clin Oncol* **17**: 1083–1085.
16. Agnew, K.L., Ruchlemer, R., Catovsky, D. et al. (2004). Cutaneous findings in chronic lymphocytic leukaemia. *Br J Dermatol* **150**: 1129–1135.
17. Meiss, F., Technau-Hafsi, K., Kern, J.S., and May, A.M. (2019). Eosinophilic dermatosis of hematologic malignancy: Correlation of molecular characteristics of skin lesions and extracutaneous manifestations of hematologic malignancy. *J Cutan Pathol* **46**: 175–181.
18. Farber, M.J., La Forgia, S., Sahu, J., and Lee, J.B. (2012). Eosinophilic dermatosis of hematologic malignancy. *J Cutan Pathol* **39**: 690–695.
19. Grandi, V., Maglie, R., Antiga, E. et al. (2019). Eosinophilic dermatosis of hematologic malignancy: a retrospective cohort of 37 patients from an Italian center. *J Am Acad Dermatol* **81**: 246–249.
20. Hull, P.R. and Saxena, A. (2000). Mycosis fungoides and chronic lymphocytic leukaemia – composite T-cell and B-cell lymphomas presenting in the skin. *Br J Dermatol* **143**: 439–444.
21. Admirand, J.H., Rassidakis, G.Z., Abruzzo, L.V. et al. (2004). Immunohistochemical detection of ZAP-70 in 341 cases of non-Hodgkin and Hodgkin lymphoma. *Mod Pathol* **17**: 954–961.
22. Chiorazzi, N., Rai, K.R., and Ferrarini, M. (2005). Chronic lymphocytic leukemia. *N Engl J Med* **352**: 804–815.
23. Apollonio, B. and Ramsay, A.G. (2016). Subclonal heterogeneity in chronic lymphocytic leukaemia: revealing the importance of the lymphoid tumour microenvironment. *Br J Haematol* **172**: 7–8.
24. Del Giudice, I., Marinelli, M., WangInter, J. et al. (2016). Inter- and intra-patient clonal and subclonal heterogeneity of chronic lymphocytic leukaemia: evidences from circulating and lymph nodal compartments. *Br J Haematol* **172**: 371–383.
25. Robak, T., Pula, A., Braun, M., and Robak, W. (2024). Extramedullary and extranodal manifestations in chronic lymphocytic leukemia – an update. *Ann Hematol* **103**: 3369–3383.
26. Porter, W.M., Sidwell, R.U., Catovsky, D., and Bunker, C.B. (2001). Cutaneous presentation of chronic lymphatic leukaemia and response to ultraviolet B phototherapy. *Br J Dermatol* **144**: 1092–1094.
27. Grey, M. (2008). Efficacy of alemtuzumab in cutaneous chronic lymphocytic leukaemia involving facial skin. *Br J Haematol* **142**: 1.
28. Kazakov, D.V., Belousova, I.E., Michaelis, S. et al. (2003). Unusual manifestation of specific cutaneous involvement by B-cell chronic lymphocytic leukemia: spontaneous regression with scar formation. *Dermatology* **207**: 111–115.
29. Robak, E., Góra-Tybor, J., Kordek, R. et al. (2005). Richter syndrome first manifesting as cutaneous B-cell lymphoma clonally distinct from primary B-cell chronic lymphocytic leukemia. *Br J Dermatol* **153**: 833–837.
30. Robertson, L.E., Pugh, W., O'Brien, S. et al. (1993). Richter's syndrome: a report on 39 patients. *J Clin Oncol* **11**: 1985–1989.
31. Ratnavel, R.C., Dunn-Walters, D.K., Boursier, L. et al. (1999). B-cell lymphoma associated with chronic lymphatic leukaemia: two cases with contrasting aggressive and indolent behaviour. *Br J Dermatol* **140**: 708–714.

32. Yamazaki, M.L., Lum, C.A., and Izumi, A.K. (2009). Primary cutaneous Richter syndrome: prognostic implications and review of the literature. *J Am Acad Dermatol* **60**: 157–161.
33. Yu, L., Bandhlish, A., Fullen, D.R. et al. (2012). Cutaneous Richter syndrome: report of 3 cases from one institution. *J Am Acad Dermatol* **67**: e187–e193.
34. Duong, T., Grange, F., Auffret, N. et al. (2010). Cutaneous Richter's syndrome, prognosis, and clinical, histological and immunohistological patterns: report of four cases and review of the literature. *Dermatology* **220**: 226–233.
35. He, R., Ding, W., Viswanatha, D.S. et al. (2018). PD-1 Expression in Chronic Lymphocytic Leukemia/Small Lymphocytic Lymphoma (CLL/SLL) and Large B-cell Richter Transformation (DLBCL-RT): A Characteristic Feature of DLBCL-RT and Potential Surrogate Marker for Clonal Relatedness. *Am J Surg Pathol* **42**: 843–854.

CHAPTER 23

# Cutaneous manifestations of myelogenous leukemia

Myelogenous leukemias and related conditions are a spectrum of diseases encompassing myeloproliferative neoplasms, myelodysplastic syndromes, myelodysplastic/myeloproliferative neoplasms, and acute myeloid leukemias and related neoplasms. The classification of these neoplasms has been considerably changed in recent times, and both the International Consensus Classification (ICC) of myeloid neoplasms and acute leukemias and the 5th edition of the World Health Organization (WHO) *Classification of Haematolymphoid Tumours* take into consideration many genetic features to define specific entities [1, 2]. In actual classifications, more than 50 entities are listed among the myeloid proliferations and neoplasms (and several discrepancies among the ICC and WHO classifications exist). A detailed discussion of these entities is beyond the scope of this book; moreover, most reports on skin involvement in acute myeloid leukemia pre-date molecular classification or do not mention molecular features, so the frequency of cutaneous involvement in the various molecular subtypes is not known. Skin manifestations can be observed in acute myeloid leukemia, as well as in a small percentage of patients with myeloproliferative neoplasms, myelodysplastic syndromes, and myelodysplastic/myeloproliferative neoplasms [3–15]. Specific skin involvement has also been observed in the context of therapy-related myeloid leukemia [16] (therapy-related myeloid leukemia is mentioned as a qualifier to the diagnosis rather than a specific disease category in the ICC classification, whereas is included as a specific category in the WHO classification). Acute myeloid leukemia is the most common form of neonatal leukemia, and skin manifestations are common in this setting [17]. Acute myeloid leukemia can also be observed in children and adolescents, representing the second most common form of leukemia after acute lymphoblastic leukemia in this group of patients; the frequency of specific cutaneous involvement has not been studied in detail [18].

Cutaneous involvement in myeloid leukemia is often referred to as "leukemia cutis." This term, however, is potentially confusing, as other types of leukemia may present with specific cutaneous manifestations (this is particularly true for B-cell chronic lymphocytic leukemia – B-CLL).

The classification of myelodysplastic and myelodysplastic/myeloproliferative disorders has changed as well [2]. In general, in patients with chronic myelogenous leukemia or myelodysplastic syndromes skin involvement is related to the transformation or progression of the chronic myeloid or myelodysplastic neoplasm. In this context, it is interesting to note that overlapping myeloid and lymphoid features may be observed in chronic myeloid leukemia, in which blast crisis in 10% of the cases reveals a B- or, more rarely, a T-cell phenotype ("transdifferentiation" – see also Chapter 1). Another interesting feature is the rare occurrence of cutaneous lesions with the phenotype of dendritic cells, clonally related to the original chronic myeloid leukemia. In rare cases, two distinct, clonally unrelated myelogenous and dendritic cell neoplasms may also be observed [19].

Cases showing isolated extramedullary tumors with myeloid differentiation have been denominated chloroma or granulocytic sarcoma in the past, and are referred to as myeloid sarcoma [20–23]. However, the term myeloid sarcoma is also widely used to refer generally to extramedullary manifestations of myeloid leukemia regardless of the number of lesions [24]. Myeloid sarcoma may precede ("de novo") or be concomitant with acute myelogenous leukemia or may follow myelodysplastic syndromes, or chronic myelogenous leukemia [25]. "De novo" cases have slightly better survival than cases associated with acute myelogenous leukemia, myelodysplastic syndromes, or chronic myelogenous leukemia [25]. Nucleophosmin 1 (*NPM1*) gene mutations can be observed in cases of myeloid sarcoma, particularly in cutaneous ones.

Some publications dealing with blastic plasmacytoid dendritic cell neoplasms showed that in some patients a relationship between this entity and myelogenous leukemia exists (see Chapter 24). In the ICC classification, blastic plasmacytoid dendritic cell neoplasm is included as a separate section within the myeloproliferative disorders, whereas in the WHO classification is included in a separate section within the histiocytic/dendritic cell neoplasms.

*Skin Lymphoma: The Illustrated Guide*, Sixth Edition. Lorenzo Cerroni.

## Acute myeloid leukemia

As already mentioned, several variants of acute myeloid leukemia (>20) are defined by genetic abnormalities or differentiation, and a detailed discussion of these entities is beyond the scope of this book. On the other hand, irrespective of the variant, cutaneous involvement is characterized by clinicopathological features that are well defined and reproducible. A precise classification of myeloid leukemia, moreover, should not be attempted on a cutaneous biopsy, but according to morphological, phenotypic, and molecular features observed in the bone marrow and the blood.

### Clinical features

The majority of patients are adults who present with multiple, localized, or generalized papules, plaques, and nodules with a characteristic reddish-brown or violaceous color in the context of known leukemia (Fig. 23.1). Involvement of the mucosal regions is common, often with typical gingival hypertrophy due to infiltrates by neoplastic cells (Fig. 23.2). Cases have been reported in children and even neonates (Fig. 23.3) [26, 27]. Interestingly, a neonate with typical "blueberry muffin" clinical presentation and skin infiltrates of myelomonocytic leukemia did not have any extracutaneous manifestation at staging, suggesting that "aleukemic" leukemia cutis may be observed in newborns, too [28]. Spontaneous regression of skin lesions without treatment has been observed in congenital myelogenous leukemia, but it is unfortunately a rare event [29].

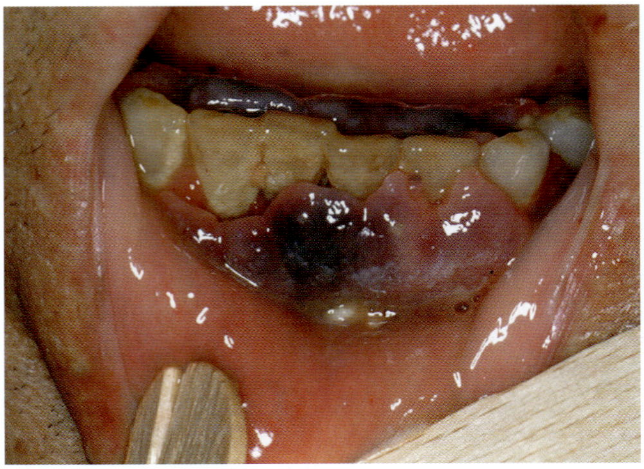

**Figure 23.2** Cutaneous manifestations of acute myeloid leukemia. Involvement of the gingiva with a characteristic violaceous swelling.

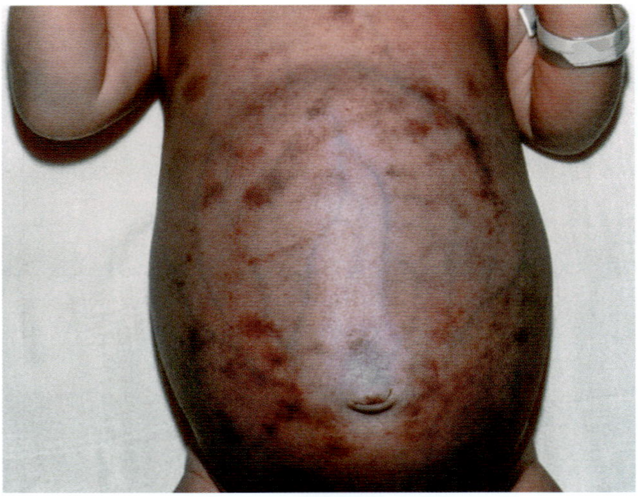

**Figure 23.3** Congenital myelogenous leukemia with cutaneous manifestations. So-called "blueberry muffin" appearance.

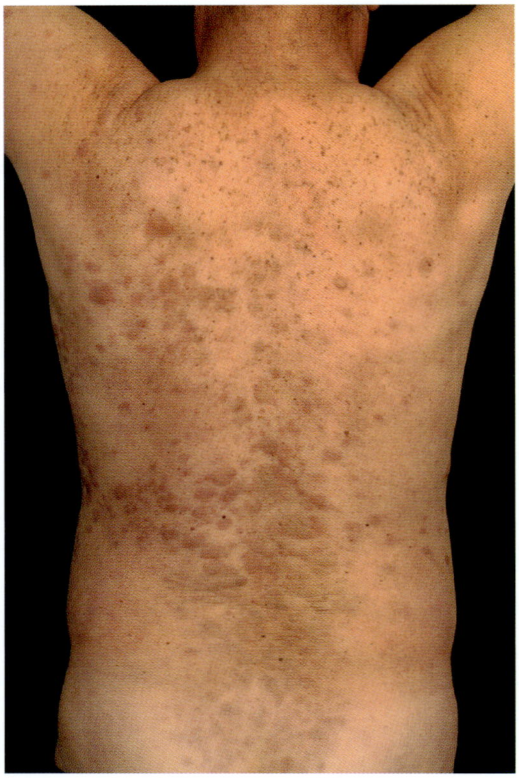

**Figure 23.1** Cutaneous manifestations of acute myeloid leukemia. Multiple erythematous-livid papules, plaques, and flat tumors on the back.

Diagnosis of specific cutaneous infiltrates may be difficult in cases presenting with unusual clinical features such as solitary skin nodules, maculopapular eruptions clinically resembling

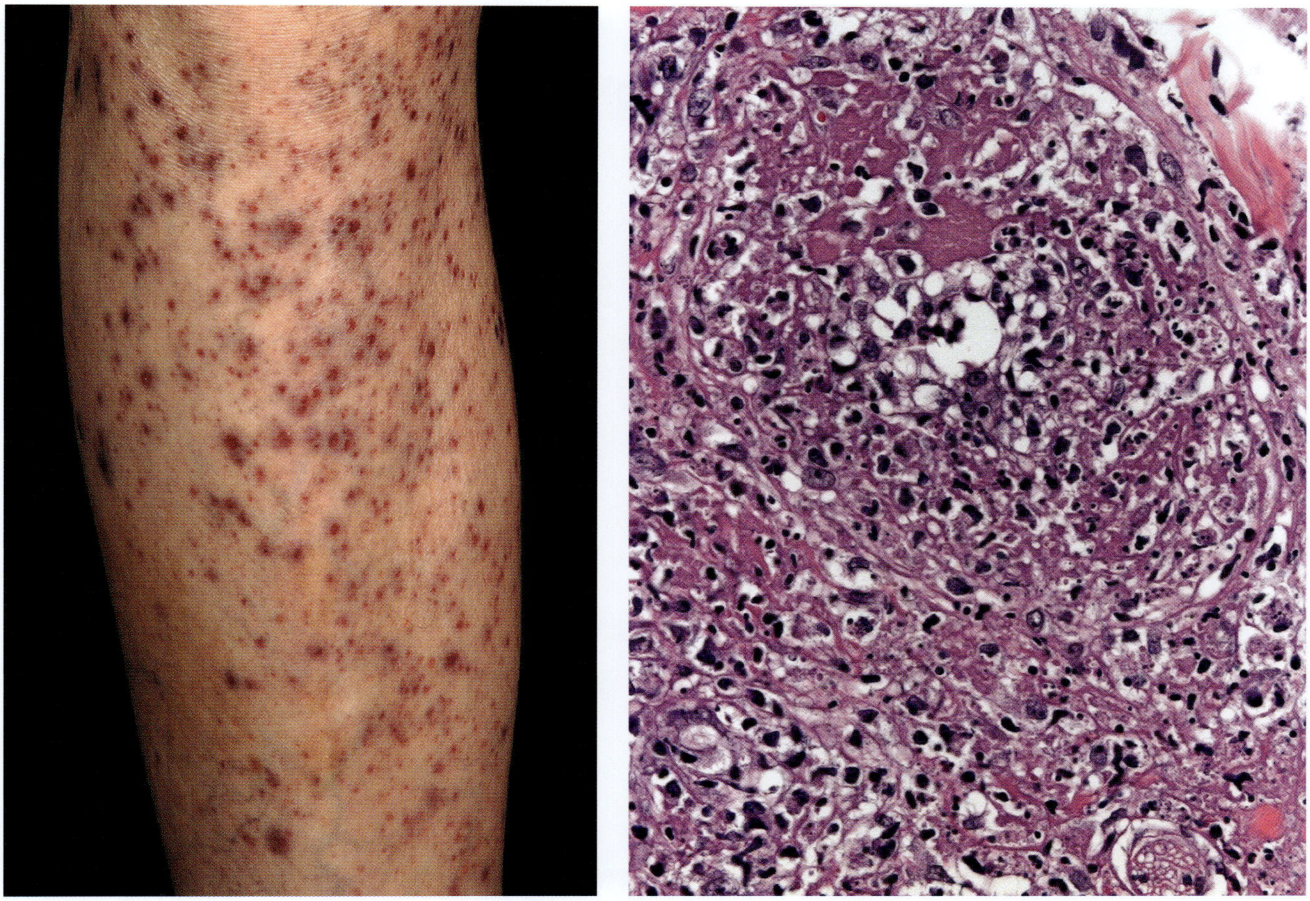


**Figure 23.4** Cutaneous manifestations of acute myeloid leukemia. (a) Multiple small hemorrhagic/purpuric papules on the leg simulating clinically the picture of a vasculitis. (b) Histology revealed a focal angiocentric pattern of atypical, pleomorphic cells with angiodestruction.

drug or viral eruptions, vasculitis, or other uncommon presentations (Figs. 23.4 and 23.5) [3]. In this context, it should be noted that in some patients "inflammatory dermatoses-like" cutaneous eruptions have been observed as the first sign of relapse of treated myelogenous leukemia, underlining the need for precise clinicopathologic correlation and for a high grade of suspicion in these patients [30].

As for other types of leukemia, specific manifestations have been observed at the site of cutaneous inflammation [31–35]. This phenomenon seems to be more frequent for lesions of Sweet syndrome (particularly so-called "histiocytoid" Sweet syndrome) (Fig. 23.6) [36, 37] (see also Chapter 29), but has been observed also at sites of psoriasis, basal cell carcinoma, needle puncture, pyoderma gangrenosum, and infusion of gabexate mesylate that had leaked from the vein among others [31–38].

Cutaneous manifestations of therapy-related acute myeloid leukemia are identical to those of acute myeloid leukemia unrelated to previous treatment or other background conditions (Fig. 23.7). I have seen specific manifestations of therapy-related acute myeloid leukemia in a young patient at the sites of herpes zoster scars (Fig. 23.8).

Myeloid sarcoma is defined as a "tumor mass involving any anatomical site other than bone marrow, that effaces tissue architecture and is composed of myeloid blasts, with or without maturation" [22]. In many publications reporting skin manifestations of myelogenous leukemia, the term myeloid sarcoma has been used irrespective of the clinical presentation (i.e., solitary or generalized lesions). Although solitary cutaneous lesions may rarely be observed (Fig. 23.9), in my experience these patients rapidly develop generalized lesions, and clinicopathological features are not dissimilar from those observed in

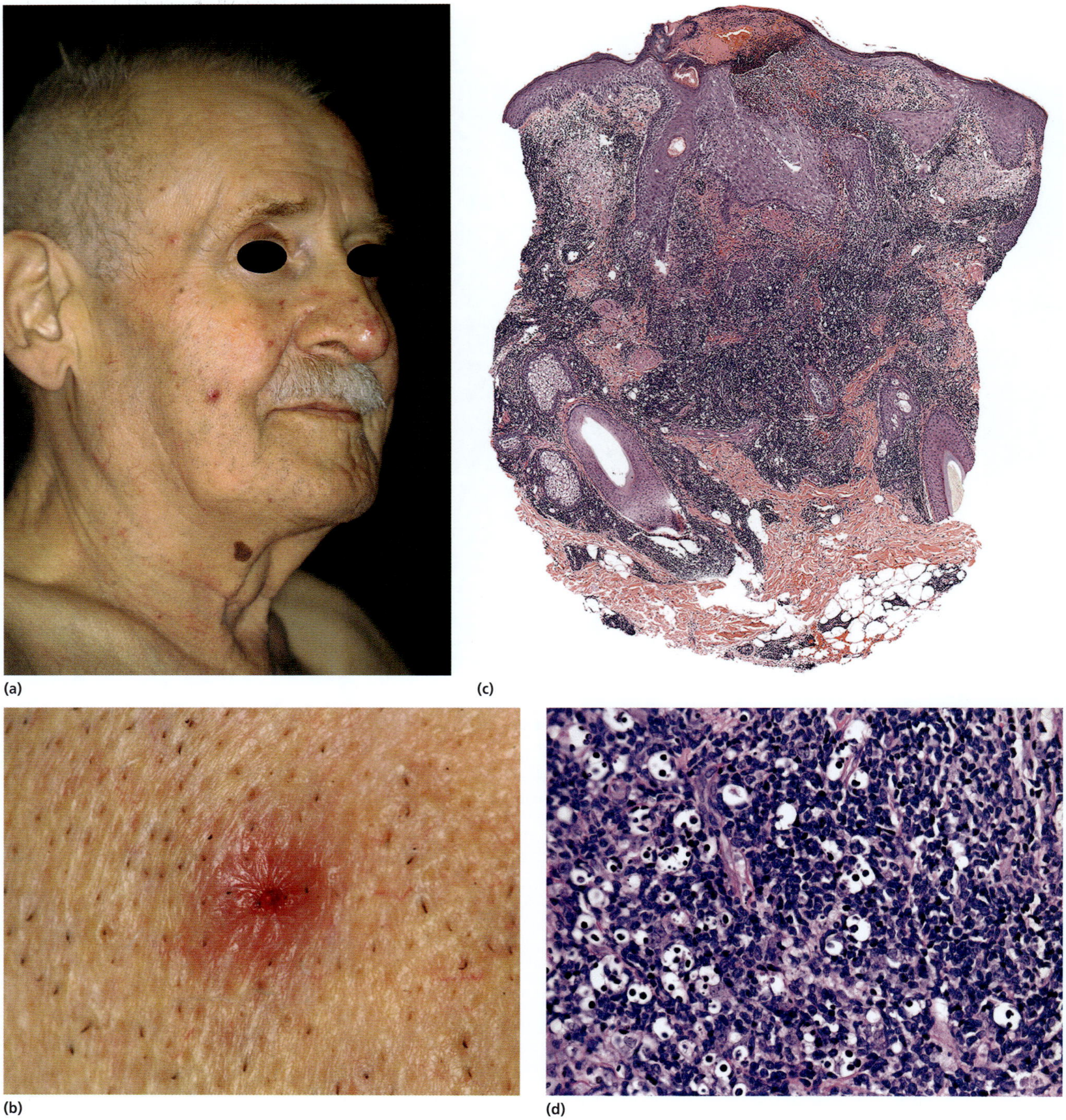

**Figure 23.5** Cutaneous manifestations of acute myeloid leukemia. (a) and (b) Small, partly crusted, hemorrhagic papules on the face mimicking vasculitis, papular rosacea, or arthropod bite reactions in a patient with known therapy-related myeloid leukemia; (c) dermal infiltrate with a “starry-sky” pattern, composed of (d) medium-sized monomorphous cells positive for (e) CD123 and (f) TdT. A repeated bone marrow biopsy confirmed the diagnosis of myeloid leukemia.

patients with more conventional skin manifestations of acute myeloid leukemia.

In a distinct proportion of patients specific skin infiltrates represent the first clinical manifestation of the disease, preceding blood and/or bone marrow involvement by weeks or even months (“aleukemic” cutaneous myeloid leukemia) [3, 39, 40]. These patients should be managed in the same way as those with cutaneous manifestations of known myelogenous leukemia.

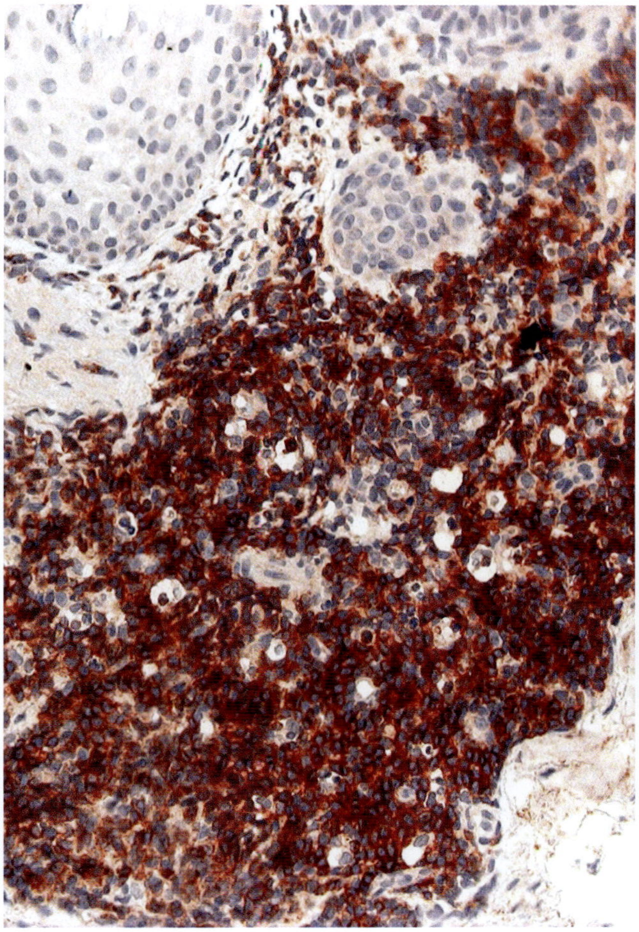

(e)

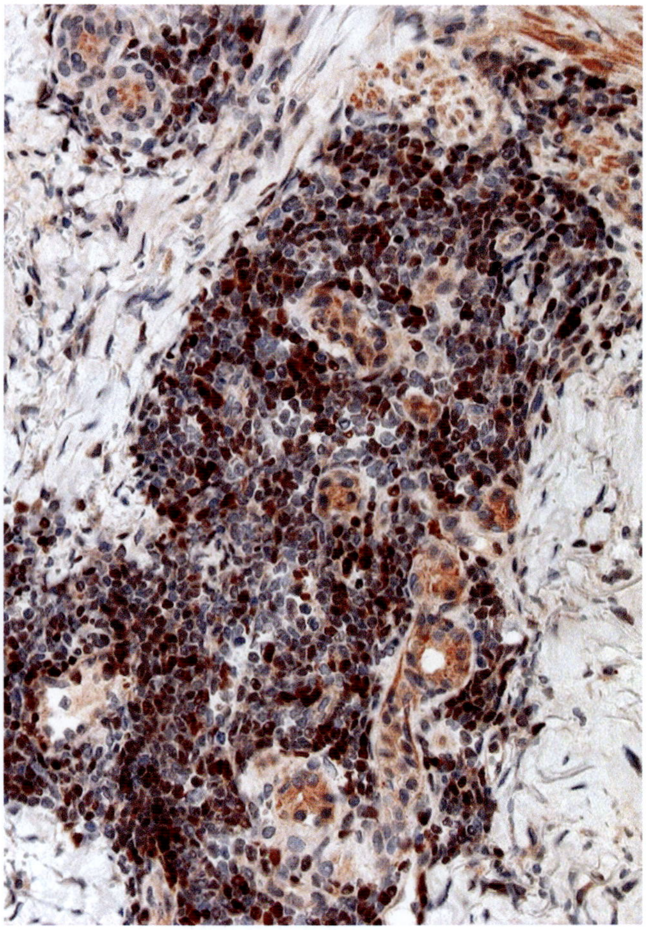

(f)

Figure 23.5 (Continued)

## Histopathology, immunophenotype, and molecular genetics

### Histopathology

In most instances, there are no major differences in the histopathologic features of specific skin involvement by acute or chronic myelogenous leukemia [3]. Cutaneous lesions show mild, moderate, or dense, diffuse, or nodular dermal infiltrates, often with perivascular and periadnexal accentuation and sparing of the upper papillary dermis (Fig. 23.10a). Involvement of the subcutis is common. In most cases, the infiltrate is composed of medium-sized, round to oval cells with slightly eosinophilic cytoplasm and distinct, sometimes indented, bilobular or kidney-shaped basophilic nuclei (atypical monocytoid cells) (Fig. 23.10b). Large cells may also be seen. In more differentiated subtypes of acute myeloid leukemia, the nuclei are smaller and the cytoplasm is less prominent, and the cells may resemble pleomorphic lymphocytes (Fig. 23.10d). Variable numbers of mitotic figures (including atypical mitoses) and apoptotic cells can be found, sometimes conferring to the infiltrate a so-called "starry sky" appearance (Figs. 23.5b and c). Reactive cells (e.g., lymphocytes, mast cells) are present in some cases but are usually not a prominent feature. A granulomatous reaction may also be observed (Fig. 23.11) [3, 41, 42].

Prominent single files of neoplastic cells between collagen bundles can be observed in the majority of cases ("Indian filing") (Figs. 23.10b and 23.12). A distinctive "figurate" pattern characterized by concentric layering of neoplastic cells around blood vessels and adnexal structures is frequently found (Fig. 23.13).

In rare cases, an angiocentric ("vasculitic") pattern with destruction of the vessels may be observed, mimicking the picture of cutaneous vasculitis or of other angiocentric/angiodestructive lymphomas (Fig. 23.4b). In some of these cases the clinical presentation, too, is reminiscent of leucocytoclastic vasculitis ("palpable purpura") (Fig. 23.4a). Phenotypic features are identical to those observed in conventional lesions of the disease, thus allowing a proper classification of these cases.

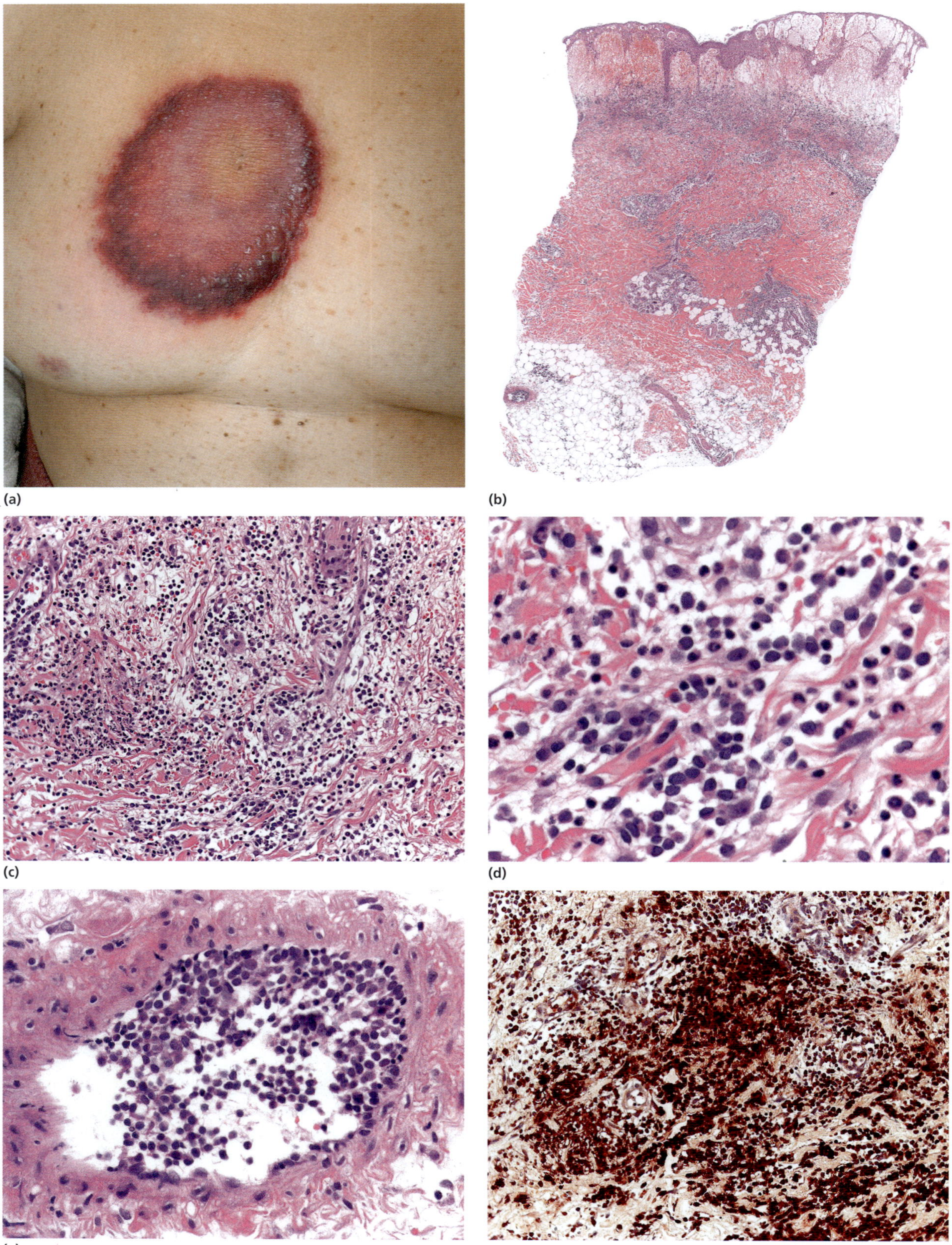

(a) (b) (c) (d) (e) (f)

Figure 23.6 Cutaneous manifestations of acute myeloid leukemia. (a) Hemorrhagic, infiltrated plaque clinically resembling hemorrhagic Sweet syndrome; (b) histology shows edematous, hemorrhagic lesions with (c, d) many mononuclear cells admixed with neutrophils; (e) one medium-sized subcutaneous vessels is filled with atypical mononuclear cells; (f) the cells are positive for myeloperoxidase.

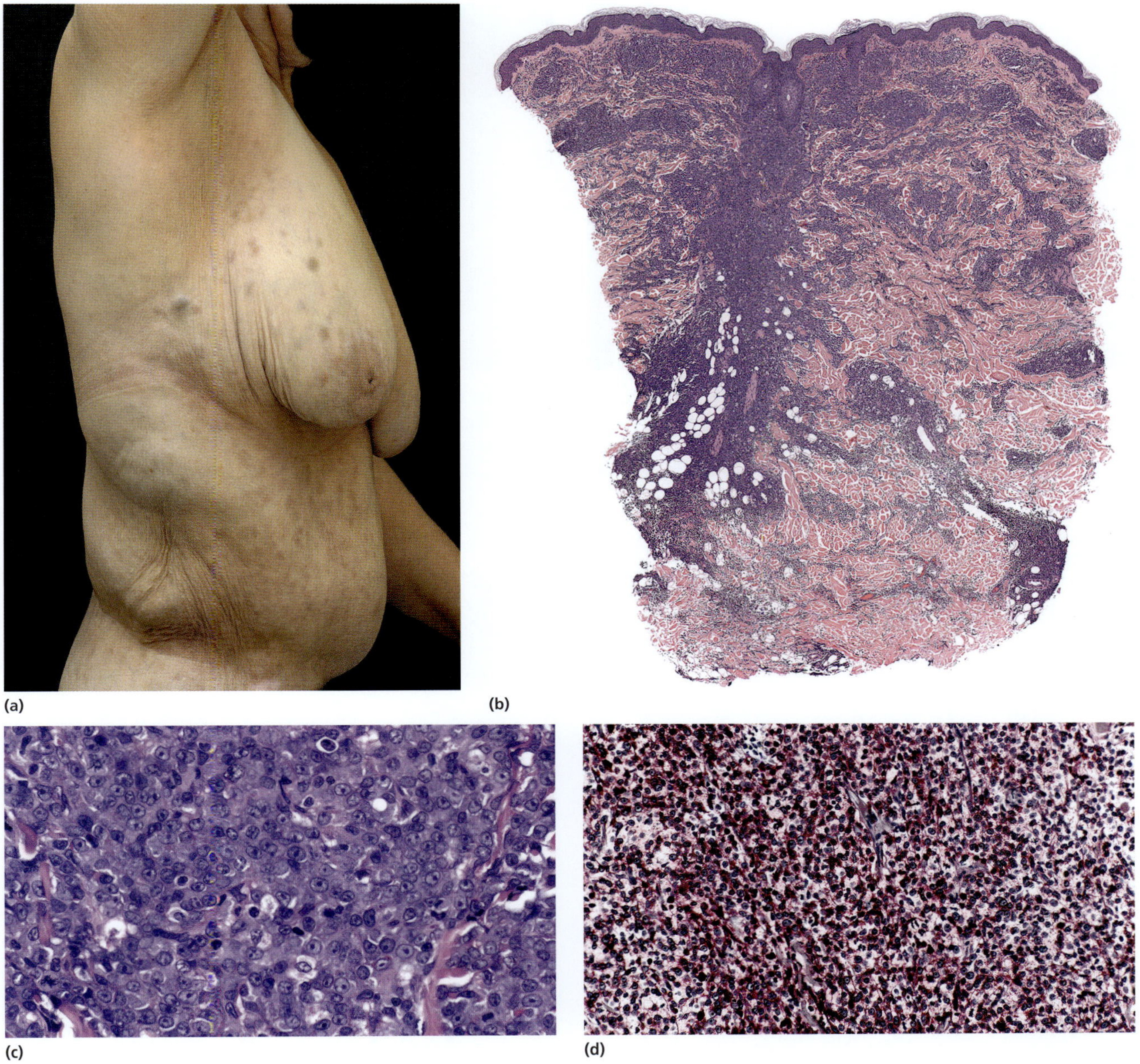


**Figure 23.7** Cutaneous manifestations of therapy-related acute myeloid leukemia. (a) Generalized violaceous papules and small nodules. (b) Histology reveals dense, diffuse dermal infiltrates characterized by (c) blastoid myeloid cells. (d) Positivity for myeloperoxidase.

Early cutaneous manifestations of myeloid leukemia may mimic an inflammatory dermatosis both clinically and histopathologically, and may be very difficult to diagnose (Fig. 23.14) [30]. Although the infiltrate may be very sparse, cytomorphological and phenotypic features allow one to make the correct diagnosis. Skin lesions with minimal infiltrates may be observed also as the first sign of relapse of myeloid leukemia in complete remission.

In some patients with a high number of recirculating neoplastic cells, specific cells of myeloid leukemia may be observed admixed with erythrocytes within cutaneous hemorrhages and/or organized hematomas (Figs. 23.15 and 23.16). Usually, the diagnosis of leukemia has already been established in these patients, but the presence of atypical myeloid blasts within areas of hemorrhage should otherwise prompt a careful evaluation for myeloid leukemia. In other cases, specific infiltrates can be observed at the site of cutaneous neoplasms or inflammatory disorders; I have observed specific infiltrates at the site of atopic dermatitis (Fig. 23.17), psoriasis (Fig. 23.18), basal cell carcinoma (Fig. 23.19), and erysipelas (Fig. 23.20).

Cutaneous lesions of myeloid sarcoma present with large cutaneous–subcutaneous tumors composed of myeloblasts or

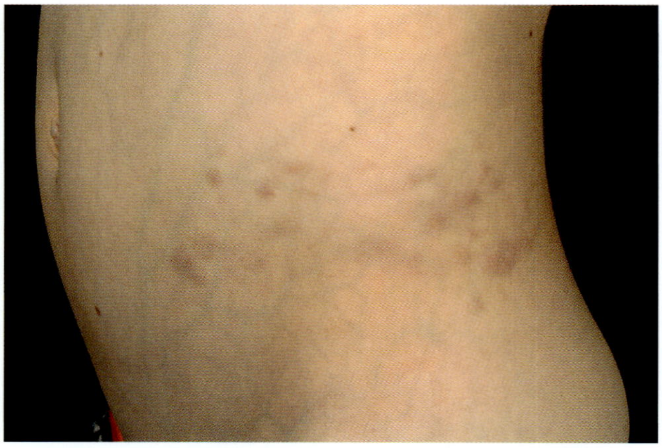

**Figure 23.8** Cutaneous manifestations of therapy-related acute myeloid leukemia at the site of a previous herpes zoster in a 12-year-old boy treated for osteosarcoma 2 years before the onset of the leukemia.

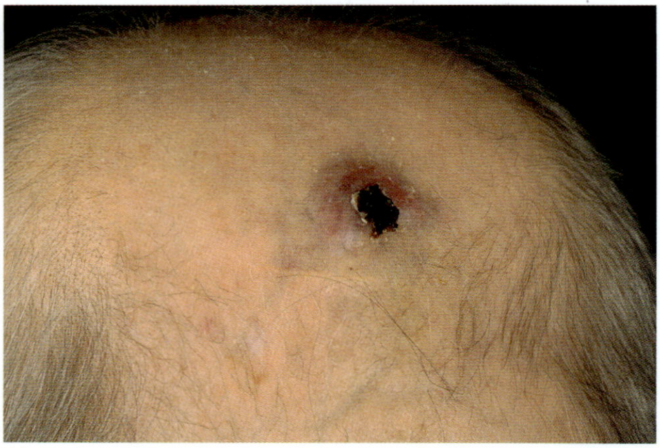

**Figure 23.9** Cutaneous myeloid sarcoma. Solitary, crusted tumor on the occipital region. The patient developed generalized cutaneous lesions 3 months after the first presentation.

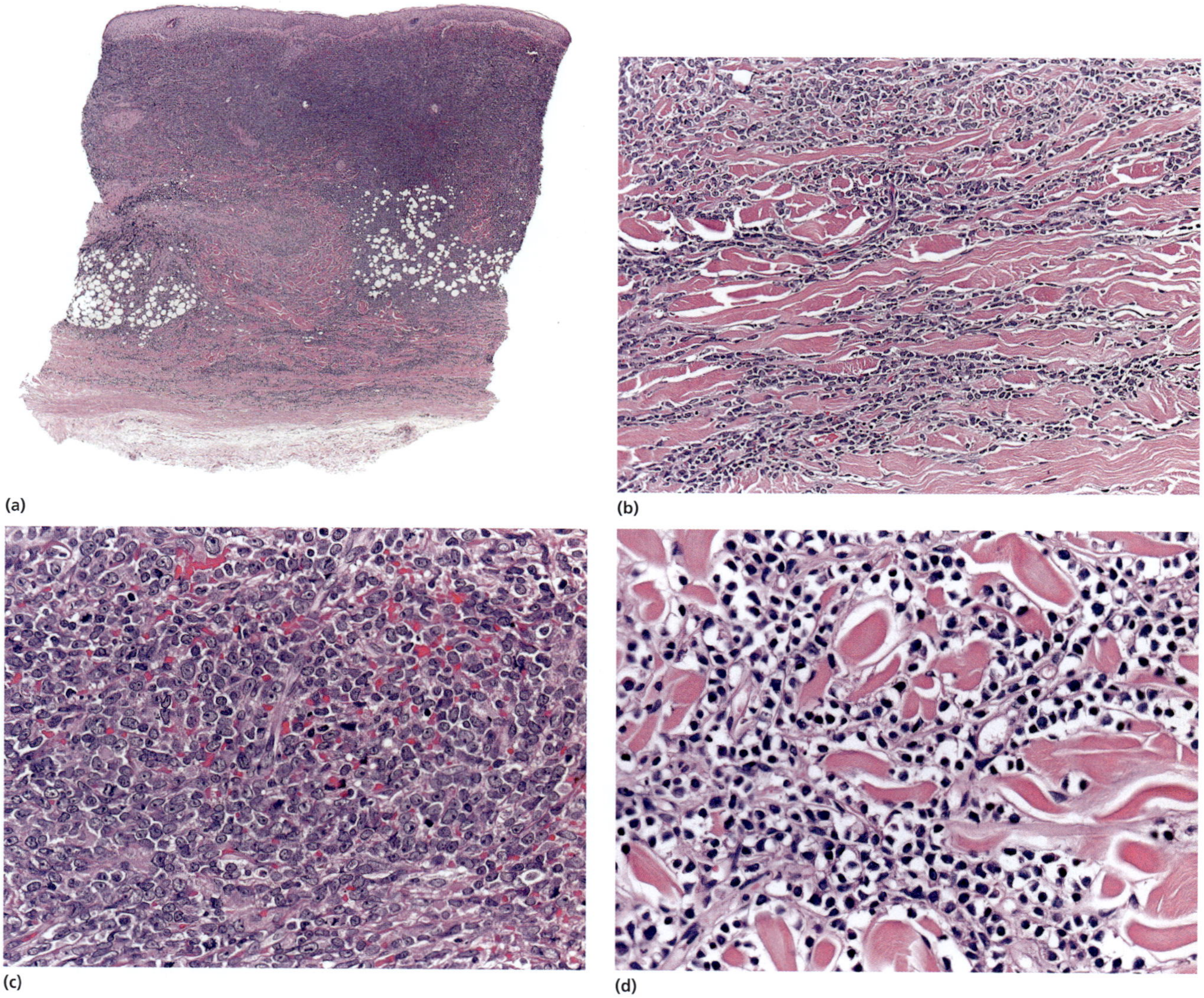


**Figure 23.10** Cutaneous manifestations of acute myeloid leukemia. (a) Dense, diffuse infiltrate within the entire dermis and subcutis with a small subepidermal grenze zone. (b) Note focal Indian filing. (c) Monomorphous infiltrate of atypical monocytoid cells. (d) Another case with more differentiated cells resembling pleomorphic lymphocytes.

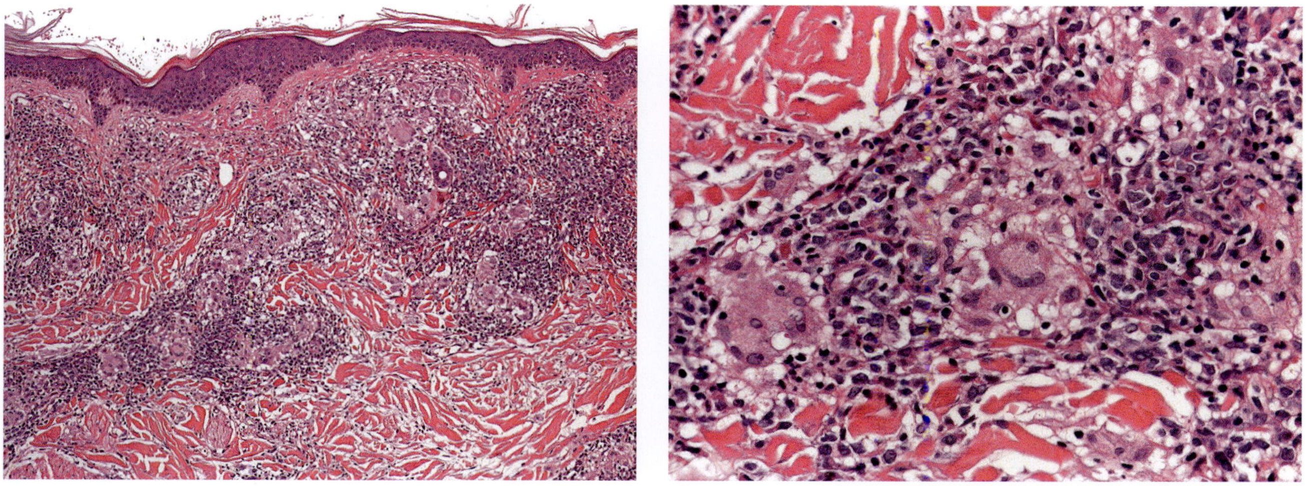

(a) (b)

Figure 23.11 Cutaneous manifestations of acute myeloid leukemia with granulomatous reaction. (a) Dense infiltrates admixed with small granulomas. (b) Note the atypical myeloid cells and histiocytic giant cells.

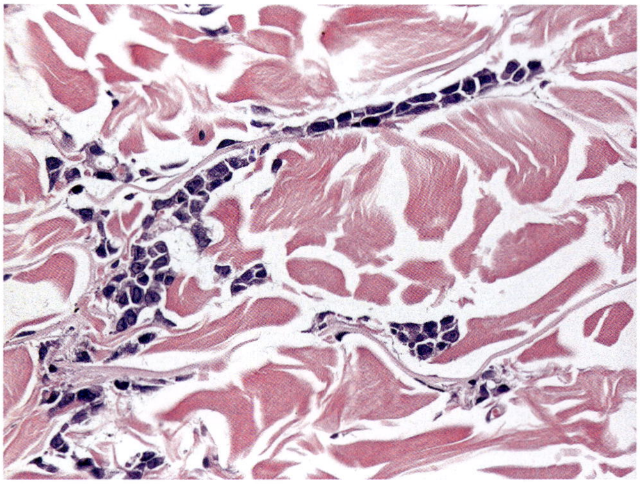

Figure 23.12 Cutaneous manifestations of acute myeloid leukemia. Linear arrangement of neoplastic cells ("Indian filing").

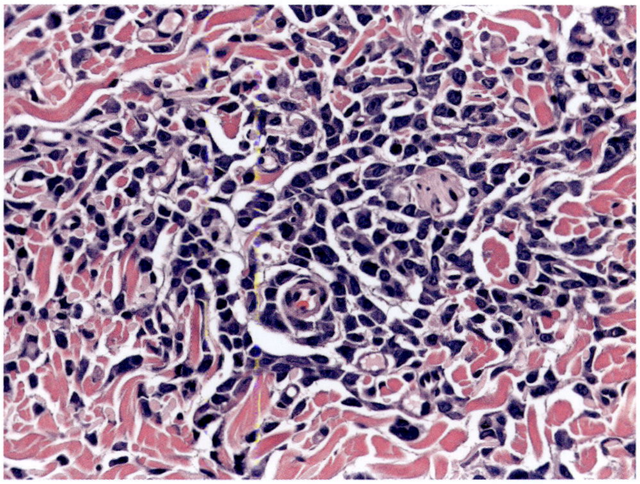

Figure 23.13 Cutaneous manifestations of acute myeloid leukemia. Typical disposition of neoplastic cells with "layering" around vessels and adnexal structures ("figurate" pattern).

monoblasts (Fig. 23.21) [23, 43]. Expression of T-cell markers (CD3, CD5 – but negative for αβ and γδ receptors) may be observed in some cases (Fig. 23.22) [25].

A segmentation anomaly of the neutrophils characterized by round, oval, or hypolobulated nuclei is known as the Pelger–Huët anomaly (observed in a genetic, autosomal dominant setting). A similar morphology of the neutrophils can be observed in a sporadic setting, mostly in myelodysplastic syndrome and acute myeloid leukemia (pseudo-Pelger–Huët anomaly) [44]. In some cases, skin infiltrates at sites of cutaneous inflammation in patients with myelodysplastic syndrome or acute myeloid leukemia may show this peculiar morphology of the neutrophils [38].

## Immunophenotype

The phenotype of cutaneous lesions depends on the type of myelogenous leukemia. Markers that are usually expressed by neoplastic cells include lysozyme, myeloperoxidase, CD13, CD14, CD15, CD33, CD43, CD45, and CD68 (Figs. 23.5–23.7, 23.14 to 23.17, 23.20), but some cases may show positivity for only a few of these antigens [45]. In particular, CD68 is positive in most cases of cutaneous myelogenous leukemia. CD163 is expressed in 30–40% of cases. CD34 and CD117 are positive in more immature forms. Staining for naphtol-ASD-chloracetate-esterase (NASDCl, Leder stain) is positive mainly in cases with

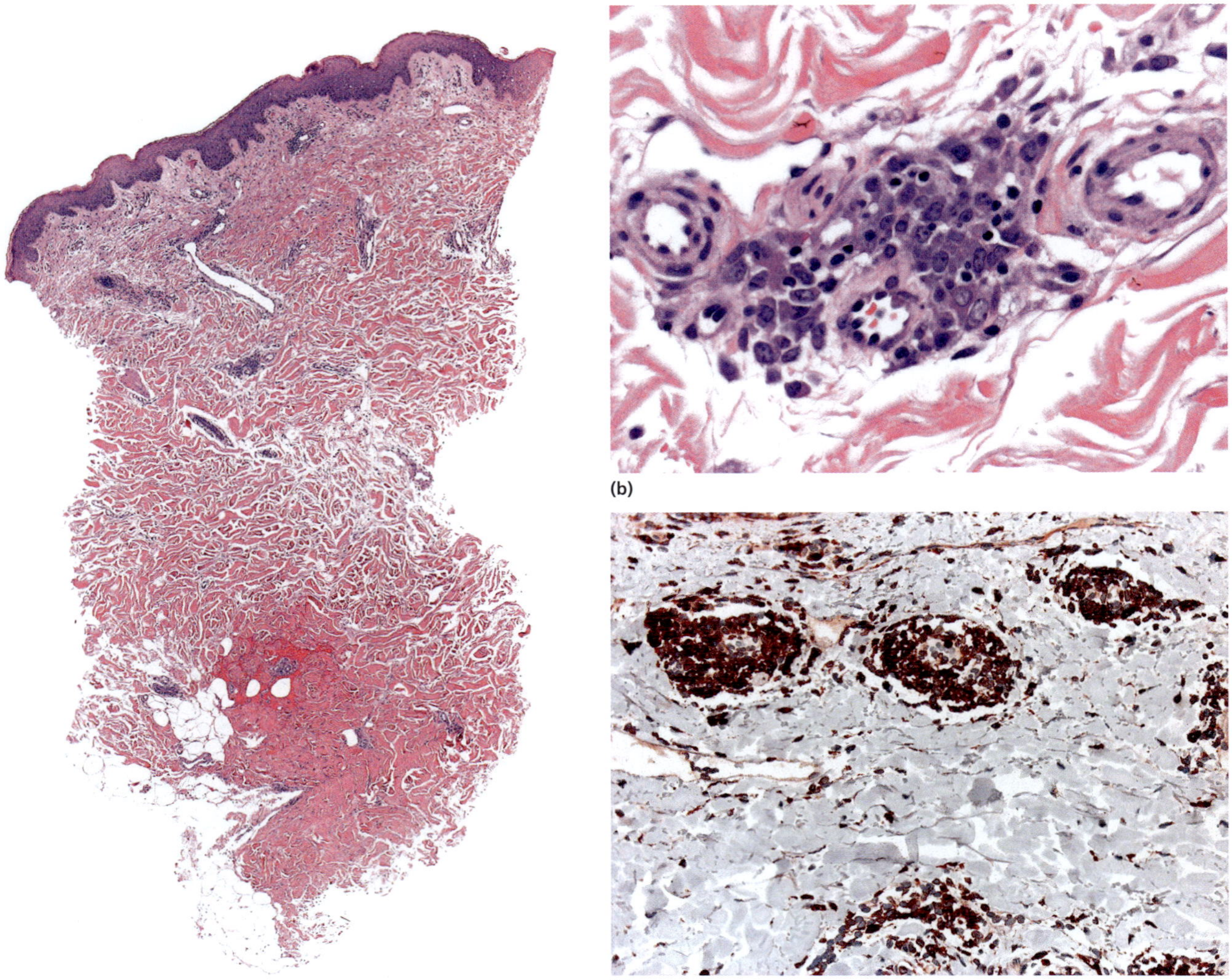

(a) (b) (c)

**Figure 23.14** Early cutaneous manifestations of acute myeloid leukemia. (a) Sparse perivascular and periadnexal infiltrates mimicking an inflammatory condition. (b) Perivascular and periadnexal cells reveal cytomorphological features of myeloid cells. (c) Most cells are positive for CD68. For practical purposes, there is no inflammatory condition that presents histopathologically exclusively with perivascular clusters of CD68⁺ cells.

a mature phenotype, but tends to be negative in more immature cells. Staining for CD56 is found in a minority of cases only; however, since positive cases exist, this marker cannot be used for reliable differentiation from lesions of blastic plasmacytoid dendritic cell neoplasm [3, 7, 46, 47]. As skin lesions of myelogenous leukemia are commonly positive for CD4 and rarely for CD123, a distinction between these two entities may be very difficult. In addition, cases of myelogenous leukemia evolving into blastic plasmacytoid dendritic cell neoplasm have been reported [48, 49].

Myeloid leukemia may show positivity for markers of precursor hematological neoplasms such as TdT (Fig. 23.5f). Neoplastic cells in some cases may also be positive for S100 protein, thus representing a pitfall in the differential diagnosis with histiocytic disorders (e.g., Langerhans cell histiocytosis). These cases represent a pitfall in the histopathological diagnosis, and only the integration of clinical, morphologic, and phenotypic features allows a proper classification.

There seems to be no clear-cut correlation between features seen in specific skin infiltrates and the subtype of the underlying myelogenous leukemia. In addition, the phenotype may be different in bone marrow and skin lesions of patients with acute myeloid leukemia involving the skin [50]. Some of the molecular aberrations defining specific subgroups may be detected by immunohistochemical stainings on paraffin sections (e.g., aberrant cytoplasmic expression of NPM1 in acute myeloid leukemia with mutated *NPM1,* which is one of the most common genetic aberrations in acute myelogenous leukemia). Patients with

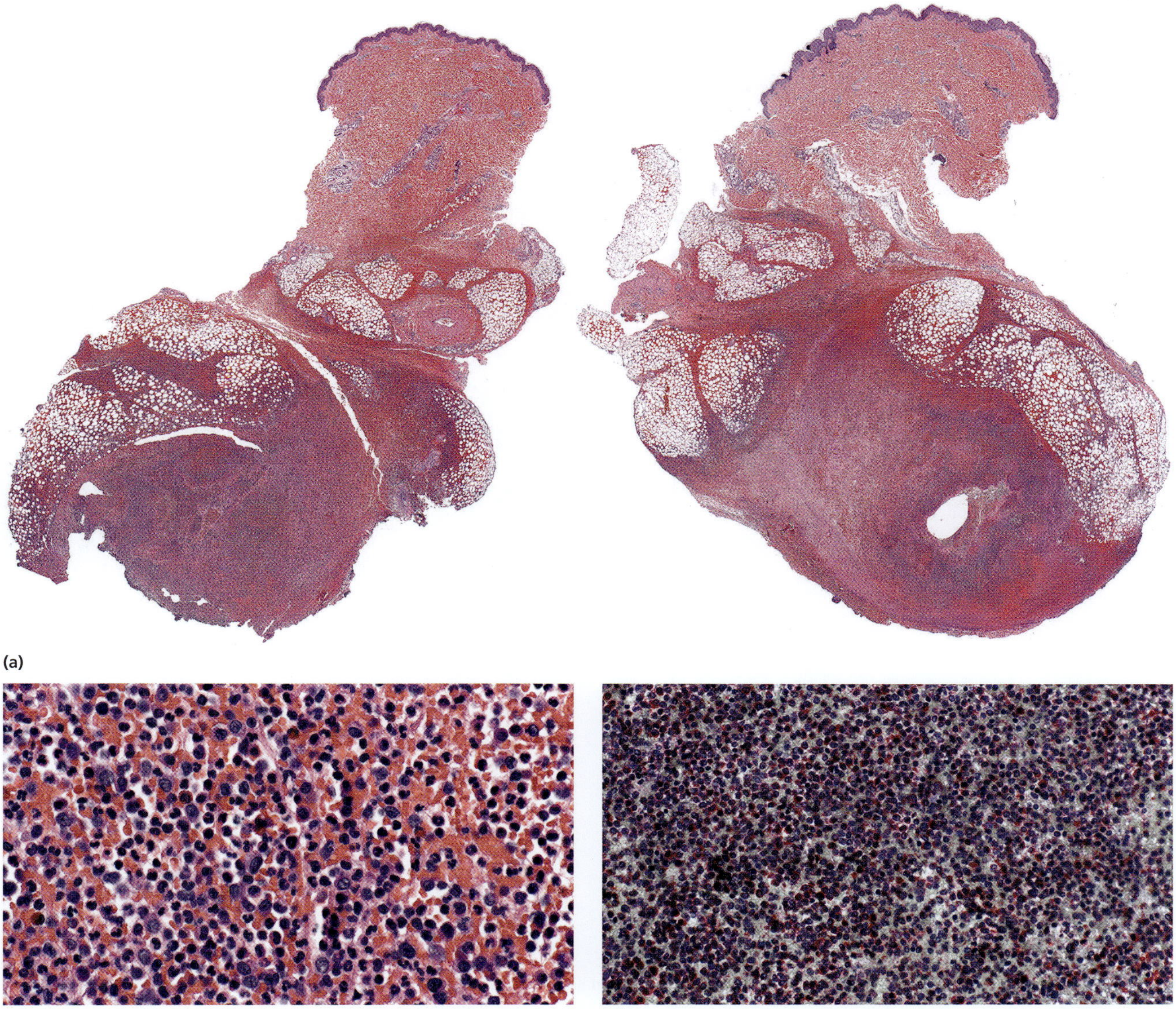

(a) (b) (c)

**Figure 23.15** Neoplastic cells of acute myeloid leukemia within an organized hematoma. (a) Large organized hematoma in the subcutaneous fat with (b) many mononuclear cells admixed with neutrophils. (c) The mononuclear cells are positive for myeloperoxidase.

*NPM1*-mutated acute myeloid leukemia may display a blastic plasmacytoid dendritic cell neoplasm-like phenotype [51].

## Molecular genetics

Many entities in the WHO classification are defined by specific genetic abnormalities. *NPM1*, *CEBPA*, *FLT3*, *RUNX1*, *IDH1*, *IDH2*, *ASXL1*, and *KIT* among others are diagnostic and prognostic molecular markers for acute myeloid leukemia. Only very limited information exist on cutaneous lesions. Interphase fluorescence in situ hybridization (FISH) analysis has been used to confirm trisomy 8 in cutaneous lesions of several patients with myelogenous leukemia. Other studies revealed similar chromosomal aberrations in the bone marrow and the skin, demonstrating the clonal nature of bone marrow and cutaneous infiltrates. The same t(15;17)(q22;q12) rearrangement has been detected in bone marrow and skin lesions of a case of acute promyelocytic leukemia, confirming that FISH may be an adjunctive tool for specific diagnosis of cutaneous infiltrates [52].

## Treatment and prognosis

The skin manifestations are managed by treating the underlying myelogenous leukemia. Treatment must be provided in a hematological setting with experience in myeloid leukemias. Patients with "aleukemic cutaneous myeloid leukemia"

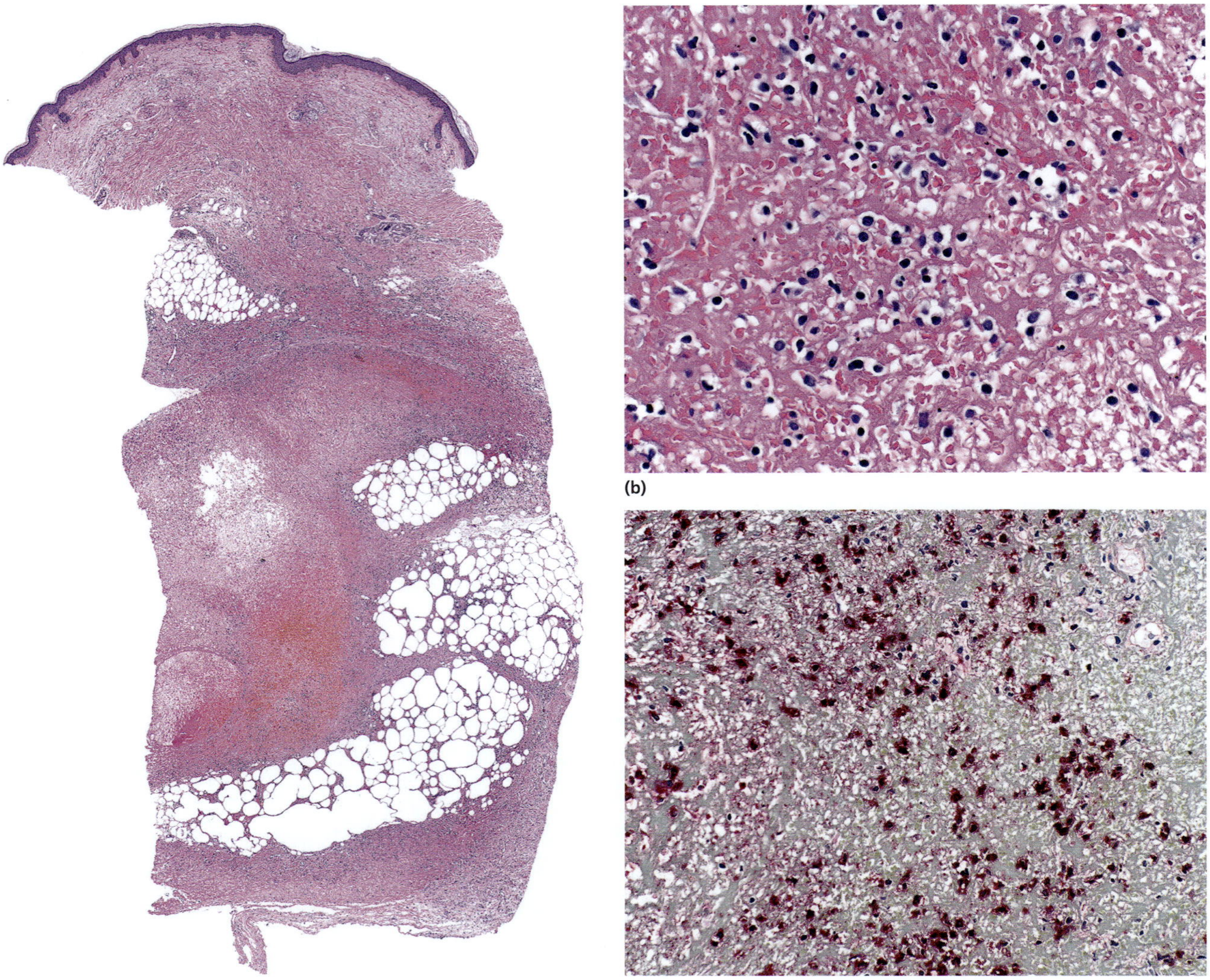

(a) (b) (c)

Figure 23.16 Neoplastic cells of acute myeloid leukemia within an organized hematoma. (a) Ill-defined area of hemorrhage in the subcutaneous fat with (b) mononuclear cells admixed with neutrophils. (c) The mononuclear cells are positive for myeloperoxidase.

should be managed in the same way as patients with blood and/or bone marrow involvement, as the disease inevitably progresses over short periods of time (usually less than 1 year, rarely longer) [53].

Induction and consolidation chemotherapy regimens are typically administered, eventually followed by stem-cell transplantation. Some mutations may be targeted by specific drugs (e.g., cases with *FLT3* gene mutation by midostaurin or gilteritinib, cases with *IDH1* of *IDH2* gene mutations by ivosidenib or enasidenib, respectively). Cases positive for CD33 may receive also gemtuzumab-ozogamicin in addition to chemotherapy.

Skin involvement represents a bad prognostic sign [54]. There seems to be no difference in survival between patients with specific skin manifestations of acute or chronic myelogenous leukemia. The course of cases with skin involvement is aggressive with poor prognosis.

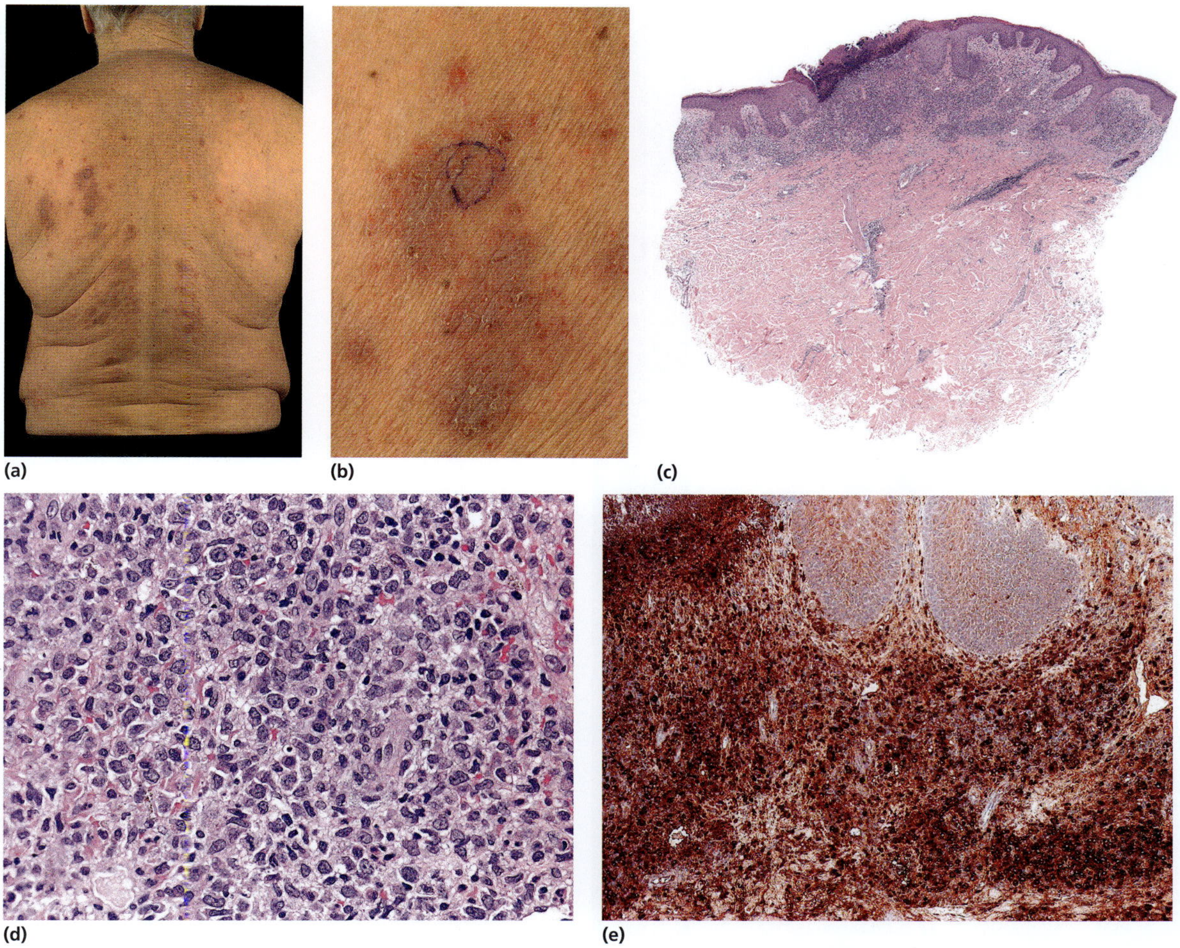


**Figure 23.17** Neoplastic cells of acute myeloid leukemia within lesions of atopic dermatitis. (a, b) Eczematous lesions on the back with scratching artifacts. (c) Histology shows hyperplastic epidermis and focal erosion with crust. (d) In the dermis there are numerous myeloid cells, (e) positive for myeloperoxidase.

## Résumé

**Cutaneous manifestations of acute myeloid leukemia**

| | | |
|---|---|---|
| **Clinical** | Adults; very rarely children and even neonates. Generalized cutaneous papules, plaques, and tumors. Common involvement of mucosal regions (gingival hypertrophy). | |
| **Morphology** | Nodular or diffuse infiltrates characterized by predominance of atypical myelomonocytic cells. "Indian filing," "figurate" pattern. | |
| **Immunohistochemistry (paraffin)** | Myeloperoxidase | +(−) |
| | NaSDCl | +(−) |
| | CD68 | +(−) |
| | CD13, CD14, CD15 | +(−) |
| | CD33, CD163 | +/− |
| | CD34, CD117 | −(+) |
| | CD56 | −/+ |
| | CD4 | + |
| | CD123 | −(+) |
| | MNDA | + |
| | NPM1 | Aberrant cytoplasmic positivity in acute myeloid leukemia with mutated *NPM1* |
| **Genetics** | Identical chromosomal alterations have been demonstrated in the skin and bone marrow in several cases. Many entities in the WHO classification are defined by specific genetic abnormalities. *NPM1*, *CEBPA*, *FLT3*, *RUNX1*, *IDH1*, *IDH2*, *ASXL1*, and *KIT* among others are diagnostic and prognostic molecular markers for acute myeloid leukemia. | |
| **Treatment guidelines** | Treatment should be offered in a hematological setting. Types of myeloid leukemia with particular genetic alterations may be treated with specific drugs. "Aleukemic" myeloid leukemia should be treated like conventional, leukemic variants of the disease. | |

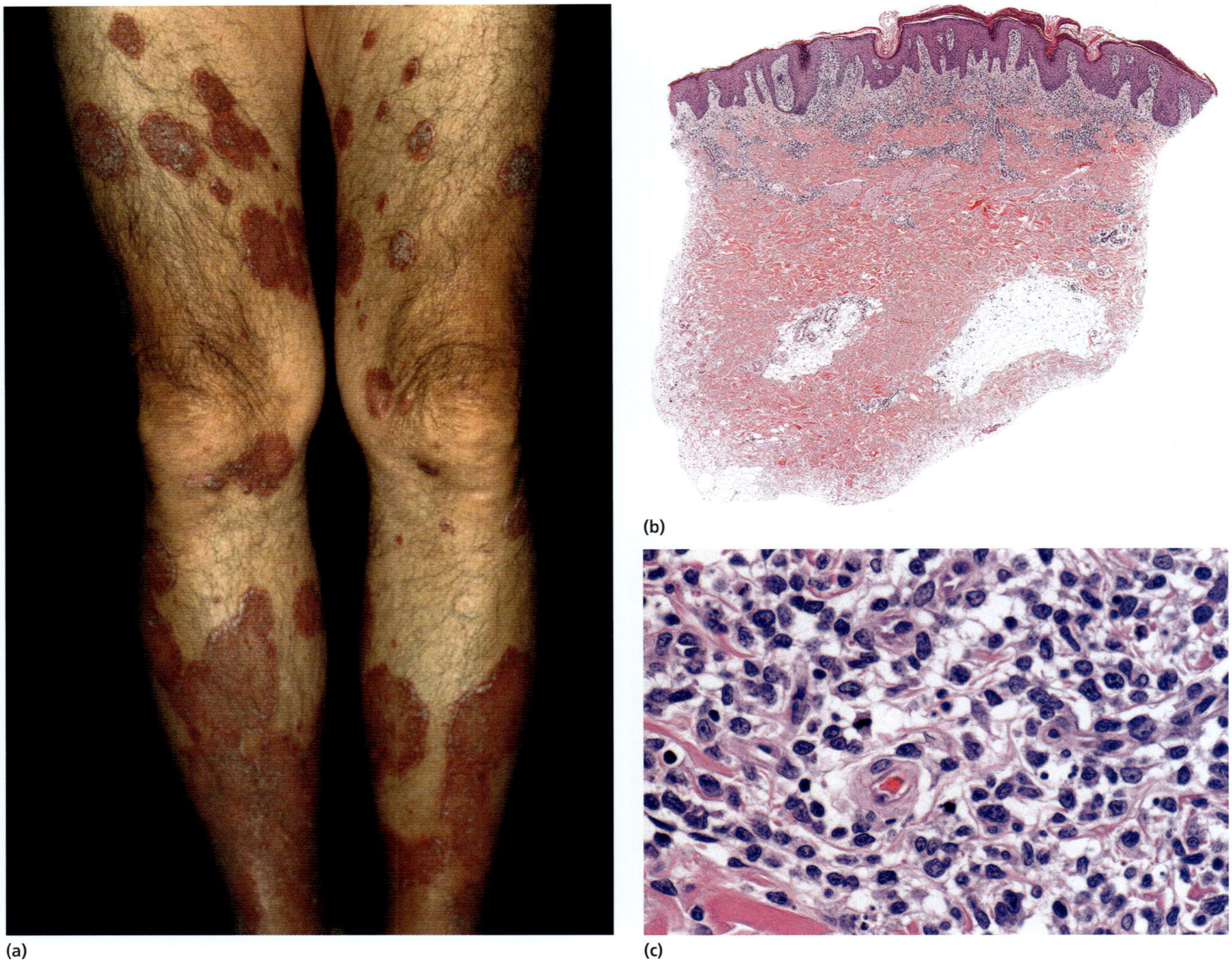

Figure 23.18 Neoplastic cells of acute myeloid leukemia within lesions of psoriasis. (a) Erythematous, scaly lesions of psoriasis on the legs. (b) Histology shows psoriasiform hyperplasia with parakeratosis. (c) In the dermis there are numerous myeloid cells.

## Chronic myelogenous leukemia

Chronic myelogenous leukemia includes two different entities: chronic myeloid leukemia (characterized by the *BCR::ABL1* fusion gene due to a t(9;22)(q34;q11.2), so-called Philadelphia chromosome), and chronic myelomonocytic leukemia, an entity characterized by a variable molecular background. Chronic myeloid leukemia is included in the group of myeloproliferative neoplasms in the WHO classification, whereas chronic myelomonocytic leukemia is listed among the myelodysplastic/myeloproliferative neoplasms. Besides acute myeloid leukemia, cutaneous involvement can occur in other types of myeloproliferative /myelodysplastic disorders, but is more common in chronic myeloid leukemia [55].

In most cases, specific skin lesions in patients with ***chronic myeloid leukemia*** have features similar to those observed in acute myeloid leukemia, and represent progression to a more aggressive stage of the disease.

In the blast phase of chronic myeloid leukemia B- or (less commonly) T-cell-derived blasts can be observed in a proportion of patients, sometimes with loss of several myeloid antigens ("transdifferentiation") (Fig. 23.23). Thus, immunophenotypic panels should include also markers for B- and T-cells (CD2, CD3, CD4, CD5, CD7, and CD8 for T-blasts, CD10, CD19, CD20, CD79a, and PAX5 for B-blasts, as well as TdT).

The essential criteria for diagnosis of chronic myeloid leukemia (>90%) are the presence of neutrophilic leukocytosis in the peripheral blood, and detection of the typical *BCR-ABL1* fusion (so-called Philadelphia chromosome) caused by the t(9;22)(q34.1;q11.2) reciprocal translocation which can be detected by cytogenetic analyses, FISH analysis and/or reverse transcriptase polymerase chain reaction (RT/PCR) (these last

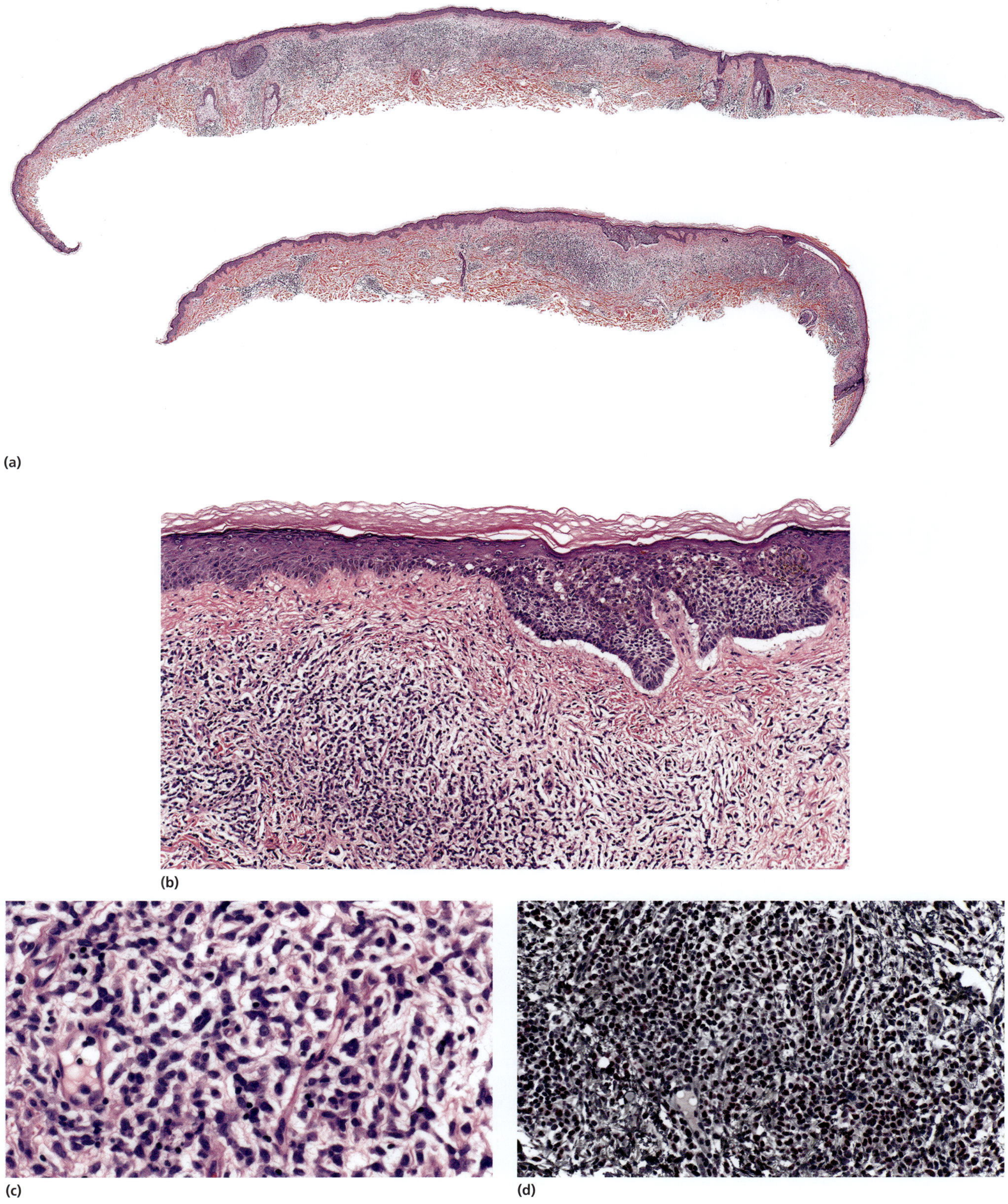

(a) (b) (c) (d)

Figure 23.19 Neoplastic cells of acute myeloid leukemia under a basal cell carcinoma. (a) Shaving biopsy showing a basaloid tumor and a dense mononuclear cell infiltrate. (b) Details of a superficial basal cell carcinoma and of the mononuclear cell infiltrate, characterized by (c) myeloid cells positive for (d) MNDA.

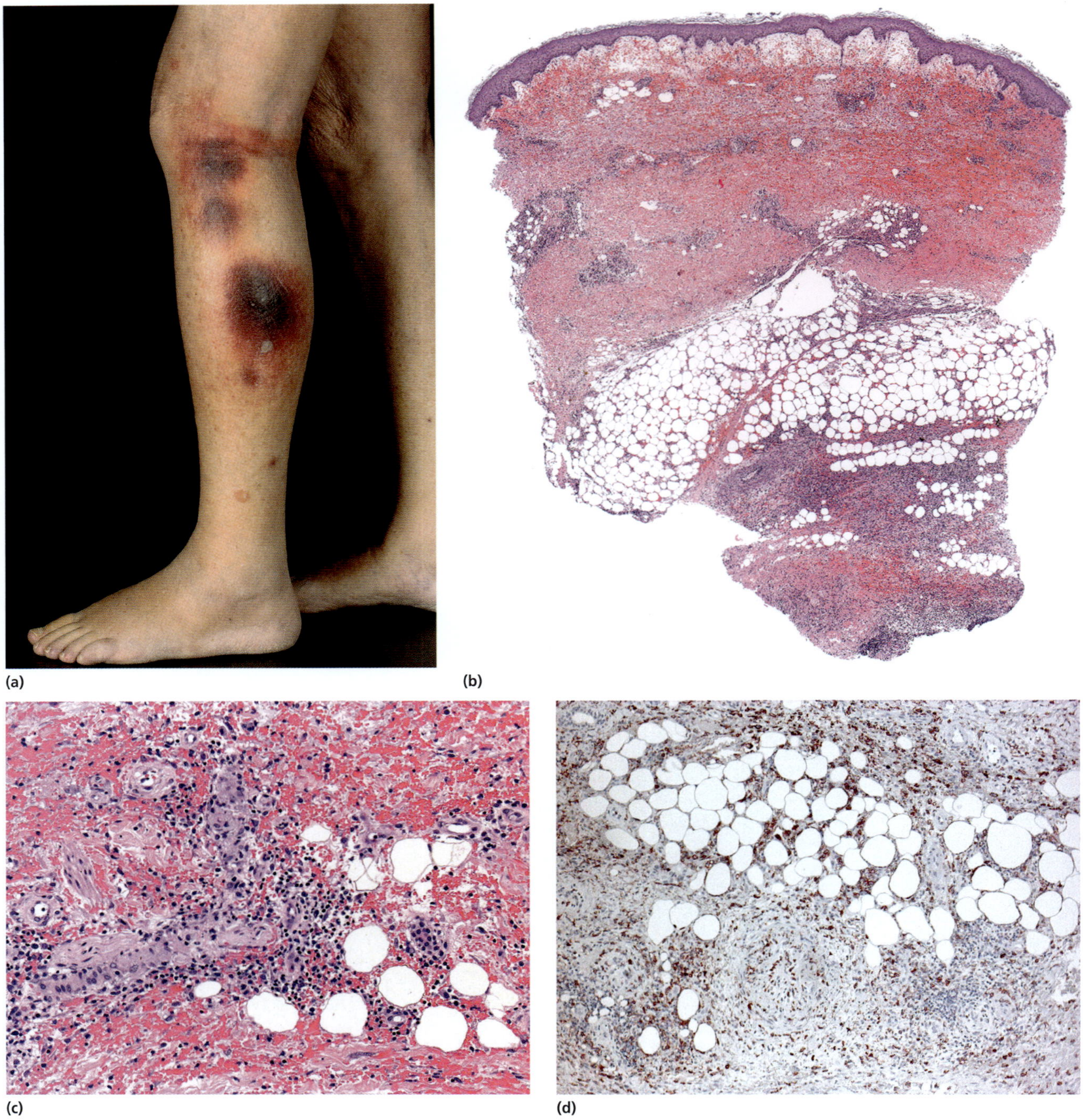

Figure 23.20 Cutaneous manifestations of acute myeloid leukemia within erysipelas. (a) Purpuric lesions on the left lower leg of an 88-year-old man presenting with fever, malaise, pancytopenia including thrombopenia, and elevated CRP and LDH. A bacterial smear showed the presence of St. aureus. In spite of antibiotic treatment, a few days later the lesions were increasing in size and a biopsy was taken, showing (b) subepidermal edema with hemorrhage in the entire dermis and subcutis, and (c) a relatively sparse dermal and subcutaneous infiltrate of neutrophils and mononuclear cells. Phenotypic analyses revealed that the mononuclear cells were positive for CD4, CD14 (d), myeloperoxidase (e), and CD68, as well as partially positive for CD13 and CD56. Three months later the patient developed systemic symptoms, and a bone marrow biopsy revealed a myelodysplastic syndrome with evolution into acute myeloid leukemia. The patient died of multiorgan failure four months after the first presentation.

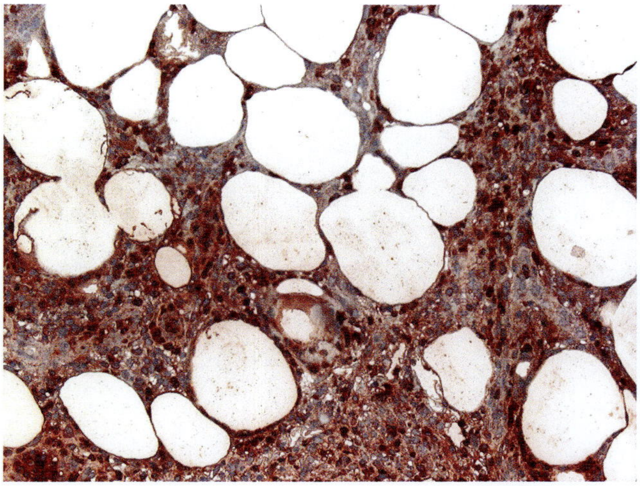

**(e)**

**Figure 23.20** (Continued)

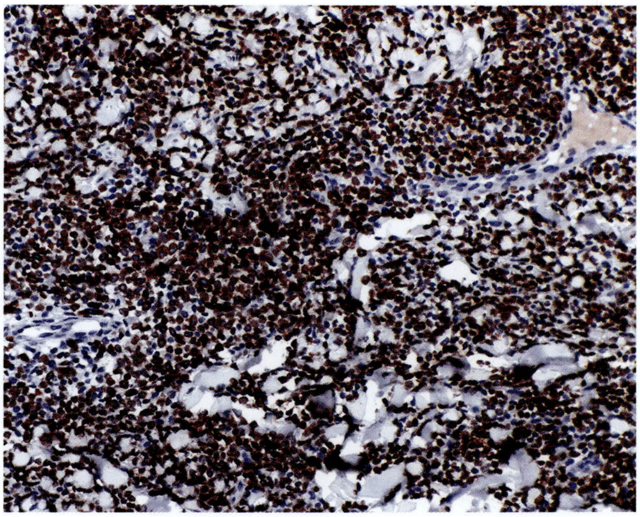

**Figure 23.22** Cutaneous myeloid sarcoma. Positivity of neoplastic cells for CD3.

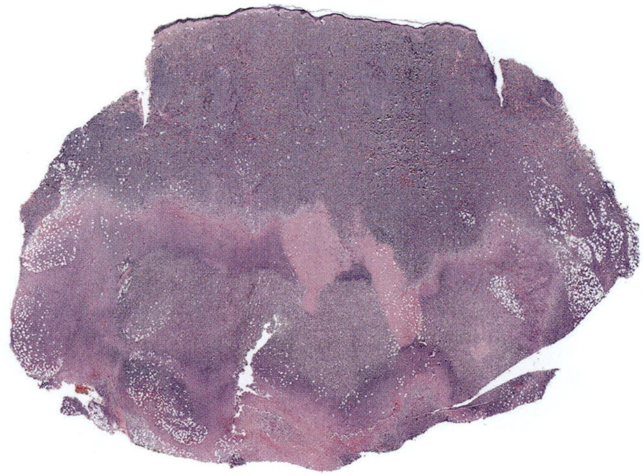

**(a)**

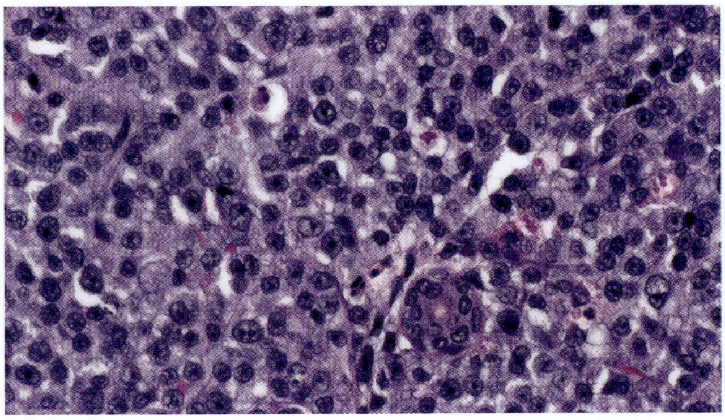

**(b)**

**Figure 23.21** Cutaneous myeloid sarcoma. (a) Dense infiltrate within the entire dermis and subcutaneous fat with large areas of necrosis, characterized by (b) sheets of atypical myeloid cells.

two methods detect also cases with variant translocations or cryptic translocations). Cutaneous manifestations are usually a sign of blast phase and portend a bad prognosis, although the introduction of treatment with imatinib has revolutionized the approach and prognosis of these patients.

In cutaneous manifestations of ***chronic myelomonocytic leukemia***, besides conventional cases showing predomination of myeloid blasts within the infiltrate, three other variants of skin lesions have been described: the first presenting with accumulations of dendritic cells with the phenotype of mature plasmacytoid dendritic cells ($CD123^+$, $TCL1^+$, $CD303^+$, $CD56^-$, $CD1a^-$, $S100^-$), the second characterized by tumors with features of blastic plasmacytoid dendritic cell neoplasm, and the third characterized by a proliferation of blastic "indeterminate" dendritic cells positive for monocytic markers and also for CD1a and S100 [15]. The subclassification according to these subtypes may be therapeutically and prognostically relevant. Compared to the other groups, patients with lesions characterized by accumulation of mature plasmacytoid dendritic cells had a better prognosis [15]. In some of these cases, the phenotype is similar to that of an indeterminate dendritic cell tumor and may mimic a histiocytic proliferation ($S100^+$, $CD1a^+$, CD207/$Langerin^-$) [56]. The cells with the "dendritic cell" phenotype in patients with skin infiltrates of chronic myeloid leukemia are clonally related to the original neoplastic cells, representing most likely trans- or de-differentiation of the original clone. More details of cutaneous tumors of mature plasmacytoid dendritic cells are provided below in this chapter.

In chronic myelomonocytic leukemia, a distinct proportion of patients are affected by autoimmune or other systemic inflammatory disorders (including skin diseases such as psoriasis) [57]. It is yet debated whether these diseases or their treatment are responsible for the onset of leukemia, or leukemia is responsible for the onset of autoimmune and other systemic inflammatory disorders, or a genetic predisposition and/or impaired immunity is responsible for the onset of both leukemia and associated diseases, but it seems likely that chronic myelomonocytic leukemia is responsible for the onset of autoimmune and other systemic inflammatory disorders [57]. In fact, a correlation between mutations in the epigenetic regulators *TET2/IDH* and *SRSF2* and T-lymphocytes imbalance has been demonstrated [58].

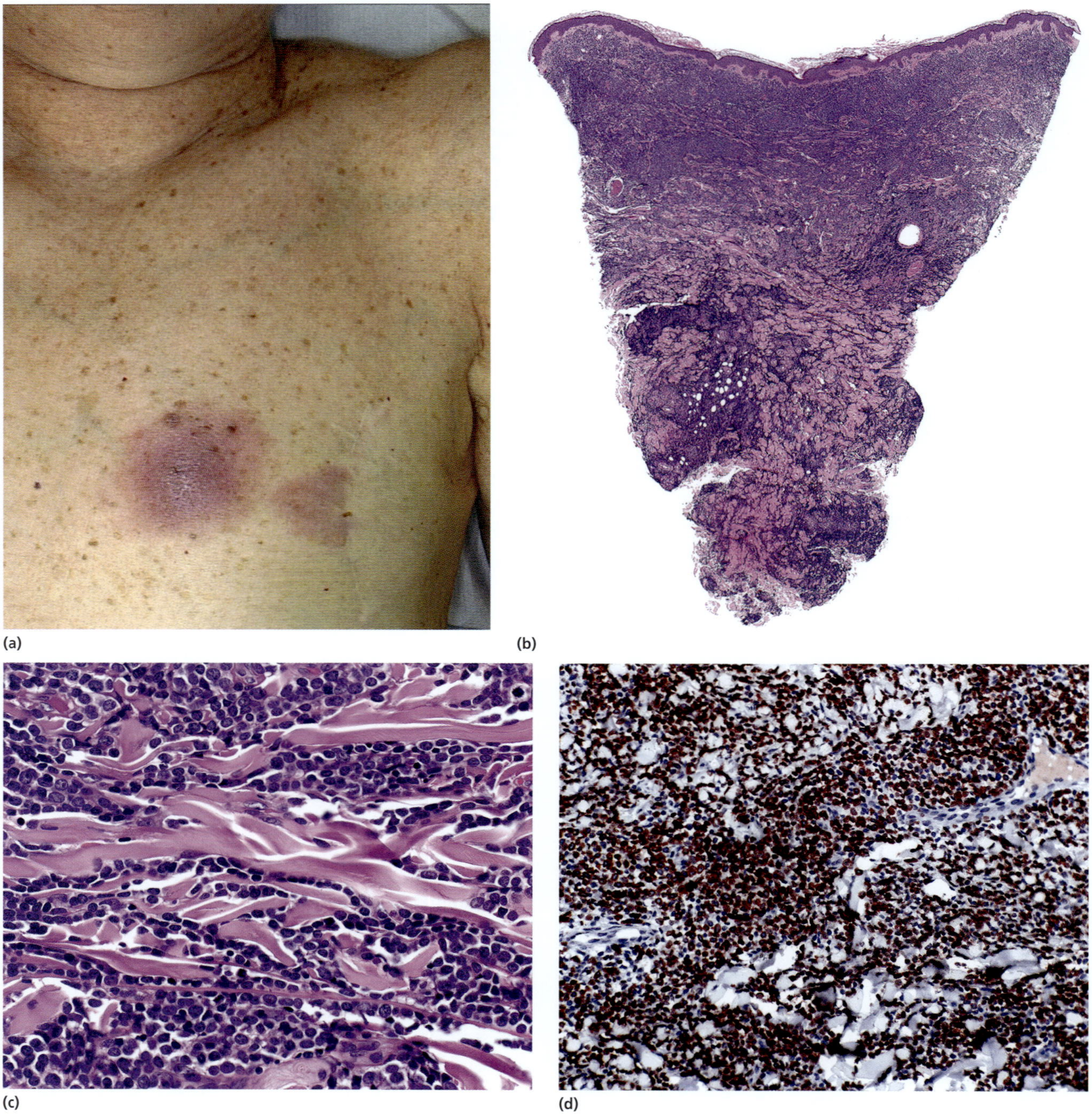

**Figure 23.23** Cutaneous manifestations of chronic myeloid leukemia with blastic phase and transdifferentiation. (a) Two localized, livid flat tumors on the chest of a patient with a history of breast carcinoma; (b) histology shows a diffuse infiltrate within the entire dermis with (c) mononuclear cells showing "indian filing"; (d) positive staining of neoplastic cells for CD3 (cytoplasmic), (e) CD34, (f) TdT, and (g) weak positivity for CD117. (h) Only focal positivity for myeloperoxidase.

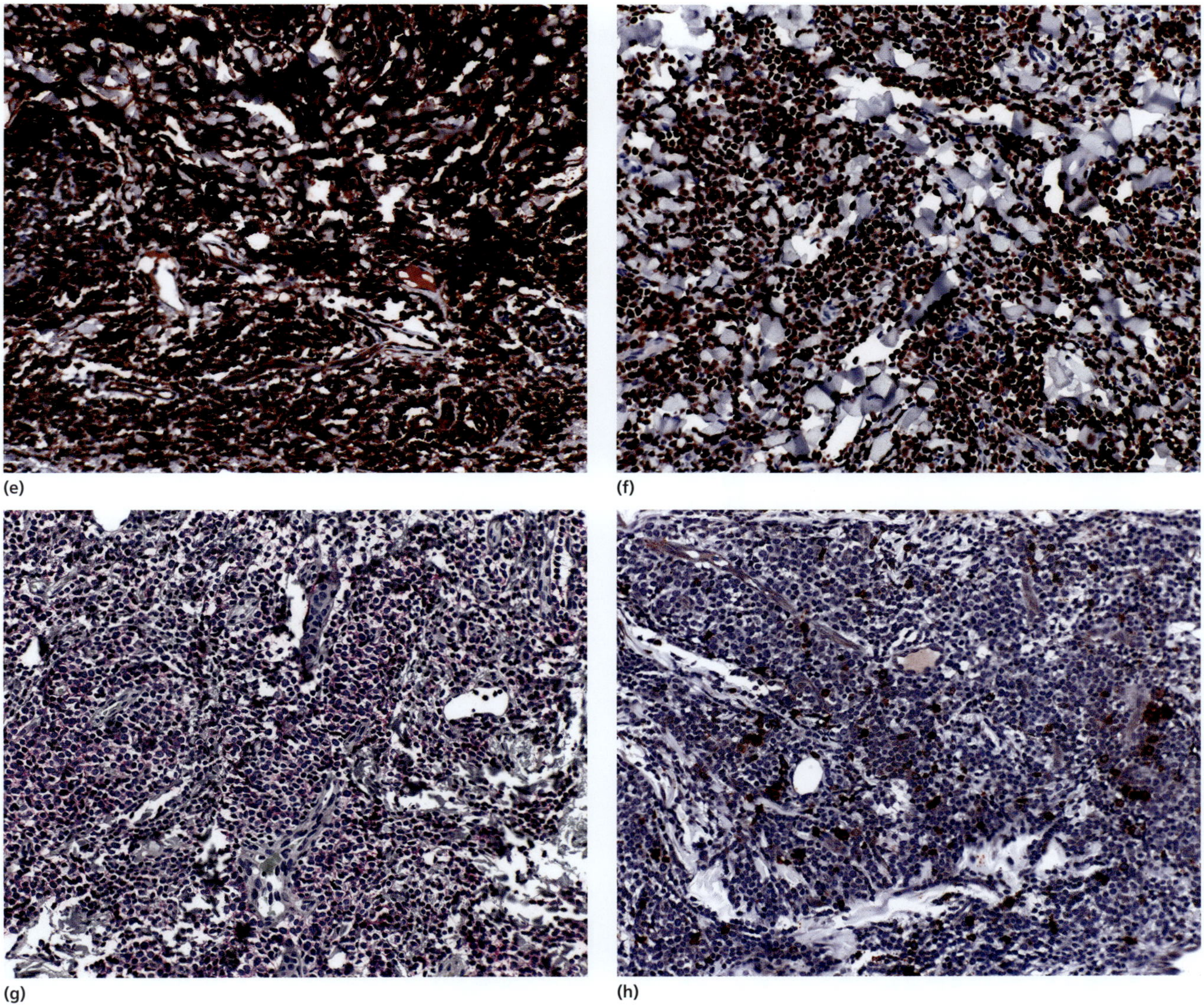


Figure 23.23 (Continued)

## Myelodysplastic syndromes (myelodysplastic neoplasms)

Myelodysplastic syndromes are a group of disorders defined as "clonal hematopoietic stem cell neoplasms, defined by cytopenias and morphological dysplasia, and clinically characterized by progressively ineffective hematopoiesis and an increased risk of acute myeloid leukemia" [59]; some variants are defined by genetic abnormalities, and other by morphological features; overlapping features with other myeloproliferative disorders exist (in the WHO classification, a total of 20 entities is included in the 3 groups of myeloproliferative neoplasms, myelodysplastic neoplasms, and myeloproliferative/myelodysplastic neoplasms). A different number of entities, but a similar concept, is adopted by the ICC *of Myeloid and Lymphoid Neoplasms* [60]. Again, a detailed discussion of all different entities is beyond the scope of this book, and I will focus only on cutaneous manifestations in myelodysplastic syndromes.

Skin manifestations in patients with myelodysplastic syndromes are usually nonspecific (e.g., Sweet syndrome, other neutrophilic dermatoses, leucocytoclastic vasculitis, etc.), that is, do not represent cutaneous involvement by the primary disease. VEXAS (vacuoles, E1 enzyme, X-linked, autoinflammatory, somatic mutations) syndrome is a recently described systemic autoinflammatory disease characterized by somatic mutations in hematopoietic progenitor cells and neutrophilic infiltrates similar to those observed in Sweet syndrome [61], and is often associated with myelodysplastic syndromes [62a].

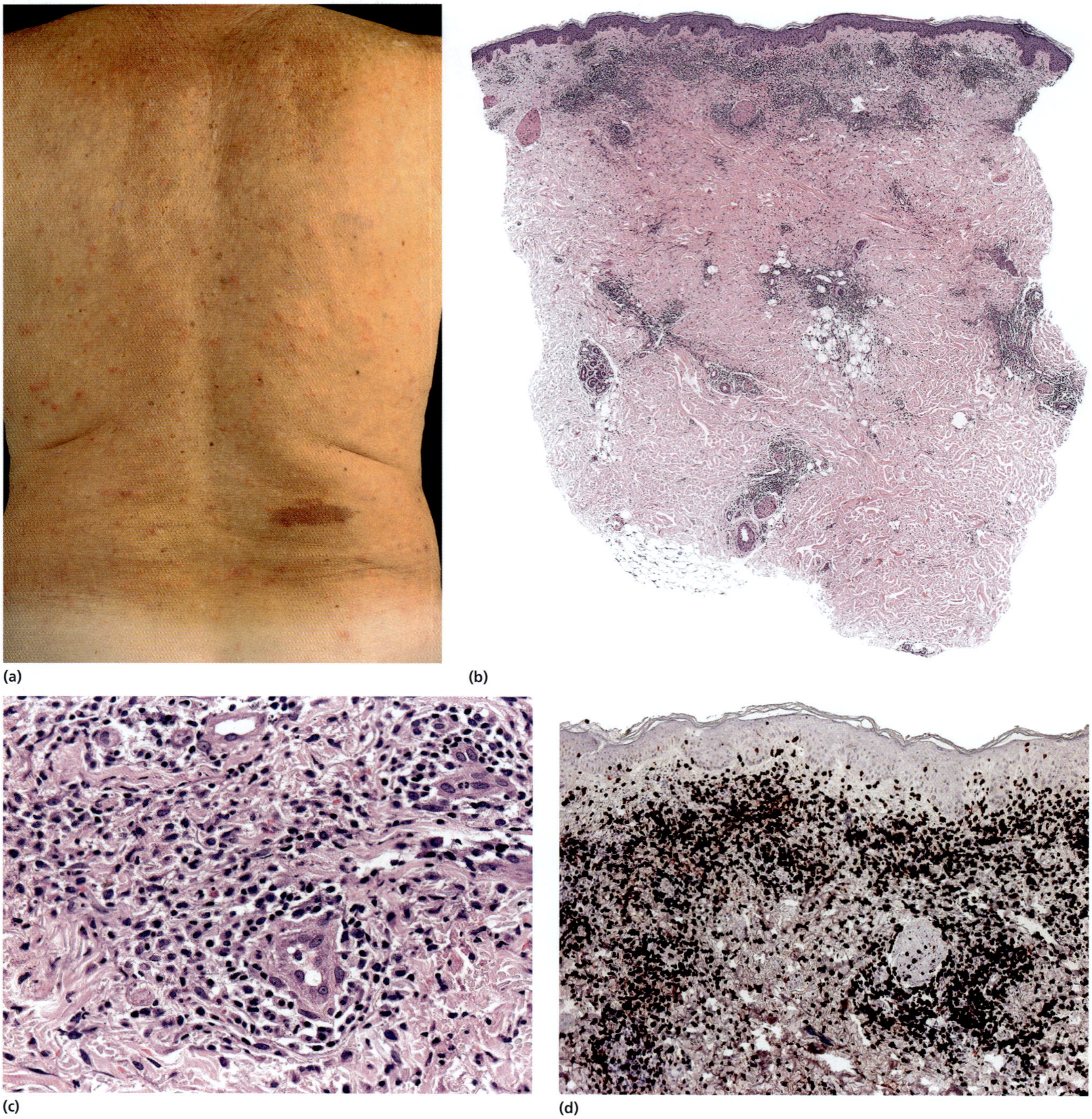

Figure 23.24 Cutaneous involvement in myelodysplastic syndrome. (a) Clinical presentation with multiple erythematous papules and small nodules on the trunk; (b) dense infiltrates in the dermis characterized by (c) many myeloid cells admixed with reactive elements. (d) Positivity of all cells for MNDA.

The presence of concomitant cutaneous lesions of histiocytoid Sweet syndrome and clonally related myelodysplastic features in the bone marrow has been termed "myelodysplasia cutis" [63, 64], suggesting that in these patients Sweet syndrome represents a specific skin manifestation of the myelodysplastic neoplasm, and may be associated with advanced disease. A recent study showed that VEXAS syndrome, myelodysplasia cutis, and Sweet syndrome are characterized by a shared inflammatory environment relying mostly on a type 1 immune response led by type 1 and 2 interferons, along with the activation of tumor necrosis factor and interleukin-1β pathways [62b].

When present, specific skin manifestations in patients with myelodysplastic syndromes are usually associated with the progression of the disease to a leukemic phase, and clinicopathologic

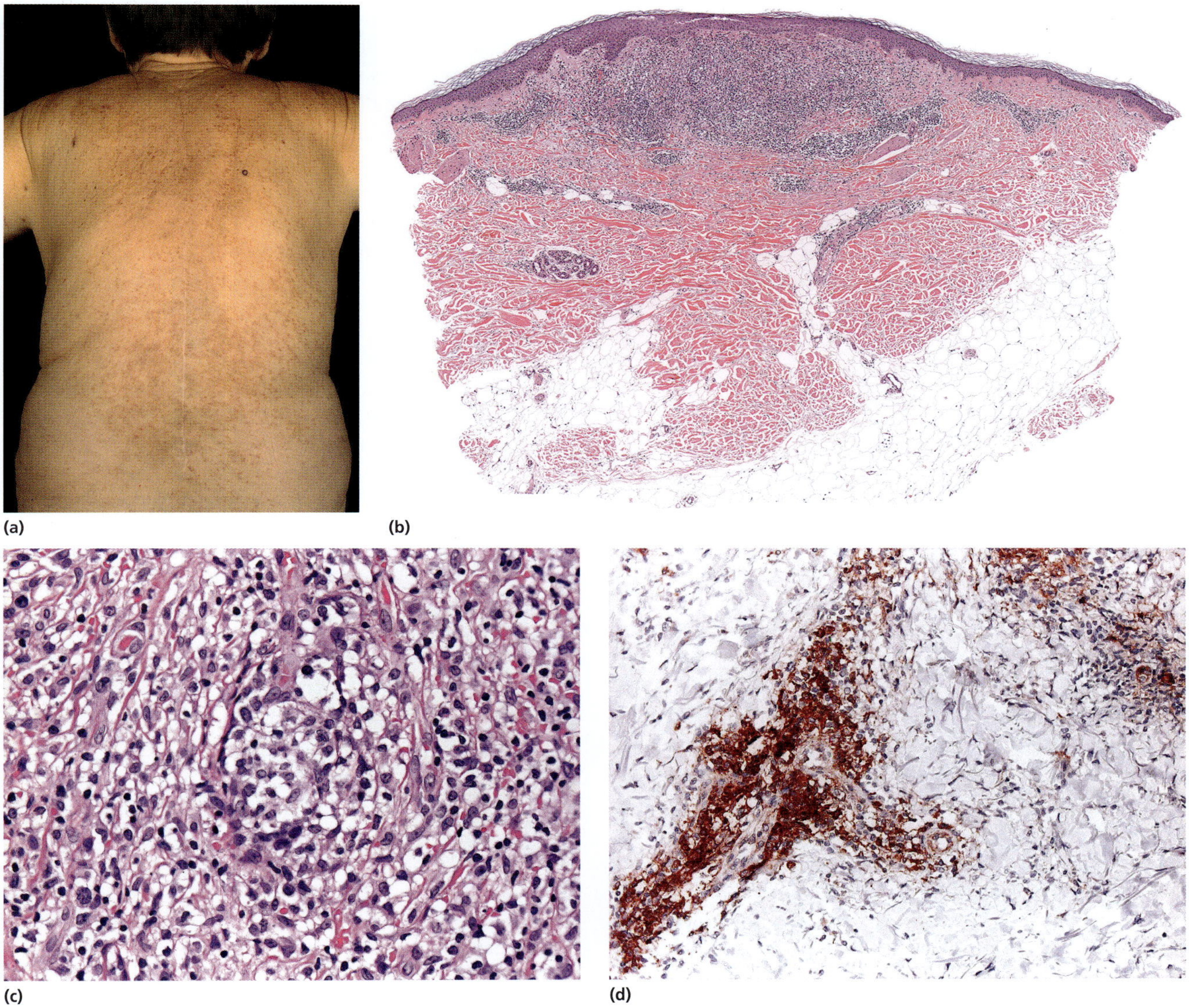


**Figure 23.25** Cutaneous mature plasmacytoid dendritic cell proliferation. (a) Nonspecific, generalized erythematous papules. (b) Histology reveals dense dermal infiltrates with (c) clusters of mature-looking plasmacytoid dendritic cells. (d) Immunohistology shows positivity for CD123.

features are similar to those observed in acute myeloid leukemia. However, in a subset of patients, skin lesions present with more discrete papules and small plaques that are characterized histopathologically by moderately dense, perivascular, and periadnexal infiltrates of lymphocytes admixed with small clusters of immature myeloid cells (these last positive for CD68 and MNDA, and only in part for lysozyme and myeloperoxidase) (Fig. 23.24). Although the infiltrates do not qualify for a clear-cut diagnosis of leukemia cutis, they also do not show features of "conventional" dermatoses that can be observed in this group of patients. The main histopathologic differential diagnosis in these cases is with so-called "histiocytoid" Sweet syndrome and VEXAS syndrome, and differentiation may be impossible without precise clinical correlation. In some patients with myelodysplastic syndromes, granulomatous skin infiltrates may be observed [65]. As for acute myeloid leukemia, also in patients with myelodysplastic syndromes skin lesions may predate the diagnosis of the disease in the bone marrow by several years [66].

Many genetic abnormalities have been detected in myelodysplastic syndromes. *TP53*, *SF3B1*, *ASXL1*, *RUNX1*, *EZH2*, and *ETV6* among others are genes involved in several cases.

Most (but not all!) patients with cutaneous manifestations of myelodysplastic syndromes eventually develop leukemic features after variable intervals of time (sometimes 1–2 years), but the management is conservative with short-term follow-up controls only [66]. It may be that these cases represent a "smoldering" form of leukemia and that a management similar to that of patients with "aleukemic" cutaneous myeloid leukemia should be considered. On the other hand, in contrast to this last group of patients, who do not have leukemia in the bone marrow or in the blood but who have skin lesions that fulfill the criteria for diagnosis of cutaneous leukemic infiltrate, the skin lesions just discussed in patients with myelodysplastic syndromes cannot be considered clearly diagnostic of leukemia, thus a more careful approach seems to be appropriate.

## Mature plasmacytoid dendritic cell proliferation associated with myeloid neoplasms

Mature plasmacytoid dendritic cell proliferations represent a clonal proliferation of plasmacytoid dendritic cells arising on the background of a myeloid neoplasm; it is included as a specific entity in the WHO, but not the ICC classification [67]. In the last edition of this book, this condition was included in the chapter on blastic plasmacytoid dendritic cell neoplasm; however, since it is closely related to myeloproliferative disorders, in this edition it has been moved to this chapter. The skin is the most frequent organ where mature plasmacytoid dendritic cell proliferation has been observed [15, 68]. The background condition is often chronic myelomonocytic leukemia, but mature plasmacytoid dendritic cell proliferations can be observed also in patients with acute myeloid leukemia, myelodysplastic neoplasms, and myeloproliferative neoplasms. Their relationship to the underlying myeloid neoplasm has been demonstrated by the finding of identical clonal chromosomal abnormalities in the two cellular components. Although the exact nosology of this proliferation is yet unclear, it should not be considered to be a "pseudolymphoma," as its neoplastic nature is confirmed by the finding of genetic aberrations similar to those of underlying leukemia.

Skin lesions are nonspecific, characterized by multiple erythematous macules, papules, or small nodules (Fig. 23.25a), resembling in some cases leukemia cutis. Histology is characterized by variably dense dermal infiltrates composed predominantly of CD123$^+$, mature-looking plasmacytoid dendritic cells admixed with reactive cells (Figs. 23.25b to d). In the skin, these tumor-forming aggregates of plasmacytoid dendritic cells may rarely mimic inflammatory conditions such as lupus erythematosus, thus representing a potential histopathological pitfall [69].

Differentiation of mature plasmacytoid dendritic cell proliferations from myelogenous leukemia and blastic plasmacytoid dendritic cell neoplasm relies mainly on morphology (nodules or irregular aggregates of cells morphologically and phenotypically similar to normal plasmacytoid dendritic cells), negativity or only focal positivity for CD56, CD117, myeloperoxidase, MNDA and TdT, low Ki-67 proliferation index (<10%), and lack of TdT. Apoptosis may be prominent, representing a further differential diagnostic clue from blastic plasmacytoid dendritic cell neoplasm.

Treatment of the underlying myeloid neoplasm may result in the regression of the cutaneous plasmacytoid dendritic cell infiltrates, but prognosis is usually poor with a median survival of 11 months, (related to the original leukemia rather than directly to the infiltrates of mature plasmacytoid dendritic cells) [15, 46]. In patients with acute myeloid leukemia, mature plasmacytoid dendritic cell proliferations are characterized by *RUNX1* mutations, and may define a subset of cases of acute myeloid leukemia potentially targeted by anti-CD123 antibodies [70].

## References

1. Solary E, Gujral S. Acute myeloid leukaemia: introduction. In: *WHO Classification of Tumours Editorial Board. Haematolymphoid Tumours*. 5th edition. Lyon: IARC, 2024: 110–111.
2. Hasserjian RP, Arber DA, Cazzola M, *et al*. Introduction to the International Consensus Classification of myeloid disorders and acute leukemias. In: Arber DA, Borowitz MJ, Cook JR, *et al*., eds. *The International Consensus Classification of Myeloid and Lymphoid Neoplasms*. Philadelphia, PA: Wolters Kluwer, 2025: 1–20.
3. Kaddu S, Zenahlik P, Beham-Schmid C, *et al*. Specific cutaneous infiltrates in patients with myelogenous leukemia: a clinicopathologic study of 26 patients with assessment of diagnostic criteria. *J Am Acad Dermatol* 1999;**40**:966–978.
4. Desch JK, Smoller BR. The spectrum of cutaneous disease in leukemias. *J Cutan Pathol* 1993;**20**:407–410.
5. Janier M, Raynaud E, Blanche P, *et al*. Leukaemia cutis and erythroleukaemia. *Br J Dermatol* 1999;**141**:372–373.
6. Kaiserling E, Horny HP, Geerts ML, Schmid U. Skin involvement in myelogenous leukemia: morphologic and immunophenotypic heterogeneity of skin infiltrates. *Mod Pathol* 1994;**7**:771–779.
7. Kuwabara H, Nagai M, Yamaoka G, *et al*. Specific skin manifestations in CD56 positive acute myeloid leukemia. *J Cutan Pathol* 1999;**26**:1–5.
8. Nagao K, Kikuchi A, Kawai Y, *et al*. Skin infiltration in acute promyelocytic leukemia. *Dermatology* 1997;**194**:168–171.
9. Namba Y, Koizumi H, Nakamura H, *et al*. Specific cutaneous lesions of the scalp in myelodysplastic syndrome with deletion of 20q. *J Dermatol* 1999;**26**:220–224.
10. Sepp N, Radaszkiewicz T, Meijer CJLM, *et al*. Specific skin manifestations in acute leukemia with monocytic differentiation: a morphologic and immunohistochemical study of 11 cases. *Cancer* 1993;**71**:124–132.
11. Stawiski MA. Skin manifestations of leukemias and lymphomas. *Cutis* 1978;**21**:814–818.
12. Ueda K, Kume A, Furukawa Y, Higashi N. Cutaneous infiltration in acute promyelocytic leukemia. *J Am Acad Dermatol* 1997;**36**:104–106.
13. Kajisawa C, Matsui C, Morohashi M. A specific cutaneous lesion revealing myelodysplastic syndrome. *Eur J Dermatol* 1998;**8**: 517–518.
14. Cho-Vega JH, Medeiros LJ, Prieto VG, Vega F. Leukemia cutis. *Am J Clin Pathol* 2008;**129**:130–142.
15. Vitte F, Fabiani B, Benet C, *et al*. Specific skin lesions in chronic myelomonocytic leukemia A spectrum of myelomonocytic and dendritic cell proliferations. A study of 42 cases. *Am J Surg Pathol* 2012;**36**:1302–1316.

16. Weinel S, Malone J, Jain D, Callen JP. Therapy-related leukaemia cutis: a review. *Australas J Dermatol* 2008;**49**:187–190.
17. Roberts I, Fordham NJ, Rao A, Bain BJ. Neonatal leukaemia. *Br J Haematol* 2018;**182**:170–184.
18. Godínez-Chaparro JA, Valencia-Herrera AM, Duarte-Abdala MR, *et al.* Leukemia cutis and other dermatological findings in pediatric patients with acute myeloid leukemia. *Bol Med Hosp Infant Mex* 2021;**78**:411–417.
19. Beckmann S, Kliffen M, Huijben A, *et al.* Concurrent langerhans cell histiocytosis and acute myeloid leukemia without clonal relationship. *JAMA Dermatol* 2024;**160**:114–116.
20. Traweek ST, Arber DA, Rappaport H, Brynes RK. Extramedullary myeloid cell tumors: an immunohistochemical and morphologic study of 28 cases. *Am J Surg Pathol* 1993;**17**:1011–1019.
21. Sisack MJ, Dunsmore K, Sidhu-Malik N. Granulocytic sarcoma in the absence of myeloid leukemia. *J Am Acad Dermatol* 1997;**37**:308–311.
22. Chen W, Madeiros JL. Myeloid sarcoma. In: *WHO Classification of Tumours Editorial Board. Haematolymphoid Tumours.* 5th edition. Lyon: IARC, 2024: 165–168.
23. Hurley MY, Ghahramani GK, Frisch S, *et al.* Cutaneous myeloid sarcoma: natural history and biology of an uncommon manifestation of acute myeloid leukemia. *Acta Derm Venereol* 2013;**93**:319–324.
24. Ullman DI, Dorn D, Jones JA, *et al.* Clinicopathological and molecular characteristics of extramedullary acute myeloid leukaemia. *Histopathology* 2019;**75** 185–192.
25. Kawamoto K, Miyoshi H, Yoshida N, *et al.* Clinicopathological, cytogenetic, and prognostic analysis of 131 myeloid sarcoma patients. *Am J Surg Pathol* 2016;**40**:1473–1483.
26. Husak R, Blume-Peytaki U, Orfanos CE. Aleukemic leukemia cutis in an adolescent boy. *N Engl J Med* 1999;**340**:893–894.
27. Canioni D, Fraitag S, Thomas C, *et al.* Skin lesions revealing neonatal acute leukemias with monocytic differentiation: a report of 3 cases. *J Cutan Pathol* 1996;**23**:254–258.
28. Torrelo A, Madero L, Mediero IG, *et al.* Aleukemic congenital leukemia cutis. *Ped Dermatol* 2004;**21**:458–461.
29. Landers MC, Malempati S, Tilford D, *et al.* Spontaneous regression of aleukemic congenital leukemia cutis. *Ped Dermatol* 2005;**22**: 26–30.
30. Martínez-Escanamé M, Zuriel D, Tee SI, *et al.* Cutaneous infiltrates of acute myelogenous leukemia simulating inflammatory dermatoses. *Am J Dermatopathol* 2013;**35**:419–424.
31. Metzler G, Cerroni L, Schmidt H, *et al.* Leukemic cells within skin lesions of psoriasis in a patient with acute myelogenous leukemia. *J Cutan Pathol* 1997;**24**:445–448.
32. Diaz-Cascajo C, Bloedern-Schlicht N. Cutaneous infiltrates of myelogenous leukemia in association with pre-existing skin diseases. *J Cutan Pathol* 1998;**25**:185–186.
33. Urano Y, Miyaoka Y, Kosaka M, *et al.* Sweet's syndrome associated with chronic myelogenous leukemia: demonstration of leukemic cells within a skin lesion. *J Am Acad Dermatol* 1999;**40**:275–279.
34. Deguchi M, Tsunoda T, Yuda F, Tagami H. Sweet's syndrome in acute myelogenous leukemia showing dermal infiltration of leukemic cells. *Dermatology* 1997;**194**:182–184.
35. Miyakura T, Yamamoto T, Kurashige Y, *et al.* Leukemia cutis originating in the extravasation site of i.v. gabexate mesilate infusion. *J Dermatol* 2008;**35**:29–32.
36. Chavan RN, Cappel MA, Ketterling RP, *et al.* Histiocytoid Sweet syndrome may indicate leukemia cutis: a novel application of fluorescence in situ hybridization. *J Am Acad Dermatol* 2014;**70**: 1021–1027.
37. Magro CM, Momtahen S, Nguyen GH, Wang X. Histiocytoid Sweet's syndrome: a localized cutaneous proliferation of macrophages frequently associated with chronic myeloproliferative disease. *Eur J Dermatol* 2015;**25**:335–341.
38. Kristensen IB, Møller H, Kjaerskov MW, *et al.* Myeloid sarcoma developing in pre-existing pyoderma gangrenosum. *Acta Derm Venereol* 2009;**89**:175–177.
39. Ohno S, Yokoo T, Ohta M, *et al.* Aleukemic leukemia cutis. *J Am Acad Dermatol* 1990;**22**:374–377.
40. Okun MM, Fitzgibbon J, Nahass GT, Forsman K. Aleukemic leukemia cutis, myeloid subtype. *Eur J Dermatol* 1995;**5**:290–293.
41. Baksh FK, Nathan D, Richardson W, *et al.* Leukemia cutis with prominent giant cell reaction. *Am J Dermatopathol* 1998;**20**:48–52.
42. Tomasini C, Quaglino P, Novelli M, Fierro MT. "Aleukemic" granulomatous leukemia cutis. *Am J Dermatopathol* 1998;**20**:417–421.
43. Tan EST, Tang MBY, Guan KYK, *et al.* A case of myeloid sarcoma with unusually extensive and rapidly progressive skin manifestations. *Ann Acad Med Singapore* 2011;**40**:424–426.
44. Sessarego M, Ajmar F. Correlation between acquired pseudo-Pelger-Huët anomaly and involvement of chromosome 17 in chronic myeloid leukemia. *Cancer Genet Cytogenet* 1987;**25**: 265–270.
45. Benet C, Gomez A, Aguilar C, *et al.* Histologic and immunohistologic characterization of skin localization of myeloid disorders: a study of 173 cases. *Am J Clin Pathol* 2011;**135**:278–290.
46. Kaddu S, Beham-Schmid C, Zenahlik P, *et al.* CD56 blastic transformation of chronic myeloid leukemia involving the skin. *J Cutan Pathol* 1999;**26**:497–503.
47. Szablewski V, Costes V, Bret C, *et al.* Cutaneous presentation preceding acute myeloid leukemia with CD4+/CD56+ expression misdiagnosed as a blastic plasmocytoid dendritic cell neoplasm: a case report. *J Cutan Pathol* 2018;**45**:610–614.
48. Cibull TL, Thomas AB, O'Malley DP, Billings SD. Myeloid leukemia cutis: a histologic and immunohistochemical review. *J Cutan Pathol* 2008;**35**:180–185.
49. Hejmadi RK, Thompson D, Shah F, Naresh KN. Cutaneous presentation of aleukemic monoblastic leukemia cutis–a case report and review of literature with focus on immunohistochemistry. *J Cutan Pathol* 2008;**3**(suppl. 1):46–49.
50. Sachdev R, George TI, Schwartz EJ, Sundram UN. Discordant immunophenotypic profiles of adhesion molecules and cytokines in acute myeloid leukemia involving bone marrow and skin. *Am J Clin Pathol* 2012;**138**:290–299.
51. Minetto P, Guolo F, Clavio M, *et al.* A blastic plasmacytoid dendritic cell neoplasm-like phenotype identifies a subgroup of NPM1-mutated acute myeloid leukemia patients with worse prognosis. *Am J Hematol* 2018;**93**:e33–e35.
52. Wrede JE, Sundram U, Kohler S, *et al.* Fluorescence in situ hybridization investigation of cutaneous lesions in acute promyelocytic leukemia. *Mod Pathol* 2005;**18**:1569–1576.
53. Chang H, Shih LY, Kuo TT. Primary aleukemic myeloid leukemia cutis treated successfully with combination chemotherapy: report of a case and review of the literature. *Ann Hematol* 2003;**82**:435–439.

54. Wang CX, Pusic I, Anadkat MJ. Association of leukemia cutis with survival in acute myeloid leukemia. *JAMA Dermatol* 2019;**155**:826–832.
55. Prieto-Torres L, Requena L, Rodríguez-Pinilla SM. Clinical, histopathological and molecular spectrum of cutaneous lesions in myelodysplastic syndrome and myeloproliferative neoplasms (MDS/MPN): an integrative review. *Cancers (Basel)* 2023;**15**:5888.
56. Loghavi S, Curry JL, Garcia-Manero G, *et al.* Chronic myelomonocytic leukemia masquerading as cutaneous indeterminate dendritic cell tumor: expanding the spectrum of skin lesions in chronic myelomonocytic leukemia. *J Cutan Pathol* 2017;**44**:1075–1079.
57. Ambinder AJ, Miller J, DeZern AE. Autoimmune disease in CMML-the chicken or the egg? *Best Pract Res Clin Haematol* 2020;**33**:101136.
58. Zhao LP, Boy M, Azoulay C, *et al.* Genomic landscape of MDS/CMML associated with systemic inflammatory and autoimmune disease. *Leukemia* 2021;**35**:2720–2724.
59. Padron E, Platzbecker U, Bejar R, *et al.* Myelodysplastic/myeloproliferative neoplasm NOS (unclassifiable). In: *WHO Classification of Tumours Editorial Board. Haematolymphoid Tumours.* 5th edition. Lyon: IARC, 2024: 108–109.
60. Hasserjian RP. Introduction to premalignant clonal cytopenias and myelodysplastic syndromes. In: Arber DA, Borowitz MJ, Cook JR, *et al.*, eds. *The International Consensus Classification of myeloid and lymphoid neoplasms.* Philadelphia, PA: Wolters Kluwer, 2025: 124–126.
61. Beck DB, Ferrada MA, Sikora KA, *et al.* Somatic mutations in UBA1 and severe adult-onset autoinflammatory disease. *N Engl J Med* 2020;**383**:2628–2638.
62. (a) Kreutzinger V, Pankow A, Boyadzhieva Z, *et al.* VEXAS and myelodysplastic syndrome: an interdisciplinary challenge. *J Clin Med* 2024;**13**:1049.(b) Grolleau C, Battistella M, Zakine E, *et al.* Inflammatory signatures in VEXAS syndrome, myelodysplasia cutis, and sweet syndrome. *JAMA Dermatol* 2025; **161**:538–543.
63. Calvo KR. Skin in the game: the emergence of myelodysplasia cutis. *Blood* 2022;**139**:1132–1134.
64. Delaleu J, Kim R, Zhao LP, *et al.* Clinical, pathological, and molecular features of myelodysplasia cutis. *Blood* 2022;**139**: 1251–1253.
65. Hagiwara A, Fujimura T, Furudate S, *et al.* Generalized granulomatous dermatitis accompanied by myelodysplastic syndrome. *Acta Derm Venereol* 2014;**94**:223–224.
66. Osio A, Battistella M, Feugeas JP, *et al.* Myelodysplasia cutis versus leukemia cutis. *J Invest Dermatol* 2015;**135**:2321–2324.
67. Khoury JD, Takeuchi K, Xiao W. Mature plasmacytoid dendritic cell proliferation associated with myeloid neoplasms. In: *WHO Classification of Tumours Editorial Board. Haematolymphoid Tumours.* 5th edition. Lyon: IARC, 2024: 224–225.
68. Facchetti F, Cigognetti M, Fisogni S, *et al.* Neoplasms derived from plasmacytoid dendritic cells. *Mod Pathol* 2016;**29**:98–111.
69. Dargent J-L, Henne S, Pranger D, *et al.* Tumor-forming plasmacytoid dendritic cells associated with myeloid neoplasms. Report of a peculiar case with histopathologic features masquerading as lupus erythematosus. *J Cutan Pathol* 2016;**43**:280–286.
70. Xiao W, Chan A, Waarts MR, *et al.* Plasmacytoid dendritic cell expansion defines a distinct subset of RUNX1-mutated acute myeloid leukemia. *Blood* 2021;**137**:1377–1391.

CHAPTER 24

# Blastic plasmacytoid dendritic cell neoplasm

Blastic plasmacytoid dendritic cell neoplasm is probably the single hematologic neoplasm that has changed more names over the years. Several synonyms have been used in the past, including "Blastic NK-cell lymphoma," "Blastic NK leukaemia/lymphoma," "NK-cell lymphoma," "Agranular CD4$^+$ NK leukaemia," "CD4$^+$ NK cell leukaemia," "Agranular CD4$^+$ CD56$^+$ haematodermic neoplasm/tumour," and "CD4$^+$/CD56$^+$ hematodermic neoplasm." All of them should be considered obsolete, mostly reflecting the wrong concept that CD56 expression was related to a natural killer derivation of tumor cells. In the International Consensus Classification (ICC)) *of Myeloid and Lymphoid Neoplasms*, blastic plasmacytoid dendritic cell neoplasm is listed as a separate entity in the section on myeloid neoplasms and acute leukemias [1], whereas it is included within the group of histiocytic and dendritic neoplasms in the 5th edition of the World Health Organization (WHO) *Classification of Haematolymphoid Tumours* [2]. Although primary cutaneous presentation without extracutaneous disease is common, blastic plasmacytoid dendritic cell neoplasm is not included in the last WHO-European Organization for Research and Treatment of Cancer (EORTC) classification of cutaneous lymphomas, and it is mentioned as a "mimicker" of lymphoma in the 2024 update [3, 4]. Neoplastic cells differentiate toward a common myeloid and lymphoid cell precursor, identified as the plasmacytoid dendritic cell (professional type I interferon-producing cell) [5–7], and a large study confirmed that the tumor originates from resting plasmacytoid dendritic cells of myeloid origin [8]. Malignant transformation occurs at a very early stage of differentiation; thus the blastic plasmacytoid dendritic cell neoplasm belongs to the precursor hematologic neoplasms.

A relationship between blastic plasmacytoid dendritic cell neoplasm and myelogenous leukemia exists [9–12]. Evolution into myeloid leukemia has been documented in some patients [13], and association with chronic myelomonocytic leukemia or myelodysplastic syndromes, including clonal hematopoiesis, is a frequent finding [14]. In spite of the putative relationship, however, studies by comparative genomic hybridization have revealed different profiles of blastic plasmacytoid dendritic cell neoplasm and cutaneous lesions of acute myeloid leukemia [15]. On the other hand, the gene signature of the cell of origin of blastic plasmacytoid dendritic cell neoplasm is much closer to that of myeloid rather than lymphoid precursors, and in elderly patients with associated clonal hematopoiesis a shared clonal origin has been demonstrated in several cases [14].

In most cases, blastic plasmacytoid dendritic cell neoplasm is confined to the skin at presentation or skin lesions represent the first manifestation of the disease [1, 2, 16–19]. Leukemic spread after variable (usually short) periods of time is the rule, indicating that primary cutaneous cases most likely represent examples of so-called "aleukemic leukemia cutis" [20]. The identification of non-neoplastic plasmacytoid monocytes within the skin provides a theoretical background to the frequent finding of lesions confined to cutaneous sites [21].

Interestingly, similar to what happens in acute myeloid leukemia, also in blastic plasmacytoid dendritic cell neoplasm neoplastic cells have been observed at the site of a cutaneous tumor (a basal cell carcinoma) [22]. Although this finding is intriguing, in my experience specific cutaneous involvement by blastic plasmacytoid dendritic cell neoplasm at the site of unrelated skin conditions is exceedingly rare, and I have never observed personally similar cases.

## Clinical features

Patients are mostly adults and elderly with a median age of 65 and with a male predominance [17–19, 23]. However, onset in children and adolescents is not rare, and even a congenital neonatal case has been reported [20, 24–30]. There is a predominance of males. Clinically, they present with solitary, localized, or generalized plaques and tumors (Figs. 24.1 to 24.4). A characteristic "bruise-like" violaceous aspect due to intratumoral hemorrhage is observed in several cases and early lesions may resemble localized areas of hemorrhage (Fig. 24.5). Ulceration is uncommon. Mucosal regions may be involved in a small minority of cases (Fig. 24.6). In some cases, the skin presentation may be characterized by the predominance of patches and ecchymotic areas, but these lesions, too, are infiltrated by variable numbers of neoplastic cells (Fig. 24.7). In a distinct proportion of patients (approximately 30–40%), skin lesions are

*Skin Lymphoma: The Illustrated Guide*, Sixth Edition. Lorenzo Cerroni.

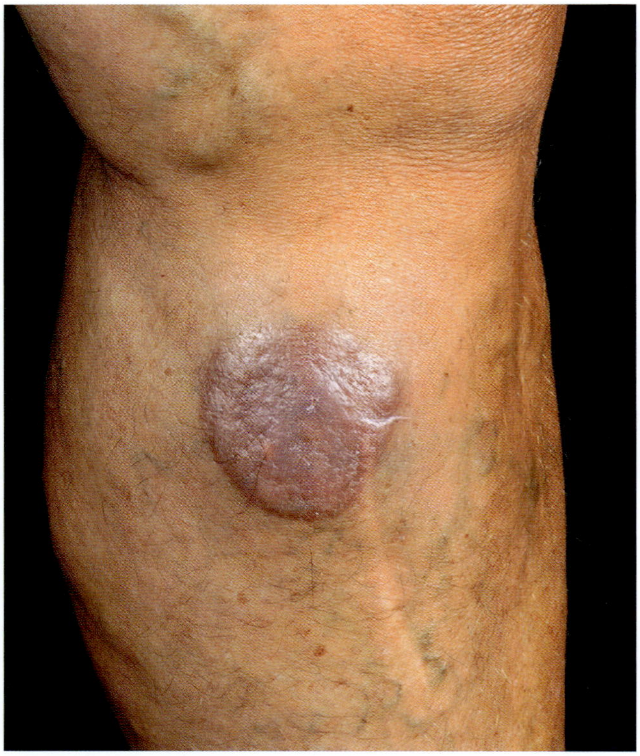

Figure 24.1 Blastic plasmacytoid dendritic cell neoplasm. Solitary tumor on the leg.

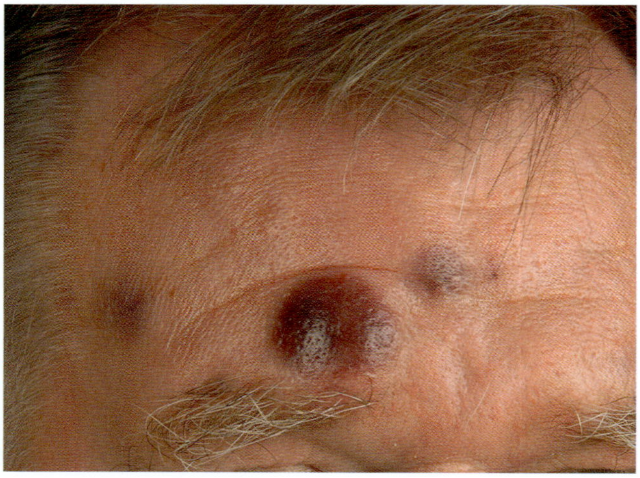

Figure 24.2 Blastic plasmacytoid dendritic cell neoplasm. Localized hemorrhagic, infiltrated plaques, and flat tumor on the forehead.

accompanied by general symptoms and extracutaneous manifestations in the blood, bone marrow, and/or other organs. Lymph nodes are involved in approximately half of the cases at presentation. Thrombocytopenia, anemia, and neutropenia are commonly found.

Cutaneous lesions are the first manifestation of the disease in over 90% of patients. In patients with primary cutaneous involvement, the time interval between the onset of skin lesions

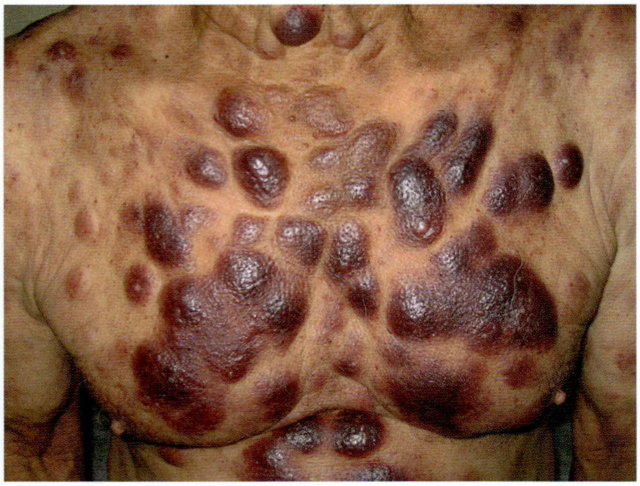

Figure 24.3 Blastic plasmacytoid dendritic cell neoplasm. Multiple plaques and tumors on the chest. Note the "bruise-like" violaceous aspect. *(Courtesy of Dr. Esmeralda Vale and Dr. Isabel Viana, Lisbon.)*

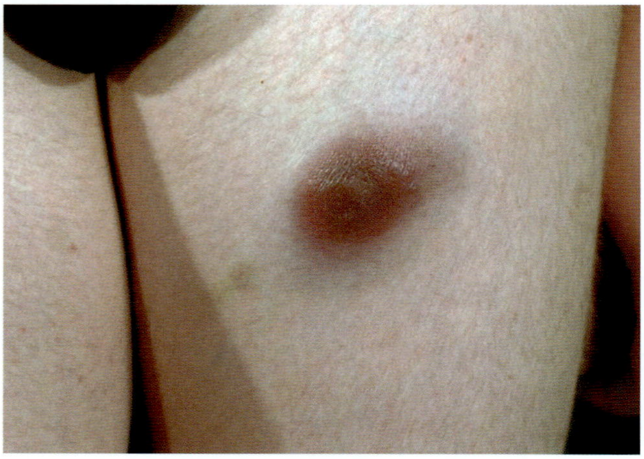

Figure 24.4 Blastic plasmacytoid dendritic cell neoplasm. Violaceous tumor on the thigh of a 13-year-old boy. *(Courtesy of Dr. Carlo Cota, Rome, Italy.)*

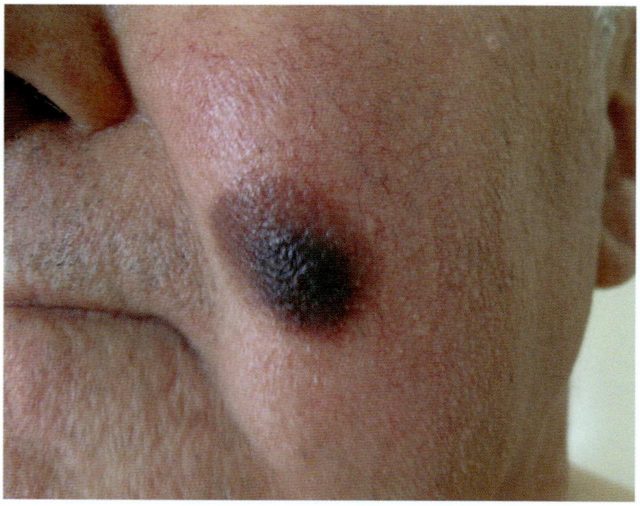

Figure 24.5 Blastic plasmacytoid dendritic cell neoplasm. Early lesion resembling localized hemorrhage. *(Courtesy of Dr. Carlo Cota, Rome, Italy.)*

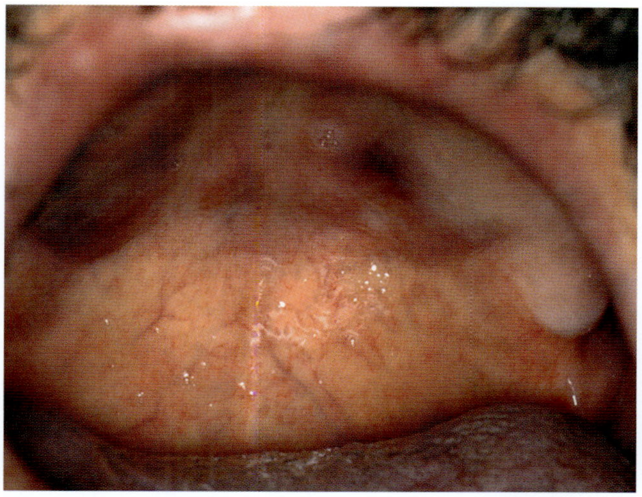

Figure 24.6 Blastic plasmacytoid dendritic cell neoplasm. Involvement of the oral mucosa with violaceous, infiltrated lesions on the hard palate.

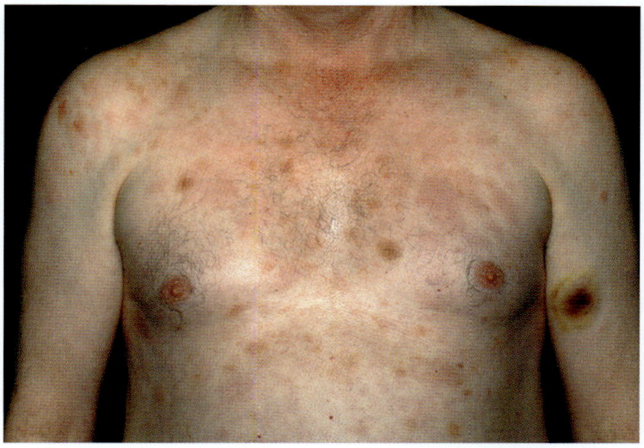

Figure 24.7 Blastic plasmacytoid dendritic cell neoplasm. Diffuse cutaneous involvement with only patches and ecchymotic lesions. *(Courtesy of Dr. Luis Requena, Madrid, Spain.)*

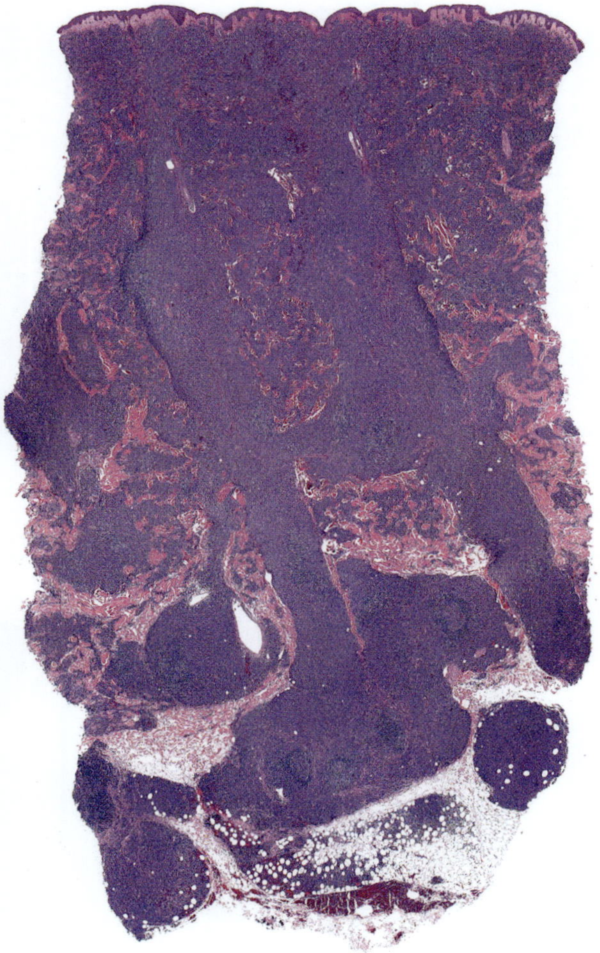

Figure 24.8 Blastic plasmacytoid dendritic cell neoplasm. Dense diffuse infiltrate involving the entire dermis and subcutaneous fat.

and leukemic spread is variable, usually between a few weeks and several months. Only rarely the disease remains confined to the skin for longer than one year (the longest period that I have observed between first cutaneous symptoms and extracutaneous involvement was 2 years).

## Histopathology, immunophenotype, and molecular genetics

### Histopathology

Histologically, blastic plasmacytoid dendritic cell neoplasm is characterized by a diffuse, monomorphous infiltrate of medium-sized neoplastic cells with a blastoid morphology (Figs. 24.8 and 24.9). The epidermis is not involved as a rule, whereas the involvement of the subcutaneous tissues is

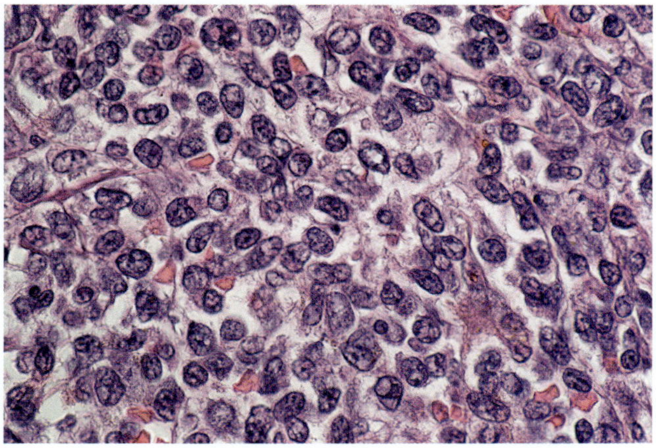

Figure 24.9 Blastic plasmacytoid dendritic cell neoplasm. Monomorphic proliferation of medium-sized blastoid cells.

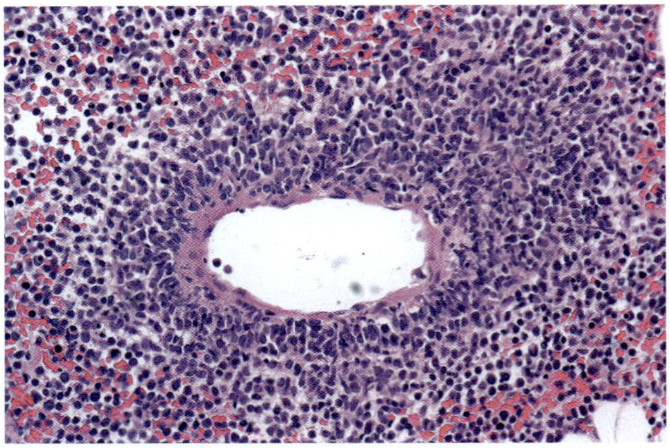

Figure 24.10 Blastic plasmacytoid dendritic cell neoplasm. Angiocentric/angiotropic infiltrate of blastoid cells.

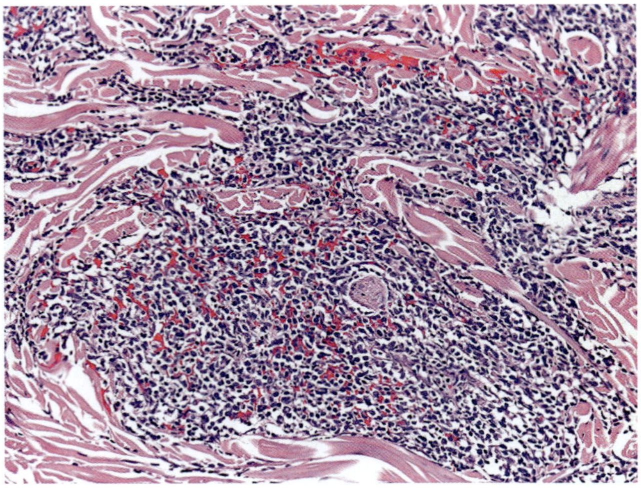

Figure 24.12 Blastic plasmacytoid dendritic cell neoplasm. Neoplastic cells admixed with many erythrocytes.

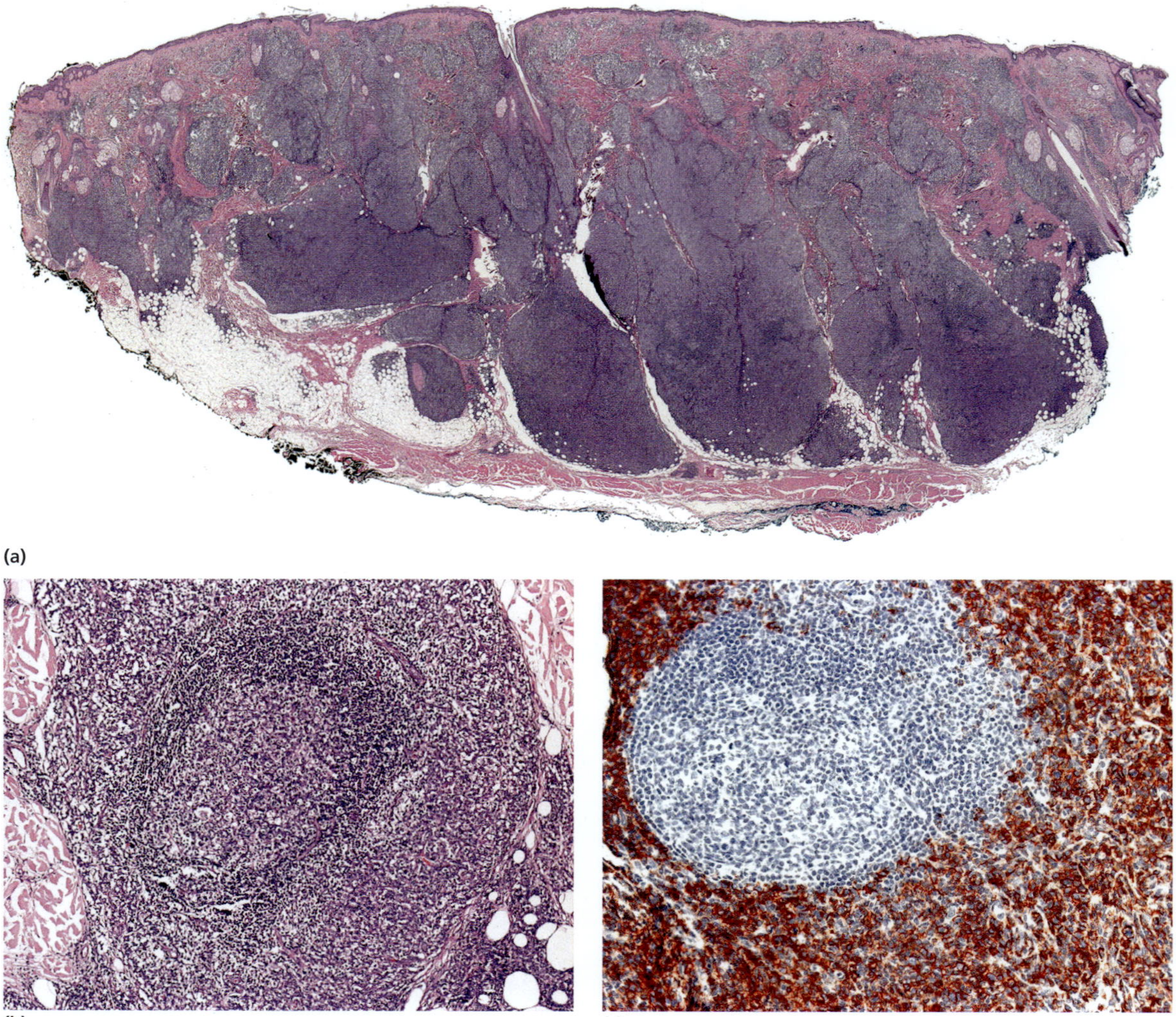

(a)

(b)

(c)

Figure 24.11 Blastic plasmacytoid dendritic cell neoplasm. (a) Nodular infiltrates within the dermis and subcutis; (b) reactive germinal centers surrounded by the neoplastic population of blastoid cells; and (c) CD56+ neoplastic cells surrounding a negative area representing a reactive germinal center.

common. Angiocentricity and/or angiodestruction, necrosis, and granulomatous reactions can be found but are uncommon (Fig. 24.10). An inflammatory infiltrate with reactive germinal centers can be observed in a minority of cases (Fig. 24.11). Intratumoral hemorrhage is common and may be prominent, and is the histological counterpart of the bruise-like presentation observed clinically (Fig. 24.12). In leukemic cases, neoplastic cells may be observed within areas of surgery-related hemorrhage (Fig. 24.13), similar to what can be seen in acute myeloid leukemia.

In early lesions there are perivascular infiltrates of blastoid cells, sometimes admixed with reactive lymphocytes (Fig. 24.14). The overall pattern may resemble that of lymphocytic infiltration (Jessner-Kanof)/lupus tumidus. As clusters of $CD123^+$ plasmacytoid dendritic cells are almost always found in lupus tumidus, care should be taken not to misdiagnose these cases for an inflammatory disorder. Complete phenotypic analyses allow an easy distinction between the two entities. These cases should also be distinguished from mature plasmacytoid dendritic cell proliferation associated with myeloid neoplasms (see Chapter 23).

Although blastic plasmacytoid dendritic cell neoplasm is considered as a rather monomorphous neoplasm, I have observed in several cutaneous cases peculiar morphologic features characterized by a pleomorphism of the neoplastic cells, which showed elongated and/or twisted nuclei resembling large centrocytes in the spindle cell variant of follicle center lymphoma (Fig. 24.15). Since Bcl-6 and multiple myeloma

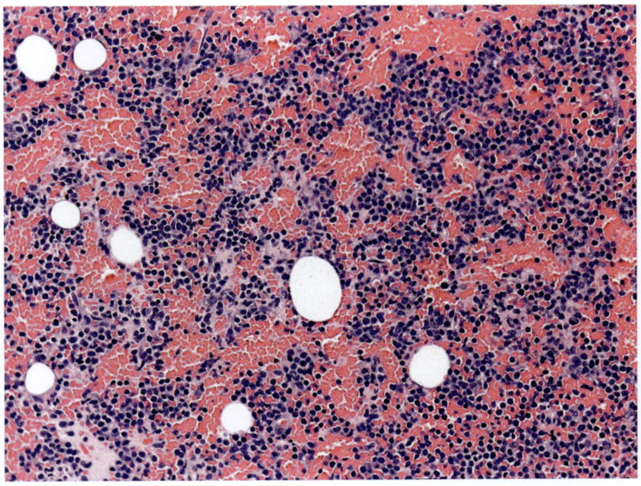

**Figure 24.13** Leukemic blastic plasmacytoid dendritic cell neoplasm. Neoplastic cells within the surgical-related hemorrhage of a skin biopsy.

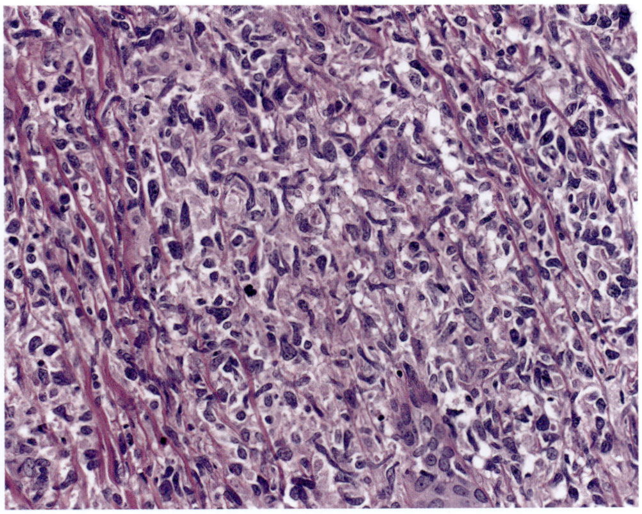

**Figure 24.15** Blastic plasmacytoid dendritic cell neoplasm. The neoplastic cells in this case reveal partly a conventional blastoid morphology and partly elongated, twisted, pleomorphic nuclei resembling large centrocytes.

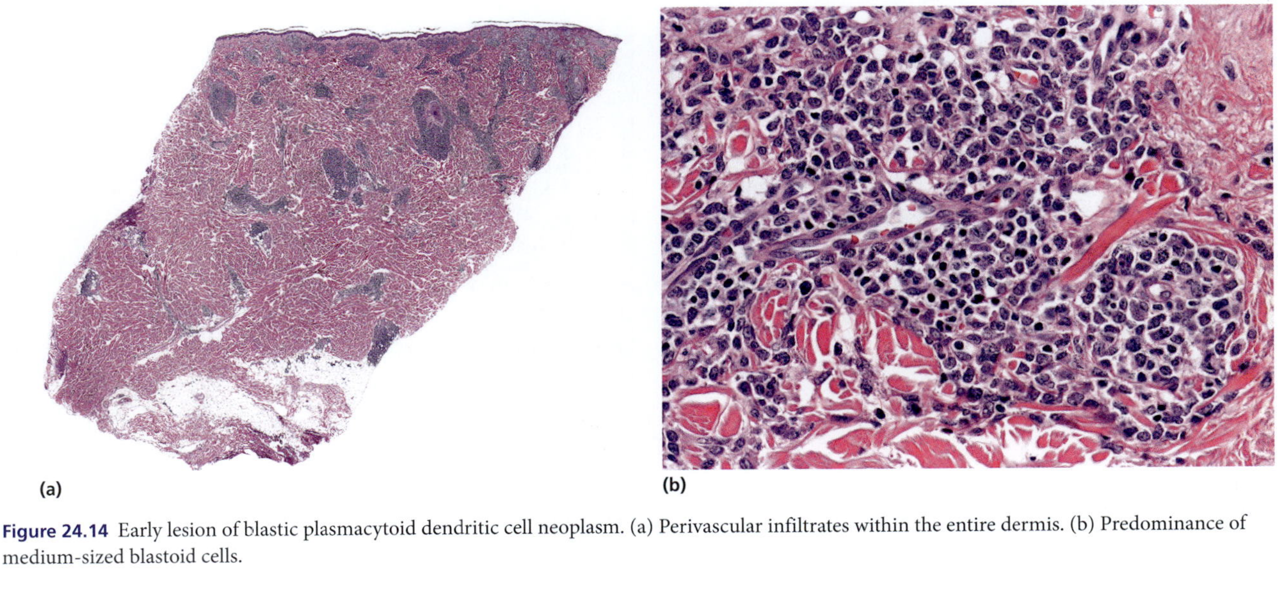

**Figure 24.14** Early lesion of blastic plasmacytoid dendritic cell neoplasm. (a) Perivascular infiltrates within the entire dermis. (b) Predominance of medium-sized blastoid cells.

oncogene 1 (MUM-1) may be positive in a proportion of cells in blastic plasmacytoid dendritic cell neoplasm, and as reactive germinal centers may be present as well (see Fig. 24.11), these morphologic features may be the source of a diagnostic pitfall.

## Immunophenotype

Blastic dendritic cell neoplasm is characterized by a recognizable phenotype. Cutaneous cases seem to be more homogeneous than noncutaneous ones [31]. Neoplastic cells express CD4, CD56, and CD123 (Figs. 24.16 and 24.17). TdT is positive in a proportion of the cells in a subset of cases (varying between one-third and two-third in different reports) (Fig. 24.18), whereas myeloid antigens, NK-cell markers, and cytotoxic proteins are negative [32, 33]. Expression of CD123 underlines the relationship with plasmacytoid dendritic cells [34]. Cases negative for CD4 have been recorded [35–37] and CD56 can be negative as well [35–39]. In addition, CD56 may be variably expressed in different lesions from a single case [40]. As CD123 may also be negative in some cases [35], the three markers most widely used for diagnosis of this rare entity should always be used together and in conjunction with a broad panel of antibodies directed toward lymphoid and myeloid antigens, keeping in mind that only integration of all stainings can allow a precise diagnosis. Myeloperoxidase, lysozyme, and the myeloid cell nuclear differentiation antigen (MNDA) are positive in myeloid leukemia and related neoplasms and negative in blastic plasmacytoid dendritic cell neoplasm, representing further immunohistochemical staining helpful for the differential diagnosis [41, 42]. In this context, it should be remembered that myeloid leukemia is also positive for CD4 and may be positive for CD56 and CD123 as well. In the differential diagnosis between skin manifestations of blastic plasmacytoid dendritic cell neoplasm from those of myeloid leukemia, these three antibodies should be used together with T-cell leukemia/lymphoma (TCL)-1, blood dendritic cell antigen 2 (BDCA-2, CD303), and CD304, which are positive in blastic plasmacytoid dendritic cell neoplasm but usually negative in myelogenous leukemia (Figs. 24.19 and 24.20) [43]. TCL-1 is a marker related to the

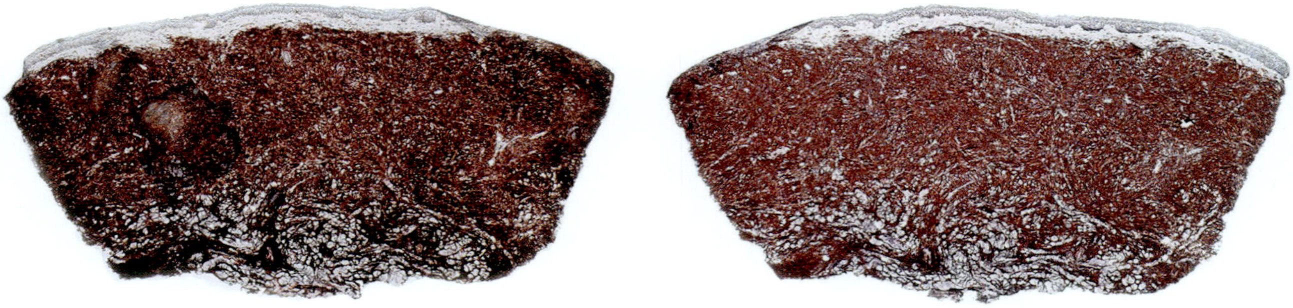

(a) (b)

**Figure 24.16** Blastic plasmacytoid dendritic cell neoplasm. Positivity for (a) CD56 and (b) CD4.

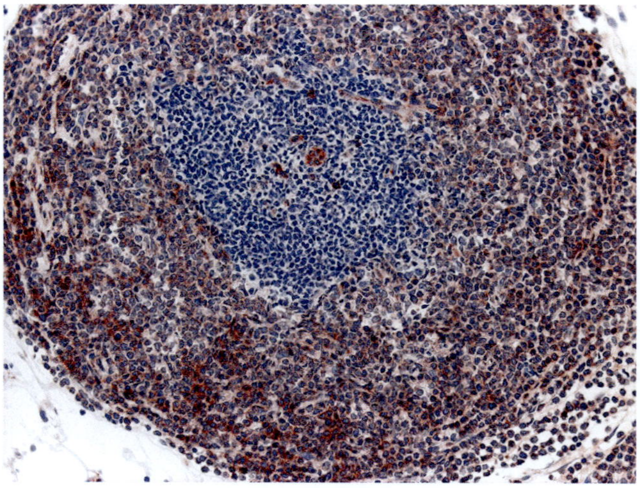

**Figure 24.17** Blastic plasmacytoid dendritic cell neoplasm. Positivity of neoplastic cells for CD123 (periphery of nodule). Negative cells in the center of the nodule represent reactive lymphocytes.

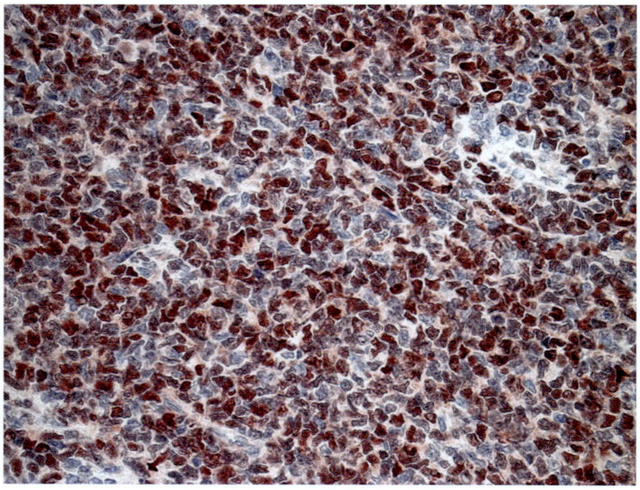

**Figure 24.18** Blastic plasmacytoid dendritic cell neoplasm. Positivity for TdT.

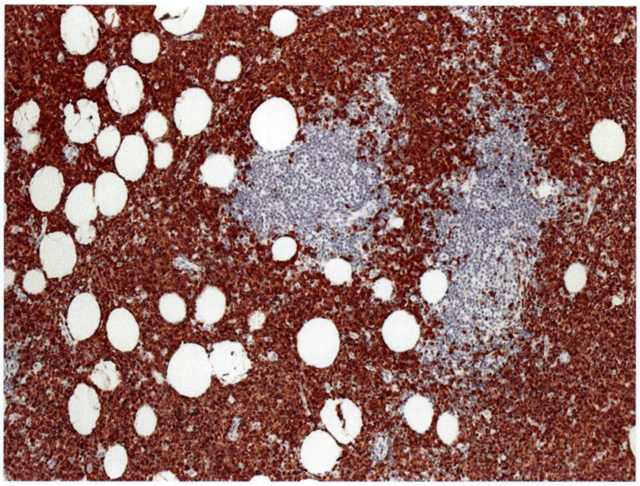

**Figure 24.19** Blastic plasmacytoid dendritic cell neoplasm with strong positivity for TCL-1. Negative areas represent reactive B lymphocytes.

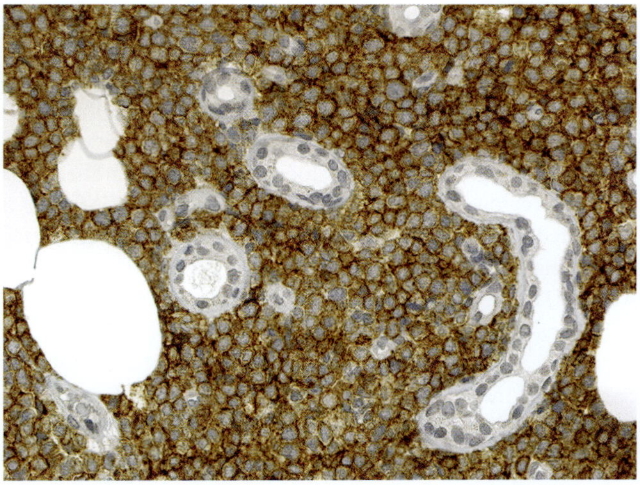

**Figure 24.20** Blastic plasmacytoid dendritic cell neoplasm. Positivity of neoplastic cells for CD303.

proto-oncogene *TCL1*, which was demonstrated in the majority of blastic plasmacytoid dendritic cell neoplasms as well as in nodal plasmacytoid dendritic cells [34, 44]. The TCF4 (E2–2) transcription factor, essential for the development of plasmacytoid dendritic cells, has been reported as a further, reliable diagnostic marker [45], and dual expression of TCF4 and CD123 has been found highly sensitive and specific for blastic plasmacytoid dendritic cell neoplasm [46]. The proliferation rate as detected by Ki-67 is variable, ranging from 20% to 30% to cases with positivity in >80% of the cells.

All phenotypic markers should be evaluated in context: CD123 can be expressed in B-cell and T-cell acute lymphoblastic leukemia as well as in acute myeloid leukemia; CD304 can be expressed in B-cell acute lymphoblastic leukemia; TCL-1 is expressed in mature lymphoid malignancies, in B-cell acute lymphoblastic leukemia and in some cases of acute myeloid leukemia; CD303 is specific, but can be lost in approximately 30% of cases of blastic plasmacytoid dendritic cell neoplasm. In short, the phenotypic evaluation must be done with a broad panel of antibodies, and results must be interpreted within the proper clinicopathologic context, keeping in mind that negative stainings (e.g. myeloperoxidase, lysozyme, CD3, CD19) are as important as positive ones.

Other markers expressed in blastic plasmacytoid dendritic cell neoplasm are Bcl-2, CD43, CD45RA, CD36, CD304, BCL11a, SPIB (a transcription factor of the E26 transformation-specific family that is expressed in mature B cells, T-cell progenitors, and plasmacytoid dendritic cells) and HLA-DR [47–50]. Neoplastic cells in a proportion of cases may be positive for any among several other antigens including CD2, CD5, CD7, CD10, CD13, CD38, CD79a, CD117, and CD2AP [51, 52]. Focal positivity for Bcl-6 and MUM-1 may also be observed, and may be misleading if not evaluated in the proper context. Granzyme B, a marker positive on normal plasmacytoid dendritic cells, is negative on blastic plasmacytoid dendritic cell neoplasm.

Cases positive for CD68 have been reported (Fig. 24.21a), but in my experience, CD68 is usually negative or positive in some cases with a single paranuclear dot (Fig. 24.21b) [7, 17, 31–33]. S100 is positive in a minority of cases, but more frequently in pediatric ones [52].

The pattern of expression of nucleophosmin, an estrogen-regulated nucleolar protein that is expressed in a mutated form in the cytoplasm in one-third of the cases of adult de novo acute myeloid leukemia, differs between blastic plasmacytoid dendritic cell neoplasms (nuclear pattern) and myelogenous leukemia (cytoplasmic pattern) [53].

## Molecular genetics

Molecular genetic studies reveal that the T-cell receptor (TCR) and immunoglobulin (Ig) genes are in germline configuration, but exceptional cases with TCR gene rearrangement have been observed [54, 55]. Thus, although for practical purposes a monoclonal rearrangement of the TCR and/or Ig genes rules out the diagnosis of blastic plasmacytoid dendritic cell neoplasm, care should be taken in the interpretation of molecular results. One potential pitfall may be represented by the presence of small oligoclonal populations of reactive T and B lymphocytes within the infiltrate.

Complex karyotypes and chromosomal abnormalities involving chromosomes 5q, 6q, 12p, 13q, 15q, and 9 have been observed in blastic plasmacytoid dendritic cell neoplasm [5]. Gain of chromosomes 7q and 22 and loss of chromosomes 3p and 13q were demonstrated by comparative genome hybridization in one study [56], while recurrent deletion of regions on chromosome 4 (4q34), chromosome 9 (9p13–p11 and 9q12–q34), and chromosome 13 (13q12–q31) was found in another study [15], and losses of 9, 9p and 13q and gain of 7 in a third [57]. The least common denominator of these studies seems to be the presence of abnormalities involving chromosomes 9 and 13,

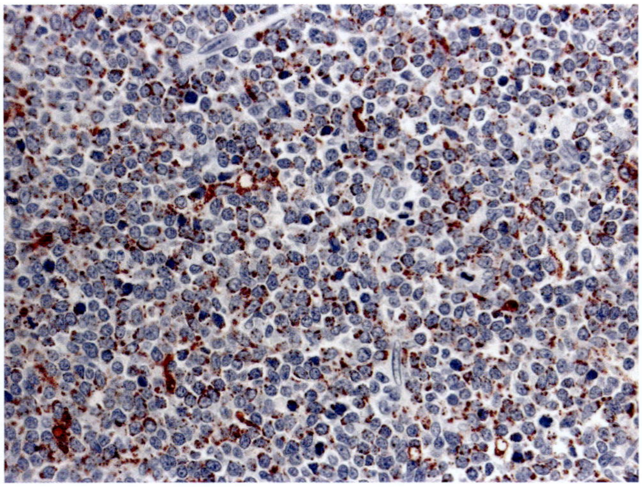

(a)

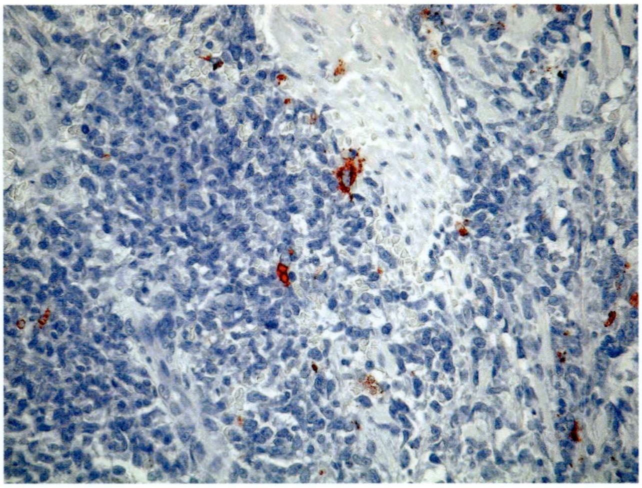

(b)

**Figure 24.21** Blastic plasmacytoid dendritic cell neoplasm. (a) This case reveals the positivity of the majority of neoplastic cells for CD68. In my experience, this pattern is the exception rather than the rule and negativity (b) is observed more frequently.

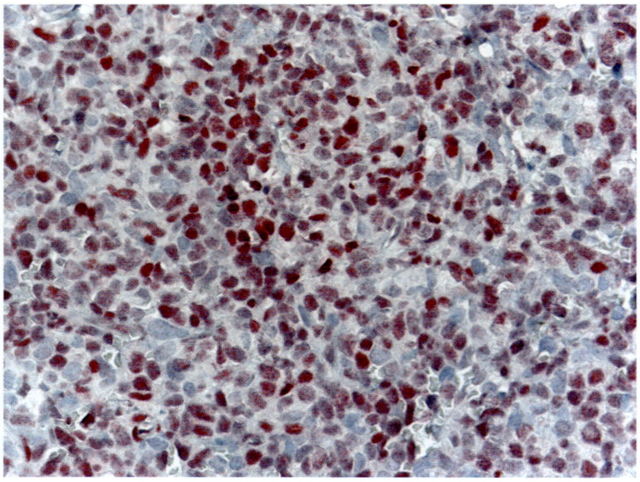

**Figure 24.22** Blastic plasmacytoid dendritic cell neoplasm. Positivity of neoplastic cells for p27.

confirmed by subsequent studies showing aberrations located at the 9p21.3 (*CDKN2A/CDKN2B*), 13q13.1-q14.3 (*RB1*), 12p13.2-p13.1 (*CDKN1B*), 13q11-q12 (*LATS2*), and 7p12.2 (*IKZF1*) regions [58–60]. 8q24/MYC rearrangement represents a recurrent cytogenetic abnormality [61], and genomic aberrations involving 12p/ETV6 may represent early clonal events [62]. The dose-dependent haploinsufficient cell-cycle inhibitor p27KIP1, encoded by *CDKN1B*, is weakly expressed in the nuclei of tumor cells in most cases (Fig. 24.22), and the cell-cycle inhibitor p16INK4a, which is encoded by *CDKN2A*, was not expressed in tumor cells, suggesting a complete loss of function. [59]. These results imply that alterations of the cell-cycle checkpoint controlling proteins p27KIP1, p16INK4a, and RB1 may exert a crucial effect in malignant transformation in blastic plasmacytoid dendritic cell neoplasms. Aberrant activation of the NF-kb pathway was demonstrated in a large study, suggesting that it may represent a therapeutic target [8]. A translocation t(6,8)(p21;q24) involving the *MYC* locus has been identified as a recurrent cytogenetic abnormality [63]. The translocation is associated with MYC expression by neoplastic cells [64]. Mutations in epigenetic modifiers (including among others *ASXL1, TET2, ZRSR2, SUZ12, ARID1A, PHF2,* and *CHD8,* with mutations in *ASXL1* being the most frequent dysregulation) may be used as a potential therapeutic target [65]. In this context, the presence of inactivating mutations in *ZRSR2* on chromosome Xp22.2, found only in male patients, may explain the male predominance of the disease [66a].

In contrast to myeloid leukemia, which in about 30% of cases is characterized by mutations of the nucleophosmin 1 (*NPM1*) gene, *NPM1* mutations are not identified in blastic plasmacytoid dendritic cell neoplasm [66b].

## Treatment

Treatment of patients with blastic plasmacytoid dendritic cell neoplasm should be carried out in a hematologic setting. Treatment with tagraxofusp, an anti-CD123 cytotoxin consisting of human interleukin-3 fused to truncated diphtheria toxin, has improved prognosis [67–70], but chemotherapy is still the first-line treatment. Anti-CD123 compounds are in general not curative, but can be used as adjuvant treatment and/or to bridge patients to stem cell transplantation. Although systemic chemotherapy is usually followed by rapid, complete primary responses, remissions are short and recurrences are the rule [71]. Good response has been observed with L-asparaginase in association with methotrexate and dexamethasone [72], and asparaginase with high-dose methotrexate is considered as a first-line treatment [73]. Bortezomib has been used with good results in some patients [74], sometimes in association with lenalidomide and dexamethasone [75]. Complete or partial response has been observed in some patients after the administration of pralatrexate and enasidenib [76].

Allogeneic stem-cell transplantation is considered as the main, potentially curative option [13, 77–81]. There seems to be a survival advantage for patients receiving total body irradiation-based myeloablative conditioning before stem cell transplantation, but this option may be unfeasible in older patients [81]. Patients presenting with primary cutaneous disorder should be treated in the same aggressive manner as those with systemic involvement.

Other treatment modalities based on the pathobiology of neoplastic cells in blastic plasmacytoid dendritic cell neoplasm include SL-401 (a recombinant protein including components of diphtheria toxin fused to interleukin-3), venetoclax (a Bcl-2 inhibitor showing activity in myeloid malignancies) [82]. Using RNAi screening, the E-box transcription factor TCF4 has been identified as a master regulator of the oncogenic program of blastic plasmacytoid dendritic cell neoplasm [45], suggesting that bromodomain and extra-terminal domain inhibitors may be used to target neoplastic cells.

Pediatric patients respond better to treatment utilizing chemotherapy regimens for high-risk acute lymphoblastic leukemia/lymphoma with central nervous system prophylaxis, and the majority of children can be cured without stem cell transplantation [27, 28]. Stem cell transplantation is recommended for children and adolescents with high-risk or refractory disease, or in patients with relapsing disease [28].

In a mouse model, the epigenetic drugs 5′-azacytidine and decitabine were able to control disease progression *in vivo* [65].

## Prognosis

Blastic plasmacytoid dendritic cell neoplasm is a very aggressive disorder and the prognosis is very poor [83]. Most patients succumb within 1 year from first diagnosis. Although presentation with solitary or localized skin lesions may be associated with a less aggressive course, at present there is no evidence that long-term survival can be achieved with conventional treatments, even for these patients. As already mentioned, allogeneic bone marrow transplantation yields better results and should be offered as a therapeutic option whenever possible [13, 77–79].

The 1-year and 5-year overall survival rates are 53%, and 20% in elderly patients (age $\geq$ 60), whereas in children and adolescents (age $\leq$ 20) are 90% and 82% [84], showing that young patients have a better prognosis [27].

TdT expression in >50% of the neoplastic cells was an independent prognostic variable associated with a better prognosis in one study [48]. Skin involvement seemed to represent an unfavorable prognostic sign both in children and adult patients in two studies [27, 85]. As already mentioned, however, cutaneous manifestations are found in the vast majority of cases, thus skin involvement is unlikely related to prognosis. Longer survival was associated with CD303 expression and high proliferative index (Ki-67) in a large study [86]. A poor outcome was observed in patients with biallelic loss of locus 9p21.3 [58].


### Résumé

**Blastic plasmacytoid dendritic cell neoplasm**

| | | |
|---|---|---|
| **Clinical** | Adults, elderly (children may be affected). Male predominance. Solitary, localized, or generalized plaques and tumors, sometimes with a "bruise-like" aspect. Ulceration uncommon. No preferential location reported. | |
| **Morphology** | Usually monomorphous infiltrate of medium-sized cells within the entire dermis and subcutis. The epidermis is spared. Cytomorphology: mid-sized blastoid cells; in skin biopsies sometimes elongated and twisted nuclei. | |
| **Immunohistochemistry** | CD4, CD56, CD123, TCL-1, CD303, CD304, TCF4, SPIB | +(−) |
| | TdT | +/− |
| | CD7, Bcl-2, MUM-1, Bcl-6 | +/− |
| | CD68 | −(+) (paranuclear dot) |
| | CD5, CD38, CD79a | −(+) |
| | CD3, CD14, CD19, CD20, Granzyme B | − |
| | Myeloperoxidase, MNDA, Lysozyme | − |
| **Genetics** | Germline configuration of the TCR and Ig genes. Complex karyotypes and chromosomal abnormalities involving chromosomes 5q, 6q, 12p, 13q, 15q, and 9. Alterations of the cell-cycle checkpoint controlling proteins p27KIP1, p16INK4a, and RB1. Inactivating mutations in *ZRSR2* on chromosome Xp22.2, found only in male patients, may explain the male predominance of the disease. | |
| **Treatment guidelines** | Systemic chemotherapy followed by allogeneic bone marrow transplantation. Anti-CD123 immunotherapies. | |

## References


1. Facchetti F, Lane AA, Lorenzi L, Pileri SA. Blastic plasmacytoid dendritic cell neoplasm. In: Arber DA, Borowitz MJ, Cook JR, *et al.*, eds. *The International Consensus Classification of Myeloid and Lymphoid Neoplasms*. Philadelphia (US): Wolters Kluver, 2025: 256–260.
2. Khoury JD, Garnache Ottou F, Gru A, *et al.* Blastic plasmacytoid dendritic cell neoplasm. In: *WHO Classification of Tumours Editorial Board. Haematolymphoid Tumours*. 5th edition. Lyon (France): IARC, 2024: 226–229.
3. Willemze R, Cerroni L, Kempf W, *et al.* The 2018 update of the WHO-EORTC classification for primary cutaneous lymphomas. *Blood* 2019;**133**:1703–1714.
4. Kempf W, Mitteldorf C, Cerroni L, *et al.* Classifications of cutaneous lymphomas and lymphoproliferative disorders: An update from the EORTC cutaneous lymphoma histopathology group. *J Eur Acad Dermatol Venereol* 2024;**38**:1491–1503.
5. Chaperot L, Bendriss N, Manches O, *et al.* Identification of a leukemic counterpart of the plasmacytoid dendritic cells. *Blood* 2001;**97**:3210–3217.
6. Leroux D, Mugneret F, Callanan M, *et al.* CD4, CD56 DC2 acute leukemia is characterized by recurrent clonal chromosomal changes affecting 6 major targets: a study of 21 cases by the Groupe Français de Cytogenetique Hematologique. *Blood* 2002;**99**:4154–4159.
7. Petrella T, Comeau MR, Maynadié M, *et al.* Agranular CD4 CD56 hematodermic neoplasm (blastic NK-cell lymphoma) originates from a population of CD56$^{+}$ precursor cells related to plasmacytoid monocytes. *Am J Surg Pathol* 2002;**26**:852–862.
8. Sapienza MR, Fuligni F, Agostinelli C, *et al.* Molecular profiling of blastic plasmacytoid dendritic cell neoplasm reveals a unique pattern and suggests selective sensitivity to NF-kB pathway inhibition. *Leukemia* 2014;**28**:1606–1616.
9. Bagot M, Bouloc A, Charue D, *et al.* Do primary cutaneous non-T non-B CD4 CD56 lymphomas belong to the myelo-monocytic lineage? *J Invest Dermatol* 1998;**111**:1242–1244.
10. Khoury JD, Medeiros LJ, Manning JT, *et al.* CD56 TdT blastic natural killer cell tumor of the skin: primitive systemic malignancy related to myelomonocytic leukemia. *Cancer* 2002;**94**:2401–2408.
11. Kazakov DV, Mentzel T, Burg G, *et al.* Blastic natural killer-cell lymphoma of the skin associated with myelodysplastic syndrome of myelogenous leukaemia: a coincidence or more? *Br J Dermatol* 2003;**149**:869–876.
12. Bekkenk MW, Jansen PM, Meijer CJLM, Willemze R. CD56+ hematological neoplasms presenting in the skin – a retrospective analysis of 23 new cases and 130 cases from the literature. *Ann Oncol* 2004;**15**:1097–1108.
13. Assaf C, Gellrich S, Whittaker S, *et al.* CD56-positive haematological neoplasms of the skin: a multicentre study of the Cutaneous Lymphoma Project Group of the European Organisation for Research and Treatment of Cancer. *J Clin Pathol* 2007;**60**:981–989.
14. Khanlari M, Yin CC, Takahashi K, *et al.* Bone marrow clonal hematopoiesis is highly prevalent in blastic plasmacytoid dendritic cell neoplasm and frequently sharing a clonal origin in elderly patients. *Leukemia* 2022;**36**:1343–1350.
15. Dijkman R, van Doom R, Szuhai K, *et al.* Gene-expression profiling and array-based CGH classify CD4/CD56 hematodermic neoplasm and cutaneous myelomonocytic leukemia as distinct disease entities. *Blood* 2007;**109**:1720–1727.
16. Bower CP, Standen GR, Pawade J, *et al.* Cutaneous presentation of steroid responsive blastoid natural killer cell lymphoma. *Br J Dermatol* 2000;**142**:1017–1020.
17. Massone C, Chott A, Metze D, *et al.* Subcutaneous, blastic natural killer (NK) NK/T-cell and other cytotoxic lymphomas of the skin: a morphologic, immunophenotypic and molecular study of 50 patients. *Am J Surg Pathol* 2004;**28**:719–735.
18. Nagatani T, Okazawa H, Kambara T, *et al.* Cutaneous monomorphous CD4- and CD56-positive large-cell lymphoma. *Dermatology* 2000;**200**:202–208.
19. Child FJ, Mitschell TJ, Whittaker SJ, *et al.* Blastic natural killer cell and extranodal natural killer cell-like T-cell lymphoma presenting in the skin: report of six cases from the UK. *Br J Dermatol* 2003;**148**:507–515.
20. Husak R, Blume-Peytaki U, Orfanos CE. Aleukemic leukemia cutis in an adolescent boy. *N Engl J Med* 1999;**340**:893–894.
21. Wollenberg A, Wagner M, Gunther S, *et al.* Plasmacytoid dendritic cells: a new cutaneous dendritic cell subset with distinct role in inflammatory skin diseases. *J Invest Dermatol* 2002;**119**:1096–1102.
22. Miedema J, Starr SR, Chan MP. Incidental diagnosis of blastic plasmacytoid dendritic cell neoplasm in skin excision for basal cell carcinoma. *J Cutan Pathol* 2018;**45**:873–875.
23. Julia F, Petrella T, Beylot-Barry M, *et al.* Blastic plasmacytoid dendritic cell neoplasm: clinical features in 90 patients. *Br J Dermatol* 2013;**169**:579–586.
24. Chang SE, Choi HJ, Huh J, *et al.* A case of primary cutaneous CD56, TdT, CD4, blastic NK-cell lymphoma in a 19-year-old woman. *Am J Dermatopathol* 2002;**24**:72–75.
25. Fass J, Tichy EH, Kraus EW, *et al.* Cutaneous tumors as the initial presentation of non-T, non-B, nonmyeloid CD4+ CD56+ hematolymphoid malignancy in an adolescent boy. *Ped Dermatol* 2005;**22**:19–22.
26. Hu SCS, Tsai KB, Chen GS, Chen PH. Infantile CD4+/CD56+ hematodermic neoplasm. *Haematologica* 2007;**92**:91–93.
27. Jegalian AG, Buxbaum NP, Facchetti F, *et al.* Blastic plasmacytoid dendritic cell neoplasm in children: diagnostic features and clinical implications. *Haematologica* 2010;**95**:1873–1879.
28. Cuglievan B, Connors J, He J, *et al.* Blastic plasmacytoid dendritic cell neoplasm: a comprehensive review in pediatrics, adolescents, and young adults (AYA) and an update of novel therapies. *Leukemia* 2023;**37**:1767–1778.
29. Li J, Wang J, Rong L, *et al.* A neonatal case of congenital blastic plasmacytoid dendritic cell neoplasm with KMT2C gene duplication. *Ann Hematol* 2023;**102**:227–229.
30. Chan G, Akintorin S, Luu M, Harter N. Blastic plasmacytoid dendritic cell neoplasm with cutaneous presentation: a case series in children. *Ped Dermatol* 2021;**38**:883–886.
31. Suzuki Y, Kato S, Kohno K, *et al.* Clinicopathological analysis of 46 cases with CD4+ and/or CD56+ immature haematolymphoid malignancy: reappraisal of blastic plasmacytoid dendritic cell and related neoplasms. *Histopathology* 2017;**71**:972–984.
32. Ko YH, Kim SH, Ree HJ. Blastic NK-cell lymphoma expressing terminal deoxynucleotidyl transferase with Homer–Wright type pseudorosettes formation. *Histopathology* 1998;**33**:547–553.
33. Nakamura S, Koshikawa T, Yatabe Y, Suchi T. Lymphoblastic lymphoma expressing CD56 and TdT. *Am J Surg Pathol* 1998;**22**:135–137.
34. Herling M, Teitell MA, Shen RR, *et al.* TCL1 expression in plasmacytoid dendritic cells (DC2s) and the related CD4 CD56 blastic tumors of skin. *Blood* 2003;**101**:5007–5009.

35. Cota C, Vale E, Viana I, *et al.* Cutaneous manifestations of blastic plasmacytoid dendritic cell neoplasm – morphologic and phenotypic variability in a series of 33 patients. *Am J Surg Pathol* 2010;**34**:75–87.
36. Argyrakos T, Rontogianni D, Karmiris T, *et al.* Blastic natural killer (NK)-cell lymphoma: report of an unusual CD4 negative case and review of the CD4 negative neoplasms with blastic features in the literature. *Leukem Lymph* 2004;**45**:2127–2133.
37. Ascani S, Massone C, Ferrara G, *et al.* CD4-negative variant of CD4+/CD56 hematodermic neoplasm: description of three cases. *J Cutan Pathol* 2008;**35**:911–915.
38. Petrella T, Teitell MA, Spiekermann C, *et al.* A CD56-negative case of blastic natural killer-cell lymphoma (agranular CD4/CD56 haematodermic neoplasm). *Br J Dermatol* 2004;**150**:174–176.
39. Marafioti T, Paterson JC, Ballabio E, *et al.* Novel markers of normal and neoplastic human plasmacytoid dendritic cells. *Blood* 2008;**111**:3778–3792.
40. Lopez AT, Shaw KS, Yamany T, *et al.* Immunophenotypic CD56 variation within a single patient with blastic plasmacytoid dendritic cell neoplasm. *JAMA Dermatol* 2018;**154**:492–494.
41. Johnson RC, Kim J, Natkunam Y, *et al.* Myeloid cell nuclear differentiation antigen (MNDA) expression distinguishes extramedullary presentations of myeloid leukemia from blastic plasmacytoid dendritic cell neoplasm. *Am J Surg Pathol* 2016;**40**:502–509.
42. Sangle NA, Schmidt RL, Patel JL, *et al.* Optimized immunohistochemical panel to differentiate myeloid sarcoma from blastic plasmacytoid dendritic cell neoplasm. *Mod Pathol* 2014;**27**:1137–1143.
43. Deconinck E, Petrella T, Garnache OF. Blastic plasmacytoid dendritic cell neoplasm: clinical presentation and diagnosis. *Hematol Oncol Clin North Am* 2020;**34**:491–500.
44. Petrella T, Meijer CJLM, Dalac S, *et al.* TCL1 and CLA expression in agranular CD4/CD56 hematodermic neoplasms (blastic NK-cell lymphomas) and leukemia cutis. *Am J Clin Pathol* 2004;**122**:307–313.
45. Ceribelli M, Hou ZE, Kelly PN, *et al.* A druggable TCF4- and BRD4-dependent transcriptional network sustains malignancy in blastic plasmacytoid dendritic cell neoplasm. *Cancer Cell* 2016;**30**:764–778.
46. Sukswai N, Aung PP, Yin CC, *et al.* Dual expression of TCF4 and CD123 is highly sensitive and specific for blastic plasmacytoid dendritic cell neoplasm. *Am J Surg Pathol* 2019;**43**:1429–1437.
47. Santucci M, Pimpinelli N, Massi D, *et al.* Cytotoxic natural killer cell cutaneous lymphomas: report of the EORTC cutaneous lymphoma task force workshop. *Cancer* 2003;**97**:610–627.
48. Meyer N, Petrella T, Poszepczynska-Guigne E, *et al.* CD4+ CD56+ blastic tumor cells express CD101 molecules. *J Invest Dermatol* 2005;**124**:668–669.
49. Jaye DL, Geigerman CM, Herling M, *et al.* Expression of the plasmacytoid dendritic cell marker BDCA-2 supports a spectrum of maturation among CD4+ CD56+ hematodermic neoplasms. *Mod Pathol* 2006;**19**:1555–1562.
50. Pilichowska ME, Fleming MD, Pinkus JL, Pinkus GS. CD4+/CD56+ hematodermic neoplasm ("blastic natural killer cell lymphoma"). Neoplastic cells express the immature dendritic cell marker BDCA-2 and produce interferon. *Am J Clin Pathol* 2007;**128**:445–453.
51. Facchetti F, Cigognetti M, Fisogni S, *et al.* Neoplasms derived from plasmacytoid dendritic cells. *Mod Pathol* 2016;**29**:98–111.
52. Sapienza MR, Pileri A, Derenzini E, et al. Blastic plasmacytoid dendritic cell neoplasm: state of the art and prospects. *Cancers (Basel).* 2019;11, pii: E595.
53. Facchetti F, Pileri SA, Agostinelli C, *et al.* Cytoplasmic nucleophosmin is not detected in blastic plasmacytoid dendritic cell neoplasm. *Haematologica* 2009;**94**:285–288.
54. Stetsenko GY, McFarlane R, Kalus A, *et al.* CD4+/CD56+ hematodermic neoplasm: report of a rare variant with a T-cell receptor gene rearrangement. *J Cutan Pathol* 2008;**35**:579–584.
55. Liu XY, Atkins RC, Feusner JH, Rowland JM. Blastic NK-cell-like lymphoma with T-cell receptor gene rearrangement. *Am J Hematol* 2004;**75**:251–253.
56. Hallermann C, Middel P, Griesinger F, *et al.* CD4+ CD56+ blastic tumor of the skin: cytogenetic observations and further evidence of an origin from plasmacytoid dendritic cells. *Eur J Dermatol* 2004;**14**:317–322.
57. Mao X, Onadim Z, Price EA, *et al.* Genomic alterations in blastic natural killer/extranodal natural killer-like T cell lymphoma with cutaneous involvement. *J Invest Dermatol* 2003;**121**:618–627.
58. Lucioni M, Novara F, Fiandrino G, *et al.* Twenty-one cases of blastic plasmacytoid dendritic cell neoplasm: focus on biallelic locus 9p21.3 deletion. *Blood* 2011;**118**:4591–4594.
59. Wiesner T, Obenauf AC, Cota C, *et al.* Alterations of the cell-cycle inhibitors p27KIP1 and p16INK4a are frequent in blastic plasmacytoid dendritic cell neoplasms. *J Invest Dermatol* 2010; **130**:1152–1157.
60. Jardin F, Callanan M, Penther D, *et al.* Recurrent genomic aberrations combined with deletions of various tumour suppressor genes may deregulate the G1/S transition in CD4+CD56+ haematodermic neoplasms and contribute to the aggressiveness of the disease. *Leukemia* 2009;**23**:698–707.
61. Boddu PC, Wang SA, Pemmaraju N, *et al.* 8q24/MYC rearrangement is a recurrent cytogenetic abnormality in blastic plasmacytoid dendritic cell neoplasms. *Leuk Res* 2018;**66**:73–78.
62. Tang Z, Li Y, Wang W, *et al.* Genomic aberrations involving 12p/ETV6 are highly prevalent in blastic plasmacytoid dendritic cell neoplasms and might represent early clonal events. *Leuk Res* 2018;**73**:86–94.
63. Sumarriva Lezama L, Chisholm KM, Carneal E, *et al.* An analysis of blastic plasmacytoid dendritic cell neoplasm with translocations involving the MYC locus identifies t(6,8)(p21;q24) as a recurrent cytogenetic abnormality. *Histopathology* 2018;**73**:767–776.
64. Sakamoto K, Katayama R, Asaka R, *et al.* Recurrent 8q24 rearrangement in blastic plasmacytoid dendritic cell neoplasm: association with immunoblastoid cytomorphology, MYC expression, and drug response. *Leukemia* 2018;**32**:2590–2603.
65. Sapienza MR, Abate F, Melle F, *et al.* Blastic plasmacytoid dendritic cell neoplasm: genomics mark epigenetic dysregulation as a primary therapeutic target. *Haematologica* 2019;**104**:729–737.
66. (a) Togami K, Sook Chung S, Madan V, *et al.* Sex-Biased *ZRSR2* mutations in myeloid malignancies impair plasmacytoid dendritic cell activation and apoptosis. *Cancer Discov* 2022;**12**:522–541.(b) Hamdan H, Siddon A, Ramia de Cap M, *et al.* NPM1 mutation frequency and protein in cutaneous blastic plasmacytoid dendritic cell neoplasms. *Hum Pathol* 2025:105766. doi: 10.1016/j.humpath.2025.105766.
67. Pemmaraju N, Lane AA, Sweet KL, *et al.* Tagraxofusp in blastic plasmacytoid dendritic-cell neoplasm. *N Engl J Med* 2019; **380**:1628–1637.
68. Economides MP, McCue D, Lane AA, Pemmaraju N. Tagraxofusp, the first CD123-targeted therapy and first targeted treatment for blastic plasmacytoid dendritic cell neoplasm. *Expert Rev Clin Pharmacol* 2019;**12**:941–946.

69. Pemmaraju N, Lane AA, Sweet KL, *et al.* Tagraxofusp in blastic plasmacytoid dendritic-cell neoplasm. *N Engl J Med* 2019;**380**:1628–1637.
70. Pemmaraju N, Kantarjian H, Sweet K, *et al.* North American blastic plasmacytoid dendritic cell neoplasm consortium: position on standards of care and areas of need. *Blood* 2023;**141**:567–578.
71. DiGiuseppe JA, Louie DC, Williams JE, *et al.* Blastic natural killer cell leukemia-lymphoma: a clinicopathologic study. *Am J Surg Pathol* 1997;**21**:1223–1230.
72. Gruson B, Vaida I, Merlusca L, *et al.* L-asparaginase with methotrexate and dexamethasone is an effective treatment combination in blastic plasmacytoid dendritic cell neoplasm. *Br J Haematol* 2013;**163**:543–545.
73. Garnache-Ottou F, Vidal C, Büchlé S, *et al.* How should we diagnose and treat blastic plasmacytoid dendritic cell neoplasm patients? *Blood Adv* 2019;**3**:4238–4251.
74. Philippe L, Ceroi A, Bôle-Richard E, *et al.* Bortezomib as a new therapeutic approach for blastic plasmacytoid dendritic cell neoplasm. *Haematologica* 2017;**102**:1861–1868.
75. Marmouset V, Joris M, Merlusca L, *et al.* The lenalidomide/bortezomib/dexamethasone regimen for the treatment of blastic plasmacytoid dendritic cell neoplasm. *Hematol Oncol* 2019;**37**:487–489.
76. Taylor J, Haddadin M, Upadhyay VA, *et al.* Multicenter analysis of outcomes in blastic plasmacytoid dendritic cell neoplasm offers a pre-targeted therapy benchmark. *Blood* 2019;**134**:678–687.
77. Hyakuna N, Toguchi S, Higa T, *et al.* Childhood blastic NK cell leukemia successfully treated with L-asparaginase and allogeneic bone marrow transplantation. *Pediatr Blood Cancer* 2004;**42**:631–634.
78. Dalle S, Beylot-Barry M, Bagot M, *et al.* Blastic plasmacytoid dendritic cell neoplasm: is transplantation the treatment of choice? *Br J Dermatol* 2010;**162**:74–79.
79. Unteregger M, Valentin A, Zinke-Cerwenka W, *et al.* Unrelated SCT induces long-term remission in patients with blastic plasmacytoid dendritic cell neoplasm. *Bone Marrow Transplant* 2013; **48**:799–802.
80. Heinicke T, Hütten H, Kalinski T, *et al.* Sustained remission of blastic plasmacytoid dendritic cell neoplasm after unrelated allogeneic stem cell transplantation--a single center experience. *Ann Hematol* 2015;**94**:283–287.
81. Kharfan-Dabaja MA, Lane AA, Pemmaraju N. How I treat blastic plasmacytoid dendritic cell neoplasm. *Blood* 2025;**145**:567–576.
82. Frankel AE, Woo JH, Ahn C, *et al.* Activity of SL-401, a targeted therapy directed to interleukin-3 receptor, in blastic plasmacytoid dendritic cell neoplasm patients. *Blood* 2014; **124**:385–392.
83. Fink-Puches R, Zenahlik P, Bäck B, *et al.* Primary cutaneous lymphomas: applicability of current classification schemes (European Organization for Research and Treatment of Cancer, World Health Organization) based on clinicopathologic features observed in a large group of patients. *Blood* 2002;**99**:800–805.
84. Lin X, Wang L, Hu Q, *et al.* Incidence, prognostic factors, and survival outcomes in patients with blastic plasmacytoid dendritic cell neoplasm: a retrospective study in the surveillance, epidemiology, and end results database. *Eur J Haematol* 2023;**110**:743–753.
85. Suzuki R, Nakamura S, Suzumiya J, *et al.* Blastic natural killer cell lymphoma/leukemia (CD56-positive) blastic tumor. Prognostication and categorization according to anatomic sites of involvement. *Cancer* 2005;**104**:1022–1031.
86. Julia F, Dalle S, Duru G, *et al.* Blastic plasmacytoid dendritic cell neoplasms. Clinico-immunohistochemical correlations in a series of 91 patients. *Am J Surg Pathol* 2014;**38**:673–680.

**CHAPTER 25**

# Cutaneous manifestations of other leukemias

Besides B-cell chronic lymphocytic leukemia (B-CLL) and myelogenous leukemias, the skin may be the site of specific manifestations in other types of leukemia. In most cases, the leukemia is already known and cutaneous lesions are not biopsied, as the diagnosis is already established. There are no exact data on the frequency of skin involvement by different types of leukemia, but B-CLL and myelogenous leukemia (covered in Chapters 22 and 23, respectively) represent by far the most frequent types.

Most cases of skin involvement by different types of leukemia present with papules, plaques, and nodules that retain, at least in part, the histopathologic and phenotypic features of the original disease [1]. Some leukemias described in the following paragraphs present with peculiar manifestations that pose problems in the differential diagnosis and are worth a brief description.

Interestingly, similar to what may be observed in B-CLL and myelogenous leukemias, in other types of leukemia, too, specific skin manifestations have been observed at sites of cutaneous inflammation, suggesting that this mechanism of skin infiltration is common to several types of leukemia, irrespective of the specific classification [2]. In this context, I have observed patients with Sézary syndrome or with late leukemic manifestations of mycosis fungoides who developed specific skin manifestations at the site of drug eruptions, conceptually similar to leukemic infiltrates at sites of skin inflammation. It seems likely that circulating leukemic cells are still at least partly capable of responding to chemotactic stimuli and to migrate to sites of inflammation, just as different subsets of normal lymphoid cells do.

## T-cell prolymphocytic leukemia

T-cell prolymphocytic leukemia (T-PLL) is a rare hematologic disease occurring mostly in elderly patients [3, 4]. Cutaneous involvement occurs in 20–30% of patients and is characterized by papules, plaques, or tumors often indistinguishable from those of mycosis fungoides/Sézary syndrome. Generalized papules may mimic clinically a drug eruption, a viral exanthema, or papular mycosis fungoides (Fig. 25.1). Erythroderma may develop and is indistinguishable from Sézary syndrome (Fig. 25.2). Skin manifestations may be the first sign of the disease [5, 6].

Histology reveals a monomorphous, superficial infiltrate of small lymphocytes, sometimes with epidermotropism (Fig. 25.3). The pattern may be indistinguishable from that of mycosis fungoides and Sézary syndrome. Immunohistology shows an α/β T-helper phenotype (βF1$^+$, CD2$^+$, CD3$^+$, CD4$^+$, CD5$^+$, CD7$^+$, CD8$^-$) in the majority of lesions, but co-expression of CD4 and CD8 is found in 25–40% of cases. CD52 is strongly expressed in most cases (Fig. 25.4), and TCL-1 is positive as well. Markers of T-lymphoblastic leukemia/lymphoma (TdT, CD1a) are negative. S100 is expressed by neoplastic cells in about one-third of cases [7].

The T-cell receptor (TCR) genes are monoclonally rearranged. The most frequent chromosomal aberrations are inversion of chromosome 14 with breakpoints in the long arm at q11 (*TCR* alpha/delta), q32 (*TCL1* gene), or Xq28 (*MTCP-1* gene), abnormalities of chromosome 8, and deletions of the long arm of chromosomes 5, 6, 11, and 13 [3, 4]. Whole-exome and targeted sequencing studies have shown recurrent genetic alterations leading to constitutive activation of the STAT signaling pathway. Cases with cutaneous involvement were associated with high tumor burden in the peripheral blood, and frequently showed *MYC*, *ATM*, and *TCL1A* alterations [8].

The disease usually runs an aggressive course and the prognosis is poor. Anti-CD52 antibody (alemtuzumab) is the treatment of choice [9]. The rationale for the treatment is provided by the strong CD52 positivity of neoplastic cells. Consolidation of remissions with autologous or allogeneic stem cell transplantation is used to prolong survival, offering a potential chance for cure. High levels of expression of TCL1 and the presence of STAT5B mutations represent poor prognostic markers.

It is interesting to note that a report described a patient with a previous "lymphomatoid contact dermatitis" who during follow-up developed a T-PLL, once more showing the difficulties in diagnosis and differential diagnosis of cutaneous lymphoproliferative diseases [10].

Differentiation of cutaneous manifestations of T-PLL from Sézary syndrome may be extremely difficult on clinicopathologic grounds alone. In contrast to T-PLL, the bone marrow is usually not involved in Sézary syndrome, but other clinicopathological features may be overlapping. Splenomegaly and hepatomegaly are found in a majority of patients with T-PLL.

*Skin Lymphoma: The Illustrated Guide*, Sixth Edition. Lorenzo Cerroni.

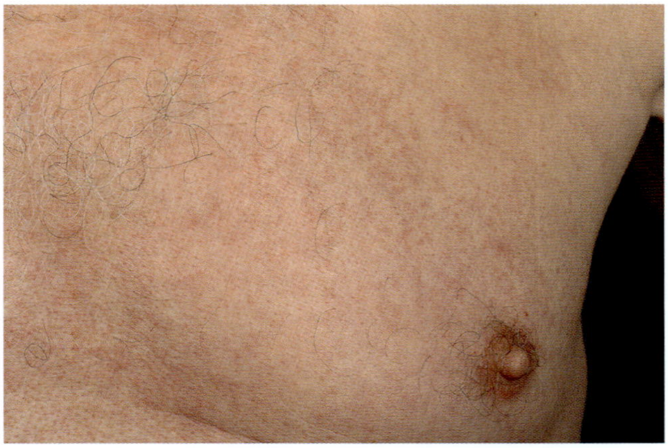

Figure 25.1 Cutaneous involvement in T-cell prolymphocytic leukemia. Generalized erythematous papules.

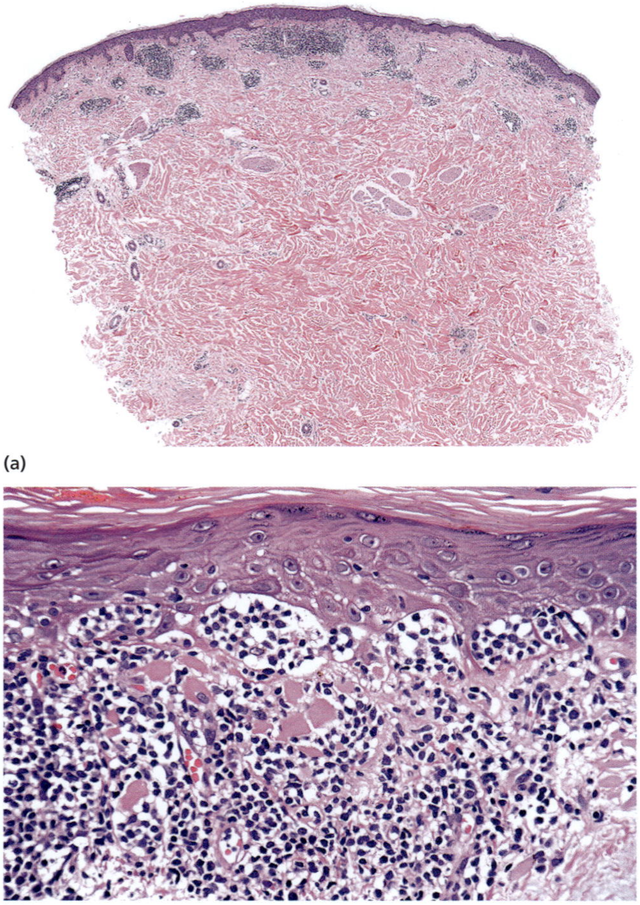

(a)

(b)

Figure 25.3 Cutaneous involvement in T-cell prolymphocytic leukemia. (a) Dense, superficial, patchy-lichenoid infiltrate of lymphocytes with (b) epidermotropism. The histopathologic features are indistinguishable from those of mycosis fungoides or Sézary syndrome.

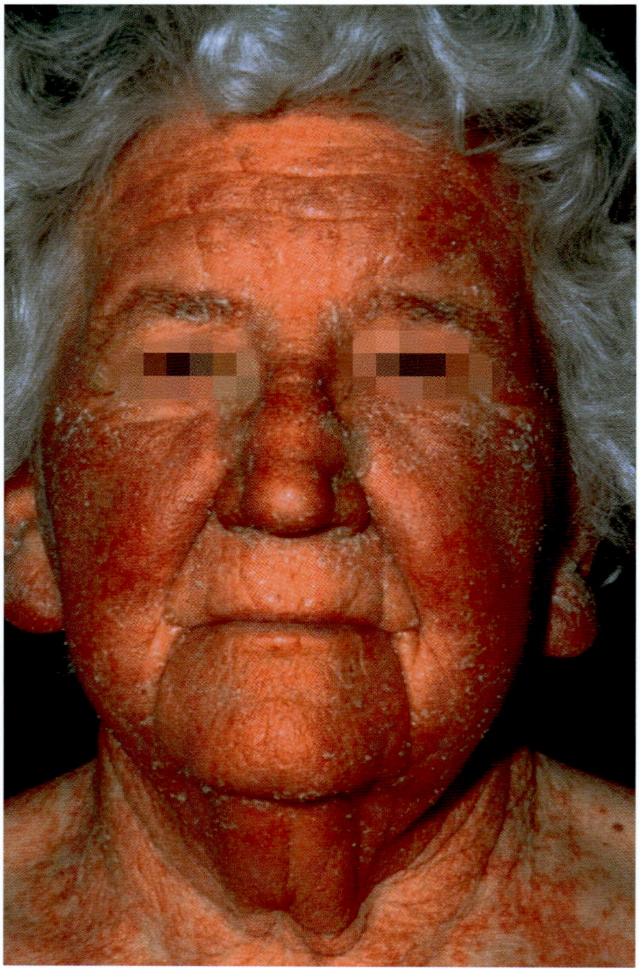

Figure 25.2 Cutaneous involvement in T-cell prolymphocytic leukemia. Erythematous, scaly lesions on the face in a patient with scaly erythroderma. The clinical picture of cutaneous T-cell prolymphocytic leukemia may be indistinguishable from that of Sézary syndrome.

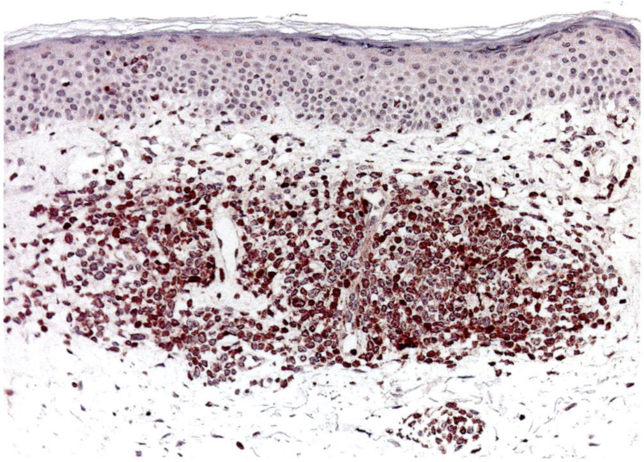

Figure 25.4 Cutaneous involvement in T-cell prolymphocytic leukemia. Strong positivity for CD52.

**Résumé**

| | | |
|---|---|---|
| **T-cell prolymphocytic leukemia** | | |
| **Clinical** | Adults. Generalized papules, plaques, and tumors. Erythroderma may develop. | |
| **Morphology** | Histopathologic features similar to those of mycosis fungoides/Sézary syndrome. | |
| **Immunohistochemistry** | CD2, CD3, CD4, CD5, CD7 | + |
| | CD52 | + |
| | CD8 | – (about 25–40% of cases CD4⁺/CD8⁺) |
| | βF1, TCL1-1 | + |
| | S100 | –/+ (about 30% of cases positive) |
| **Genetics** | Monoclonal rearrangement of the TCR genes. Inversion of chromosome 14 with breakpoints in the long arm at q11 and q32. Frequent *MYC*, *ATM*, and *TCL1A* alterations. | |
| **Treatment guidelines** | Alemtuzumab (anti-CD52 antibody); autologous or allogeneic stem cell transplantation. | |

## Aggressive natural killer cell leukemia

Aggressive natural killer (NK) cell leukemia is characterized by a proliferation of NK cells, observed predominantly in young and middle-aged adult Asian patients [11–13]. There is a strong association with Epstein–Barr virus (EBV) infection and a distinct overlap with extranodal NK cell lymphomas arising at different sites [14]. The skin may be involved, usually concurrently with blood and bone marrow manifestations. The liver and spleen are also frequently affected. Patients present with overt leukemic picture, fever, and systemic symptoms.

Skin manifestations present histopathologically with diffuse infiltration of the dermis and the subcutaneous tissue, showing nodules or sheets with accentuation around the vessels and the adnexal structures [15]. Neoplastic cells show variable morphology (Fig. 25.5) and have a phenotype identical to extranodal NK-cell lymphomas, characterized by expression of CD2, CD56, CD43, and cytotoxic proteins, negativity for CD3, and positivity for CD3ε. In contrast to extranodal NK/T-cell lymphoma, CD16 is positive in the majority of cases. In situ hybridization for EBV is positive as a rule (Fig. 25.6). TCR genes are in germline configuration.

In spite of the phenotypic similarities, genetic studies by array comparative genomic hybridization showed differences between aggressive NK-cell leukemia (frequent losses in 7p and 17p as well as gains in 1q) and extranodal NK/T-cell lymphoma (frequent deletions in 6q) [16]. Activating *STAT5B* mutations have been observed in a small percentage of cases [15].

The prognosis is very poor, as the disease usually runs a fulminant course. Treatment should be administered in a hematologic setting. Relapses are commonly observed also in patients who underwent complete remission after stem cell transplantation. Some patients have partially responded to gemcitabine.

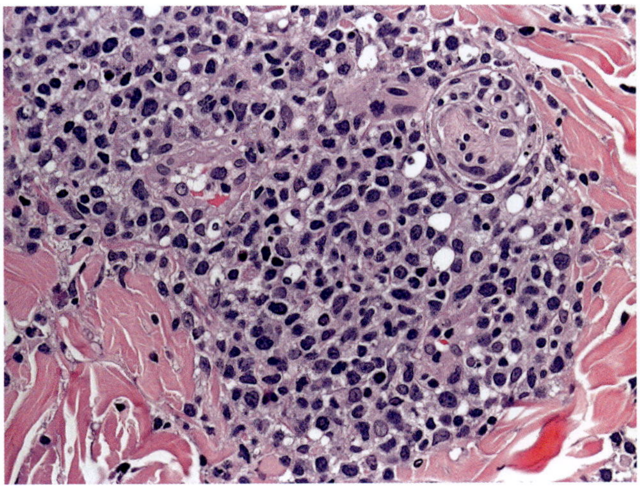

**Figure 25.5** Cutaneous aggressive NK cell leukemia. Perivascular infiltrates of small- and medium-sized pleomorphic cells admixed with large cells.

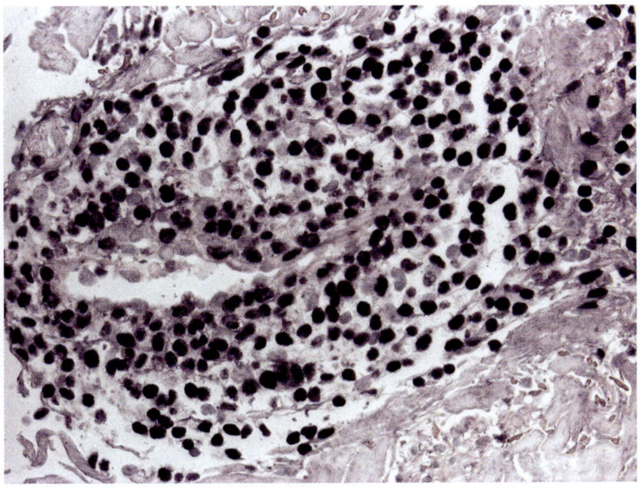

**Figure 25.6** Cutaneous aggressive NK cell leukemia. Positive signal upon in situ hybridization for EBV (EBER-1).

| Résumé | |
|---|---|
| **Aggressive NK cell leukemia** | |
| **Clinical** | Adolescents, young, and middle-aged adults; mostly Asian patients. Generalized papules, plaques, and tumors. |
| **Morphology** | Histopathologic features similar to those of extranodal NK/T-cell lymphomas. |
| **Immunohistochemistry** | CD2, CD56 + <br> CD3 − <br> CD3ε, CD43 + <br> EBER-1 + |
| **Genetics** | TCR genes in germline configuration. Frequent losses in 7p and 17p as well as gains in 1q. |
| **Treatment guidelines** | Systemic chemotherapy (usually a fulminant course in spite of treatment). |

## Specific skin manifestations of other types of leukemia

Besides T-PLL and aggressive NK-cell leukemia, other leukemias (and leukemic phases of non-Hodgkin lymphomas) may involve the skin secondarily. Clinical features are characterized usually by generalized papules, plaques, and/or small tumors. All these cases are managed in a hematologic setting and treatment is tailored to the background condition.

***Hairy cell leukemia.*** Cutaneous infiltrates may be observed in some cases of hairy-cell leukemia [17], a low-grade neoplasm of mature B lymphocytes. Neoplastic cells are positive for CD20, surface immunoglobulins, CD11c, and CD22. Staining for annexin A1 (encoded by the ANXA1 gene which is upregulated in hairy-cell leukemia) shows membranous or sometimes cytoplasmic expression and is considered a specific marker for diagnosis. Other positive markers are CD25, CD103, CD123, CD200, and cyclin D1, whereas CD5 is expressed only rarely. The BRAF V600E mutation is present in virtually all cases, leading to constitutional activation of the MAPK pathway, thus immunohistochemical staining for BRAF may be helpful for diagnosis. The disease shows an excellent response to interferon-α or purine analogs (e.g., pentostatin), eventually in association with rituximab. BRAF inhibitors can be used in refractory and/or relapsing cases.

***B-cell prolymphocytic leukemia.*** Cutaneous involvement may occur rarely in B-cell prolymphocytic leukemia [18], a disease involving primarily the bone marrow, peripheral blood, and spleen. The disease is no longer listed as a specific entity in the 5th edition of the World Health Organization (WHO) Classification of Haematolymphoid Tumors (in which it is listed as the prolymphocytic progression of B-CLL or of small lymphocytic lymphoma) [19], but it is still included as a specific entity in the International Consensus Classification (ICC) of mature lymphoid and histiocytic/dendritic cell neoplasms [20], and re-inclusion as a distinct disorder in the WHO classification has been advocated [21]. Neoplastic cells are positive for B-cell markers and for IgM. Differentiation between B-CLL and mantle cell lymphoma may be difficult. The prognosis is bad and the disease responds poorly to therapy (usually done with regimens utilized for B-CLL, such as ibrutinib and rituximab).

***T-large granular lymphocytic leukemia.*** Cutaneous lesions have been reported in T-cell large granular lymphocytic leukemia, both in the $CD8^+$ and in the less frequent $CD4^+$ variant [22]. The disease involves mostly the peripheral blood, bone marrow, liver, and spleen. Most cases are characterized by an α/β T-cytotoxic phenotype ($CD3^+$, $CD8^+$, $TIA\text{-}1^+$, Granzyme $B^+$, $ßF1^+$, $CD57^+$). I have rarely observed patients presenting with specific skin infiltrates on the background of hypersensitivity reactions related to drugs (Fig. 25.7), similar to other leukemic infiltrates at the site of skin inflammation. T-cell large granular lymphocytic leukemia is characterized by an indolent course. Low-dose methotrexate, cyclophosphamide, cyclosporine A, and systemic steroids may be used to control the disease.

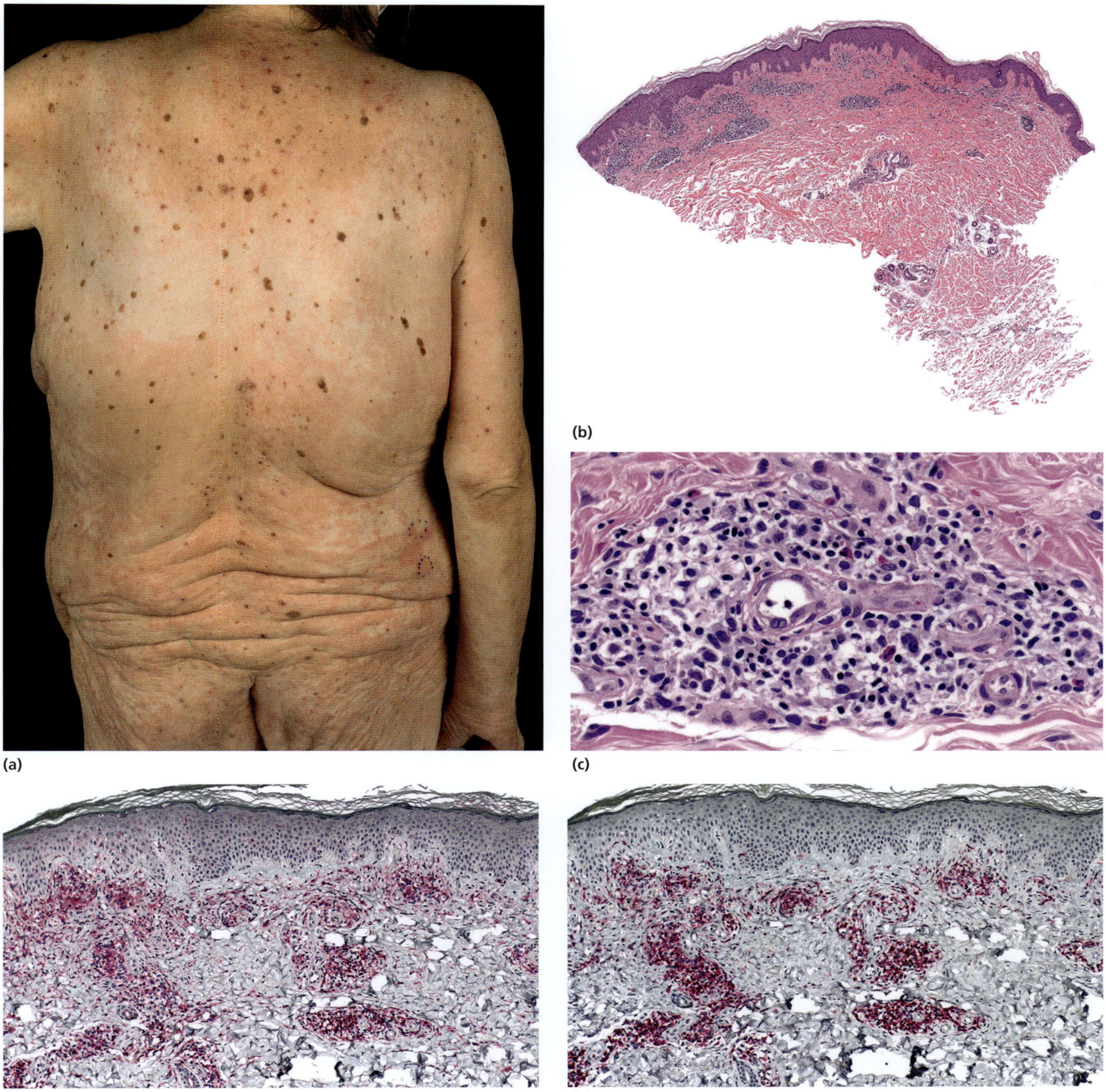

(a) (b) (c) (d) (e)

Figure 25.7 T-large granular lymphocytic leukemia. (a) Exanthematic erythematous skin lesions. (b) Histology reveals dense, superficial perivascular infiltrates composed of (c) large cells with granular cytoplasm admixed with small lymphocytes and a few eosinophils. Positivity of large cells for both CD4 (d) and CD8 (e).

## References


1. Cerroni L. Cutaneous lymphomas and cutaneous signs of systemic lymphomas. In: Callen JP, Jorizzo JL, Zone JJ, *et al.*, eds. *Dermatological Signs of Systemic Disease*. 5th edition. Edinburgh: Elsevier, 2017: 159–170. (ISBN: 978-0-323-35829-3).
2. Kim JE, Kim MY, Kim HO, Park YM. Plasma cell leukaemia cutis preferentially localized to recent puncture sites. *Br J Dermatol* 2004;**151**:237–238.
3. Elenitoba-Johnson KSJ, Chen X, Herling M. T-prolymphocytic lekaemia. In: *WHO Classification of Tumours Editorial Board. Haematolymphoid Tumours*. 5th edition. Lyon: IARC, 2024: 659–661.
4. Dearden C, Bechy E, Lopez C, Wang SA. T-cell prolymphocytic leukemia. In: Arber DA, Borowitz MJ, Cook JR, *et al.*, eds. *The International Consensus Classification of Myeloid and Lymphoid Neoplasms*. Philadelphia, PA: Wolters Kluwer, 2025: 588–593.
5. Serra A, Estrach MT, Marti R, *et al.* Cutaneous involvement as the first manifestation in a case of T-cell prolymphocytic leukaemia. *Acta Derm Venereol (Stockh)* 1998;**78**:198–200.
6. Ventre MO, Bacelieri RE, Lazarchick J, *et al.* Cutaneous presentation of T-cell prolymphocytic leukemia. *Cutis* 2013;**91**:87–91.
7. Aggarwal N, Pongpruttipan T, Patel S, *et al.* Expression of S100 protein in CD4-positive T-cell lymphomas is often associated with T-cell prolymphocytic leukemia. *Am J Surg Pathol* 2015;**39**:1679–1687.
8. Hsi AC, Robirds DH, Luo J, *et al.* T-cell prolymphocytic leukemia frequently shows cutaneous involvement and is associated with gains of MYC, Loss of ATM, and TCL1A rearrangement. *Am J Surg Pathol* 2014;**38**:1468–1483.
9. Dearden C. How I treat prolymphocytic leukemia. *Blood* 2012; **120**:538–551.
10. Abraham S, Braun RP, Matthes T, *et al.* Follow-up: previously reported apparent lymphomatoid contact dermatitis, now followed by T-cell prolymphocytic leukaemia. *Br J Dermatol* 2006;**155**:633–634.
11. Suzuki R, Ng SB, Cheng CL, *et al.* Aggressive NK-cell leukaemia. In: *WHO Classification of Tumours Editorial Board. Haematolymphoid Tumours*. 5th edition. Lyon: IARC, 2024: 677–679.
12. Chan WC, Kim WS, Ko YH, Pittaluga S. Aggressive natural killer-cell leukemia. In: Arber DA, Borowitz MJ, Cook JR, *et al.*, eds. *The International Consensus Classification of Myeloid and Lymphoid Neoplasms*. Philadelphia, PA: Wolters Kluwer, 2025: 635–639.
13. Zhang Y, Lee D, Gesiotto Q, Sokol L. Aggressive natural killer cell leukemia: diagnosis, treatment recommendations, and emerging therapies. *Expert Rev Hematol* 2021;**14**:731–740.
14. Takahashi E, Ohshima K, Kimura H, *et al.* Clinicopathological analysis of the age-related differences in patients with Epstein–Barr virus (EBV)-associated extranasal natural killer (NK)/T-cell lymphoma with reference to the relationship with aggressive NK cell leukaemia and chronic active EBV infection-associated lymphoproliferative disorders. *Histopathology* 2011;**59**:660–671.
15. Gao LM, Zhao S, Liu WP, *et al.* Clinicopathologic characterization of aggressive natural killer cell leukemia involving different tissue sites. *Am J Surg Pathol* 2016;**40**:836–846.
16. Nakashima Y, Tagawa H, Suzuki R, *et al.* Genome-wide array-based comparative genomic hybridization of natural killer cell lymphoma/leukemia: different genomic alteration patterns of aggressive NK-cell leukemia and extranodal Nk/T-cell lymphoma, nasal type. *Genes Chromosomes Cancer* 2005;**44**:247–255.
17. Colović N, Perunicić M, Jurisić V, Colović M. Specific skin lesions in hairy cell leukemia at presentation: case report and review of literature. *Med Oncol* 2010;**27**:559–561.
18. Bachmeyer C, Hunault M, Bazarbachi A, *et al.* Specific cutaneous involvement in B-cell prolymphocytic leukaemia. *Br J Dermatol* 1996;**134**:979–980.
19. Naresh KN, Rawstron AC, Akinola NO, *et al.* Chronic lymphocytic leukaemia/lymphoma. In: *WHO Classification of Tumours Editorial Board. Haematolymphoid Tumours*. 5th edition. Lyon: IARC, 2024: 368–377.
20. Sander B, Campo E, Dreyling M, Matutes E. B-cell prolymphocytic leukemia. In: Arber DA, Borowitz MJ, Cook JR, *et al.*, eds. *The International Consensus Classification of Myeloid and Lymphoid Neoplasms*. Philadelphia, PA: Wolters Kluwer, 2025: 348–350.
21. Menakuru SR, Roepke J, Siddiqui S. De-novo B-cell prolymphocytic leukemia. *J Hematol* 2023;**12**:82–86.
22. Kim J, Park CJ, Jang S, *et al.* A case of CD4(+)T-cell large granular lymphocytic leukemia. *Ann Lab Med* 2013;**33**:196–199.

## CHAPTER 26

# Cutaneous lymphoblastic lymphomas

Lymphoblastic lymphomas are precursor hematologic neoplasms with aggressive behavior and relatively frequent skin involvement. In spite of extensive staging investigations, the skin may appear as the only involved site in some patients, particularly in the B-cell variant of the disease [1–12]. These cases resemble conceptually so-called "aleukemic" leukemia cutis or primary cutaneous blastic plasmacytoid dendritic cell neoplasm, where apparent exclusive skin involvement is invariably followed by overt leukemic manifestations, usually in a matter of a few weeks or months.

The distinction between leukemic and lymphomatous forms depends on the involvement of the peripheral blood and bone marrow, and is sometimes arbitrary. Although lymphoblastic lymphomas are divided into B and T types, rarely neoplastic cells do not express B- or T-cell markers, thus having a so-called "null-cell" phenotype. Distinction of these cases from other precursor neoplasms (e.g., natural killer [NK], myeloid) is extremely difficult, as some degree of overlapping phenotypic features may be observed. In fact, in the 5th edition of the World Health Organization (WHO) *Classification of Haematolymphoid Tumours* there are two groups of "myeloid/lymphoid neoplasms" (including cases with rearrangement of *PDGFRA*, *PDGFRB*, *FGFR1*, and *JAK2* among others), and of "acute leukemias of mixed or ambiguous lineage" showing overlapping myeloid/lymphoid differentiation and including cases that do not show differentiation along a single lymphoid or myeloid lineage [13]. Compared to the WHO classification, the International Consensus Classification (ICC) contains more molecular variants for both B and T lymphoblastic lymphoma/leukemia (a comparison of the entities included in the two classification schemes is summarized in Table 26.1) [14, 15]. These genetic aberrations are associated with multilineage differentiation, and cases of concomitant lymphoblastic lymphoma and myelogenous leukemia sharing this genetic background have been reported. Cutaneous involvement has been described in one case with a *PDGFRA* rearrangement [16]. A trisomy of chromosome 4 was found in three cases of primary cutaneous lymphoblastic lymphoma (two of B-cell and one of T-cell type) [2].

According to the WHO classification, the term B-lymphoblastic leukemia/lymphoma not otherwise specified (NOS) should not be used for cases showing specific recurrent genetic abnormalities associated with distinctive clinical and phenotypic properties or with important prognostic implications, or showing evidence that they are mutually exclusive of other entities [17]. These cases should be rather classified according to their genetic abnormalities (see Table 26.1). However, most reports on skin involvement by B-lymphoblastic lymphoma predate the WHO classification and are case reports or very small series, thus data on the relative incidence of cutaneous involvement in various types of precursor lymphoid neoplasms are lacking. Even in cases published recently, genetic data are often not included. In particular, it would be very interesting to study cases with "primary cutaneous" involvement to ascertain whether they are characterized by a particular molecular pattern.

Although in general histologic features alone do not allow one to differentiate lymphoblastic lymphomas of B phenotype from those of T-cell lineage, in skin lesions a starry sky pattern is more common in the B-cell type of the disease and neoplastic cells in the T-cell type display a more pleomorphic morphology.

## Cutaneous B-Lymphoblastic Lymphoma

B-lymphoblastic lymphoma is a malignant proliferation of precursor B lymphocytes. Cutaneous involvement is not rare but exact data are not available. Although patients usually have secondary skin manifestations of acute lymphoblastic leukemia with bone marrow and peripheral blood involvement, primary skin involvement has been observed occasionally [1–11].

*Skin Lymphoma: The Illustrated Guide*, Sixth Edition. Lorenzo Cerroni.

**Table 26.1** Classification of precursor lymphoid neoplasms according to the WHO [13] and ICC [14, 15]

| B-lymphoblastic leukemia/lymphoma (WHO) | B- lymphoblastic leukemia/lymphoma (ICC) |
|---|---|
| B-ALL/LBL with high hyperdiploidy | B-ALL/LBL, hyperdiploidy |
| B-ALL/LBL with hypodiploidy | B-ALL/LBL, low hypodiploidy |
| | B-ALL/LBL, near haploid |
| B-ALL/LBL with iAMP21 | B-ALL/LBL with iAMP21 |
| B-ALL/LBL with *BCR::ABL1* fusion | B-ALL/LBL with BCR::ABL1 with lymphoid only involvement |
| | B-ALL/LBL with *BCR::ABL1* with multilineage involvement |
| B-ALL/LBL with *BCR::ABL1*-like features | B-ALL/LBL with *BCR::ABL1*-like features |
| | B-ALL/LBL with *BCR::ABL1*-like, *ABL1*-class rearranged |
| | B-ALL/LBL with *BCR::ABL1*-like, JAK–STAT activated |
| | B-ALL/LBL with *BCR::ABL1*-like, not otherwise specified |
| B-ALL/LBL with *KMT2A* rearrangement | B-ALL/LBL with *KMT2A* rearrangement |
| B-ALL/LBL with *ETV6::RUNX1* fusion | B-ALL/LBL with *ETV6::RUNX1* fusion |
| B-ALL/LBL with *ETV6::RUNX1*-like features | |
| B-ALL/LBL with *TCF3::PBX1* fusion | B-ALL/LBL with *TCF3::PBX1* fusion |
| B-ALL/LBL with *IGH::IL3* fusion | B-ALL/LBL with *IGH::IL3* fusion |
| B-ALL/LBL with *TCF3::HLF* fusion | |
| B-ALL/LBL with other defined genetic alterations | B-ALL/LBL with *DUX4*-rearrangement |
| | B-ALL/LBL with *ZNF384*-rearrangement |
| | B-ALL/LBL with *MEF2D*-rearrangement |
| | B-ALL/LBL with *MYC*-rearrangement |
| | B-ALL/LBL with *NUTM1*-rearrangement |
| | B-ALL/LBL with *UBTF::ATXN723/PAN3, CDX2 (CDX"/UBTF)* |
| | B-ALL/LBL with *HLF*-rearrangement |
| | B-ALL/LBL with PAX5 P80R |
| | B-ALL/LBL with IKZF1 N159Y |
| B-ALL/LBL NOS | B-ALL/LBL NOS |
| | B-ALL/LBL, provisional entities |
| **T-lymphoblastic leukemia/lymphoma** | **T-lymphoblastic leukemia/lymphoma** |
| T-ALL/LBL NOS | T-ALL/LBL NOS |
| Early T-precursor ALL/LBL | Early T-precursor ALL/LBL, *BCL11B*-activated |
| | Early T-precursor ALL/LBL, NOS |
| | T-ALL/LBL: provisional entities |

WHO: World Health Organization; ICC: International Consensus Classification; ALL/LBL: lymphoblastic leukemia/lymphoma; T-ALL/LBL: T-lymphoblastic leukemia/lymphoma.

## Clinical features

Children and young adults are usually affected, but cases in neonates have been also observed [1–12, 16, 18–20]. Clinically patients present with large erythematous tumors, usually solitary, commonly located on the head and neck (Figs. 26.1 and 26.2). In patients with precursor B-lymphoblastic leukemia, cutaneous involvement may be the first sign of recurrence after successful first-line treatment. In these cases, skin manifestations may be characterized by solitary or localized papules and small tumors that may be impossible to recognize clinically (Fig. 26.3).

## Histopathology, immunophenotype, and molecular genetics

### Histopathology

Dense, diffuse monomorphous infiltrates are found within the dermis and the subcutaneous fat (Fig. 26.4). Cytomorphologically, the lymphoblasts are medium-sized cells with round, oval or convoluted nuclei, fine chromatin, inconspicuous nucleoli, and scant cytoplasm (Fig. 26.5). Mitoses and necrotic ("apoptotic") cells are frequent, and "starry sky" or "mosaic stone"-like patterns may be seen (Figs. 26.6 and 26.7). In some cases of secondary skin involvement from B-lymphoblastic leukemia,

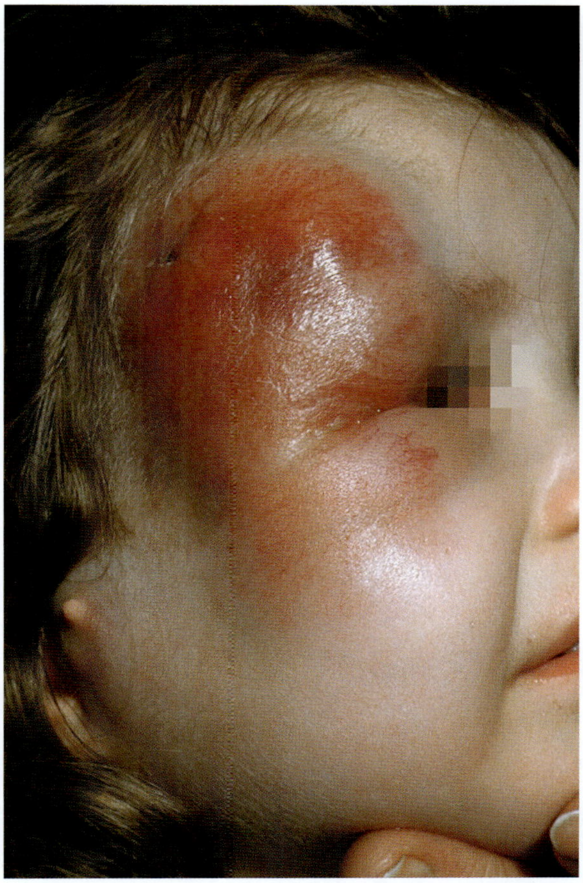

Figure 26.1 Cutaneous B-lymphoblastic lymphoma. Large tumor on the face of an 18-month-old child.

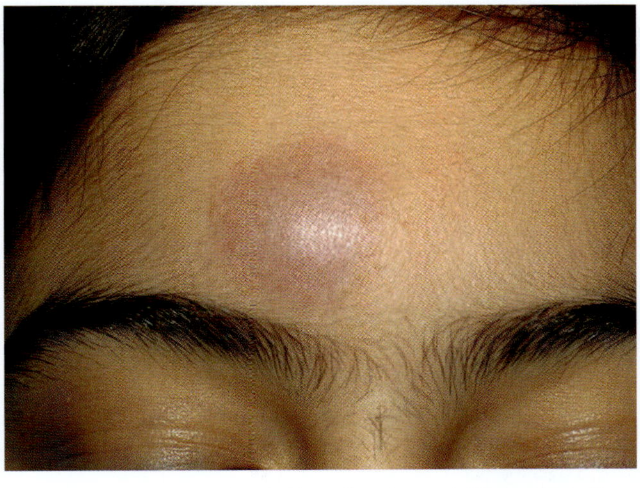

Figure 26.2 Cutaneous B-lymphoblastic lymphoma. Infiltrate plaque/flat tumor on the forehead of a 10-year-old boy. Note the complete absence of epidermal involvement. (*Courtesy of Prof. Ernesto Bonifazi, Bari, Italy.*)

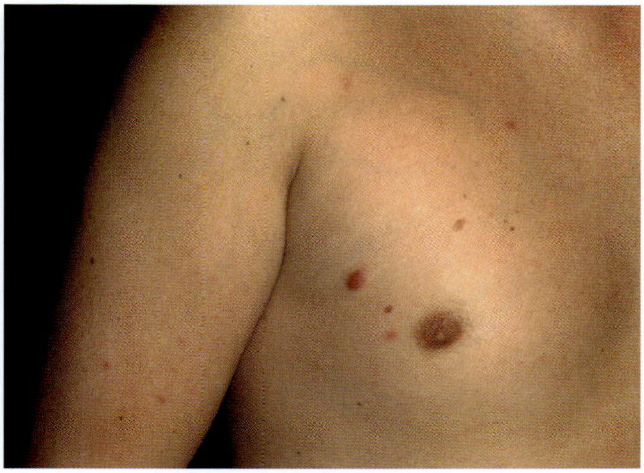

Figure 26.3 Cutaneous B-lymphoblastic lymphoma. A small erythematous papule on the chest is the first sign of recurrence of acute lymphoblastic leukemia in a 28-year-old man (histopathologic and immunophenotypical features are depicted in Fig. 23.8).

the pattern at low power may mimic that of an inflammatory skin condition, emphasizing the need for careful histologic and immunohistochemical examination to make a confident diagnosis (Figs. 26.8a and b).

## Immunophenotype

Cutaneous B-lymphoblastic lymphoma expresses usually CD79a, TdT, CD10 (common acute lymphoblastic leukemia/lymphoma antigen – CALLA), paired box gene (PAX)-5, and cytoplasmic μ heavy chain without surface immunoglobulins (Igs) (Figs. 26.8c and 26.9). CD20 is positive in the majority of cases. A proportion of cases are also positive for CD99 and CD34 (Fig. 26.8d). Expression of the various markers is related to the stage of differentiation of the cells, and B-cell markers may be negative in some cases.

## Molecular genetics

Molecular genetics shows a monoclonal rearrangement of the Ig genes in virtually all cases. Although a polyclonal pattern of the T-cell receptor (TCR) genes is more commonly found, in a variable proportion of cases a concomitant monoclonal rearrangement of TCR and Ig genes can be observed, giving rise to potential pitfalls in the molecular diagnosis of the tumor.

Several genetic aberrations have been described in B-lymphoblastic lymphoma, resulting in the identification of specific variants listed in the WHO and ICC classifications (Table 26.1) [13]. Two cases of primary cutaneous B-lymphoblastic lymphoma with different genetic changes have been reported in adult patients (one with rearrangement of the *MLL* gene and the

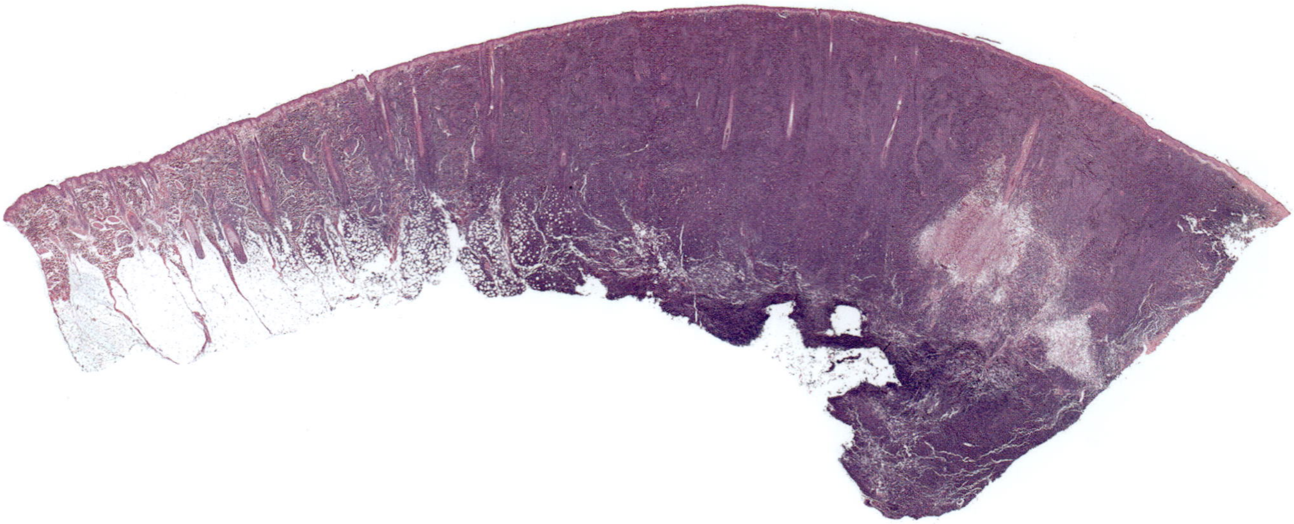

**Figure 26.4** Cutaneous B-lymphoblastic lymphoma. The entire dermis and subcutaneous fat are replaced by a dense, diffuse proliferation of neoplastic cells.

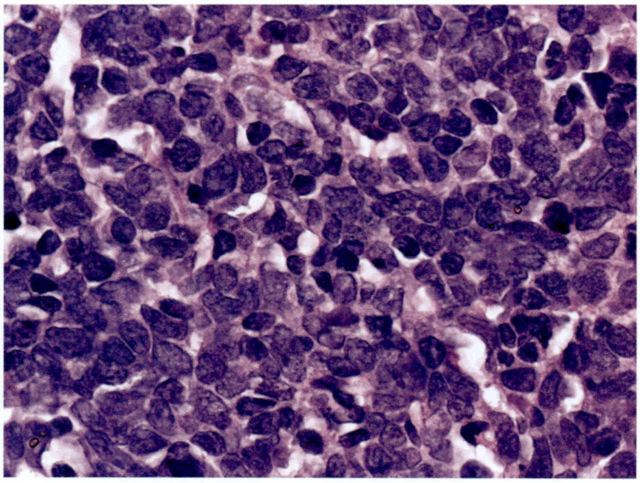

**Figure 26.5** Cutaneous B-lymphoblastic lymphoma. B lymphoblasts with finely dispersed chromatin.

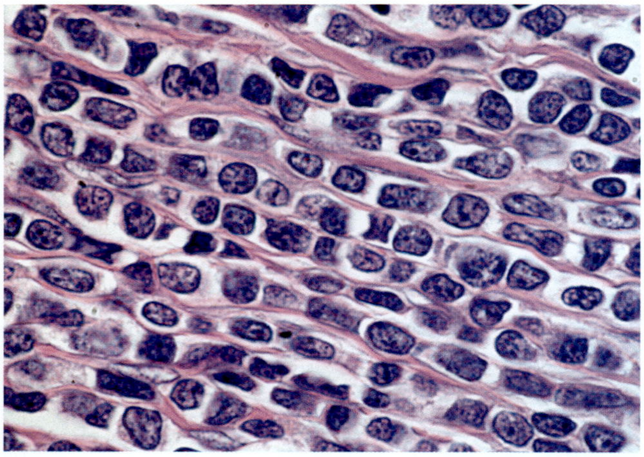

**Figure 26.7** Cutaneous B-lymphoblastic lymphoma. Note the "mosaic stone"-like arrangement of neoplastic cells.

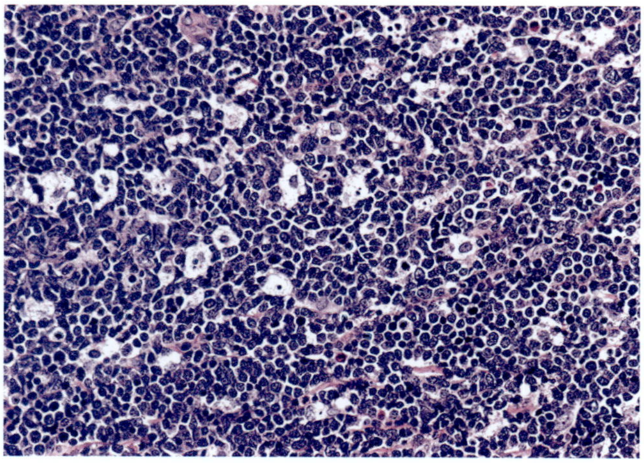

**Figure 26.6** Cutaneous B-lymphoblastic lymphoma. Monomorphous proliferation of medium-sized cells. Note the "starry sky" pattern.

other with hyperdiploidy), showing that various molecular subtypes of lymphoblastic leukemia/lymphoma may involve the skin [21]. However, comprehensive molecular data on cutaneous cases, particularly those arising "primary" in the skin, are still lacking.

## Differential diagnosis

The differential diagnosis of cutaneous B-lymphoblastic lymphoma includes several entities that may show similar morphologic features. Mantle cell lymphoma contains cells with more cleaved or irregularly shaped nuclei and with a characteristic immunophenotype ($CD5^+$, cyclin-$D1^+$, $CD10^-$, $TdT^-$) (see Chapter 20). Myelogenous leukemia shows a proliferation of immature myeloid cells with figurate or "Indian-line" patterns that stain positive for myeloid markers (e.g., CD68

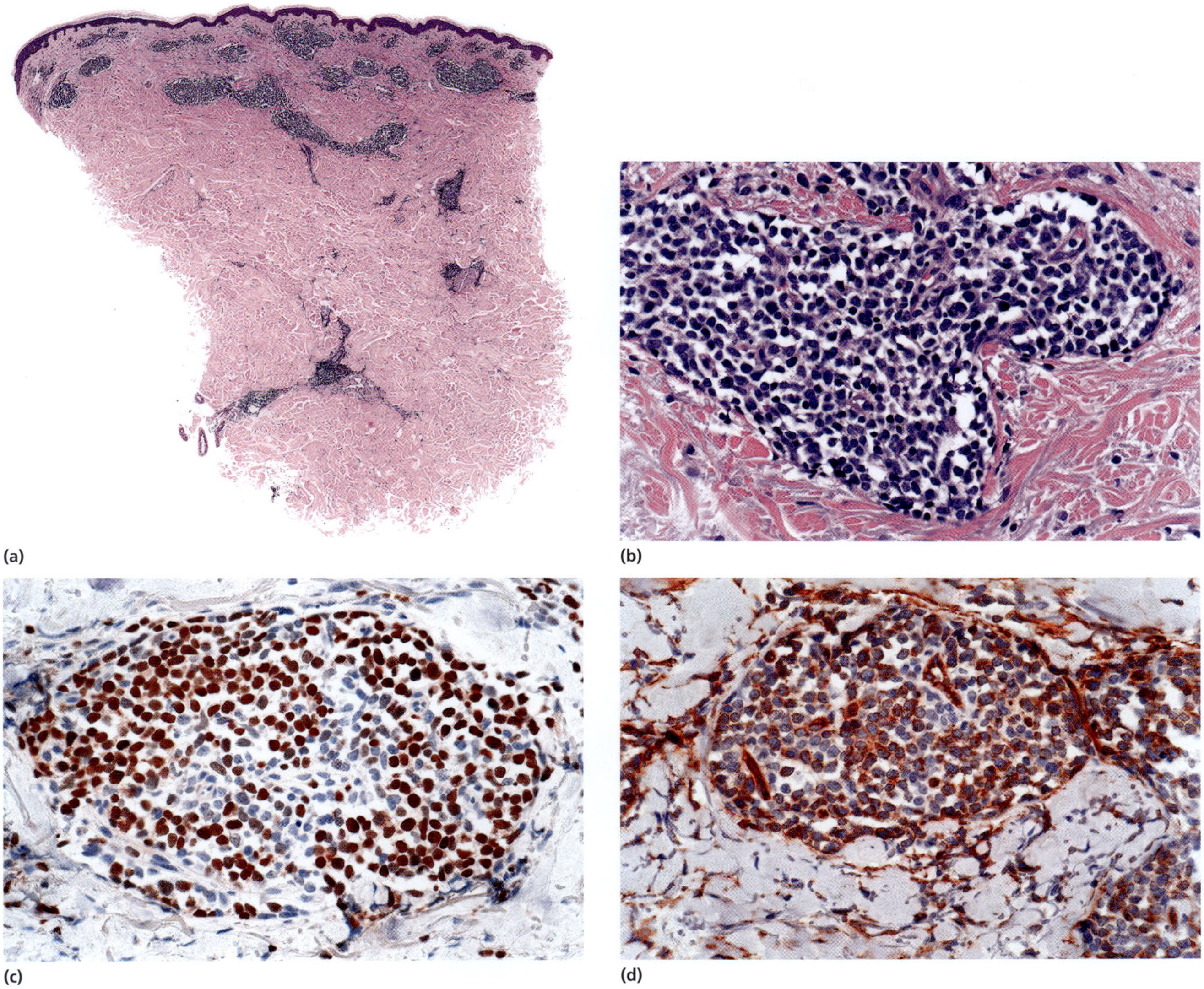

Figure 26.8 Cutaneous B-lymphoblastic lymphoma (same case as Fig. 23.3). (a) Dense perivascular infiltrates in the superficial and mid-dermis. (b) Monomorphous, medium-sized cells predominate. Most neoplastic cells show positivity for (c) TdT and (d) CD34.

and myeloperoxidase among others) and do not reveal a monoclonal rearrangement of the Ig genes (see Chapter 23). Blastic plasmacytoid dendritic cell neoplasm is characterized by a strong positivity for CD4, CD56, and CD123 in addition to a variable positivity for TdT, as well as by lack of rearrangement of the Ig genes (see Chapter 24). The differential diagnosis may also include cutaneous Merkel cell carcinoma and metastatic neuroendocrine carcinomas, which are characterized by the co-expression of cytokeratin filaments, neurofilament proteins, and various other neuroendocrine markers (e.g., chromogranin-A, synaptophysin). A subset of cases of Merkel cell carcinoma are positive for the Merkel cell polyoma virus. Cases of Merkel cell carcinoma showing a phenotype overlapping with B-cell precursor neoplasms have been observed [22].

## Treatment and prognosis

These patients should be managed in a hematologic setting. The treatment of choice is systemic chemotherapy, often followed by stem cell transplantation. Children have a better prognosis than adults, with complete remission in >90% of cases managed with new treatment strategies tailored to different genetic abnormalities. Patients with localized skin disease appear to have a relatively good prognosis and seem to respond well to systemic chemotherapic regimens, but treatment strategies should be the same as for the systemic variants of the disease. In a large series, patients with only cutaneous involvement had a better prognosis (yet not statistically significant), and children had a better prognosis than adults [23].

**Résumé**

| | | |
|---|---|---|
| **Cutaneous B-lymphoblastic lymphoma** | | |
| **Clinical** | Children, young adults. Solitary tumors. Preferential location: head and neck. | |
| **Morphology** | Nodular or diffuse infiltrates characterized by monomorphous proliferations of lymphoblasts. | |
| **Immunohistochemistry** | CD19, CD79a | + |
| | CD20 | +(−) |
| | CD10 | + |
| | PAX5 | + |
| | CD34 | +/− |
| | TdT | + |
| **Genetics** | Monoclonal rearrangement of the Ig genes detected in the majority of cases. TCR genes may be clonally rearranged as well. Different genetic aberrations correspond to distinct subtypes included in the ICC and WHO classifications (Table 26.1). | |
| **Treatment guidelines** | Systemic chemotherapy; stem cell transplantation. Management tailored to specific genetic aberrations. | |

## Cutaneous T-Lymphoblastic Lymphoma

T-lymphoblastic lymphoma is a malignant proliferation of precursor T lymphocytes [15, 24]. The exact incidence of specific cutaneous involvement is not known. In the skin, T-lymphoblastic lymphoma almost always represents a secondary manifestation of primary extracutaneous disease, but rare primary cutaneous cases have been reported [1, 2, 25–27]. In a large series of patients with cutaneous involvement by T-lymphoblastic lymphoma, all of them had extracutaneous disease (in contrast, 4/38 patients with B-lymphoblastic lymphoma had disease limited to the skin) [23].

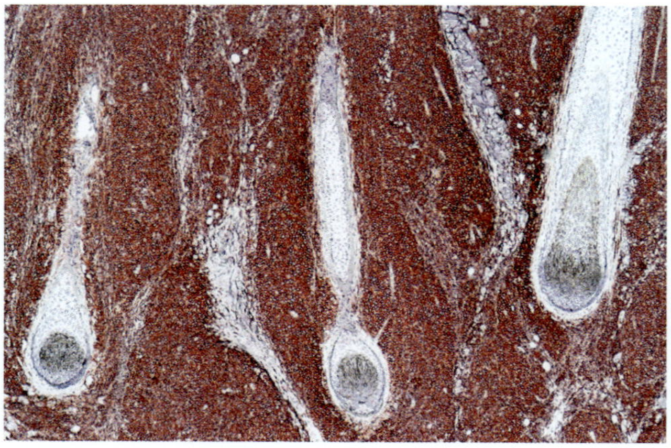

**Figure 26.9** Cutaneous B-lymphoblastic lymphoma. Neoplastic cells show strong positivity for CD10.

### Clinical features

Although T-lymphoblastic lymphoma is observed mainly in children and adolescents, reports of cutaneous involvement are mainly in young adults or adults [1, 3, 28], and only rare

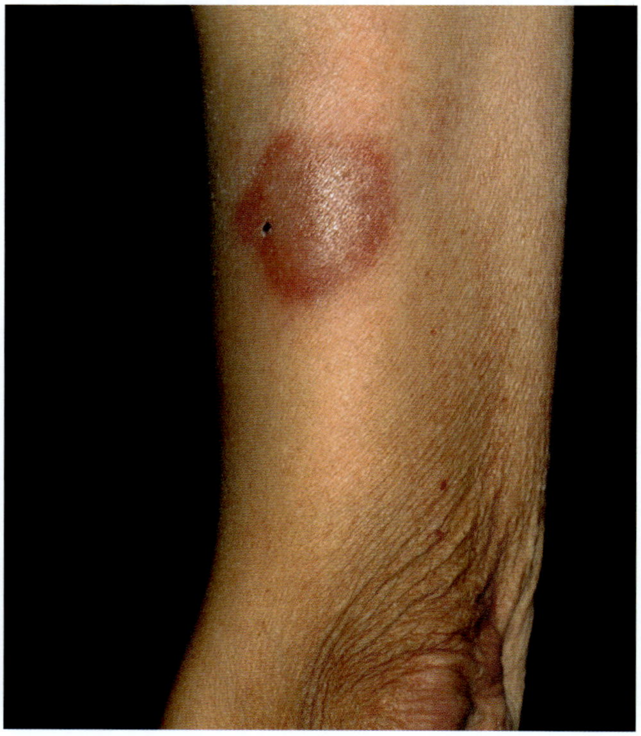

**Figure 26.10** Cutaneous T-lymphoblastic lymphoma. Infiltrated plaque on the upper arm.

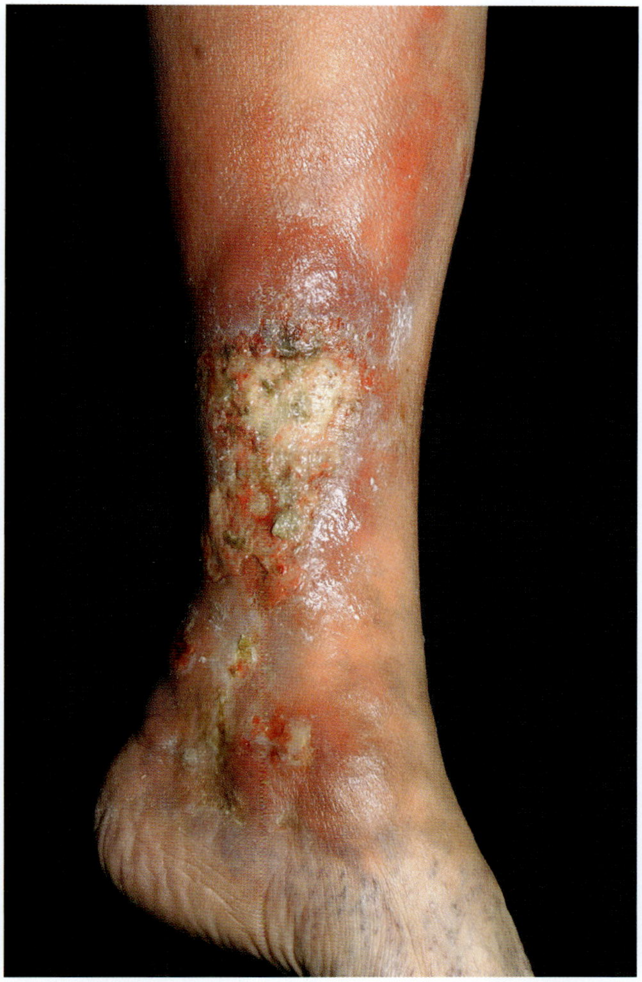

Figure 26.11 Cutaneous T-lymphoblastic lymphoma. Ulcerated, infiltrated lesions on the lower leg.

primary cutaneous cases in children have been reported [25]. Clinically, patients present with nondescript, localized, or generalized cutaneous–subcutaneous plaques and tumors (Fig. 26.10) [1, 3]. In contrast to B-lymphoblastic lymphoma, ulcerated lesions are not rare (Fig. 26.11). Involvement of the mediastinum (thymus) is common and the central nervous system may be involved as well.

## Histopathology, immunophenotype, and molecular genetics

Tumor aggregates may be diffuse in the entire dermis or show a more infiltrative pattern between the collagen bundles with "Indian filing" (reminiscent of that observed in myelogenous leukemia) (Figs. 26.12 and 26.13). In some cases, histology of cutaneous infiltrates reveals a monomorphous proliferation of medium-sized cells similar to that observed at extracutaneous sites, characterized by round or convoluted nuclei with finely dispersed chromatin and scanty cytoplasm. Morphologic features, however, often appear more pleomorphic than in the nodal counterpart (Fig. 26.14). A "starry sky" pattern is much less common than in skin lesions of B-lymphoblastic lymphoma. Particularly when the infiltrate does not form sheets of cells, the morphologic appearance can be indistinguishable from that of other cutaneous NK/T-cell lymphomas.

Cutaneous T lymphoblastic lymphoma may be characterized rarely by epidermotropism of neoplastic cells [29]. Cases with pagetoid epidermotropism indistinguishable from that of pagetoid reticulosis have also been reported (Fig. 26.15) [30].

The immunophenotype of neoplastic cells is variable, depending also upon their degree of differentiation. TdT is positive as a rule (Fig. 26.16) and most cases express cytoplasmic CD3 and CD7 as well. Both CD4 and CD8 can be positive or negative. CD1a, CD2, CD5, CD99, and CD34 are other useful markers, but are not constantly positive. Expression of B-cell (CD79a) or myeloid cell markers (CD13, CD33) is present in a minority of cases and may be the source of diagnostic pitfalls. Cases of early T-cell precursor lymphoblastic leukemia are positive for CD7, cytoplasmic CD3, and CD34, variably positive for CD2 and CD4, but lack CD1a and CD8 expression.

Molecular genetics usually shows monoclonally rearranged TCR and germline Ig genes, but clonal rearrangements of both TCR and Ig genes can be observed in a minority of cases. Several genetic abnormalities have been detected in T-lymphoblastic leukemia/lymphoma, involving particularly the *TCR* loci at 14q11.2 (TCR $\alpha$ and $\delta$), 7q35 (TCR $\beta$), and 7p14–15 (TCR $\gamma$) [24]. A case of primary cutaneous T-lymphoblastic lymphoma showed trisomy of chromosome 4 and a gain of 1p36.33-p22.1 [2]. Several other molecular aberrations may be observed in precursor T-cell lymphomas/leukemias which are beyond the scope of this chapter.

## Treatment and prognosis

The treatment of choice is systemic chemotherapy, possibly followed by stem cell transplantation. Patients are managed with schemes similar to those for other types of acute lymphoblastic leukemia/lymphoma. One patient with primary cutaneous T-lymphoblastic lymphoma showed rapid progression in spite of systemic polychemotherapy [2], underlining the need for aggressive treatment regardless of the results of staging investigations. As for B-lymphoblastic lymphoma, for T-lymphoblastic lymphoma, too, the prognosis is better in children than in adults.

## Résumé

**Cutaneous T-lymphoblastic lymphoma**

| | | |
|---|---|---|
| **Clinical** | Skin involvement mainly in adults. Localized or generalized large cutaneous or subcutaneous tumors. | |
| **Morphology** | Proliferation of medium-sized cells with round or convoluted nuclei showing finely dispersed chromatin and scanty cytoplasm. A Starry sky pattern is less common than in the B-cell variant. | |
| **Immunohistochemistry** | TdT | + |
| | Cytoplasmic CD3 | + |
| | CD1a, CD2, CD7 | + |
| | CD5 | − (+) |
| | CD34, CD99, CD117 | + (−) |
| | CD99 | +/− |
| **Genetics** | Monoclonal rearrangement of the TCR genes. In a minority of cases clonal rearrangement of both TCR and Ig genes. Common aberrations involving the *TCR* loci. | |
| **Treatment guidelines** | Systemic chemotherapy, stem cell transplantation. | |

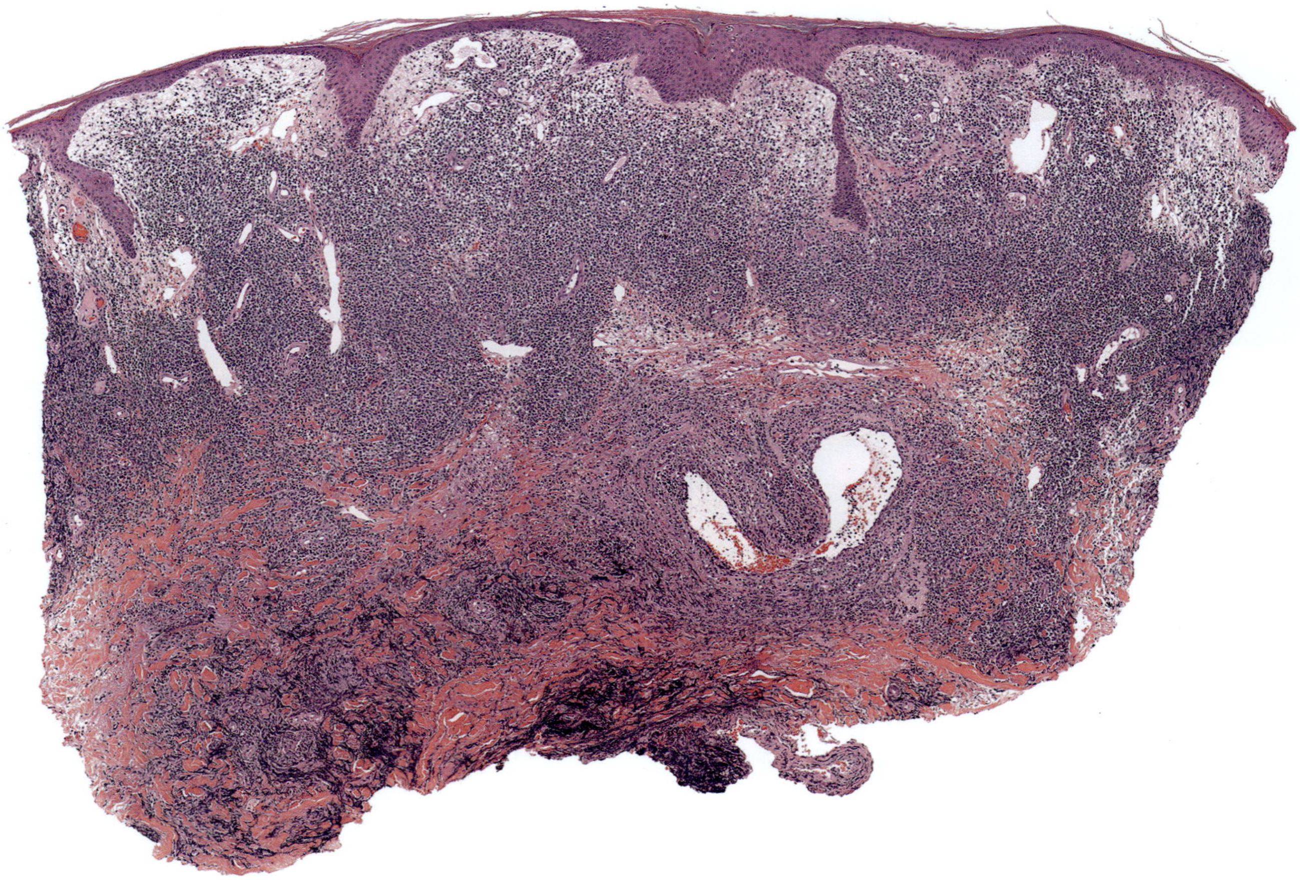

**Figure 26.12** Cutaneous T-lymphoblastic lymphoma. Dense, diffuse dermal infiltrate. Note the absence of a "starry sky" pattern.

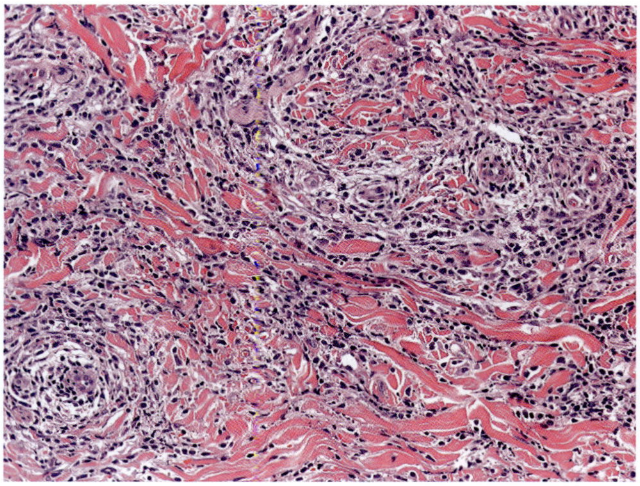

Figure 26.13 Cutaneous T-lymphoblastic lymphoma. Infiltrating cells dissecting the collagen bundles with some "Indian filing."

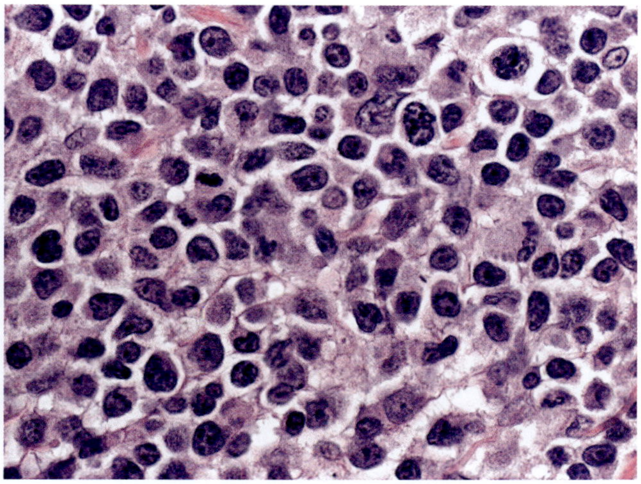

Figure 26.14 Cutaneous T-lymphoblastic lymphoma. Predominance of medium-sized cells. Note pleomorphic nuclei and less monomorphous appearance than in B-lymphoblastic lymphoma.

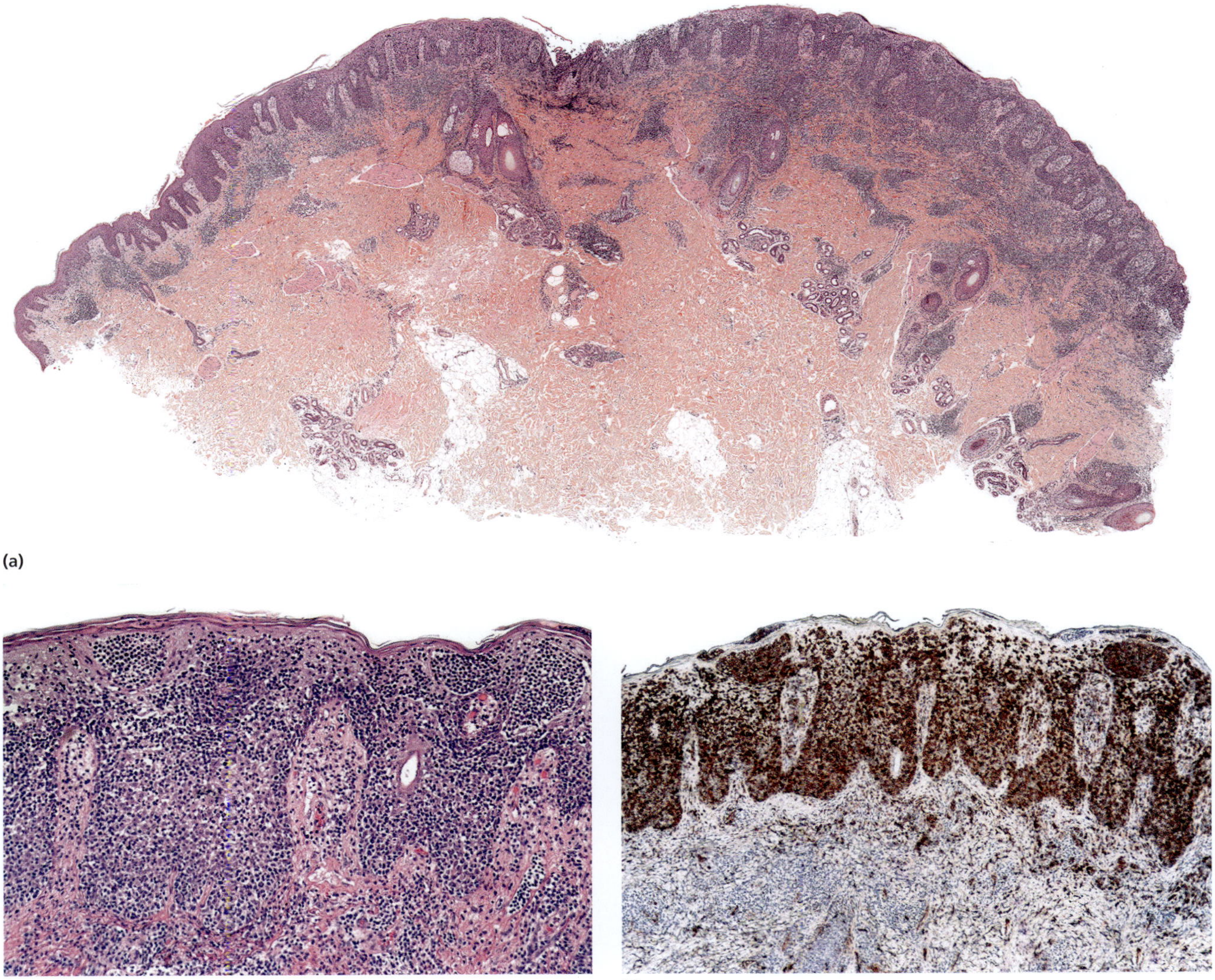

(a)

(b)

(c)

Figure 26.15 Cutaneous T-lymphoblastic lymphoma. (a) Dense, mainly superficial lymphoid infiltrates with (b) prominent acanthosis and marked epidermotropism indistinguishable from pagetoid reticulosis. (c) Neoplastic cells are positive for CD34.

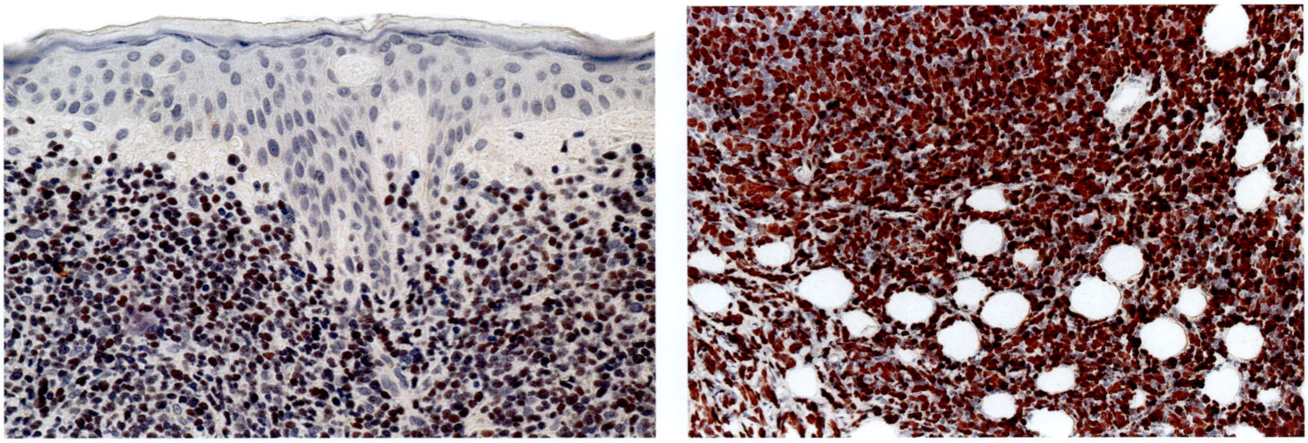


**Figure 26.16** Cutaneous T-lymphoblastic lymphoma. (a) Positive nuclear staining for TdT. (b) Almost all cells are positive for Ki-67.

## References


1. Chimenti S, Fink-Puches R, Peris K, *et al*. Cutaneous involvement in lymphoblastic lymphoma. *J Cut Pathol* 1999;**26**:379–385.
2. Vezzoli P, Novara F, Fanoni D, *et al*. Three cases of primary cutaneous lymphoblastic lymphoma: microarray-based comparative genomic hybridization and gene expression profiling studies with review of literature. *Leuk Lymphoma* 2012;**53**:1978–1987.
3. Sander CA, Medeiros LJ, Abruzzo LV, *et al*. Lymphoblastic lymphoma presenting in cutaneous sites: a clinicopathologic analysis of six cases. *J Am Acad Dermatol* 1991;**25**:1023–1031.
4. Schmitt IM, Manente L, Di Matteo A, *et al*. Lymphoblastic lymphoma of the pre-B phenotype with cutaneous presentation. *Dermatology* 1997;**195**:289–292.
5. Trupiano JK, Bringelsen K, Hsi E. Primary cutaneous lymphoblastic lymphoma presenting in an 8-week old infant. *J Cutan Pathol* 2002;**29**:107–112.
6. Grümayer ER, Ladenstein RL, Slavc I, *et al*. B-cell differentiation pattern of cutaneous lymphomas in infancy and childhood. *Cancer* 1988;**61**:303–308.
7. Kamps WA, Poppema S. Pre-B-cell non-Hodgkin's lymphoma in childhood. *Am J Clin Pathol* 1988;**90**:103–107.
8. Kim JY, Kim YC, Lee ES. Precursor B-cell lymphoblastic lymphoma involving the skin. *J Cutan Pathol* 2006;**33**:649–653.
9. Choi JE, Ahn H, Kye YC, Kim SN. Precursor B-cell lymphoblastic lymphoma presenting as solitary infiltrative plaque in a child. *Acta Derm Venereol (Stockh)* 2008;**88**:282–284.
10. Kawakami T, Kimura S, Kinoshita A, *et al*. Precursor B-cell lymphoblastic lymphoma with only cutaneous involvement. *Acta Derm Venereol* 2009;**89**:540–541.
11. Boccara O, Laloum-Grynberg E, Jeudy G, *et al*. Cutaneous B-cell lymphoblastic lymphoma in children: a rare diagnosis. *J Am Acad Dermatol* 2012;**66**:51–57.
12. Kahwash SB, Qualman SJ. Cutaneous lymphoblastic lymphoma in children: report of six cases with precursor B-cell lineage. *Pediatr Dev Pathol* 2002;**5**:45–53.
13. WHO Classification of Tumours Editorial Board. *Haematolymphoid Tumours*. 5th edition. Lyon (France): IARC, 2024.
14. Duffield A, Borowitz MJ, Cherian S, *et al*. B-lymphoblastic lekemias/lymphomas. In: Arber DA, Borowitz MJ, Cook JR, *et al*., eds. *The International Consensus Classification of Myeloid and Lymphoid Neoplasms*. Philadelphia (US): Wolters Kluwer, 2025: 289–314.
15. Duffield A, Borowitz MJ, Cherian S, *et al*. T-lymphoblastic lekemias/lymphomas. In: Arber DA, Borowitz MJ, Cook JR, *et al*., eds. *The International Consensus Classification of Myeloid and Lymphoid Neoplasms*. Philadelphia (US): Wolters Kluwer, 2025: 315–322.
16. Behdad A, Allen P, Lu X, *et al*. Cutaneous T-cell lymphoma, a novel manifestation of PDGFRA-rearranged neoplasm. *Am J Dermatopathol* 2018;**40**:610–613.
17. Wood BL, Akkary Y, Gujral S. B-lymphoblastic leukaemias/lymphomas: introduction. In: *WHO Classification of Tumours Editorial Board. Haematolymphoid Tumours*. 5th edition. Lyon (France): IARC, 2024: 328–329.
18. Maitra A, McKenna RW, Weinberg AG, *et al*. Precursor B-cell lymphoblastic lymphoma. A study of nine cases lacking blood and bone marrow involvement and review of the literature. *Am J Clin Pathol* 2001;**115**:868–875.
19. Lin P, Jones D, Dorfman DM, Medeiros LJ. Precursor B-cell lymphoblastic lymphoma: a predominantly extranodal tumor with low propensity for leukemic involvement. *Am J Surg Pathol* 2000; **24**:1480–1490.
20. Yen A, Sanchez R, Oblender M, Raimer S. Leukemia cutis: Darier's sign in a neonate with acute lymphoblastic leukemia. *J Am Acad Dermatol* 1996;**34**:375–378.
21. Shafer D, Wu H, Al-Saleem T, *et al*. Cutaneous precursor B-cell lymphoblastic lymphoma in 2 adult patients. Clinicopathologic and molecular cytogenetic studies with a review of the literature. *Arch Dermatol* 2008;**144**:1155–1162.
22. Papalas JA, McKinney MS, Kulbacki E, *et al*. Merkel cell carcinoma with partial B-cell blastic immunophenotype: a potential mimic of cutaneous Richter transformation in a patient with chronic lymphocytic lymphoma. *Am J Dermatopathol* 2014;**36**:148–152.
23. Bontoux C, de Masson A, Boccara O, *et al*. Outcome and clinicophenotypical features of acute lymphoblastic leukemia/lymphoblastic lymphoma with cutaneous involvement: a multicenter case series. *J Am Acad Dermatol* 2020;**83**:1166–1170.

24. Czader M, Miles RR, Chandy M, *et al.* T-lymphoblastic leukaemia/lymphoma NOS. In: *WHO Classification of Tumours Editorial Board. Haematolymphoid Tumours.* 5th edition. Lyon (France): IARC, 2024: 651–655.
25. Najem N, Zadeh VB, Badawi M, *et al.* Aleukemic leukemia cutis in a child preceding T-cell acute lymphoblastic leukemia. *Pediatr Dermatol* 2011;**28**:535–537.
26. van Zuuren EJ, Wintzen M, Jansen PM, Willemze R. Aleukaemic leukaemia cutis in a patient with acute T-cell lymphoblastic leukaemia. *Clin Exp Dermatol* 2003;**28**:330–332.
27. Nascimbeni C, Chantepie S, Brugiere C, *et al.* Cutaneous involvement in T-lymphoblastic lymphoma. *Ann Dermatol Venereol* 2017;**144**:268–274.
28. Lee WJ, Moon HR, Won CH, *et al.* Precursor B- or T-lymphoblastic lymphoma presenting with cutaneous involvement: a series of 13 cases including 7 cases of cutaneous T-lymphoblastic lymphoma. *J Am Acad Dermatol* 2014;**70**:318–325.
29. Mansoori P, Taheri A, SS ON, Sangueza OP. T-lymphoblastic leukemia/lymphoma with annular skin rash and epidermotropism. *Am J Dermatopathol* 2018;**40**:676–678.
30. Leinweber B, Chott A, Kerl H, Cerroni L. Epidermotropic precursor T-cell lymphoma with highly aggressive clinical behavior simulating localized pagetoid reticulosis. *Am J Dermatopathol* 2007;**29**:392–394.

SECTION 5

# Cutaneous manifestations of other lymphomas and non-neoplastic cutaneous signs of systemic lymphomas

CHAPTER 27

# Cutaneous manifestations of Hodgkin lymphoma

Hodgkin lymphoma is a distinct malignant lymphoma characterized by the presence of neoplastic Reed–Sternberg cells in association with different patterns of reactive cells. In the World Health Organization (WHO), *Classification of Haematolymphoid Tumours* is subdivided into two distinct entities: classic Hodgkin lymphoma (about 90% of cases) and nodular lymphocyte predominant Hodgkin lymphoma (about 10% of cases) (this last probably representing a variant of mature B-cell non-Hodgkin lymphoma rather than of Hodgkin lymphoma, thus for this entity the term "nodular lymphocyte predominant B-cell lymphoma" has been added as a synonym in the WHO classification) [1]. In the International Consensus Classification (ICC) *of Myeloid and Lymphoid Neoplasms*, nodular lymphocyte-predominant B-cell lymphoma has been separated from classic Hodgkin lymphoma [2]. Classic Hodgkin lymphoma is traditionally classified into four subtypes: nodular sclerosis, mixed cellularity, lymphocyte-rich, and lymphocyte-depleted, but their prognostic value is no longer considered as relevant [1, 2]. The Epstein–Barr virus (EBV) is detected in a variable proportion of cases in all four subtypes of classic Hodgkin lymphoma, whereas is uncommon in nodular lymphocyte-predominant Hodgkin lymphoma.

Skin manifestations of nodal Hodgkin lymphoma were not uncommon in the past [3–8]. Modern treatment modalities have resulted in a dramatic decrease in cutaneous involvement, although occasional cases are still reported [9–11]. The incidence is probably less than 1%, but exact figures are missing. All types of classic Hodgkin lymphoma may present with specific skin manifestations; in a recent study on 25 patients, 15 of them (60%) had classic Hodgkin lymphoma not otherwise specified, 6 (24%) the nodular sclerosis type, 3 (12%) the mixed cellularity type, and 1 (4%) the lymphocyte depleted type [12]. In exceptional cases, the diagnosis of the underlying Hodgkin lymphoma is not known, and skin lesions represent the first clinical manifestation of the disease [13].

Besides specific involvement by neoplastic cells, as in all systemic lymphomas, the skin may be the site of nonspecific cutaneous manifestations, including various dermatoses and so-called "pruritus sine materia," among others (see Chapter 29). This last condition is a characteristic (albeit not pathognomonic) prodromic sign of the disease, and the diagnosis of Hodgkin lymphoma should always be considered when evaluating patients with chronic pruritus of unknown etiology.

Nodal Hodgkin lymphoma may be preceded by, concomitant with, or followed by other cutaneous lymphoproliferative disorders including mycosis fungoides, lymphomatoid papulosis, and anaplastic large-cell lymphoma (see also Chapters 3 and 5) [14–18]. Cases of Hodgkin lymphoma associated with granulomatous slack skin have also been described [19, 20]. These last may represent examples of mycosis fungoides-associated granulomatous slack skin in patients with Hodgkin lymphoma rather than true specific cutaneous manifestations of the disease. Similarly, the patient reported as having "follicular mucinosis" in association with Hodgkin lymphoma [21] may have had co-existent mycosis fungoides-associated follicular mucinosis. It must be underlined that many reports on the association of Hodgkin lymphoma and mycosis fungoides antedated the introduction of precise phenotypic and molecular studies. In this context, it may be possible that at least some of the reported cases represented examples of nodal anaplastic large-cell lymphoma or nodal involvement by mycosis fungoides rather than of genuine Hodgkin lymphoma. In exceptional cases, cutaneous cells of nodal Hodgkin lymphoma have been observed at the site of cutaneous inflammation [22] and at the site of mycosis fungoides [23], representing in this last case an example of cutaneous composite lymphoma.

Exclusively cutaneous relapse of Hodgkin lymphoma in patients who were treated for nodal disease and who are otherwise in complete remission should be regarded as highly unlikely. I have seen several such putative cases, all of them representing examples of cutaneous anaplastic large-cell lymphoma or of lymphomatoid papulosis. In publications on this subject, it is often impossible to ascertain whether the skin lesions did indeed represent specific cutaneous manifestations of Hodgkin lymphoma or not [24]. Treatment in these cases should be tailored to the cutaneous disease, as skin lesions in this particular setting are most likely unrelated to the nodal Hodgkin lymphoma and do not represent a sign of relapse.

The onset of cutaneous manifestations of Hodgkin lymphoma has been observed in an human immunodeficiency virus (HIV)-infected patient [25] and nodal Hodgkin lymphoma may arise in the setting of immune suppression

*Skin Lymphoma: The Illustrated Guide*, Sixth Edition. Lorenzo Cerroni.

(see Chapter 21). Distinction from other EBV-associated lymphomas may be extremely difficult in that setting.

## Clinical features

Clinically, skin lesions in Hodgkin lymphoma are usually confined to the drainage area of affected lymph nodes (retrograde lymphatic spread) [7, 26]. Papules, plaques, and tumors may all be observed (Figs. 27.1 and 27.2) [26, 27]. Ulceration is not uncommon. In some cases, lesions are generalized.

## Histopathology, immunophenotype, and molecular genetics

Histology shows the typical features of Hodgkin lymphoma with Reed–Sternberg and Hodgkin cells on a diffuse background of small lymphocytes, histiocytes, eosinophils, and plasma cells

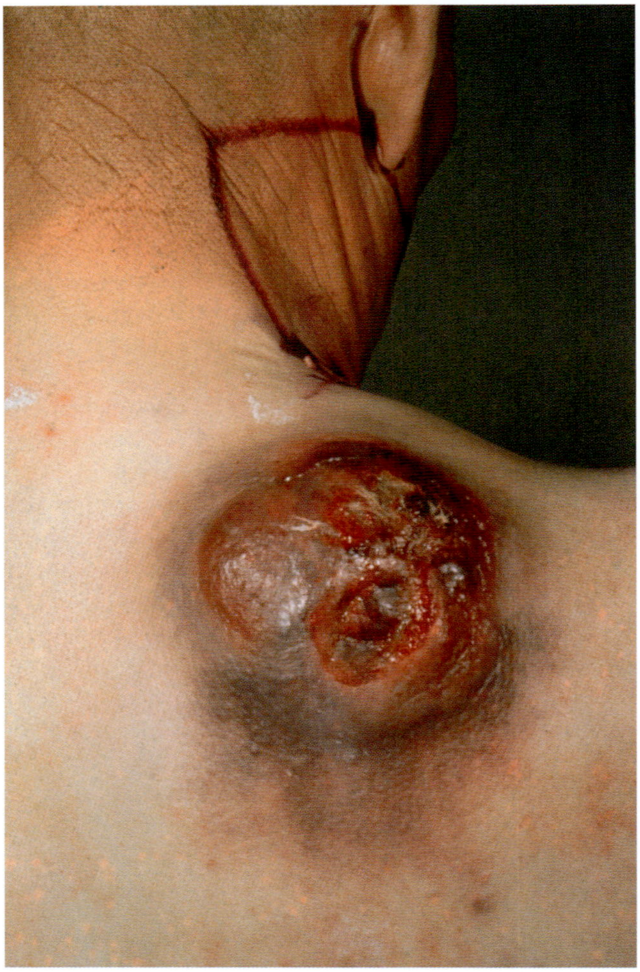

Figure 27.1 Cutaneous Hodgkin lymphoma. Large ulcerated tumor on the right shoulder.

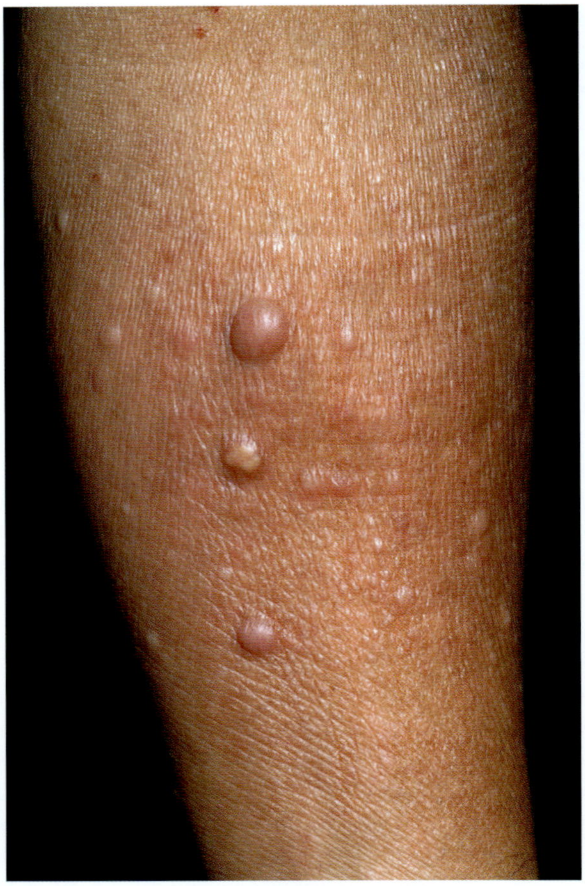

Figure 27.2 Cutaneous Hodgkin lymphoma. Several papules and small nodules in the drainage area of an affected lymph node.

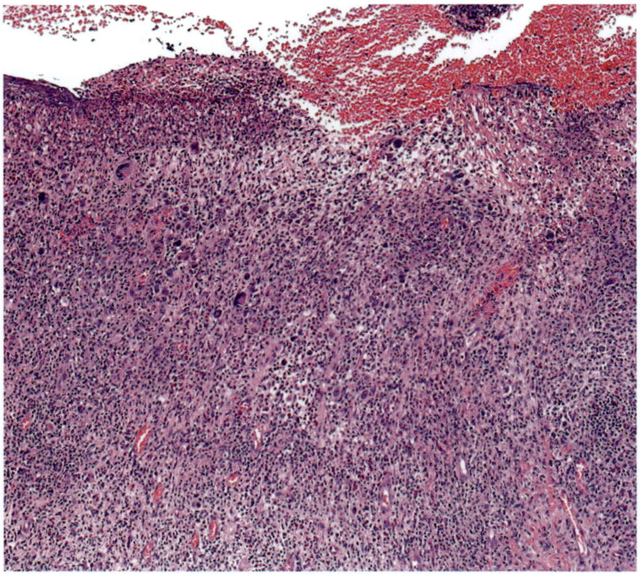

Figure 27.3 Cutaneous Hodgkin lymphoma. Ulcerated epidermis and sheets of cells in the dermis. Note large atypical cells.

(Figs. 27.3 and 27.4) [26]. Reed–Sternberg cells may be absent in some cutaneous lesions. It should be noted that Hodgkin and Reed–Sternberg-like cells may be found in a variety of other conditions including mainly lymphomatoid papulosis and cutaneous anaplastic large-cell lymphoma, and thus cannot be considered specific for the diagnosis of cutaneous Hodgkin lymphoma. The presence of mummified cells (cells with condensed cytoplasm and pyknotic eosinophilic or basophilic nuclei) represents a diagnostic clue [28] (Fig. 27.4c).

In the lymph nodes, neoplastic cells in nodular lymphocyte-predominant Hodgkin lymphoma are positive for CD45, CD20, CD79a, and Bcl-6. CD30, and CD15 are usually negative in this subtype. A diagnosis of specific skin manifestations in this subtype of Hodgkin lymphoma may be very subjective and can only be made upon knowledge of nodal disease, as distinction from a cutaneous "Hodgkin-like" follicle center lymphoma and from T-cell/histiocyte-rich B-cell lymphoma may be impossible (see Chapters 13 and 17).

In classic Hodgkin lymphoma, which represent about 90% of all cases, Reed–Sternberg and Hodgkin cells are always positive for CD30 (Fig. 27.5a). The small lymphocytes are of both B- and T-cell lineages.

In the four subtypes of classic Hodgkin lymphoma neoplastic cells in the lymph nodes are only rarely positive for CD20 or CD79a. Staining for CD15 is usually positive in a proportion of the cells in the lymph nodes, but it may be negative in cutaneous lesions (Fig. 27.5b) [26, 29]. Paired box gene (PAX)-5 is almost always positive in these subtypes, although sometimes with a weak staining pattern, confirming differentiation toward the B-cell lineage. Positivity for EBER-1 and PAX-5 can also be observed in specific cutaneous lesions (Figs. 27.5c and d), representing a good clue for differentiation of cutaneous classical Hodgkin lymphoma from other CD30+ T-cell lymphomas [30]. However, it must be underlined that in the lymph nodes, EBER-1 positivity is found only in a subset of cases (particularly in lymphocyte-depleted and mixed cellularity classic Hodgkin lymphoma). MUM-1 expression is also observed in neoplastic cells, but positivity cannot be used for differentiation of Hodgkin lymphoma from simulators of it, as both lymphomatoid papulosis and cutaneous anaplastic large-cell lymphoma are commonly positive. Zeta-chain-associated protein kinase 70 (ZAP-70), a protein that is part of the T-cell receptor, is positive in the majority of cases of anaplastic large-cell lymphoma, but is consistently negative in Reed–Sternberg and Hodgkin cells of classic Hodgkin lymphoma [31]. Oct-2 and BOB.1, two markers that are usually strongly expressed in diffuse large B-cell lymphoma, are only focally and/or weakly expressed in cutaneous cases of classic Hodgkin lymphoma [30].

There are no molecular data on specific cutaneous manifestations of Hodgkin lymphoma. In the classic type, molecular analyses on microdissected Reed–Sternberg cells reveal clonal rearrangements of the immunoglobulin genes (molecular analyses of the entire biopsy specimen usually fail to reveal any clonality).

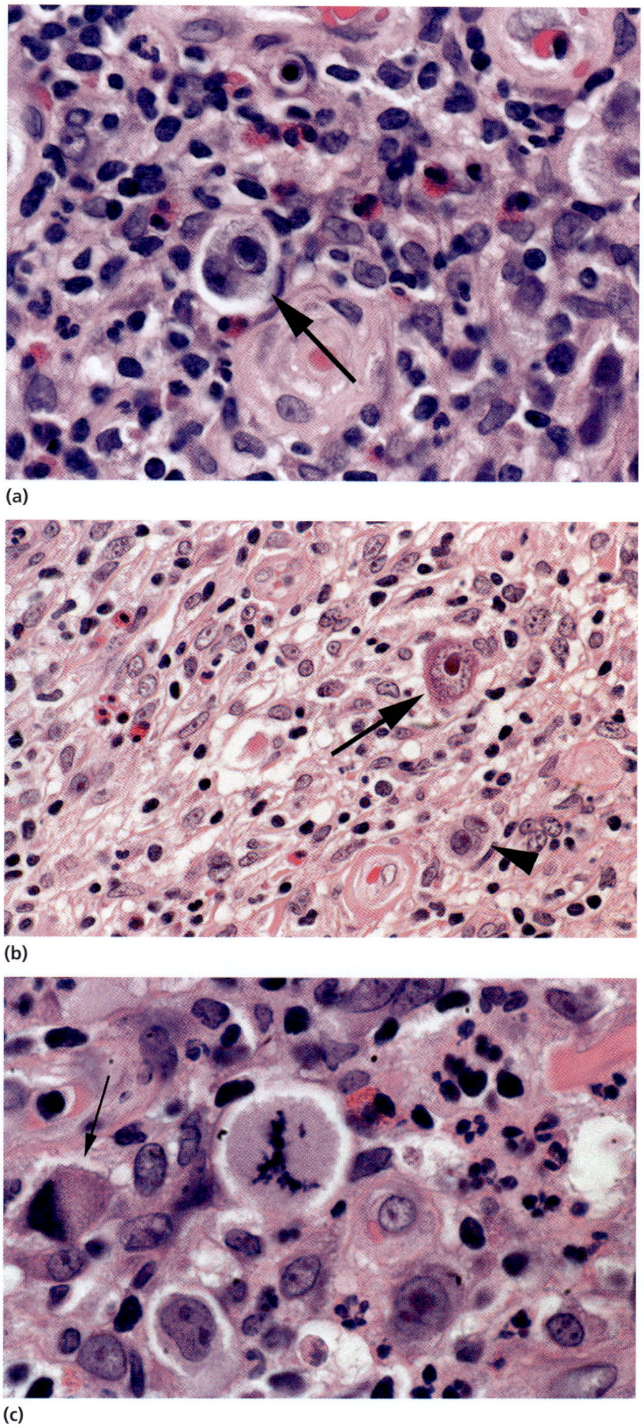


**Figure 27.4** Cutaneous Hodgkin lymphoma. (a) Reed–Sternberg cell (arrow) on the background of small lymphocytes, histiocytes, and eosinophils. (b) Large Hodgkin cell with eosinophilic nucleolus (arrow) admixed with small lymphocytes, histiocytes, and eosinophils. Note a Reed–Sternberg cell (arrowhead). (c) A large, atypical mitosis and a mummified cell (arrow), as well as large, atypical cells on the background of small lymphocytes, histiocytes, and neutrophils.

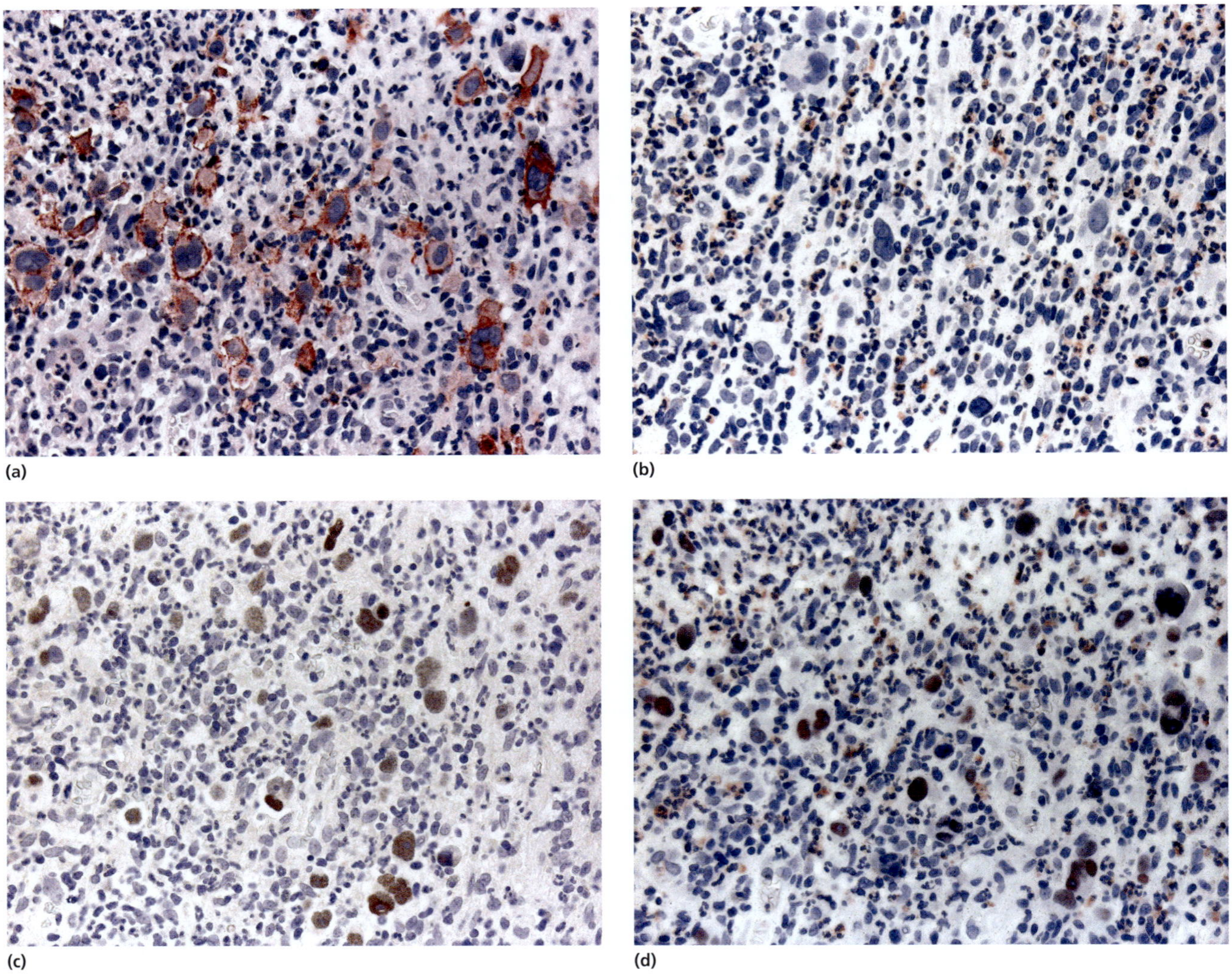

Figure 27.5 Cutaneous Hodgkin lymphoma. (a) Positivity of the large cells for CD30; (b) negativity for CD15; (c) positivity for EBV (EBER-1); and (d) for PAX-5.

## Treatment and prognosis

Patients with specific cutaneous manifestations of Hodgkin lymphoma should be treated in a hematologic setting according to schemes tailored for the underlying disease. In the past, the prognosis for patients with skin manifestations of nodal Hodgkin lymphoma was poor in spite of aggressive treatment. Modern treatment modalities have resulted in a steady decline in the onset of specific skin manifestations, but cutaneous involvement has been reported rarely, even after successful allogeneic stem cell transplantation [9]. Since only occasional patients present with cutaneous involvement, there is little information on which to base both prognostic evaluation and therapeutic options. However, cutaneous Hodgkin lymphoma usually represents advanced (stage IV) disease and carries a bad prognosis. One case responded well to treatment [30]. Radiotherapy can be used to treat solitary or localized skin tumors.

As already mentioned, patients with "primary cutaneous" Hodgkin lymphoma most likely have lymphomatoid papulosis or cutaneous anaplastic large-cell lymphoma, and thus should be managed conservatively with treatment modalities used for these conditions. One case with a phenotype strongly suggestive of primary cutaneous Hodgkin lymphoma responded to treatment with ABVD chemotherapy (doxorubicin, bleomycin, vinblastine, and dacarbazine) [32].

## Primary cutaneous Hodgkin lymphoma

Rare cases of Hodgkin lymphoma presenting primarily in the skin without concomitant nodal disease have been described, even in recent years [32–37]. Although some of these cases may indeed represent a primary cutaneous Hodgkin lymphoma, particularly those reported in the past, in my opinion, represent examples of lymphomatoid papulosis or cutaneous anaplastic large-cell lymphoma (Fig. 27.6). Although it cannot be excluded that in exceptional cases Hodgkin lymphoma arises primary in the skin without concomitant extracutaneous disease, on a practical level such a diagnosis should not be accepted unless alternative explanations can be ruled out by compelling evidence.

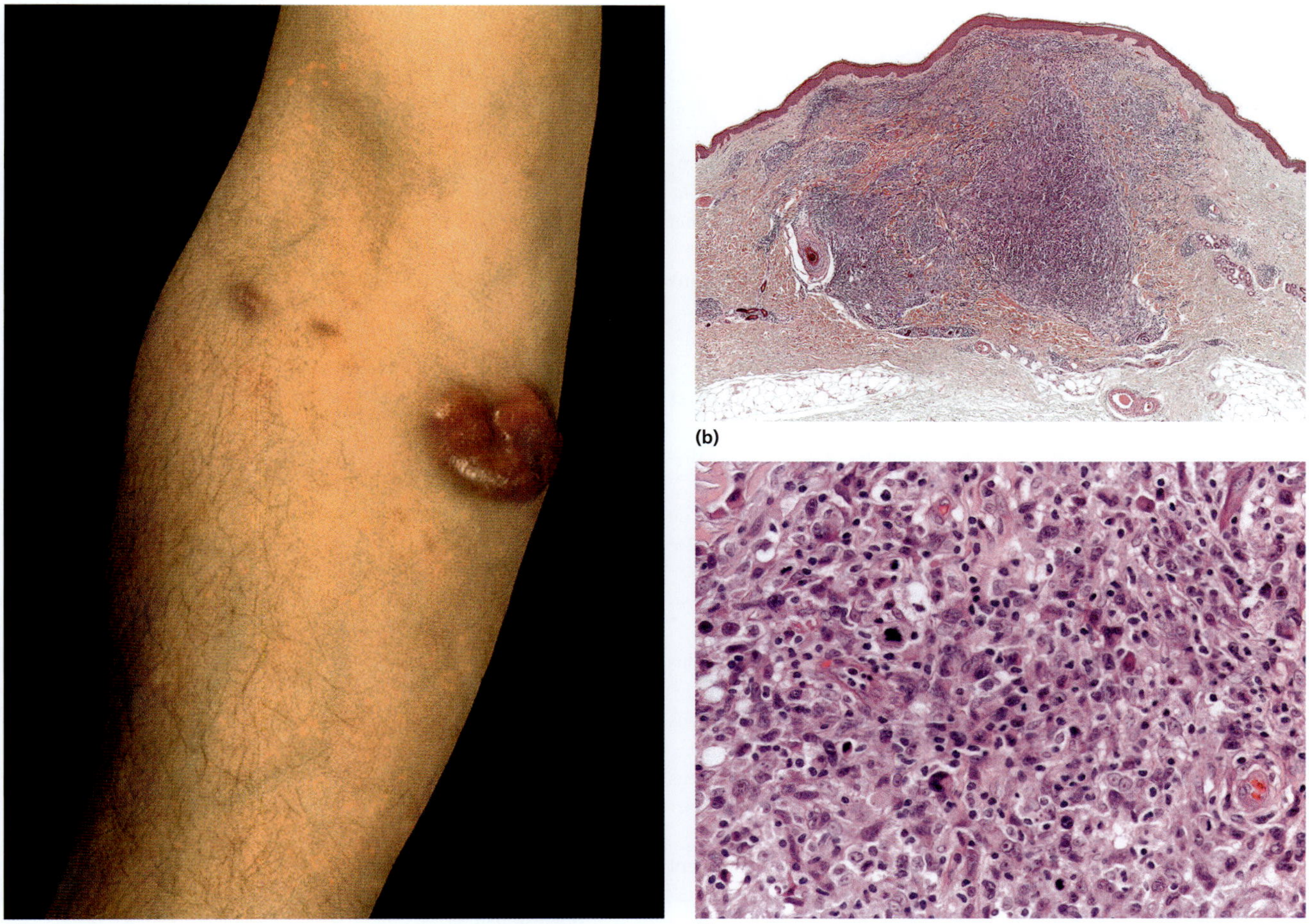

(a) (b) (c)

**Figure 27.6** Lymphomatoid papulosis previously reported as primary cutaneous Hodgkin lymphoma [33]. (a) Large, reddish-brown tumor and a few smaller papules on the right forearm. (b) Histology shows nodular lymphoid infiltrates with (c) Reed–Sternberg-like and Hodgkin-like cells. The patient subsequently developed several new papules and nodules on the same arm over a period of >20 years, always with similar histopathologic features and without systemic involvement ("regional" lymphomatoid papulosis).

**Résumé**

**Cutaneous manifestations of Hodgkin lymphoma**

| | | |
|---|---|---|
| **Clinical** | Adults. Solitary, grouped, or rarely, generalized cutaneous papules, plaques, and tumors. Lesions are commonly located at the drainage area of affected lymph nodes. "Primary" cutaneous cases are exceedingly rare; such a diagnosis should not be accepted unless alternative explanations can be ruled out by compelling evidence. | |
| **Morphology** | Nodular or diffuse infiltrates characterized by the presence of Reed–Sternberg and Hodgkin cells on a background of small lymphocytes, histiocytes, neutrophils, and eosinophils. "Mummified" cells. | |
| **Immunohistochemistry (neoplastic cells)** | CD30 | + |
| | CD15 | +/– |
| | PAX-5 | + (rarely –) |
| | EBER-1 | +/– |
| | MUM-1 | + |
| | CD19, CD20, CD79a | –/+ |
| | BOB.1, Oct-2 | (–) |
| | ZAP-70 | – |
| **Genetics** | Data on molecular features of specific skin manifestations are not available. | |
| **Treatment guidelines (skin lesions)** | Treatment is planned on the basis of the underlying disease. Radiotherapy of isolated skin tumors. | |

## References


1. De Jong D, Gujral S. Hodgkin lymphoma: introduction. In: *WHO Classification of Tumours Editorial Board. Haematolymphoid Tumours*. 5th edition. Lyon (France): IARC, 2024: 579.
2. Brousset P, Ansell SM, LaCasce A, *et al*. Classic Hodgkin lymphoma. In: Arber DA, Borowitz MJ, Cook JR, *et al*., eds. *The International Consensus Classification of Myeloid and Lymphoid Neoplasms*. Philadelphia (US): Wolters Kluwer, 2025: 573–585.
3. Gordon RA, Lookingbill DP, Abt AB. Skin infiltration in Hodgkin's disease. *Arch Dermatol* 1980;**116**:1038–1040.
4. Silverman CL, Strayer DS, Wasserman TH. Cutaneous Hodgkin's disease. *Arch Dermatol* 1982;**118**:918–921.
5. Smith JL, Butler JJ. Skin involvement in Hodgkin's disease. *Cancer* 1980;**45**:354–361.
6. White RM, Patterson JW. Cutaneous involvement in Hodgkin's disease. *Cancer* 1985;**55**:1136–1145.
7. Benninghoff DL, Medina A, Alexander LL, Camiel MR. The mode of spread of Hodgkin's disease to the skin. *Cancer* 1970;**26**: 1135–1140.
8. Tassies D, Sierra J, Montserrat E, *et al*. Specific cutaneous involvement in Hodgkin's disease. *Hematol Oncol* 1992;**10**:75–79.
9. Introcaso CE, Kantor J, Porter DL, Junkins-Hopkins JM. Cutaneous Hodgkin's disease. *J Am Acad Dermatol* 2008;**58**:295–298.
10. Dhull AK, Soni A, Kaushal V. Hodgkin's lymphoma with cutaneous involvement. *BMJ Case Rep* 2012. doi: 10.1136/bcr-2012-007599.
11. Gru AA, Lu D. Concurrent malignant melanoma and cutaneous involvement by classical Hodgkin lymphoma (CHL) in a 63 year-old man. *Diagn Pathol* 2013;**8**:135.
12. Gru AA, Bacchi CE, Pulitzer M, *et al*. Secondary skin involvement in classic Hodgkin lymphoma: results of an international collaborative cutaneous lymphoma working group study of 25 patients. *J Cutan Pathol* 2021;**48**:1367–1378.
13. Goyal A, Casillo C, Narayanan D, *et al*. Initial diagnosis of classic Hodgkin lymphoma with skin biopsy: a rare case and review of diagnostic considerations. *Am J Dermatopathol* 2023;**45**:577–581.
14. Caya JG, Choi H, Tieu TM, *et al*. Hodgkin's disease followed by mycosis fungoides in the same patient: case report and review of the literature. *Cancer* 1984;**53**:463–467.
15. Clement M, Bhakri H, Monk B, *et al*. Mycosis fungoides and Hodgkin's disease. *J R Soc Med* 1984;**77**:1037–1038.
16. Davis TH, Morton CC, Miller-Cassman R, *et al*. Hodgkin's disease, lymphomatoid papulosis, and cutaneous T-cell lymphoma derived from a common T-cell clone. *N Engl J Med* 1992;**326**:1115–1122.
17. Hawkins KA, Schinella R, Schwartz M, *et al*. Simultaneous occurrence of mycosis fungoides and Hodgkin disease. *Am J Hematol* 1983;**14**:355–362.
18. Simrell CR, Boccia RV, Longo DL, Jaffe ES. Coexisting Hodgkin's disease and mycosis fungoides. *Arch Pathol Lab Med* 1986;**110**:1029–1034.
19. DeGregorio R, Fenske NA, Glass LF. Granulomatous slack skin: a possible precursor of Hodgkin's disease. *J Am Acad Dermatol* 1995;**33**:1044–1047.
20. Noto G, Pravatà G, Miceli S, Aricò M. Granulomatous slack skin: report of a case associated with Hodgkin's disease and a review of the literature. *Br J Dermatol* 1994;**131**:275–279.
21. Stewart M, Smoller BR. Follicular mucinosis in Hodgkin's disease: a poor prognostic sign? *J Am Acad Dermatol* 1991;**24**:784–785.
22. Facheris P, Valenti M, Pavia G, *et al*. Specific infiltrate of Hodgkin lymphoma at site of cellulitis mimicking secondary cutaneous involvement. *J Cutan Pathol* 2020;**47**:462–465.
23. Chen Y, Nong L, Li X, Wang Y. Cutaneous composite lymphoma of mycosis fungoides and Hodgkin lymphoma: response to sequential therapy. *J Cutan Pathol* 2020;**47**:829–833.
24. Jurisic V, Bogunovic M, Colovic N, Colovic M. Indolent course of the cutaneous Hodgkin's disease. *J Cutan Pathol* 2005;**32**:176–178.
25. Shaw MT, Jacobs SR. Cutaneous Hodgkin's disease in a patient with human immunodeficiency virus infection. *Cancer* 1989; **64**:2585–2587.
26. Cerroni L, Beham-Schmid C, Kerl H. Cutaneous Hodgkin's disease: an immunohistochemical analysis. *J Cutan Pathol* 1995; **22**:229–235.
27. Hayes TG, Rabin VR, Rosen T, Zubler MA. Hodgkin's disease presenting in the skin: case report and review of the literature. *J Am Acad Dermatol* 1990;**22**:944–947.
28. Kastnerova L, Belousova IE, Hadravsky L, *et al*. Mummified cells are a common finding in cutaneous Hodgkin lymphoma and can be used as a diagnostic clue. *Am J Dermatopathol* 2020;**42**:24–28.
29. Moretti S, Pimpinelli N, Di Lollo S, *et al*. In situ immunologic characterization of cutaneous involvement in Hodgkin's disease. *Cancer* 1989;**63**:661–666.
30. Cho RJ, McCalmont TH, Ai WZ, *et al*. Use of an expanded immunohistochemical panel to distinguish cutaneous Hodgkin lymphoma from histopathologic imitators. *J Cutan Pathol* 2012;**39**:651–658.
31. Admirand JH, Rassidakis GZ, Abruzzo LV, *et al*. Immunohistochemical detection of ZAP-70 in 341 cases of non-Hodgkin and Hodgkin lymphoma. *Mod Pathol* 2004; **17**:954–961.
32. Huong G, Olson LC, Rippis GE, Magro CM. An index case of cutaneous Hodgkin lymphoma and review of the literature. *Am J Dermatopathol* 2016;**38**:739–743.
33. Sioutos N, Kerl H, Murphy SB, Kadin ME. Primary cutaneous Hodgkin disease: unique clinical, morphologic and immunophenotypic findings. *Am J Dermatopathol* 1994;**16**:2–8.
34. Kumar S, Kingma DW, Weiss WB, *et al*. Primary cutaneous Hodgkin's disease with evolution to systemic disease: association with Epstein–Barr virus. *Am J Surg Pathol* 1996;**20**:754–759.
35. Guitart J, Fretzin D. Skin as the primary site of Hodgkin's disease: a case report of primary cutaneous Hodgkin's disease and review of its relationship with non-Hodgkin's lymphoma. *Am J Dermatopathol* 1998;**20**:218–222.
36. Pranteda G, Osti MF, Cox MC, *et al*. Primary cutaneous Hodgkin lymphoma. *J Am Acad Dermatol* 2010;**62**:e52–e53.
37. Mukesh M, Shuttleworth D, Murray P. Primary cutaneous Hodgkin's lymphoma. *Clin Exp Dermatol* 2009;**34**:e673–e675.

CHAPTER 28

# Cutaneous composite lymphomas

Composite lymphomas are defined as two distinct subtypes of lymphoma occurring at a single anatomic site; in the case of the skin, two malignant lymphomas are found in one and the same biopsy specimen. According to this definition, a patient with a specific cutaneous infiltrate of B-cell chronic lymphocytic leukemia (B-CLL) within a lesion of mycosis fungoides has a composite lymphoma in that particular body area. On the other hand, a patient with both cutaneous follicle center lymphoma and mycosis fungoides at different cutaneous sites does not have a composite, but a concurrent lymphoma. In the same way, a patient with B-CLL in the blood and bone marrow and mycosis fungoides in the skin does not have a composite lymphoma (patients with more than one malignant lymphoma arising either sequentially or at the same time, but involving different sites, are well known, and are not considered as having a composite lymphoma). In this context, cases of mycosis fungoides, lymphomatoid papulosis, and cutaneous anaplastic large cell lymphoma, which may coexist in the same patient and rarely within the same lesion and show a clonal relationship [1], do not represent examples of composite lymphoma either. Concurrent lymphomas of the skin characterized by the onset of two different types of cutaneous lymphoma/lymphoproliferative disorder at different skin sites or at different times have been described [2]. True cutaneous composite lymphomas are exceedingly rare, and only a few examples have been reported (Table 28.1). Parenthetically, a primary cutaneous lymphoma with lymph node involvement may be part of a composite lymphoma within the lymph node [31].

Composite lymphomas are rarely found in other organs, particularly the lymph nodes, often involving Hodgkin lymphoma with different non-Hodgkin lymphoma types [32]. Two separate and distinct lymphoma types are necessary for the diagnosis of composite lymphoma: for example, a patient with follicular lymphoma with focal transformation into diffuse large B-cell lymphoma does not have a composite lymphoma. It must also be underlined that the molecular finding of two different clones *per se* does not define a composite lymphoma [33], and several cases reported as such represent in fact one lymphoma type with clonal diversity [22, 34].

Cutaneous composite lymphomas may reflect the presence of two distinct systemic lymphomas, or of one systemic lymphoma and one primary cutaneous lymphoma, or of two primary cutaneous lymphomas. One of the most frequent associations is between B-CLL and mycosis fungoides or Sézary syndrome [3–6]. This is not surprising, as B-CLL is the most common leukemia in Western countries, and often colonizes the skin at sites of cutaneous "inflammation," and mycosis fungoides is the most common cutaneous lymphoma. B-CLL has been observed also at the site of lymphomatoid papulosis [24], and of cutaneous follicle center lymphoma [6, 17–19]. A combination of mycosis fungoides with a $CD5^{+}$ small B-cell lymphoma without extracutaneous involvement has also been reported [7, 8].

Other combinations of distinct lymphoma entities in the same cutaneous biopsy showed variable associations of CD8-positive peripheral T-cell lymphoma and in situ follicular lymphoma, diffuse large B-cell lymphoma, leg-type and subcutaneous panniculitis-like T-cell lymphoma, peripheral T-cell lymphoma, not otherwise specified (NOS) and follicle center lymphoma, peripheral T-cell lymphoma, NOS and clonal plasma cell proliferation, secondary mantle cell and primary cutaneous anaplastic large cell lymphoma, secondary mantle cell lymphoma and primary cutaneous marginal zone lymphoproliferative disorder, mycosis fungoides and diffuse large B-cell lymphoma, leg-type, primary cutaneous anaplastic large cell lymphoma and primary cutaneous follicle center lymphoma, small lymphocytic lymphoma and primary cutaneous follicle center lymphoma, small-medium pleomorphic $CD4^{+}$ T-cell lymphoproliferative disorder and clonal plasma cell proliferation, and mycosis fungoides and Hodgkin lymphoma [6, 19, 21, 25, 27, 29].

In some cases, cutaneous composite lymphomas have been observed in the setting of immunodeficiency and/or in association with Epstein–Barr virus infection, particularly under treatment with methotrexate, representing a rare variant of the cutaneous lymphomas in immune deficiency/dysregulation [10, 11, 28, 30].

Finally, in a few instances, patients with cutaneous composite lymphomas had two distinct primary cutaneous lymphomas

*Skin Lymphoma: The Illustrated Guide*, Sixth Edition. Lorenzo Cerroni.

Table 28.1 Cases of cutaneous composite lymphoma observed at the Research Unit Dermatopathology of the Medical University of Graz (Austria) or reported in the literature (some of the cases reported in patients with immunodeficiency)

| References or institution | Type of composite lymphoma |
|---|---|
| [3–6], Graz | MF or Sèzary syndrome and B-CLL |
| [7, 8] | MF and primary cutaneous CD5$^+$ small B-cell lymphoma |
| [9] | MF and DLBCL |
| Graz | MF and EBV$^+$ DLBCL |
| [10–12], Graz | MF and primary cutaneous FCL |
| [13] | MF and Hodgkin lymphoma |
| [6, 14], Graz | MF and primary cutaneous MZLD |
| Graz | MF and splenic MZL |
| [15] | MF and low grade B-cell lymphoma with plasmacytic differentiation |
| [16] | MF and Hodgkin lymphoma |
| [6, 17–19] | Primary cutaneous FCL and B-CLL |
| [20] | Primary cutaneous FCL and PTCL-NOS |
| [21] | Primary cutaneous FCL and small lymphocytic lymphoma |
| [22] | Primary cutaneous FCL and ALCL |
| [23] | Primary cutaneous FCL and secondary cutaneous CD8$^+$ PTCL-NOS |
| [24] | Lymphomatoid papulosis and B-CLL |
| Dr. Kutzner, Friedrichshafen (Germany) | IVNK/TLCL and B-CLL |
| [9, 25] | SPTCL and DLBCL |
| [26] | Primary cutaneous ALCL and Mantle cell lymphoma |
| [27] | Mantle cell lymphoma and cutaneous MZLD |
| [28] | Primary cutaneous PTCL-NOS and EBV$^+$ DLBCL |
| [29] | Primary cutaneous PTCL-NOS and cMPCP |
| [30] | EBV$^+$ DLBCL and secondary PTCL-NOS |
| [29] | CD4$^+$SMTCLD and cMPCP |

***Legend:*** Graz: Research Unit Dermatopathology, Department of Dermatology, Medical University of Graz, Austria; MF: Mycosis fungoides; B-CLL: B-cell chronic lymphocytic leukemia; DLBCL: diffuse large B-cell lymphoma; EBV: Epstein–Barr virus; MZL: marginal zone lymphoma; MZLD: marginal zone lymphoproliferative disorder; FCL: follicle center lymphoma; PTCL-NOS: peripheral T-cell lymphoma, not otherwise specified; ALCL: anaplastic large cell lymphoma; IVNK/TLCL: intravascular NK/T-large cell lymphoma; SPTCL: subcutaneous panniculitis-like T-cell lymphoma; cMPCP: cutaneous monoclonal plasma cell proliferation; CD4$^+$SMTCLD: small-medium pleomorphic CD4$^+$ T-cell lymphoproliferative disorder

occurring at the same site (involving particularly mycosis fungoides as one of the two components), representing a pitfall in diagnosis and differential diagnosis from reactive infiltrates within mycosis fungoides [7, 9, 11, 12, 14–16, 28].

## Clinical features

Cutaneous composite lymphomas have been reported only in adult patients. The exact incidence is unknown; one study addressing cases of mycosis fungoides associated with B-cell malignancies reported the presence of a composite lymphoma in 2/398 patients [6]. Clinical features depend on the lymphoma entities involved. When mycosis fungoides represents one component of a cutaneous composite lymphoma, typical lesions of the disease are usually found (Fig. 28.1a).

The main pitfall in the clinical evaluation of cutaneous composite lymphomas, particularly when mycosis fungoides represents one of the two entities, is the possibility of upgrading the clinical stage to tumor stage. In fact, lesions are commonly nodular due to the presence of more lymphoma types, and only histopathological evaluation allows a precise diagnosis. Cutaneous composite lymphomas are usually characterized by a single lesion; that is, a patient with mycosis fungoides may develop a second lymphoma in one of the original lesions of mycosis fungoides. The main exception is represented by B-CLL colonizing mycosis fungoides, where neoplastic cells of both lymphomas may be seen at different cutaneous sites.

Staging investigations are mandatory in all cases of cutaneous composite lymphoma; however, staging investigations may be difficult to interpret, particularly if both lymphomas show extracutaneous manifestations.

## Histopathology, immunophenotype, and molecular genetics

Histopathological features of cutaneous composite lymphomas depend on the entities involved. It should be stressed that punch biopsies, shaving biopsies, or biopsies with crush, drying, or fixation artifacts do not allow a precise characterization of the infiltrate in these complicated cases, as the substrate may be missing in small, partial biopsies, and a precise correlation of

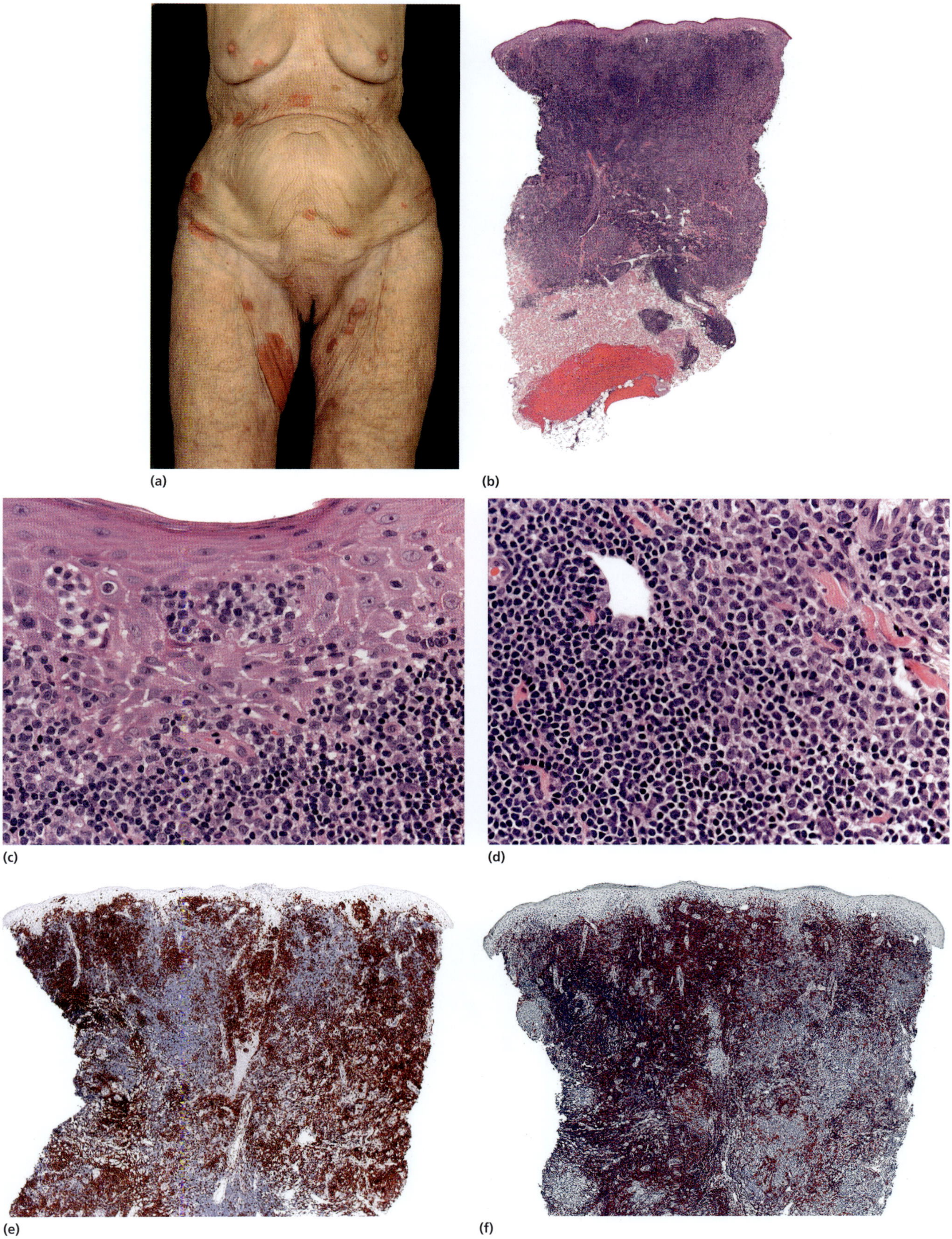

**Figure 28.1** Composite lymphoma consisting of mycosis fungoides and B-CLL. (a) 92-year-old woman with a history of B-CLL presenting with generalized cutaneous patches and plaques; (b) Dense lymphoid infiltrates within the entire dermis with (c) epidermotropism with formation of Darier's nests and (d) dermal infiltrate composed of small hyperchromatic lymphocytes admixed with nodules of medium-sized, pleomorphic cells; immunohistology shows (e) positivity for $CD3^{+}$ of most cells, including epidermotropic lymphocytes and medium-sized cells, and (f) positivity for CD20 of the small, hyperchromatic lymphocytes (which were also positive for CD23 and CD43), representing neoplastic cells of the known B-CLL.

phenotype with morphological features is not possible on specimens showing surgical artifacts (see also Chapter 1).

As mycosis fungoides commonly represents one of the two entities of cutaneous composite lymphomas, typical features of the disease with epidermotropic T-lymphocytes are detected in these cases (Figs. 28.1b and c). Neoplastic cells of the two lymphoma entities are usually at least partially intermingled (Fig. 28.1d), but epidermotropic cells usually correspond only to the T-cell counterpart. As cutaneous T-cell lymphomas may show aberrant expression of CD20, and as a B-cell reaction, sometimes with the formation of germinal centers, can be observed in mycosis fungoides and in other T-cell lymphomas [12], diagnosis of composite lymphomas is possible only with large panels of antibodies, and should be made only when unequivocal features of both lymphoma entities can be demonstrated. In this context, it should be reminded that populations of reactive lymphocytes are common in most low-grade and also in high-grade cutaneous lymphomas, and care should be taken not to misinterpret a florid inflammatory reaction for a second lymphoma.

The combination of B-CLL and mycosis fungoides is one of the most reported cutaneous composite lymphoma. In such cases, biopsy specimens reveal aspects of mycosis fungoides (epidermotropic, $CD4^+$ T lymphocytes) admixed with a B-cell component with an aberrant phenotype ($CD3^-$, $CD5^+$, $CD20^+$, $CD23^+$) (Figs. 28.1e and f). B-CLL can also be associated with other entities, and Dr. Kutzner (Friedrichshafen, Germany) showed me a unique case with coexisting intravascular NK/T-cell lymphoma (Fig. 28.2). In my experience, another common cutaneous composite lymphoma is characterized by the combination of mycosis fungoides and cutaneous marginal zone lymphoproliferative disorder. This last entity can be confirmed by the finding of a monoclonal population of lymphoplasmacytoid cells/plasma cells. Follicular lymphoma as a component of cutaneous composite lymphoma is identified by the presence of a population of $CD20^+/Bcl6^+/Bcl2^{-(+)}$ lymphocytes. As already discussed, care should be taken not to misinterpret reactive germinal centers as a cutaneous follicle center lymphoma, and morphological as well as molecular data must be used in conjunction with the phenotype in order to establish the diagnosis. Diffuse large B-cell lymphoma coexisting with mycosis fungoides is characterized by the typical histopathological picture of mycosis fungoides and by variably large, nodular-diffuse infiltrates of large cells with phenotypic features of diffuse large B-cell lymphoma (Fig. 28.3).

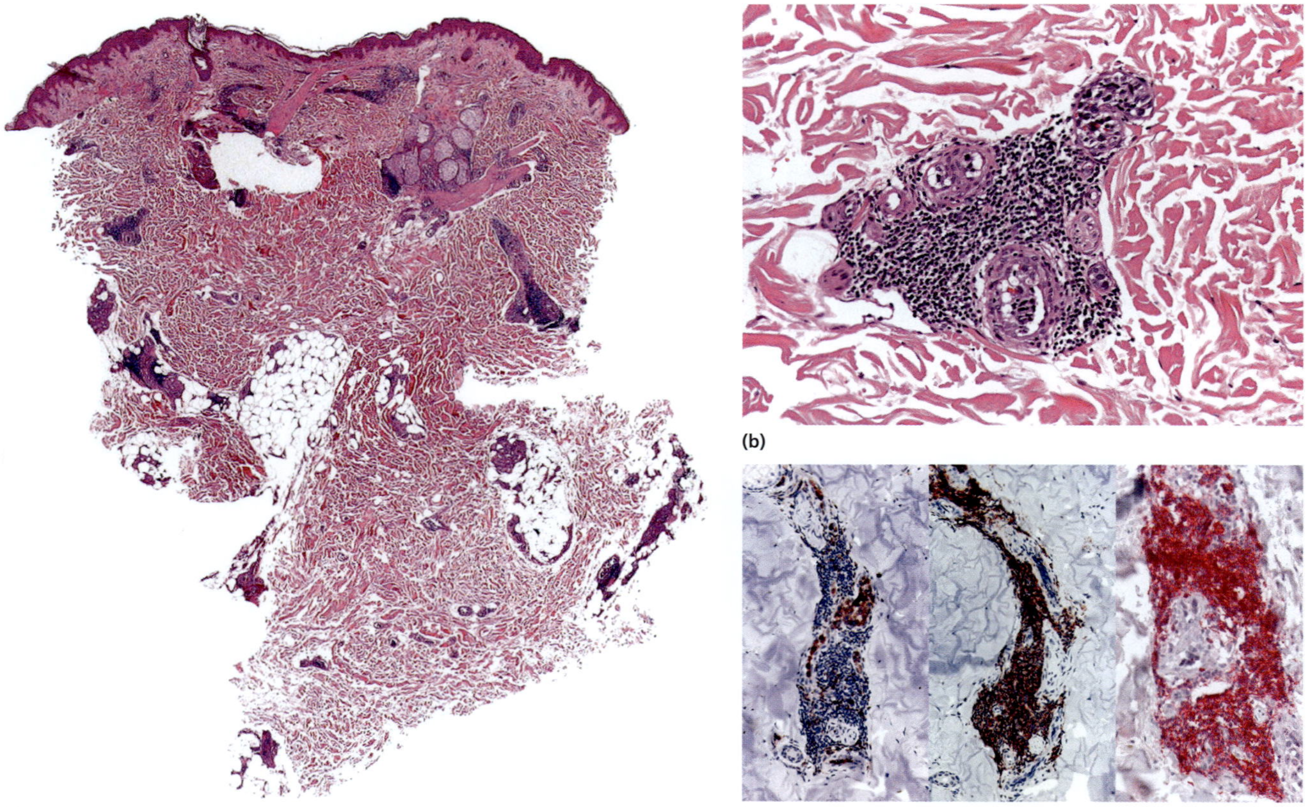

(a) (b) (c)

**Figure 28.2** Composite lymphoma consisting of B-CLL and intravascular NK/T-cell lymphoma. (a) Lymphoid infiltrates within the entire dermis and visible subcutaneous fat, consisting of (b) perivascular aggregates of small, hyperchromatic lymphocytes and intravascular large cells; immunohistology reveals (c, left) positivity of the intravascular cells for CD3; (c, middle) both intravascular and perivascular cells are positive for CD5, whereas (c, right) CD20 is only positive on the perivascular component of the infiltrate. (*Courtesy of Dr. Heinz Kutzner, Friedrichshafen, Germany.*)

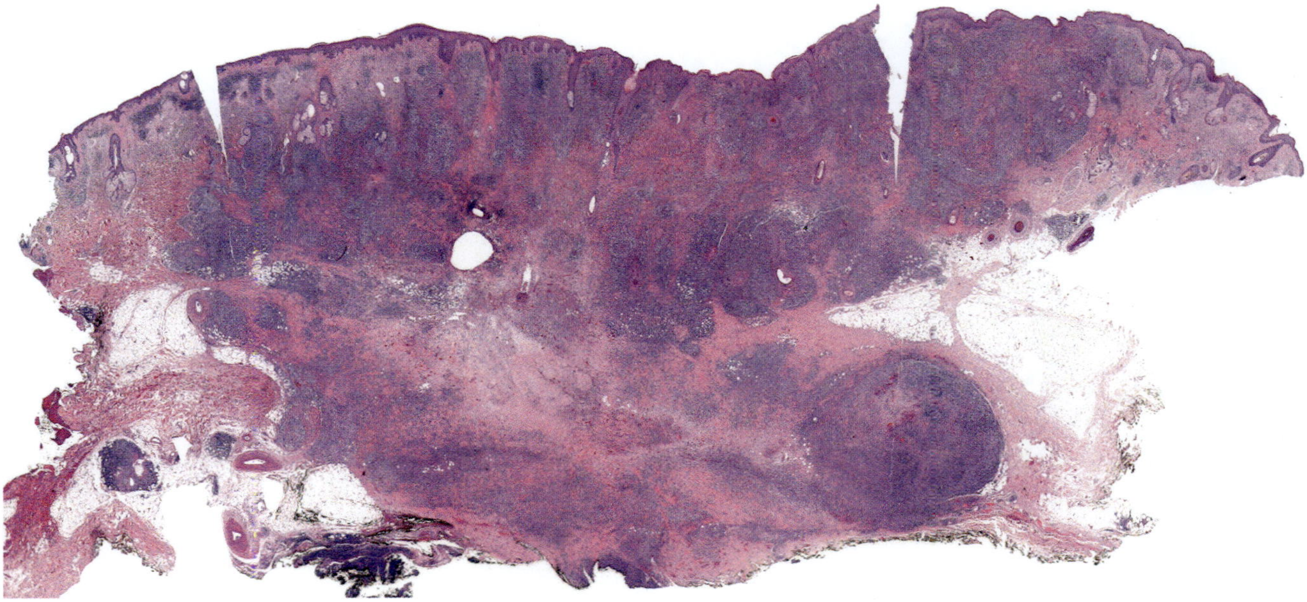

(a)

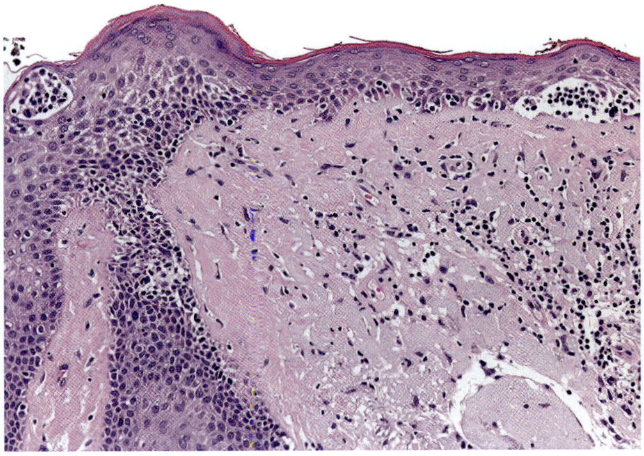

(b)

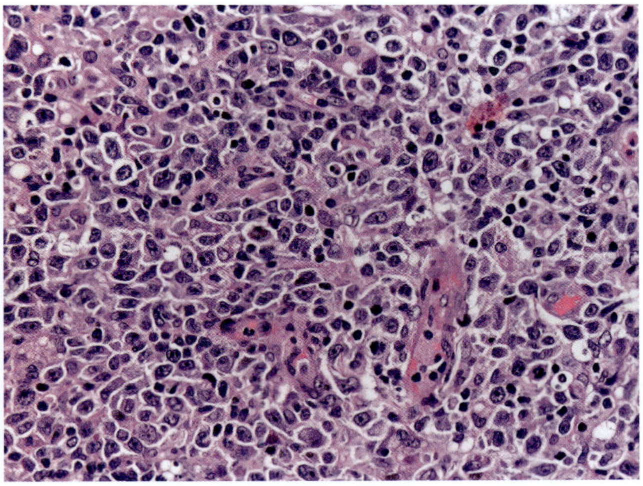

(c)

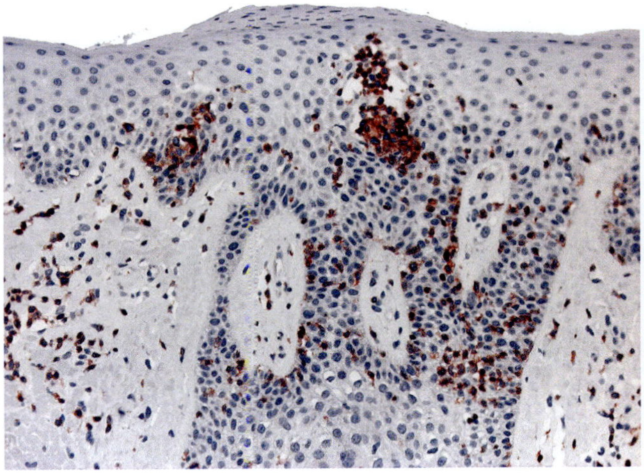

(d)

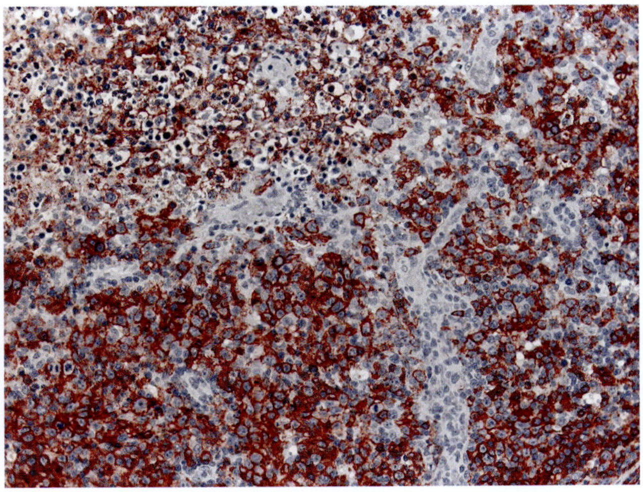

(e)

Figure 28.3 Composite lymphoma consisting of mycosis fungoides and EBV+ diffuse large B-cell lymphoma, NOS. (a) Dense, diffuse infiltrate involving the dermis and subcutis, showing (b) epidermotropism of small and medium-sized lymphocytes with formation of Darier's nests as well as (c) a second population of large cells with features of immunoblasts and centroblasts. Immunohistology shows (d) positivity of the epidermotropic cells for CD3, and (e) of the large cells for CD20. (f) The population of B lymphocytes, but not the T cells, is positive for EBV (EBER-1).

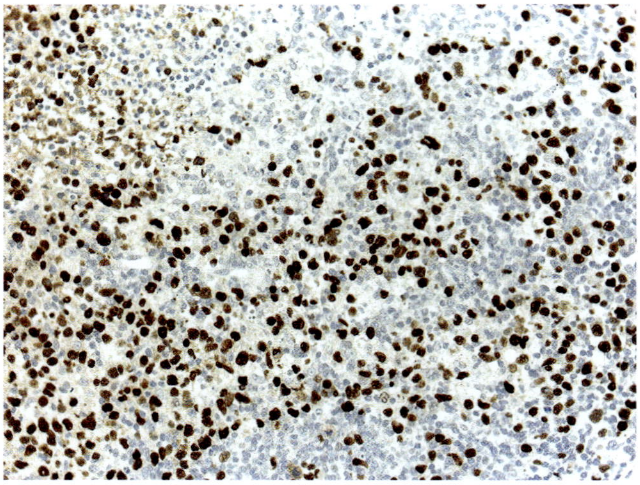

(f)

Figure 28.3 (Continued)

When a cutaneous composite lymphoma is composed of a T- and a B-cell lymphoma, then gene rearrangement studies will show a clonal population in both components, thus confirming the diagnosis. However, even in these cases the interpretation of molecular results is not devoid of pitfalls [35]. Two different clones may be observed in cases harboring either two T- or two B-cell lymphomas. Molecular characterization of the original clones is important in order to better monitor recurrences (which are often restricted to only one of the two lymphoma types).

## Treatment and prognosis

There are no guidelines for management of patients with cutaneous composite lymphomas, and treatment is selected on a case-by-case basis. If one aggressive and one indolent entity are involved, treatment is tailored to the more aggressive of the two entities. When one of the two components is represented by early mycosis fungoides, this should be treated with conventional skin-directed schemes irrespective of the treatment adopted for the second lymphoma (see Chapter 3).

Pegylated liposomal encapsulated doxorubicin has been used in a case of cutaneous composite lymphoma (peripheral T-cell lymphoma, NOS, and cutaneous follicle center lymphoma), but the patient relapsed a few months after treatment and eventually succumbed to the disease [20].

Recognition of the two lymphoma types is crucial in order to assess the prognosis of patients with cutaneous composite lymphomas. In general, as for other cases of extracutaneous lymphomas involving the skin secondarily, prognosis is bad when one or both components are primarily extracutaneous (B-CLL may represent an exception, due to the frequent involvement of the skin at sites of cutaneous "inflammation" without prognostic relevance). When both components are primary cutaneous, then prognosis is dictated by the more aggressive among the two entities, and the course may be indolent if both are low grade (e.g., patch-stage mycosis fungoides associated with cutaneous marginal zone lymphoproliferative disorder).

| Résumé | |
|---|---|
| Clinical | Depending on the lymphomas involved. B-CLL colonizing mycosis fungoides may present as the development of nodular lesions within pre-existent lesions of mycosis fungoides ("pseudo-tumor stage"). |
| Morphology | Depending on the lymphomas involved. Epidermotropism restricted to the T-cell component in cutaneous composite B and T-cell lymphoma. |
| Immunohistochemistry | Depending on the lymphomas involved. Mycosis fungoides is usually $CD4^+$; if B-CLL represents the second lymphoma presence of a B-cell component with a $CD5^+$, $CD20^+$, $CD23^+$ phenotype. Marginal zone lymphoproliferative disorder is identified by the presence of monoclonal plasmacytoid cells and plasma cells. Follicular lymphoma identified by the presence of $CD20^+$, $Bcl6^+$, $Bcl2^{-(+)}$ follicular lymphocytes. Other lymphoma types show characteristic features of the involved entity. |
| Genetics | Presence of a clonal rearrangement of both T and B lymphocytes (composite B- and T-cell lymphomas), or of two different clones of B or T lymphocytes (composite lymphomas with two different B- or T-cell lymphomas). |
| Treatment guidelines | Treatment tailored to the most aggressive of the two lymphomas. |

## References


1. Cieza-Díaz DE, Prieto-Torres L, Rodríguez-Pinilla SM, *et al.* Mycosis fungoides associated with lesions in the spectrum of primary cutaneous CD30+ lymphoproliferative disorders: the same process or 3 coexisting lymphomas? *Am J Dermatopathol* 2019;**41**:846–850.
2. Prieto-Torres L, Machan S, Haro R, *et al.* Concurrent presentation of mycosis fungoides and primary cutaneous marginal zone LPD: clinicopathological study of 4 cases and literature review. *Am J Dermatopathol* 2023;**45**:163–169.
3. Volk AL, Vannucci SA, Cook W, *et al.* Composite mycosis fungoides and B-cell chronic lymphocytic leukemia. *Ann Diagn Pathol* 2002;**6**:172–182.
4. Hull PR, Saxena A. Mycosis fungoides and chronic lymphocytic leukaemia–composite T-cell and B-cell lymphomas presenting in the skin. *Br J Dermatol* 2000;**143**:439–444.
5. Liu YC, Tomashefski JF Jr, Cleveland RP, *et al.* Composite cutaneous T-cell lymphoma and small B-cell lymphocytic lymphoma: morphologic, immunologic, and molecular genetic documentation of concurrent lymph node involvement. *Mod Pathol* 1994;**7**:641–646.
6. Barzilai A, Trau H, David M, *et al.* Mycosis fungoides associated with B-cell malignancies. *Br J Dermatol* 2006;**155**:379–386.
7. Whitling NA, Shanesmith RP, Jacob L, *et al.* Composite lymphoma of mycosis fungoides and cutaneous small B-cell lymphoma in a 73-year-old male patient. *Hum Pathol* 2013;**44**:670–675.
8. Wang E, Papavassiliou P, Wang AR, *et al.* Composite lymphoid neoplasm of B-cell and T-cell origins: a pathologic study of 14 cases. *Hum Pathol* 2014;**45**:768–784.
9. Suefuji N, Niino D, Arakawa F, *et al.* Clinicopathological analysis of a composite lymphoma containing both T- and B-cell lymphomas. *Pathol Int* 2012;**62**:690–698.
10. Makis W, Ciarallo A, Wang B, *et al.* Composite cutaneous lymphoma (iatrogenic immunodeficiency-associated lymphoproliferative disorder) in a patient with rheumatoid arthritis treated with methotrexate: staging and evaluation of response to therapy with 18F-FDG PET/CT. *Nucl Med Mol Imaging* 2017;**51**:261–265.
11. Huwait H, Wang B, Shustik C, Michel RP. Composite cutaneous lymphoma in a patient with rheumatoid arthritis treated with methotrexate. *Am J Dermatopathol* 2010;**32**:65–70.
12. Jullie ML, Carlotti M, Vivot A Jr, *et al.* CD20 antigen may be expressed by reactive or lymphomatous cells of transformed mycosis fungoides: diagnostic and prognostic impact. *Am J Surg Pathol* 2013;**37**:1845–1854.
13. Park CS, Chung HC, Lim HY, *et al.* Coexisting mycosis fungoides and Hodgkin's disease as a composite lymphoma: a case report. *Yonsei Med J* 1991;**32**:362–369.
14. Sluzevich JC, Tun H, Jacks DS, Jiang L. A case of exuberant cutaneous lymphomagenesis in the setting of chronic patch mycosis fungoides. *JAAD Case Rep* 2015;**1**:46–48.
15. Chen S, Boyer D, Hristov AC. Primary cutaneous composite lymphomas. *Arch Pathol Lab Med* 2018;**142**:1352–1357.
16. Chen Y, Nong L, Li X, Wang Y. Cutaneous composite lymphoma of mycosis fungoides and hodgkin lymphoma: response to sequential therapy. *J Cutan Pathol* 2020;**47**:829–833.
17. Ricci C, Ambrosi F, Agostinelli C, *et al.* Cutaneous composite lymphoma consisting of chronic lymphocytic leukemia/small lymphocytic lymphoma and follicular lymphoma: a unique entity and a putative pathological mechanism for cutaneous composite lymphomas. *G Ital Dermatol Venereol* 2021;**156**(suppl. 1):18–19.
18. Boiocchi L, Witter RE, He B, *et al.* Composite chronic lymphocytic leukemia/small lymphocytic lymphoma and follicular lymphoma are biclonal lymphomas: a report of two cases. *Am J Clin Pathol* 2012;**137**:647–659.
19. Jelloul FZ, Chen QH, Yang T, *et al.* Composite small lymphocytic lymphoma/chronic lymphocytic leukemia and follicular lymphoma: a clinicopathological study of six cases. *Int J Surg Pathol* 2018;**26**:135–144.
20. Wollina U, Langner D, Hansel G, Haroske G. Pegylated liposomal-encapsulated doxorubicin in cutaneous composite lymphoma: a case report. *Medicine (Baltimore)* 2016;**95**:e4796.
21. Wang HY, Hinds BR. Cutaneous composite small lymphocytic lymphoma and primary cutaneous follicle center lymphoma. *Blood* 2019;**134**:717.
22. Ahmed A, Aragao AP, Mudaliar K, *et al.* The conundrum of diagnosing cutaneous composite lymphoma in the molecular age. *Am J Dermatopathol* 2019;**41**:757–766.
23. Sagasta A, Molina-Urra R, Martinez D, *et al.* CD8-positive peripheral T-cell lymphoma with aberrant expression of CD20 and concurrent in situ follicular lymphoma. *J Cutan Pathol* 2015;**42**:66–72.
24. Hibler J, Salavaggione AL, Martin A, Gru AA. A unique case of concurrent chronic lymphocytic leukemia/small lymphocytic lymphoma and lymphomatoid papulosis in the same biopsy. *J Cutan Pathol* 2015;**42**:276–284.
25. Szablewski V, Costes-Martineau V, René C, *et al.* Composite cutaneous lymphoma of diffuse large B-cell lymphoma-leg type and subcutaneous panniculitis-like T-cell lymphoma. *J Cutan Pathol* 2018;**45**:716–720.
26. Leduc C, Blandino II, Alhejaily A, *et al.* Composite mantle cell and primary cutaneous anaplastic large cell lymphoma: case report and review of the literature. *Am J Dermatopathol* 2015;**37**:232–236.
27. Wehkamp U, Pott C, Unterhalt M, *et al.* Skin involvement of mantle cell lymphoma may mimic primary cutaneous diffuse large B-cell lymphoma, leg type. *Am J Surg Pathol* 2015;**39**:1093–1101.
28. Yang SF, Chang WY, Lan CC, *et al.* Composite primary cutaneous peripheral T-cell lymphoma and Epstein-Barr virus-positive large B-cell lymphoma. *Leuk Lymphoma* 2011;**52**:2027–2030.
29. Balagué O, Martínez A, Colomo L, *et al.* Epstein-Barr virus negative clonal plasma cell proliferations and lymphomas in peripheral T-cell lymphomas: a phenomenon with distinctive clinicopathologic features. *Am J Surg Pathol* 2007;**31**:1310–1322.
30. Papalas JA, Puri PK, Sebastian S, Wang E. Primary cutaneous, composite, Epstein-Barr virus-associated, diffuse large B-cell

lymphoma and peripheral T-cell lymphoma. *Am J Dermatopathol* 2011;**33**:719–725.
31. Steinhoff M, Hummel M, Assaf C, *et al.* Cutaneous T cell lymphoma and classic Hodgkin lymphoma of the B cell type within a single lymph node: composite lymphoma. *J Clin Pathol* 2004;**57**:329–331.
32. Gonzalez CL, Medeiros LJ, Jaffe ES. Composite lymphoma: a clinicopathologic analysis of nine patients with Hodgkin's disease and B-cell non-Hodgkin's lymphoma. *Am J Clin Pathol* 1991;**96**:81–89.
33. Kazakov DV, Kutzner H, Palmedo G, *et al.* Primary cutaneous lymphoproliferative disorders with dual lineage rearrangement. *Am J Dermatopathol* 2006;**28**:399–409.
34. Tokunaga M, Tokudome T, Shimizu S, *et al.* Biclonality of composite B- and T-cell lymphomas. *A case report. Acta Pathol Jpn* 1990; **40**:522–530.
35. Symes E, Dominiak N. Primary cutaneous B-cell lymphoma complicated by clonal T-cell populations: a diagnostic dilemma. *Am J Dermatopathol* 2021;**43**:454–458.

# CHAPTER 29

# Non-neoplastic cutaneous signs of systemic lymphomas

In addition to specific skin manifestations of hematological malignancies, many non-neoplastic cutaneous conditions may be associated with variable frequency to systemic lymphomas [1, 2]. The most important of them will be briefly discussed in this chapter; a list of non-neoplastic skin manifestations and related conditions in hematological malignancies is summarized in Table 29.1.

Patients with systemic lymphomas may present different skin diseases unrelated to direct colonization by neoplastic cells (that is, "non-specific" cutaneous manifestations of systemic lymphomas). These skin disorders may precede, arise concomitant with, or be subsequent to the systemic lymphoma. Some of them are very common skin conditions observed often in non-paraneoplastic settings as well, thus do not represent helpful diagnostic clues (e.g., erythema nodosum). Other conditions, on the other hand, are frequently related to nodal Hodgkin or non-Hodgkin lymphomas, and may represent useful clues for diagnosis and/or for monitoring disease activity.

Deposition of paraproteins in the skin, in some instances precipitated by cold, is one of the specific complications of immunoglobulin-producing hematological neoplasms [3, 4]. The deposition may be related either to an intact paraprotein (nodular and bullous macroglobulinosis, light chain disease, heavy chain disease), or to modified paraproteins (amyloid, cryoglobulins, and crystalglobulins). ***Cryoglobulinemic obstructive vasculopathy*** in hematological neoplasms is associated mostly with monoclonal cryoglobulins (type I) or with a mixture of monoclonal and polyclonal cryoglobulins (type II) (a third type, observed mostly in the setting of chronic inflammatory disorders, consists of two or more polyclonal cryoglobulins) [3–5]. Type I cryoglobulinemia is due to a monoclonal protein (IgG, IgM, IgA, or rarely a light chain) that reversibly precipitates within small vessels when the serum temperature goes below 37°. It is usually seen in association with monoclonal gammopathy of undetermined significance, Waldenström's macroglobulinemia, multiple myeloma, or rarely other immunoglobulin-producing B-cell lymphomas. Patients present clinically with purpura, acrocyanosis, and livedo racemosa mostly located at acral sites (particularly the distal parts of the extremities and the ears), often with areas of cutaneous infarction (Fig. 29.1a). Histological examination in type I cryoglobulinemia reveals intraluminal PAS+ thrombi within the small vessels of the dermis and subcutaneous fat (Figs. 29.1b and c). Subsequent reactive endothelial proliferation may lead to the histopathological picture of reactive angioendotheliomatosis. Mixed cryoglobulinemia (types II and III) presents histopathologically with features of a small-vessel vasculitis without thrombi.

Intravascular crystalline deposits within small vessels, precipitated by cold, can be observed in the rare ***crystalglobulinemia (cryocrystalglobulinemia)***, characterized by purpura, skin infarction, and hemorrhagic blisters on acral sites, and associated mostly with multiple myeloma. The intravascular crystals are positive for PAS and are composed of monoclonal immunoglobulins. Crystalglobulinemia is a severe, life-threatening condition with systemic involvement (kidney failure, lung, gastrointestinal, and central nervous system manifestations) [6].

Deposition of cryoglobulins can be observed also in the rare but distinct entity known as ***cryokeratotic spicules***, which is specific for immunoglobulin-producing hematological neoplasms [7]. Clinically, patients present with tiny, filiform spicules protruding from the follicular openings, particularly on the nose and face. Histology shows dilated follicular infundibula with eosinophilic deposits around the keratinocytes of the inner half of the infundibular wall and extending to the surface of the hair follicle, representing here a mixture of cryoglobulins, parakeratotic corneocytes, and rudimentary hair keratin. Cryokeratotic spicules may be a marker of recurrence or disease progression of the underlying hematological neoplasm [8].

Besides cryoprecipitated immunoglobulins, crystallized immunoglobulins may be observed in the skin in other settings including crystal storing histiocytosis and interstitial crystalglobulinosis. ***Crystal storing histiocytosis*** is characterized by crystalloid intracytoplasmic inclusions within histiocytes and macrophages, representing intracellular deposits of immunoglobulins with peculiar geometric shapes (Fig. 29.2) [9, 10]. Crystal storing histiocytosis is mostly related to multiple myeloma, but cases have been observed also in association with other conditions such as lymphoplasmacytic lymphoma, MALT lymphoma, and monoclonal gammopathy of undetermined

*Skin Lymphoma: The Illustrated Guide*, Sixth Edition. Lorenzo Cerroni.

**Table 29.1** Mucocutaneous signs and symptoms that may be associated with systemic lymphomas and leukemias[#]

| |
|---|
| ***Associated with tumor-induced or treatment-related bone marrow suppression and resulting cytopenia*** |
| Pallor |
| Bruising; Ecchymoses; Persistent hemorrhages; Purpura, especially petechial |
| Gingival hemorrhage; Epistaxis; Prolonged bleeding after minor injuries |
| Oral ulcerations in neutropenic patients |
| ***Associated with either tumor-specific or treatment-related immune dysregulation*** |
| Opportunistic infections; Unusual presentations of common infections (e.g., vegetating lesions, severe demodicosis – demodex folliculitis; prolonged duration of self-limited infections; severe manifestations of otherwise banal infections) |
| Trichodysplasia spinulosa |
| Infection-induced panniculitis |
| Septic vasculitis (either bacterial or fungal, particularly *aspergillus* sepsis) |
| Neutrophilic eccrine hidradenitis |
| Gout due to hyperuricemia in tumor lysis syndrome (after chemotherapy for a rapidly dividing chemosensitive malignancy) (elevated levels of uric acid in the urine are associated with uric acid nephrolithiasis and may cause acute renal failure)[$] |
| Development of multiple melanocytic nevi after chemotherapy |
| ***Associated with autoantibodies produced by the hematologic neoplasm*** |
| Paraneoplastic pemphigus[$] |
| ***Associated with deposition of amyloid protein*** |
| Cutaneous amyloidosis |
| ***Associated with paraproteinemia with deposition of M-protein*** |
| Nodular and bullous macroglobulinosis (IgM storage papules)[$] |
| Light- and heavy-chain deposition disease[$] |
| Crystal storing histiocytosis[$] |
| Reactive angioendotheliomatosis |
| Acquired cutis laxa (binding of immunoglobulins to the elastic fibers)[$] |
| ***Associated with paraproteinemia with deposition of cryoglobulins***[$] |
| Cryoglobulinemic obstructive vasculopathy (type I/II cryoglobulinemia) |
| Crystalglobulinemia (cryocrystalglobulinemia) |
| Interstitial crystalglobulinosis |
| Cryokeratotic follicular spicules |
| ***Often / constantly associated with paraproteinemia (without deposition of M-protein)***[$] |
| Scleromyxedema |
| Scleredema (type 2) |
| Normolipemic plane xanthomas |
| Necrobiotic xanthogranuloma |
| POEMS syndrome *(Polyneuropathy, Organomegaly, Endocrinopathy, Monoclonal gammopathy, and Skin changes – particularly hyperpigmentation and angiomas)* |
| AESOP syndrome *(Adenopathy and Extensive Skin Patch Overlying a Plasmacytoma)* |
| TEMPI syndrome *(Telangiectasias, Elevated erythropoietin and erythrocytosis, Monoclonal gammopathy, Perinephric fluid collection, and Intrapulmonary shunting)* |
| Schnitzler's syndrome |
| Subepidermal bullous dermatosis associated with IgM gammopathy |
| Systemic capillary leak syndrome (Clarkson syndrome) |
| ***Occasionally associated with paraproteinemia (without deposition of M-protein)*** |
| Sneddon-Wilkinson disease |
| Localized lichen myxedematosus in HIV-infected patients |
| ***Other cutaneous conditions often or occasionally associated with hematological malignancies*** |
| Generalized "pruritus sine materia" (particularly in Hodgkin lymphoma) |
| Sweet syndrome (acute febrile neutrophilic dermatosis), especially the "histiocytoid" variant (particularly in myeloid leukemia)[$] |
| VEXAS (vacuoles, E1 enzyme, X-linked, autoinflammatory, somatic mutations) syndrome[$] |
| Bullous pyoderma gangrenosum |
| Eosinophilic dermatosis of hematological malignancy (exaggerated insect bite-like reaction) ($) |
| Wells syndrome |
| Juvenile xanthogranuloma |
| Generalized eruptive histiocytoma |
| Xanthoma disseminatum |
| Langerhans cell histiocytosis |
| Indeterminate cell histiocytosis |
| Erythema annulare centrifugum |
| Urticaria vasculitis |
| Erythema nodosum |

Table 29.1 (Continued)

| |
|---|
| Polyarteritis (panarteritis) nodosa (especially in patients with hairy cell leukemia) |
| Cutaneous and/or systemic sarcoidosis[ϕ] |
| Erythema elevatum et diutinum |
| Cutaneous small vessel vasculitis |
| Eosinophilic folliculitis |
| Deficiency dermatitis |
| Acquired ichthyosis |
| Spiny keratoderma |
| Acquired angioedema due to C1 esterase inhibitor dysfunction |
| Linear IgA bullous dermatosis |
| Epidermolysis bullosa acquisita |
| Calcinosis cutis |
| Annular elastolytic giant cell granuloma |
| Cutis verticis gyrate |
| Paraneoplastic scleroderma-like syndrome (similar to systemic sclerosis, but older age at onset; seen in association with a monoclonal gammopathy, hairy cell leukemia, and solid tumors (e.g., breast, lung) |
| Papuloerythroderma of Ofuji (in some patients with B-cell chronic lymphocytic leukemia, acute myeloid leukemia, Hodgkin lymphoma, or other systemic lymphomas)[$] |
| ***Familial cancer syndromes most commonly associated with systemic hematological malignancies presenting with cutaneous manifestations (main cutaneous signs in brackets)*** |
| Ataxia–telangiectasia (telangiectasia on sun-exposed areas, premature graying of hairs, vitiligo) |
| Bloom syndrome (Photosensitivity, butterfly erythema, telangiectasia) |
| Dyskeratosis congenita (reticulate hyperpigmentation, nail changes, oral leukoplakia) |
| Fanconi anemia (widespread areas of hyper- and/or hypopigmentation) |
| Li-Fraumeni syndrome (skin tumors related to a mutation in *TP53*) |
| Neurofibromatosis (Café-au-lait spots, axillary freckling, multiple neurofibromas) |
| Trisomy 21 [Down syndrome] (single transverse palmar crease, dry skin, fissured tongue, increased susceptibility to cutaneous bacterial and fungal infections) |

[#] Most of these conditions may be observed also in settings other than hematological neoplasms.
[$] Observed mostly in the setting of hematological malignancies.
[ϕ] Sarcoidosis may antedate the diagnosis of non-Hodgkin lymphoma ("sarcoidosis-lymphoma syndrome") or arise during the course of the disease.
[§] Neoplastic cells clonally related to the underlying myeloid neoplasm can be found within the cutaneous infiltrate.

significance, and rarely without association with an underlying lymphoproliferative disorder.

Besides the aforementioned conditions, related to direct deposition of paraproteins in the skin, patients with paraproteinemia due to hematological conditions may present with other peculiar skin conditions, some of which are rarely, if ever, observed in other settings (e.g., necrobiotic xanthogranuloma and scleromyxedema, among others). ***Schnitzler's syndrome*** (chronic urticarial lesions, intermittent fever, malaise, bone pain, arthralgia, and monoclonal IgM gammopathy) is another disorder with peculiar skin manifestations ("neutrophilic urticaria") associated to paraproteinemia, possibly representing an autoinflammatory condition related to the paraproteinemia. ***POEMS syndrome*** (polyneuropathy, organomegaly, endocrinopathy, monoclonal gammopathy [M protein], and skin changes) and ***AESOP syndrome*** (adenopathy and extensive skin patch overlying a plasmacytoma), too, are almost always related to paraproteinemia.

Cutaneous deposition of fibrils composed of low-molecular-weight protein subunits derived from immunoglobulins (AL-amyloid) is observed in systemic AL amyloidosis. Besides cases of localized amyloid deposition observed in so-called cutaneous amyloidoma (see Chapter 17), cutaneous deposition of AL amyloid can be observed in several B-cell malignancies in the setting of ***primary systemic AL amyloidosis***. Primary systemic AL amyloidosis is associated with immunoglobulin-producing proliferation of plasma cells, particularly monoclonal gammopathies and less frequently multiple myeloma.

Clinically, the amyloid deposition may be diffuse or localized. Involvement of the mucosal regions may result in a markedly enlargement of the tongue (Fig. 29.3). On the fingers and palms, waxy nodules may be the consequence of local amyloid deposition (Fig. 29.4), and on the scalp swelling of the tissue may result in a picture similar to cutis verticis gyrata. Diffuse infiltration of the skin may confer a sclerodermoid appearance. Petechiae, purpura, and ecchymoses are common, and the area of amyloid deposition may be purpuric as well (Fig. 29.5); a peculiar periorbital hemorrhage described as the "raccoon sign" may be precipitated by coughing. Histology shows deposition of an amorphous, eosinophilic substance in the dermis and often in the subcutis, with concentric accentuation of the deposits around the blood vessels (Fig. 29.6). AL amyloid shows a bright fluorescence with stainings for thyoflavin, and is positive for Congo red (leading to green birefringence under polarized light). With the exception of cutaneous amyloidoma (which does not belong to the spectrum of primary systemic AL

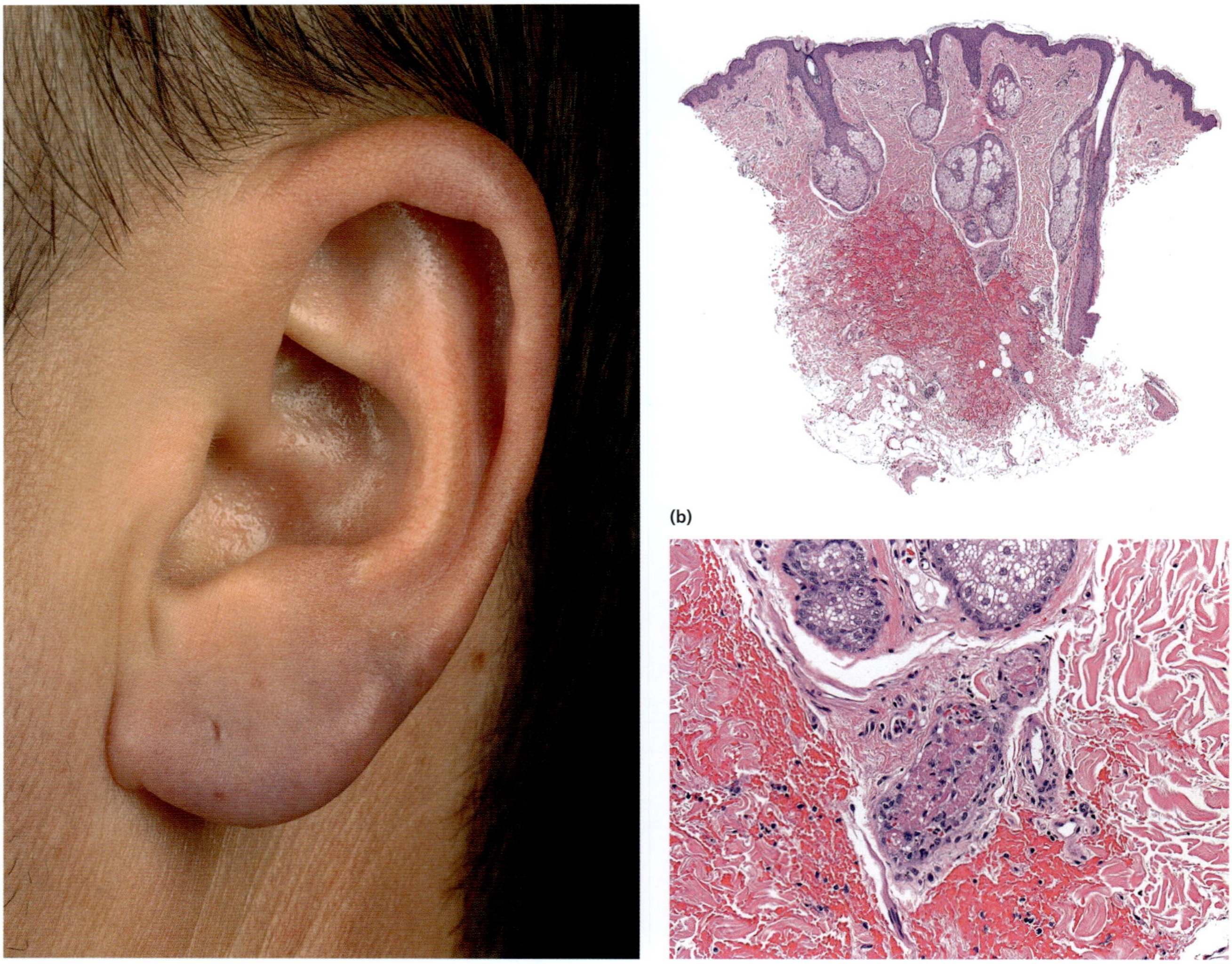

(a) (b) (c)

**Figure 29.1** Monoclonal cryoglobulinemia in a patient with a diffuse large B-cell lymphoma, NOS diagnosed after the onset of cutaneous lesions. (a) Purpuric lesions on the ear; (b) Histopathology shows hemorrhage without relevant inflammatory infiltrates and with (c) fibrin thrombi within small and medium-sized vessels.

amyloidosis), only exceedingly rarely a plasma cell tumor is found in the vicinity of the cutaneous amyloid deposition (in such cases usually representing a secondary cutaneous manifestation of a multiple myeloma) (see Chapter 20, Fig. 20.16).

Besides skin biopsies of clinically apparent amyloid deposits, the presence of amyloid can be demonstrated histopathologically in the majority of patients with systemic amyloidosis by abdominal subcutaneous fat aspirates. Random rectal mucosal biopsies also show amyloid deposition, but are associated with the risk of bleeding. In order to facilitate classification of the amyloidosis, cutaneous amyloid deposits can be stained with antibodies directed to pan-cytokeratin, AA amyloid, amyloid P-component, fibrinogen, lysozyme, transthyretin, λ-light chain, and κ-light chain with high specificity and sensitivity [11]. In my experience, in-situ hybridization for the immunoglobulin light chains κ and λ is not feasible for staining AL amyloid deposits, and conventional immunohistology should be used instead.

A peculiar condition described as "***exaggerated arthropod bite-like reaction***" has been described originally in patients with B-cell chronic lymphocytic leukemia (B-CLL) [12]. It has subsequently been shown that it can arise in different hematological malignancies besides B-CLL, including acute lymphoblastic leukemia, acute monocytic leukemia, mantle-cell lymphoma, large-cell lymphoma, and myelofibrosis, among others [13]. Hypersensitivity to mosquito bites is a well-known feature of systemic hydroa vacciniforme lymphoproliferative disorder and of some forms of natural killer (NK)-cell lymphoma occurring in some populations (see also Chapter 15), but the condition described as exaggerated arthropod bite-like

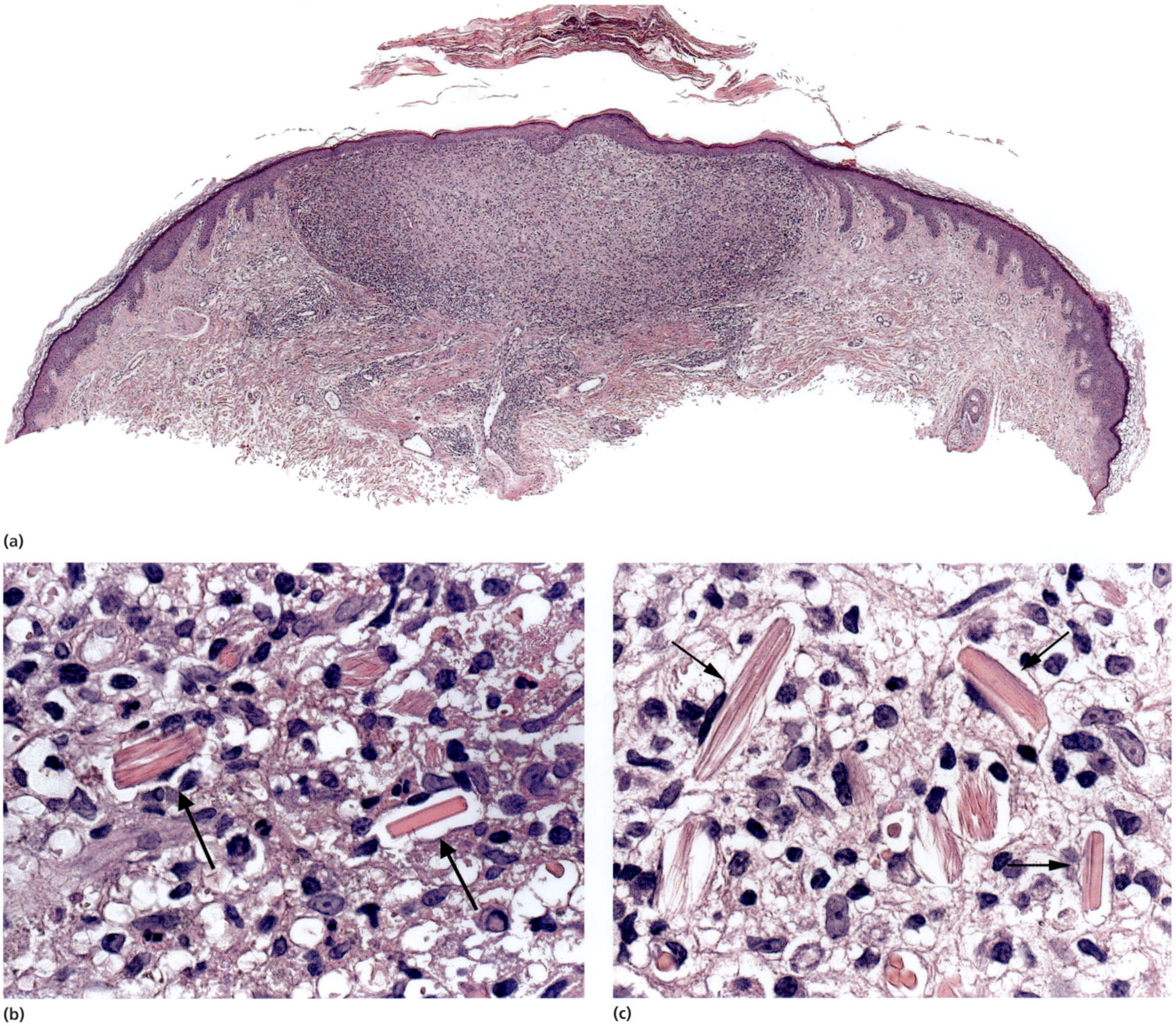

Figure 29.2 Crystal storing histiocytosis. (a) Circumscribed infiltrate in the dermis, composed of (b, c) small lymphocytes, plasma cells, and histiocytes, these last with large, geometric crystalloid intracytoplasmic inclusions (arrows).

reaction has no relationship with the entity described as "severe mosquito bite allergy". Although a link to insect bites has been postulated in some patients [14], in many patients with B-CLL and other types of non-Hodgkin lymphoma the direct link to an arthropod bite cannot be established with certainty, and clinical features sometimes are not those of arthropod bites (Fig. 29.7). For these reasons, the term ***"eosinophilic dermatosis of hematological malignancy"*** has been proposed as a better name for this condition [15, 16]. Eosinophilic dermatosis of hematological malignancy may be observed in different B- and T-cell non-Hodgkin lymphomas with a median latency of 40 months after the hematological malignancy [16]. The lesions are unrelated to laboratory findings, disease course, therapy, or prognosis, and usually resolve within a few weeks. Clinically, eosinophilic dermatosis of hematological malignancy is characterized by solitary, localized, or generalized erythematous or hemorrhagic areas of skin infiltration, often showing tense bullae (Figs. 29.7–29.9) [17]. Some cases show clinicopathological features similar to those of Wells syndrome. Particularly in lesions arising in B-CLL patients, neoplastic cells are sometimes found within the biopsy specimen admixed with large numbers of eosinophils and with reactive T and B lymphocytes (Fig. 29.10) [18]. Flame figures may be present.

***Paraneoplastic pemphigus*** is an autoimmune blistering disorder mainly associated with non-Hodgkin lymphomas (particularly B-cell lymphomas and leukemias, but also other types, as

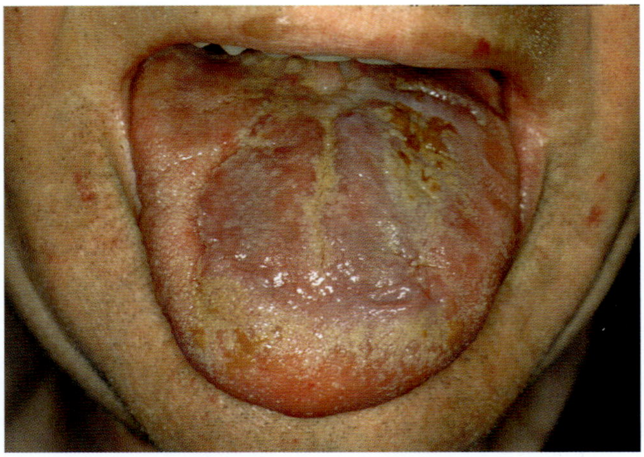

Figure 29.3 Macroglossia in a male patient with multiple myeloma and systemic AL amyloidosis. Note also focal erosions.

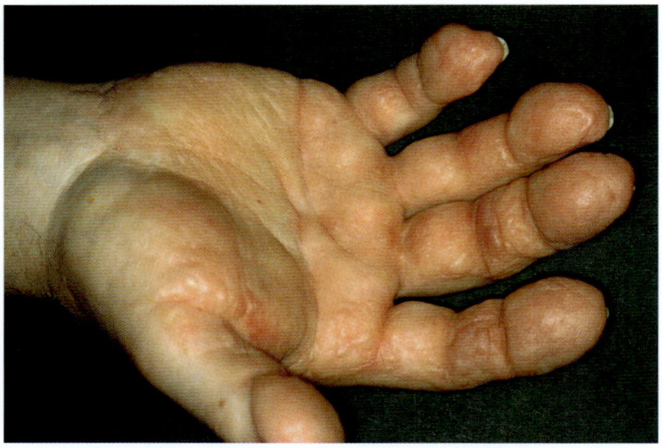

Figure 29.4 Deposition of AL amyloid on the palm and fingers in a patient with multiple myeloma (same patient of figure 26.2X1). Note waxy, partly confluent papules.

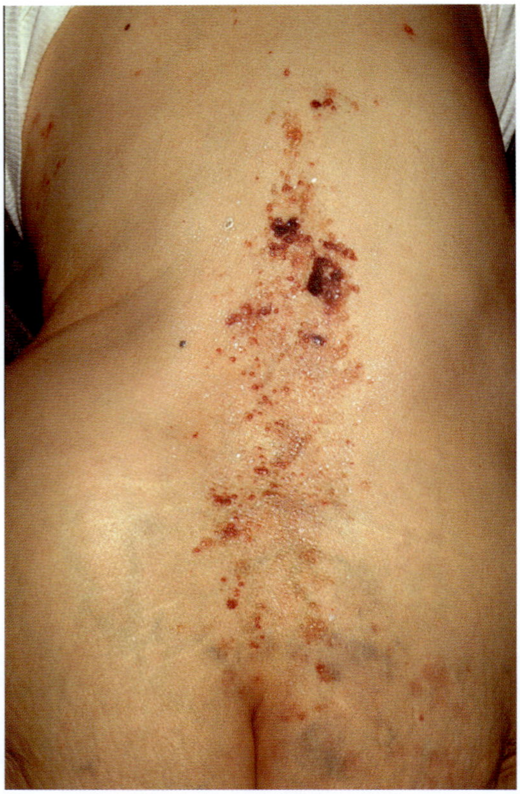

Figure 29.5 Purpuric, partly confluent papules on the back of a woman with multiple myeloma and systemic AL amyloidosis.

well as thymoma and Castleman's disease). It is characterized by polymorphous skin lesions with features of both erythema multiforme and pemphigus vulgaris; in some cases the lesions are not erosive and have a different clinical aspect than those of conventional forms of pemphigus (Fig. 29.11). Histologically, too, paraneoplastic pemphigus shows features of a multiforme-like condition rather than of an acantholytic dermatosis (Fig. 29.12). Paraneoplastic pemphigus may precede the diagnosis of the underlying hematologic condition. Antibodies directed against multiple skin antigens can be detected, including members of the plakin family as well as the desmogleins. Besides skin lesions, severe involvement of the oral mucosa can often be observed in patients with paraneoplastic pemphigus (Fig. 29.13), as well as the presence of ocular involvement and of severe pulmonary manifestations.

Patients with paraneoplastic pemphigus should always be screened for a hematologic malignancy. The therapy is very difficult, and the disease is resistant to most treatment options. Management of the underlying non-Hodgkin lymphoma is paramount, and the anti-CD20 antibody (rituximab) has been used in cases of B-cell lymphoma-associated paraneoplastic pemphigus in order to target specifically the antibody-producing tumor cells (although with variable efficacy).

The onset of ***sarcoidal granulomas*** may be observed in patients with non-Hodgkin lymphoma. The term ***"sarcoidosis-lymphoma syndrome"*** has been used for patients with systemic sarcoidosis who subsequently developed non-Hodgkin lymphoma, but sarcoidal granulomas may develop also after the diagnosis of the lymphoma, and the skin may represent one of the sites of involvement. Cutaneous sarcoidal granulomas may represent a sign of activity of the underlying lymphoma, and in some cases may be used to monitor the disease.

***Pyoderma gangrenosum*** is characterized by the rapid development of pustules evolving into large, undermined ulcerative lesions, often following minor trauma or after surgical procedures (so-called "pathergy"). In some cases pyoderma gangrenosum, especially the bullous variant, may be associated with hematological malignancies (particularly myeloid leukemia and variants). In these patients, lesions may have a bullous appearance and may show overlapping features with bullous Sweet syndrome. Similar to Sweet syndrome, also in

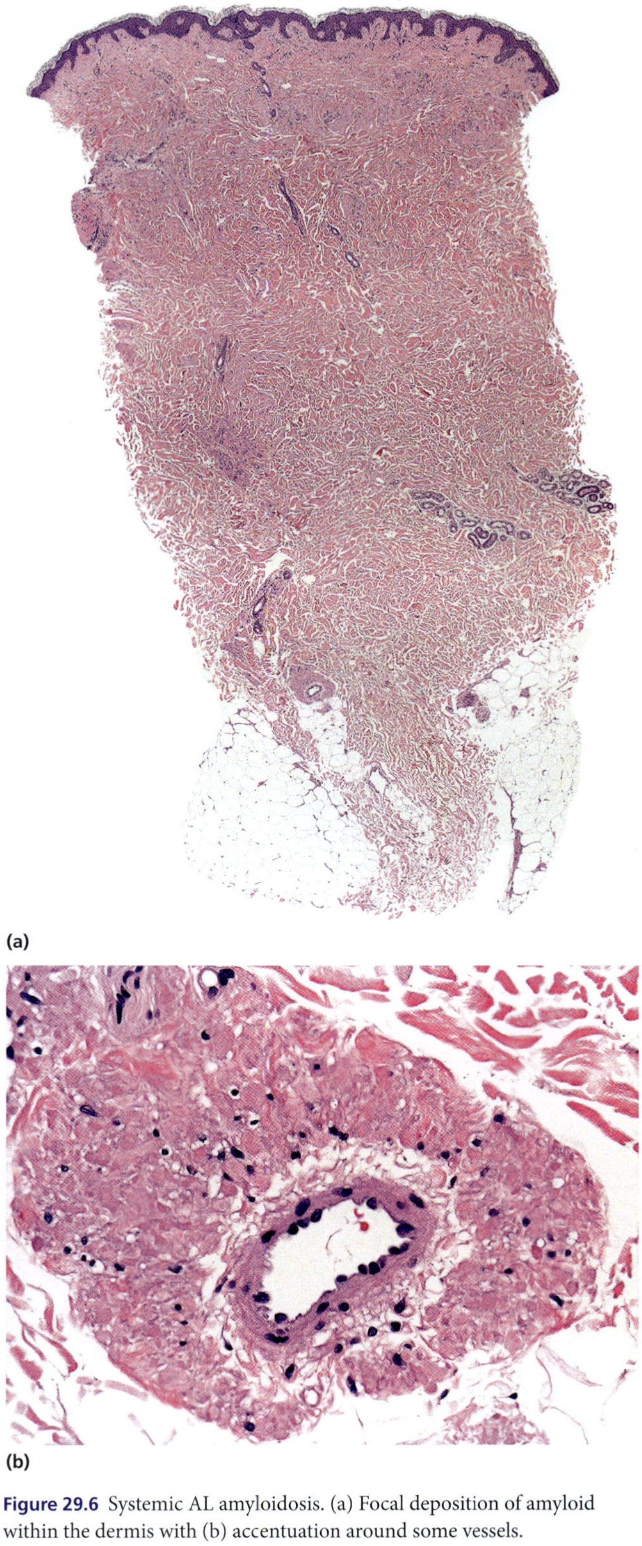

(a)

(b)

**Figure 29.6** Systemic AL amyloidosis. (a) Focal deposition of amyloid within the dermis with (b) accentuation around some vessels.

patients with pyoderma gangrenosum extensive screening investigations in search of an underlying hematological disorder are not necessary if other signs and/or symptoms are not present (bullous pyoderma gangrenosum, though, is more frequently associated with hematological malignancies than other variants of the disease, and these patients should be managed carefully).

***Pruritus*** is a very common cutaneous symptoms and can be associated with myriads of cutaneous and systemic disorders. Chronic pruritus without evidence of skin lesions ("pruritus sine materia") may be a cutaneous sign of Hodgkin or non-Hodgkin lymphomas, and can antedate the diagnosis of the nodal disease by several months or years. Although pruritus sine materia may be observed also in several other conditions unrelated to hematological malignancies, screening for an underlying lymphoma belongs to the standard management of these patients. The pitfall of overlooking a serious condition associated with persistent itching has been the subject of an episode of "Caro Diario," a movie by Nanni Moretti for which he won the Best Director Award at the 1994 Cannes Film Festival. In this episode, he tells of his own struggle with persistent itching accompanied by sleep disturbances; he describes the many visits to several physicians, who only gave various symptomatic treatments and did not perform any relevant investigation, and who did not realize for almost one year that the itching and sleep disturbances were symptoms of mediastinal Hodgkin disease.

***Acquired ichthyosis*** is a skin condition similar to ichthyosis vulgaris both clinically and histopathologically, but it appears during adult life and usually associated with an underlying malignancy, particularly a non-Hodgkin lymphoma. A similar clinicopathologic presentation may be observed also as a drug eruption (clofazimine, pravastatin, allopurinol and cimetidine, among others), or in association with other conditions such as malnutrition, hypothyroidism, and infections, among others. It should be remembered that features of ichthyosis vulgaris are present in a subset of patients with atopic dermatitis as well. As acquired ichthyosis can be observed in several settings, in the absence of other signs and/or symptoms, patients should not undergo extensive screening investigations for an underlying hematological disorder.

***Sweet syndrome***, particularly the histiocytoid variant, may be associated with myeloid leukemias or myelodysplastic syndromes (see also Chapter 23). Histiocytoid Sweet syndrome was described by Requena and coworkers in 2005 [19]. In subsequent years, besides cases associated with various non-neoplastic conditions (including administration of drugs, autoimmune diseases, inflammatory bowel disease, and rheumatoid arthritis, among others), some reports described the presence within the infiltrate of malignant cells of an associated myelogenous leukemia [20, 21]. The association with myelogenous disorders had already been described in "conventional" Sweet syndrome [22, 23]. Although it has been suggested that histiocytoid Sweet syndrome is almost always associated with a myelogenous hematological disorder [21], a large study demonstrated that this is present only in a minority of patients [24]. Nonetheless,

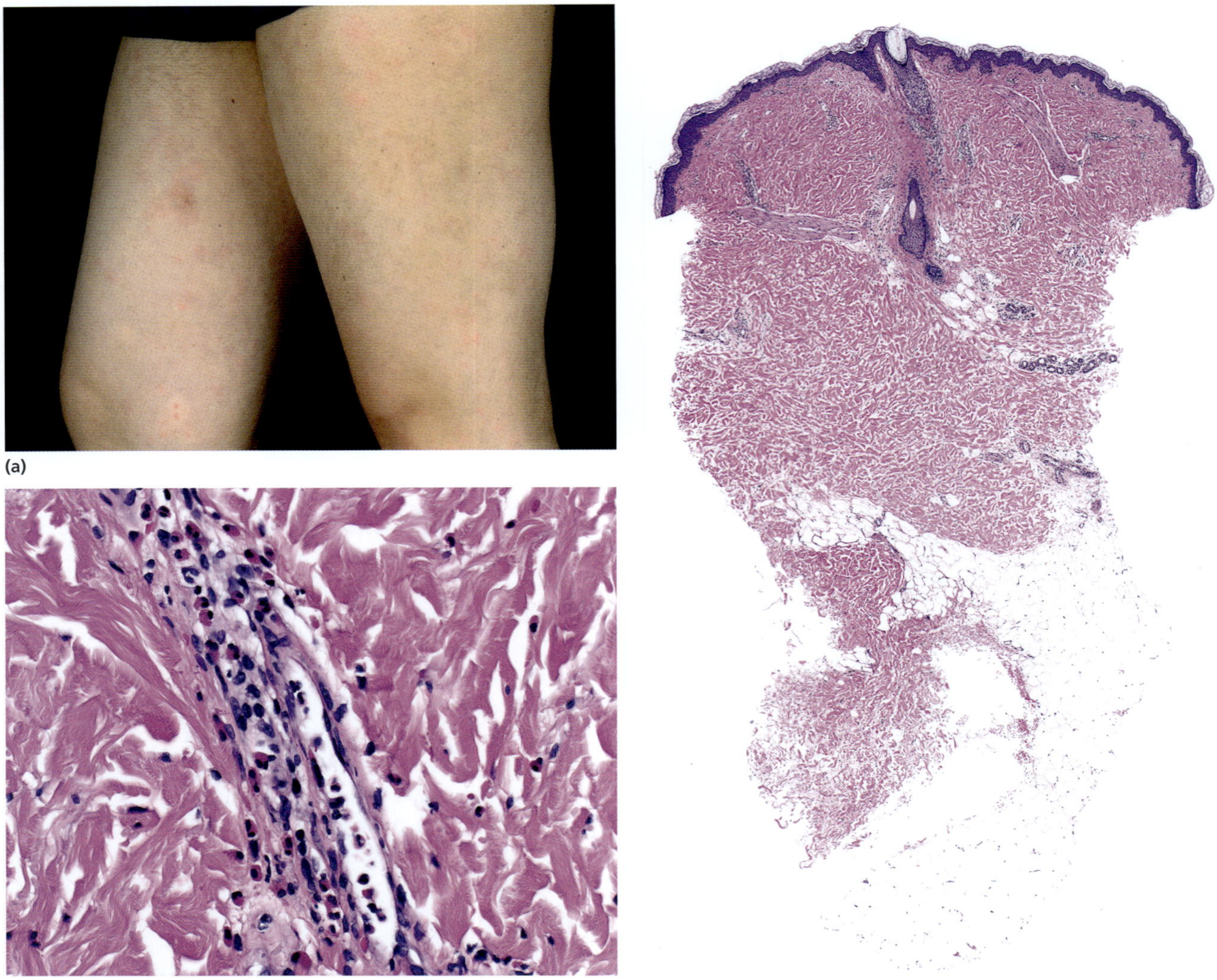

(a)

(c)

(b)

Figure 29.7 Eosinophilic dermatosis of hematological malignancy. (a) Urticarial patches and plaques on the legs. (b) The infiltrate is more sparse than in "exaggerated insect bite-like reaction," but (c) eosinophils are prominent as well.

careful clinical investigations are warranted in all these patients, and the concept of ***"myelodysplasia cutis"*** has been recently proposed to describe the association of Sweet syndrome and bone marrow myelodysplasia [25, 26]. Patients with histiocytoid Sweet syndrome present with fever (may be absent), neutrophilia (may be absent as well), and rapid onset of generalized cutaneous erythematous, infiltrated plaques that may have an edematous or bullous appearance. Recurrences can be observed (Fig. 29.14). Histopathology shows variable amounts of subepidermal edema (may be missing), and dense dermal infiltrates characterized by variable numbers of neutrophils admixed with a predominant population of histiocytoid cells positive for myeloperoxidase and MNDA (Fig. 29.15). Eosinophils may be observed. In several cases, the cells of the infiltrate are clonally related to those of the underlying myeloid leukemia/myelodysplastic syndrome. A recent study showed that ***VEXAS*** (vacuoles, E1 enzyme, X-linked, autoinflammatory, somatic mutations) syndrome, myelodysplasia cutis, and Sweet syndrome are characterized by a shared inflammatory

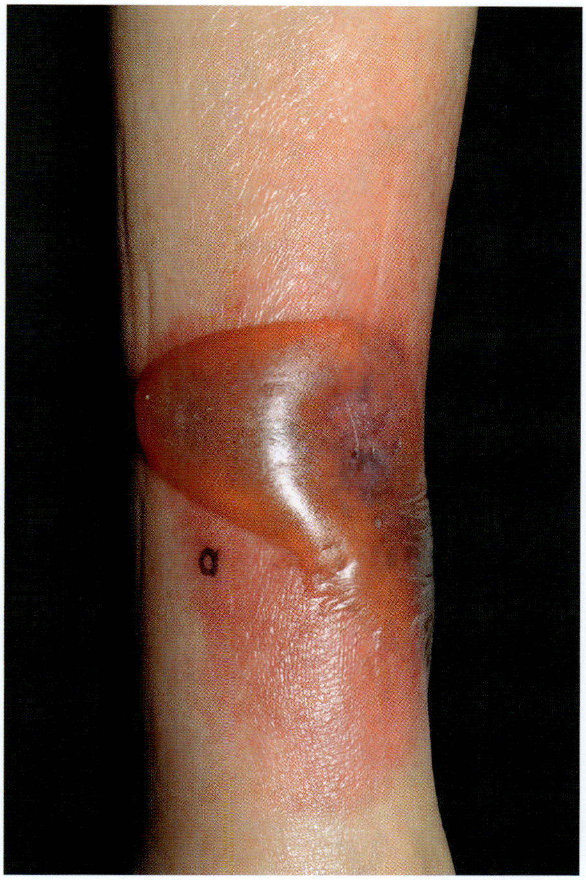

Figure 29.8 Exaggerated insect bite-like reaction in a patient with B-CLL. Solitary, infiltrated, erythematous lesion on the leg with a large, hemorrhagic bulla.

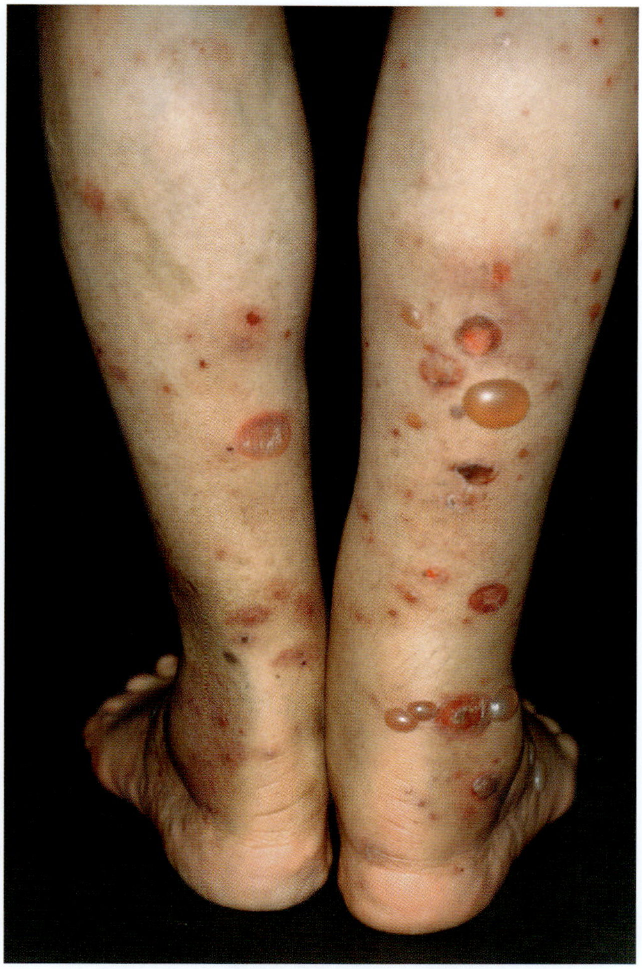

Figure 29.9 Exaggerated insect bite-like reaction in a patient with B-CLL. Several, partly bullous, partly erosive lesions on both legs.

environment relying mostly on a type 1 immune response led by type 1 and 2 interferons, along with the activation of tumor necrosis factor and interleukin-1β pathways [27].

Many other non-specific cutaneous manifestations may be observed in patients with hematological malignancies, either related to substances produced by the malignant tumor (e.g. paraproteins in scleromyxedema) or to bone marrow suppression due to the neoplasm (e.g., pallor, purpura, ecchymosis), or to the decreased immune competence related to both the hematological malignancy and the treatment (e.g., opportunistic infections such as aspergillosis, disseminated candidiasis) (Fig. 29.16), or to the side effects of treatment (e.g., exanthematic drug eruptions, palmar erythema). Common infections may present with clinical features different from conventional presentations (e.g., vegetating or ulcerative lesions) (Fig. 29.17). The histopathological features in such cases may deviate from the conventional presentation of these disorders. For example, ulcerated lesions of vegetating herpes infection may show only subtle histopathological features of herpes virus masked by prominent inflammation (Fig. 29.18). A more detailed discussion of all these conditions, on the other hand, is beyond the scope of this book.

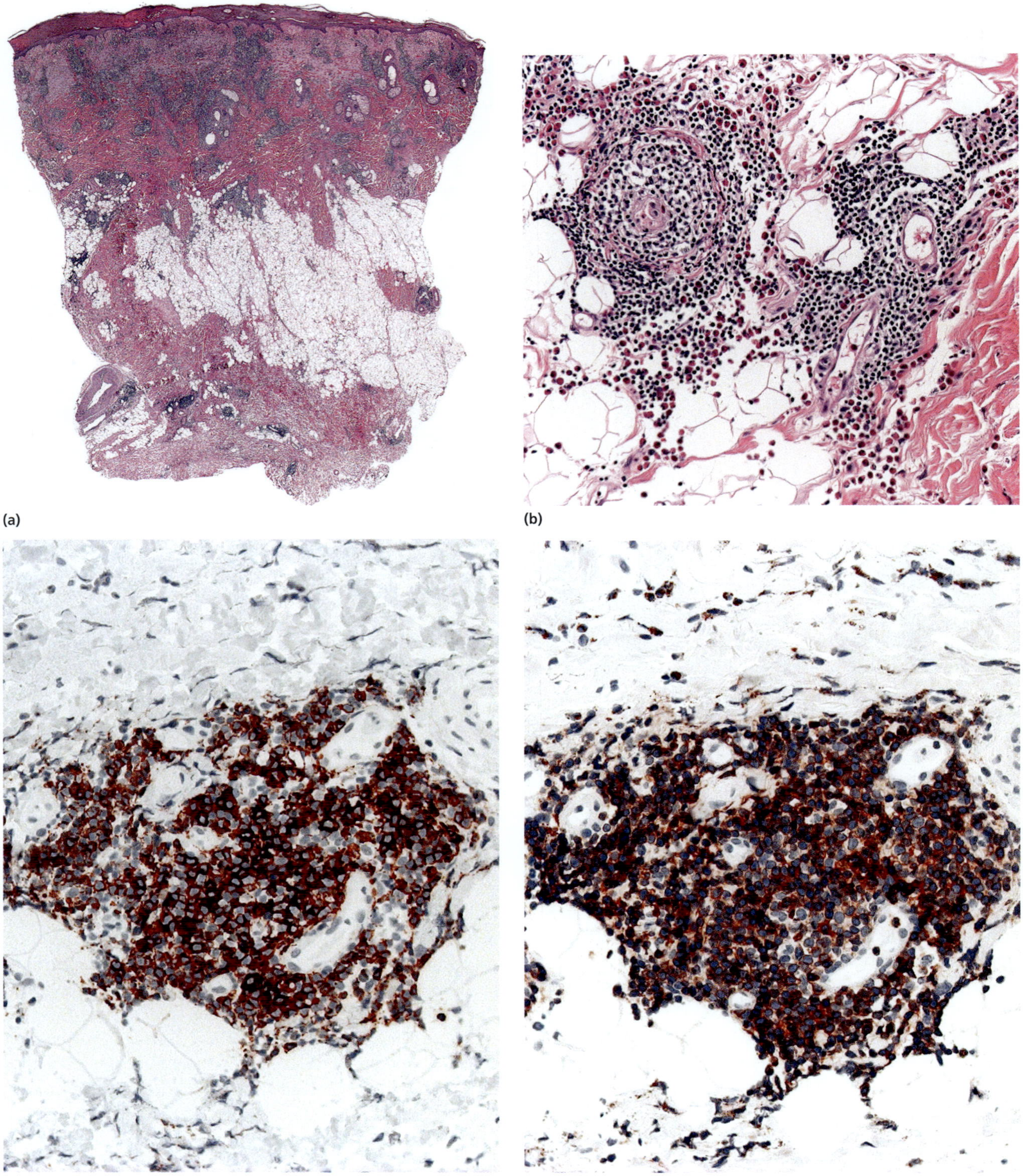

(a) (b) (c) (d)

Figure 29.10 Exaggerated insect bite-like reaction in a patient with B-CLL. (a) Patchy lymphoid infiltrates within the dermis and subcutaneous fat, composed of (b) small lymphocytes admixed with numerous eosinophils. Most lymphocytes are positive for both (c) CD20 and (d) CD5, representing neoplastic cells of the B-CLL.

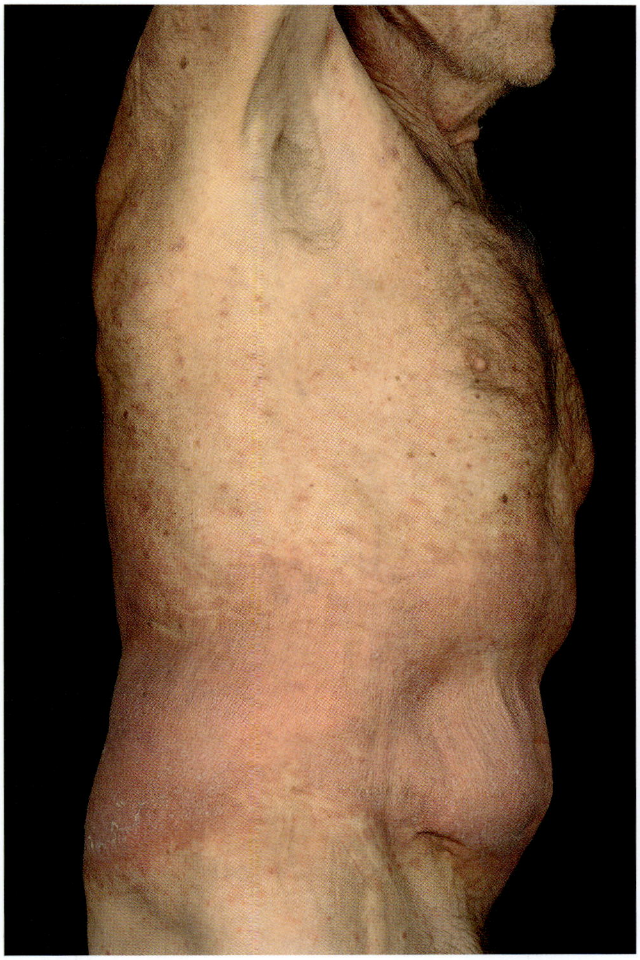

Figure 29.11 Paraneoplastic pemphigus in a patient with B-CLL. Generalized erythematous, partly scaly lesions.

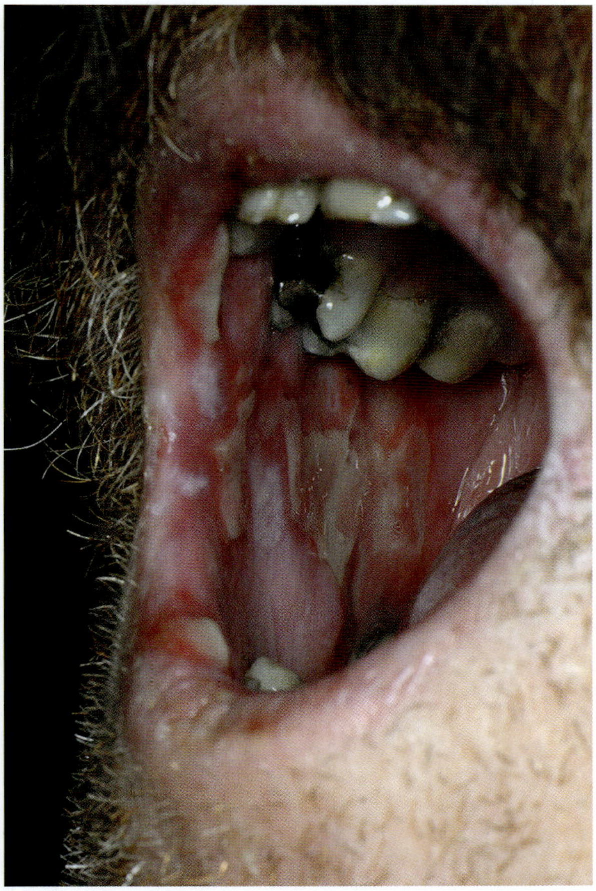

Figure 29.13 Paraneoplastic pemphigus showing severe involvement of the oral mucosa.

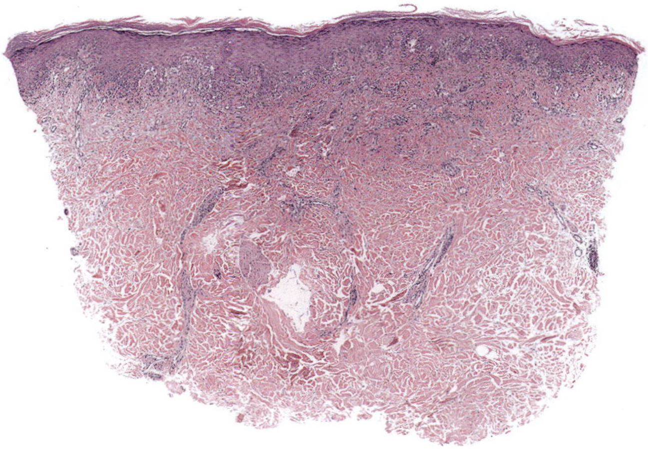

(a)

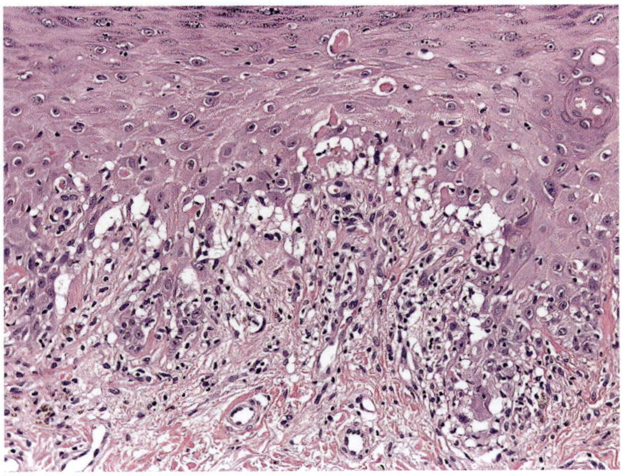

(b)

Figure 29.12 Paraneoplastic pemphigus (same patient of figure 26.5X1). Histology shows (a) a lichenoid dermatitis with (b) several apoptotic keratinocytes. There are no acantholytic aspects.

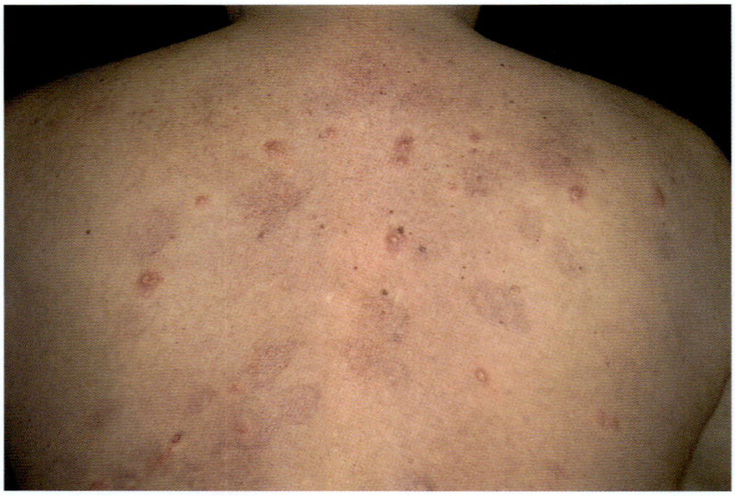

Figure 29.14 Recurrent histiocytoid Sweet syndrome in a patient with acute myeloid leukemia. New infiltrated, elevated lesions on the back admixed with flat, erythematous ones representing resolution of a previous eruption 5 weeks earlier.

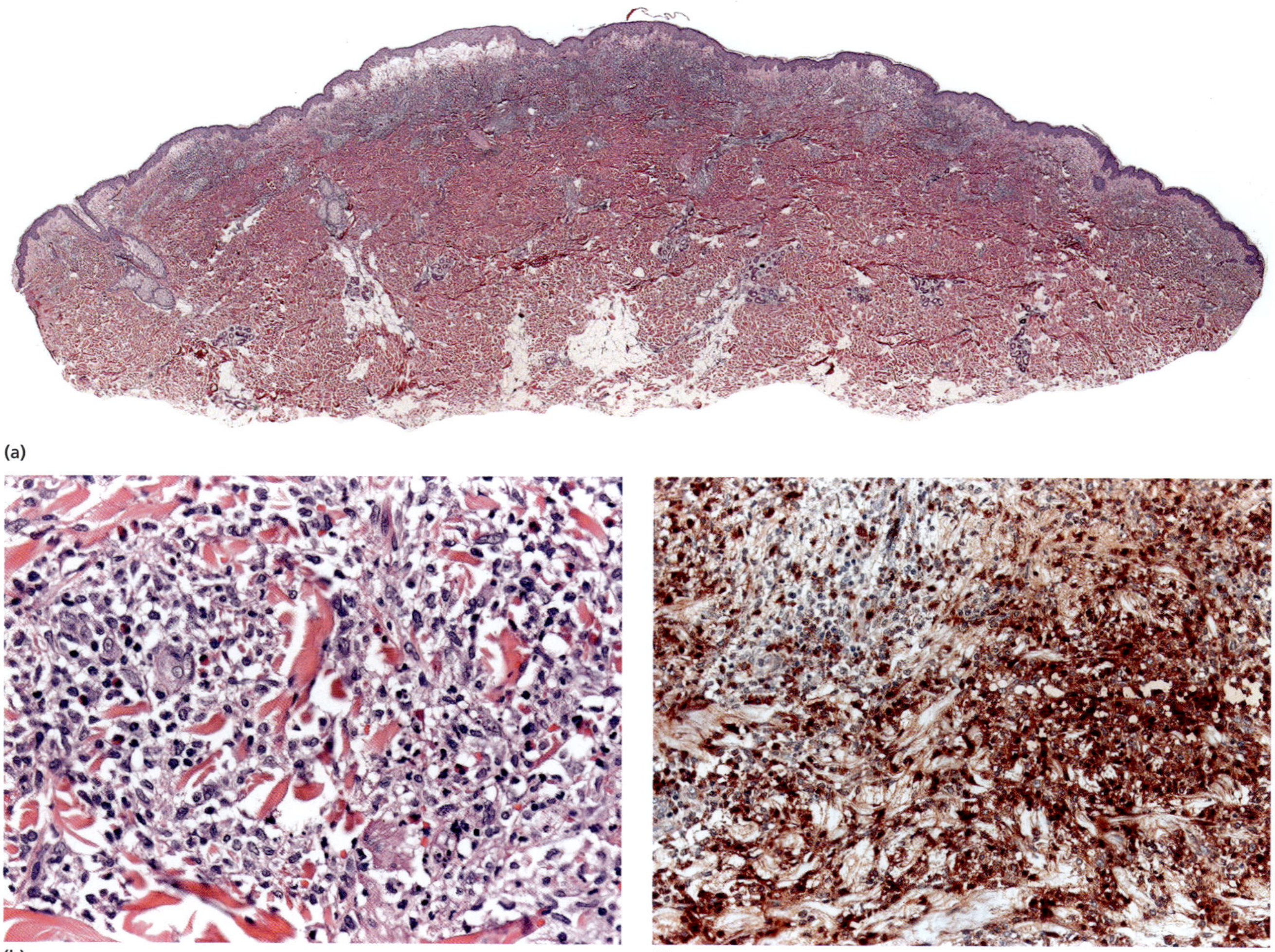

(a)

(b)

(c)

Figure 29.15 Histiocytoid Sweet syndrome in a patient with acute myeloid leukemia. Histopathology shows (a) focal subepidermal edema and dense infiltrates in the superficial and mid-dermis, composed (b) of histiocytoid cells admixed with neutrophils and eosinophils. (c) The histiocytoid cells are positive for myeloperoxidase.

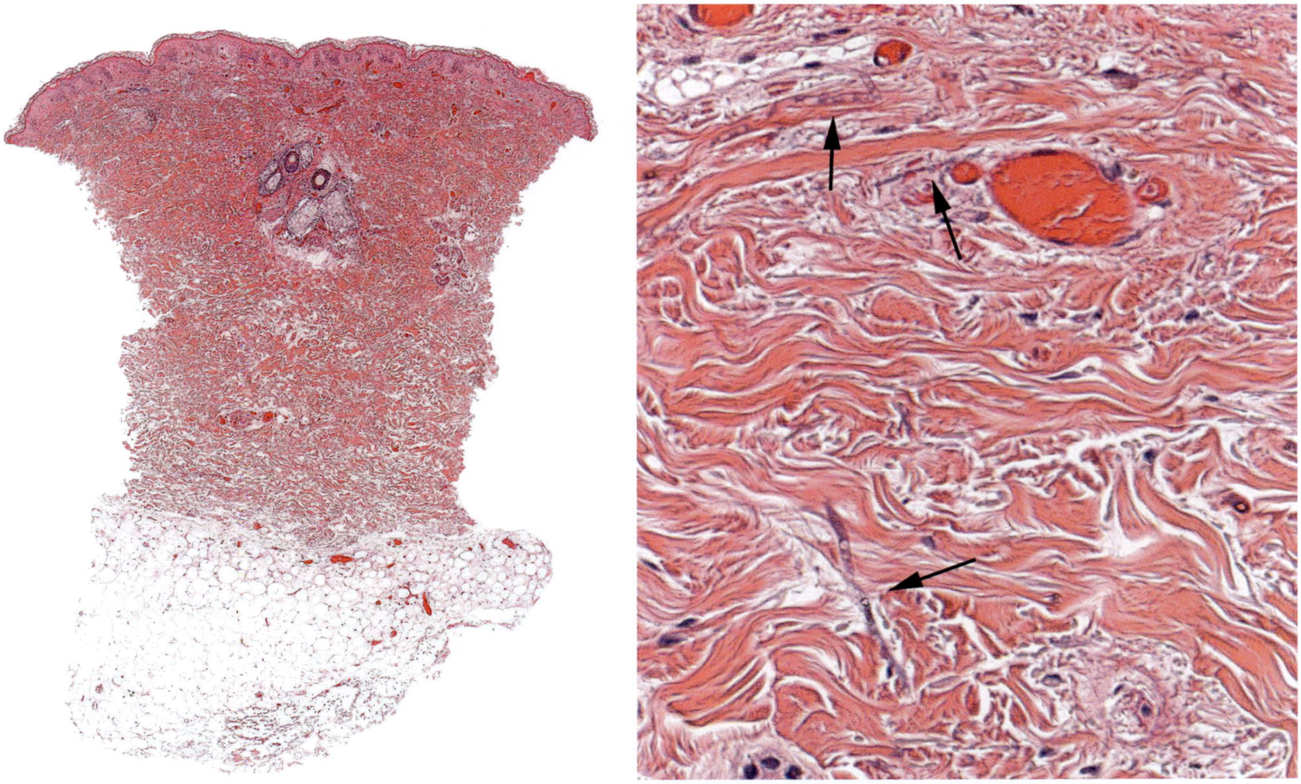

(a) (b)

**Figure 29.16** Sepsis caused by *aspergillus* in a patient with myeloid leukemia. (a) Congested vessels in the dermis an subcutis without relevant inflammation; (b) High power shows several hyphae within the vessels and free in the dermis.

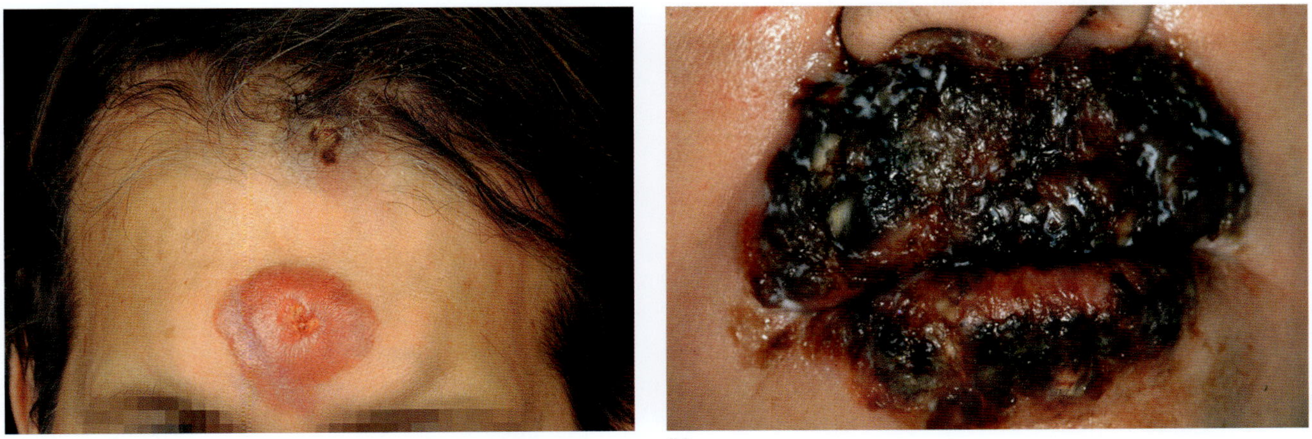

(a) (b)

**Figure 29.17** Herpes infection in patients with hematological malignancies. (a) Herpes zoster in a patient with acute myeloid leukemia. Large, flat tumor with central ulceration and a second, smaller, erosive lesion on the forehead. (b) Large, hemorrhagic, necrotizing, vegetating lesion of herpes simplex in a patient with acute myeloid leukemia.

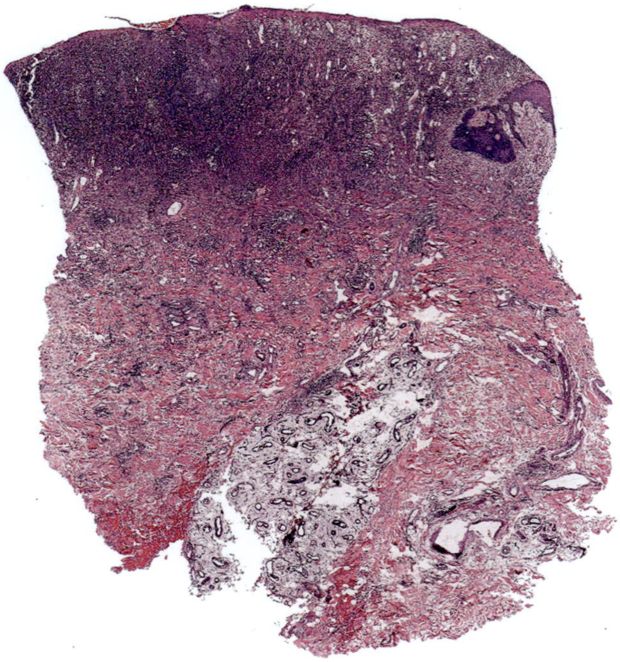

(a)

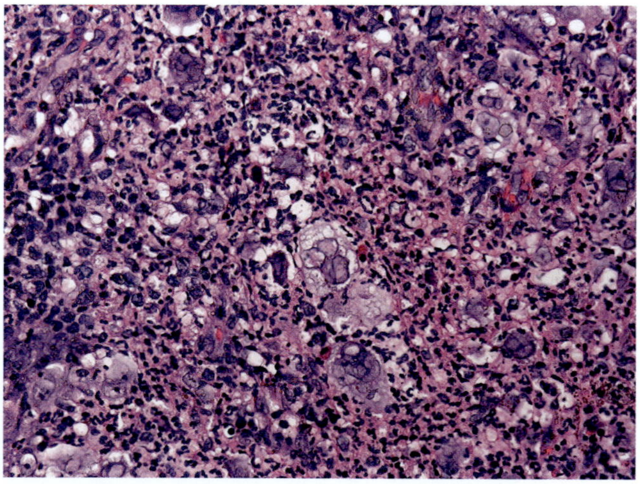

(b)

**Figure 29.18** Vegetating herpes simplex infection in a patient with B-CLL. (a) Ulcerated plaque with pronounced inflammation and with (b) only scattered large, ballooned cells representing remnants of infected keratinocytes.

## References


1. Cerroni L. Cutaneous lymphomas and cutaneous signs of systemic lymphomas. In: Callen JP, Jorizzo JL, Zone JJ, *et al.*, eds. *Dermatological signs of systemic disease*. 5th edition. Elsevier, Edinburgh, 2017: 159–170. (ISBN: 978-0-323-35829-3).
2. Desch JK, Smoller BR. The spectrum of cutaneous disease in leukemias. *J Cutan Pathol* 1993;**20**:407–410.
3. Alegría-Landa V, Cerroni L, Kutzner H, Requena L. Paraprotein deposits in the skin. *J Am Acad Dermatol* 2017;**77**:1145–1158.
4. Walsh NM, Kutzner H, Requena L, Cerroni L. Plasmacytic cutaneous pathology: a review. *J Cutan Pathol* 2019;**46**:698–708.
5. Retamozo S, Brito-Zerón P, Bosch X, *et al.* Cryoglobulinemic disease. *Oncology (Williston Park)* 2013;**27**(1098–1105):1110–1116.
6. DeLyria PA, Avedschmidt SE, Yamada C, Farkash EA. Fatal cryocrystalglobulinemia with intravascular and renal tubular crystalline deposits. *Am J Kidney Dis* 2016;**67**:787–791.
7. Requena L, Sarasa JL, Masllorrens FO, *et al.* Follicular spicules of the nose: a peculiar cutaneous manifestation of multiple myeloma with cryoglobulinemia. *J Am Acad Dermatol* 1995;**32**:834–839.
8. Tay LK, Lim FL, Ng HJ, *et al.* Cutaneous follicular hyperkeratotic spicules-the first clinical sign of multiple myeloma progression or relapse. *Int J Dermatol* 2010;**49**:934–936.
9. Jenkins RE, Calonje E, Fawcett H, *et al.* Cutaneous crystalline deposits in myeloma. *Arch Dermatol* 1994;**130**:484–488.
10. Dogan S, Barnes L, Cruz-Vetrano WP. Crystal-storing histiocytosis: report of a case, review of the literature (80 cases) and a proposed classification. *Head Neck Pathol* 2012;**6**:111–120.
11. Schönland SO, Hegenbart U, Bochtler T, *et al.* Immunohistochemistry in the classification of systemic forms of amyloidosis: a systematic investigation of 117 patients. *Blood* 2012;**119**:488–493.
12. Weed RI. Exaggerated delayed hypersensitivity to mosquito bites in chronic lymphocytic leukemia. *Blood.* 1965;**26**:257–268.
13. Barzilai A, Shpiro D, Goldberg I, *et al.* Insect bite-like reaction in patients with hematologic malignant neoplasms. *Arch Dermatol* 1999;**135**:1503–1507.
14. Michelerio A, Rubatto M, Roccuzzo G, *et al.* Eosinophilic dermatosis of hematologic malignancy: emerging evidence for the role of insect bites-a retrospective clinico-pathological study of 35 cases. *J Clin Med* 2024;**16**(13):2935.
15. Farber MJ, La Forgia S, Sahu J, Lee JB. Eosinophilic dermatosis of hematologic malignancy. *J Cutan Pathol* 2012;**39**:690–695.
16. Grandi V, Maglie R, Antiga E, *et al.* Eosinophilic dermatosis of hematologic malignancy: a retrospective cohort of 37 patients from an Italian center. *J Am Acad Dermatol* 2019;**81**:246–249.
17. Stingl G, Cerroni L, Wolf P. *Eosinophils in Skin Disease: Bystanders or Pathogenic Players? Skin Deep* 2025 (in press)
18. Meiss F, Technau-Hafsi K, Kern JS, May AM. Eosinophilic dermatosis of hematologic malignancy: correlation of molecular characteristics of skin lesions and extracutaneous manifestations of hematologic malignancy. *J Cutan Pathol* 2019;**46**:175–181.
19. Requena L, Kutzner H, Palmedo G, *et al.* Histiocytoid Sweet syndrome: a dermal infiltration of immature neutrophilic granulocytes. *Arch Dermatol* 2005;**141**:834–842.
20. Magro CM, Momtahen S, Nguyen GH, Wang X. Histiocytoid Sweet's syndrome: a localized cutaneous proliferation of macrophages frequently associated with chronic myeloproliferative disease. *Eur J Dermatol* 2015;**25**:335–341.
21. Chavan RN, Cappel MA, Ketterling RP, *et al.* Histiocytoid Sweet syndrome may indicate leukemia cutis: a novel application of fluorescence In situ hybridization. *J Am Acad Dermatol* 2014;**70**:1021–1027.
22. Urano Y, Miyaoka Y, Kosaka M, *et al.* Sweet's syndrome associated with chronic myelogenous leukemia: demonstration of leukemic cells within a skin lesion. *J Am Acad Dermatol* 1999;**40**:275–279.

23. Deguchi M, Tsunoda T, Yuda F, Tagami H. Sweet's syndrome in acute myelogenous leukemia showing dermal infiltration of leukemic cells. *Dermatology* 1997;**194**:182–184.
24. Alegría-Landa V, Rodríguez-Pinilla SM, Santos-Briz A, *et al.* Clinicopathologic, immunohistochemical, and molecular features of histiocytoid sweet syndrome. *JAMA Dermatol* 2017;**153**: 651–659.
25. Calvo KR. Skin in the game: the emergence of myelodysplasia cutis. *Blood* 2022;**139**:1132–1134.
26. Delaleu J, Kim R, Zhao LP, *et al.* Clinical, pathological, and molecular features of myelodysplasia cutis. *Blood* 2022;**139**:1251–1253.
27. Grolleau C, Battistella M, Zakine E, *et al.* Inflammatory signatures in VEXAS syndrome,myelodysplasia cutis, and sweet syndrome. *JAMA Dermatol* 2025;**161**:538–543.

SECTION 6

# Cutaneous lymphomas and lymphoproliferative disorders in children and adolescents

**CHAPTER 30**

# Cutaneous lymphomas and lymphoproliferative disorders in children and adolescents

In the literature on cutaneous lymphomas, data on children and adolescents are often lumped together with those of adult patients. Although clinicopathologic features may indeed be similar, sometimes in young individuals cutaneous lymphomas present with peculiar aspects. This chapter offers an overview of cutaneous lymphomas arising in children and adolescents. A detailed discussion of each lymphoma entity is beyond the scope of this section, as it can be found in the corresponding chapters of the book; data pertinent to children and adolescents are summarized in this chapter.

In medicine in general, and in cutaneous lymphomas in particular, the definition of "childhood" has been used variably. For the purpose of this chapter, childhood ends with puberty and adolescence (somehow artificially, I have to admit) with the age of 18. Cutaneous lymphomas in children and adolescents are listed in Table 30.1, together with available data on relative frequency (based on the Graz experience on 221 patients and on the only five other large series published). In this context, it must be underlined that the incidence and prevalence of different types of cutaneous lymphomas in pediatric patients vary in different reports. Some of the discrepancies may be due, at least in part, to the author's affiliations, as some lymphomas observed commonly in departments of dermatology may be rare in those of pediatric hematology, and vice versa. In addition, most of the published articles deal with specific entities (particularly mycosis fungoides), and only a few studies on the relative frequency of all cutaneous lymphomas in children and adolescents are available [1–6]. One of these studies [3] has some unclear data, like one case of "secondary cutaneous" mycosis fungoides; thus, data from this publication should be interpreted with great caution. A recent small series, too, includes cases that are not classified according to standard schemes (e.g., "CD30-negative anaplastic large cell lymphoma") [7]. A further study from the Cutaneous Lymphoma Registry of the Spanish Academy of Dermatology and Venereology included only 10 patients: 7 with mycosis fungoides (2 of which adnexotropic), and 3 with marginal zone lymphoproliferative disorder [8], thus in my opinion not reflecting the real distribution of cases in Spain (and for this reason not included in Table 30.1). The overrepresentation of systemic hydroa vacciniforme lymphoproliferative disorder observed in Graz is due to the inclusion of 9 cases received in consultation from Mexico and Brazil; no case has been observed in the pediatric population in Graz.

## Mycosis fungoides

In my experience, as well as in that of others, this is the most common cutaneous lymphoma in children and adolescents (about one-third of cases) [1, 2, 4]. More important, it is the most reported cutaneous lymphoma in different parts of the globe [2, 4, 9–23], showing that high incidence is not due to a geographical bias. The low incidence (10%) reported by Boccara *et al.* [1] may be explained by selection bias, as cases were observed at a children's hospital located in a large city with many other dermatological facilities that may have managed other cases of mycosis fungoides in the pediatric population. In addition, aggressive cases (e.g., acute leukemia) are overrepresented in the study by Boccara *et al.* [1], providing a further explanation for the low percentage of cases of mycosis fungoides. The same considerations apply to the series published by Colmant et al. as well [6].

Children and adolescents may present with conventional lesions of mycosis fungoides identical to those observed in adults (Figs. 30.1a to d) [11, 12, 24–28]. A cytotoxic phenotype is more common in young than in adult patients, and double positivity for CD8 and CD56 may be observed in these cases [29, 30].

Follicular mucinosis has been observed often in children, adolescents, and even neonates (Figs. 30.1e and f) [31–33]. Many of these cases represent the so-called "benign" type of follicular mucinosis, but association with mycosis fungoides has been reported in the pediatric population [31, 34, 35]. Localized pagetoid reticulosis (Woringer–Kolopp) is another rare variant of mycosis fungoides that is probably more frequent in children and adolescents than in adults (Figs. 30.1g and h) [36–39]. Indeed, the first description by Woringer and Kolopp concerned

*Skin Lymphoma: The Illustrated Guide*, Sixth Edition. Lorenzo Cerroni.

**Table 30.1** Relative frequency of cutaneous lymphomas in children and adolescents (% of total cases observed) (including entities not observed in the Research Unit Dermatopathology, Medical University of Graz, Austria, and not included in the three other studies, but reported sporadically in the literature, with pertinent references in brackets)

| Entity | Graz# | Boccara *et al.** [1] | Kempf *et al.*† [2] | Moon *et al.*• [3] | Alberti-Violetti *et al.*$ [5] | Colmant *et al.*¥ [6] |
|---|---|---|---|---|---|---|
| Mycosis fungoides | 34.4 (35.8)# | 9.8 | 38.7 | 22.0 | 30.7 | 16.7 |
| Sézary syndrome [52, 53] | 0 | 0 | 0 | 0 | 1 | 0 |
| Lymphomatoid papulosis | 19.0 (19.8) | 47.1 | 32.6 | 24.4 | 47.5 | 27.8 |
| Anaplastic large cell lymphoma | 4.5 (4.7) | 0 | 9.7 | 19.5 | 5 | 11.1 |
| Subcutaneous T-cell lymphoma | 3.2 (3.3) | 2 | 0 | 2.4 | 2 | 0 |
| Extranodal NK/T-cell lymphoma, nasal type | 0.9 (0.9) | 2 | 0 | 4.9 | 0 | 2.8 |
| Cutaneous $\gamma/\delta$ T-cell lymphoma | 1.8 (1.9) | 2 | 0 | 0 | 0 | 0 |
| Aggressive epidermotropic CD8+ cytotoxic T-cell lymphoma [70, 71] | 0 | 0 | 0 | 0 | 0 | 0 |
| Adult T-cell lymphoma/leukemia (ATLL) [75] | 0 | 0 | 0 | 0 | 0 | 0 |
| CD4+ small/medium T-cell lymphoproliferative disorder | 7.7 (8.0) | 0 | 3.2 | 2.4 | 6.9 | 2.8 |
| Cutaneous peripheral T-cell lymphoma, NOS [73] | 0.9 (0.9) | 0 | 0 | 0 | 1 | 0 |
| Cutaneous angioimmunoblastic T-cell lymphoma [88] | 0 | 0 | 0 | 0 | 0 | 0 |
| Systemic hydroa vacciniforme lymphoproliferative disorder | 4.1 (0) | 0 | 0 | 0 | 0 | 2.8 |
| Marginal zone lymphoproliferative disorder | 11.8 (12.3) | 0 | 9.7 | 2.4 | 3 | 11.1 |
| Follicle center lymphoma | 3.2 (3.3) | 0 | 0 | 0 | 2 | 0 |
| Immune deficiency-associated lymphomas | 0.5 (0.5) | 7.8 | 0 | 0 | 0 | 0 |
| Cutaneous Burkitt lymphoma [96] | 0 | 0 | 0 | 0 | 0 | 0 |
| B lymphoblastic lymphoma/leukemia | 2.7 (2.8) | 13.7 | 6.5 | 14.6 | 1 | 16.7 |
| Acute myelogenous leukemia | 0.9 (0.9) | 11.8 | not searched | 0 | 0 | 8.3 |
| Blastic plasmacytoid dendritic cell neoplasm | 2.3 (2.4) | 0 | not searched | 7.3 | 0 | 0 |
| Unclassified | 0.9 (0.9)$ | 3.9§ | 0 | 0 | 0 | 0 |

# Total of 221 cases recorded in the Dermatopathology Unit of the Medical University of Graz (Austria) (including 57 cases published previously [4], and including cases sent in consultation for second expert opinion); overrepresentation of systemic hydroa vacciniforme lymphoproliferative disorder due to inclusion of consultation cases from Mexico and Brazil; no case has been observed in Caucasian children and adolescents (percentage values in brackets are calculated on 212 patients, excluding the 9 cases of systemic hydroa vacciniforme lymphoproliferative disorder).
† Total of 31 cases observed in Zürich (Switzerland), Pilsen (Czech Republic), and Saint Petersburg (Russia).
• Total of 41 cases observed in Korea; some data are unclear (e.g., 1 case of "secondary cutaneous" mycosis fungoides).
$ Total of 101 cases observed in Milan (Italy).
¥ Total of 36 cases observed in Montreal (Canada).
$ One unclassified blastoid T-cell lymphoma and one unclassified cytotoxic NK/T-cell lymphoma.
§ One unclassified T-cell lymphoma and one unclassified EBV+ lymphoproliferative disorder in an immunocompetent patient.
* Total of 51 cases observed in Paris (France).

a 13-year-old boy. One case of granulomatous slack skin was reported in a 16-year-old boy, showing fatal outcome a few months after first presentation [40]. The clinical and histopathological pictures are convincing of granulomatous slack skin; however, the patient died of unknown causes after having developed sudden hypotension, and a systemic involvement was never proven by biopsy.

A peculiar type of mycosis fungoides in young patients simulates pityriasis lichenoides (personally, I don't make distinction between pityriasis lichenoides et varioliformis acuta and pityriasis lichenoides chronica, as clinicopathological presentation is indistinguishable) (Fig. 30.1i) [41–46]. Some authors pointed at a possible relationship between the two disorders [1], and cases of "transformation" of pityriasis lichenoides chronica into mycosis fungoides have been reported [47]. I have observed many cases of otherwise conventional mycosis fungoides showing histopathological features that were indistinguishable from those of pityriasis lichenoides, and it may be that cases with "transformation" represented in truth mycosis fungoides from the outset (for a detailed discussion, see also Chapter 31, section on pityriasis lichenoides, and Chapter 3, section on pityriasis lichenoides-like mycosis fungoides).

Hypopigmentation is a common variant of mycosis fungoides in children and adolescents (Figs. 30.1j and k), particularly in dark-skinned individuals and in patients from Middle-Eastern countries. In fact, hypopigmented mycosis fungoides is much more common in young individuals than in adults. Other morphological presentations observed in children and adolescents reflect the protean nature of the disease, similarly to what is found in adult patients (Figs. 30.1l).

It is important to underline that in children and adolescents the clinicopathologic differential diagnosis of mycosis fungoides

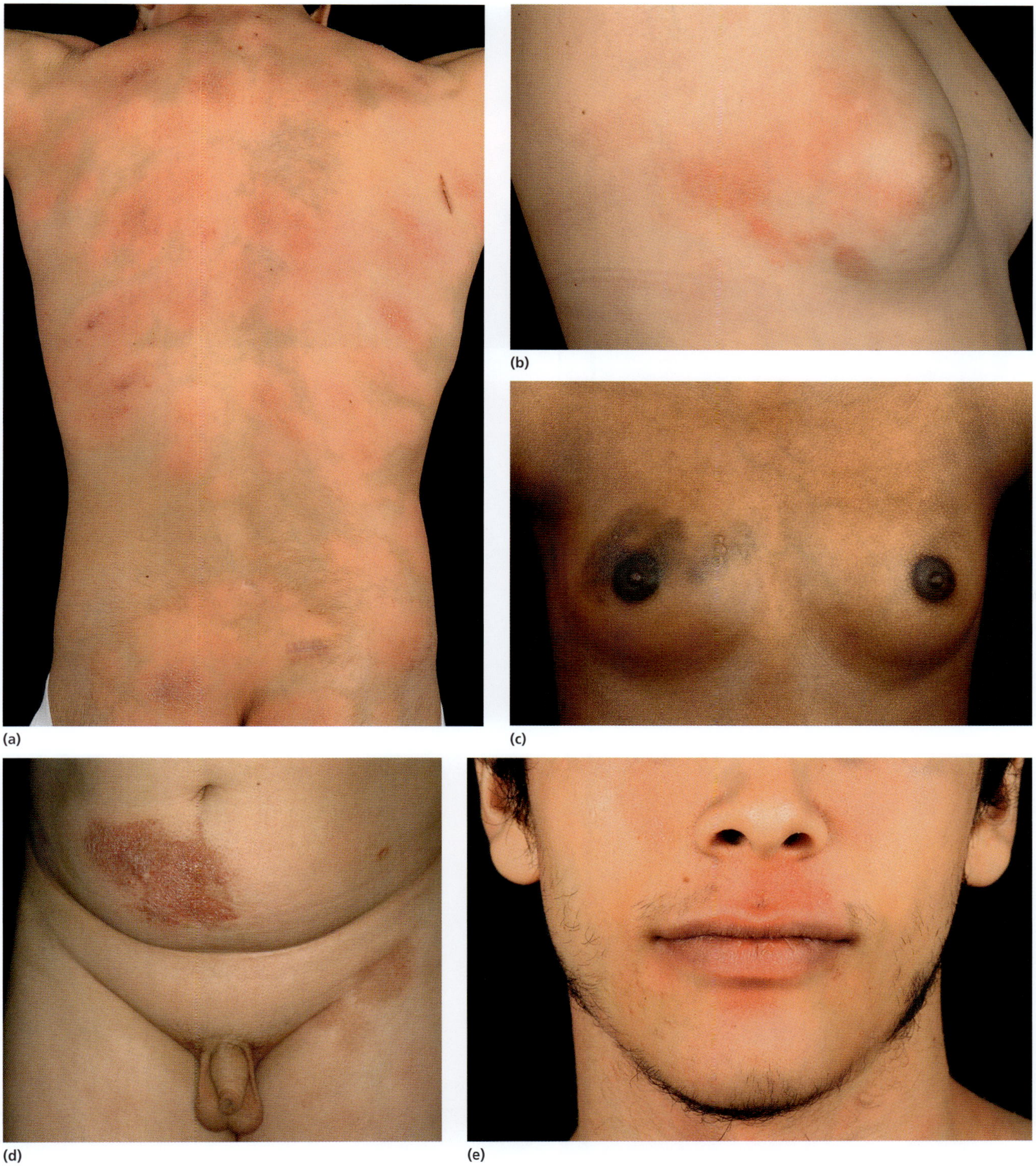

**Figure 30.1** Various clinical presentations of mycosis fungoides in children and adolescents. (a) 17-year-old boy with "conventional" mycosis fungoides. (b) 13-year-old girl with lesions localized on the breast; (c) Similar lesions on the same location in a 17-year-old girl with dark skin resulting clinically in hyperpigmentation; (d) Partly poikilodermatic lesion in a 14-year-old boy with sexual underdevelopment; (e) Follicular involvement with focal alopecia on the upper lip in a 17-year-old boy; (f) Pilotropic mycosis fungoides with patchy alopecia of the extremities in a 16-year-old boy; (g) Localized pagetoid reticulosis in a 5-year-old girl with small verrucous lesions on the foot, (h) clinically mimicking viral warts; (i) Pityriasis lichenoides-like lesions in a 13-year-old boy (*Courtesy of Dr. Guido Massi, Rome, Italy.*); (j) Hypopigmented mycosis fungoides with only minimal erythema in an 11-year-old boy (*Courtesy of Dr. Belfrage, Skane.*); (k) Hypopigmented lesions of mycosis fungoides with also areas of erythema on the shoulder of a 7-year-old Caucasian boy (*Courtesy of Prof. Ernesto Bonifazi, Bari, Italy.*); (l) Confluent papules with a "cobblestone" appearance in an 11-year old boy *(Courtesy of Dermatology Service, University Hospital of Paraná, Curitiba, Brazil.)*

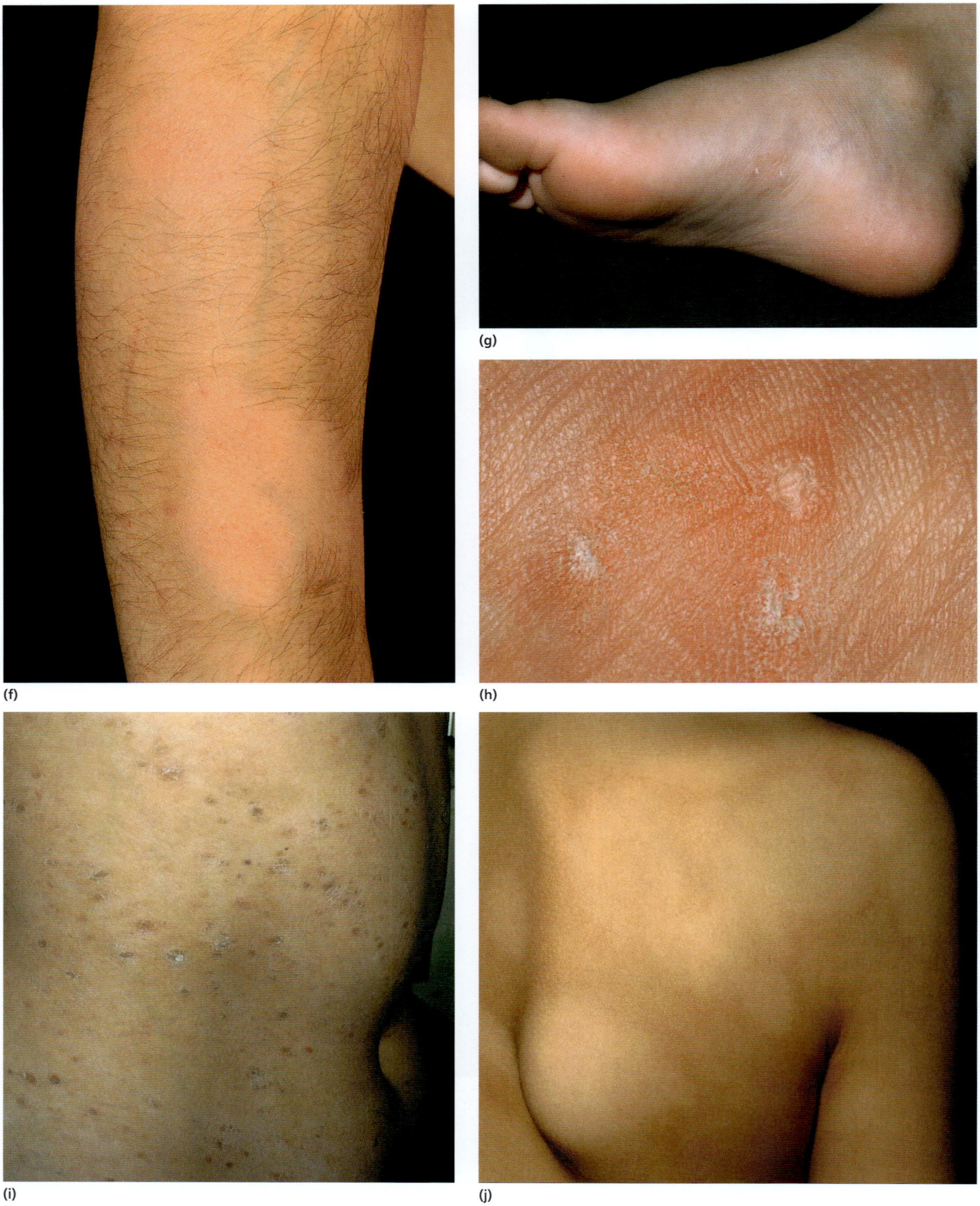


**Figure 30.1** (Continued)

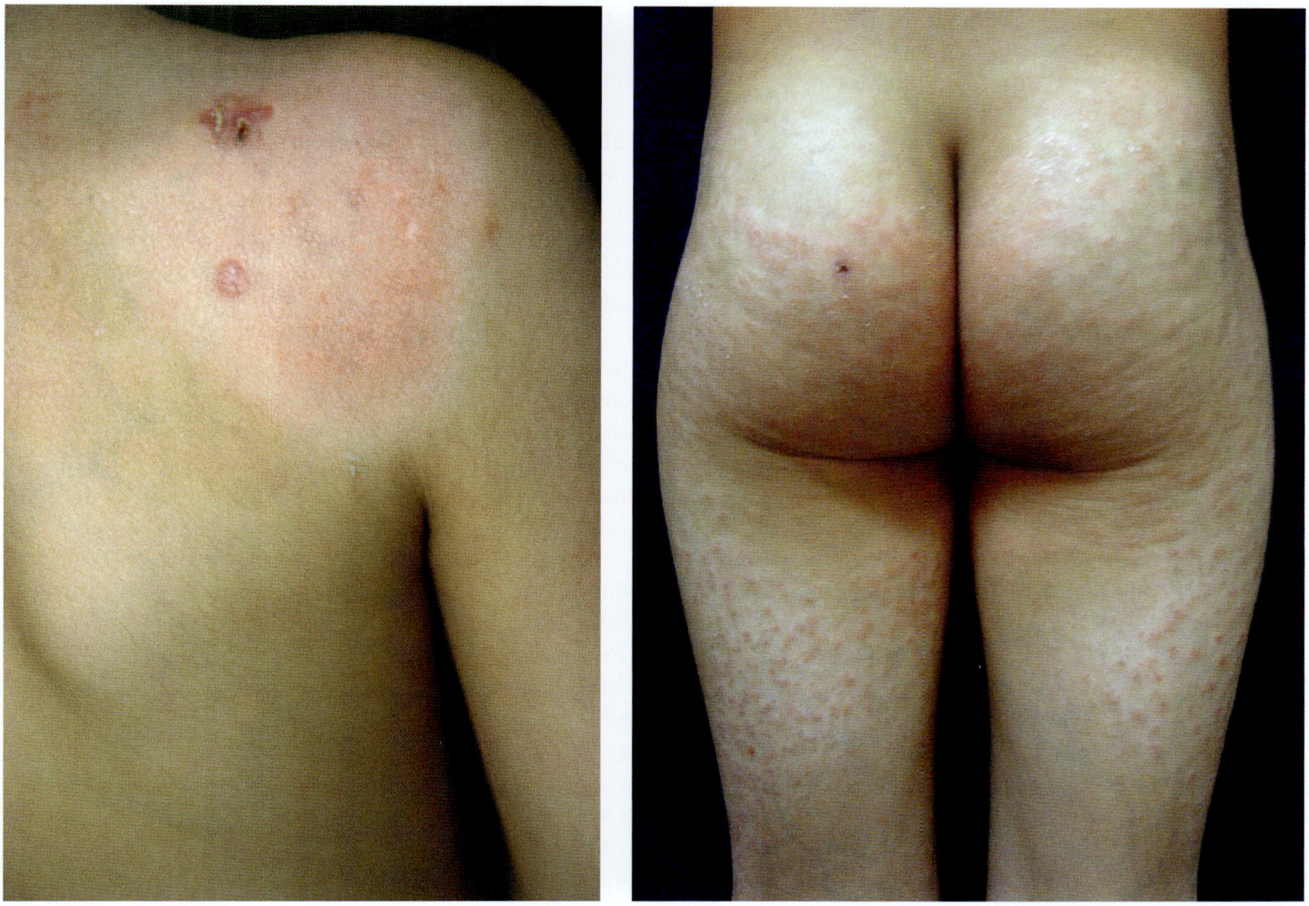

(k) (l)

Figure 30.1 (Continued)

is not identical to that of adult patients. Some types of pseudolymphoma are mostly restricted to young individuals (e.g., annular lichenoid dermatitis of youth), and others arise only in adults (e.g., lichenoid {lymphomatoid} keratosis). I have never seen cases of pseudolymphomatous atopic dermatitis in pediatric patients, even if the disease is common in this age group. Although infection by *Borrelia* species occurs often in children and adolescents, and *Borrelia*-induced lymphocytoma is common in young patients, acrodermatitis chronica atrophicans is exceptional in the pediatric population, and the mycosis fungoides-like presentations of this variant of *Borreliosis* have never been observed.

The prognosis of mycosis fungoides in children and adolescents seems to be similar to that of adult patients [4, 11, 13, 26, 48, 49], and only one report pointed at a more aggressive course [50]. On the other hand, early onset of the disease allows time for progression during the lifetime of patients. Poikilodermatous clinical presentation was associated with onset of progressive disease in one study [51a]. Recommendations for the diagnosis, staging, and treatment of early-stage pediatric (i.e., <18 years of age) mycosis fungoides have been recently issued by a panel of lymphoma experts from the International Society of Cutaneous Lymphomas (ISCL), the European Organization for Research and Treatment of Cancer-Cutaneous Lymphoma Tumour Group (EORTC-CLTG), and the United States Cutaneous Lymphomas Consortium (USCLC) [51b, 51c]. The panelists underlined the high prevalence of hypopigmented and adnexotropic variants of the disease in the pediatric population and recommended that while the staging approach is similar to that in adults, imaging for early-stage pediatric mycosis fungoides, if indicated, should rely on ultrasound of the lymph nodes rather than computer tomography (CT)/positron emission tomography-CT. There was also consensus on the indolent nature of the disease in the pediatric age, with only rare progression to the advanced stage [51b]. The therapeutic approach suggested by these guidelines is similar to that of adult patients with early-stage disease, with the exception of oral psoralen and ultraviolet A (PUVA), for which other UVA-based therapies are preferred, such as topical PUVA, UVA1, or a combination of UVA and narrow-band UVB [51c].

## Sézary syndrome

Only two cases of Sézary syndrome have been reported in pediatric patients, one in an 11-year-old girl [52], and a second one in a 17-year-old boy [5], showing that the disease is exceedingly rare in young patients and should not be considered as a serious differential diagnosis when evaluating erythroderma in children and adolescents. A third case was reported as having "erythrodermic follicular mucinosis" possibly related to Sézary syndrome [53]. In this context, erythroderma in neonates evokes a spectrum of differential diagnoses among which Sézary syndrome has no place at all, including mainly ichthyosis, Netherton syndrome, primary immune deficiency syndromes ("inborn error of immunity"), seborrheic dermatitis, psoriasis, metabolic diseases, and atopic dermatitis [54].

## Lymphomatoid papulosis

In my experience and that of others [2], this is the second most common cutaneous lymphoma in children and adolescents, but it was the most frequent in the series by Boccara *et al.*, Alberti-Violetti *et al.*, and Colmant *et al.* [1, 5, 6]. However, I think that in these three series, the distribution of cases is affected by selection bias. In fact, although lymphomatoid papulosis is not uncommon in pediatric patients, in my opinion it cannot be considered more frequent than mycosis fungoides in this population.

As for adult patients, multiple lesions in different stages of evolution are usually seen (Fig. 30.2a, b). Non-ulcerated lesions may be difficult to distinguish from other causes of papular eruptions (Fig. 30.2c). Mucosal surfaces can be involved (Fig. 30.2d). There are no specific clinicopathologic features of lymphomatoid papulosis in young patients that warrant a detailed discussion beyond what has already been written in Chapter 5 [55]. Progression into a second lymphoma has not been reported in one study on young patients [56], but I have observed children with lymphomatoid papulosis and a second nodal lymphoma (Hodgkin lymphoma or anaplastic large cell lymphoma), and other cases are reported as well [57].

## Cutaneous anaplastic large cell lymphoma

Children and adolescents may be affected by both primary and secondary cutaneous anaplastic large cell lymphoma. As well as in adult cases, staging investigations should always be carried out in young patients, too.

In contrast to primary cutaneous anaplastic large cell lymphoma arising in adults, several cases occurring in pediatric patients are positive for ALK-1 and show the t(2,5)(q23;q35) translocation, suggesting that ALK-1+ cutaneous anaplastic large cell lymphoma is not infrequent in young individuals (Fig. 30.3) [58–61]. An association with insect bites has been reported in some patients [62], but it is debatable whether the history is reliable enough to establish a precise link in these cases.

The prognosis in children and adolescents seems to be similar to that of conventional cutaneous anaplastic large cell lymphoma in adults.

## Subcutaneous panniculitis-like T-cell lymphoma

This type of lymphoma has been described in young patients, but is rare in this age group [1, 63–65]. The clinicopathologic features are similar to those observed in adults (Fig. 30.4). A hemophagocytic syndrome has been observed in pediatric cases with an aggressive course [66].

The differential diagnoses of subcutaneous panniculitis-like T-cell lymphoma in children are in part different from those considered for adult patients. In fact, although lupus erythematosus panniculitis can be observed in childhood, it is rare in this age group [67]. On the other hand, in young children with immune deficiency disorders a lobular panniculitis indistinguishable from that of subcutaneous panniculitis-like T-cell lymphoma may be observed, even with clonality of the T lymphocytes, representing an important differential diagnosis. Histopathologic features similar to those observed in subcutaneous panniculitis-like T-cell lymphoma have also been described in a macrophage activating syndrome presenting in pediatric patients [68] and in lipoatrophic panniculitis of the ankles in childhood [69]. For practical purposes, a diagnosis of subcutaneous panniculitis-like T-cell lymphoma in children should be accepted only if other causes of lobular panniculitis have been excluded.

## Primary cutaneous aggressive epidermotropic CD8+ cytotoxic T-cell lymphoma

Only exceptional cases of cutaneous aggressive epidermotropic CD8+ cytotoxic T-cell lymphoma have been reported in young patients [70, 71]. Differentiation from CD8+ mycosis fungoides (a common phenotype in children and adolescents) and from lymphomatoid papulosis, type D, may be very difficult, and only follow-up data may be diriment. As a general rule, a diagnosis of primary cutaneous aggressive epidermotropic CD8+ cytotoxic T-cell lymphoma in children and adolescents should be made only if mycosis fungoides and lymphomatoid papulosis can be ruled out by compelling clinicopathologic evidence.

## Primary cutaneous $\gamma/\delta$ T-cell lymphoma

This lymphoma is rare in the pediatric population, but sporadic cases are reported [1, 72]. There are no relevant clinicopathologic differences from adult cases, and patients can present with "mycosis fungoides-like" lesions (Fig. 30.5a) and/or ulcerated tumors (Fig. 30.5b). Differentiation from mycosis fungoides with $\gamma/\delta$ phenotype is crucial, as prognosis and management are completely different. As a rule, a diagnosis of cutaneous $\gamma/\delta$ T-cell lymphoma in pediatric patients should be made only when mycosis fungoides and lymphomatoid papulosis, as well as reactive infiltrates, can be excluded with certainty.

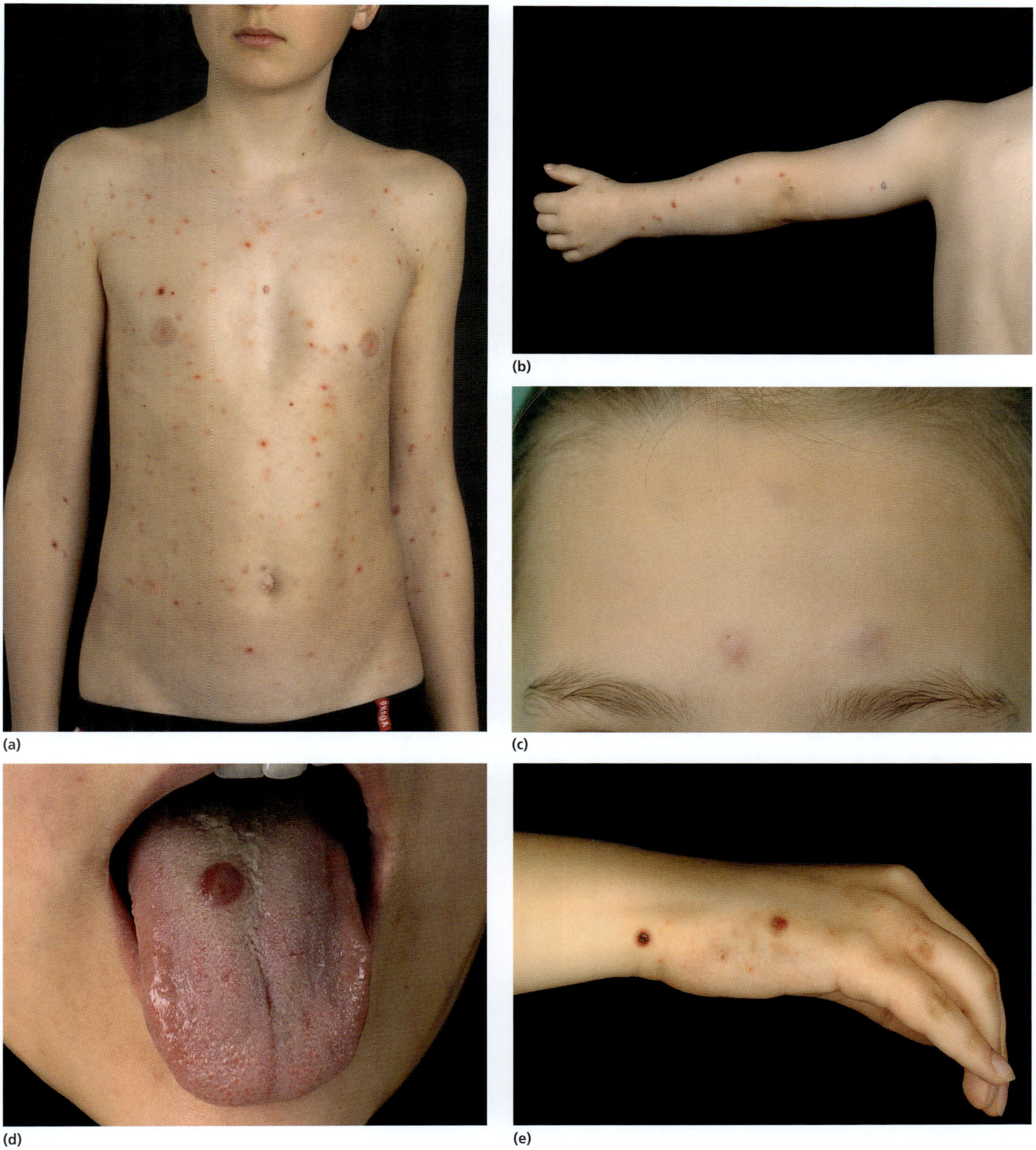

(a) (b) (c) (d) (e)

**Figure 30.2** Lymphomatoid papulosis in pediatric patients. (a, b) Generalized, partly crusted papules in different stages of evolution; (c) Two lesions on the forehead, one almost completely resolved; (d) Single lesion on the tongue *(Courtesy of Prof. Chott, Vienna, Austria)*; (e) lesions on the hand.

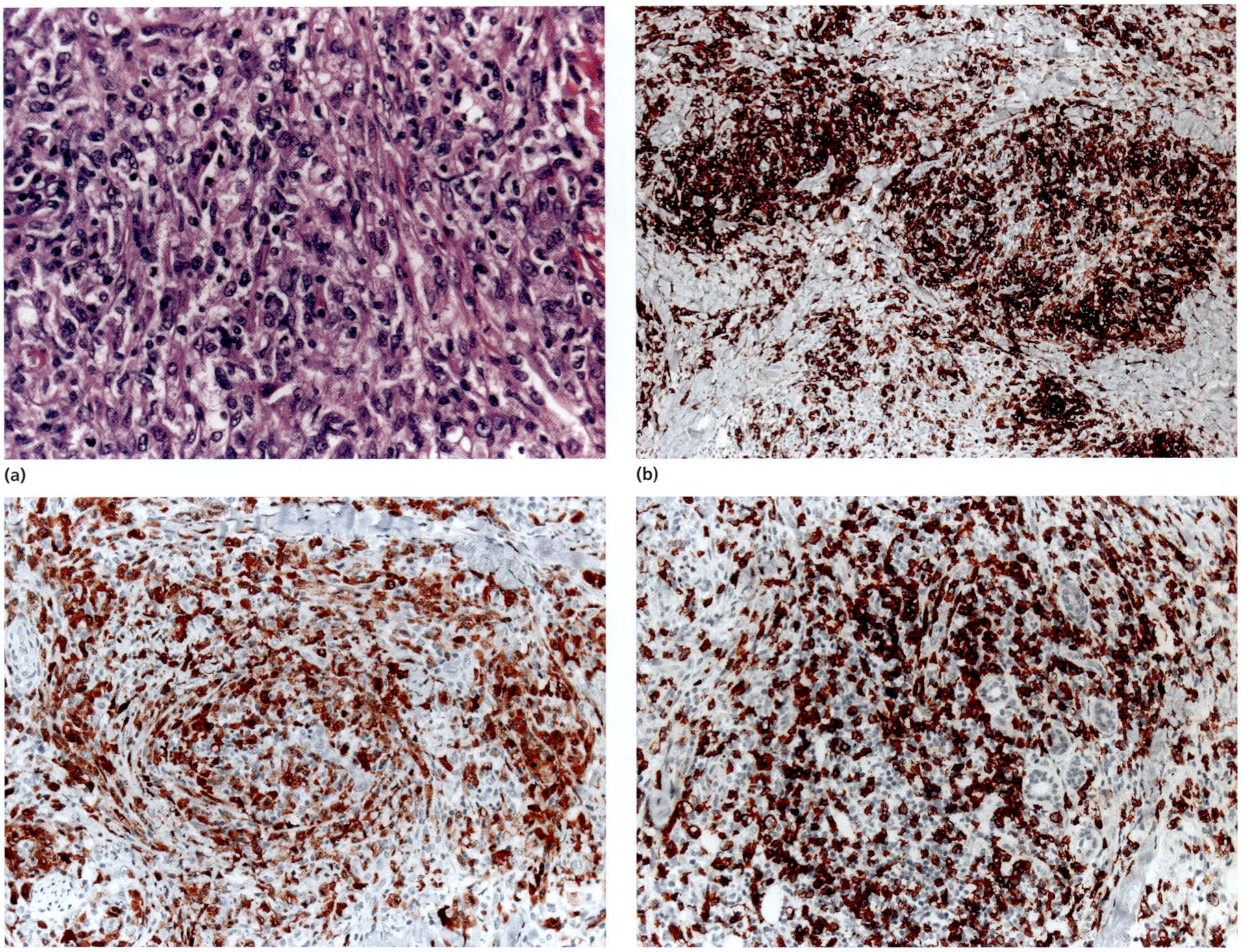

(a) (b) (c) (d)

Figure 30.3 ALK+ anaplastic large cell lymphoma on the thigh of a 14-year-old girl. (a) Large, pleomorphic cells, which are positive for (b) CD30, (c) ALK-1, and (d) CD8.

## Cutaneous extranodal NK/T-cell lymphoma, nasal type

Only a few cases of pediatric cutaneous extranodal natural killer (NK)/T-cell lymphoma, nasal type, have been reported [1, 3, 6]. I have seen rare cases arising in adolescents presenting with the clinical picture of "lethal midline granuloma," who eventually succumbed to their disease (at times antecedent modern targeted therapies) (Fig. 30.6a), and others with a presentation characterized by swelling of the cheeks and puffy eyelids (Fig. 30.6b). The clinicopathologic features are similar to those observed in adults.

## Primary cutaneous peripheral T-cell lymphoma, not otherwise specified (NOS)

There are reports on children and adolescents with cutaneous peripheral T-cell lymphoma, not otherwise specified (NOS), but it is unclear whether patients presented with primary cutaneous manifestations or with secondary skin involvement of a nodal lymphoma [73]. One further case has been reported by Alberti-Violetti *et al.* [5]. However, in my opinion, primary cutaneous cases are exceptional, if they exist at all.

## Cutaneous CD4+ small/medium T-cell lymphoproliferative disorder

In my experience, cutaneous CD4+ small/medium T-cell lymphoproliferative disorder represents a relatively common entity of cutaneous lymphoproliferative disorder in children and adolescents [4]. Several cases have been reported [4–6, 74]. The clinicopathologic features are similar to those observed in adults (Fig. 30.7), and prognosis of solitary lesions located on the head and neck region is excellent. For a detailed discussion about the

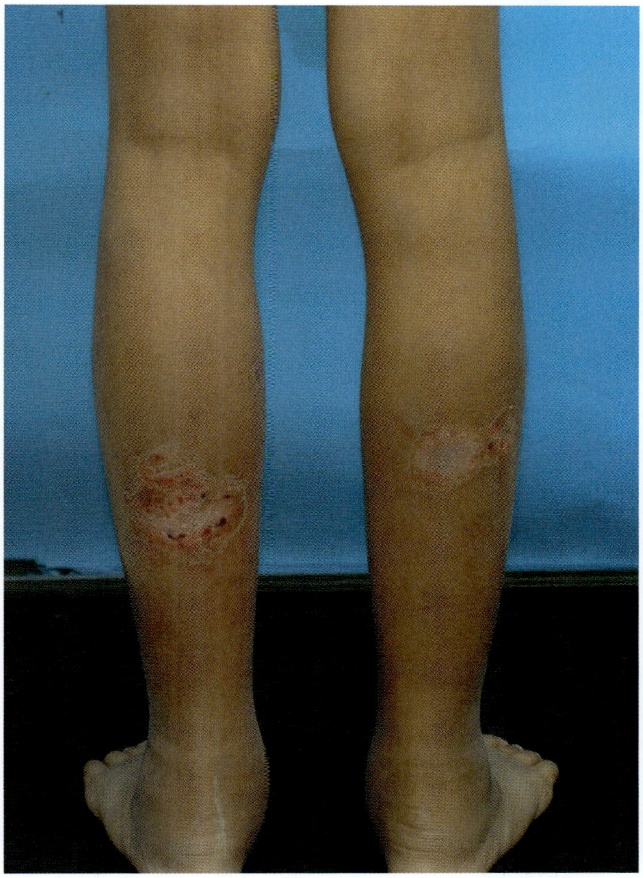

(a)

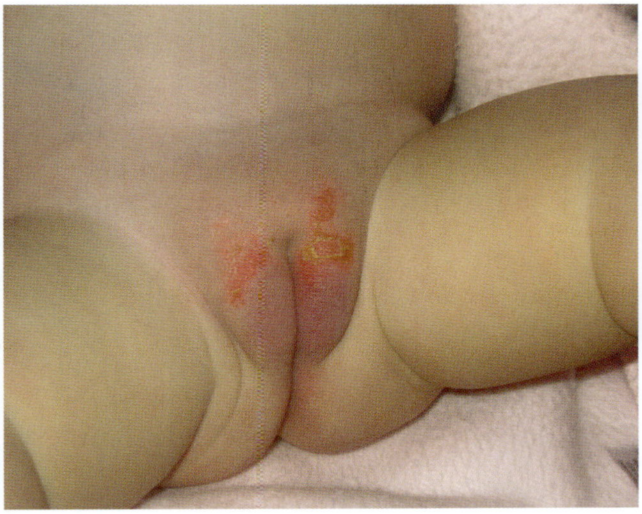

(b)

**Figure 30.4** Subcutaneous panniculitis-like T-cell lymphoma. (a) Partly erosive, infiltrated lesions on the lower legs *(Courtesy of Dr. Bugum, Kuala Lumpur, Malaysia.)* (b) Infiltrated lesions of the external genital area *(Courtesy of Dr. Bruecks and Dr. Campbell, Calgary, Canada.)*

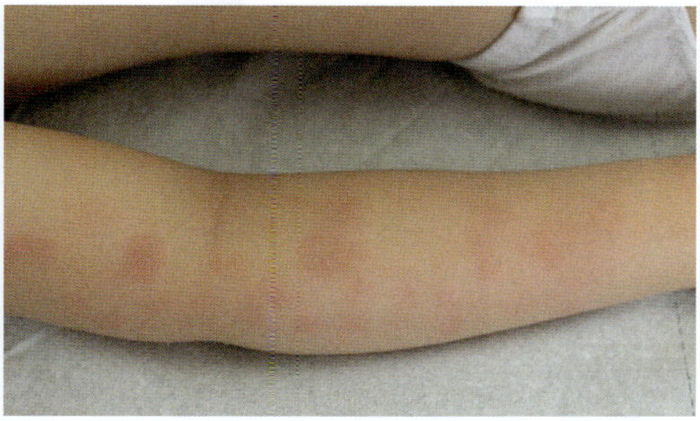

(a)

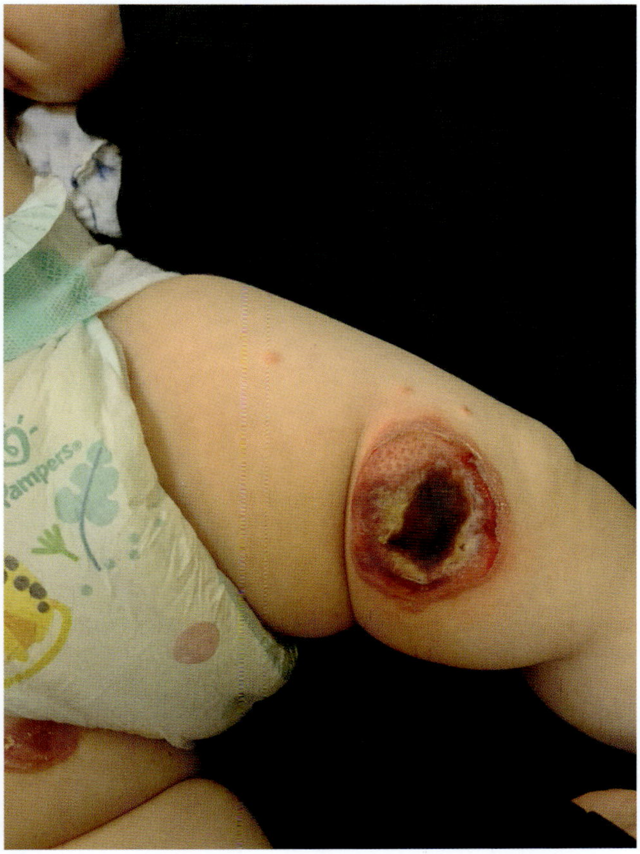

(b)

**Figure 30.5** Cutaneous gamma/delta T-cell lymphoma. (a) Infiltrated macules and plaques similar to those observed in mycosis fungoides *(Courtesy of Dr. Boccaletti, Parma, and Dr. D'Amore, Vicenza, Italy.)* (b) Large ulcerated tumor on the thigh *(Courtesy of Dr. Werner, Curitiba, Brazil.)*

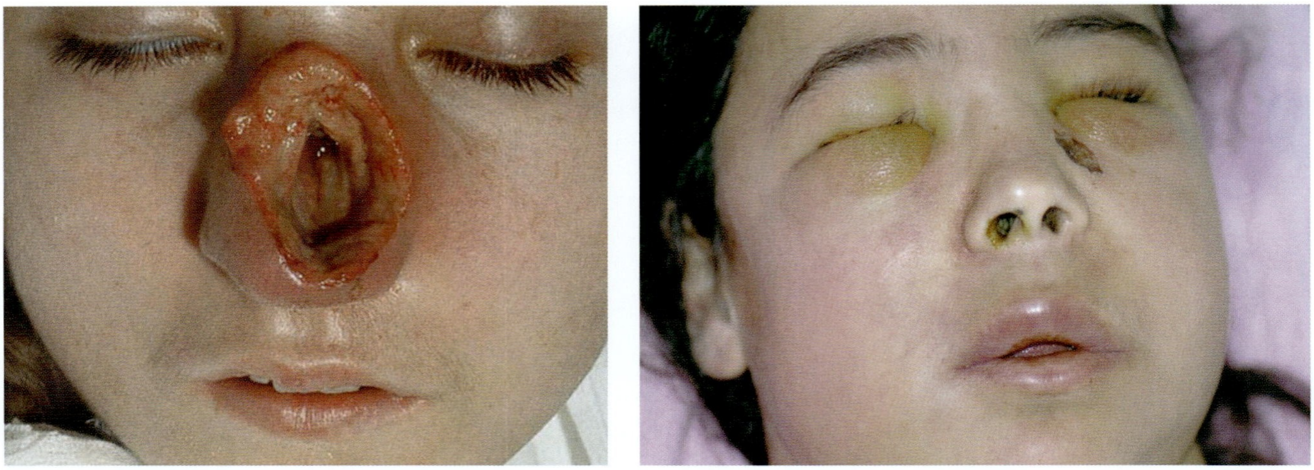

(a) (b)

Figure 30.6 Cutaneous involvement in extranodal NK/T-cell lymphoma, nasal-type. (a) "Lethal midline granuloma" in a young girl. (b) Swelling of the face with "puffy" eyelids as presenting manifestation of the disease *(Courtesy of Dr. Sahin, Ankara, Turkey.)*

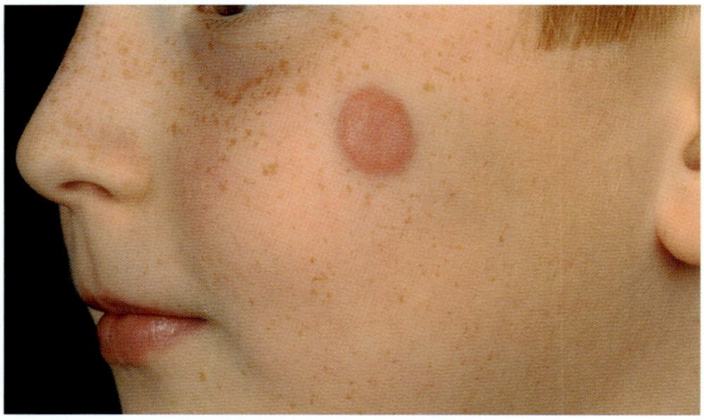

Figure 30.7 Cutaneous small-medium pleomorphic CD4+ lymphoproliferative disease presenting as a reddish nodule on the cheek of a young boy.

nosologic classification of this condition (as a low-grade lymphoma or pseudolymphoma), see Chapter 11.

### Acral CD8+ T-cell lymphoproliferative disorder

This indolent cutaneous T-cell lymphoproliferative disorder has been observed only in adult patients.

## Adult T-cell lymphoma/leukemia

Most patients with adult T-cell lymphoma/leukemia (ATLL) are adults and the elderly, but the disease has been observed rarely in adolescents [75]. Clinicopathologic features are indistinguishable from those of mycosis fungoides; thus, demonstration of infection with human T-cell lymphotropic virus I (HTLV-I) is mandatory in order to confirm the diagnosis.

## Epstein–Barr virus (EBV)-positive T-cell and NK-cell lymphoproliferative diseases of childhood (systemic hydroa vacciniforme lymphoproliferative disorder, severe mosquito bite allergy)

A detailed discussion of these entities is presented in Chapter 15. Systemic hydroa vacciniforme lymphoproliferative disorder arises almost exclusively in children and adolescents [76]. Although originally reported in Latin American countries [77–80], several cases have been observed in Asiatic countries as well [81–86]. Onset in Caucasians is exceptional. Severe mosquito bite allergy, too, is a condition occurring in the same racial backgrounds and commonly arising in children [87]. Classic hydroa vacciniforme is a rare cutaneous photodermatosis observed in all ethnicities, but in my opinion "progression" to systemic hydroa vacciniforme lymphoproliferative disorder and extracutaneous lymphoma is exceptional, if it occurs at all.

## Cutaneous nodal T-follicular helper cell lymphoma, angioimmunoblastic type

This type of lymphoma is exceedingly rare in children and adolescents, and only anecdotal cases have been reported [88]. The involvement of the skin represents a secondary manifestation of an extracutaneous (nodal) lymphoma. Care should be taken to distinguish skin manifestations of T-follicular helper cell lymphoma, angioimmunoblastic type or of other T-follicular helper lymphomas from the more common cases of cutaneous CD4+ small/medium T-cell lymphoproliferative disorder presenting with phenotypic features of T-follicular helper lymphocytes.

## Cutaneous follicle center lymphoma

Cutaneous follicle center lymphoma is very rare in children and adolescents, and only a few cases have been reported [89]. One patient presented with the spindle cell variant of the disease [90]. With the exception of the clinical picture of so-called Crosti lymphoma, which is not found in pediatric patients, clinico-pathologic features are similar irrespective of the age of onset.

## Cutaneous marginal zone lymphoproliferative disorder

This is a relatively frequent cutaneous lymphoproliferative disorder in children and adolescents, and several patients have been observed [4, 91–93]. Cases reported as primary cutaneous plasmacytoma probably represented examples of the plasmacytic variant of cutaneous marginal zone lymphoproliferative disorder [92]. The clinicopathologic features are similar to those observed in adults, and the prognosis is excellent (Fig. 30.8).

In a study on marginal zone lymphomas from different organs in young patients, several cases were located within the lymph nodes or the conjunctiva, but only one within the skin [94], suggesting that in the pediatric population, cutaneous cases are less frequent than extracutaneous ones. On the other hand, in my experience, cutaneous marginal zone lymphoproliferative disorder represents the third most common entity of cutaneous lymphoproliferative disorder in children and adolescents.

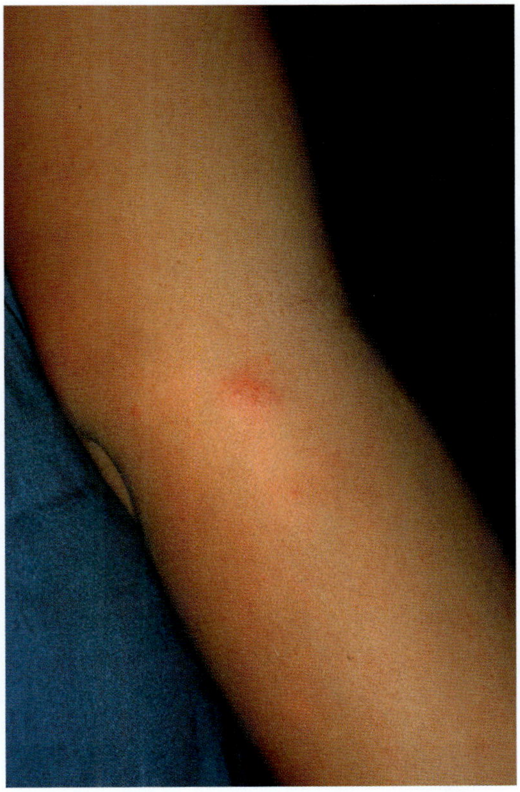

**Figure 30.8** Cutaneous marginal zone lymphoproliferative disease presenting as a small nodule on the arm of a young girl. The lesion was positive for Borrelia DNA and was treated with antibiotics with complete remission.

## Cutaneous diffuse large B-cell lymphoma, leg-type

This aggressive cutaneous B-cell lymphoma has been observed only in adult patients, mostly the elderly.

## Cutaneous intravascular large cell lymphoma

Both the more frequent B-cell and the exceedingly rare NK/T-cell type of intravascular large cell lymphoma arise almost exclusively in adults or elderly patients. One congenital case of intravascular NK/T-cell lymphoma was detected at autopsy [95]; in spite of involvement of multiple organs, tumor complexes were not present in the skin in this case.

## Cutaneous Burkitt lymphoma

Although many cases of extracutaneous Burkitt lymphoma arise in pediatric patients, most reports on cutaneous involvement concern adults, and only a few children with cutaneous Burkitt lymphoma have been described [96, 97]. It is unclear whether the low incidence is due to underreporting or if it represents a true phenomenon in young individuals. Clinicopathologic features are similar, irrespective of age.

## Cutaneous lymphomatoid granulomatosis

Lymphomatoid granulomatosis is a lymphoproliferative disorder observed more often in adults, but children may be affected, particularly immunosuppressed ones [98]. The clinicopathologic features are similar to those observed in adults. A diagnosis of cutaneous lymphomatoid granulomatosis should not be made if the typical lung involvement is not present.

## Cutaneous lymphomas in immune suppressed children and adolescents

A few cases of cutaneous lymphoma associated with EBV infection have been reported in children with immune suppression due to different causes (congenital immune deficiencies, post-transplantation setting, HIV infection) [1, 99, 100]. Post-transplant lymphoproliferative disorders are the most common complication in children who receive a solid organ transplantation or a stem cell transplantation [100]. The clinicopathologic features are similar to those described in immunocompromised adults.

## EBV+ mucocutaneous ulcer

EBV+ mucocutaneous ulcer is a disease of elderly patients with a median age of >70. Cases in children have not been reported.

## Cutaneous B-cell chronic lymphocytic leukemia

This B-cell leukemia is observed only in adult patients, particularly the elderly.

## Cutaneous manifestations of myelogenous leukemia

Most cases of myeloid leukemia in children are congenital (5/6 in the study by Boccara *et al.*) and of monoblastic type [1].

The clinical presentation is that of so-called "blueberry muffin" neonates (see Chapter 23). Although isolated cases with spontaneous remission have been observed, the disease usually runs an aggressive course.

### Blastic plasmacytoid dendritic cell neoplasm

Cutaneous cases arising in children and adolescents are well documented [4, 101–104]. In the database of the Dermatopathology Unit of the University of Graz, Austria, cases in patients <18 years of age represent approximately 10% of all recorded cases (including consultation cases) (Fig. 30.9).

Although cutaneous involvement is common in this rare hematological malignancy, it seems to be less frequent in children affected by the disease [101]. The clinicopathologic and prognostic features are similar to those observed in adults.

### Cutaneous lymphoblastic lymphoma/leukemia (B- or T-cell)

Cases of B-lymphoblastic lymphoma with primary cutaneous presentation are well documented in children and adolescents [1, 3, 4, 105–107]. Considering primary and secondary cases together, cutaneous lymphoblastic lymphoma is not uncommon in pediatric patients and represents an important differential diagnosis of rapidly growing tumors, particularly on the head and neck area. Cutaneous B-lymphoblastic lymphoma is much more common than cutaneous T-lymphoblastic lymphoma (both in adults and in children).

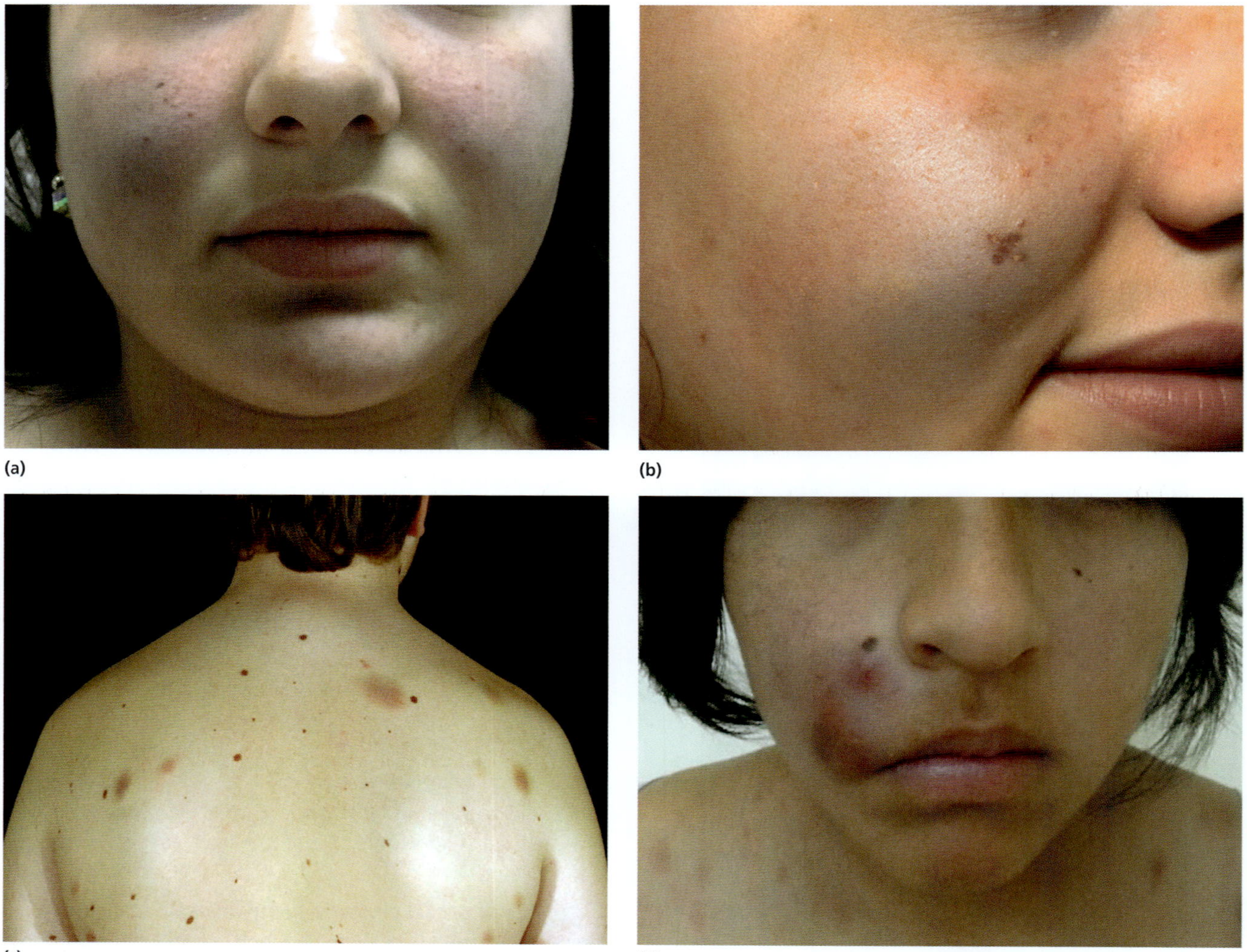

(a) (b) (c) (d)

**Figure 30.9** Cutaneous blastic plasmacytoid dendritic cell neoplasm. (a, b) Livid swelling of both cheeks (*Courtesy of Dr. Theriault, Quebec, Canada*); (c) Infiltrated, livid nodules on the back (*Courtesy of Dr. Cota, Rome, Italy*); (d) Infiltrated tumor on the upper lip (*Courtesy of Dr. Nunzi, Genova, Italy*).

## References


1. Boccara O, Blanche S, de Prost Y, *et al.* Cutaneous hematologic disorders in children. *Pediatr Blood Cancer* 2012;**58**:226–232.
2. Kempf W, Kazakov DV, Belousova I, *et al.* Paediatric cutaneous lymphomas: a review and comparison with adult counterparts. *J Eur Acad Dermatol Venereol* 2015;**29**:1696–1709.
3. Moon HR, Lee WJ, Won CH, *et al.* Paediatric cutaneous lymphoma in Korea: a retrospective study at a single institution. *J Eur Acad Dermatol Venereol* 2014;**8**:1798–1804.
4. Fink-Puches R, Chott A, Ardigó M, *et al.* The spectrum of cutaneous lymphomas in patients less than 20 years of age. *Ped Dermatol* 2004;**21**:525–533.
5. Alberti-Violetti S, Avallone G, Colonna C, *et al.* Paediatric cutaneous lymphomas including rare subtypes: A 40-year experience at a tertiary referral centre. *J Eur Acad Dermatol Venereol* 2025;**39**: 161–170.
6. Colmant C, Demers MA, Hatami A, *et al.* Pediatric cutaneous hematologic disorders: cutaneous lymphoma and leukemia cutis-experience of a tertiary-care pediatric institution and review of the literature. *J Cutan Med Surg* 2022;**26**:349–360.
7. DeLost GR, Giesey RL, Christensen LF, *et al.* Cutaneous lymphomas in adolescents and young adults. Clinical spectrum and physician-reported and patient-reported outcomes. *J Am Acad Dermatol* 2020;**82**:751–753.
8. Torre-Castro J, Estrach T, Penate Y, *et al.* Primary cutaneous lymphomas in children: a prospective study from the Spanish Academy of Dermatology and Venereology (AEDV) primary cutaneous lymphoma registry. *Ped Dermatol* 2021;**38**:1506–1509.
9. Nanda A, AlSaleh QA, Al-Ajmi H, *et al.* Mycosis fungoides in Arab children and adolescents: a report of 36 patients from Kuwait. *Ped Dermatol* 2010;**27**:607–613.
10. Yazganoglu KD, Topkarci Z, Buyukbabani N, *et al.* Childhood mycosis fungoides: a report of 20 cases from Turkey. *J Eur Acad Dermatol Venereol* 2013;**27**:295–300.
11. Heng YK, Koh AMJ, Giam YC, *et al.* Pediatric mycosis fungoides in Singapore: a series of 46 children. *Ped Dermatol* 2014;**31**: 477–482.
12. Boulos S, Vaid R, Aladily TN, *et al.* Clinical presentation, immunopathology, and treatment of juvenile-onset mycosis fungoides: a case series of 34 patients. *J Am Acad Dermatol* 2014;**71**: 1117–1126.
13. Quaglino P, Zaccagna A, Verrone A, *et al.* Mycosis fungoides in patients under 20 years of age: report of 7 cases, review of the literature and study of the clinical course. *Dermatology* 1999;**199**: 8–14.
14. Jung JM, Lim DJ, Won CH, *et al.* Mycosis fungoides in children and adolescents. A systematic review. *JAMA Dermatol* 2021; **157**: 431–438.
15. Jacob JS, Hunt RD. Increasing incidence of pediatric mycosis fungoides from 2000 to 2017: a national population-based study of the surveillance, epidemiology, and end results database and texas cancer registry. *J Am Acad Dermatol* 2023;**88**:185–187.
16. Wohlmut-Wieser I. Primary cutaneous T-cell lymphomas in childhood and adolescence. *J Deutsch Dermatol Ges* 2021; **19**:563–581.
17. Çaytemel C, Gürbüz BÇ. Linear, blaschkoid, hypopigmented and childhood mycosis fungoides. *Indian J Dermatol* 2023;**68**:727.
18. Welfringer-Morin A, Barroil M, Fraitag S, *et al.* Clinical features, histological characteristics, and disease outcomes of mycosis fungoides in children and adolescents: a nationwide multicentre cohort of 46 patients. *Dermatology* 2023;**239**:132–139.
19. Ben-Amitai D, David M, Feinmesser M, *et al.* Juvenile mycosis fungoides diagnosed before 18 years of age. *Acta Derm Venereol (Stockh)* 2003;**83**:451–456.
20. Kim ST, Sim HJ, Jeon YS, *et al.* Clinicopathological features and T-cell receptor gene rearrangement findings of mycosis fungoides in patients younger than age 20 years. *J Dermatol* 2009; **36**: 392–402.
21. Pope E, Weitzman S, Ngan B, *et al.* Mycosis fungoides in the pediatric population: report from an international childhood registry of cutaneous lymphoma. *J Cut Med Surg* 2010;**14**:1–6.
22. Zackheim HS, Mc Calmont TH, Deanovic FW, Odom RB. Mycosis fungoides with onset before 20 years of age. *J Am Acad Dermatol* 1997;**36**:557–562.
23. Peters MS, Thibodeau SN, White JW Jr, Winkelmann RK. Mycosis fungoides in children and adolescents. *J Am Acad Dermatol* 1990;**22**:1011–1018.
24. Tan E, Tay YK, Giam YC. Profile and outcome of childhood mycosis fungoides in Singapore. *Ped Dermatol* 2000;**17**:352–356.
25. Whittam LR, Calonje E, Orchard G, *et al.* CD-8-positive juvenile onset mycosis fungoides: an immunohistochemical and genotypic analysis of six cases. *Br J Dermatol* 2000;**143**:1199–1204.
26. Wain EM, Orchard GE, Whittaker SJ, *et al.* Outcome in 34 patients with juvenile-onset mycosis fungoides. A clinical, immunophenotypic, and molecular study. *Cancer* 2003;**98**:2282–2290.
27. El Shabrawi-Caelen L, Cerroni L, Medeiros LJ, McCalmont TH. Hypopigmented mycosis fungoides: frequent expression of a CD8 T-cell phenotype. *Am J Surg Pathol* 2002;**26**:450–457.
28. Ardigó M, Borroni G, Muscardin L, *et al.* Hypopigmented mycosis fungoides in Caucasian patients: a clinicopathologic study of 7 cases. *J Am Acad Dermatol* 2003;**49**:264–270.
29. Poppe H, Kerstan A, Böckers M, *et al.* Childhood mycosis fungoides with a CD8+ CD56+ cytotoxic immunophenotype. *J Cutan Pathol* 2015;**42**:258–264.
30. Rovaris M, Colato C, Girolomoni G. Pediatric CD8+/CD56+ mycosis fungoides with cytotoxic marker expression: a variant with indolent course. *J Cutan Pathol* 2018;**45**:782–785.
31. Cerroni L, Fink-Puches R, Bäck B, Kerl H. Follicular mucinosis: a critical reappraisal of clinicopathologic features and association with mycosis fungoides and Sézary syndrome. *Arch Dermatol* 2002;**138**:182–189.
32. Dalle S, Marrou K, Balme B, *et al.* Neonatal follicular mucinosis. *Br J Dermatol* 2007;**157**:609–610.
33. Zvulunov A, Shkalim V, Ben-Amitai D, *et al.* Clinical and histopathologic spectrum of alopecia mucinosa/follicular mucinosis

and its natural history in children. *J Am Acad Dermatol* 2012;**67**:1174–1181.

34. Alikhan A, Griffin J, Nguyen N, *et al.* Pediatric follicular mucinosis: presentation, histopathology, molecular genetics, treatment, and outcomes over an 11-year period at the mayo clinic. *Pediatr Dermatol* 2013;**30**:192–198.
35. Santos-Briz A, Cañueto J, García-Dorado J, *et al.* Pediatric primary follicular mucinosis: further evidence of its relationship with mycosis fungoides. *Pediatr Dermatol* 2013;**30**:e218–e220.
36. Matsuzaki Y, Kimura K, Nakano H, *et al.* Localized pagetoid reticulosis (Woringer–Kolopp disease) in early childhood. *J Am Acad Dermatol* 2009;**61**:120–123.
37. Corbeddu M, Ferreli C, Pilloni L, *et al.* Pagetoid reticulosis (Woringer-Kolopp disease) in a 2-year-old girl—Case report and review of the literature. *JAAD Case Reports* 2019;**5**:104–107.
38. Torre-Castro J, Carrasco Santos L, Rodriguez-Pinilla SM, Requena L. Pagetoid reticulosis in a 13-year old female. A unique immunohistochemical profile. *J Cutan Pathol* 2020;**47**:466–469.
39. Osto M, Atify O, Musa A, *et al.* Woringer-Kolopp disease (localized pagetoid reticulosis): a systematic review. *Int J Dermatol* 2023;**62**:312–321.
40. Rambhia KD, Haldar S, Dongre AM, Khopkar US. Granulomatous slack skin with systemic involvement and a fatal outcome in an adolescent. *Clin Exper Dermatol* 2014;**39**:653–654.
41. Fortson JS, Schroeter AL, Esterly NB. Cutaneous T-cell lymphoma (parapsoriasis en plaque). An association with pityriasis lichenoides et varioliformis acuta in young children. *Arch Dermatol* 1990;**126**:1449–1453.
42. Fraitag S, Boccara O, Brousse N, *et al.* Mycosis fungoides following pityriasis lichenoides: an exceptional event or a potential evolution? *Pediatr Blood Cancer* 2012;**58**:307.
43. Ko JW, Seong JY, Suh KS, *et al.* Pityriasis lichenoides-like mycosis fungoides in children. *Br J Dermatol* 2000;**142**:347–352.
44. Byul E, Hwan S, Joo E, *et al.* CD8-positive pityriasis lichenoides-like mycosis fungoides. *Eur J Dermatol* 2012;**22**:415–416.
45. Pileri A, Neri I, Raone B, *et al.* Mycosis fungoides following pityriasis lichenoides: an exceptional event or a potential evolution? *Pediatr Blood Cancer* 2012;**58**:306.
46. Borra T, Custrin A, Saggini A, *et al.* Pityriasis lichenoides, atypical pityriasis lichenoides, and related conditions: a study of 66 cases. *Am J Surg Pathol* 2018;**42**:1101–1112.
47. Niemczyk UM, Zollner TM, Wolter M, *et al.* The transformation of pityriasis lichenoides chronica into parakeratosis variegata in an 11-year-old girl. *Br J Dermatol* 1997;**137**:983–987.
48. Crowley JJ, Nikko A, Varghese A, *et al.* Mycosis fungoides in young patients: clinical characteristics and outcome. *J Am Acad Dermatol* 1998;**38**:696–701.
49. Zvulunov A, Neale H, Stern J, *et al.* Approach to mycosis fungoides in children: consensus-based recommendations. *J Am Acad Dermatol* 2024;**91**:1078–1085.
50. Sun G, Berthelot C, Li Y, *et al.* Poor prognosis in non-Caucasian patients with early-onset mycosis fungoides. *J Am Acad Dermatol* 2009;**60**:231–235.
51. (a) Virmani P, Levin L, Myskowski PL, *et al.* Clinical outcome and prognosis of young patients with mycosis fungoides. *Pediatr Dermatol* 2017;**34**:547–553.(b) Hodak E, Amitay-Laish I, Bagot M, *et al.* ISCL/EORTC-CLTG/USCLC recommendations for the diagnosis, staging and treatment of early-stage paediatric mycosis fungoides - a modified Delphi consensus. Part 1: Diagnosis and staging. *Br J Dermatol* 2025;**193**:405–414. (c) Hodak E, Amitay-Laish I, Bagot M, *et al.* ISCL/EORTC-CLTG/USCLC recommendations for the diagnosis, staging and treatment of early-stage paediatric mycosis fungoides - a modified delphi consensus. Part 2: treatment. *Br J Dermatol* 2025;**193**:653–661.
52. Meister L, Duarte AM, Davis J, *et al.* Sezary syndrome in an 11-year-old girl. *J Am Acad Dermatol* 1993;**28**:93–95.
53. LeBoit PE, Abel EA, Cleary ML, *et al.* Clonal rearrangement of the T cell receptor beta gene in the circulating lymphocytes of erythrodermic follicular mucinosis. *Blood* 1988;**71**:1329–1333.
54. Fraitag S, Bodemer C. Neonatal erythroderma. *Curr Opin Pediatr* 2010;**22**:438–444.
55. Blanchard M, Morren MA, Busschots AM, *et al.* Paediatric-onset lymphomatoid papulosis: results of a multicentre retrospective cohort study on behalf of the EORTC Cutaneous Lymphoma Tumours Group (CLTG). *Br J Dermatol* 2024;**191**:233–242.
56. van Neer FJMA, Toonstra J, van Voorst Vader PC, *et al.* Lymphomatoid papulosis in children: a study of 10 children registered by the Dutch cutaneous lymphoma working group. *Br J Dermatol* 2001;**144**:351–354.
57. Nijsten T, Curiel-Lewandrowski C, Kadin ME. Lymphomatoid papulosis in children. A retrospective cohort study of 35 cases. *Arch Dermatol* 2004;**140**:306–312.
58. Gould JW, Eppes RB, Gilliam AC, *et al.* Solitary primary cutaneous CD30+ large cell lymphoma of natural killer cell phenotype bearing the t(2,5)(p23;q35) translocation and presenting in a child. *Am J Dermatopathol* 2000;**22**:422–428.
59. Hinshaw M, Trowers AB, Kodish E, *et al.* Three children with CD30+ cutaneous anaplastic large cell lymphomas bearing the t(2,5)(q23;q35) translocation. *Ped Dermatol* 2004;**21**:212–217.
60. Oschlies I, Lisfeld J, Lamant L, *et al.* ALK-positive anaplastic large cell lymphoma limited to the skin: clinical, histopathological and molecular analysis of 6 pediatric cases. A report from the ALCL99 study. *Haematologica* 2013;**98**:50–56.
61. Pulitzer M, Ogunrinade O, Lin O, Steinherz P. ALK-positive (2p23 rearranged) anaplastic large cell lymphoma with localization to the skin in a pediatric patient. *J Cutan Pathol* 2015;**42**:182–187.
62. Lamant L, Pileri S, Sabattini E, *et al.* Cutaneous presentation of ALK-positive anaplastic large cell lymphoma following insect bites: evidence for an association in five cases. *Haematologica* 2010;**95**:449–455.
63. Huppmann AR, Xi L, Raffeld M, *et al.* Subcutaneous panniculitis-like T-cell lymphoma in the pediatric age group: a lymphoma of low malignant potential. *Pediatr Blood Cancer* 2013;**60**:1165–1170.
64. Shani-Adir A, Lucky AW, Prendiville J, *et al.* Subcutaneous panniculitic T-cell lymphoma in children: response to combination therapy with cyclosporine and chemotherapy. *J Am Acad Dermatol* 2004;**50**:s18–s22.
65. Taniguchi S, Kono T. Subcutaneous T-cell lymphoma in a child with eosinophilia. *Br J Dermatol* 2000;**142**:183–184.
66. Koh MJA, Sadarangani SP, Chan YC, *et al.* Aggressive subcutaneous panniculitis-like T-cell lymphoma with hemophagocytosis in two children (subcutaneous panniculitis-like T-cell lymphoma). *J Am Acad Dermatol* 2009;**61**:875–881.

67. Weingartner JS, Zedek DC, Burkhart CN, Morrell DS. Lupus erythematosus panniculitis in children: report of three cases and review of previously reported cases. *Pediatr Dermatol* 2012;**29**: 169–176.
68. Bader-Meunier B, Fraitag S, Janssen C, *et al.* Clonal cytophagic histiocytic panniculitis in children may be cured by cyclosporine A. *Pediatrics* 2013;**132**:e545–e549.
69. Santonja C, Gonzalo I, Feito M, *et al.* Lipoatrophic panniculitis of the ankles in childhood: differential diagnosis with subcutaneous panniculitis-like T-cell lymphoma. *Am J Dermatopathol* 2012;**34**: 295–300.
70. Kikuchi Y, Kashii Y, Gunji Y, *et al.* Six-year-old girl with primary cutaneous aggressive epidermotropic CD8+ T-cell lymphoma. *Pediatr Int* 2011;**53**:393–396.
71. Wang L, Gao T, Wang G. Primary cutaneous CD8+ cytotoxic T-cell lymphoma involving the epidermis and subcutis in a young child. *J Cutan Pathol* 2015;**42**:271–275.
72. Merrill ED, Agbay R, Miranda RN, *et al.* Primary cutaneous T-cell lymphomas showing gamma-delta (gammadelta) phenotype and predominantly epidermotropic pattern are clinicopathologically distinct from classic primary cutaneous gammadelta T-cell lymphomas. *Am J Surg Pathol* 2017;**41**:204–215.
73. Kobayashi R, Yamato K, Tanaka F, *et al.* Retrospective analysis of non-anaplastic peripheral T-cell lymphoma in pediatric patients in Japan. *Pediatr Blood Cancer* 2010;**54**:212–215.
74. Baum CL, Link BK, Neppalli VT, *et al.* Reappraisal of the provisional entity primary cutaneous CD4+ small/medium pleomorphic T-cell lymphoma: a series of 10 adult and pediatric patients and review of the literature. *J Am Acad Dermatol* 2011;**65**: 739–748.
75. Lucas CT, Gillis KJ, Ness JM, *et al.* Adult T-cell leukemia/lymphoma in an adolescent presenting with skin lesions. *Ped Dermatol* 2008;**25**:373–377.
76. Kimura H, Plaza JA, Araujo I, *et al.* Hydroa vacciniforme lymphoproliferative disorder. In: *WHO Classification of Tumours Editorial Board. Haematolymphoid Tumours.* 5th edition. Lyon (France): IARC, 2024: 774–776.
77. Ruiz-Maldonado R, Parrilla F, Orozco-Covarrubias M, *et al.* Edematous, scarring vasculitic panniculitis: a new multisystemic disease with malignant potential. *J Am Acad Dermatol* 1995;**32**:37–44.
78. Barrionuevo C, Anderson VM, Zevallos-Giampietri E, *et al.* Hydroa-like cutaneous T-cell lymphoma: a clinicopathologic and molecular genetic study of 16 pediatric cases from Peru. *Appl Immunohistochem Mol Morph* 2002;**10**:7–14.
79. Sangueza M, Plaza JA. Hydroa vacciniforme-like cutaneous T-cell lymphoma: clinicopathologic and immunohistochemical study of 12 cases. *J Am Acad Dermatol* 2013;**69**:112–119.
80. Magana M, Sangueza P, Gil-Beristain J, *et al.* Angiocentric cutaneous T-cell lymphoma of childhood (hydroa-like lymphoma): a distinctive type of cutaneous T-cell lymphoma. *J Am Acad Dermatol* 1998;**38**:574–579.
81. Feng S, Jin P, Zeng X. Hydroa vacciniforme-like primary cutaneous CD8-positive T-cell lymphoma. *Eur J Dermatol* 2008;**18**: 364–365.
82. Xu Z, Lian S. Epstein–Barr virus-associated hydroa vacciniforme-like cutaneous lymphoma in seven Chinese children. *Ped Dermatol* 2010;**27**:463–469.
83. Zhang X, Wang T, Wang L. Hydroa vacciniforme-Like lymphoma in tibetan children: 2 cases and a literature review. *Am J Dermatopathol* 2018;**40**:358–361.
84. Zhang Y, Liu Y, Xu J, *et al.* Hydroa vacciniforme lymphoproliferative disorder: a retrospective study of 42 paediatric cases. *Eur J Dermatol* 2024;**34**:144–149.
85. Liu Y, Ma C, Wang G, Wang L. Hydroa vacciniforme-like lymphoproliferative disorder: clinicopathologic study of 41 cases. *J Am Acad Dermatol* 2019;**81**:534–540.
86. Guo N, Chen Y, Wang Y, *et al.* Clinicopathological categorization of hydroa vacciniforme-like lymphoproliferative disorder: An analysis of prognostic implications and treatment based on 19 cases. *Diagn Pathol* 2019;**14**:82.
87. Kimura H, Araujo I, Kato S, Ng SB. Severe mosquito bite allergy. In: *WHO Classification of Tumours Editorial Board. Haematolymphoid Tumours.* 5th edition. Lyon (France): IARC, 2024: 772–773.
88. Schotte U, Megahed M, Jansen T, *et al.* Angio-immunoblastische Lymphadenopathie mit kutanen manifestationen bei einem 13jährigen Mädchen. *Hautarzt* 1992;**43**:728–734.
89. Ghislanzoni M, Gambini D, Perrone T, *et al.* Primary cutaneous follicular center cell lymphoma of the nose with maxillary sinus involvement in a pediatric patient. *J Am Acad Dermatol* 2005;**52**:s73–s75.
90. Amitay-Laish I, Feinmesser M, Ben-Amitai D, *et al.* Juvenile onset of primary low-grade cutaneous B-cell lymphoma. *Br J Dermatol* 2009;**161**:140–147.
91. Sharon V, Mecca PS, Steinherz PG, *et al.* Two pediatric cases of primary cutaneous B-cell lymphoma and review of the literature. *Ped Dermatol* 2009;**26**:34–39.
92. Koletsa T, Patsatsi A, Kostopoulos I, *et al.* A case of primary cutaneous plasmacytoma presenting in adolescence. *Am J Dermatopathol* 2012;**34**:537–540.
93. Amitay-Laish I, Tavallaee M, Kim J, *et al.* Paediatric primary cutaneous marginal zone B-cell lymphoma: does it differ from its adult counterpart? *Br J Dermatol* 2017;**176**:1010–1020.
94. Rizzo KA, Streubel B, Pittaluga S, *et al.* Marginal zone lymphomas in children and the young adult population; characterization of genetic aberrations by FISH and RT-PCR. *Mod Pathol* 2010;**23**:866–873.
95. Tateyama H, Eimoto T, Tada T, *et al.* Congenital angiotropic lymphoma (intravascular lymphomatosis) of the T-cell type. *Cancer* 1991;**67**:2131–2136.
96. Gogia A, Sharma MC, Bakhshi S. Subcutaneous nodules as initial presentation of Burkitt lymphoma in HIV-negative child. *J Pediatr Hematol Oncol* 2013;**35**:e326–e328.
97. Thakkar D, Lipi L, Misra R, Yadav SP. Skin involvement in Burkitt's lymphoma. *Hematol Oncol Stem Cell Ther* 2018;**11**:251–252.
98. Sebire NJ, Haselden S, Malone M, *et al.* Isolated EBV lymphoproliferative disease in a child with Wiskott–Aldrich syndrome manifesting as cutaneous lymphomatoid granulomatosis and responsive to anti-CD20 immunotherapy. *J Clin Pathol* 2003;**56**:555–557.
99. Wallet-Faber N, Bodemer C, Blanche S, et al. Primary cutaneous Epstein–Barr virus-related lymphoproliferative disorders in 4 immunosuppressed children. *J Am Acad Dermatol* 2008;**58**:74–80.
100. Rogers TS, McGevna L, Cook DL. Pediatric cutaneous T-cell post-transplant lymphoproliferative disorder: case report and review of the literature. *J Cutan Pathol* 2018;**45**:858–863.

101. Jegalian AG, Buxbaum NP, Facchetti F, *et al.* Blastic plasmacytoid dendritic cell neoplasm in children: diagnostic features and clinical implications. *Haematologica* 2010;**95**:1873–1879.
102. Cuglievan B, Connors J, He J, *et al.* Blastic plasmacytoid dendritic cell neoplasm: a comprehensive review in pediatrics, adolescents, and young adults (AYA) and an update of novel therapies. *Leukemia* 2023;**37**:1767–1778.
103. Li J, Wang J, Rong L, *et al.* A neonatal case of congenital blastic plasmacytoid dendritic cell neoplasm with KMT2C gene duplication. *Ann Hematol* 2023;**102**:227–229.
104. Chan G, Akintorin S, Luu M, Harter N. Blastic plasmacytoid dendritic cell neoplasm with cutaneous presentation: a case series in children. *Ped Dermatol* 2021;**38**:883–886.
105. Sander CA, Medeiros LJ, Abruzzo LV, *et al.* Lymphoblastic lymphoma presenting in cutaneous sites: a clinicopathologic analysis of six cases. *J Am Acad Dermatol* 1991;**25**:1023–1031.
106. Lee WJ, Moon HR, Won CH, *et al.* Precursor B- or T-lymphoblastic lymphoma presenting with cutaneous involvement: a series of 13 cases including 7 cases of cutaneous T-lymphoblastic lymphoma. *J Am Acad Dermatol* 2014;**70**:318–325.
107. Bontoux C, de Masson A, Boccara O, *et al.* Outcome and clinicophenotypical features of acute lymphoblastic leukemia/lymphoblastic lymphoma with cutaneous involvement: a multicenter case series. *J Am Acad Dermatol* 2020;**83**:1166–1170.

SECTION 7

# Pseudolymphomas of the skin

CHAPTER 31

# Pseudolymphomas of the skin

Pseudolymphomas of the skin are a heterogeneous group of disorders that simulate cutaneous malignant lymphomas clinically and/or histopathologically. Although "pseudolymphoma" is usually considered a synonym for a benign condition, some non-lymphoid malignant tumors of the skin may also simulate the picture of a cutaneous lymphoma ("malignant" pseudolymphomas – see Chapter 32). In this context, it must be underlined that the term "pseudolymphoma" is not a diagnosis per se and should not be used to classify given cases, as it encompasses skin conditions with different etiologies, pathogeneses, clinicopathologic presentations, and behavior, requiring targeted management according to the specific condition.

Reading the pertinent literature, one gets the impression that the number of cutaneous "pseudolymphomas" increases regularly. Some of the published cases represent reactive conditions, that in rare exceptions, may simulate histopathologically a cutaneous lymphoma, usually mycosis fungoides. This problem is discussed in the section on other "accidental" pseudolymphomas in this chapter, in order to underline that these conditions do not represent in general a pseudolymphoma, but rather may simulate a lymphoma (usually histopathologically) in exceptional cases only. Pseudolymphomas are reactive, inflammatory conditions and should not be lumped together with cases considered to be at the edge between benign and malignant disorders (e.g., small-patch parapsoriasis). In this context, it must be underlined that true "progression" from a clear-cut cutaneous pseudolymphoma into a malignant lymphoma of the skin is exceptionally rare.

There are no data concerning the incidence, prevalence, and geographic distribution of cutaneous pseudolymphomas, and only Mitteldorf and Kempf reported their experience on the distribution of different types [1]. My personal experience is summarized in Fig. 31.1. Cutaneous pseudolymphomas associated with infectious organisms (such as *Borrelia burgdorferi*-related lymphocytoma, for example) commonly arise in regions with endemic infection for the responsible organisms (however, *Borrelia*-associated pseudolymphomas are due to specific strains of the microorganism, and are frequent in Europe but rare in the United States). On the other hand, there has been a rise in the number of cases of *Borrelia* lymphocytoma in countries where *Borrelia* species are absent, in patients returning from travels in endemic regions. In the context of *Borrelia* infection, it should be reminded that the microorganism has been convincingly linked to some cases of cutaneous B-cell lymphoma as well; thus, detection of *Borrelia* DNA within a lesion is not equivalent to a diagnosis of benignancy (see Chapters 16 and 17).

The clinical manifestations of cutaneous pseudolymphomas are protean. The lesions are often solitary or regionally clustered, but may also be generalized in distribution, and even erythroderma may be observed. The course varies considerably. The lesions may persist for weeks, months, or even years; they may resolve spontaneously and they may recur unpredictably.

Histologic criteria for the diagnosis of cutaneous pseudolymphomas include two main features: (i) the architectural pattern of the infiltrates and (ii) the cellular composition of those infiltrates, which frequently show a mixed character. These histologic features need to be integrated carefully with the immunophenotypic data. Analysis of the rearrangement of the T-cell receptor (TCR) and immunoglobulin (Ig) genes allows to check the clonality of cutaneous T- and B-cell infiltrates. Although, as a rule, malignant lymphomas reveal a monoclonal population of lymphocytes, whereas pseudolymphomas show a polyclonal infiltrate, it must be underlined that demonstration of monoclonality may be lacking in true malignant lymphomas, and that a distinct proportion of cutaneous pseudolymphomas harbor a monoclonal T- or B-cell population. In addition, pseudoclonality represents a pitfall in cutaneous infiltrates, particularly when results are interpreted without knowledge of other data [2]. Although next-generation sequencing may be more sensitive for analysis of clonal populations of T lymphocytes [3–5], data on reactive cutaneous conditions are still lacking; thus, specificity has not yet been tested adequately. In this context, it must be clearly stated that differentiation of benign from malignant lymphoid infiltrates of the skin is possible only after careful synthesis and integration of the clinical, histopathologic, immunophenotypic, and molecular features. In some cases, the true diagnosis will be revealed only at follow-up. It is important not to overdiagnose cutaneous malignant lymphomas, and a

*Skin Lymphoma: The Illustrated Guide*, Sixth Edition. Lorenzo Cerroni.

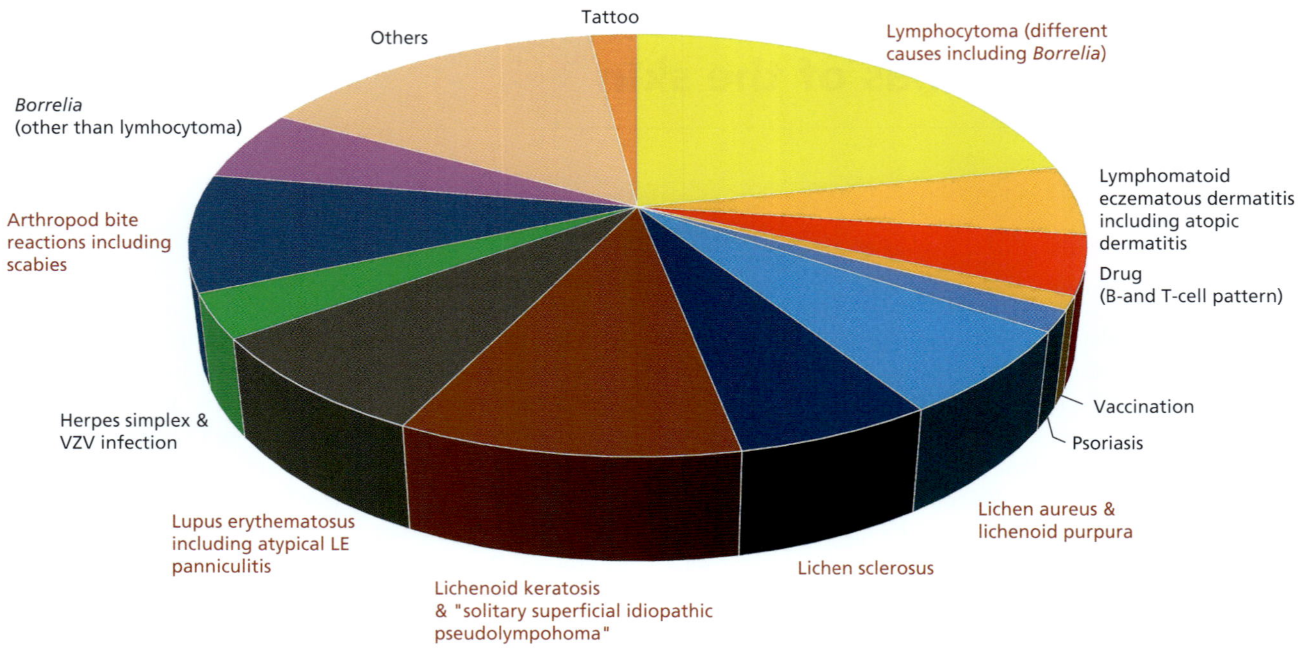


**Figure 31.1** Distribution of pseudolymphomas based on my personal experience on >1200 cases.

descriptive term such as "cutaneous atypical lymphoid proliferation" may be a useful working diagnosis for unclear cases (see Chapter 33).

Cutaneous pseudolymphomas are traditionally divided into T- and B-cell variants according to the histopathologic and immunophenotypic features, but in many conditions this distinction is artificial. For example, pseudolymphomas induced by drugs may present with either a T- or a B-cell pattern, and the same drug may induce different patterns in different patients. In addition, in many instances both T and B lymphocytes are present within the infiltrate of a given pseudolymphoma. Thus, in what follows cutaneous pseudolymphomas will be classified according to specific clinicopathologic entities (Table 31.1).

## Chronic actinic dermatitis (actinic reticuloid)

Although actinic reticuloid is considered to be one of the classical simulators of mycosis fungoides both clinically and histopathologically, in truth in many instances the histopathologic picture is more similar to a chronic eczematous dermatitis than to a cutaneous T-cell lymphoma. In addition, the disease is one of the rarest among the pseudolymphomas; thus, the diagnosis should be made only when compelling evidence is present, and can be accepted only when confirmed by pathologic phototesting. Although "progression" into T-cell lymphoma has been reported, it seems more likely that these cases represented examples of undiagnosed mycosis fungoides or Sézary syndrome from the onset, and that actinic reticuloid is not a potential precursor of cutaneous T-cell lymphomas [6].

Actinic reticuloid is a severe, persistent photodermatitis that usually affects older men. The disease is characterized by extreme photosensitivity to a broad spectrum of UV radiation [7]. Clinically, patients present with variably scaly erythema, lichenification, and scratching artifacts on the face and neck and on the back of the hands and distal part of the arms (Fig. 31.2). Ectropion is a common complication (Fig. 31.3). In some areas, the lesions may consist of lichenoid papules. Confluence of lesions may result in large, lichenified plaques. Recurrent erythroderma is common in these patients [8]. A "leonine" face with deep furrowing of markedly thickened skin as well as diffuse alopecia can also be seen. Pruritus is generally severe and intractable and may lead to attempts at suicide. The disease is chronic and shows no tendency to spontaneous remission [9].

Histologic examination reveals a hyperplastic epidermis and variably dense, superficial or deep perivascular infiltrates of lymphocytes, histiocytes, plasma cells, and eosinophils, as well as some atypical mononuclear cells with hyperchromatic, lobulated nuclei (Fig. 31.4). In the upper part of the dermis, the infiltrate may be band-like or patchy. The papillary dermis is usually thickened. Stellate and multinucleated fibroblasts are present. Exocytosis of lymphocytes within the hyperplastic epidermis can be found. When present, the features of lichen simplex chronicus superimposed upon an inflammatory process are helpful in distinguishing actinic reticuloid from mycosis fungoides and Sézary syndrome. Immunohistology is characterized by the predominance of $CD8^+$ T cells [10, 11].

The clinical differentiation of actinic reticuloid from mycosis fungoides and Sézary syndrome can be difficult because

**Table 31.1** Classification of cutaneous pseudolymphomas (excluding "malignant" pseudolymphomas)

| Clinicopathologic entity | Simulated malignant lymphoma |
|---|---|
| Chronic actinic dermatitis (actinic reticuloid) | Mycosis fungoides/Sézary syndrome |
| Lymphomatoid contact dermatitis | |
| Pseudolymphomatous atopic dermatitis and other eczematous dermatoses | |
| Pseudolymphomatous psoriasis | |
| Pseudolymphomatous lichen planus | |
| Non-mycosis fungoides-associated follicular mucinosis and other mimickers of pilotropic/adnexotropic mycosis fungoides | *(adnexotropic mycosis fungoides)* |
| Non-neoplastic erythroderma in adult patients | |
| Cutaneous pseudolymphoma associated with mogamulizumab treatment | |
| Lichenoid/lymphomatoid keratosis (including "solitary idiopathic T/B-cell pseudolymphoma") | |
| Pityriasis lichenoides | |
| Lichen aureus / Lichenoid pigmented purpuric dermatitis | |
| Lichen sclerosus | |
| Other pseudolymphomas in genital skin and mucosal regions | |
| Vitiligo (inflammatory stage) | |
| Annular lichenoid dermatitis of youth | |
| Pseudolymphomatous acrodermatitis chronica atrophicans (superficial type) | |
| Superficial CD8+ cutaneous infiltrates in HIV-infected patients or in other immune deficiencies | |
| Lymphomatoid drug reaction, lichenoid type | |
| Pseudolymphomas in tattoos, lichenoid type | |
| Pseudolymphomas after vaccination, lichenoid type | |
| Syphilis, secondary (superficial type) | |
| Lupus erythematosus (superficial variant) | |
| Nevoid hyperkeratosis of the nipple | |
| Immune response in epithelial tumors | |
| Occasional pseudolymphomatous infiltrates in other inflammatory disorders (e.g., bullous pemphigoid) | |
| Pseudolymphomas in herpes simplex or herpes zoster infections | Cytotoxic NK/T-cell lymphomas or lymphomatoid papulosis/cutaneous anaplastic large cell lymphoma |
| Pityriasis lichenoides, including the ulceronecrotic variant | |
| Lupus erythematosus, angiocentric variant | |
| Syphilis, secondary, plasma cell-poor | |
| Atypical lymphoid infiltrates (CD30+) associated with: orf, milker's nodule, molluscum contagiosum, and other infectious or non-infectious disorders | Lymphomatoid papulosis/cutaneous anaplastic large cell lymphoma |
| Persistent arthropod bite reactions (including nodular scabies) | |
| Syphilis, primary | |
| Lupus panniculitis | Subcutaneous panniculitis-like T-cell lymphoma |
| Lipoatrophic panniculitis of the ankles | |
| Lobular panniculitis in children with congenital immune deficiencies | |
| Angiomatoid pseudolymphoma (Acral pseudolymphomatous angiokeratoma in children (APACHE), T-cell-rich angiomatoid polypoid pseudolymphoma, pre-tibial lymphoplasmacytic plaque in children) | Cutaneous CD4+ small/medium T-cell lymphoproliferative disorder |
| Nodular pseudolymphomatous cutaneous infiltrates in congenital immune deficiencies | |
| Pseudolymphomas in tattoo (T-cell-rich nodular variant) | |
| Conventional hydroa vacciniforme | Systemic hydroa vacciniforme lymphoproliferative disorder |
| Lymphocytoma cutis (*Borrelia*-associated) | Follicle center lymphoma or diffuse large B-cell lymphoma |
| Lymphocytoma cutis due to several causes (non-*Borrelia*-associated) | Follicle center lymphoma |
| Pseudolymphoma after vaccination, B-cell type | |
| Lymphomatoid drug reaction, B-cell type | |
| Cutaneous plasma cell granuloma | Marginal zone lymphoproliferative disorder |
| Pseudolymphoma in tattoos, B-cell type | |
| Pseudolymphomatous acrodermatitis chronica atrophicans, nodular plasmacytic type | |
| Pseudolymphomatous drug eruptions with prominent plasma cell population | |
| Syphilis, secondary (plasma cell-rich nodular type) | |
| Localized scleroderma/morphea, inflammatory stage | |
| Cutaneous and systemic plasmacytosis | |
| Lupus tumidus/lymphocytic infiltration of the skin (Jessner–Kanof) | Cutaneous manifestations of B-cell chronic lymphocytic leukemia |
| Cutaneous extramedullary hematopoiesis | Cutaneous manifestations of myeloid leukemia |
| Histiocytoid Sweet syndrome[#] | |
| Intralymphatic histiocytosis | Intravascular diffuse large cell lymphoma, intralymphatic anaplastic large cell lymphoma, or intralymphatic lymphomatoid papulosis |
| Benign intralymphatic proliferation of T-cell lymphoid blasts | |

[#] in some cases, neoplastic cells of a myeloid leukemia are present within the infiltrate of histiocytoid Sweet syndrome.

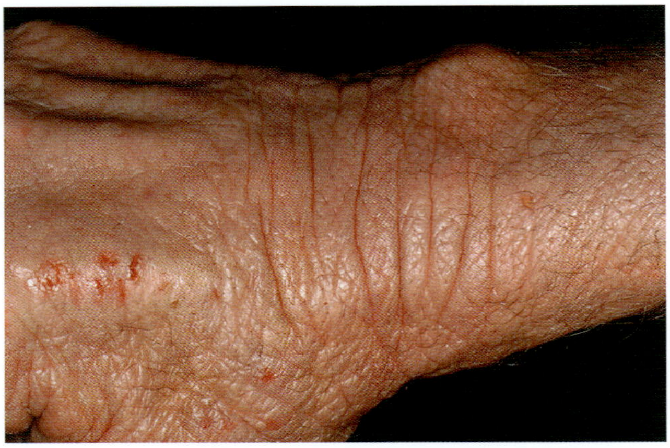

Figure 31.2 Actinic reticuloid. Erythematous, scaly, lichenified lesions with scratching artifacts on the arm and back of hand.

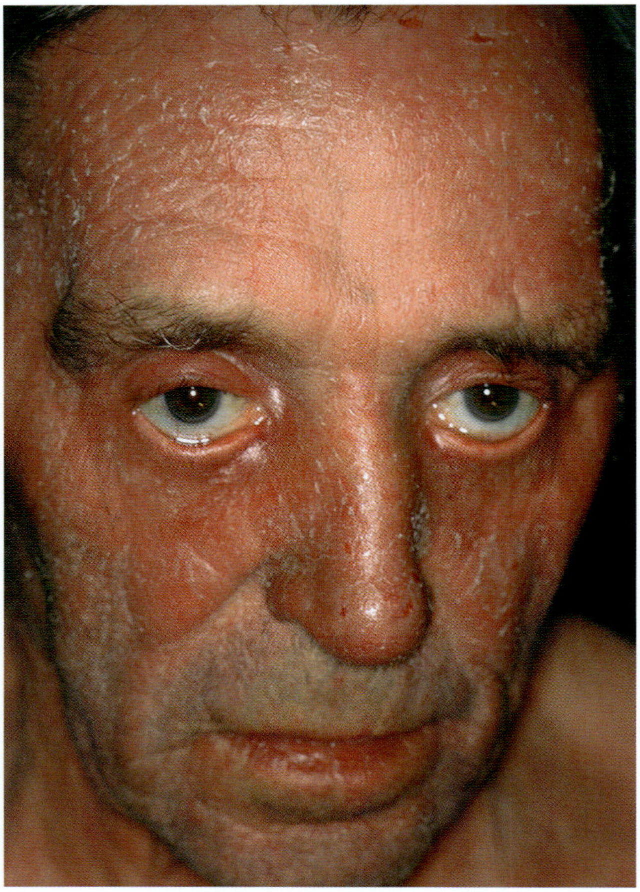

Figure 31.3 Actinic reticuloid. Suberythroderma causing complete involvement of the face by erythematous, scaly lesions. Note ectropion.

circulating cerebriform lymphocytes may be found in the peripheral blood of patients with actinic reticuloid [12]. T-helper lymphocytes are invariably predominating in Sézary syndrome, whereas T-cytotoxic cells are numerous in actinic reticuloid. A low helper-to-suppressor ratio in the peripheral blood has been found in patients with erythrodermic actinic reticuloid, as opposed to the high ratio commonly observed in patients with Sézary syndrome [13]. Unlike patients with mycosis fungoides and Sézary syndrome, on phototesting patients with chronic actinic dermatitis are sensitive to UV-B, UV-A, and, in most instances, to visible light. Fluorescent light may lead to an exacerbation of the disease. In patients with actinic reticuloid, the minimal erythema dose is lower than normal.

Treatment of chronic actinic dermatitis is difficult, and numerous therapeutic approaches have been proposed [14]. Photoprotection is crucial. Any relevant associated contact or photocontact allergens have to be identified and avoided. Some patients have been reported to respond to corticosteroids, photochemotherapy with psoralen and UV-A (PUVA), interferon-α, or a combination treatment with azathioprine, hydroxychloroquine, and prednisone. Cyclosporine (sometimes combined with bath PUVA) or topical tacrolimus ointment (especially for facial lesions) also appears to be effective. Tofacitinib, a JAK 1/3 inhibitor with activity in helper T cell 1- and helper T cell 2-mediated cutaneous diseases including psoriasis, atopic dermatitis, dermatomyositis, and alopecia areata, has been used with success in one patient [15], and dupilumab in other ones (reviewed in [16]).

## Lymphomatoid contact dermatitis

The term lymphomatoid contact dermatitis was coined by Gomez Orbaneja *et al.* in 1976 [17]. These authors described four patients with persistent allergic contact dermatitis proved by patch tests. The clinical picture and histologic features in their patients were highly suggestive of mycosis fungoides. Clinically, lymphomatoid contact dermatitis is characterized by pruritic, confluent erythematous papules and plaques that may mimic a cutaneous lymphoma (Fig. 31.5). Generalized plaques or exfoliative erythroderma can be observed rarely. In some cases, lymphomatoid contact dermatitis is limited to a small area of the body where antigen exposure has taken place; in these cases the clinical features do not mimic those of a lymphoma (Fig. 31.6a).

The lesions undergo phases of exacerbation and remission. Although lymphomatoid contact dermatitis has been reported to evolve into true malignant lymphoma, it is more likely that such patients had malignant lymphoma from the outset.

Histologically, lymphomatoid contact dermatitis shows dense, band-like lymphoid infiltrates resembling mycosis fungoides (Figs. 31.6b and c) [18]. The differentiation is determined mainly on the basis of changes within the epidermis, which shows variable acanthosis and spongiosis. In lymphomatoid contact dermatitis, there are usually only a few intraepidermal atypical lymphocytes that have no tendency to form "Darier nests." Small intraepidermal collections of keratinocytes admixed with Langerhans cells and lymphocytes are

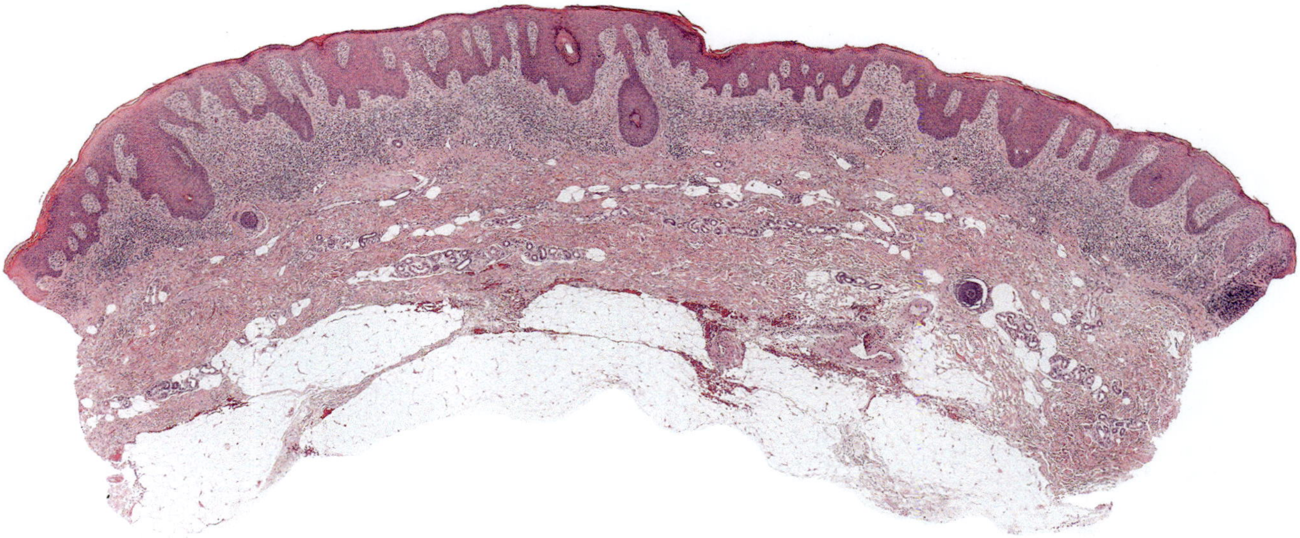

(a)

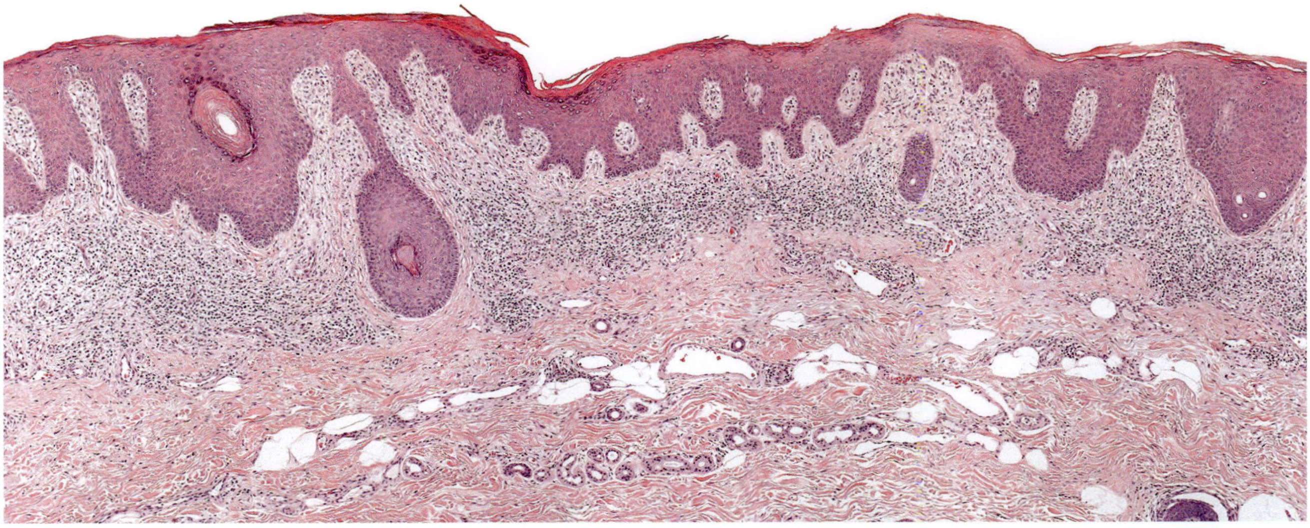

(b)

**Figure 31.4** Actinic reticuloid. (a) Psoriasiform epidermal hyperplasia with band-like infiltrate of lymphocytes in the upper dermis. (b) Detail of epidermal hyperplasia and lymphoid infiltrate.

common, and should not be misinterpreted as true "Darier nests." In contrast to mycosis fungoides, lymphocytes in these collections are small and without any atypical features, and staining for CD1a highlights Langerhans cells admixed with variables numbers of lymphocytes (Fig. 31.6c). A unique case due to methylisothiazolinone and the mixture of methyl chloroisothiazolinone/methylisothiazolinone revealed dermal infiltrates with predominance of B-lymphocytes and formation of germinal centers [19].

Analysis of TCR genes rearrangement commonly shows a polyclonal population of T lymphocytes in the skin lesions of lymphomatoid contact dermatitis. However, monoclonality can be observed in the majority of patch test lesions in patients with conventional contact dermatitis, demonstrating that the finding of a clonal population of T lymphocytes in such patients does not have any diagnostic implications [20].

Patch tests for a variety of common antigens can give a positive reaction in lymphomatoid contact dermatitis, and the diagnosis should be reserved for patients in whom the lymphomatoid skin lesions are caused by a positively reacting antigen. For the management of patients, a thorough search for antigens is necessary in order to interrupt the process. When contact with the responsible allergens is avoided, the lesions heal in a relatively short time.

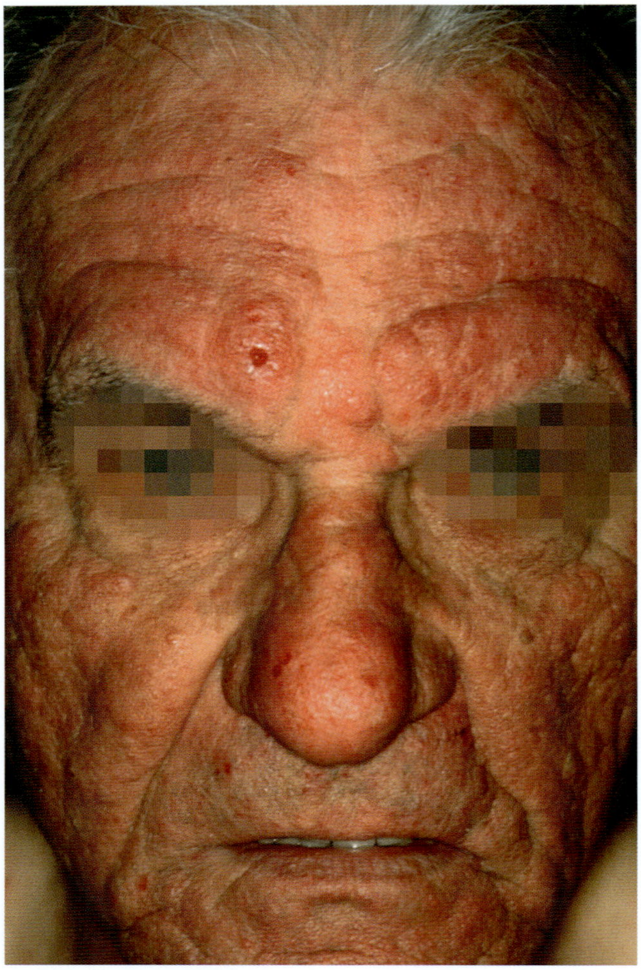

**Figure 31.5** Lymphomatoid contact dermatitis. Confluent, partly erosive erythematous papules and plaques on the forehead.

## Pseudolymphomatous atopic dermatitis and other eczematous dermatoses

Besides contact dermatitis, pseudolymphomatous clinical and/or histopathological features can be observed in other eczematous dermatoses as well, including atopic dermatitis. Atopic dermatitis is a relatively common, chronic, itchy condition that presents with eczematous, scaly patches and areas of lichenification due to chronic rubbing. The disease is usually diagnosed easily on clinical grounds, and biopsies are performed only seldom. On the other hand, some patients may develop erythroderma, and others may present with infiltrated plaques and even tumors that resemble lesions of mycosis fungoides clinically (Fig. 31.7). Because of the problems related to the use of immunomodulatory drugs and the risk of rapid progression of undiagnosed mycosis fungoides (see Chapter 3), in these cases a biopsy will often be performed before treatment is started.

Pseudolymphomatous atopic dermatitis shows clinically irregular, infiltrated, partly scaly patches and plaques associated with areas of lichenification at typical sites (flexural sites of elbows and knees) or at other sites of the body (Fig. 31.8). The patients have always a long history of atopic dermatitis. Histology reveals acanthosis of the epidermis with variable spongiosis and, particularly in areas of lichenification, compact orthohyperkeratosis alternating with parakeratosis. Dense, sometimes band-like infiltrates of lymphocytes and histiocytes are present in the dermis (Fig. 31.9). Eosinophils may be observed, but their number is variable. Epidermotropic lymphocytes are commonly found, but in most cases there is no disproportionate epidermotropism (i.e., marked epidermotropism unrelated to the amount of epidermal spongiosis). However, some cases are characterized by the presence of a prominent population of epidermotropic lymphocytes (usually $CD8^+$), which can be better visualized with immunohistochemical stainings (Fig. 31.10). Analysis of the TCR genes rearrangement shows a polyclonal pattern.

A peculiar histopathologic presentation of atopic dermatitis is characterized by pilotropic infiltrates and variable deposition of mucin within the hair follicles, mimicking pilotropic mycosis fungoides. I have seen this presentation exclusively in biopsies from lesions on the face (Fig. 31.11). The infiltrate is not as dense as in pilotropic mycosis fungoides, and the lesions clear within a few days with appropriate local treatment.

As a general rule, in order to differentiate atopic dermatitis from mycosis fungoides, it is advisable to take several biopsies from different body sites. When more biopsies are available, some of them invariably show the picture of a spongiotic dermatitis with less prominent lymphoid infiltrates, consistent with the pattern of conventional atopic dermatitis. On a single biopsy, on the other hand, differentiation may be extremely difficult or even impossible.

Treatment of pseudolymphomatous atopic dermatitis is similar to that of other severe forms of the disease (PUVA, immunomodulatory drugs).

### Pseudolymphomatous psoriasis

In the last years, I have observed a marked increase in the number of biopsies taken from patients with psoriasis, mostly due to the need to confirm diagnosis before expensive immunomodulatory drugs are prescribed, and to rule out other diseases for which these drugs would have no therapeutic (or a detrimental) effect. In this way, I came across many cases of psoriasis presenting histopathologically with features that deviate from those conventionally described in textbooks, and in particular cases with pseudolymphomatous aspects that mimic the histopathological features of mycosis fungoides. In this context, I now believe that most, if not all cases of the condition described in the literature as "palmo-plantar mycosis fungoides" [21–24] represent in truth cases of psoriasis with pseudolymphomatous infiltrates (see Chapter 3 for a detailed discussion on palmo-plantar mycosis fungoides).

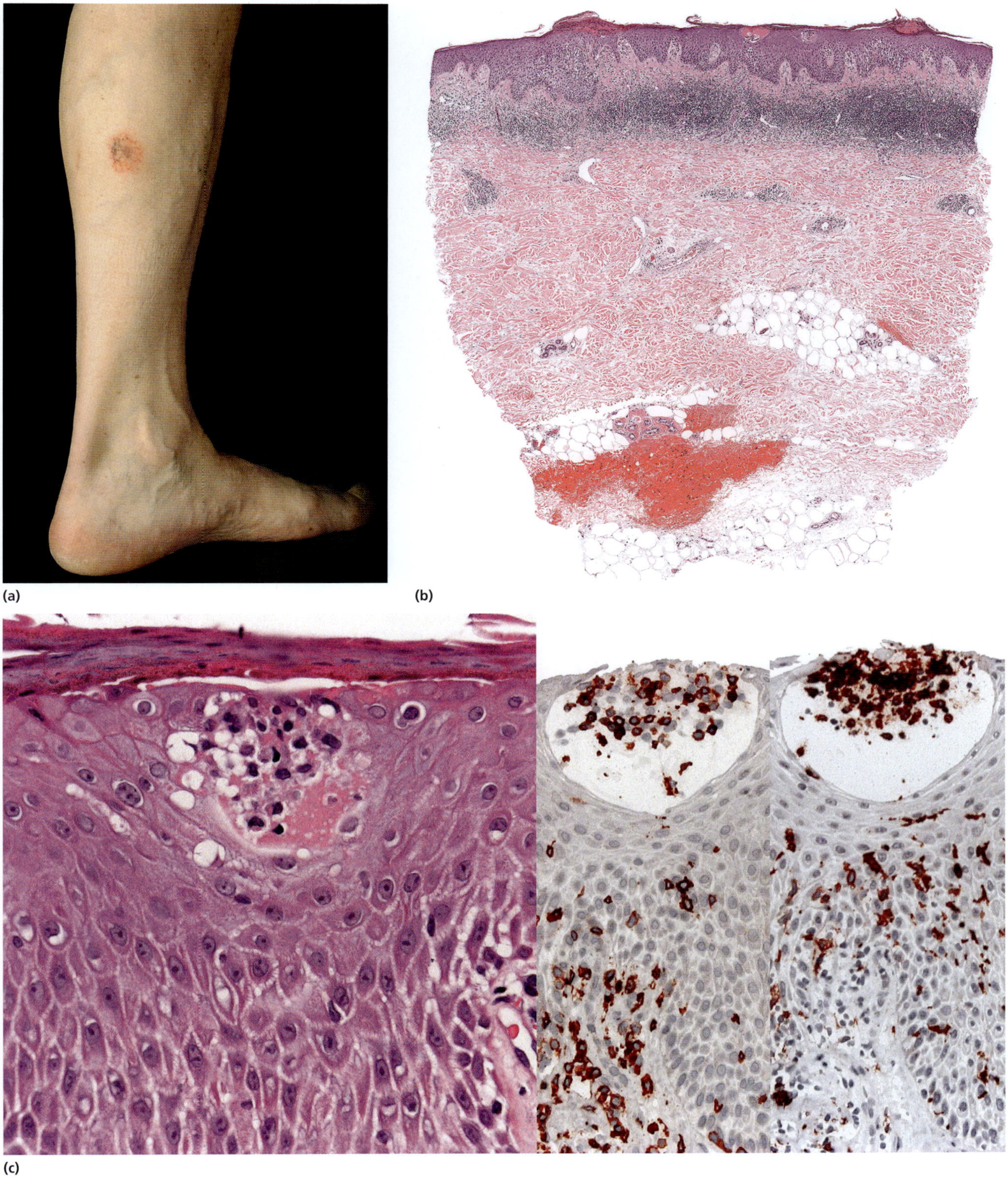

(a) (b) (c)

**Figure 31.6** Lymphomatoid contact dermatitis. (a) Circumscribed eczematous lesion on the left lower leg. (b) Histology shows a hyperplastic, spongiotic epidermis with a band-like infiltrate in the superficial dermis and with (c, left) small intraepidermal collections of lymphocytes admixed with Langerhans cells; (c, middle) the lymphocytes are positive for CD3, whereas (c, right) the Langerhans cells are positive for CD1a.

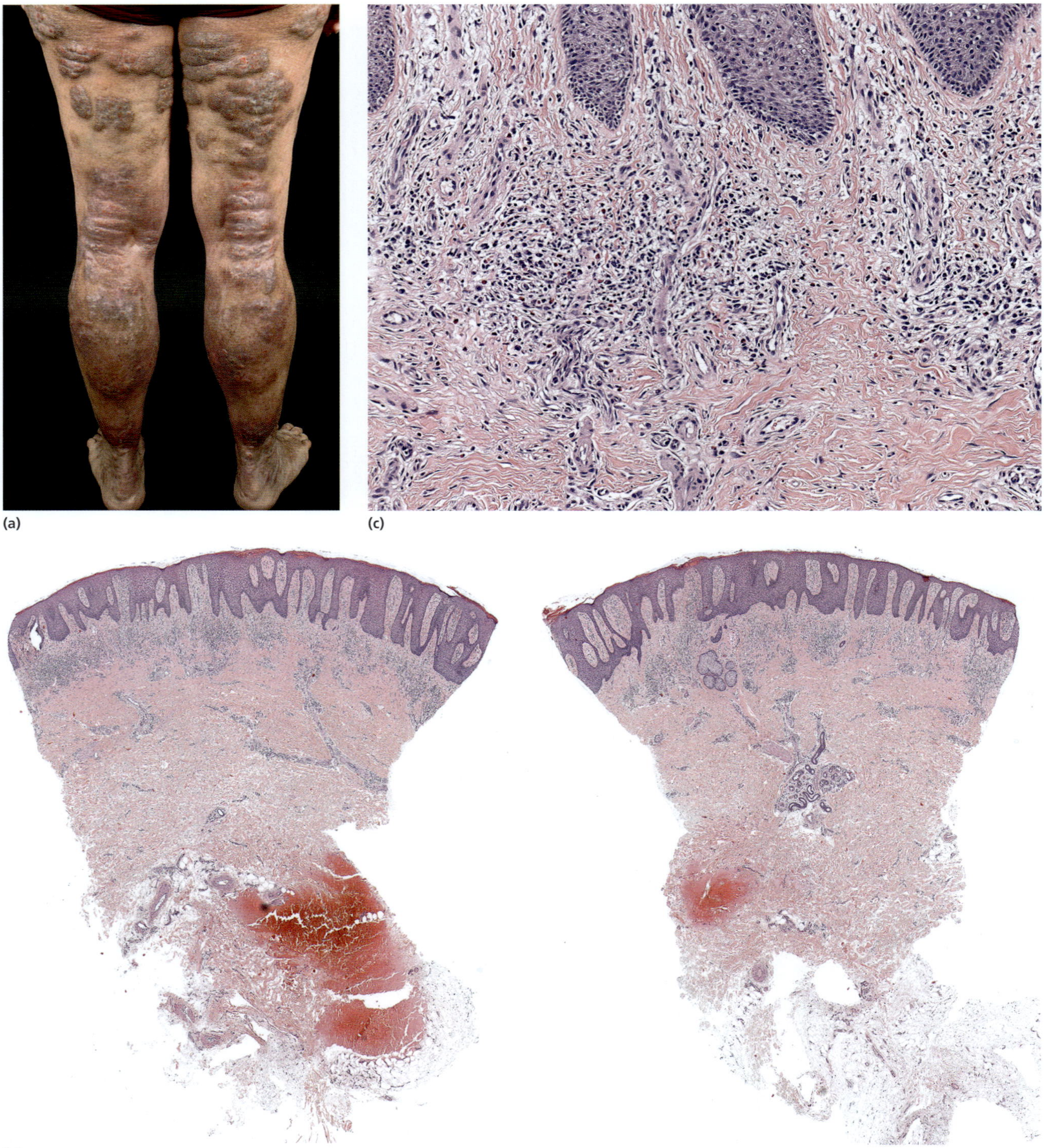

(a) (c)

(b)

Figure 31.7 Atopic dermatitis with tumoral lesions. (a) Infiltrated plaques and tumors on the legs; note several small excoriations due to scratching *(Courtesy of Dr. Thomas Wiesner, Vienna, Austria.)* (b) Histology shows a pronounced hyperplasia of the epidermis with spongiosis, parakeratosis and small, beginning excoriations; (c) in the superficial and focally in the mid-dermis there is an inflammatory infiltrate admixed with eosinophils.

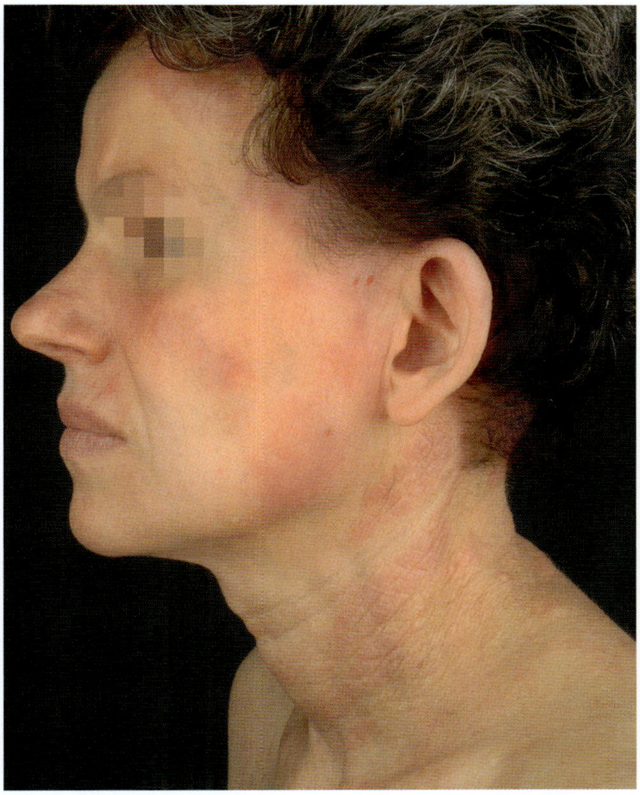

Figure 31.8 Atopic dermatitis. Infiltrated, erythematous patches and plaques on the head and neck. Note lichenification on the neck.

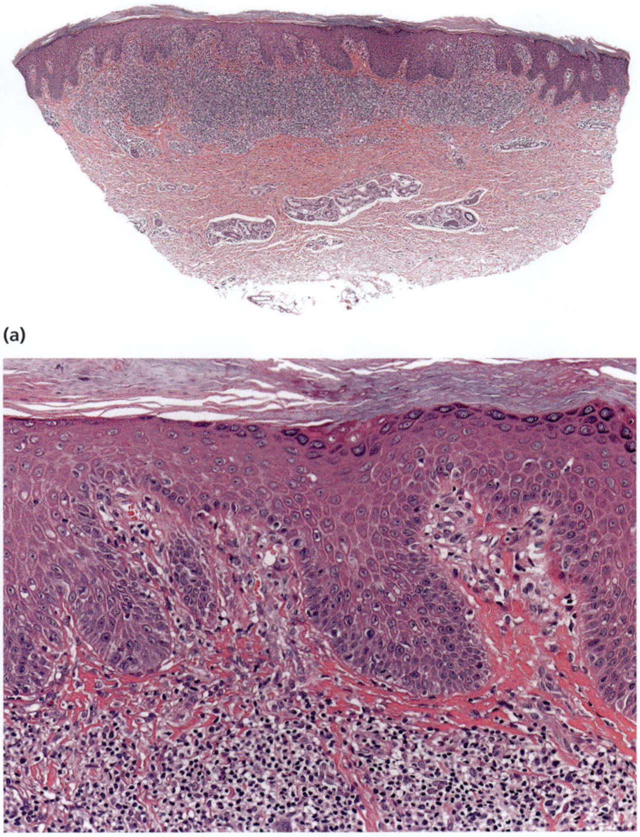

(a)

(b)

Figure 31.9 Atopic dermatitis. (a) Epidermal hyperplasia and compact orthohyperkeratosis (features of lichen simplex chronicus) in association with dense lymphoid infiltrates in the dermis. (b) Detail of epidermal features and of the lymphoid infiltrate without cytomorphologic atypia.

Pseudolymphomatous psoriasis is observed mostly on the palms and soles, and presents histopathologically with band-like lymphocytic infiltrates showing also epidermotropic cells (Fig. 31.12). The number of epidermotropic lymphocytes is variable and can be quite high. In my experience, in the vast majority of cases the epidermotropic lymphocytes are positive for CD8 (Fig. 31.12e), and are admixed with variable numbers of neutrophils and of mononuclear, elongated cells positive for MNDA (Fig. 31.12f). These cells may represent "histiocytoid" cells, similar to what can be observed in other neutrophilic dermatoses (e.g., Sweet syndrome). Band-like lymphocytic infiltrates in psoriasis are not restricted to cases arising on the palms and soles, and can occasionally be observed also in lesions located at other sites of the body (Figs. 31.13 and 31.14). In all cases that I have seen, clinical features as well as follow-up data clearly pointed at the diagnosis of psoriasis, showing that clinicopathological correlation is crucial to confirm the correct diagnosis, and suggesting also that great caution should be exerted before making a histopathological diagnosis of mycosis fungoides if lesions are restricted to the palms and soles.

## Pseudolymphomatous lichen planus

Of particular interest are cases of lichen planus mimicking histopathologically mycosis fungoides. Although lichen planus is characterized by a "band-like" (lichenoid) infiltrate, the histopathological pattern only rarely creates confusion or differential diagnostic concerns with mycosis fungoides. In some instances of atrophic lichen planus, however, I have observed dense, band-like infiltrates that were histologically and phenotypically indistinguishable from those observed in mycosis fungoides (Fig. 31.15), and some of these cases had received a previous histopathological diagnosis of cutaneous T-cell lymphoma (Fig. 31.16) [25]. In addition, one case of lichen planus with pronounced syringotropism mimicking syringotropic mycosis fungoides has been reported [26]. Interestingly, hypopigmented macules have been observed in lichen planus and lichen planopilaris, thus representing a clinical pitfall as well [27]. In these cases, clinicopathological correlation is of paramount importance in order to achieve the correct diagnosis, and one should always consider performing more than one biopsy from different lesions.

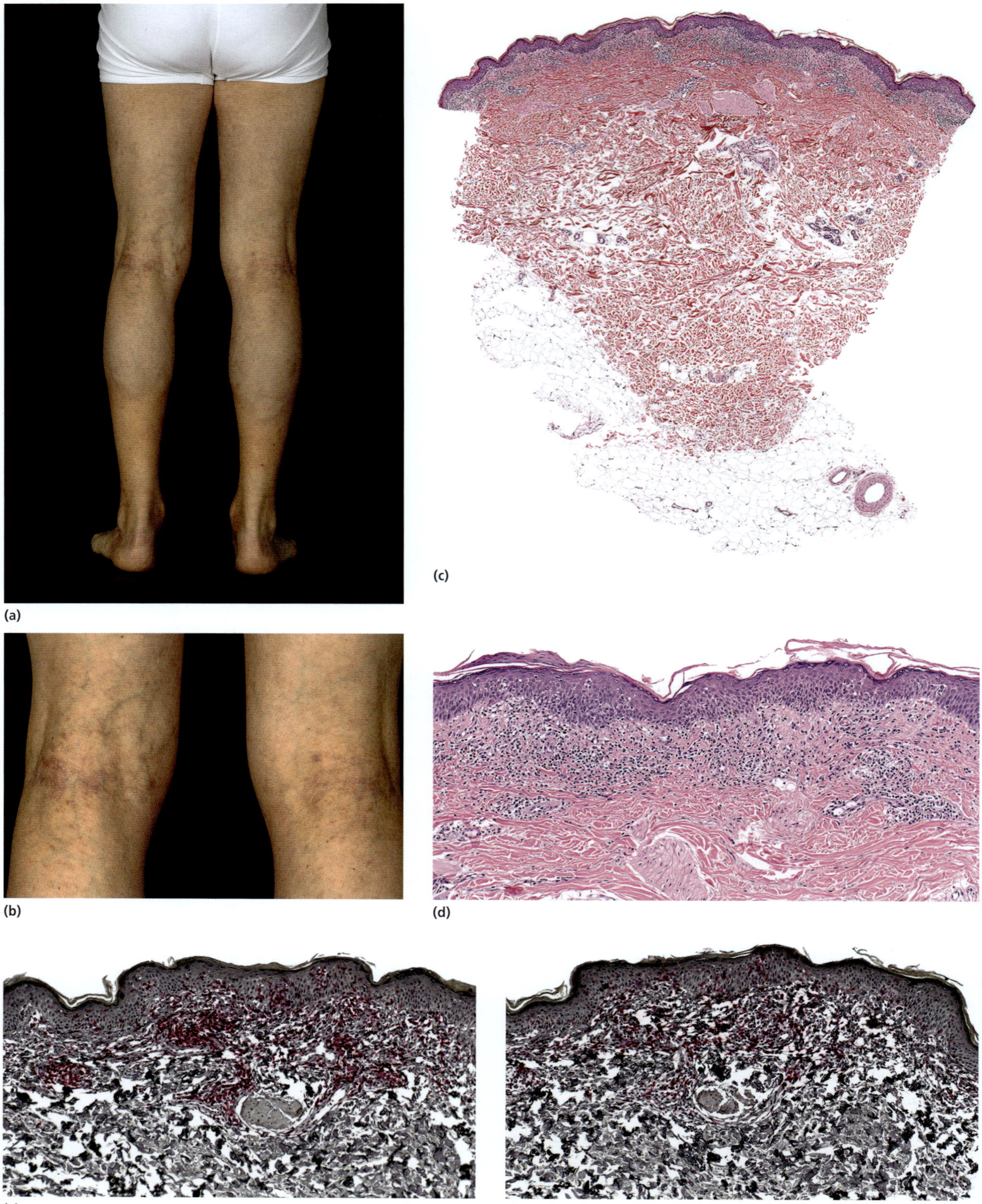

(a) (b) (c) (d) (e) (f)

**Figure 31.10** Atopic dermatitis. (a, b) Eczematous lesions on the flexural aspect of both knees. (c) Histology reveals a band-like inflammatory infiltrate with (d) epidermotropic lymphocytes; note also epidermal spongiosis. The epidermotropic cells are better visualized with stainings for (e) CD3 and (f) CD8.

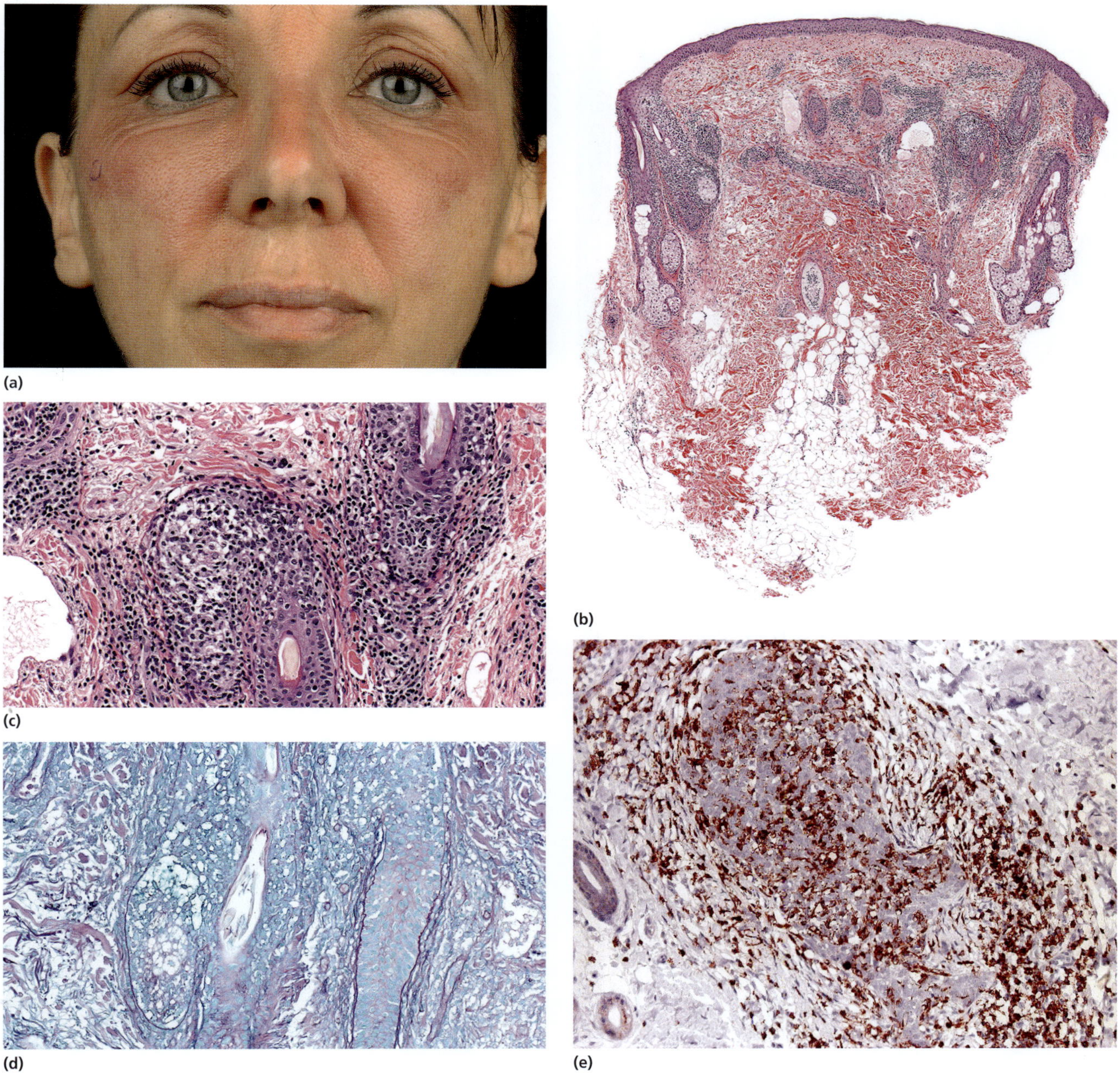

Figure 31.11 Atopic dermatitis with follicular mucinosis. (a) Eczematous lesions on the face with accentuation in the periocular region. (b) Histology reveals dermal inflammatory infiltrates (c) with numerous pilotropic lymphocytes and (d) deposition of mucin within the hair follicles. (e) Staining for CD2 highlights the pilotropic lymphocytes.

## Non-mycosis fungoides-associated follicular mucinosis and other mimickers of pilotropic/adnexotropic mycosis fungoides

Although the discussion on the exact nosology of "idiopathic" follicular mucinosis (alopecia mucinosa) is far from being settled (see Chapter 3), it should be reminded that the finding of mucin deposition within a hair follicle *per se* does not represent a feature of mycosis fungoides-associated or idiopathic alopecia mucinosa. In fact, to a certain extent follicular mucinosis may be regarded as a cutaneous histopathological pattern, akin to other non-specific findings such as epidermolytic hyperkeratosis or acantholytic dyskeratosis among many others. Isolated follicles with features of follicular mucinosis may be observed in unrelated inflammatory and neoplastic skin conditions such as squamous cell carcinoma, insect bite reactions, and acne vulgaris, among many others [28]. The features of the background condition dominate the histopathological pattern (Fig. 31.17). In some cases, I have observed

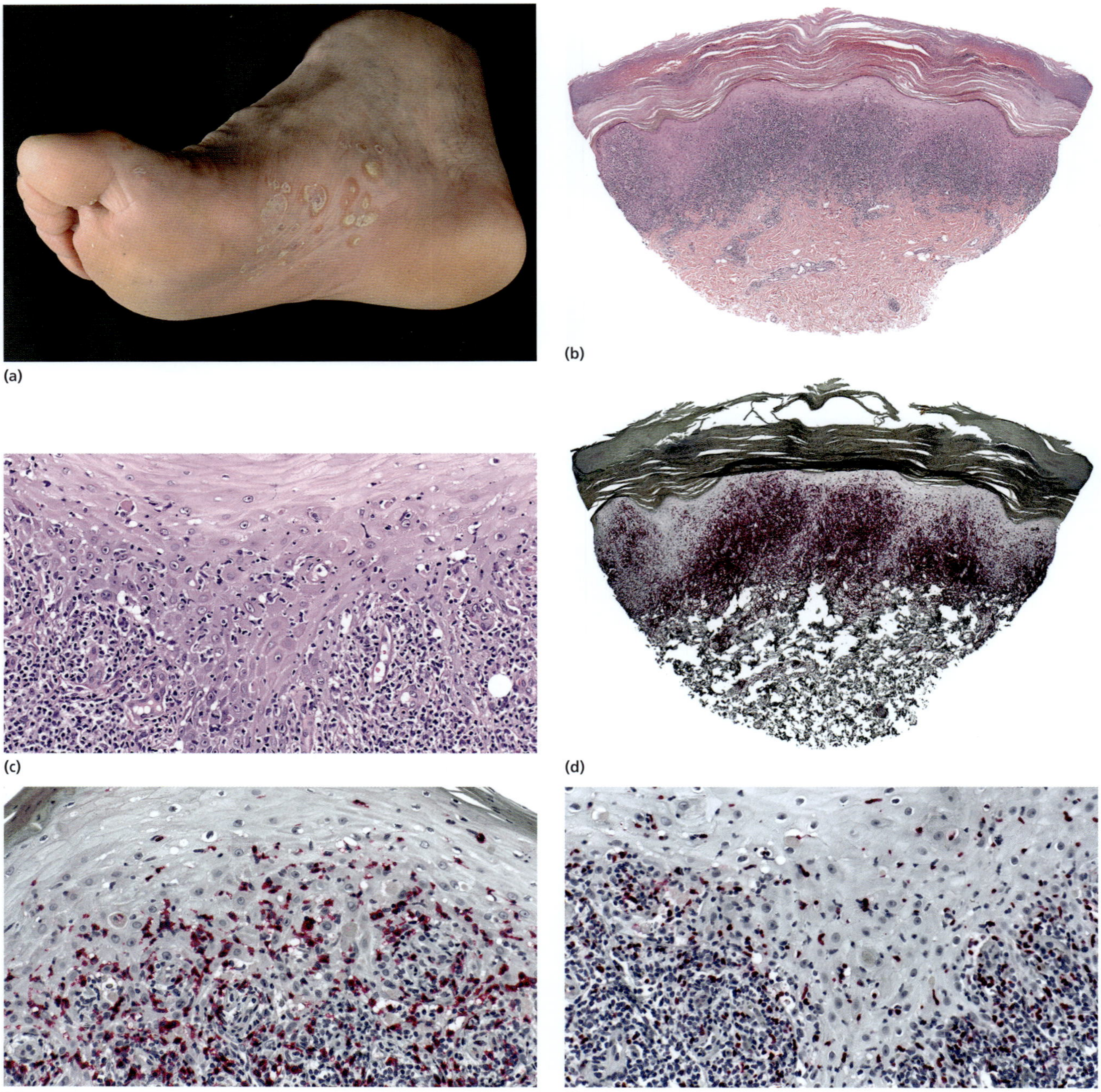


**Figure 31.12** "Pseudolymphomatous" infiltrate in psoriasis. (a) Typical lesions of psoriasis on the sole. (b) Histology reveals a dense, band-like inflammatory infiltrate (c) with numerous epidermotropic lymphocytes admixed with neutrophils and with elongated, "histiocytoid" cells. (d) The lymphocytes are positive for CD3; (e) Most intraepidermal lymphocytes are positive for CD8; (f) The "histiocytoid" cells are positive for MNDA.

follicular mucinosis also in the context of cutaneous lesions of other lymphoid malignancies such as B-CLL, and cases arising in several other hematological malignancies, including Hodgkin lymphoma, acute and chronic myelogenous leukemia, myelodysplastic syndrome, mantle cell lymphoma, diffuse large B-cell lymphoma, multiple myeloma, and lymphoplasmacytic lymphoma, have been reported as well [29]. In addition, follicular mucinosis has been observed as a drug reaction after administration of different drugs, including infliximab, imatinib, oxcarbamazepine, captopril, and dextromorphan [30, 31], and in patients undergoing immunosuppressive therapy [32]. In short, predicting the nature of follicular mucinosis (i.e., associated or not with mycosis fungoides) has been defined as a "sticky situation" [31].

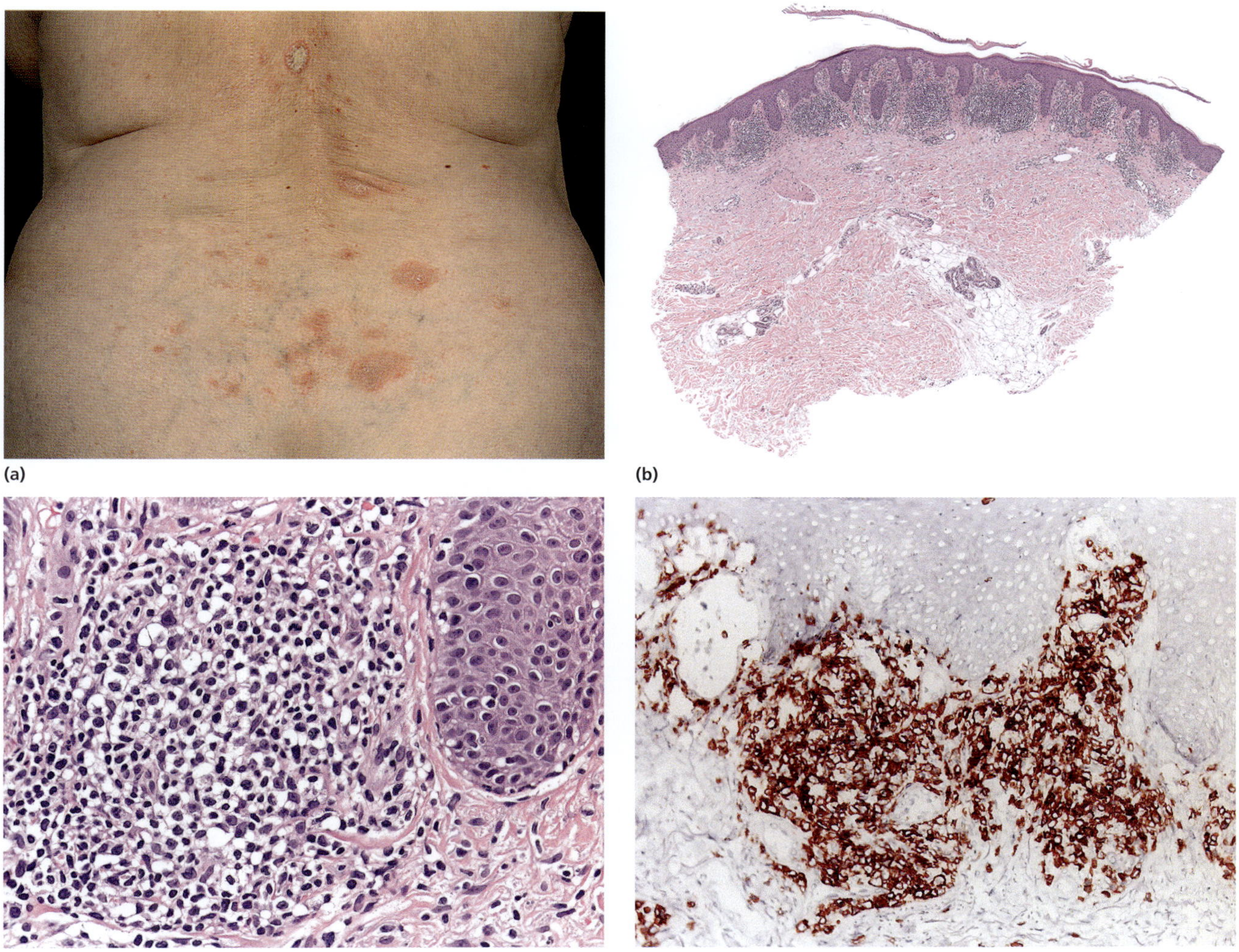

(a) (b) (c) (d)

**Figure 31.13** "Pseudolymphomatous" infiltrate in psoriasis. (a) Psoriasiform plaques on the back. Histology shows (b) psoriasiform hyperplasia with a dense, band-like lymphoid infiltrate, showing (c) many mid-sized, pleomorphic lymphocytes. (d) Staining for CD5 highlights the T lymphocytes and shows only minimal epidermotropism.

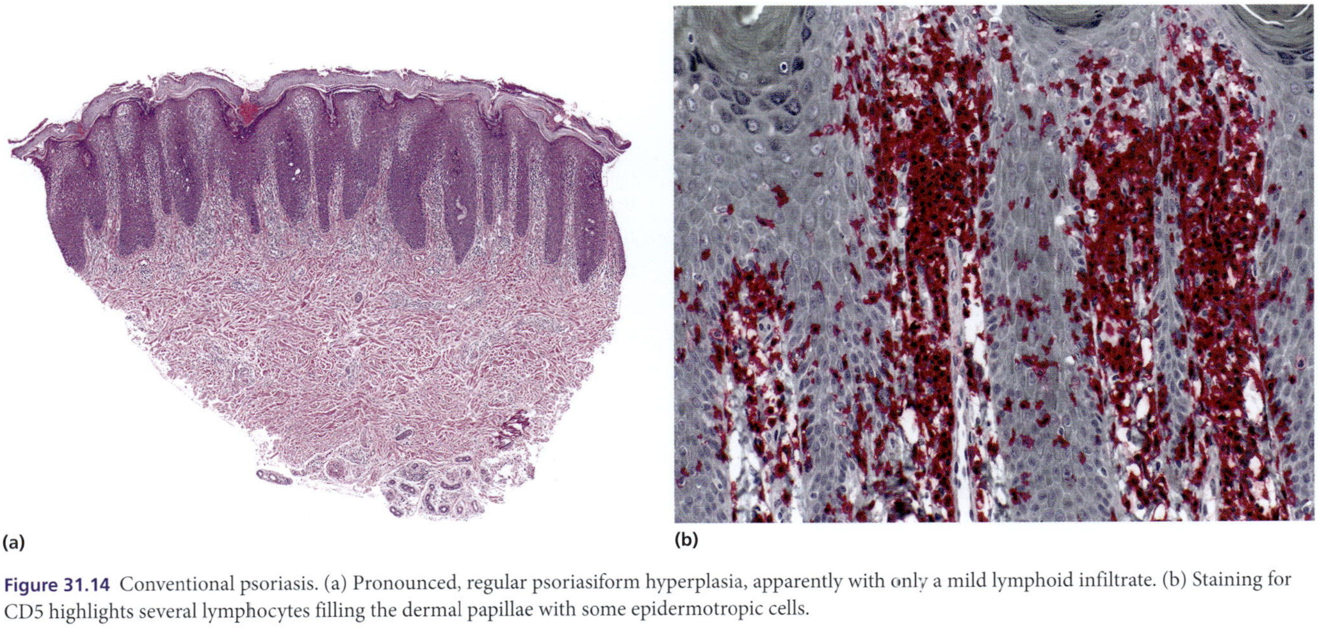

(a) (b)

**Figure 31.14** Conventional psoriasis. (a) Pronounced, regular psoriasiform hyperplasia, apparently with only a mild lymphoid infiltrate. (b) Staining for CD5 highlights several lymphocytes filling the dermal papillae with some epidermotropic cells.

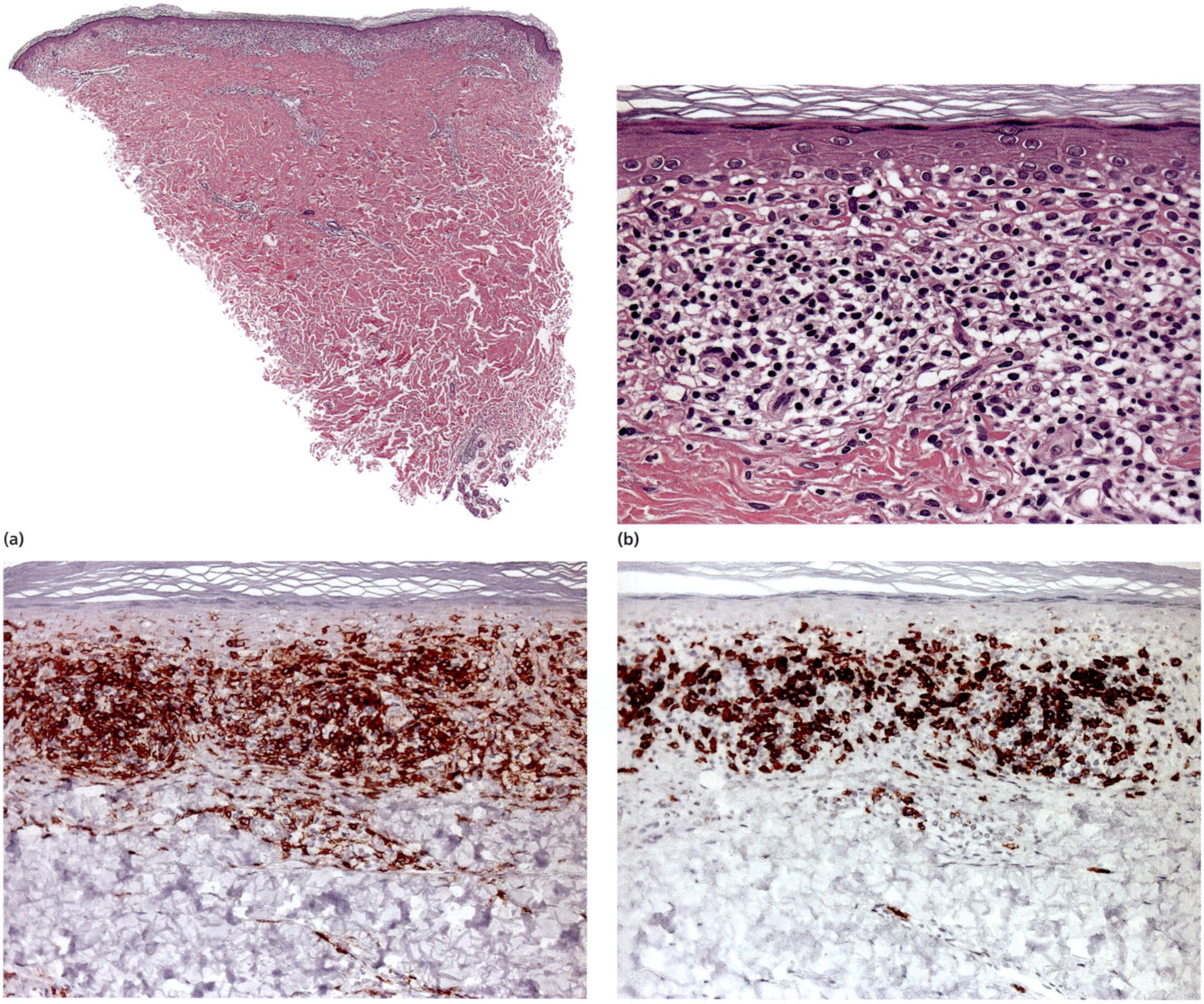

(a) (b) (c) (d)

**Figure 31.15** "Pseudolymphomatous" infiltrate in lichen planus. (a) Dense, band-like infiltrate without the characteristic epidermal changes of lichen planus. (b) Detail of the infiltrate with some medium-sized cells and without clear-cut lichenoid changes. (c) The lymphocytes are predominantly positive for CD4, (d) admixed with several CD8+ cytotoxic T cells.

From a clinical perspective, I have rarely observed patients with pityriasis rubra pilaris presenting at onset of the disease with mostly follicular, partly confluent lesions that resembled clinically follicular mycosis fungoides (Fig. 31.18). Histopathological features, however, allow to clearly distinguish between the two conditions. Another condition that resembles pilotropic mycosis fungoides clinically (and sometimes histopathologically) is lichen spinulosus, a disorder of unknown etiology considered to be a variant of keratosis pilaris. In fact, cases reported in the literature as "lichen spinulosus with follicular mucinosis" [33] may represent in truth examples of juvenile follicular mycosis fungoides, and cases of juvenile follicular mycosis fungoides mimicking lichen spinulosus have been reported [34], underlying the need for long-term follow-up in these patients. Milia-en-plaque is a reactive condition characterized by localized, grouped small milia. It can be observed in inflammatory disorders such as lichen planus or lupus erythematosus, among others, and rarely in patients with pilotropic mycosis fungoides. In this last condition, milia-en-plaques is usually observed in concomitance with other typical manifestations of the disease, and does not represent a problem in the differential diagnosis.

From a histopathological perspective, dense infiltrates with pilotropic and/or syringotropic lymphocytes observed in inflammatory conditions also represent a mimic of adnexotropic mycosis fungoides. I have seen similar, deceptive infiltrates in the setting of atopic

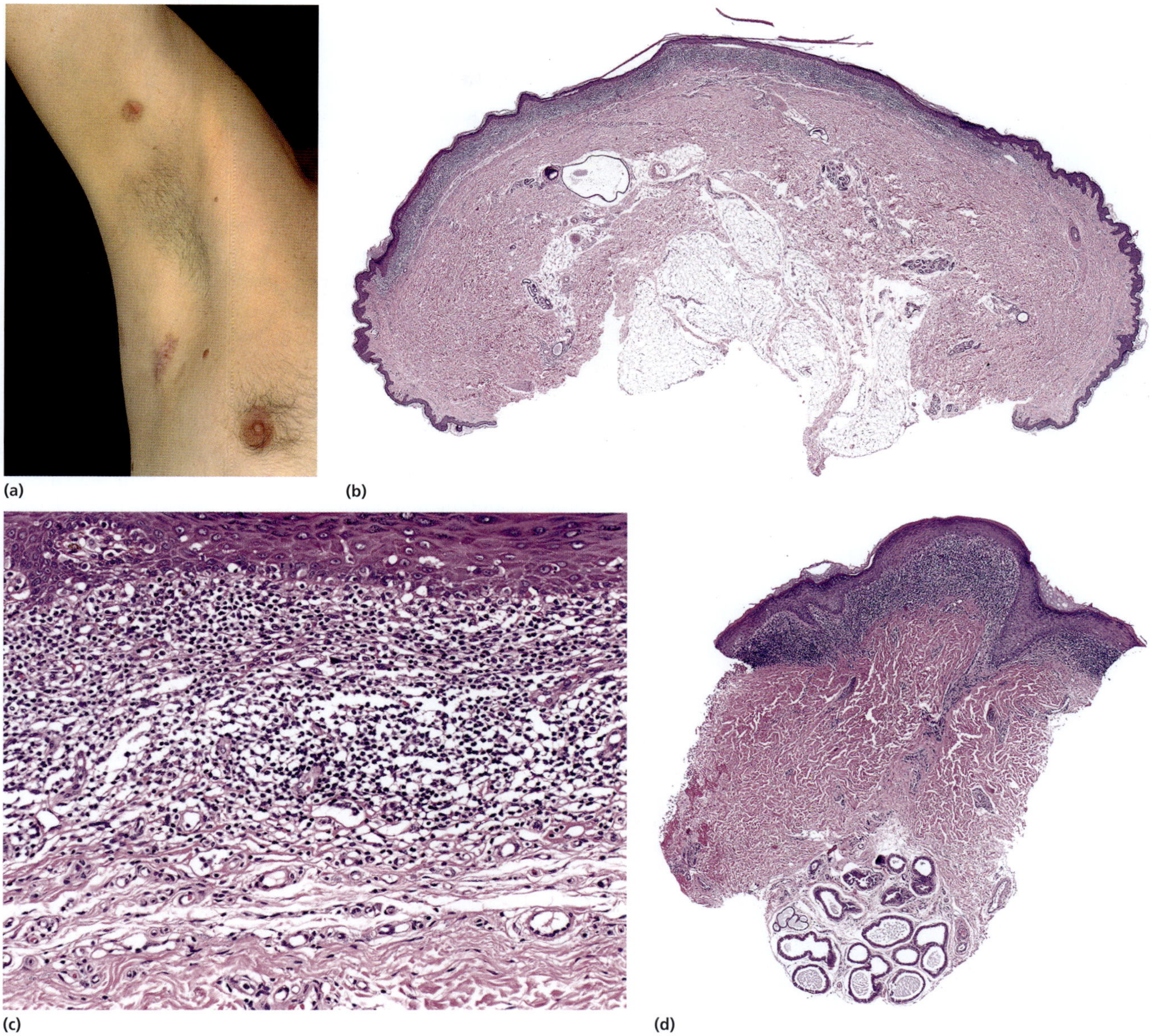

Figure 31.16 "Pseudolymphomatous" infiltrate in lichen planus previously diagnosed as cutaneous T-cell lymphoma on a previous biopsy. (a) Axillary lesions of atrophic pigmented lichen planus; note scar due to the complete excision of one lesion following previous diagnosis of cutaneous T-cell lymphoma. (b) Complete excision specimen showing a dense, band-like infiltrate. (c) Detail of the infiltrate. (d) A second punch biopsy from a different lesion shows more conventional features of lichen planus.

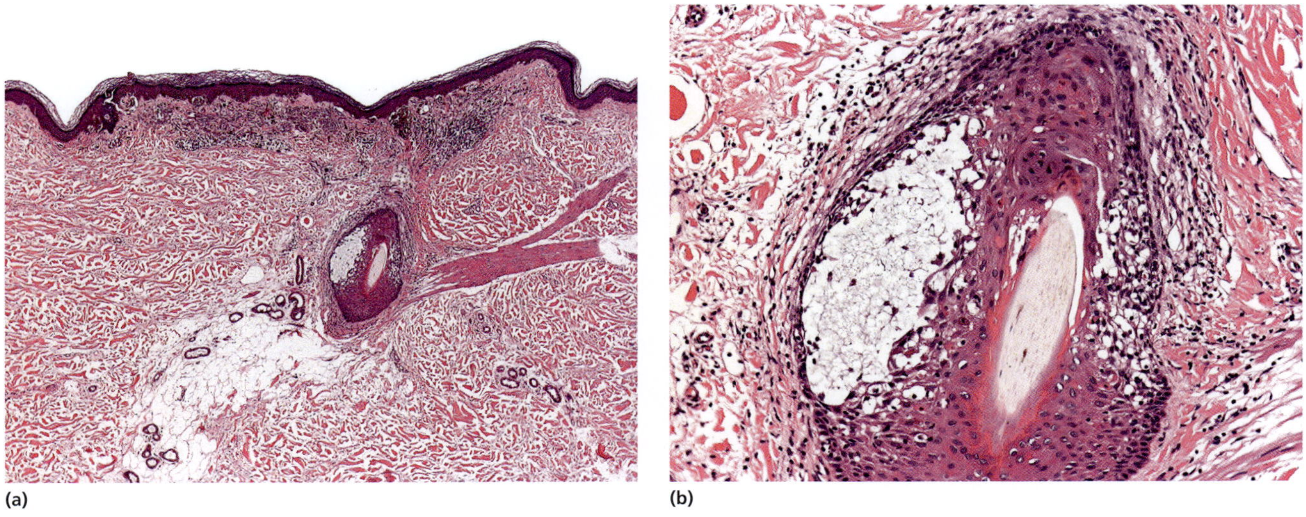

Figure 31.17 Follicular mucinosis within a melanocytic nevus. (a) Symmetrical melanocytic tumor without atypical features and with mucin deposition within a hair follicle. (b) Detail of the hair follicle with mucin deposition.

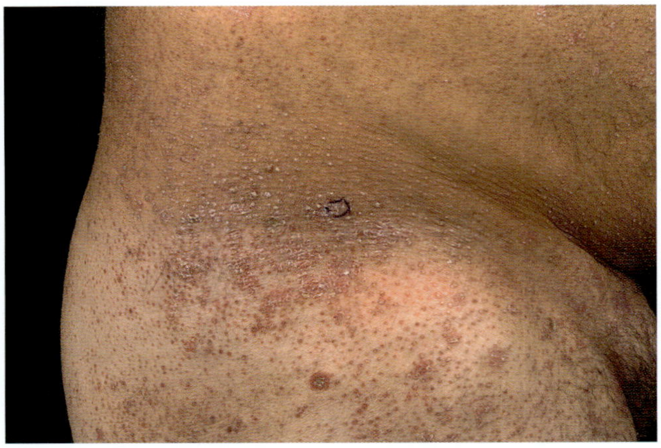

Figure 31.18 Pityriasis rubra pilaris. Prominent involvement of the hair follicles is unusual and may mimic clinically the picture of pilotropic mycosis fungoides.

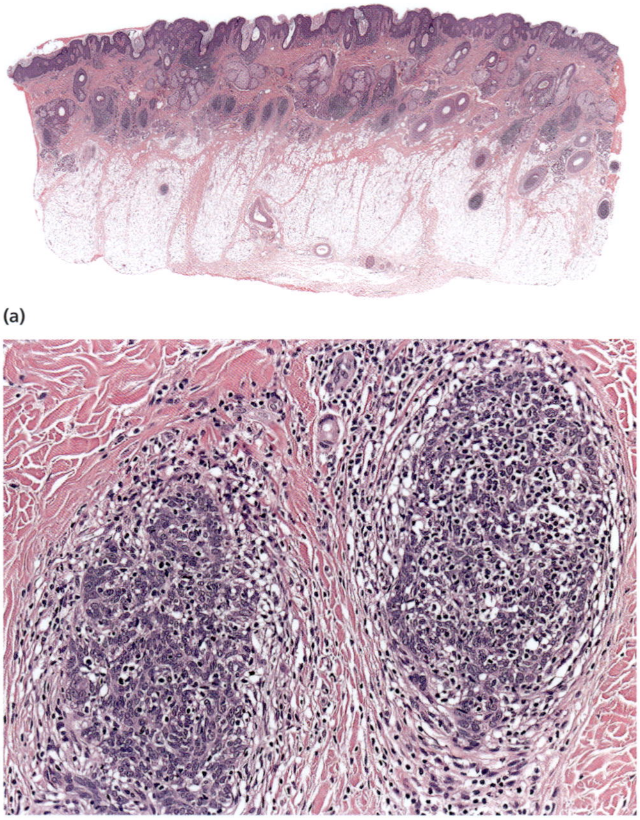

(a)

(b)

Figure 31.19 Nevus sebaceous with adnexotropic lymphocytes. (a) Irregular epidermal hyperplasia with a papillomatous surface; (b) Prominent syringometaplasia with numerous epitheliotropic lymphocytes.

dermatitis (see the specific section above in this chapter and Fig. 31.11), epidermal nevus, nevus sebaceous (Fig. 31.19), and rhinophyma (Fig. 31.20), and similar findings have been described in other cutaneous inflammatory and neoplastic disorders as well [28]. As adnexotropic mycosis fungoides in several cases does not show follicular deposition of mucin, these cases, too, represent a pitfall in the histopathological diagnosis. In addition, atopic dermatitis may be a differential diagnosis of mycosis fungoides clinically, thus representing a further problem in the correct classification of these cases. However, adnexotropic infiltrates in inflammatory conditions are uncommon, and in my experience, accurate clinicopathological correlation is sufficient to avoid a misdiagnosis of mycosis fungoides. Pilotropic lymphoid infiltrates have been observed also in patients receiving anti-TNFα treatment [35].

As neoplastic cells of mycosis fungoides may colonize skin lesions of other conditions, the theoretical possibility of a specific manifestation of the disease at the site of an inflammatory dermatosis cannot be ruled out completely at time of first diagnosis, and the final diagnosis must be confirmed by follow-up data. For practical purposes, however, the finding of hair follicles showing follicular mucinosis in otherwise different diseases and without skin signs of mycosis fungoides should not be overdiagnosed as follicular mycosis fungoides, and rather interpreted as a non-specific histopathological pattern. The same applies for lymphocytic infiltrates showing syringotropism, that can occasionally be observed in conditions other than mycosis fungoides (see above the section on pseudolymphomatous lichen planus).

## Non-neoplastic erythroderma in adult patients

The evaluation of adult patients with erythroderma represents one of the more vexing problems in dermatology and dermatopathology, and erythroderma may be considered as a kind of paradoxical pseudolymphoma (discussion of neonatal and childhood erythroderma is beyond the scope of this section, but a list of entities and differential diagnostic criteria of erythroderma in neonates and young patients is provided in several reviews; see also Chapter 30) [36, 37]. If it is true that benign conditions may present with a clinical picture mimicking that of Sézary syndrome, it is also true that Sézary syndrome often presents with nonspecific histopathological features similar to those of a benign dermatosis ("pseudodermatitis"). In this context, it should also be reminded that patients with Sézary syndrome may not present the clinical picture of erythroderma [38]. In addition, although emphasis in the diagnosis of erythroderma is usually put on differentiation of benign inflammatory dermatoses from malignant lymphoma, in erythrodermic patients severe systemic complications may arise irrespective of the background condition, including particularly hypothermia and loss of fluid, electrolytes, and albumin with subsequent cardiac failure and, if untreated, even death. Thus, this is a "pseudolymphoma" that may run a fatal course.

One of the problems in diagnosing different types of erythroderma is the very definition of it. In clinical practice (as well as in many publications), the percentage of the "red" body area

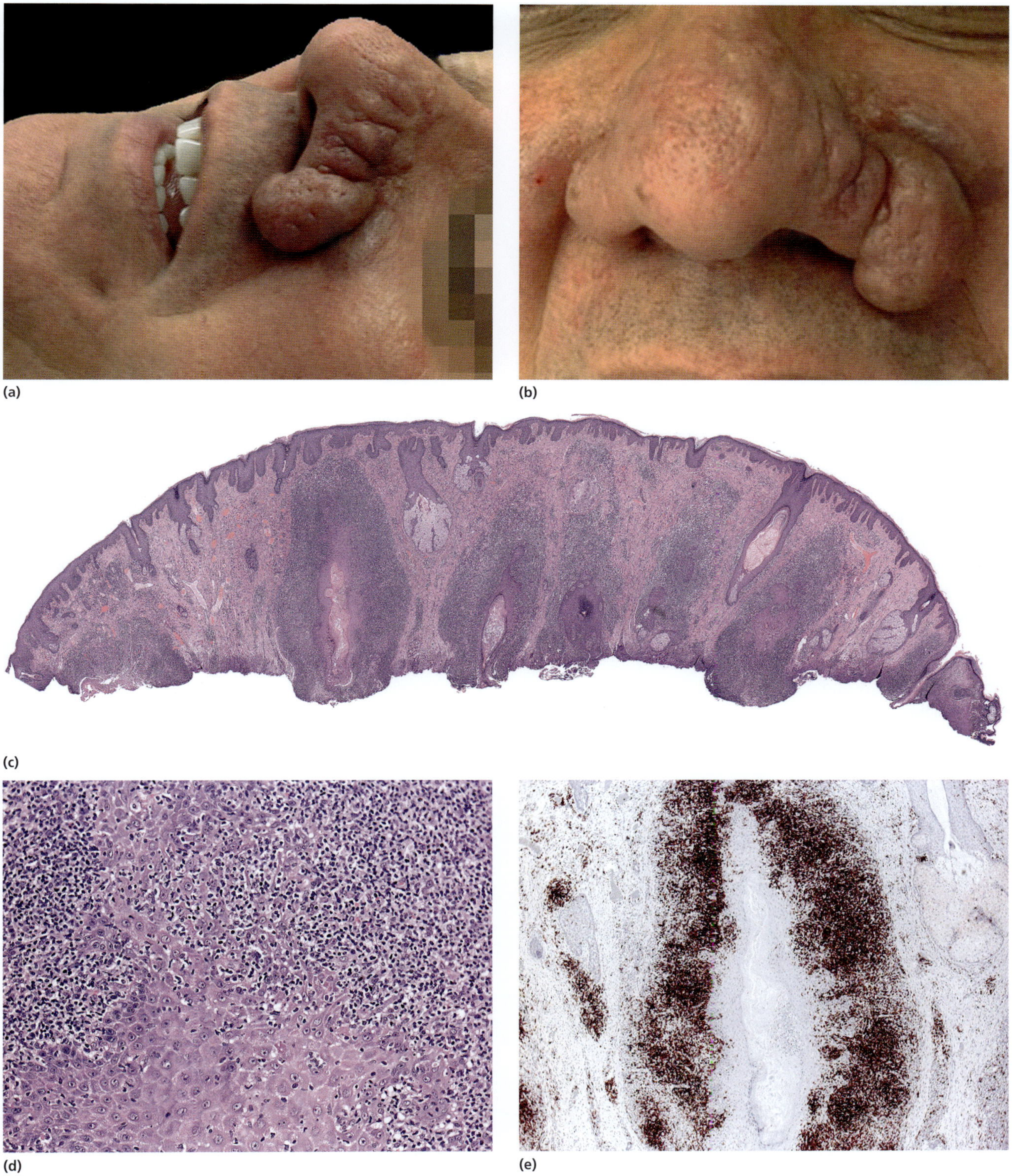


**Figure 31.20** Pilotropic infiltrates in rhinophyma. (a, b) Typical clinical picture of rhinophyma *(Photo courtesy of Dr. Jason Williams and Dr. Noreen Walsh, Halifax, Canada.)* (c) Dense perifollicular inflammatory infiltrates with (d) pilotropic lymphocytes which are (e) positive for CD5 and show approximately equal numbers of (f) CD4+ and (g) CD8+ cells.

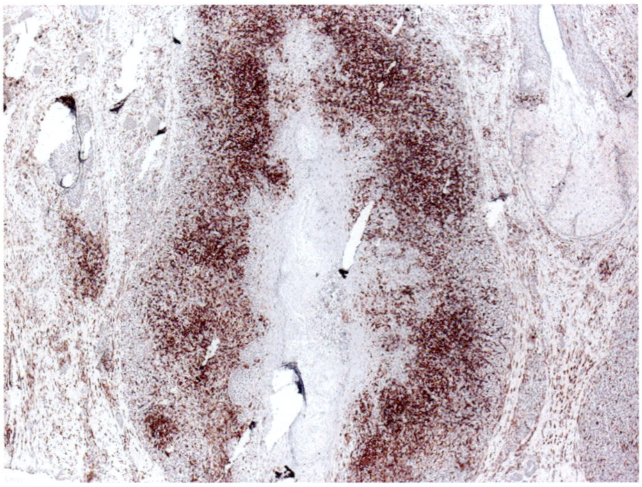

(f)

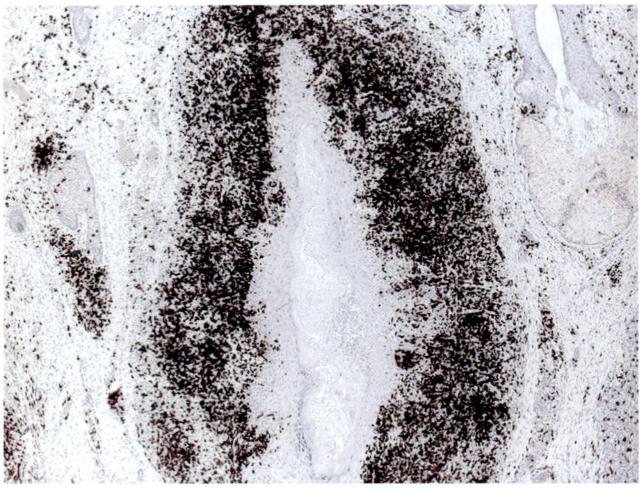

(g)

**Figure 31.20** (Continued)

necessary for a diagnosis of erythroderma can vary markedly. In medical dictionaries, erythroderma is defined variously as "widespread reddening of the skin," or "abnormal reddening of the entire skin surface," or "intense and usually widespread reddening of the skin," thus leaving ample margins for personal interpretation as to what is really erythroderma. In the consensus statement of the International Society of Cutaneous Lymphoma (ISCL) and EORTC–Cutaneous Lymphoma Task Force, erythroderma is defined as erythema covering ≥80% of the body area [39].

Some of the conditions that may give rise to erythroderma are listed in specific paragraphs in this chapter (i.e., atopic dermatitis, actinic reticuloid, psoriasis, lymphomatoid drug eruption – T-cell type, lymphoid proliferations in HIV+ patients). Other benign dermatoses may present with erythroderma, such as pityriasis rubra pilaris, for example. The presence of pruritus does not provide differential diagnostic clues, as it is observed in >90% of cases of erythroderma, irrespective of the etiology. In patients with erythroderma, differential diagnosis from Sézary syndrome is achieved by precise history (e.g., previous diagnosis of a condition known to have the potential to eventuate in erythroderma, drug ingestion, known malignant neoplasm), identification of clinical clues (e.g., lichenification of skin in the flexural aspects of the knees and elbows in atopic dermatitis, presence of some pustules, often in the flexural areas, in psoriasis, islands of spared skin, follicular hyperkeratosis, and palmar keratoderma in pityriasis rubra pilaris), and evaluation of biopsy specimens including morphologic, phenotypic, and molecular criteria. The most important criterion for the diagnosis of Sézary syndrome, thus also for differentiation of non-neoplastic erythroderma from it, is the examination of the peripheral blood (see Chapter 4 for details). If differentiation is not possible, the term used for unclassifiable cases is "idiopathic" erythroderma – in the past they were also termed "red man syndrome" in the Anglo-American literature or "syndrome de l'homme rouge" in the French literature, this last being a term that has also been used for an allergic reaction to vancomycin. A list of conditions that may present with erythroderma with the main clinical differential diagnostic features is presented in Table 31.2. The main histopathological, immunohistochemical, and molecular criteria for differentiation of Sézary syndrome from inflammatory erythroderma are summarized in Table 31.3.

Many publications over the years tried to address the differential diagnosis of erythroderma at a clinical, histopathological, phenotypical, or molecular level, but it is fair to say that results have been, at least in part, disappointing. No matter how good a clinician is, and no matter how good a dermatopathologist is, some cases of erythroderma will evolve into a direction that both had neither predicted nor expected. Histologically, there is a variable overlap between different types of erythroderma, and finding or not specific features may also be influenced by previous treatment. In particular, spongiosis is common to many types of erythroderma, possibly due to the intense pruritus that all these patients usually have, with consequent scratching. In this context, spongiosis cannot be considered as a histopathological differential diagnostic criterion. However, this is not to say that in patients with erythroderma a precise diagnosis is not possible: many cases can indeed be classified correctly with accurate clinicopathological correlation (Figs. 31.21, 31.22, and 31.23). However, particularly in erythroderma presenting as a first manifestation of a given disease, the final diagnosis may be possible only upon follow-up data. In addition, many dermatopathologists do not have access to precise clinical data, thus rendering the histopathological diagnosis more difficult. In a large study, a correct histopathological diagnosis (without clinical or laboratory data) could be made in only

**Table 31.2** Main causes of erythroderma in adult patients and clinical differential diagnostic features

| Disorder | Frequency | Main differential diagnostic features |
|---|---|---|
| Sézary syndrome | Rare | Slowly evolving erythroderma; sparing of large skin folds; no history of previous inflammatory skin disorders; palmo-plantar hyperkeratosis; enlarged lymph nodes; patchy, irregular alopecia. |
| Psoriasis | Common | History of psoriasis and/or onset after withdrawal of systemic steroids or of methotrexate; focal pustulation; face may be spared. |
| Atopic dermatitis* | Common | History of atopic dermatitis; focal areas of lichenification, particularly in the flexural areas of elbows and knees; elevated serum IgE. |
| Drug eruption | Common | Sudden onset, sometimes preceded by an exanthematic eruption; history of ingestion of drug(s). |
| Pityriasis rubra pilaris | Uncommon | Islands of spared skin ("nappes claires"); palmar keratoderma; hyperkeratotic follicular papules. |
| Actinic reticuloid / Chronic actinic dermatitis | Rare | Intractable pruritus (yet pruritus common to the vast majority of erythrodermic patients!); photosensitivity, pathologic phototesting. |
| Paraneoplastic erythroderma | Rare | History of malignant tumor; cachexia. |
| Superficial pemphigus† | Rare | History of pemphigus; impetiginization due to frequent superficial erosions. |

* Similar changes may be observed in generalized, erythrodermic eczema unrelated to atopic dermatitis.
† Other bullous disorders such as bullous pemphigoid and paraneoplastic pemphigus may rarely present with erythroderma; clinical differential diagnostic features are similar to those listed for superficial pemphigus.

**Table 31.3** Histopathological, immunohistochemical and molecular criteria for differentiation of Sézary syndrome from inflammatory erythroderma

| Histopathological / Immunohistological Criterion | Sézary syndrome | Inflammatory erythroderma |
|---|---|---|
| Cellular atypia | May be present | Absent |
| Darier nests (Pautrier microabscesses) | Present in a small number of cases | Always absent |
| Marked thinning of suprapapillary epidermis | Absent | Present (psoriasis) |
| Follicular hyperkeratosis | Absent | Present (some cases of pityriasis rubra pilaris) |
| Acantholysis | Absent | Present (pemphigus) |
| Numbers of CD8+ reactive cells | Low | High |
| Ki-67 index | High* | Low* |
| CD7 expression | Reduced | Normal |
| Expression of PD-1 | Present in CD4+ neoplastic cells | Lower number of positive cells, and present in CD8+ reactive lymphocytes |
| TCR rearrangement studies | Same clone in the skin and blood | May be clonal in the skin, but never shows the same clone in the blood |
| Altered expression of *STAT4*, *TWIST1*, and *DNM3* or *PLS3* | Found in the majority of cases | Not found |

* The KI-67 index sometimes may be very high in erythrodermic drug eruptions, and low in Sézary syndrome.

51% of cases of Sézary syndrome, and in 80% of cases of inflammatory erythroderma [40]. Multivariate analysis of histopathological criteria identified increased numbers of small cerebriform lymphocytes, loss of CD7 expression, low numbers of $CD8^+$ lymphocytes and increased proliferation (as detected by Ki-67) as the strongest indicators predicting the correct diagnosis of Sézary syndrome [40]. However, a selection bias may have influenced the results of this study, as Darier nests could be observed in 23% of cases of Sézary syndrome; in my experience, they are not as common in early stages of the disease (on the other hand, of course, the diagnosis is easy when they are present). Reduction of CD7 expression in Sézary syndrome was found useful in the differential diagnosis with inflammatory erythroderma also in another study [41]. Expression of JunB by T lymphocytes seems to be more common in Sézary syndrome than in non-neoplastic erythroderma, but is present only in a minority of cases [42]. PD-$1^+$ T lymphocytes are almost always found in Sézary syndrome, but are less frequent in other types of erythroderma [41]. In addition, PD-1 is expressed by most neoplastic $CD4^+$ T cells in Sézary syndrome, but predominantly expressed by dermal and epidermal $CD8^+$ T cells in inflammatory erythroderma, thus providing a further diagnostic clue [41].

The presence of the same T-cell clone in the skin and in the blood is considered one of the main diagnostic criteria of Sézary syndrome, and rules out all inflammatory erythrodermas. Although next-generation sequencing may provide clues for identifying clonal populations of T lymphocytes in skin biopsies of neoplastic erythroderma [3–5], sufficient data on other types of erythroderma are not available. Molecular biomarkers may be helpful in the differential diagnosis of neoplastic from inflammatory erythroderma. Analyzing molecular markers to distinguish Sézary syndrome from inflammatory dermatoses, two

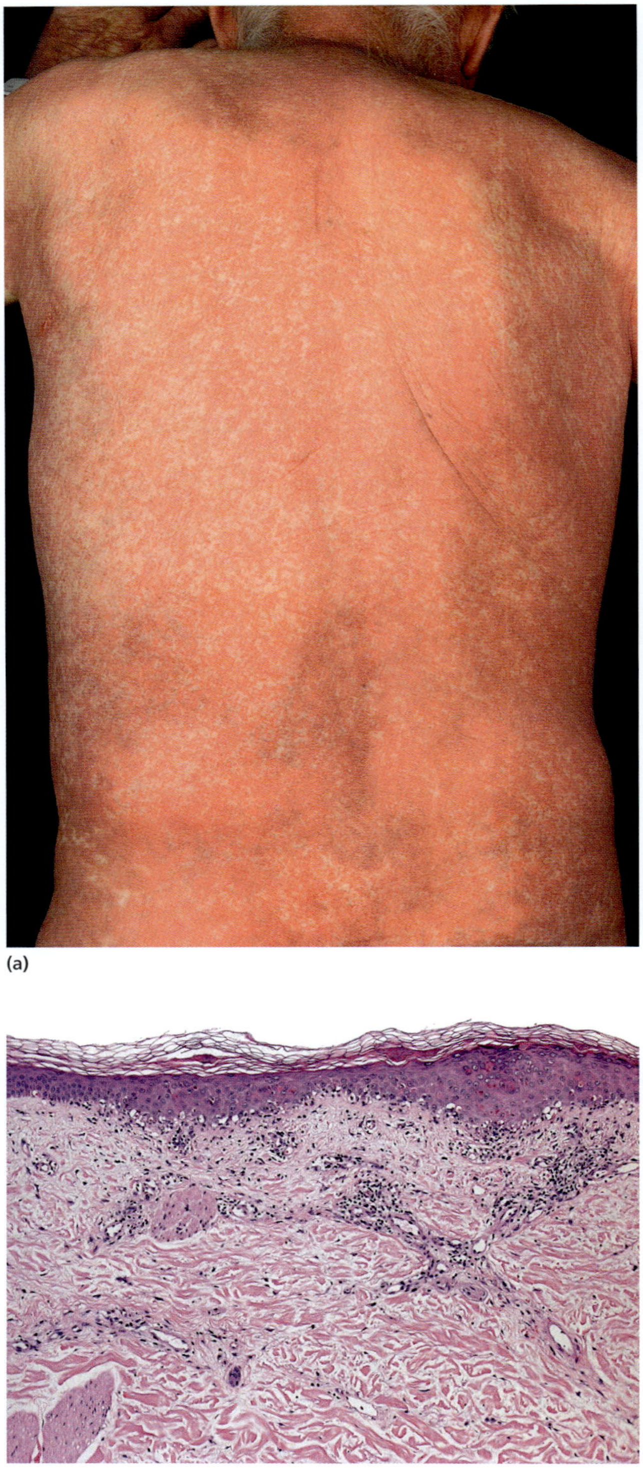

(a)

(b)

**Figure 31.21** Erythroderma in drug eruption. (a) Erythroderma with small, irregular areas of uninvolved skin. (b) Interface-lichenoid dermatitis with some necrotic keratinocytes.

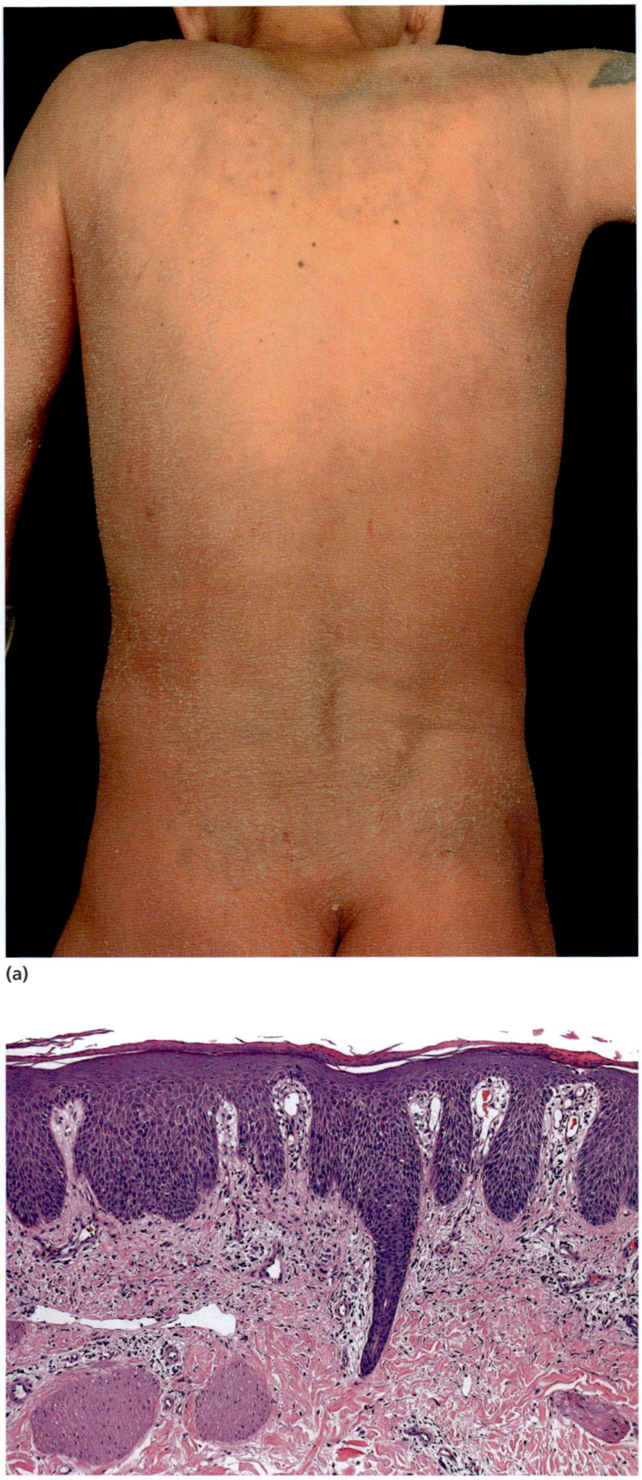

(a)

(b)

**Figure 31.22** Erythroderma in psoriasis. (a) Diffuse erythroderma with focal scaling. (b) Psoriasiform epidermal hyperplasia with parakeratosis and focal loss of granular layer.

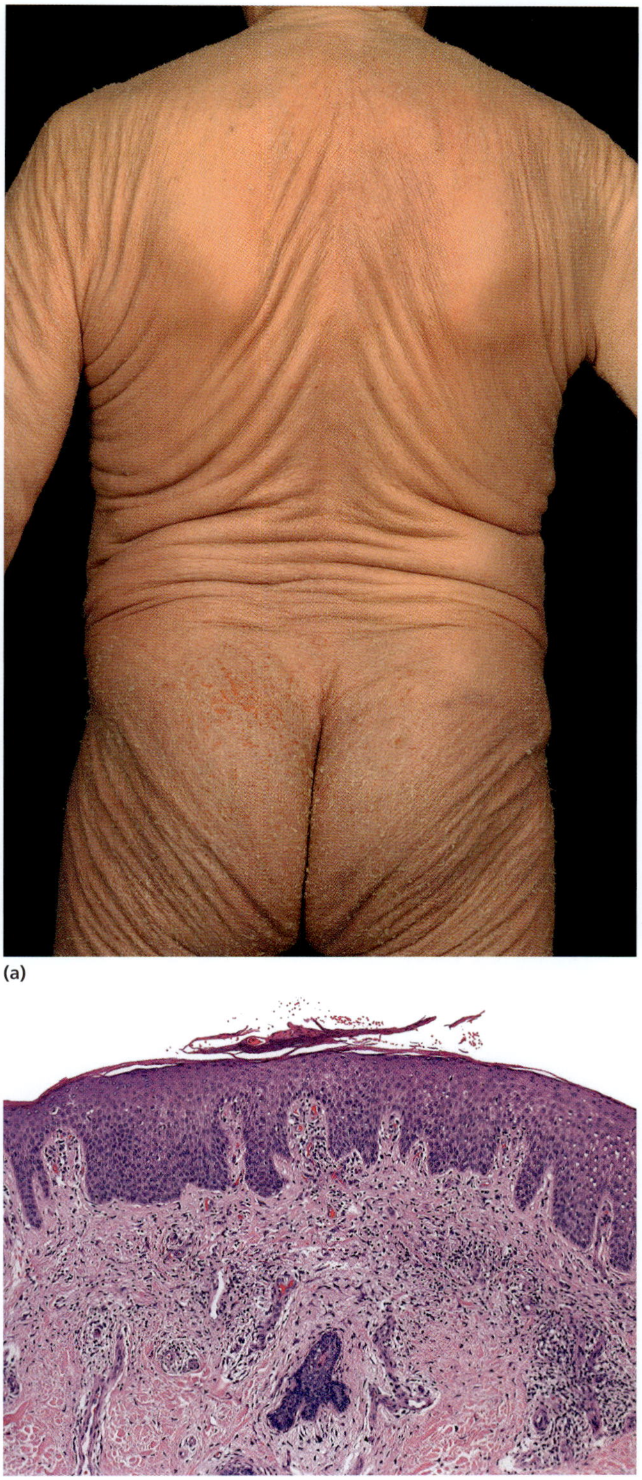

(a)

(b)

Figure 31.23 Erythroderma in atopic dermatitis. (a) Diffuse erythroderma with focal scaling and erosions. (b) Irregular epidermal hyperplasia with focal parakeratosis and dense dermal lymphoid infiltrates.

combinations of genes were identified: (1) *STAT4, TWIST1*, and *DNM3* or (2) *STAT4, TWIST1*, and *PLS3*, that showed high sensitivity and specificity for the diagnosis of Sézary syndrome [43].

Besides skin biopsy, examination of the peripheral blood is routinely performed in diagnostic algorithms of erythroderma [44]. However, cerebriform lymphocytes ("Sézary cells") may be observed in reactive conditions in patients with actinic reticuloid or atopic dermatitis, among others. For a discussion of blood markers in Sézary syndrome and their value in differential diagnosis, see Chapter 4.

Treatment of erythroderma depends on the background condition.

## Cutaneous pseudolymphoma associated with mogamulizumab treatment

Cases of $CD8^+$ pseudolymphoma characterized by plaque and tumors arising in patients treated with mogamulizumab have been reported [45–48]. Mogamulizumab is a monoclonal antibody that selectively targets the chemokine receptor type 4, and is used for management of mycosis fungoides and particularly of Sézary syndrome (see also Chapters 3 and 4). One of the most common side effects is the so-called mogamulizumab-associated rash, affecting a distinct proportion of patients and sometimes leading to discontinuation of the treatment. In some cases, mogamulizumab-associated rash shows pseudolymphomatous features that may mimic those of the very same disease that is being treated, thus posing a differential diagnostic problem between side effect of the drug and disease recurrence/persistence.

The clinical presentation and time between the beginning of treatment and onset of mogamulizumab-associated rash are variable [46]. The lesions are frequently (but not exclusively) located on the head and neck area (Fig. 31.24). The rash is more common in patients with Sézary syndrome, and in many cases is related to the efficacy of the treatment [49], thus underlying the crucial importance of the differential diagnosis between mogamulizumab-associated rash and recurrent/persistent disease.

The histopathological features in mogamulizumab-associated rash are variable, and pseudolymphomatous aspects are observed only in a subset of cases (Fig. 31.25). In a large study, histopathological characteristics that allowed to distinguish mogamulizumab-associated rash from Sézary syndrome were the inverted or normalized intraepidermal CD4:CD8 ratio (i.e., $CD8^+$ cells are more or equal in number to $CD4^+$ ones) (Fig. 31.25c), and the demonstration of absent or nondominant levels of disease-associated TCR sequences [50]. An interesting aspect of this study was the finding in 43.5% of the cases of low-level of the patient's previously identified neoplastic clone as detected by high-throughput sequencing of the T-cell receptor genes, showing that mogamulizumab-associated rash is a side

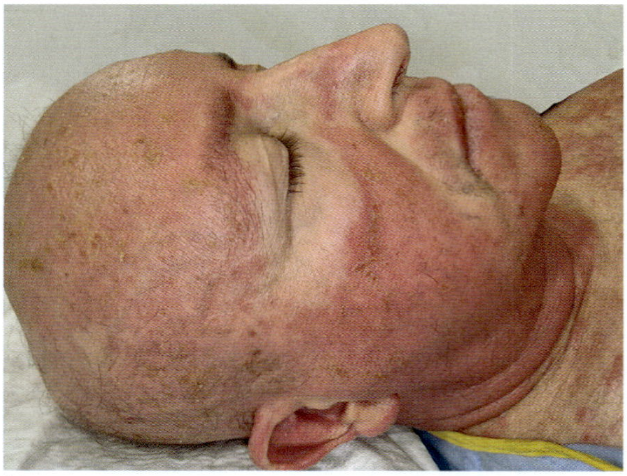

(a)

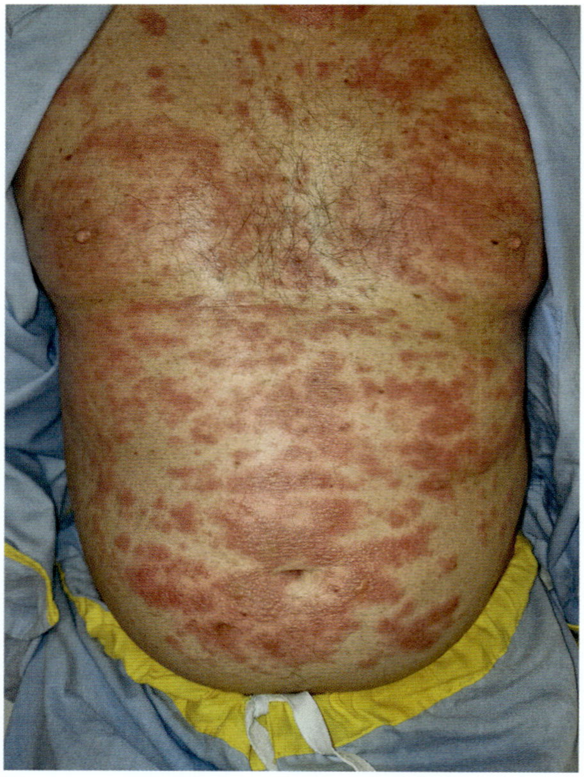

(b)

Figure 31.24 Skin eruption under mogamulizumab treatment ("mogamulizumab-associated rash") *(Courtesy of Dr. Laura Najera, Madrid, Spain.)* (a) Erythematous lesions on the face and (b) trunk.

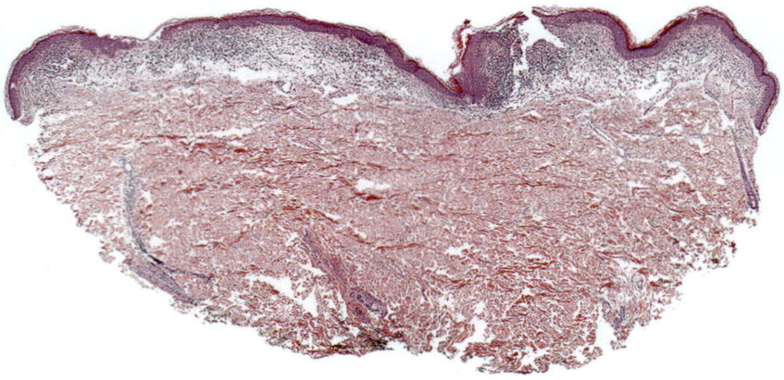

(a)

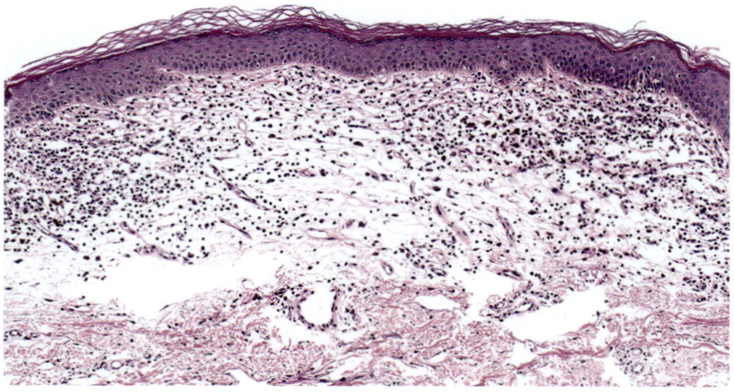

(b)

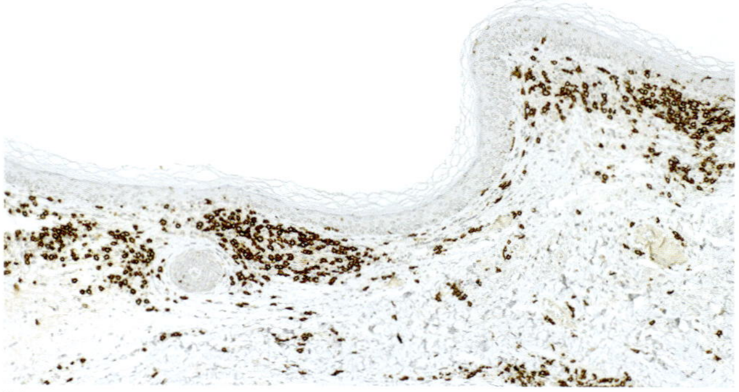

(c)

Figure 31.25 Skin eruption under mogamulizumab treatment ("mogamulizumab-associated rash") *(Courtesy of Dr. Luis Requena, Madrid, Spain.)* (a) Dense, band-like infiltrate within a partly edematous papillary dermis; (b) only a few epidermotropic lymphocytes are present; (c) Staining for CD8 reveals positivity of most lymphocytes.

effect of the drug characterized in almost half of the cases by the presence of some neoplastic lymphocytes as well, similar to what can be observed in other leukemic conditions in which neoplastic cells "colonize" the skin at sites of inflammation.

Interestingly, a similar cutaneous eruption, also posing differential diagnostic problems with mycosis fungoides histopathologically, can be observed during treatment with brentuximab vedotin [51].

## Solitary idiopathic T/B-cell pseudolymphoma

In the past, a category of "solitary idiopathic T-cell pseudolymphoma" has been used frequently to classify cases that do not fit precisely within other entities of cutaneous pseudolymphoma. As a distinct population of B lymphocytes is invariably present in biopsy specimens from these lesions, the term "solitary idiopathic T/B-cell pseudolymphoma" seems to be more appropriate. Two different patterns have been described for "solitary idiopathic T/B-cell pseudolymphoma." One is characterized by superficial lesions with clinicopathologic features similar to those observed in mycosis fungoides, arising in patients who are not taking any drug (thus ruling out the diagnosis of lymphomatoid drug eruption; see the corresponding section in this chapter) [52]. In the original description by Van der Putte and coworkers, absence of epidermotropism was the distinguishing feature from mycosis fungoides [52], but I have seen several cases with epidermotropic lymphocytes, and rarely even with small intraepidermal Darier nests containing medium-sized lymphocytes (Fig. 31.26). The second is characterized by nodular lesions and reveals overlapping clinicopathologic features with cutaneous CD4⁺ small/medium T-cell lymphoproliferative disorder. Similar cases have also been reported as "pseudolymphomatous folliculitis" [53].

As a matter of fact, solitary idiopathic T/B-cell pseudolymphoma is probably one of the most controversial types of pseudolymphoma, as definition and differential diagnostic criteria are not clear. The superficial pattern is indistinguishable from lichenoid (lymphomatoid) keratosis, and will be discussed in that context (see below in this chapter). The nodular pattern is indistinguishable from cutaneous CD4⁺ small/medium T-cell lymphoproliferative disorder (see Chapter 11). Although in the past it was unclear whether these cases represented a

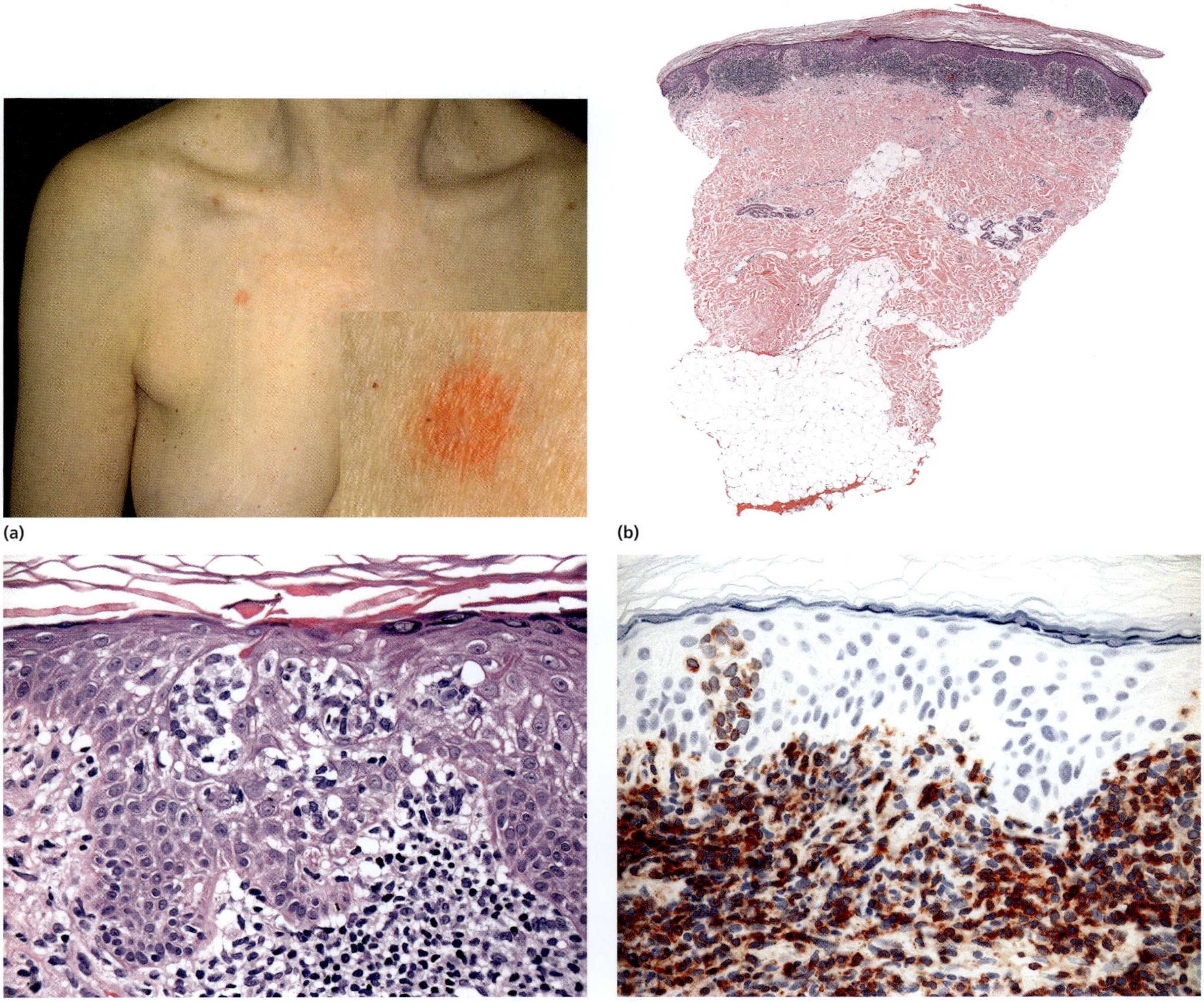

(a) (b) (c) (d)

Figure 31.26 Solitary idiopathic T/B-cell pseudolymphoma. (a) Small, solitary erythematous plaque on the thorax of a 70-year-old woman (insert: detail of the lesion). (b) Histology shows a dense, band-like lympho-histiocytic infiltrates with (c) small intraepidermal collections of medium-sized cells identical to Darier nests. (d) Staining for CD3 is positive in the majority of the cells within the intraepidermal collection.

reactive process or a low-grade malignant T-cell lymphoma [54, 55], the term lymphoma has been replaced by "lymphoproliferative disorder" in the 2018 and 2024 update classification of cutaneous lymphomas by the European Organization for Research and Treatment of Cancer (EORTC) / World Health Organization (WHO) [56, 57], and the same terminology has been adopted in the most recent International Consensus Classification (ICC) of lymphomas and 5th edition of the WHO *Classification of Haematolymphoid Tumours* [58, 59]. Besides other phenotypic similarities, increased numbers of PD-1$^+$ lymphocytes have been reported in both CD4$^+$ small/medium T-cell lymphoproliferative disorder and solitary idiopathic T/B-cell pseudolymphoma, thus showing an overlapping phenotype [60].

In short and in sum, to my eyes the category of solitary idiopathic T/B-cell pseudolymphoma is somewhat artificial. Many cases showing superficial, mycosis fungoides-like infiltrates can be classified as lichenoid (lymphomatoid) keratosis; many of those with nodular infiltrates located on the head and neck area can be classified as cutaneous CD4$^+$ small/medium T-cell lymphoproliferative disorder. Most cases presenting with solitary lesions located at sites other than the head and neck and showing histopathologically nodular infiltrates can be included into more specific categories (e.g., pseudolymphomatous arthropod bite reaction, reactions to infectious agents), and only uncommonly a non-specific category of solitary idiopathic T/B-cell pseudolymphoma is needed.

## Lichenoid/lymphomatoid keratosis

Lichenoid/lymphomatoid keratosis is defined as a circumscribed lichenoid reactive infiltrate, often related to a benign epithelial neoplasm (mostly seborrheic keratosis or lentigo actinica undergoing regressive changes) [61, 62]. The relationship to seborrheic keratosis or lentigo actinica has been confirmed by the finding of *FGFR3*, *PIK3CA*, and *RAS* mutations (previously observed in the latter conditions) in approximately 50% of cases of lichenoid keratosis [63]. As already discussed, differentiation of lichenoid/lymphomatoid keratosis from the superficial variant of solitary idiopathic T/B-cell pseudolymphoma is impossible, and in my opinion the two conditions represent variations of the same process.

Patients are elderly adults presenting with small scaly plaques located usually on the trunk, particularly the breast in women (Fig. 31.27), often diagnosed clinically as seborrheic keratosis, actinic keratosis, Bowen disease, or superficial basal cell carcinoma. The histopathologic features show dense, band-like inflammatory lymphoid infiltrates that may be indistinguishable from those of mycosis fungoides [61]. Besides the focal epithelial hyperplasia related to the pre-existent epithelial tumor (if present), another histopathologic clue is the sharp lateral circumscription of the lymphoid infiltrate in lichenoid keratosis

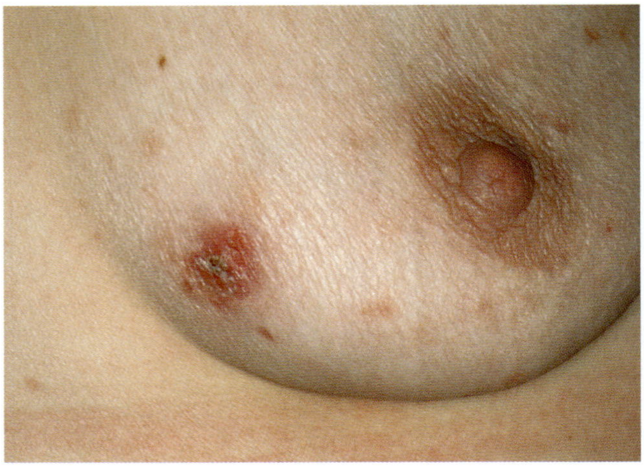

**Figure 31.27** Lichenoid (lymphomatoid) keratosis. Small scaly plaque on the breast.

(Fig. 31.28a). Although epidermotropism may be striking (Figs. 31.28b and c), even mimicking Darier nests (Fig. 31.29a), intraepidermal collections are usually characterized by a mixture of Langerhans cells, keratinocytes, and only a few T-lymphocytes (Fig. 31.29b), in contrast to true Darier nests observed in mycosis fungoides. However, true Darier nests can be observed rarely in benign conditions such as lichenoid/lymphomatoid keratosis or nevoid hyperkeratosis of the nipple (see Fig. 31.26 and below in this chapter). In fact, in some cases the histopathologic diagnosis may be extremely difficult or even impossible without accurate correlation with the clinical presentation, particularly in small, partial biopsies. The T-cell infiltrate is admixed with variable numbers of B-lymphocytes, which in some instances may be as numerous as the T-cells. In some patients a monoclonal rearrangement of the TCR genes may be observed. Surgical excision results in complete remission, and recurrences are uncommon (the lesions never recur if completely excised).

Although many cases of lichenoid/lymphomatoid keratosis indubitably represent a histopathologic diagnostic challenge, they can be compared conceptually to seborrheic keratoses with heavy inflammatory infiltrates, a common situation where variable numbers of intraepidermal ("epidermotropic") lymphocytes do not represent a diagnostic problem (Fig. 31.30).

Some of the cases reported in the past as "unilesional" or "solitary" mycosis fungoides (excluding pagetoid reticulosis) probably represent examples of lichenoid/lymphomatoid keratosis or solitary idiopathic T/B-cell pseudolymphoma. Checking the follow-up of 15 patients included in a previous study on solitary mycosis fungoides published by our group in 1999 [64], only two of them developed further lesions of mycosis fungoides, whereas all others were free of disease after a median time of 176 months (mean: 137), suggesting that these lesions were reactive rather than malignant. In fact, clinical presentation of some of these cases was typical of what I would classify today as

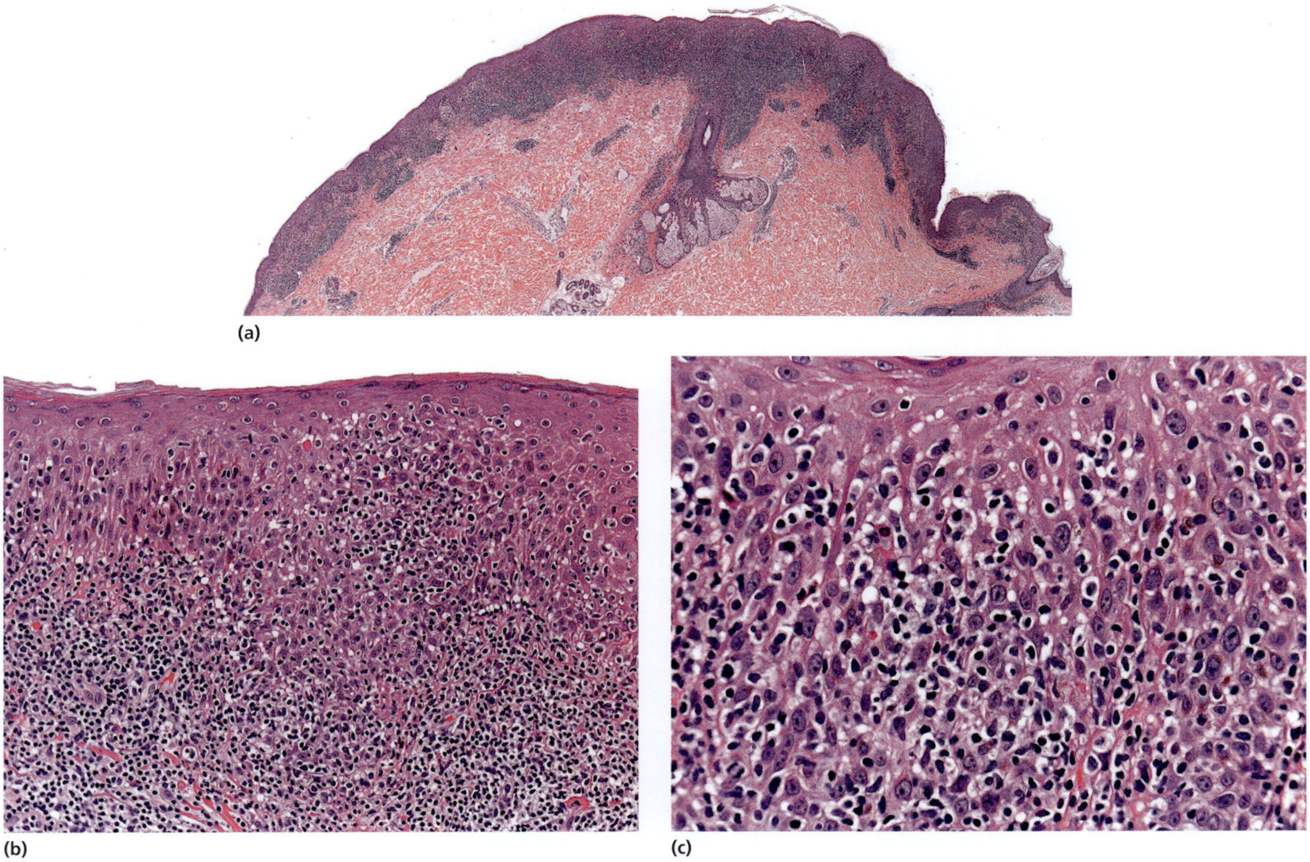


Figure 31.28 Lichenoid (lymphomatoid) keratosis. (a) Band-like infiltrate of lymphocytes with sharp lateral circumscription. (b) Note prominent epidermotropism. (c) Detail of intraepidermal lymphocytes.

lichenoid/lymphomatoid keratosis or solitary idiopathic T/B-cell pseudolymphoma (Fig. 31.31).

## Pityriasis lichenoides

Pityriasis lichenoides et varioliformis acuta (PLEVA) (Mucha–Habermann disease) and pityriasis lichenoides chronica represent two variants of pityriasis lichenoides that are indistinguishable on clinical or histopathological grounds; hence, they will be referred to as pityriasis lichenoides in this section. It is important to underline that conventional cases of pityriasis lichenoides should be considered as a benign disorder of unknown etiology without relationship to cutaneous lymphomas. A viral infection has long been suspected as the cause of the disease, and different viruses have been demonstrated in some cases (including parvovirus B19, herpes simplex, herpes varicella/zoster, and measles, among others), yet the precise etiology is still unknown, and a study investigating several viruses did not show repeatable associations [65]. On the other hand, in some cases the T lymphocytes of pityriasis lichenoides are monoclonally rearranged [66, 67]; evolution of pityriasis lichenoides into cytotoxic mycosis fungoides has been reported, and some authors suggested that the disease may represent yet another variant of the cutaneous T-cell lymphomas [68]. Some cases reported in the literature had a peculiar phenotype with positivity for $\gamma/\delta$ T-cell markers [69, 70]. Patients with pityriasis lichenoides are predominantly children, adolescents, and young adults, presenting clinically with generalized, scaly papules (Fig. 31.32). In contrast to lymphomatoid papulosis, the lesions in pityriasis lichenoides are usually monomorphous (i.e., are in the same stage of evolution). Histology is characterized by superficial or wedge-shaped lymphoid infiltrates with marked involvement of the epidermis (necrotic keratinocytes, intraepidermal lymphocytes, parakeratosis, and neutrophils in the horny layer – "busy" stratum corneum) (Fig. 31.33). There are variable numbers of extravasated erythrocytes in the papillary dermis. Adnexotropism is common [71]. The infiltrate is composed predominantly of $CD8^+$ T lymphocytes, which are negative for CD30. Clonality of the T-cell population can be demonstrated in a majority of cases [72].

In a large study, we demonstrated that conventional cases of pityriasis lichenoides have an invariably benign behavior [67], and a similar course has been observed by others [73, 74]. On

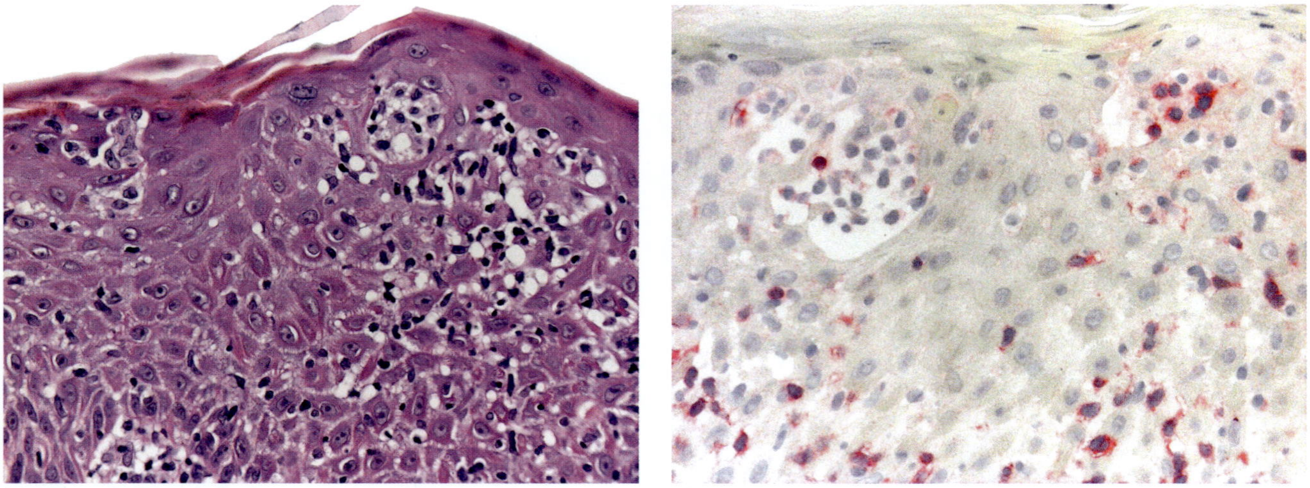

(a) (b)

**Figure 31.29** Lichenoid (lymphomatoid) keratosis. (a) Intraepidermal collections of cells simulating Darier nests. (b) Staining for CD3 reveals only a few lymphocytes within the intraepidermal collections.

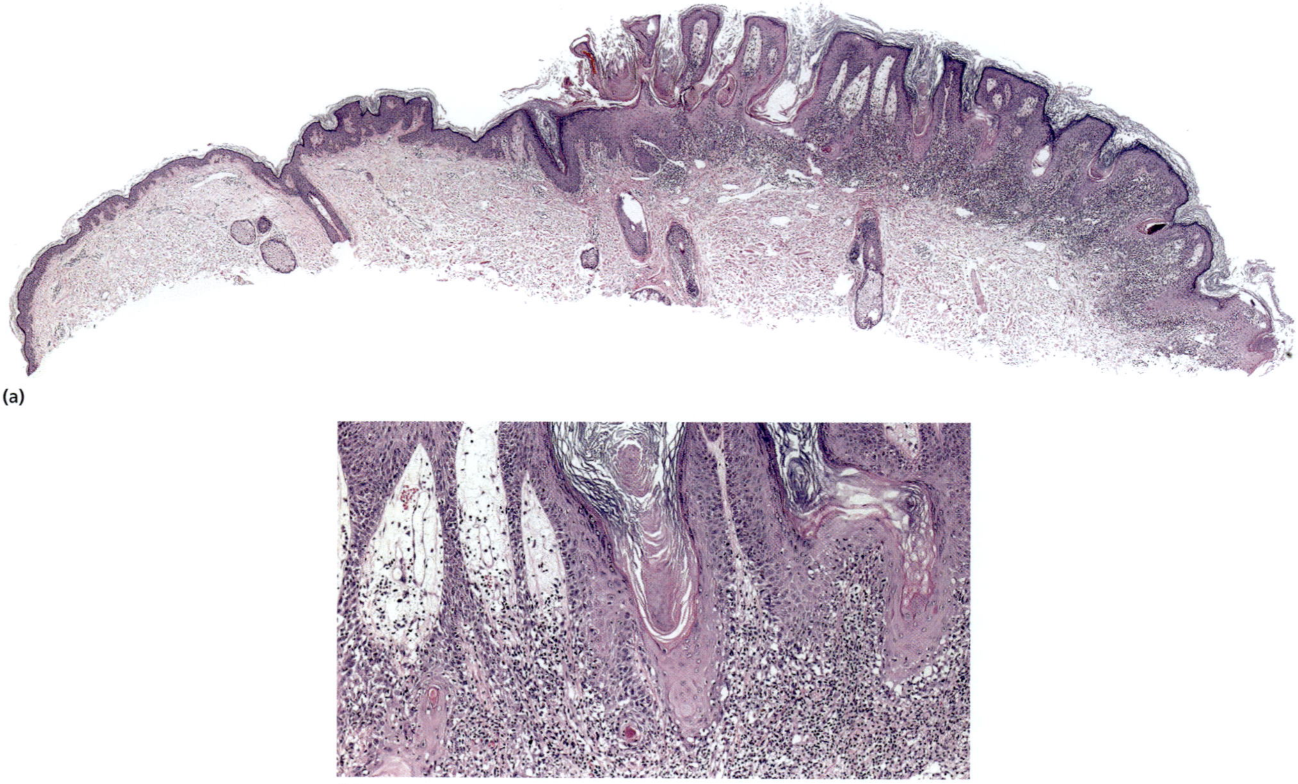

(a)

(b)

**Figure 31.30** Seborrheic keratosis with inflammatory infiltrates. (a) Low-power magnification shows typical features of seborrheic keratosis. The heavy inflammatory infiltrate is characterized (b) by many intraepidermal ("epidermotropic") lymphocytes.

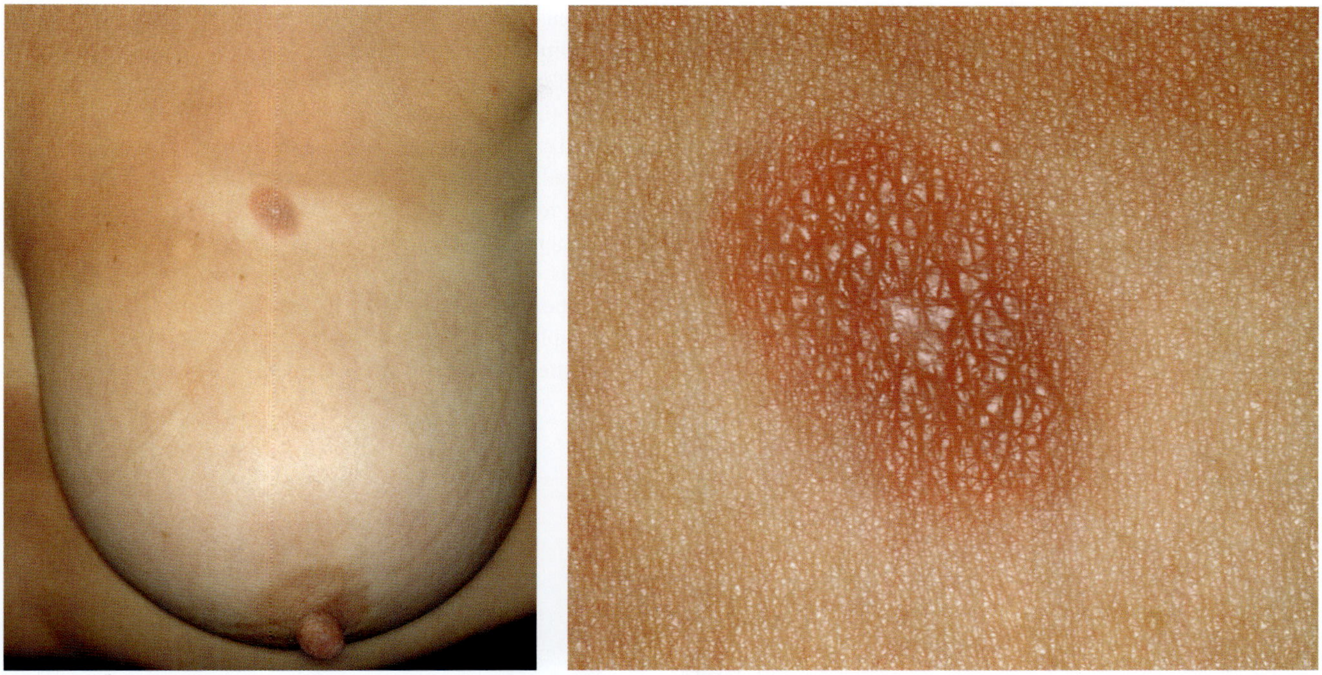

(a) (b)

Figure 31.31 Lichenoid (lymphomatoid) keratosis *(this case was previously published as an example of solitary mycosis fungoides* [64]; *see text for explanation)*. (a) Solitary lesion on the breast. (b) Detail of the lesion.

the other hand, a group of "atypical" pityriasis lichenoides, defined by the presence of an aberrant phenotype, may be linked to mycosis fungoides and in a minority of the cases shows progression to it (see also Chapter 3) [67, 75]. The phenotypic aberrations defining atypical pityriasis lichenoides include one or more of the following: loss of a pan-T-cell antigen (CD2, CD3, or CD5); double positivity or double negativity for CD4 and CD8; $CD4^+$ phenotype; positivity for CD56 or for TCR-$\gamma/\delta$ [67]. The presence of a monoclonal population of T lymphocytes was not diriment in distinguishing conventional from atypical pityriasis lichenoides [67]. In this context, it should also be reminded that clinically as well as histopathologically mycosis fungoides may present with features similar or indistinguishable from those of pityriasis lichenoides; thus, accurate clinicopathological correlation and complete phenotypic investigations are crucial for a precise diagnosis [67, 76]. A diagnosis of "atypical" pityriasis lichenoides made according to the above listed criteria should be considered with great caution, and patients should be followed up.

One peculiar variant of pityriasis lichenoides, the so-called febrile ulcero-necrotic type, presents with multiple, large, ulcerating lesions that may be become generalized, thus simulating a cutaneous lymphoma clinically (Fig. 31.34). Histology reveals lymphoid infiltrates located predominantly in the superficial and mid-dermis, slightly denser than those observed in conventional pityriasis lichenoides (Figs. 31.35a and b). Prominent ulceration is observed in biopsies taken from the center of the lesions. Atypical cells may be present, sometimes arranged in small clusters (Fig. 31.35c). In this type of pityriasis lichenoides, too, the infiltrating cells reveal a T-cytotoxic phenotype (Fig. 31.35d). The phenotype may correspond to the atypical form of pityriasis lichenoides, showing some aberrant features. A relationship of ulcero-necrotic pityriasis lichenoides to cutaneous cytotoxic lymphomas has been postulated [77]. Patients may die of the disease, but not from lymphoma-specific causes, and transition between "conventional" pityriasis lichenoides and the febrile ulcero-necrotic form has been reported [78]. In Graz we have had patients starting with ulcero-necrotic pityriasis lichenoides who, after complete response to methotrexate, relapsed with lesions of "conventional" pityriasis lichenoides upon discontinuation of the drug.

Patients with the febrile ulcero-necrotic variant of pityriasis lichenoides should be monitored carefully and require more aggressive treatment. Low-dose methotrexate is usually administered; high-dose immunoglobulins and extracorporeal photochemotherapy have also been used [79]. Death from complications may ensue in spite of aggressive, early treatment [80].

The presence of $CD30^+$ cells within lesions of pityriasis lichenoides has been the source of considerable debate, as this immunohistochemical staining is traditionally considered a valid tool for the differential diagnosis of the disease from lymphomatoid papulosis. Although some of the published cases of $CD30^+$ pityriasis lichenoides probably represented in truth examples of lymphomatoid papulosis, some convincing cases

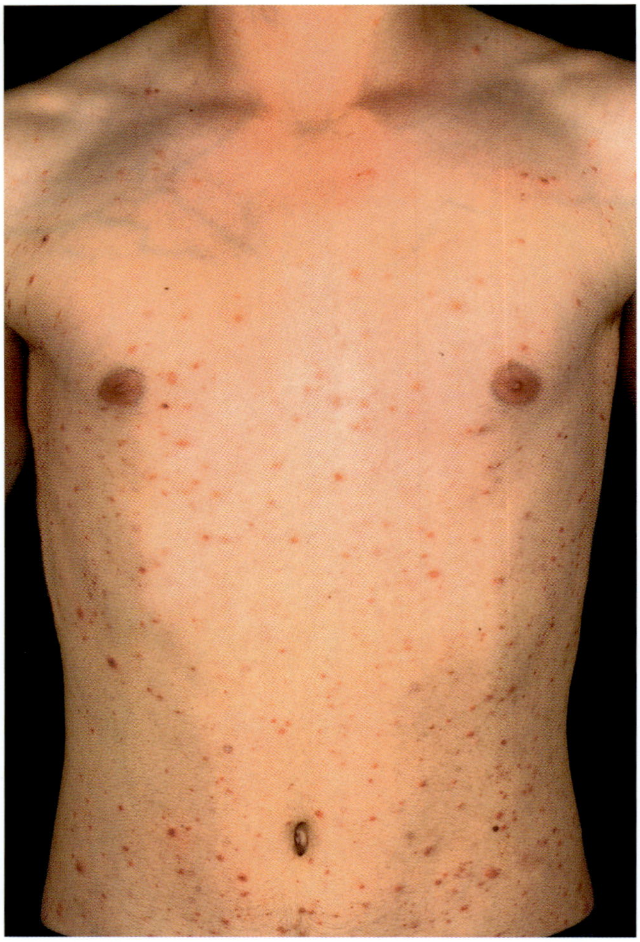

Figure 31.32 Pityriasis lichenoides. Multiple erythematous, partly crusted papules on the trunk.

have been reported [81]. A large series of pityriasis lichenoides with prominent epidermotropism of $CD30^+$ cells has been published [82], and parvovirus B19 has been identified in lesional skin in 40% of patients in this series. However, most of the reported cases displayed complete or partial loss of one or more pan-T-cell marker expression, or other phenotypic aberrations such as double positivity for CD4 and CD8, and others had a $CD4^+$ phenotype, suggesting that a diagnosis of lymphomatoid papulosis or papular mycosis fungoides may be an alternative explanation in these cases. In my experience, $CD30^+$ cells are completely absent or present only in minimal numbers within the infiltrate of the vast majority of cases of pityriasis

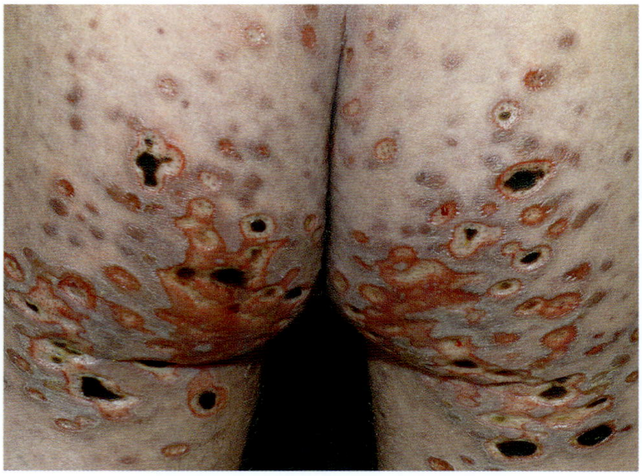

Figure 31.34 Pityriasis lichenoides et varioliformis acuta, ulceronecrotic variant. Multiple, confluent, ulcerated lesions on the buttocks and thighs.

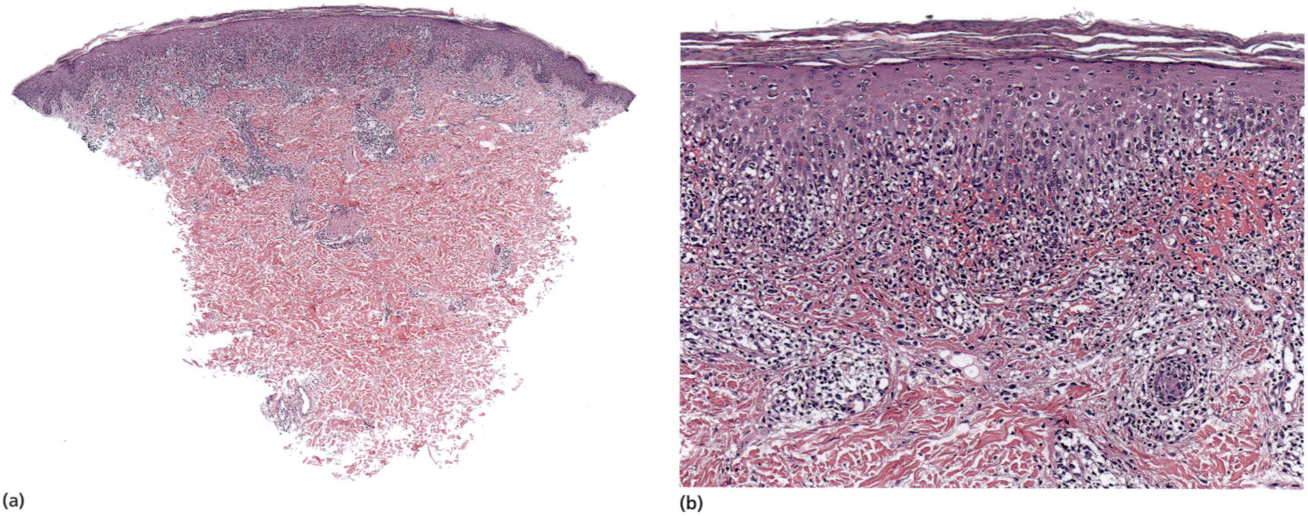

(a) (b)

Figure 31.33 Pityriasis lichenoides. (a) Superficial, wedge-shaped infiltrate with parakeratotic horny layer as well as (b) necrotic keratinocytes, intraepidermal lymphocytes, and superficial haemorrhages.

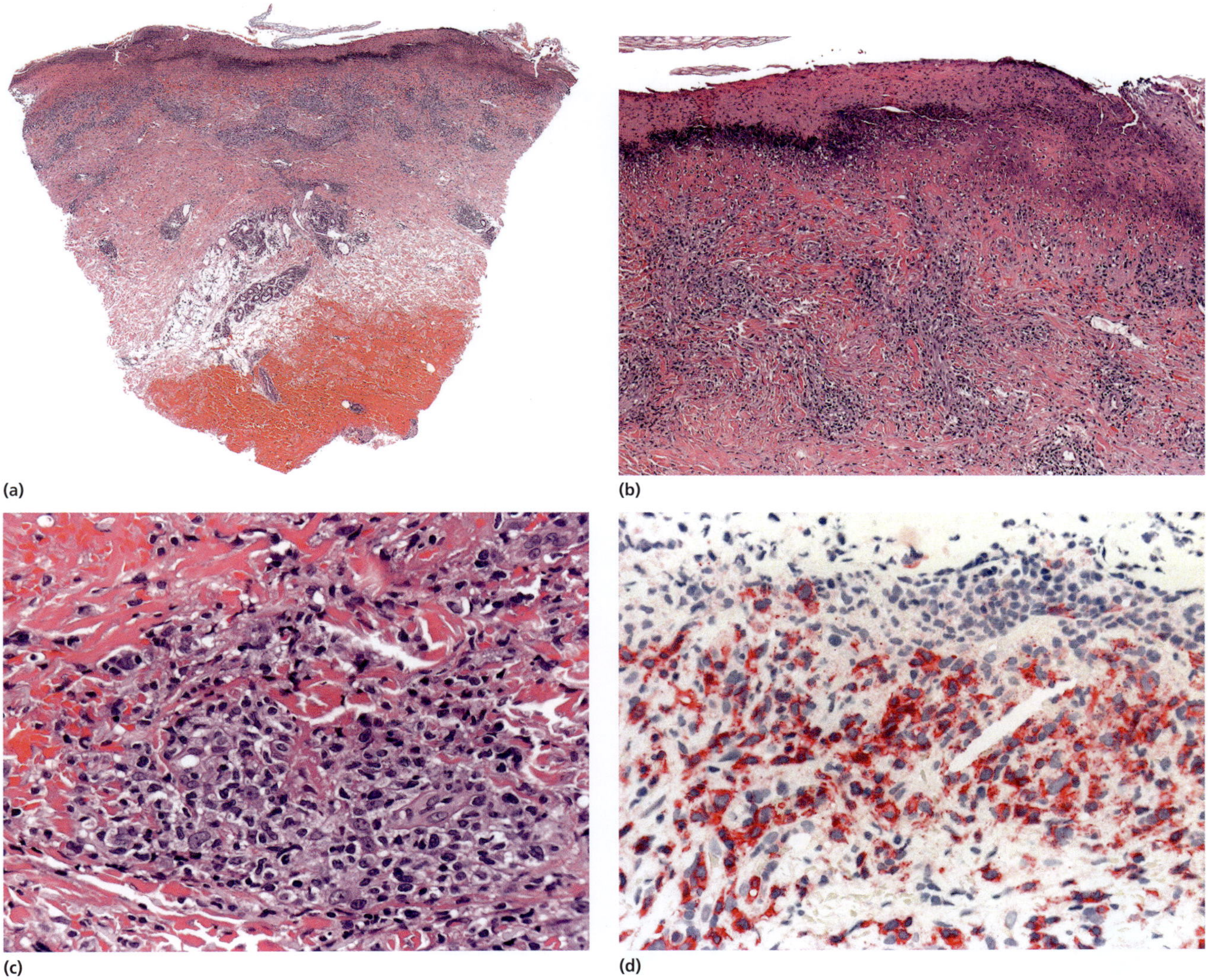

Figure 31.35 Pityriasis lichenoides et varioliformis acuta, ulceronecrotic variant. (a, b) Ulcerated lesion with dense lymphoid infiltrates and hemorrhagic crust. (c) Note mid-sized pleomorphic lymphocytes. (d) Staining for CD8 reveals positivity of most lymphocytes.

lichenoides (Fig. 31.36). If compelling clinicopathologic features of pityriasis lichenoides are present, however, the finding of a few $CD30^+$ cells should not be a reason for changing the diagnosis. On the other hand, in my opinion, CD30-positivity observed in many cells should be considered with great caution, and the diagnosis of pityriasis lichenoides, though not impossible, should be questioned.

## Lichen aureus/lichenoid pigmented purpuric dermatitis

Lichen aureus is a benign skin condition characterized by asymmetric, persistent purpuric skin macules and thin plaques with a typical golden-brown color clinically (Fig. 31.37), and by a variably dense, band-like lymphocytic infiltrate that may simulate mycosis fungoides histopathologically, particularly the purpuric variant of it (Fig. 31.38) [83, 84]. The lesions are usually localized. Interface/lichenoid changes at the dermo-epidermal junction and variable numbers of erythrocytes are always present in lichen aureus; exocytosis of lymphocytes (epidermotropism) may be observed (Figs. 31.38b and c), but is usually minimal or absent. Molecular analyses may reveal T-lymphocyte clonality in some cases [83, 85a]. Accurate clinicopathologic correlation is crucial to establish a correct diagnosis. Local steroid ointments or PUVA therapy can be used to treat lichen aureus, but the disease may persist in spite of treatment.

Exacerbation of a pre-existing pigmented purpuric dermatitis under pembrolizumab treatment has been reported, with onset of widesprerad lesions and mycosis fungoides-like histopathological features [85b].

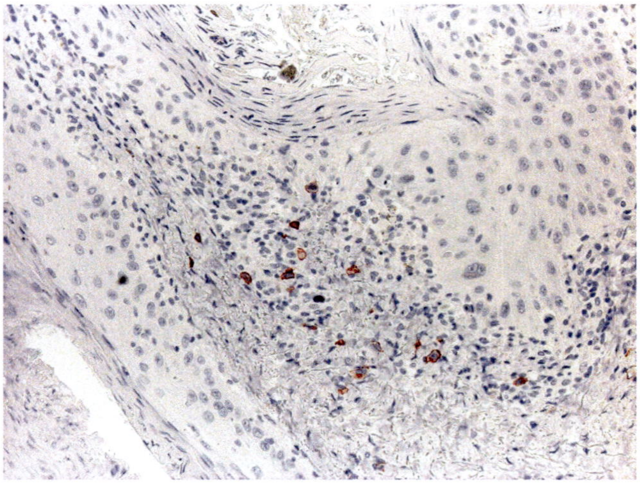

**Figure 31.36** Pityriasis lichenoides. Staining for CD30 shows only a few positive cells.

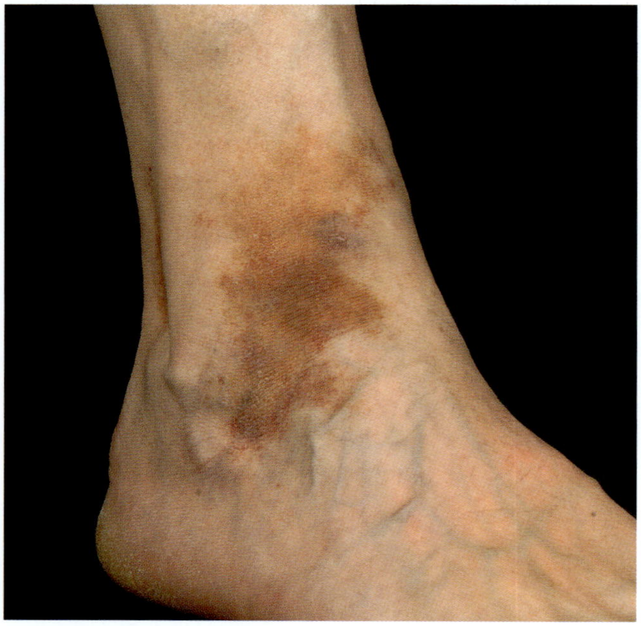

**Figure 31.37** Lichen aureus. Localized, irregular macules with characteristic brown-orange color on the ankle.

A relationship between lichen aureus or lichenoid pigmented purpuric dermatitis and mycosis fungoides has been postulated [86, 87]. In a large group of patients with long follow-up data, however, we could not observe any progression from conventional lichen aureus to mycosis fungoides [83]. On the other hand, some patients showed persistent lesions with clonal populations of T lymphocytes after many years of follow-up, suggesting that lichen aureus may belong to the spectrum of clonal dermatoses. Nonetheless, I believe that lichen aureus is a benign inflammatory disorder without any relationship with cutaneous lymphomas, and that cases of mycosis fungoides preceded by "pigmented purpuric dermatitis" probably represented examples of mycosis fungoides from the outset. Evaluation of the literature, however, is complicated by the inclusion in this group of patients with different clinicopathologic features, including some with clear-cut features of mycosis fungoides.

## Lichen sclerosus

Cases of lichen sclerosus on genital skin may reveal histopathologic features characterized by dense band-like lymphoid infiltrates and epidermotropism of lymphocytes that may be indistinguishable from those of mycosis fungoides (Fig. 31.39) [88, 89]. I have seen many such examples in specimens of preputial skin excised for surgical treatment of phimosis in children. In a considerable proportion of such cases, typical histopathological features of lichen sclerosus (i.e., hyalinization and sclerosis of the papillary dermis) are missing or present only focally, and the histopathological picture is dominated by the inflammatory, mycosis fungoides-like changes (Fig. 31.40) [89]. The intraepidermal cells often show "haloed," slightly larger nuclei resembling the epidermotropic lymphocytes of mycosis fungoides. Sometimes the histopathological pattern may even resemble so-called "pagetoid" epidermotropism. As lichen sclerosus is a pruriginous disease, the epidermis shows almost invariably a compact ortho-hyperkeratosis like that observed in lichen simplex chronicus, representing a good histopathological clue to the diagnosis. Immunohistochemical stainings reveal many intraepidermal T lymphocytes with a cytotoxic phenotype ($CD8^+$, $CD4^-$) (Fig. 31.41). T-lymphocyte clonality can be found in some cases of pseudolymphomatous lichen sclerosus [88, 90].

Accurate clinicopathologic correlation is required to establish a correct diagnosis. In this context, a diagnosis of mycosis fungoides on genital skin should never be made without a precise correlation between histopathologic and clinical features, even in cases that show monoclonality of the infiltrate. More specifically, I have never come across patients with solitary mycosis fungoides located on the genital skin.

This peculiar pseudolymphomatous variant of lichen sclerosus is encountered almost exclusively on genital skin and particularly in young males, and only exceptional cases arising in the context of extragenital lichen sclerosus have been reported [91]. Although extragenital lichen sclerosus is often associated to morphea, pseudolymphomatous lichen sclerosus never shows dermal changes typical of localized scleroderma.

The treatment of "pseudolymphomatous" lichen sclerosus does not differ from that of the conventional variant of the disease (e.g., surgical excision, topical or intralesional corticosteroids, topical calcineurin inhibitors, UV radiation, among others).

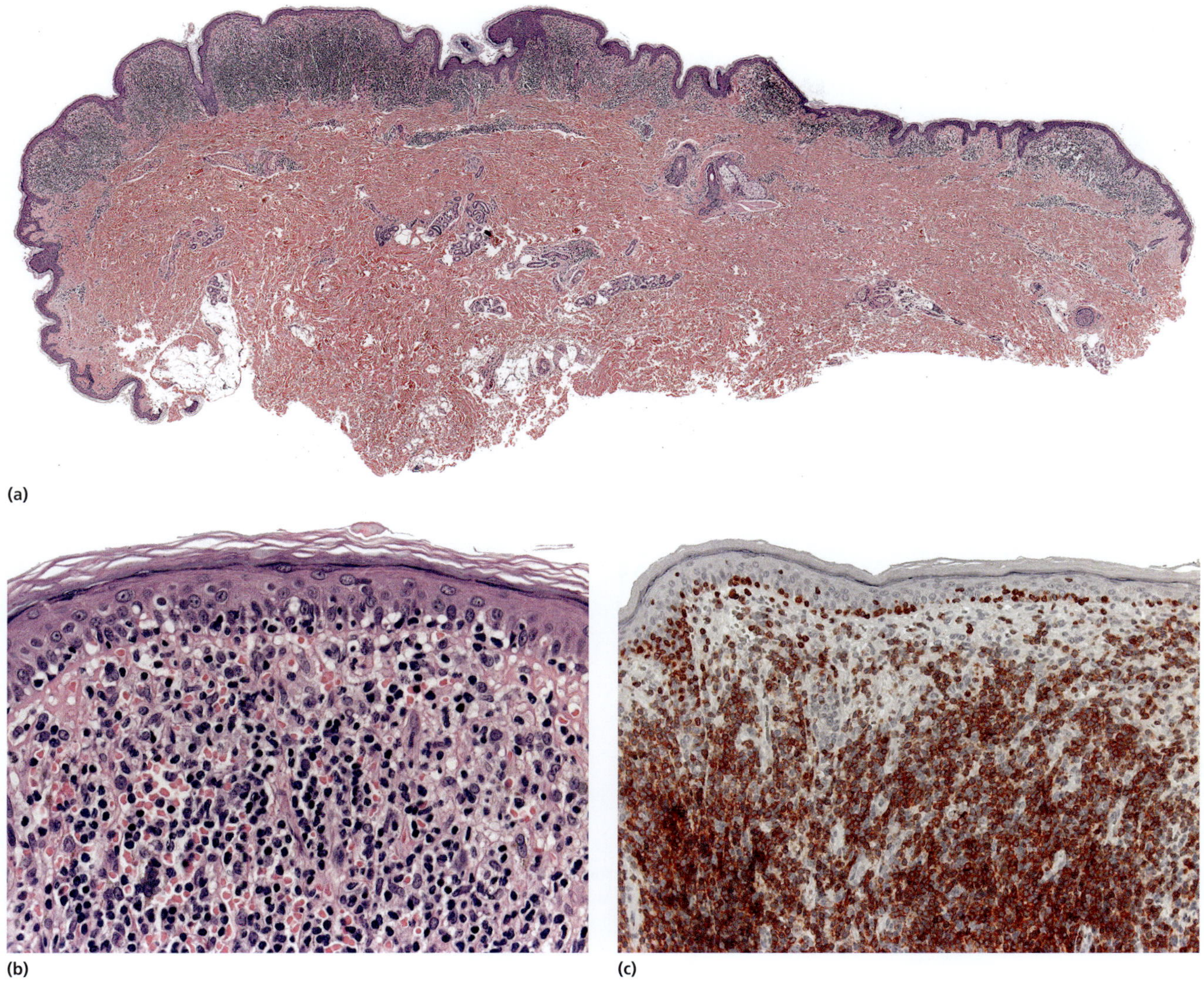

Figure 31.38 Lichen aureus. (a) Dense, band-like infiltrate of lymphocytes with (b) many extravasated erythrocytes and several intraepidermal lymphocytes. (c) The intraepidermal lymphocytes are highlighted by an immunohistochemical staining for CD3.

## Other pseudolymphomas in genital skin and mucosal regions

Interestingly, lesions mimicking mycosis fungoides may be observed on genital skin also in the context of common balanoposthitis or vulvitis, and in the absence of lichen sclerosus, showing similar epitheliotropic features and an identical $CD8^+$ phenotype, suggesting that this particular area of the body may be prone to this peculiar histopathological presentation (Fig. 31.42). Some of these cases present with epitheliotropic infiltrates that are indistinguishable from those observed in mycosis fungoides or pagetoid reticulosis [92]. Prominent epitheliotropism of $CD8^+$ lymphocytes is observed only in rare specimens of balanoposthitis or vulvitis, and most cases of these conditions present histopathologically with conventional, non-epitheliotropic inflammatory infiltrates admixed with variable number of plasma cells. The reason for the presence of pseudolymphomatous aspects in some cases is unknown, and they do not present any peculiar clinical feature or a different clinical history.

Besides genital skin, I have rarely observed mycosis fungoides-like histopathological features with prominent epidermotropism in biopsies of inflammatory cheilitis as well (Fig. 31.43). In this setting, too, the reason for this peculiar histopathological presentation is unknown.

In sum, a histopathological diagnosis of mycosis fungoides in patients who have lesions restricted to mucosal surfaces or to the lips is most likely a misdiagnosis, and careful examination of the patient as well as a critical discussion of alternative diagnoses are needed.

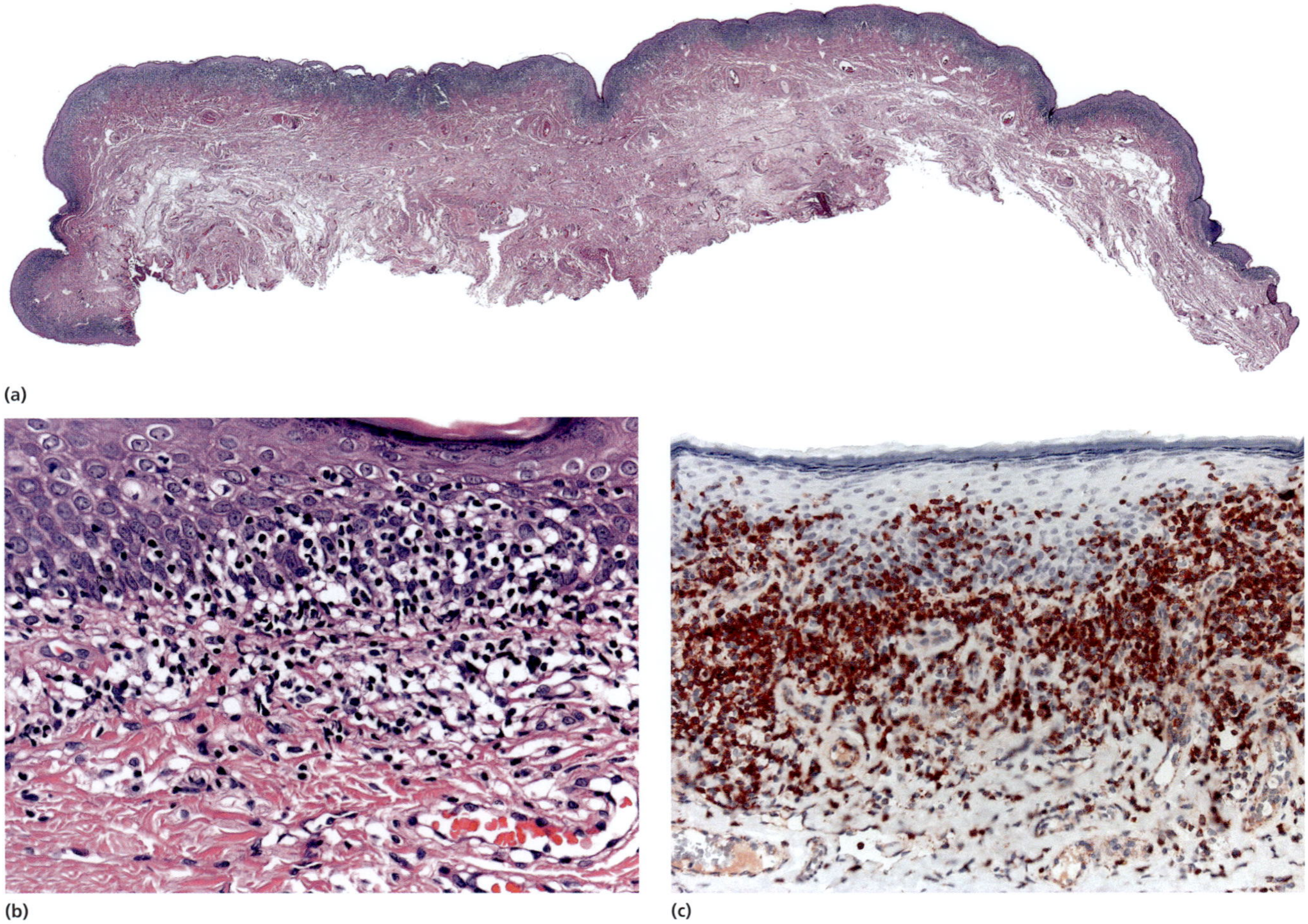


**Figure 31.39** Lichen sclerosus. (a) Dense, band-like infiltrate of lymphocytes with prominent epidermotropism. (b) Intraepidermal lymphocytes with perinuclear halo ("haloed lymphocytes") mimicking mycosis fungoides. (c) Most cells are positive for CD8.

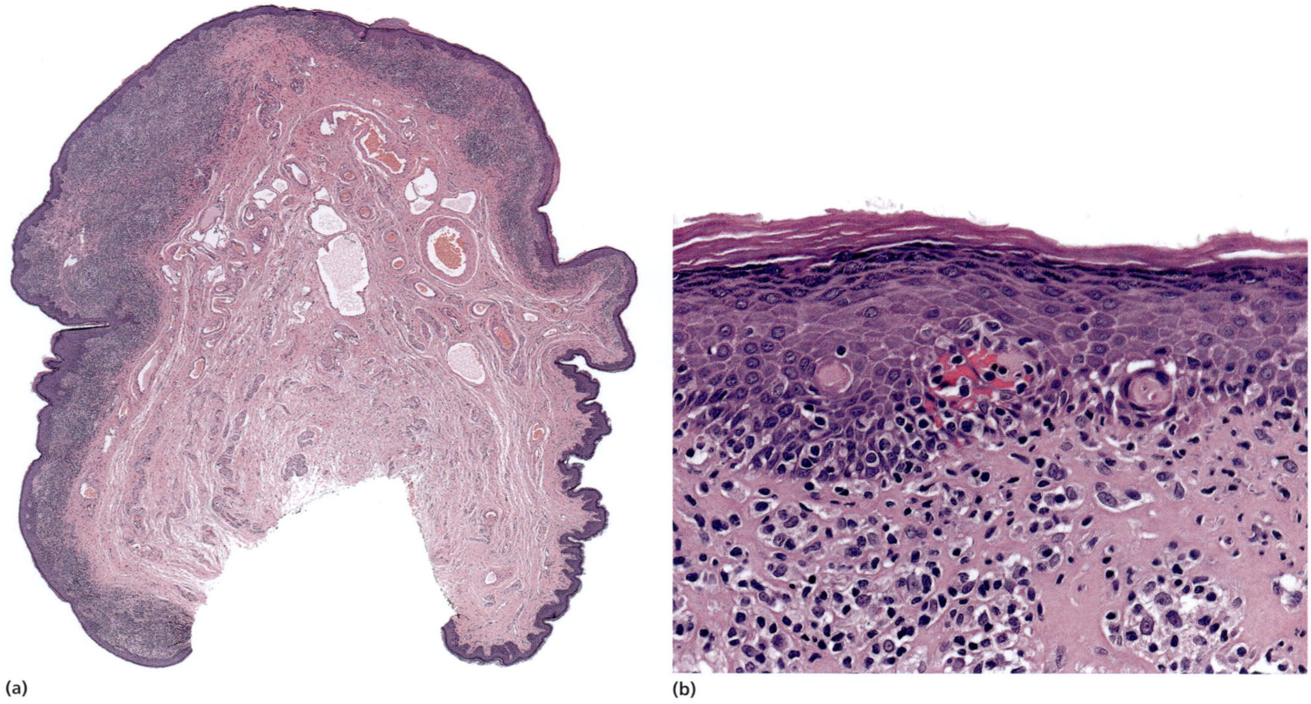


**Figure 31.40** Lichen sclerosus. (a) Dense, band-like infiltrate of lymphocytes with epidermotropism and with only (b) focal hyalinization of the papillary dermis. Note compact orthohyperkeratosis as a sign of chronic mechanic irritation.

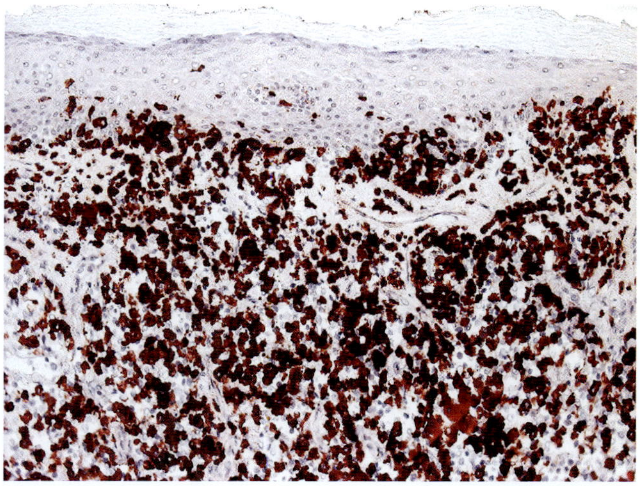

Figure 31.41 Lichen sclerosus. Staining for CD8 is positive by the vast majority of dermal as well as intraepidermal lymphocytes.

## Vitiligo (inflammatory stage)

A lichenoid inflammation can be observed in the early (inflammatory) stage of vitiligo. Some of these cases present with clinical and histopathologic features mimicking those of mycosis fungoides [93]. Clinically there are erythematous, scaly patches, whereas typical hypopigmented lesions of vitiligo are missing (Figs. 31.44a, 31.45a, b). Even when depigmentation occurs, the differential diagnosis with hypopigmented mycosis fungoides can be very difficult. In fact, in my professional life I have missed the histopathological diagnosis in all cases of inflammatory vitiligo that I have seen, and could only revise the diagnosis when follow-up data showed the development of clear-cut lesions of vitiligo in the same areas or in other parts of the body.

Histopathologically, pseudolymphomatous lesions of vitiligo show dense, band-like infiltrates of lymphocytes with exocytosis of cells within the lower part of the epidermis (Figs. 31.44b and c). The histopathological features may rarely resemble those of pagetoid reticulosis (Fig. 31.45c–f), and the number of epidermotropic lymphocytes may be high. Most cells are $CD8^+$ cytotoxic lymphocytes, thus mimicking both the hypopigmented variant of mycosis fungoides observed frequently in children and pagetoid reticulosis (Fig. 31.44d). CD30 can be expressed, representing a further confounding factor (Fig. 31.45f). The number of intraepidermal melanocytes as detected by immunohistochemical staining may be helpful in distinguishing vitiligo (melanocytes almost completely or completely absent) from hypopigmented mycosis fungoides (melanocytes reduced in number but present) [94, 95]. However, some melanocytes may still be present in early inflammatory lesions of vitiligo.

Sometimes only the onset of conventional lesions of vitiligo during follow-up allows the correct diagnosis. In this context, it should be underlined that in children a diagnosis of mycosis fungoides should be established only upon compelling clinicopathologic evidence, and that a delay of a few months is probably better than a wrong diagnosis of "cancer."

The treatment of the inflammatory stage of vitiligo has never been investigated in detail, as in many cases the diagnosis is established only retrospectively.

## Annular lichenoid dermatitis of youth

A condition termed "annular lichenoid dermatitis of youth" has been reported as a simulator of mycosis fungoides [96–101]. Although the original publication included only children and adolescents (hence the term "of youth"), subsequent reports pointed at the presence of similar clinicopathologic findings in adults as well [98, 99]. Patients present with annular erythematous macules that evolve into round or oval annular patches with elevated erythematous borders and central depigmentation (Fig. 31.46). Lesions occur mostly on the trunk. Histology reveals a band-like lymphocytic infiltrate with vacuolar alterations at the dermo-epidermal junction (Fig. 31.47) and many necrotic keratinocytes at the tip of the rete ridges (the rete ridges are "squared off" by the lichenoid infiltrate) (Fig. 31.48). The histopathological picture may resemble lichen planus [102]. Immunohistology reveals predominance of cytotoxic T lymphocytes positive for T-cell markers as well as for CD8 and TIA-1 (Fig. 31.49). A link to *Borrelia* infection has been proposed [103], but in my opinion, infection by *Borrelia* does not play any role in this condition. Cases with similar features have been termed "lymphomatoid annular erythema" [104], and have been considered as a variant of mycosis fungoides in young patients. However, they may represent examples of annular lichenoid dermatitis of youth.

Annular lichenoid dermatitis of youth can be treated by local steroids or local tacrolimus ointment and usually shows complete resolution within a matter of weeks.

Although this condition has been described as a simulator of mycosis fungoides, genuine cases of mycosis fungoides may present with identical histopathological features (see Chapter 3). A diagnosis of annular lichenoid dermatitis of youth can be accepted only when the histopathological features are found in conjunction to the typical clinical aspects. Patients should be carefully followed up.

## Pseudolymphomatous cutaneous infiltrates in human immunodeficiency virus (HIV)-infected patients and in other immune deficiencies

The onset of aggressive non-Hodgkin lymphomas, including skin lymphomas, has been described in patients with advanced HIV infection (see Chapter 21). Besides true lymphomas, in some patients a cutaneous eruption clinically and histopathologically similar to mycosis fungoides and characterized by the

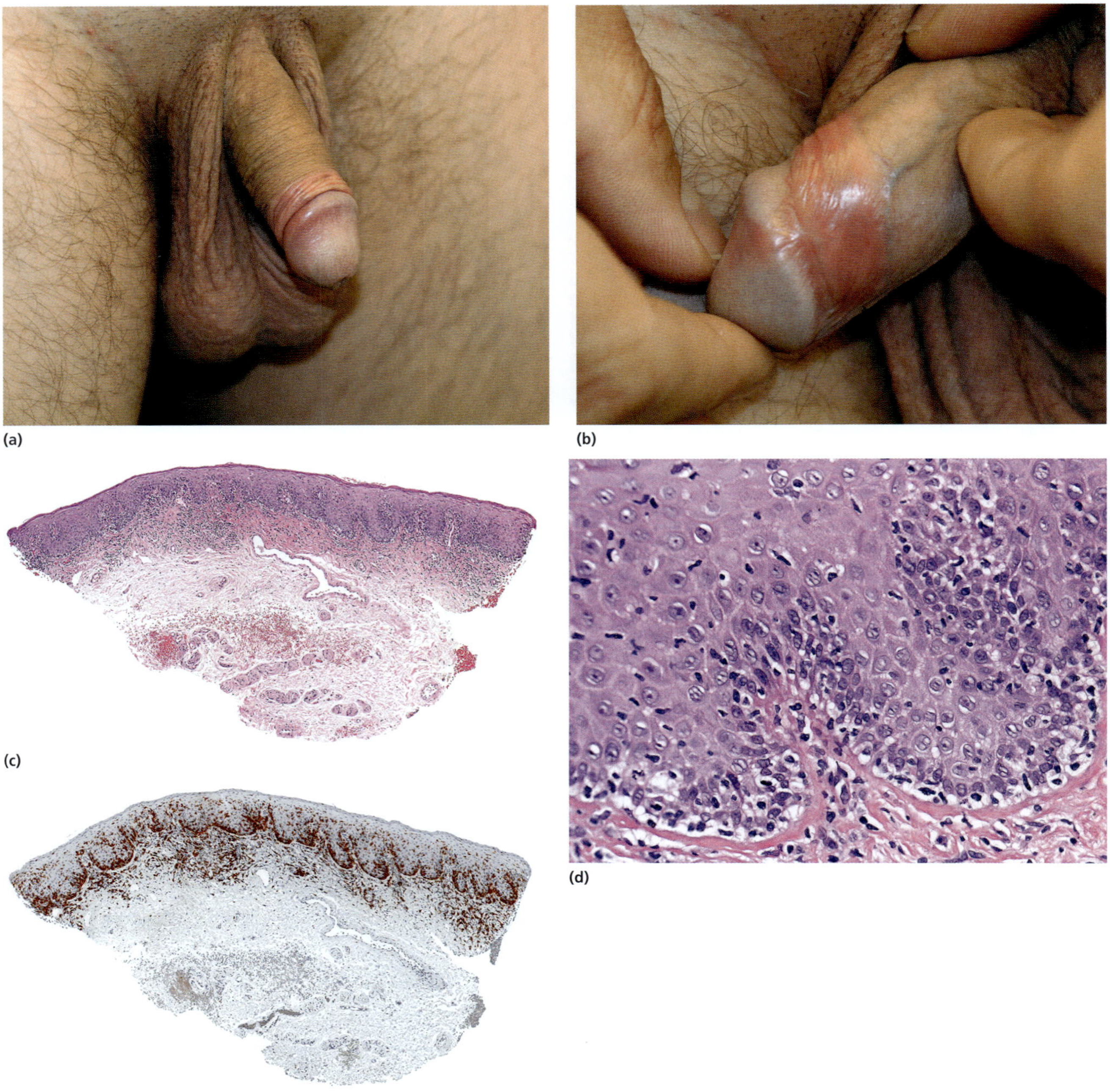

**Figure 31.42** Pseudolymphomatous balanoposthitis. (a, b) Erythematous lesions of recent onset located on the glans and foreskin of a 39-year-old man. (c) Histology showed a superficial, band-like lymphoid infiltrate with (d) many intraepithelial lymphocytes, partly aligned along the dermo-epidermal junction. (e) Immunohistology revealed positivity for CD8. The lesions resolved completely after 3 weeks of local treatment, and the patient did not develop local recurrences or other skin lesions during a follow-up period of >8 years.

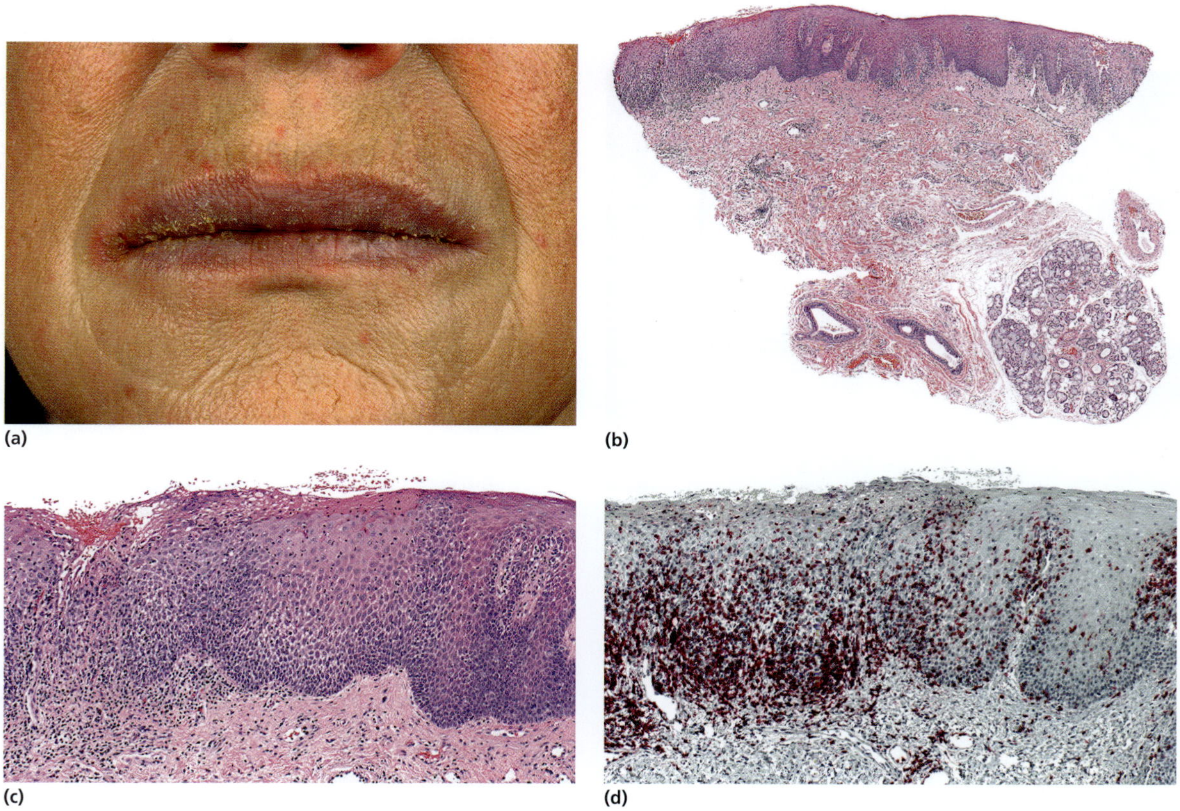

**Figure 31.43** Pseudolymphomatous cheilitis. (a) Partly crusted lesions on the lips. (b) Histology showed a superficial, band-like lymphoid infiltrate with (c) numerous intraepithelial lymphocytes. (d) Staining for CD3 highlights the intraepithelial lymphocytes.

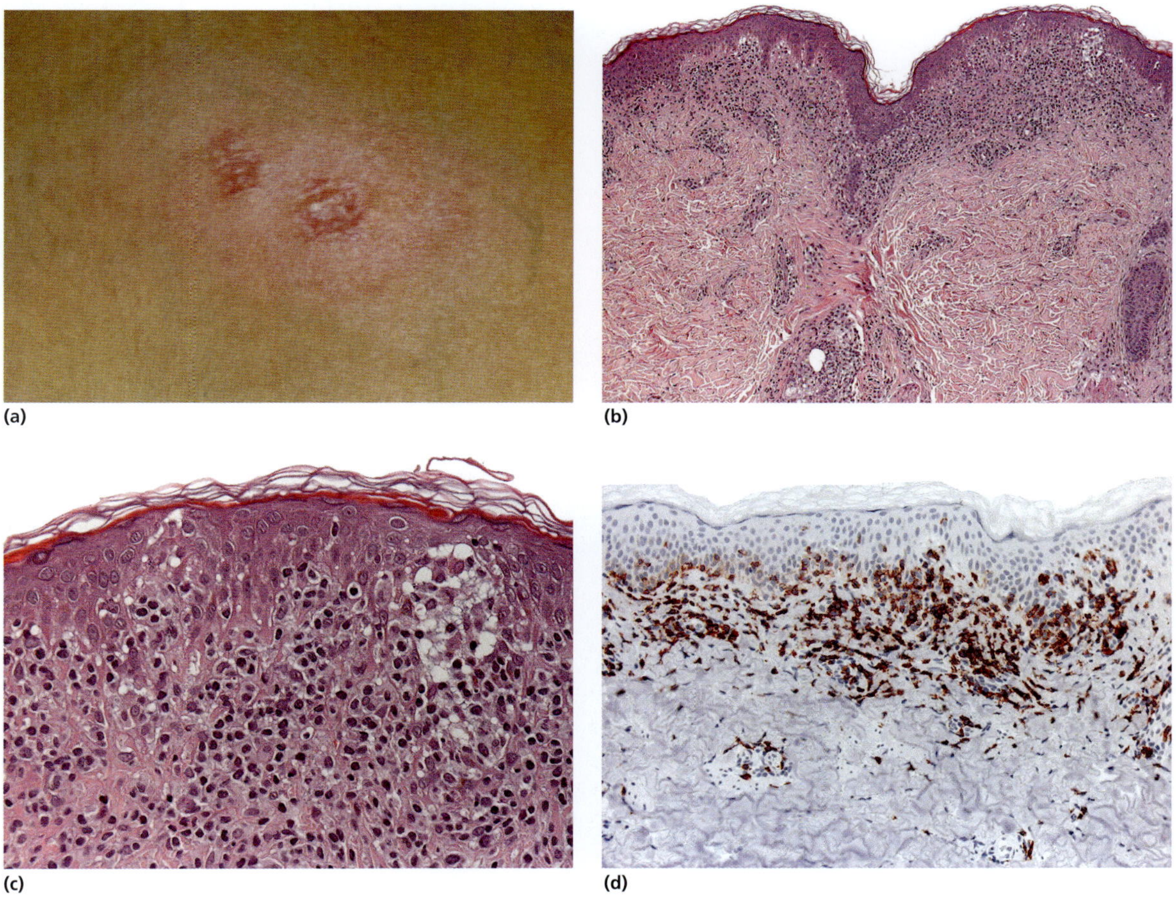

**Figure 31.44** Vitiligo, inflammatory stage. (a) Irregular erythematous patch; note signs of two previous punch biopsies. (b) Band-like infiltrate with many intraepidermal lymphocytes. (c) Detail of intraepidermal lymphocytes. (d) Staining for CD8 reveals positivity of most lymphocytes.

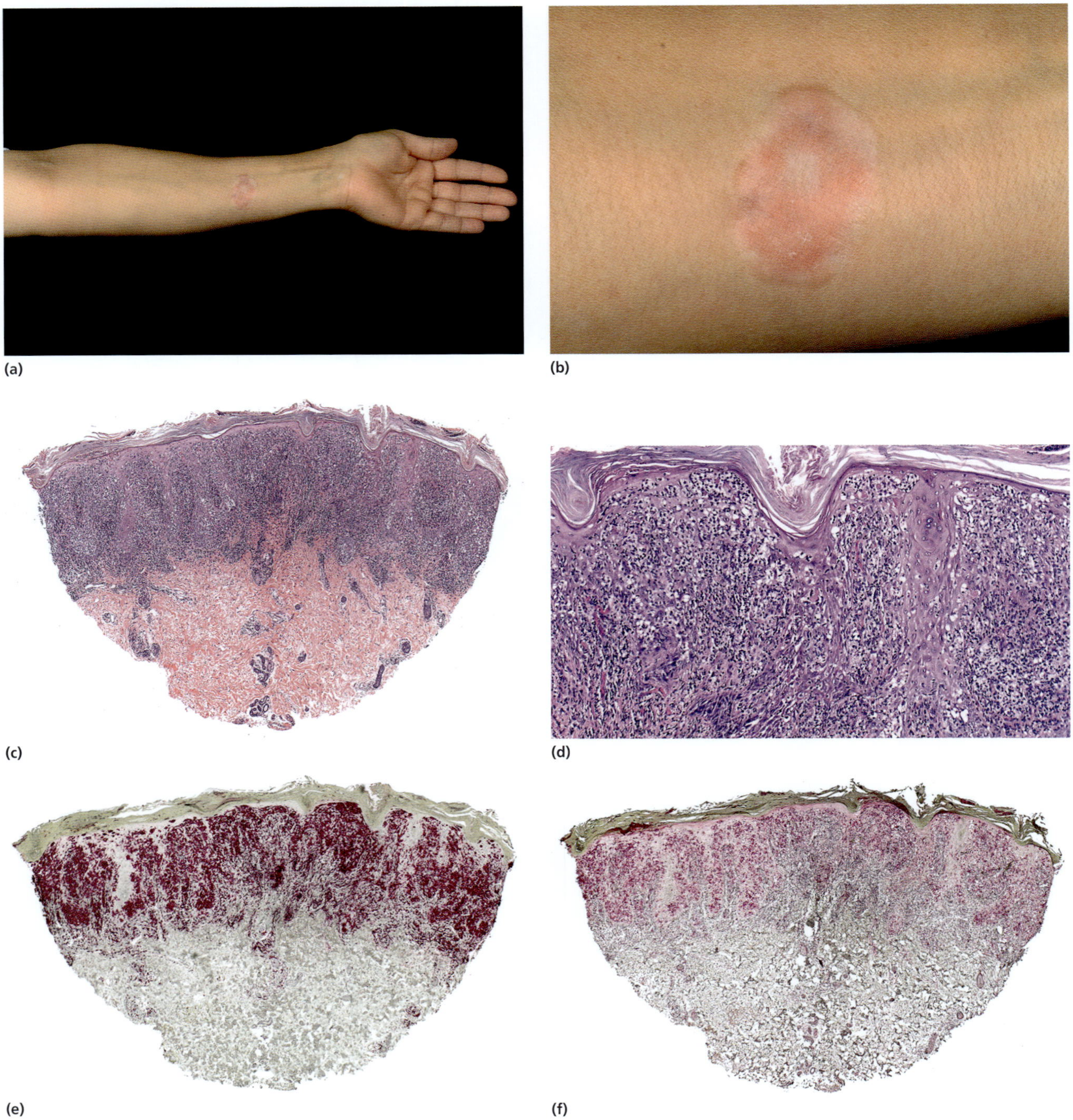

(a) (b) (c) (d) (e) (f)

Figure 31.45 Vitiligo, inflammatory stage. (a, b) Irregular, partly erythematous, partly hypopigmented plaque. (c) Hyperplastic epidermis and dense, band-like infiltrate with (d) many intraepidermal lymphocytes. (e) Staining for CD8 reveals positivity of most lymphocytes; (f) Many lymphocytes are positive for CD30.

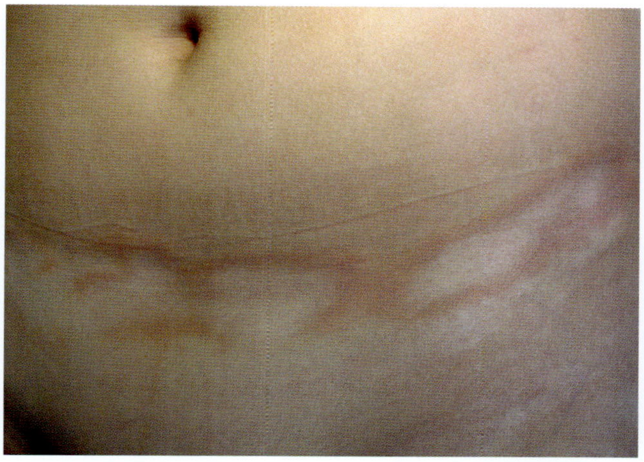

**Figure 31.46** Annular lichenoid dermatitis of youth. Confluent, annular lesions with erythematous border simulating clinically morphea in an 11-year-old girl. *(Courtesy of Dr. Piana, Reggio Emilia, Italy.)*

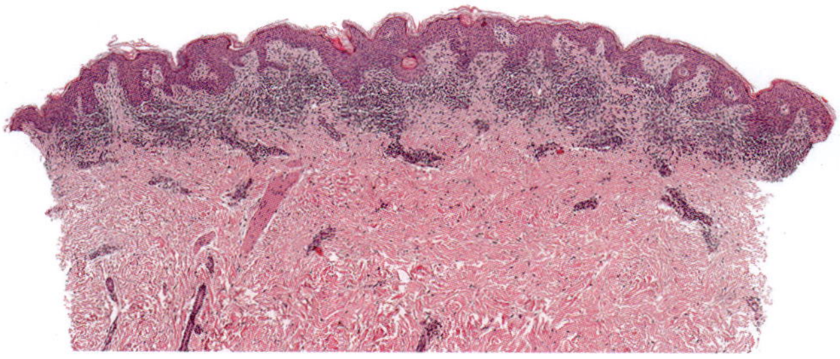

**Figure 31.47** Annular lichenoid dermatitis of youth. Dense band-like infiltrate in the superficial dermis.

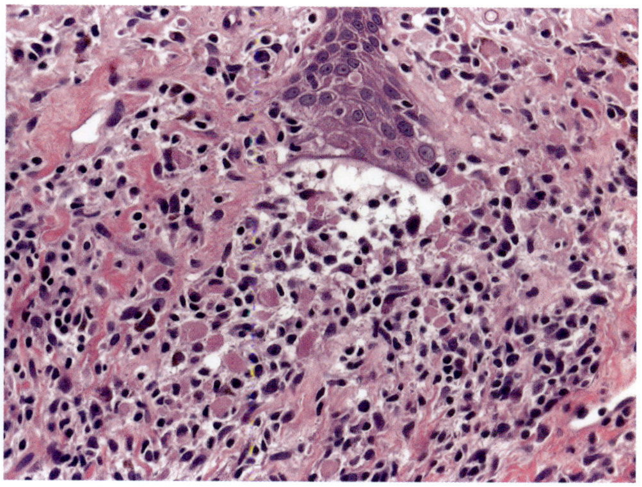

**Figure 31.48** Annular lichenoid dermatitis of youth. Prominent necrosis of keratinocytes at the tip of rete ridges ("squaring" of rete ridges).

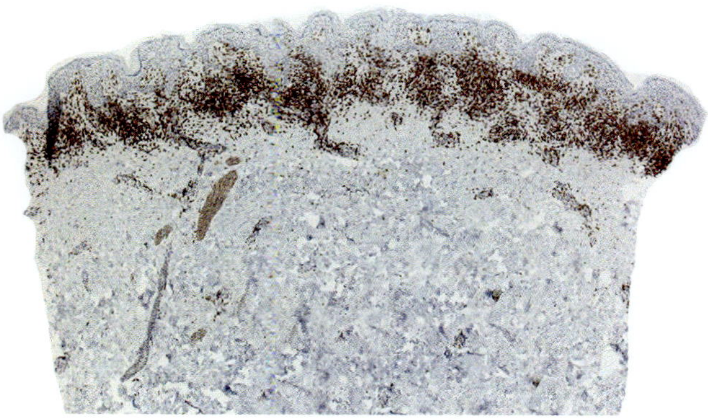

**Figure 31.49** Annular lichenoid dermatitis of youth. Staining for CD3 shows strong positivity of the infiltrate.

predominance of CD8$^+$ T lymphocytes has been observed [105–108]. This condition was not uncommon in the past, but has become very rare due to the remarkable improvements in the treatment of HIV patients with antiretroviral therapy (antiretroviral treatment – ART). Indeed, disappearance of the cutaneous lesions has been reported after complete response to ART [109]. On the other hand, a cutaneous CD8$^+$ pseudolymphoma may be the first sign of an unknown HIV infection.

Patients present with patches or with papulo-nodular lesions, often in photoexposed areas. Erythroderma may be observed rarely. Histology reveals dense lymphoid infiltrates of CD8$^+$ T lymphocytes with a band-like arrangement and variable epidermotropism (Fig. 31.50). In all reported cases the lymphocytes were polyclonal, suggesting that this eruption is more likely to be reactive rather than a cytotoxic variant of mycosis fungoides. On the other hand, genuine mycosis fungoides may arise in HIV patients as well; thus, precise classification may be difficult in given cases.

CD8$^+$ cutaneous infiltrates arise usually in HIV-infected patients with a profound CD4 lymphopenia and are considered as a bad prognostic sign for the underlying disease (the bad prognosis, however, is likely to be due to the very low CD4 count rather than to the skin lesions per se). PUVA, topical or systemic steroids, and even chemotherapy have been used for the treatment of this uncommon condition [105]. Regression upon antiviral triple treatment has been observed [110]. Detection of the HIV p24-gag viral capsid (P24) is possible by immunohistochemistry on fixed biopsy specimens. In the skin, positivity is found in epidermal and dermal Langerhans cells (in the lymph nodes mainly within follicular dendritic cells) [111]. Positivity for P24 can be observed in Langerhans cells before seroconversion and may be considered equivalent to serological tests.

A similar condition to that described in HIV patients, but with monoclonal CD8$^+$ T lymphocytes, has been observed in ***common variable immunodeficiency***. In fact, in children and neonates with congenital immunodeficiencies erythroderma may develop and is rarely characterized by dense, band-like infiltrates of T lymphocytes (Fig. 31.51). Particularly in severe combined

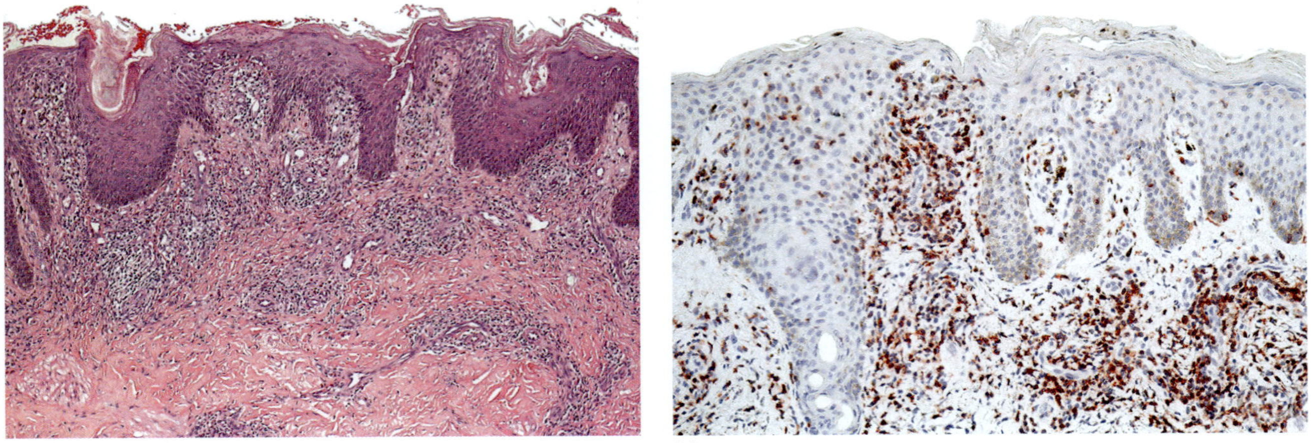

(a) (b)

Figure 31.50 Atypical CD8+ lymphoid proliferation in AIDS. (a) Irregular epidermal hyperplasia with dense, band-like dermal lymphoid infiltrates and intraepidermal lymphocytes, which are (b) mostly positive for CD8.

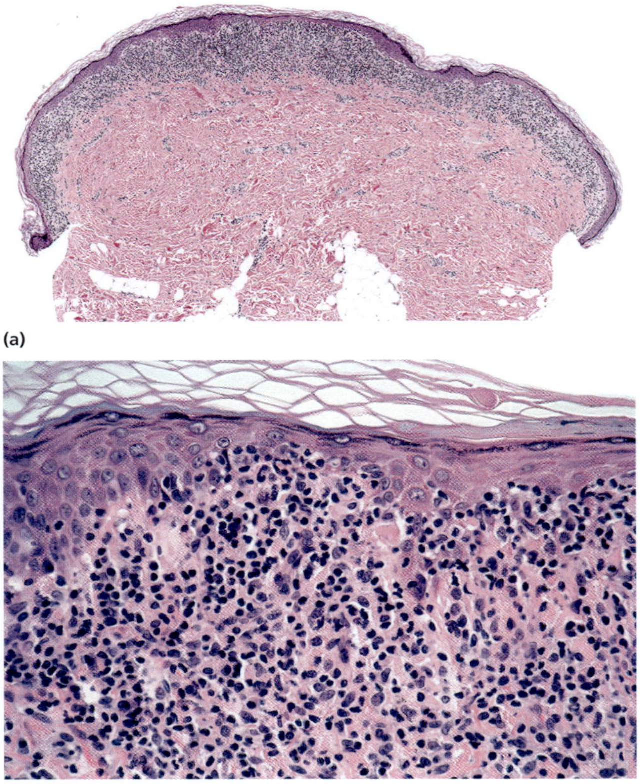

(a) (b)

Figure 31.51 Erythroderma in congenital immunodeficiency. (a) Dense, band-like lymphoid infiltrate in the superficial dermis. (b) Detail showing some intraepidermal lymphocytes and necrotic keratinocytes.

immunodeficiency disorders, a graft-versus-host-disease-like pattern is common, characterized by epidermotropism, folliculotropism, and the presence of apoptotic keratinocytes. The infiltrate in these cases is usually not very dense, but it may mimic early lesions of mycosis fungoides or Sézary syndrome. Atypical lymphoid infiltrates may be observed also in adults with congenital immunodeficiency syndromes (Fig. 31.52).

Another pseudolymphomatous presentation in young children with congenital immune deficiencies shows features that may be indistinguishable from those of subcutaneous panniculitis-like T-cell lymphoma, sometimes with the presence of a monoclonal population of T-lymphocytes as well. For practical purposes, even if a monoclonal population of T-lymphocytes is present, atypical lymphoid proliferations arising in neonates or in young children should not be considered malignant unless compelling evidence is present, and thorough investigations to detect a possible immunodeficiency should be carried out (the obvious exceptions are cutaneous lymphoblastic lymphoma and other high-grade lymphomas and leukemias with skin involvement, but in these cases the histopathologic appearance is that of a high-grade lymphoma).

The occurrence of $CD8^+$ pseudolymphomatous infiltrates has been observed also in a ***renal transplant*** patient at acral sites [112], clinically and histopathologically similar to the papular eruption of atypical $CD8^+$ lymphocytes described in HIV+ patients. This patient healed after topical treatment with corticosteroids and alteration of immunosuppressive therapy, supporting the role of immunosuppression in the pathogenesis of the disease [112].

In the context of pseudolymphomas associated with different types of immune deficiency, it should be reminded once again that any malignant lymphoma may arise in this setting as well (see Chapter 21), sometimes even with unusual histopathological features similar to reactive conditions [113].

## $CD30^+$ T-cell pseudolymphomas

$CD30^+$ T-cells are not restricted to a disease or a specific group of disorders but may be observed in practically all cutaneous infiltrates characterized by the presence of activated

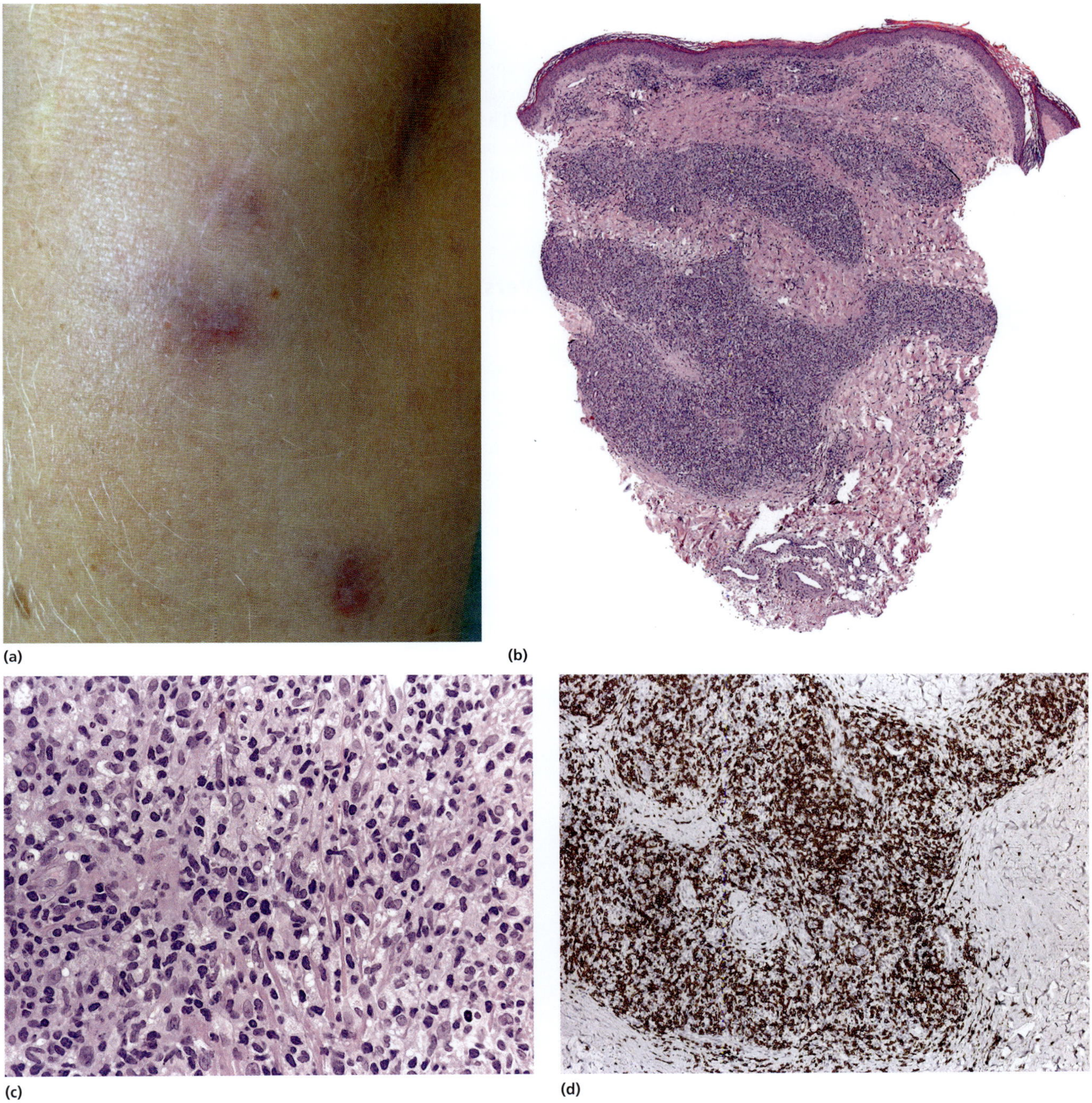

Figure 31.52 Pseudolymphoma in congenital immunodeficiency. (a) Several infiltrated lesions on one arm in a young adult female with FAS-related autoimmune lymphoproliferative syndrome (*Photo courtesy of Dr. Gniadecki and Dr. Rahbek-Gjerdrum, Copenhagen.*) (b) Dense dermal infiltrates, composed predominantly of (c) small and medium-sized lymphocytes, (d) mostly positive for CD8.

lymphocytes; thus the term "CD30$^+$ T-cell pseudolymphoma" completely lacks specificity. Some of the entities characterized by the presence of CD30$^+$ large lymphocytes are discussed in other specific sections in this chapter (herpes infections, persistent arthropod bite reactions, and primary syphilis).

CD30$^+$ T-cell pseudolymphomas encompass skin disorders that have as least common denominator the histopathologic similarity to cutaneous CD30$^+$ lymphoproliferative diseases, particularly lymphomatoid papulosis. Thus, diagnostic and differential diagnostic criteria for this group of pseudolymphomas are, at least conceptually, similar. In fact, any reactive condition showing large, activated lymphoid cells may reveal positivity of the latter for CD30, and this marker *per se* should never be considered specific for any diagnosis. Even criteria used in the past for distinguishing lymphomatoid papulosis from reactive disorders do not work in routine conditions:

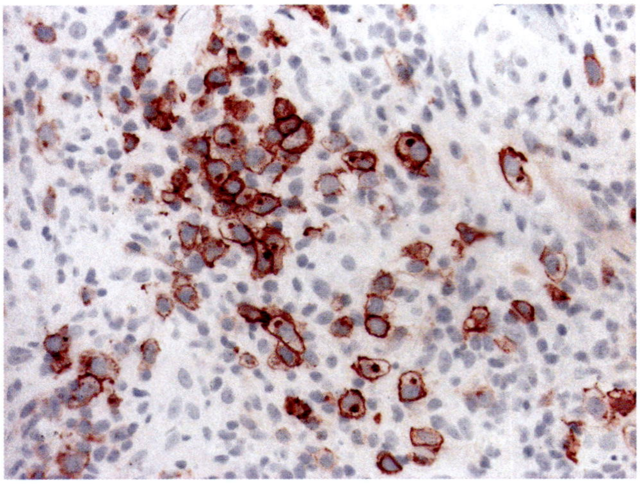

**Figure 31.53** Clusters of CD30+ lymphocytes with accentuation in the Golgi area in a pseudolymphomatous reaction to herpes simplex infection. The distribution of the cells and staining pattern are indistinguishable from those observed in cutaneous CD30+ lymphoproliferative disorders.

although CD30+ cells in lymphomatoid papulosis are often arranged in clusters, the presence of such clusters should not be regarded as synonymous with lymphomatoid papulosis, as they can be observed in benign infiltrates as well; presence of accentuation of the staining in the Golgi area, too, can be observed in CD30+ cells in many reactive infiltrates (Fig. 31.53). Positivity for clusterin has been reported more frequently in lymphomatoid papulosis than in its simulators [114], but in my opinion this marker is of very little value for differential diagnosis.

The most frequent causes of cutaneous CD30+ T-cell pseudolymphomas are infections, particularly viral ones (orf, milker's nodule, molluscum contagiosum, viral warts, herpes simplex, and herpes zoster, among others), as well as reactions to arthropod bites, scabies, and drug eruptions (see also specific sections in this chapter) [115, 116]. Cases may be observed also in disparate conditions such as cysts and perniosis (Fig. 31.54) [115, 117]. Besides the presence of large atypical CD30+ cells, the histology in cutaneous CD30+ T-cell pseudolymphomas reveals the typical changes of the specific underlying disorder, allowing a precise diagnosis in most cases [115]. Sometimes deeper sections are needed to disclose these changes, and special stainings and/or PCR analyses for microbial DNA may be helpful in solving unclear cases.

The presence of dense lymphoid infiltrates with scattered CD30+ cells has been observed also in skin lesions of non-viral infectious disorders, such as mycotic infections and Leishmaniasis, among others (Fig. 31.55) (see also Fig. 31.91) [118]. One case characterized by a monoclonal population of CD30+ T lymphocytes has been reported in a patient with hypereosinophilic syndrome, possibly representing a lymphocytic population related to the hypereosinophilic syndrome [119]. Unlike the situation in lymphomatoid papulosis and cutaneous anaplastic large cell lymphoma, gene rearrangement studies in CD30+ T-cell pseudolymphomas reveal the presence of a polyclonal population of T lymphocytes.

The therapy of CD30+ T-cell pseudolymphomas depends on the specific diagnosis and includes surgical excision, cryotherapy, and specific treatment modalities for the underlying infectious disorders.

## Persistent nodular arthropod bite reactions and nodular scabies

Persistent nodular arthropod bite reactions and nodular scabies belong to the group of CD30+ T-cell pseudolymphomas. Clinically, in nodular scabies, multiple, elevated, round or oval bright reddish papules and nodules occur most frequently on the genitalia, elbows, and in the axillae (Fig. 31.56). The lesions are found in approximately 7% of patients with scabies. The nodules are very pruritic and may persist for many months. The mite and its parts are almost never identified in the long-standing papules or nodules of scabies. The clinical differential diagnosis includes mainly prurigo nodularis and lymphomatoid papulosis.

Persistent arthropod bite reactions present with solitary, localized, or rarely generalized lesions, and usually do not resemble a conventional arthropod bite clinically. Variably large, irregular, erythematous plaques, or nodules are commonly found at the site of the previous bite (Fig. 31.57).

Histopathologically, both nodular scabies and persistent arthropod bite reactions present with dense, superficial, and deep perivascular lympho-histiocytic infiltrates with plasma cells and varying numbers of eosinophils (Figs. 31.58 and 31.59). Eosinophils are also scattered among collagen bundles, and are particularly numerous in lesions of scabies. Large activated ("atypical") lymphocytes are observed as a rule. Prominent vessels with thickened walls lined by plump endothelial cells are nearly always found. The epidermis may be slightly spongiotic, hyperplastic, and hyperkeratotic. The histologic features may mimic those of mycosis fungoides, lymphomatoid papulosis, or rarely Hodgkin lymphoma. Occasionally, a B-cell pattern analogous to lymphocytoma cutis can be recognized as well.

Immunohistologic investigations reveal that T lymphocytes predominate, almost always admixed with B cells. The CD30 antigen is expressed by the large lymphoid cells as a rule. One case of cutaneous infiltrate after a tick bite was characterized by a predominant $\gamma/\delta$ T-cell infiltrate [120].

Large nodules of persistent arthropod bite reaction or nodular scabies may be excised surgically. Intralesional injection of corticosteroids may be helpful. Antiscabietic therapy is usually ineffective in nodular scabies. Spontaneous resolution in time is the rule for all persistent arthropod bite reactions.

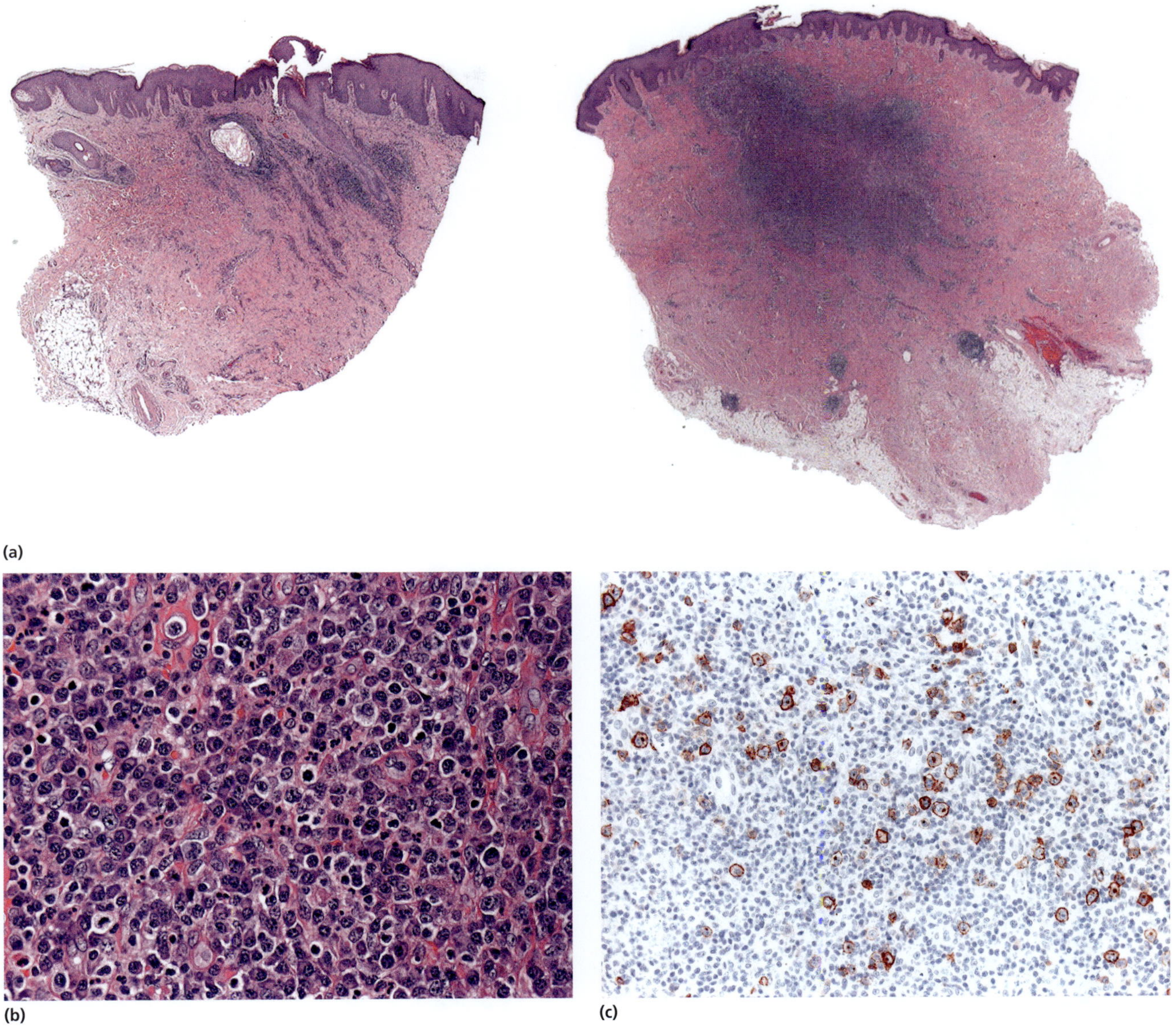


**Figure 31.54** Pseudolymphomatous infiltrate around a ruptured infundibular cyst. (a) A bisected biopsy specimen of a lesion diagnosed clinically as inflamed cyst shows a small infundibular cyst and focally dense inflammatory infiltrates, (b) characterized by large, activated lymphoid cells admixed with many plasma cells. (c) The large lymphocytes are positive for CD30; note the accentuation of the staining in the Golgi area, similar to what is observed in cutaneous CD30+ lymphoproliferative disorders.

## Molluscum contagiosum

Molluscum contagiosum is a disorder caused by infection with the molluscum contagiosum virus (referred to also as molluscipoxvirus), a variant of the poxviruses [121]. The disease is mostly observed in children, and in the vast majority of cases is transmitted by human-to-human contact.

In molluscum contagiosum, lesions that are histopathologically pseudolymphomatous are clinically inflamed as well, and if solitary are usually biopsied, as the diagnosis of molluscum contagiosum has not been suspected (Fig. 31.60). Histopathology reveals dense lymphoid infiltrates with many large, blastoid, "activated" lymphocytes (Fig. 31.61) that are positive for T-cell markers and for CD30 (Fig. 31.61d) [115]. The percentage of cases of molluscum contagiosum that present histopathologically with pseudolymphomatous features has not been evaluated in detail, but in contrast to parapoxvirus infections (milker's nodule and orf, see the section below in this chapter) I have seen this pattern only uncommonly, and most biopsies show only minimal or no inflammation. Sporadic case reports have been published [122–126], but in a histopathological study on 578 cases of molluscum contagiosum a "pseudolymphomatous" variant was not mentioned [127]. The diagnostic finding of

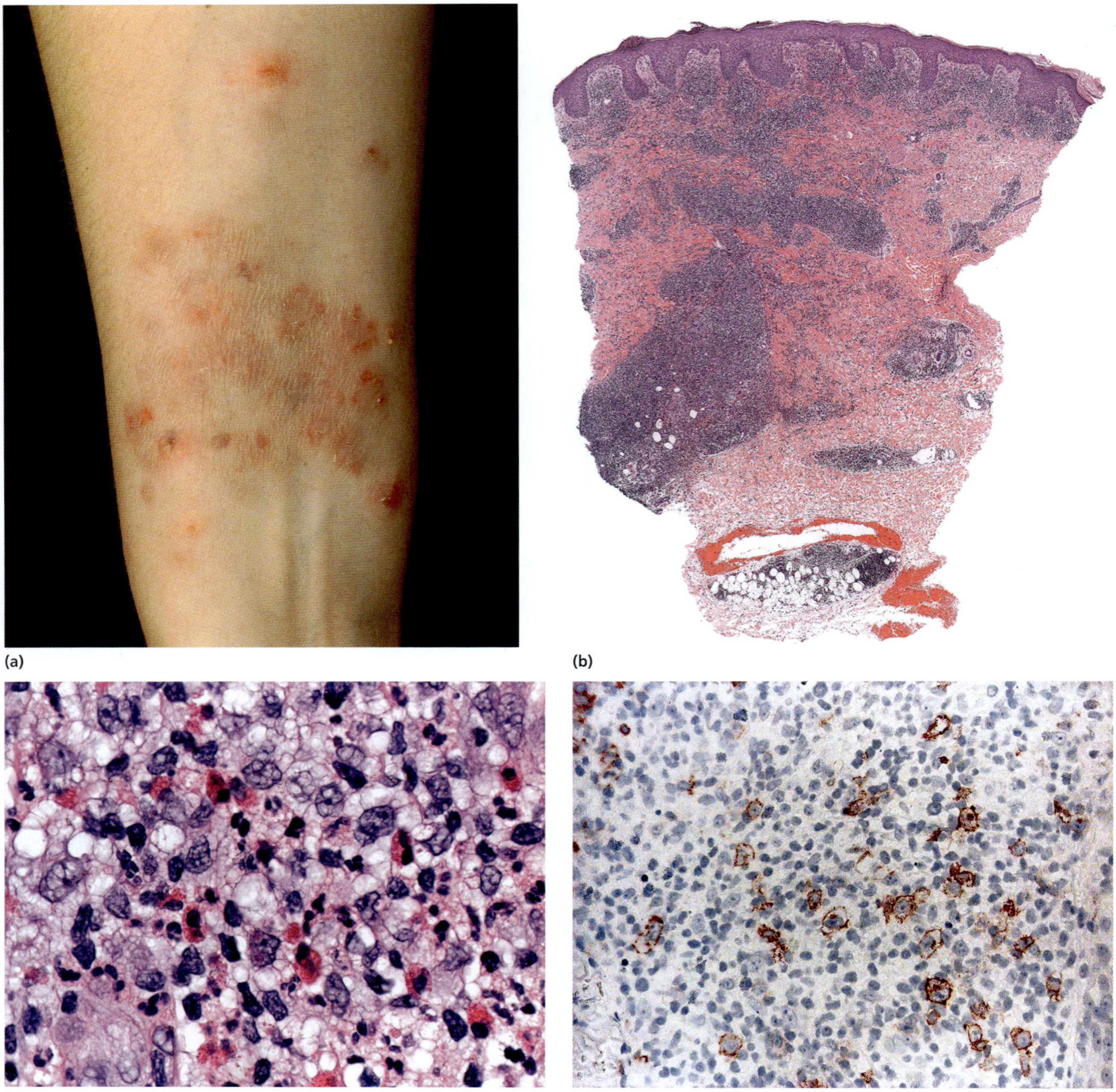

(a) (b) (c) (d)

Figure 31.55 Pseudolymphomatous trichophytia (culture: *Trichophyton rubrum*). (a) Infiltrated, erythematous, scaly lesions on the distal part of the arm. (b) Dense lymphoid infiltrates within the entire dermis reaching into the subcutaneous fat. (c) Large, activated lymphocytes admixed with several neutrophils and eosinophils. (d) Several lymphocytes are positive for CD30.

molluscum contagiosum, that is, the presence of large intracytoplasmic eosinophilic inclusions within the keratinocytes (known also as molluscum bodies, representing the largest intracellular viral inclusion in human pathology), is never prominent in cases with pseudolymphomatous infiltrates, and may be visible only in deeper sections (Fig. 31.61c). In the past, one case of molluscum contagiosum had been misinterpreted as "leukemia cutis" even by an experienced dermatopathologist like A. Bernard Ackerman, who wrote in the report of that case: "Perplexed by the contradiction between the dire histologic interpretation and the negative clinical and other laboratory findings, we obtained the original block of the cutaneous

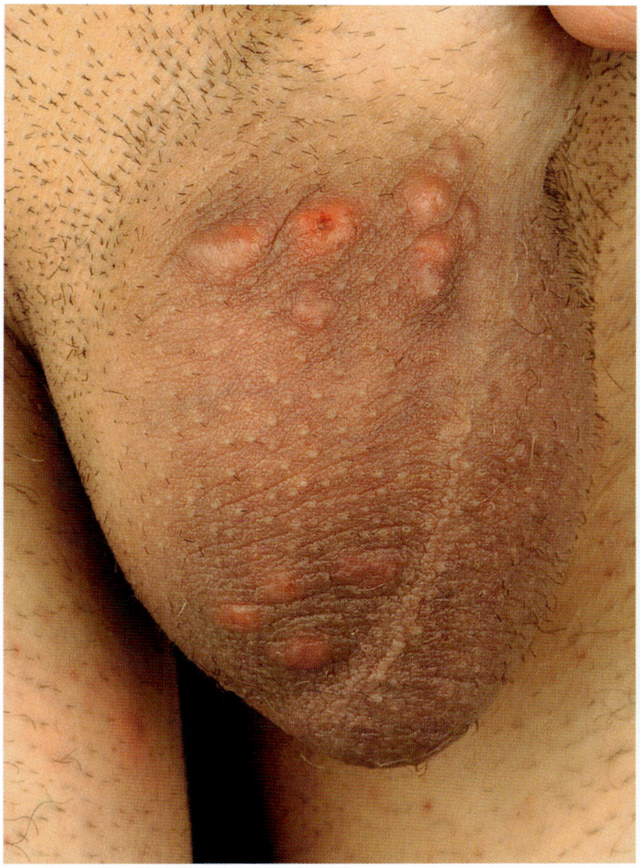

Figure 31.56 Nodular scabies. Erythematous papules on the scrotum with focal excoriation.

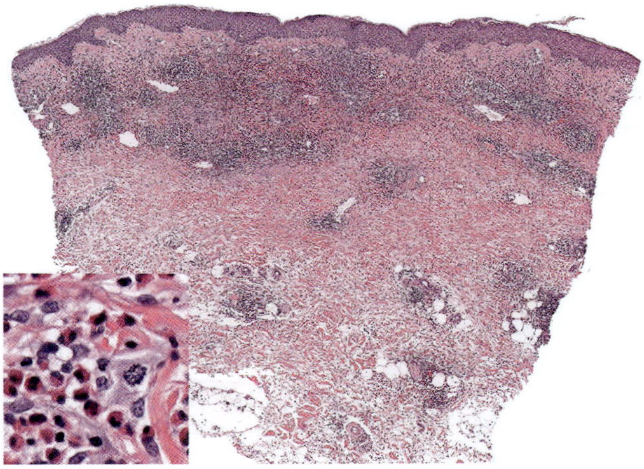

Figure 31.58 Nodular lesions of scabies. Dense lymphoid infiltrate reaching into the deep dermis. Note a mitotic figure and several eosinophils (inset).

specimen and cut deeper sections through it. To our amazement and embarassment, those sections revealed molluscum bodies within the cornified cells of an epithelial, cyst-like structure that had ruptured" [128].

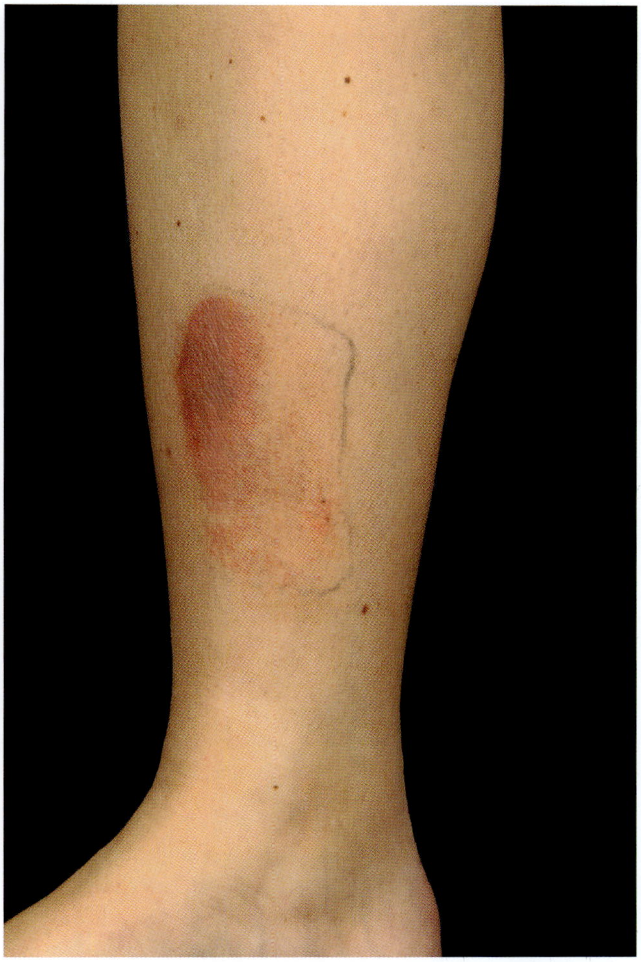

Figure 31.57 Persistent arthropod bite reaction. Infiltrated erythematous plaque on the leg.

## Milker's nodule and orf

Milker's nodule and orf are infectious diseases caused by transmission of a parapoxvirus from infected cattle (cows in milker's nodule, sheep and goats in orf) to people attending the infected animal or working with contaminated flesh [121]. The infection is caused by direct contact with the infected cattle, but in some cases can been acquired from contaminated surfaces as well. The orf virus is responsible for orf, and the pseudocowpox virus for milker's nodule. Clinical and histopathological features are similar in both diseases. Clinically, lesions are restricted to the skin sites that came in contact with the infected animal, thus confined mostly to the hands (yet other sites of the body that came in direct contact with the virus can be affected). The disease presents with sudden onset of multiple hemorrhagic, partly bullous, partly necrotic lesions that resolve spontaneously over a period of some weeks (Fig. 31.62). Solitary lesions may be observed in some cases (Fig. 31.63). Six consecutive clinical stages have been described: maculopapular, targetoid, acute weeping, nodular, papillomatous, and regressive. Each stage

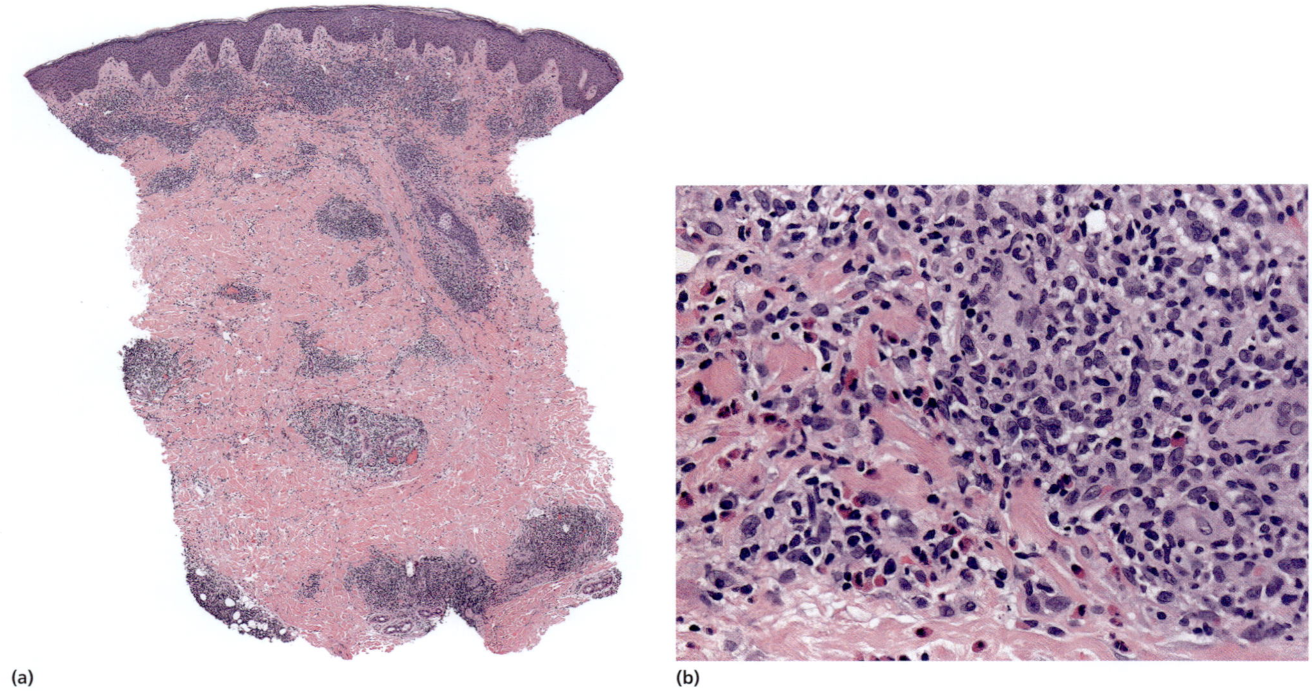

Figure 31.59 Persistent arthropod bite reaction. (a) Dense lymphoid infiltrates reaching into the subcutaneous fat. (b) Detail of large, activated (atypical-looking) lymphocytes admixed with several eosinophils.

lasts approximately for one week. Histopathologically, cases presenting with a pseudolymphomatous infiltrate are characterized by necrosis of the epidermis, subepidermal edema, and variably dense lymphoid infiltrates containing numerous large, blastoid lymphocytes strongly positive for CD30 (Fig. 31.64) [115]. Variable numbers of eosinophils are commonly found. The epidermal necrosis is usually characterized by a characteristic fenestrated ("reticulated") pattern (Fig. 31.65). Cytoplasmic and/or nuclear viral inclusions may be present within the epidermis (Fig. 31.66) [129], but their demonstration may be difficult due to the presence of apoptotic keratinocytes, as well as of intraepidermal erythrocytes and eosinophils.

The histopathological picture of milker's nodule and orf may be indistinguishable from that observed in cutaneous anaplastic large cell lymphoma or in lymphomatoid papulosis (Fig. 31.67). Mitotic figures are numerous (Fig. 31.67b), and staining for Ki-67 usually shows a high proliferation rate (Fig. 31.67d). Pan-T-cell markers (CD2, CD3, CD5) are not lost, a distinguishing feature from many cases of cutaneous anaplastic large cell lymphoma (see also Chapter 5, Fig. 5.39). Another peculiar feature is the presence of blastoid rather than pleomorphic lymphocytes, a feature observed in several viral-induced CD30$^+$ pseudolymphomas (besides orf and milker's nodule, they can be observed also in molluscum contagiosum and herpes infections, among others).

The percentage of cases of milker's nodule and orf presenting histopathologically with pseudolymphomatous infiltrates is not known, but I have seen such features in most of the biopsies of these conditions that I have observed. Precise history taking is paramount for a correct diagnosis, and the presence of CD30$^+$ lesions restricted to the hands should prompt one to consider orf and milker's nodule in the differential diagnosis.

## Pseudolymphomas in herpes simplex and herpes zoster infections

In some instances, skin lesions of herpes simplex or herpes zoster infection may present with dense, atypical lymphoid infiltrates that simulate a cutaneous lymphoma, usually aggressive cytotoxic natural killer (NK)/T-cell lymphomas, or cutaneous CD30$^+$ lymphoproliferative disorders [130–132]. These features may be observed both in immunocompetent and immunocompromised patients. In most of these cases a variable population of large CD30$^+$ cells can be observed. In the lymph nodes, reactive features associated with herpes infection may simulate Richter syndrome in patients with B-cell chronic lymphocytic leukemia (B-CLL) [133]; I have never seen comparable cases in the skin, although it is well known that specific infiltrates of B-CLL may colonize cutaneous lesions of herpes simplex or herpes zoster [134], and Richter syndrome may arise in lesions of previous herpes zoster (see Chapter 22). In fact, in the context of the discussion on cutaneous

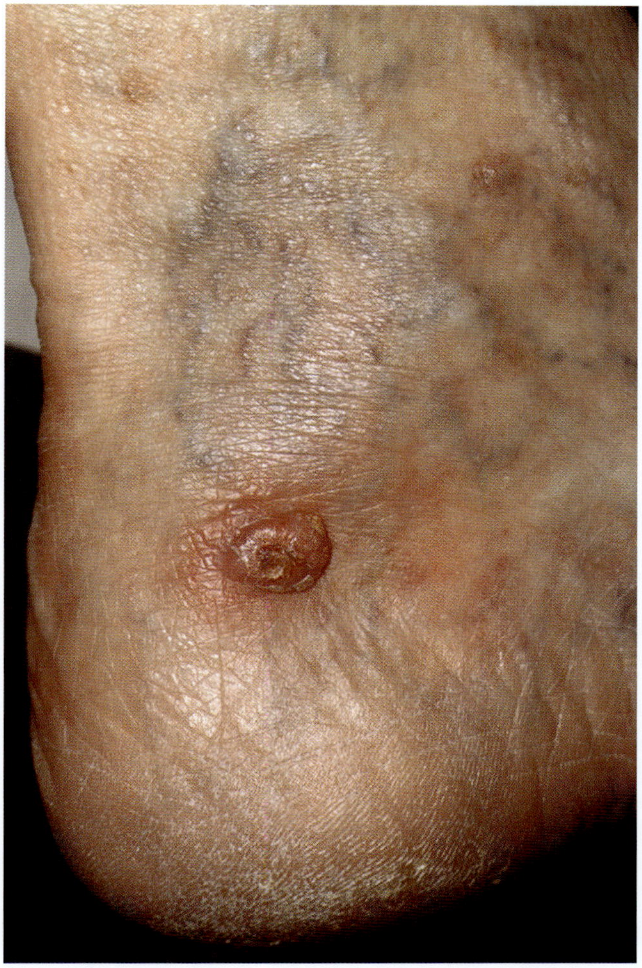

**Figure 31.60** Molluscum contagiosum with pseudolymphomatous infiltrates. Solitary, inflamed papule on the foot of an elderly man. Similar lesions are usually not diagnosed clinically as molluscum contagiosum, and due to persistence may be biopsied.

pseudolymphomas arising at the site of herpes simplex or herpes zoster infection, it should be underlined that most of the cases reported in the past as pseudolymphoma at the site of herpes zoster scar in patients with B-CLL actually represent specific infiltrates of B-CLL at sites of previous herpes infections (see Chapter 22).

Lining-up of $CD8^+$ lymphocytes at the dermo-epidermal junction but predominance of $CD4^+$ lymphocytes in the dermal infiltrate (inverse CD8:CD4 ratio) was observed in some cases of pseudolymphoma associated with herpes simplex 1 infection [135].

Clinical features deviate from conventional presentations of herpes simplex or herpes zoster, as lesions are papules rather than vesicles (Fig. 31.68), and in immunocompromised patients may be vegetating (Fig. 31.69). Histology shows dense, dermal infiltrates with variable involvement of epithelial structures and with large numbers of activated, atypical lymphocytes (Fig. 31.70). A reassuring histopathologic feature is represented by the presence of different cell types other than the large blastic elements (mixed cell infiltrate). The typical cytopathic changes of herpes simplex and herpes varicella/zoster infections may be absent ("herpes incognito") or be present only focally, and several levels may be necessary to reveal them (Fig. 31.71) [130, 136]. A histopathological clue for the varicella/zoster virus is the presence of necrosis localized at the level of hair follicles and/or sebaceous glands only. Immunohistologic investigations are less sensitive than molecular ones in confirming the viral etiology.

Treatment of pseudolymphomas arising at sites of previous herpes simplex or herpes zoster should be achieved with conventional antiviral strategies used for these infections.

## Pseudolymphomas associated with lupus erythematosus

Several variants of cutaneous lupus erythematosus may present histopathologically with dense infiltrates simulating different types of cutaneous T- or B-cell lymphoma [137]. Although in most instances a precise diagnosis is possible without ancillary techniques, in some cases only complete phenotypic and molecular studies may allow the distinction of lupus erythematosus from cutaneous lymphoma. If a previous diagnosis of lupus erythematosus is known the distinction is made easier, but sometimes patients present with pseudolymphomatous infiltrates as the first manifestation of the disease. In addition, antinuclear antibodies (ANA) and their subsets, as well as direct immunofluorescence studies, may be negative in cases of cutaneous lupus erythematosus. Atypical lymphoid infiltrates associated with lupus erythematosus may be observed in lesions arising in the skin and rarely also in those located in the oral mucosa [138, 139], and occasionally within the lymph nodes as well. Although the lymphadenopathy that can be associated with systemic lupus erythematosus usually does not represent a problem in the histopathological differentiation from lymphomas, Prof. Andreas Chott, an outstanding hematopathologist from Vienna, Austria, once showed me a case of lymph node involvement by lupus erythematosus that resembled morphologically a lymphoma due to the presence of very large aggregates of mid-sized plasmacytoid dendritic cells.

In what follows, the different cutaneous pseudolymphomatous presentation of various types of cutaneous lupus erythematosus will be summarized.

### Lupus tumidus and lymphocytic infiltration of the skin (*Jessner-Kanof*)

The most common histopathological presentation of pseudolymphomatous lupus erythematosus is that of lupus tumidus and lymphocytic infiltration of the skin (Jessner–Kanof), this last considered by many authors to be a variant of lupus

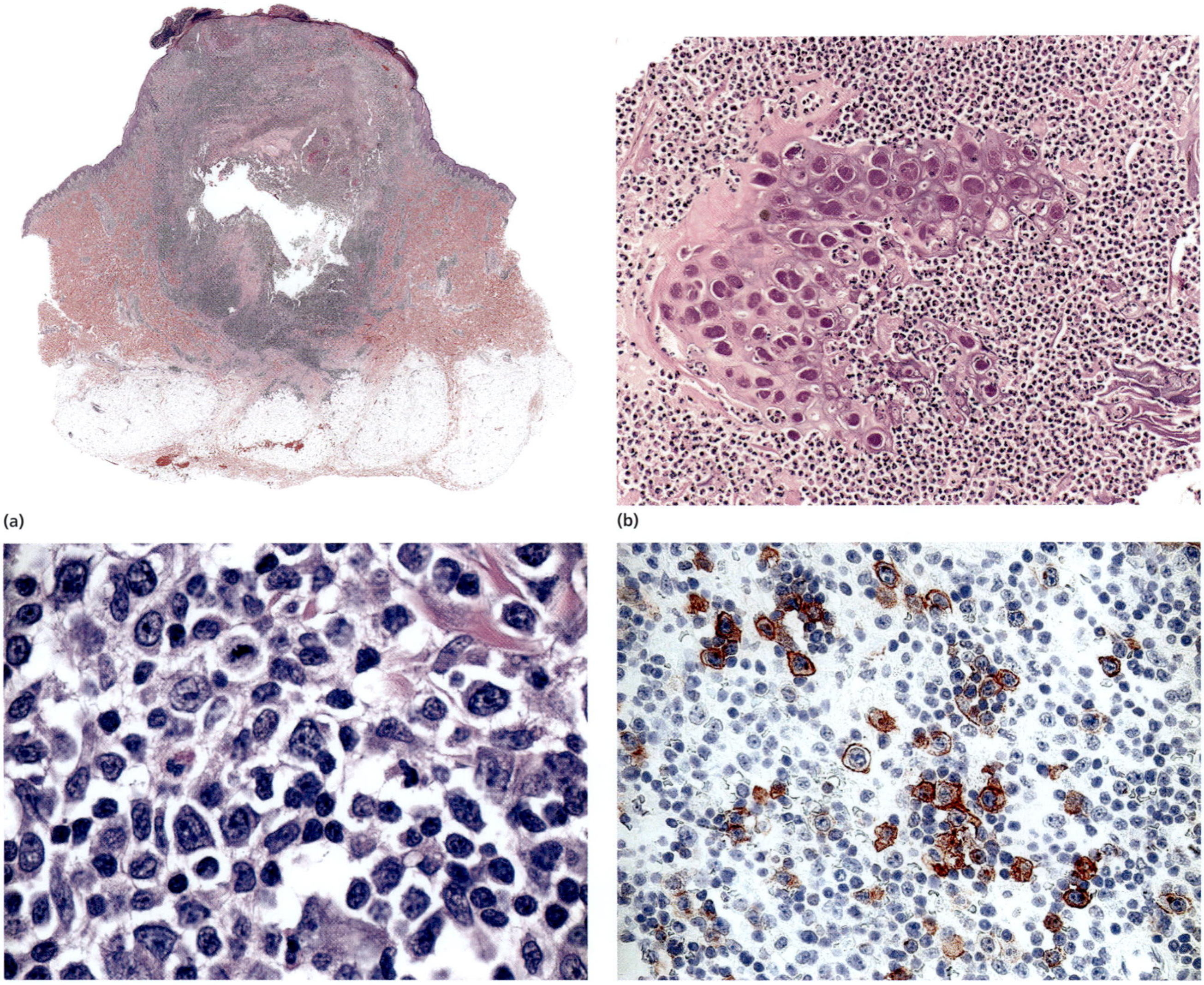



**Figure 31.61** Molluscum contagiosum with pseudolymphomatous infiltrates. (a) Partly cystic lesion with dense lymphoid infiltrates, (b) characterized by the presence of several blastoid, atypical-looking lymphocytes. (c) Molluscum bodies may not be readily visible at scanning magnification, but can be observed at higher power or in step sections. (d) Several atypical cell, some in clusters, strongly positive for CD30 and with accentuation of the staining in the Golgi area.

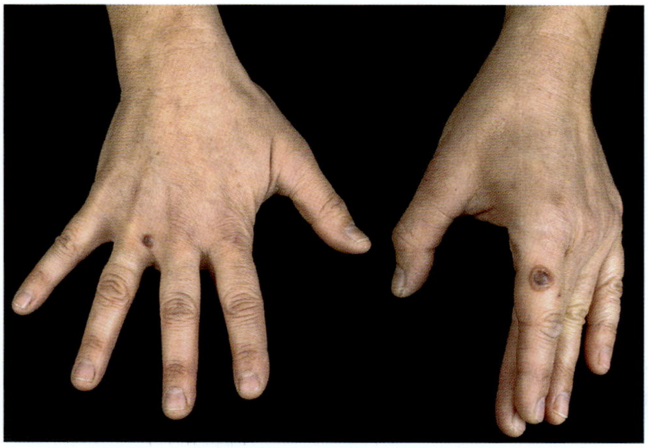

**Figure 31.62** Milker's nodule. Two hemorrhagic nodules on the hands.

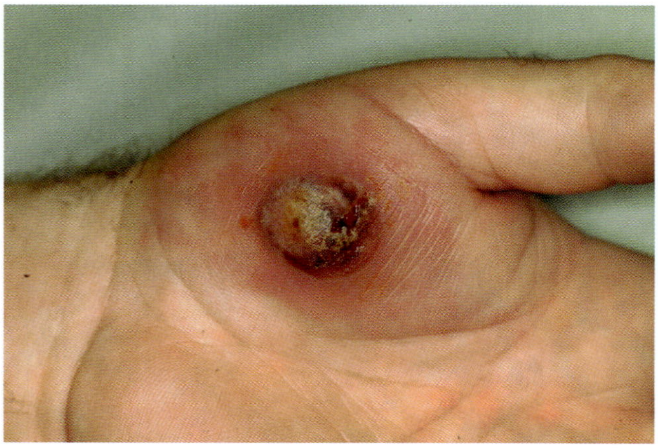

**Figure 31.63** Milker's nodule. Solitary, ulcerated nodule on the palm.

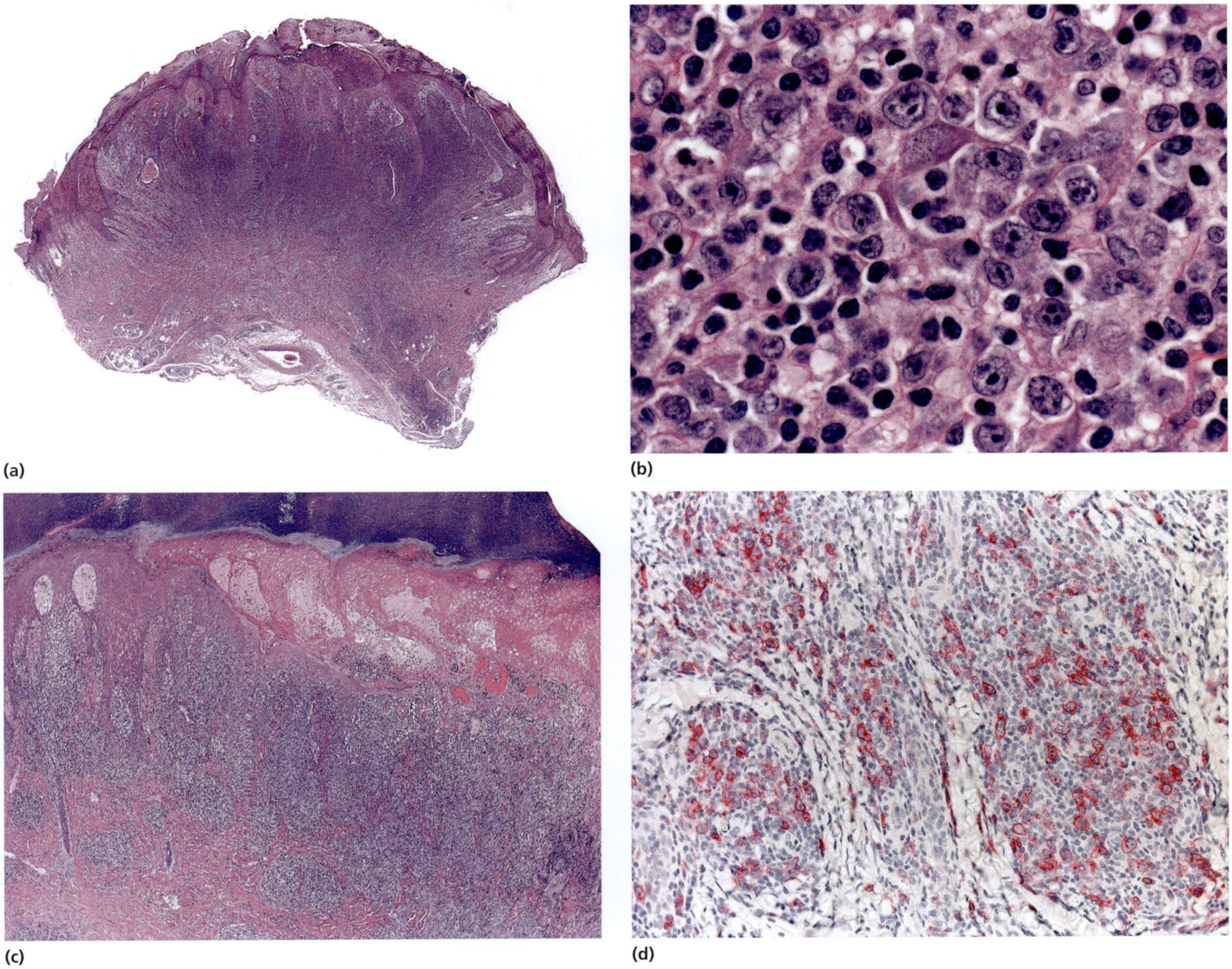


Figure 31.64 Milker's nodule. (a) Epidermal hyperplasia with crust, hemorrhage, and dense infiltrate of lymphocytes. (b) Note the presence of large blastoid cells. (c) Another case showing epidermal necrosis and dilated superficial blood vessels in association with dense lymphoid infiltrates. (d) Positivity of the large cells for CD30.

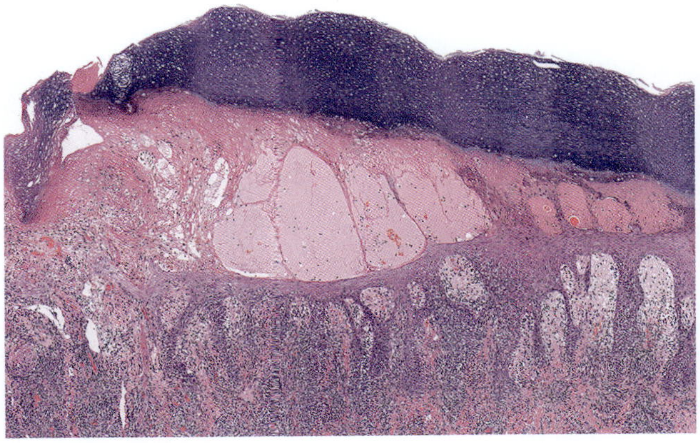

Figure 31.65 Milker's nodule. Fenestrated (reticulated) pattern of epidermal necrosis.

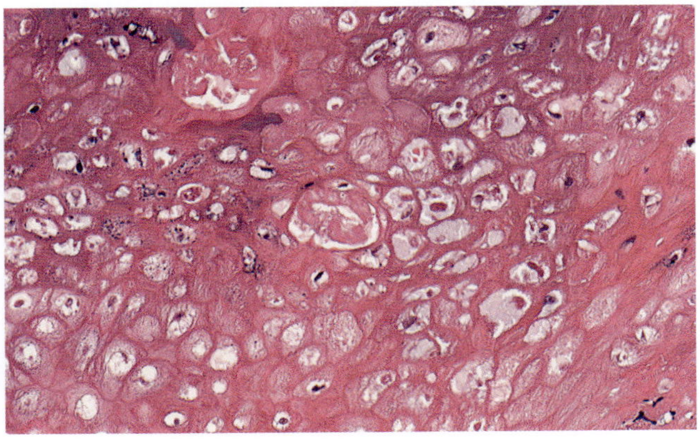

Figure 31.66 Milker's nodule. Nuclear and cytoplasmic inclusions in several keratinocytes.

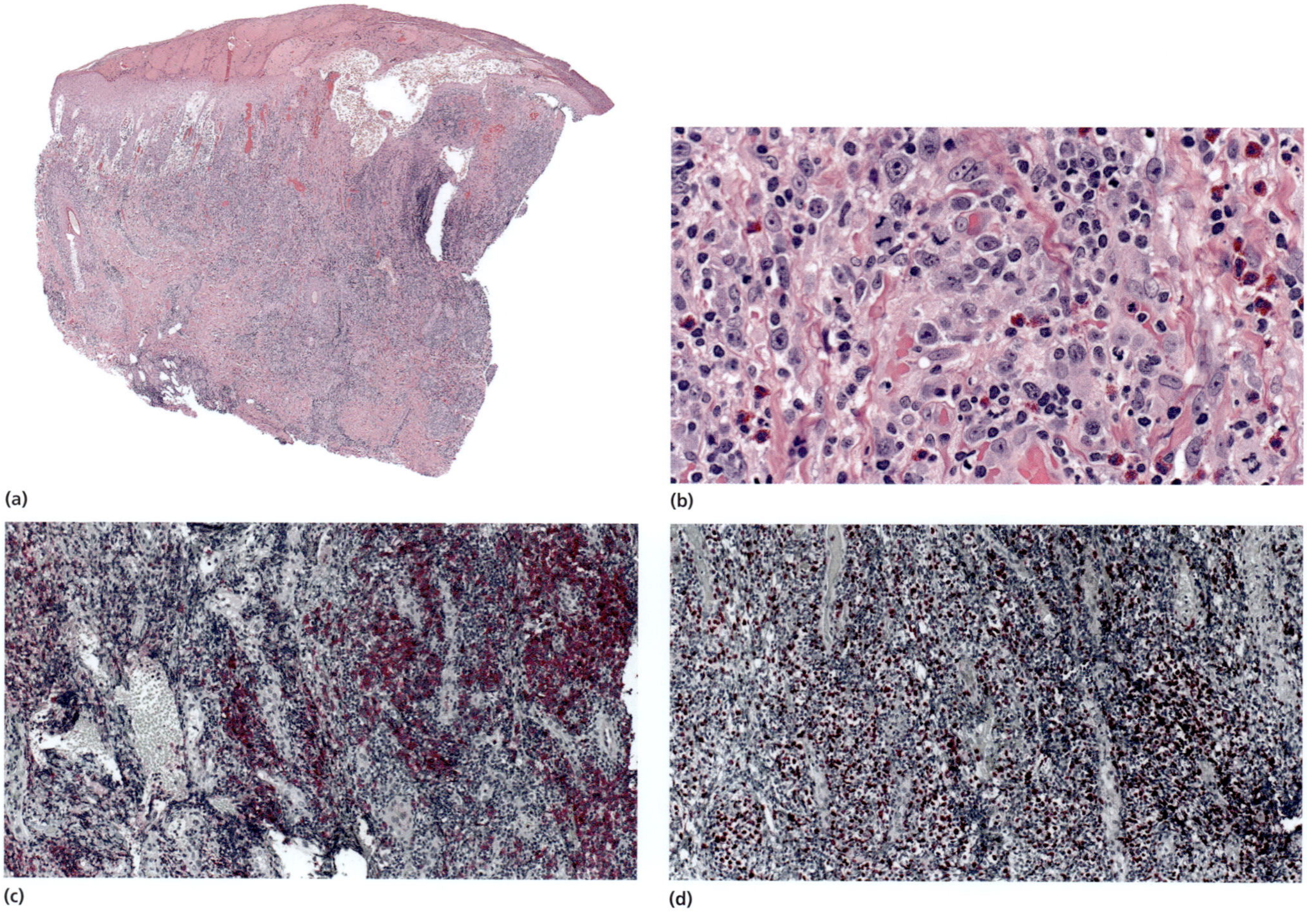

Figure 31.67 Milker's nodule. (a) Epidermal hyperplasia with focal necrosis and serum crust; (b) clusters of large, blastoid cells with several mitoses are present within the infiltrate, admixed with many eosinophils; (c) staining for CD30 shows sheets of positive large lymphocytes, a pattern indistinguishable from that observed in cutaneous CD30+ lymphoproliferative disorders. (d) High proliferation rate demonstrated by staining for Ki-67.

tumidus [140]. Histology shows dense, perivascular, and periadnexal lymphoid infiltrates, sometimes with scattered large, activated lymphocytes (Figs. 31.72a and b). In addition, features of an interface dermatitis may be detected focally. Clusters of $CD123^+$ plasmacytoid dendritic cells are present in lupus tumidus as a rule (Fig. 31.72c). These clusters may be confused with atypical lymphoid follicles morphologically (Fig. 31.73), but are easily distinguished immunohistochemically. On pure morphologic grounds, the main histopathologic differential diagnosis of lupus tumidus/lymphocytic infiltration of the skin is with specific cutaneous manifestations of B-CLL. The co-expression of CD20, CD5, and CD23 by neoplastic cells of B-CLL as well as the detection of a monoclonal rearrangement of the Ig genes, in contrast to the predominance of polyclonal T lymphocytes admixed with $CD123^+$ plasmacytoid dendritic cells in lupus tumidus, allows an easy distinction between these diseases.

## Lupus panniculitis

Patients with lupus erythematosus may present with prominent involvement of the subcutaneous tissues, a condition that has been termed lupus panniculitis or lupus erythematosus profundus. A detailed discussion on differential diagnosis between the two entities is provided in Chapter 6.

Lupus panniculitis presents with subcutaneous plaques and indurations, mostly located on the extremities, which can simulate clinically and histopathologically those observed in subcutaneous panniculitis-like T-cell lymphoma (Fig. 31.74) [141]. Severe atrophy may develop upon resolution of the lesions, and the overlying skin may show features identical to those of chronic discoid lupus erythematosus (Fig. 31.75). ANA and other clinical and/or serologic criteria for the diagnosis of systemic lupus erythematosus are absent in many cases of lupus panniculitis. Histology shows a predominantly lobular panniculitis, often with concomitant presence of broadened fibrotic

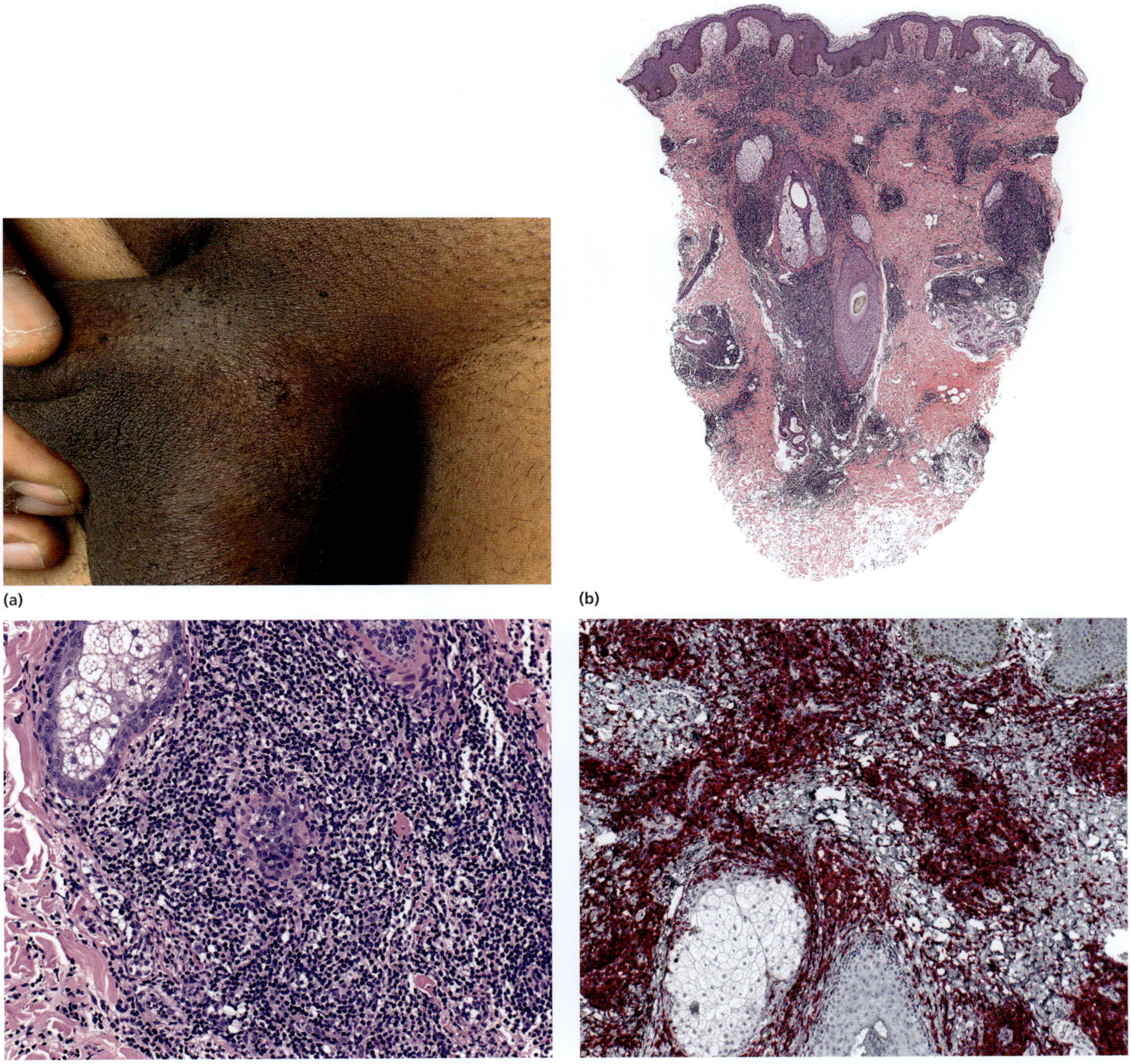

(a) (b) (c) (d)

Figure 31.68 Pseudolymphomatous herpes simplex presenting with (a) small, clustered papules on the scrotum. (b) Histology revealed dense lymphoid infiltrates (c) composed predominantly of small lymphocytes, which (d) are positive for CD3.

septa (Fig. 31.76a). The lymphocytes are of small size without atypical features. In older lesions, degenerative changes of the subcutaneous fat and focal areas of necrosis are prominent features. So-called "rimming" of fat cells by pleomorphic, atypical T lymphocytes that are positive for proliferation markers is seen only in subcutaneous panniculitis-like T-cell lymphoma but not in lupus panniculitis (rimming of the adipocytes by different cell types, including lymphocytes, histiocytes, and plasma cells, may be observed in lupus panniculitis, and mimic genuine neoplastic rimming – "pseudo-rimming") (Fig. 31.76c).

A useful clue for the differentiation of subcutaneous panniculitis-like T-cell lymphoma from lupus panniculitis is the presence in the latter of a mixed cell infiltrate with plasma cells (Fig. 31.76b) and of variably large nodules of B-lymphocytes, sometimes with the formation of germinal centers (Fig. 31.77). The B-cell nodules are typically located at the periphery of the

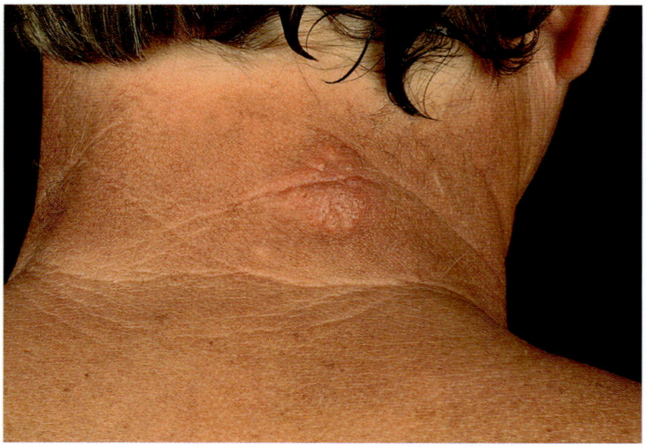

Figure 31.69 Pseudolymphomatous herpes simplex presenting with infiltrated, clustered lesions on the neck.

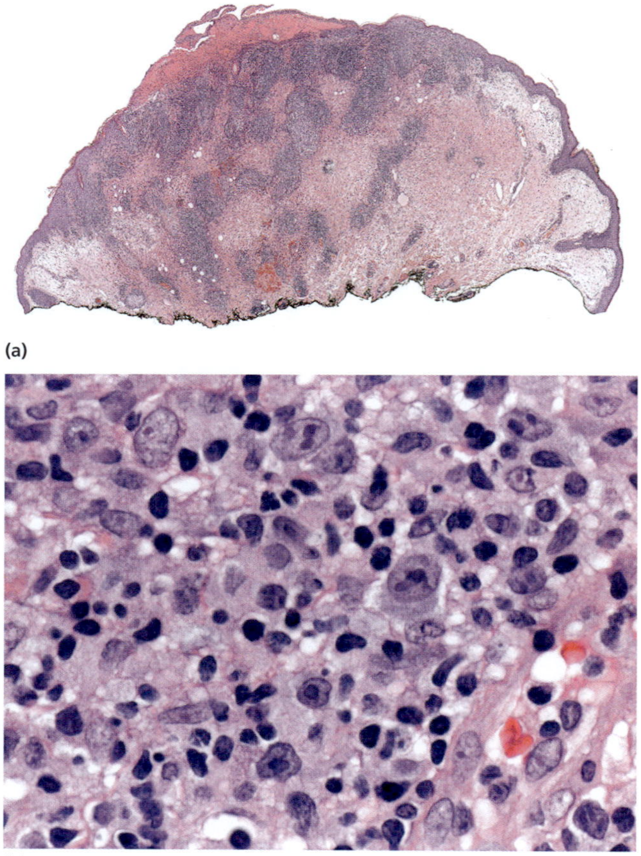

(a)

(b)

Figure 31.70 Pseudolymphomatous herpes simplex. (a) Ulcerated lesion with dense lymphoid infiltrates. (b) Note several large, activated, atypical-looking lymphocytes.

fat lobules. For practical purposes, the finding of clusters of B lymphocytes rules out the diagnosis of subcutaneous panniculitis-like T-cell lymphoma. In lupus panniculitis, the dermo-epidermal junction may show features of lupus

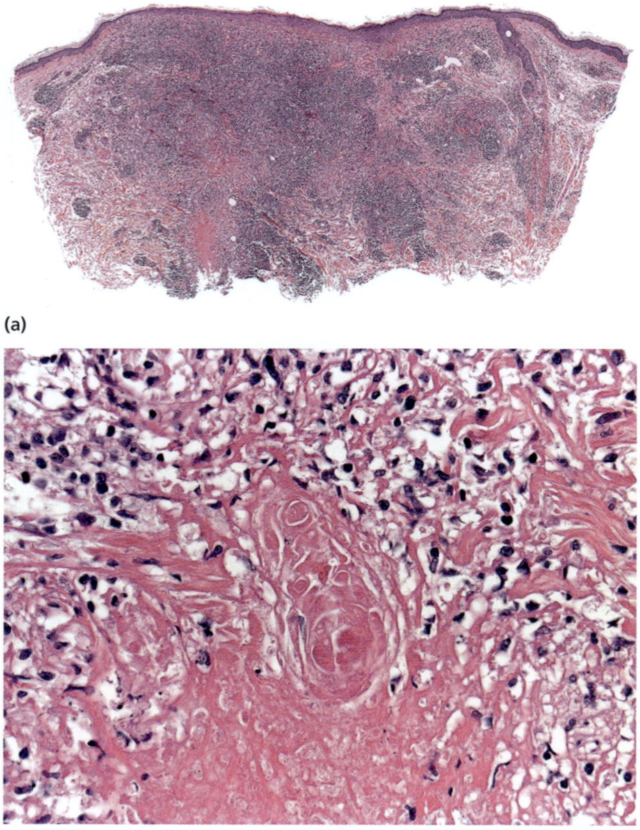

(a)

(b)

Figure 31.71 Pseudolymphomatous herpes zoster. (a) Dense lymphoid infiltrates within the entire dermis. (b) Focal, small area of necrosis of the hair follicle and surrounding tissue.

erythematosus (interface dermatitis) [141]. Another criterion for the diagnosis of lupus panniculitis is the presence of clusters of plasmacytoid dendritic cells positive for CD123 (Fig. 31.78) [142–144]. The T lymphocytes in lupus panniculitis are a mixture of $CD4^+$ helper and $CD8^+$ cytotoxic lymphocytes, with $CD4^+$ cells often being the predominant ones. The proliferation rate is low and proliferating cells are not arranged around the adipocytes (Fig. 31.79) [145]. Different numbers of c-myc + cells have been described in the infiltrate in the two conditions (more numerous in subcutaneous panniculitis-like T-cell lymphoma) [146]. Analysis of TCR genes rearrangement reveals polyclonal populations of T lymphocytes in lupus panniculitis, in contrast to subcutaneous panniculitis-like T-cell lymphoma where monoclonality of T lymphocytes is found in most cases.

Although lupus panniculitis and subcutaneous panniculitis-like T-cell lymphoma can be differentiated in most cases, some patients may present with clinical features suggestive of lupus erythematosus (e.g., positivity of ANA and/or subsets, features of lupus erythematosus in organs other than the skin such as lupus nephritis), and at the same time skin lesions with histopathological features indistinguishable from those of subcutaneous

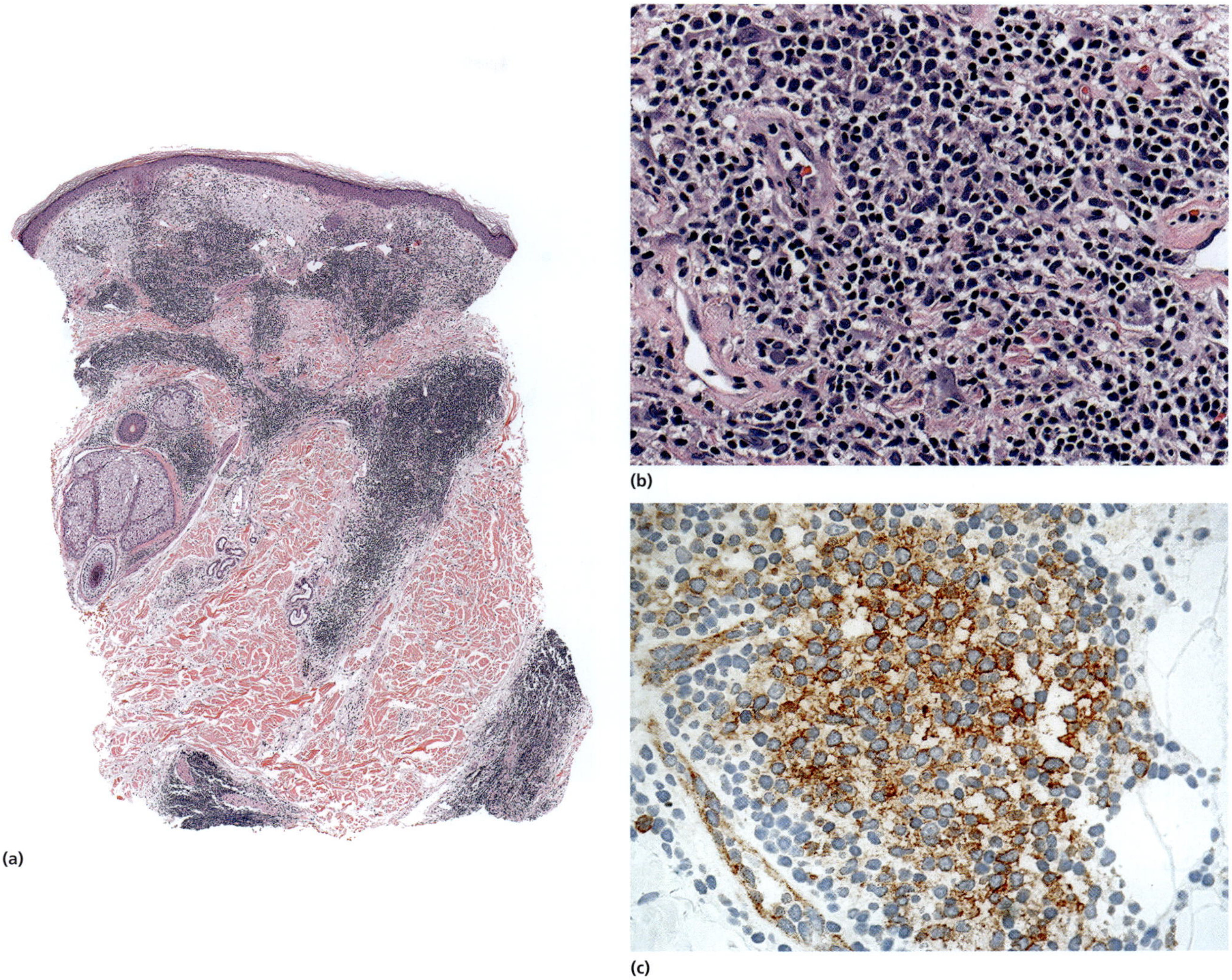

Figure 31.72 Lupus erythematosus, tumidus type (so-called lymphocytic infiltration of Jessner–Kanof). (a) Dense lymphoid infiltrates around the vessels and appendageal structures in the entire dermis and visible subcutaneous fat. (b) Predominance of small lymphocytes admixed with some larger, activated cells. (c) Staining for CD123 highlights a large cluster of plasmacytoid dendritic cells.

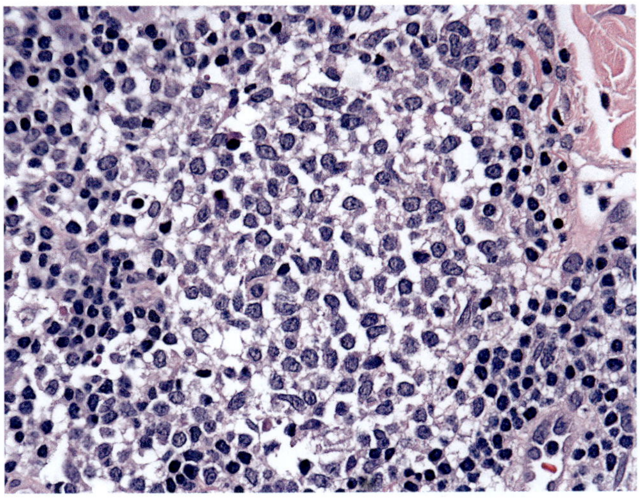

Figure 31.73 Lupus erythematosus, tumidus type. A large cluster of plasmacytoid dendritic cells. Clusters of plasmacytoid dendritic cells may mimic germinal centers morphologically.

panniculitis-like T-cell lymphoma [147]. In addition, in some patients, biopsy specimens reveal histopathological features of lupus panniculitis in some areas of the specimen, but suggestive of subcutaneous panniculitis-like T-cell lymphoma in other areas [148]. The term "atypical" lupus panniculitis may be used for such cases. A detailed discussion of these cases is presented in Chapter 6.

A condition similar to lupus panniculitis and subcutaneous panniculitis-like T-cell lymphoma can be observed in children with congenital immunodeficiencies, even with monoclonality of the T-cell infiltrate (see the section on pseudolymphomatous cutaneous infiltrates in human immunodeficiency virus (HIV)-infected patients and in other immune deficiencies in this chapter). Lipoatrophic panniculitis of the ankles in childhood is another rare disease of young patients that may simulate histopathologically a subcutaneous panniculitis-like T-cell lymphoma [149]. Differential diagnostic features in these cases are similar to those discussed for lupus panniculitis. Although

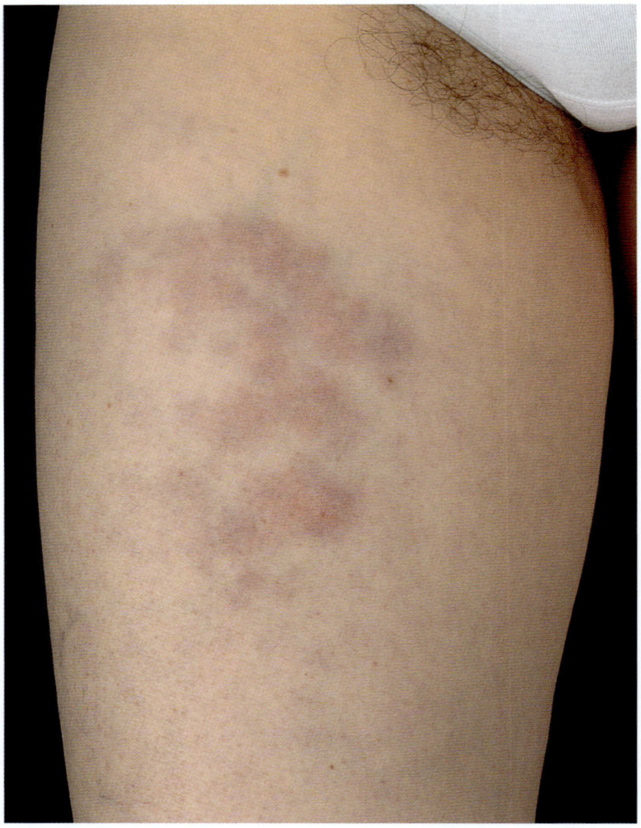

Figure 31.74 Lupus panniculitis. Erythematous, infiltrated plaques on the right thigh.

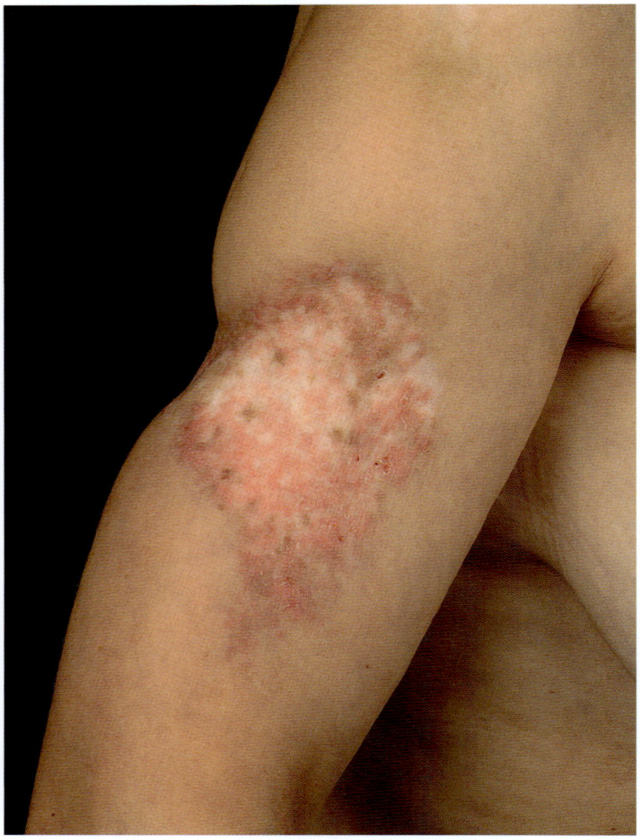

Figure 31.75 Lupus panniculitis. Late lesion showing pronounced subcutaneous atrophy and skin features identical to those of chronic cutaneous lupus erythematosus.

subcutaneous panniculitis-like T-cell lymphoma can occur in children, care should be taken not to overdiagnose the disease in this age group.

### Other pseudolymphomas associated with cutaneous lupus erythematosus

Besides the pseudolymphomatous presentations just described, in patients with cutaneous lupus erythematosus angiocentric/angiodestructive infiltrates characterized by the presence of mid-sized and large atypical cells have been described (Fig. 31.80) [137]. Some of the vessels show thrombotic occlusions. In contrast to lymphomas with angiodestructive features, the affected vessels are located mostly in the superficial and mid-dermis, and the overlying epidermis reveals features of an interface dermatitis. Immunohistology shows that the cells have a predominant T-helper phenotype with negativity for cytotoxic granules, thus ruling out the diagnosis of cytotoxic lymphoma by definition. Many of the perivascular cells are $CD123^+$ plasmacytoid dendritic cells. In situ hybridization for EBV is negative. Clinically, the lesions do not deviate from those observed in various types of cutaneous lupus erythematosus. Some of the patients presenting with these unusual features have an elevated titer of anti-cardiolipin antibodies, even in the absence of other clinical manifestations of the antiphospholipid syndrome. Particularly if the patients are under immunosuppressive treatment, concern for a lymphoproliferative disorder may arise; thus, careful analysis of the skin biopsy, in situ hybridization for EBV, and correlation with the clinical picture are mandatory.

Another pseudolymphomatous presentation of lupus erythematosus mimics mycosis fungoides histopathologically, and it is characterized by dense, band-like infiltrates of lymphocytes with several intraepidermal cells and with large cells within the infiltrate (Figs. 31.81a and b) [137]. Most of the large cells are $CD123^+$ plasmacytoid dendritic cells located within the infiltrate and also at the dermo-epidermal junction and/or within the epidermis (Figs. 31.81c). In some cases, small intraepidermal collections of cells admixed with keratinocytes may resemble Darier nests (Fig. 31.82). The phenotype of the lymphocytes may be indistinguishable from that observed in mycosis fungoides, but as already mentioned, staining for CD123 invariably shows the presence of many positive cells at the dermo-epidermal junction and within the epidermis, representing a very valuable diagnostic clue [144, 150]. Lupus erythematosus can also present with the clinical picture of milia en plaques, thus simulating histopathologically pilotropic mycosis fungoides [151]; as in other unusual presentations of the disease, the presence of clusters of $CD123^+$ plasmacytoid dendritic cells in lupus erythematosus represents a good clue for the differential diagnosis.

Treatment of pseudolymphomas associated with lupus erythematosus is similar to that of other variants of cutaneous

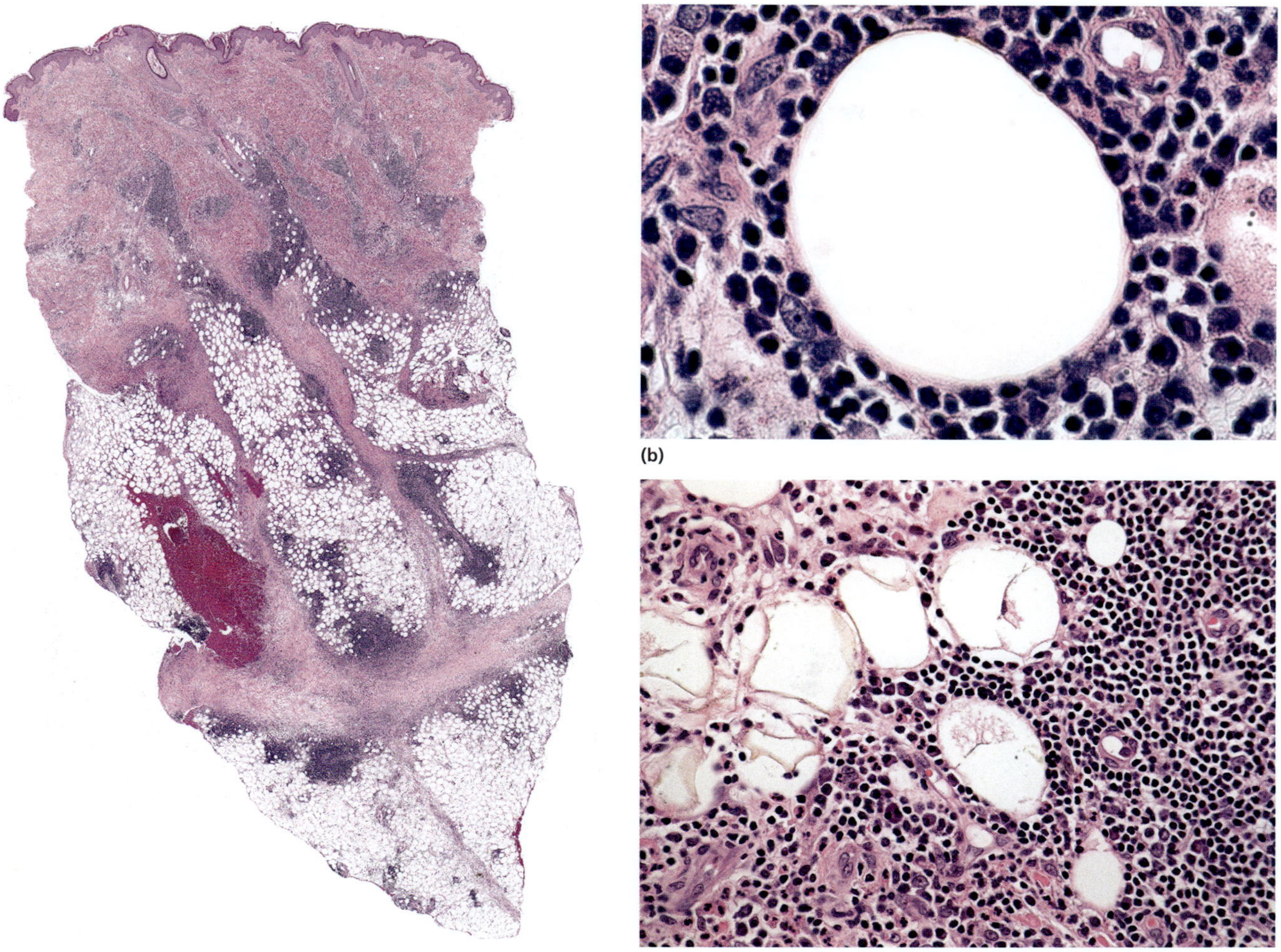

(a) (b) (c)

**Figure 31.76** Lupus panniculitis. (a) Lobular panniculitis with dense lymphoid infiltrates and fibrotic septa. Note lymphoid infiltrates also in the dermis. (b) Mixed-cell infiltrate with lymphocytes, histiocytes, neutrophils, and several plasma cells. (c) “Pseudo-rimming” of the adipocytes surrounded by small lymphocytes, histiocytes and plasma cells rather than by neoplastic, pleomorphic lymphocytes as in genuine rimming.

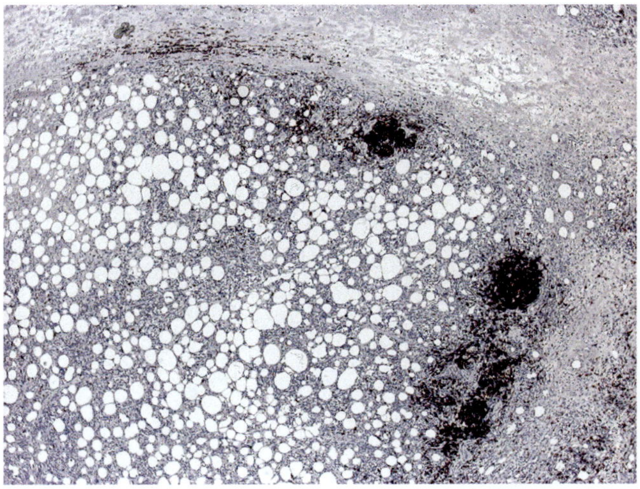

**Figure 31.77** Lupus panniculitis. Clusters of CD20+ B lymphocytes at the periphery of the fat lobules.

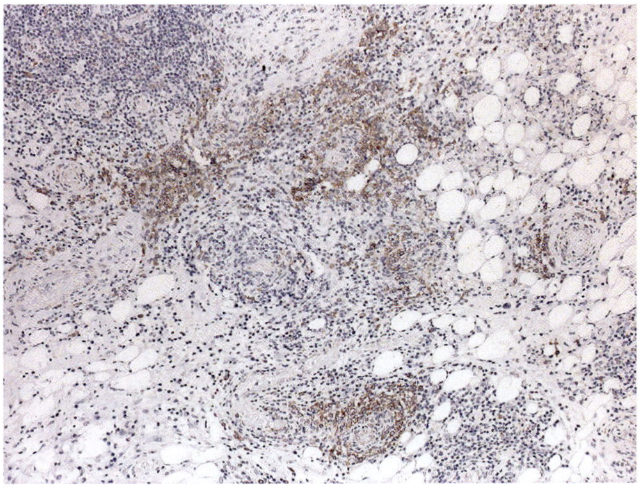

**Figure 31.78** Lupus panniculitis. Staining for CD123 shows several clusters of plasmacytoid dendritic cells.

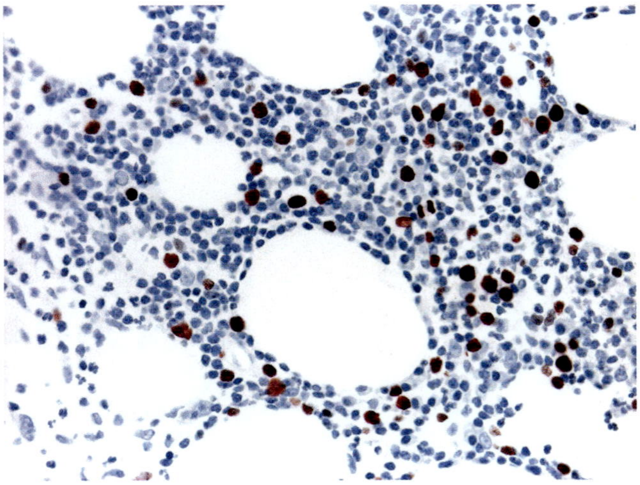

Figure 31.79 Lupus panniculitis. Staining for Ki-67 shows proliferation of a small minority of the cells. Note absence of "rimming" of proliferating cells around the adipocytes.

lupus erythematosus. The lesions respond well to antimalarics, systemic steroids, or other systemic therapies, but upon discontinuation of the treatment recurrences (not necessarily with the same pseudolymphomatous features!) are common.

## Lymphomatoid drug reactions

A pseudolymphoma syndrome characterized by generalized lymphadenopathy, hepatosplenomegaly, leukocytosis, fever, malaise, arthralgia, severe edema of the face, and cutaneous lesions such as erythematous pruritic macules, papules, and nodules has been described in patients treated with anticonvulsants, particularly hydantoin derivatives. Many other drugs may induce lymphoid infiltrates in the skin that simulate malignant lymphoma clinically and/or histopathologically [152–155]. The external use of etheric plant oils may also cause lymphoproliferative reactions that mimic malignant lymphomas, both clinically and histopathologically.

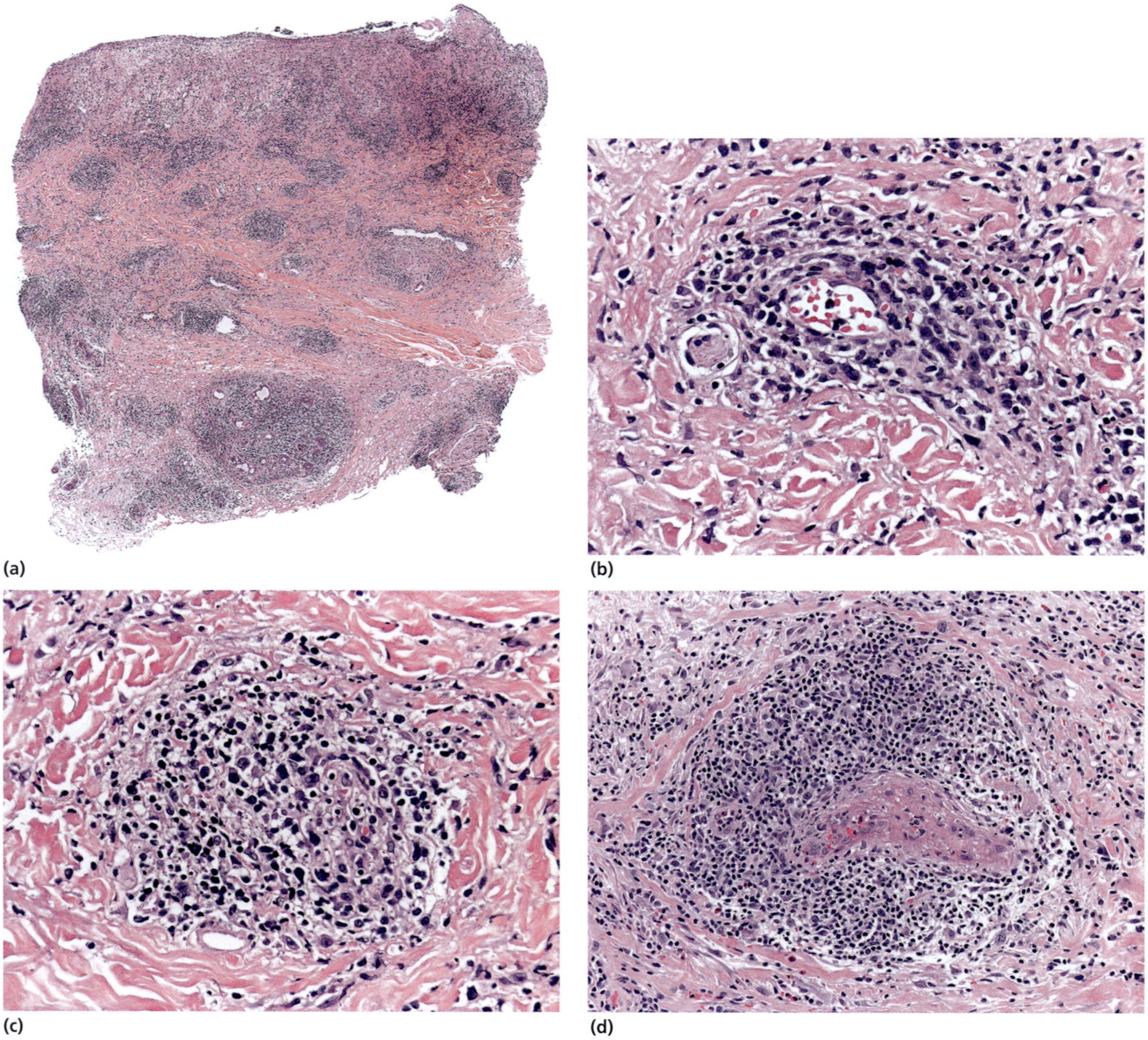

Figure 31.80 Lupus erythematosus. (a) Dense lymphoid infiltrates around the vessels in the entire dermis, with (b, c) several large lymphocytes within the infiltrate mimicking the picture of an "angiotropic" lymphoma. (d) In another case one vessel is occluded by a fibrin thrombus.

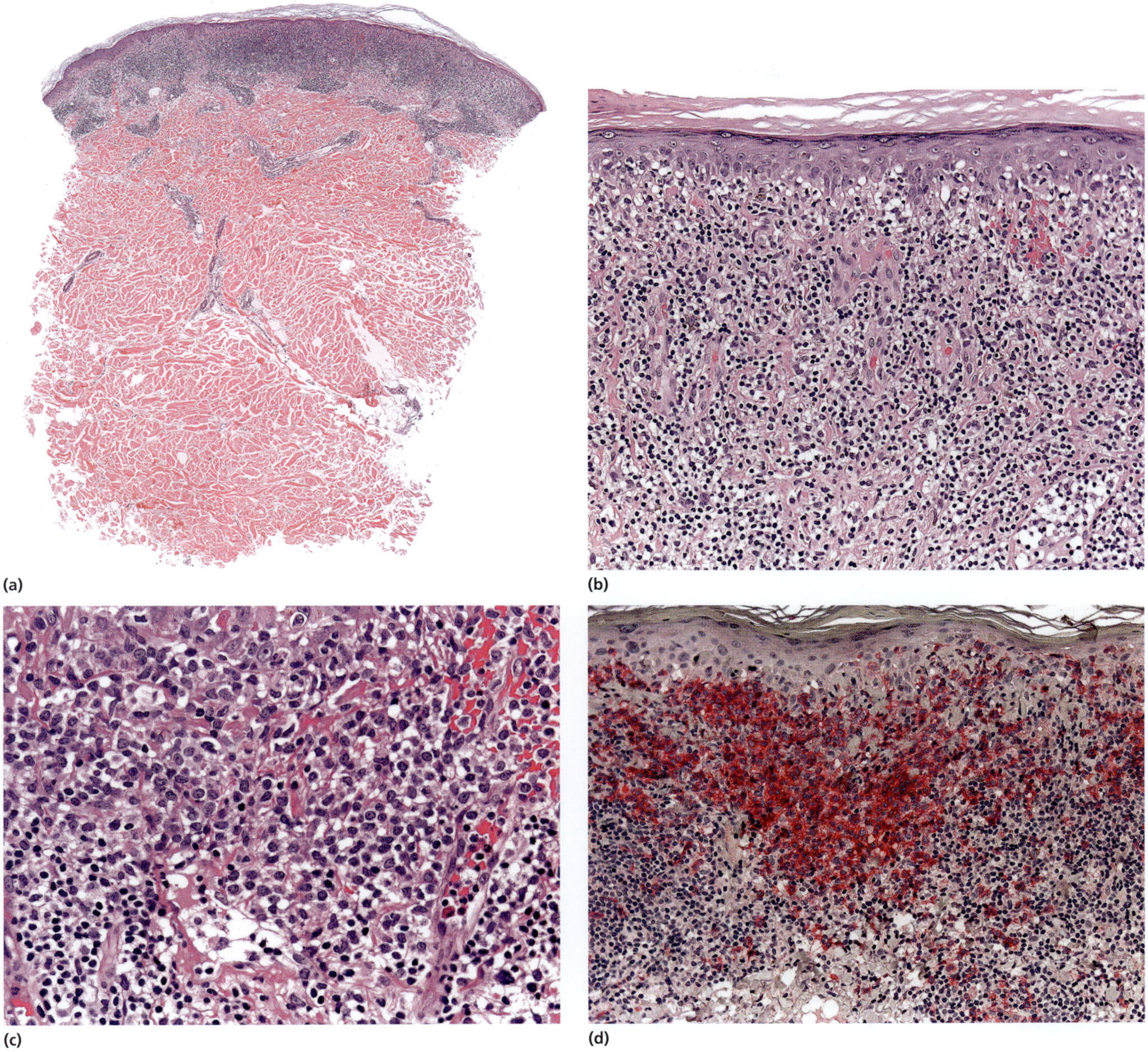

Figure 31.81 Lupus erythematosus. (a, b) Dense band-like infiltrate in the superficial dermis with (c) several mid-sized and large cells. (d) Staining for CD123 reveals the presence of numerous plasmacytoid dendritic cells (representing the majority of mid-sized and large cells).

Lymphomatoid drug eruptions may present with a T- or B-cell pattern, simulating either mycosis fungoides, Sézary syndrome, follicle center lymphoma, or marginal zone lymphoproliferative disorder [154, 155]. A rare type of lymphomatoid drug eruption with many $CD30^+$ cells may mimic the $CD30^+$ cutaneous lymphoproliferative disorders [156, 157]. It should be noted that the same drug may be responsible for cutaneous lesions with different histopathologic features and phenotypes in different patients.

Pseudolymphomatous drug eruptions with a T-cell pattern are characterized clinically by an exanthematic, generalized eruption or even by erythroderma (Fig. 31.83). Accentuation of skin changes in sun-exposed areas ("photoaggravation") may occur, and, when present, is a clue to differentiate these lesions from mycosis fungoides. Histology reveals dense, band-like infiltrates of small lymphocytes admixed with mid-sized and large activated ("atypical") T-lymphocytes (Figs. 31.84a and b). Eosinophils are usually present (but do not represent a differential diagnostic clue). Follicular mucinosis has been detected rarely [158]. The activated lymphocytes are usually positive for CD30 and may be the source of diagnostic concern (Fig. 31.84c). Paradoxically, the

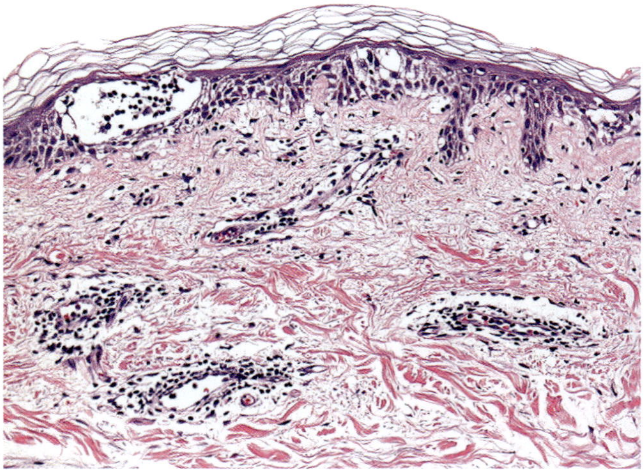

Figure 31.82 Lupus erythematosus. Aggregates of intraepidermal cells mimicking Darier nests.

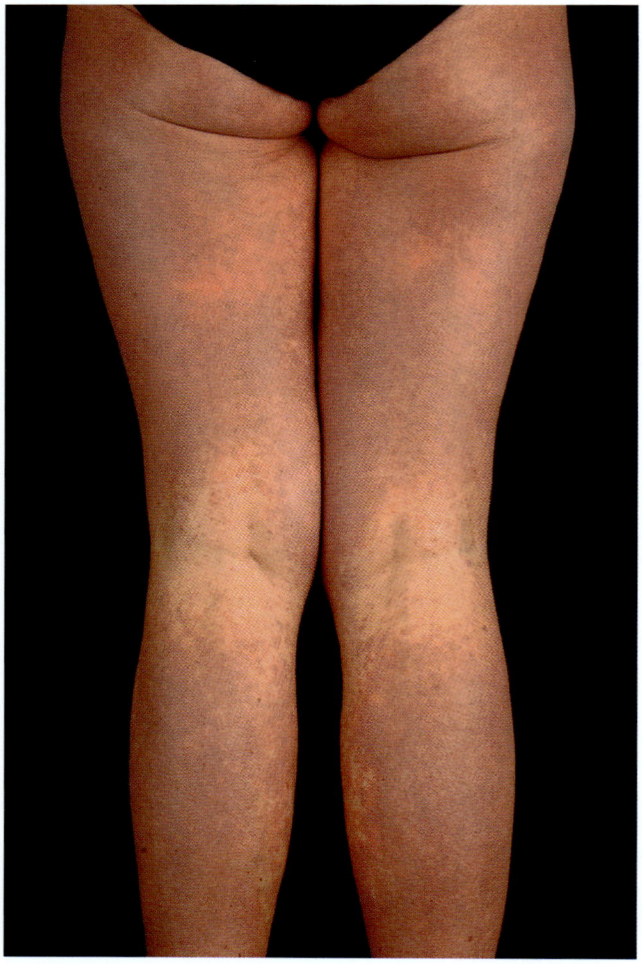

Figure 31.83 Lymphomatoid drug eruption, T-cell type. Confluent erythematous-livid macules on both legs.

cytomorphological atypia and the very high proliferation that is found in many of these cases (sometimes close to 100% – Fig. 31.84d) are a good clue to distinguish them from early mycosis fungoides, in which the proliferation rate is never that high and cytomorphologic atypia is mild or even absent. Molecular analysis of TCR genes usually shows a polyclonal pattern, but monoclonality may be observed.

Pseudolymphomatous drug eruptions revealing a B-cell pattern are characterized clinically by multiple, sometimes generalized papules or small nodules (Fig. 31.85). In these cases, the histopathologic changes are those of lymphadenosis benigna cutis (lymphocytoma cutis) with the formation of reactive germinal centers (Fig. 31.86). Eosinophils may or may not be present. Molecular analysis of Ig genes shows a polyclonal pattern.

I have observed rarely a peculiar type of pseudolymphomatous drug eruption with a B-cell pattern mimicking cutaneous marginal zone lymphoproliferative disorder in patients with metastatic melanoma, at the injection site of talimogene laherparepvec (T-VEC) (a genetically engineered herpes simplex virus type 1 – HSV-1). Biopsies taken at several sites of previous cutaneous metastases injected with T-VEC showed large nodules of plasma cells with monotypic expression of one immunoglobulin light chain (Fig. 31.87). Distinction from marginal zone lymphoproliferative disorder was impossible on pure histopathological grounds. None of these lesions progressed to overt lymphoma, and complete resolution was achieved with local treatment only [159]. A similar cutaneous reaction mimicking histopathologically marginal zone lymphoproliferative disorder was observed also in a patient receiving neoadjuvant cemiplimab therapy for squamous cell carcinoma [160]. Interestingly, a pseudolymphomatous T-cell infiltrate has been observed also in the re-excision specimen of a nodular melanoma before any systemic or local treatment, other than the previous surgical excision, was administered [161].

Lymphomatoid drug reactions invariably regress when the offending drug is withdrawn and recur if the same or a similar compound is reintroduced. In exceptional cases, the development of a true cutaneous lymphoma has been observed in relation to the use of drugs that commonly induce lymphomatoid drug eruptions [162]. On the other hand, patients with systemic leukemias/lymphomas (or cutaneous lymphomas in advanced stages) may present with drug eruptions characterized by colonization of the skin lesions by neoplastic cells admixed with the inflammatory infiltrate (see the section on mogamulizumab in this chapter). In short, the interplay between the immune system (in both normal and neoplastic conditions) and drugs that induce immunologic reactions is probably much more complicated than the dichotomy benign/malignant implies, and patients with lymphomatoid drug eruptions characterized histopathologically by markedly atypical infiltrates should be evaluated in order to exclude the presence of an occult hematologic disease.

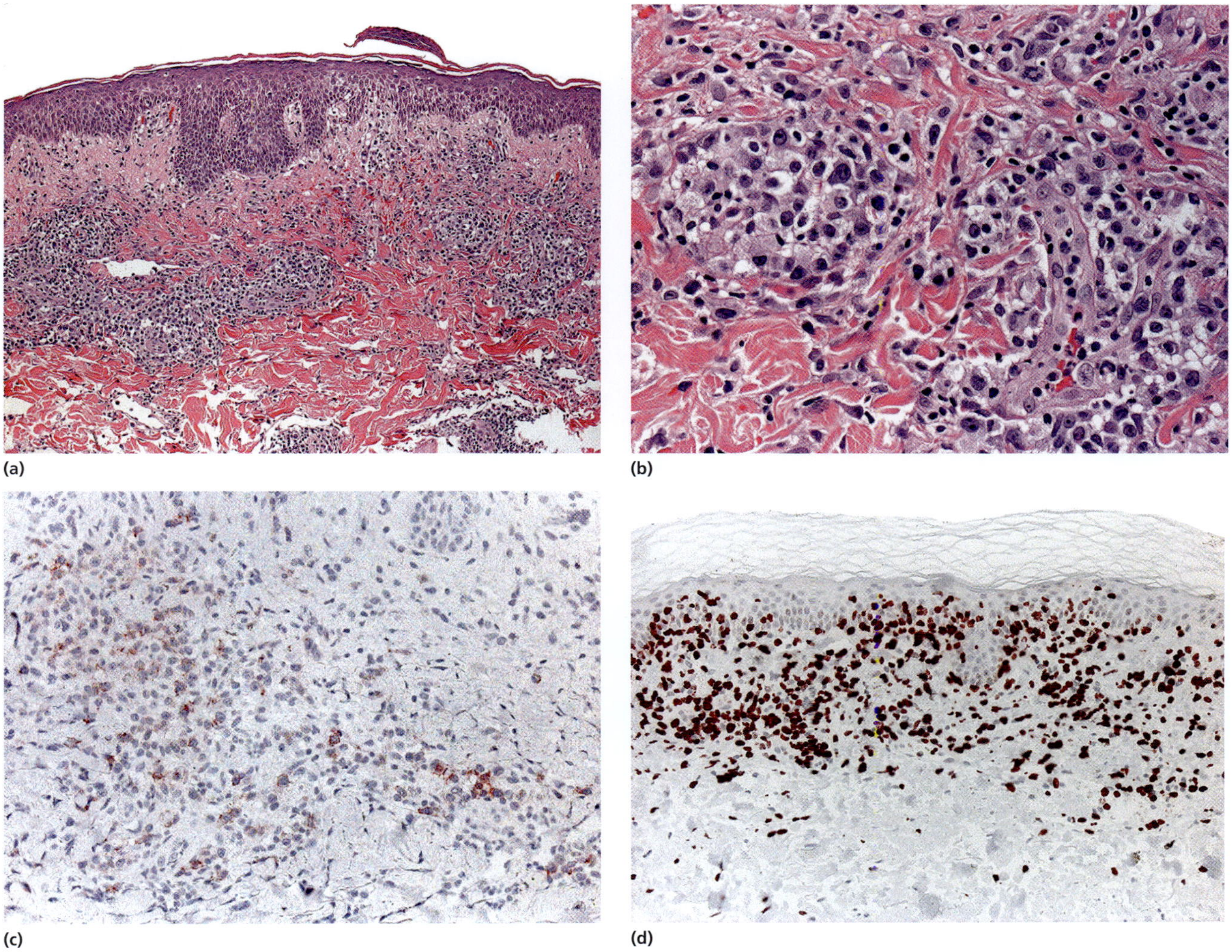

**Figure 31.84** Lymphomatoid drug eruption, T-cell type. (a) Patchy lichenoid infiltrate of lymphocytes within the superficial dermis. (b) Note several pleomorphic lymphocytes. (c) Staining for CD30 reveals positivity of the larger cells. (d) Staining for Ki-67 shows proliferation of almost all lymphocytes.

## Lymphocytoma cutis

Lymphocytoma cutis is a generic term used to describe cutaneous pseudolymphomas of different etiology, characterized histopathologically by the presence of reactive germinal centers. Several synonyms have been used for lymphocytoma cutis, including lymphadenosis benigna cutis, cutaneous lymphoplasia, cutaneous lymphoid hyperplasia, and pseudolymphoma of Spiegler–Fendt. Most of the cases reported in the literature are associated with infection by different species of *B. burgdorferi*; *Borrelia*-associated lymphocytoma cutis is discussed in detail in a specific section in this chapter. Various other antigenic stimuli can induce lymphocytoma cutis, including insect bites, drugs, vaccinations, acupuncture, wearing of gold pierced earrings, medicinal leech therapy, and tattoos, among others. A similar histopathological picture has been observed also in cutaneous lesions associated with cutaneous *Leishmania* infection [163, 164]. Finally, a pseudolymphomatous infiltrate with numerous reactive germinal centers may be observed rarely also in cases of angiolymphoid hyperplasia with eosinophilia.

Lymphocytoma cutis can occur in both genders of any age. Clinically, a solitary nodule is a frequent presentation, but lesions may be clustered in a region or, rarely, be scattered widely (Fig. 31.88). Besides nodules or small tumors, papules or plaques may also be observed. A miliary pattern of the lesions has been reported [165]. The color varies from reddish brown to reddish purple. Scaling and ulceration are usually absent.

Histologic examination of cases of lymphocytoma cutis that are not related to *B. burgdorferi* shows "top-heavy," nodular mixed cell infiltrates with the formation of reactive lymphoid follicles (Fig. 31.89a). The germinal centers display benign

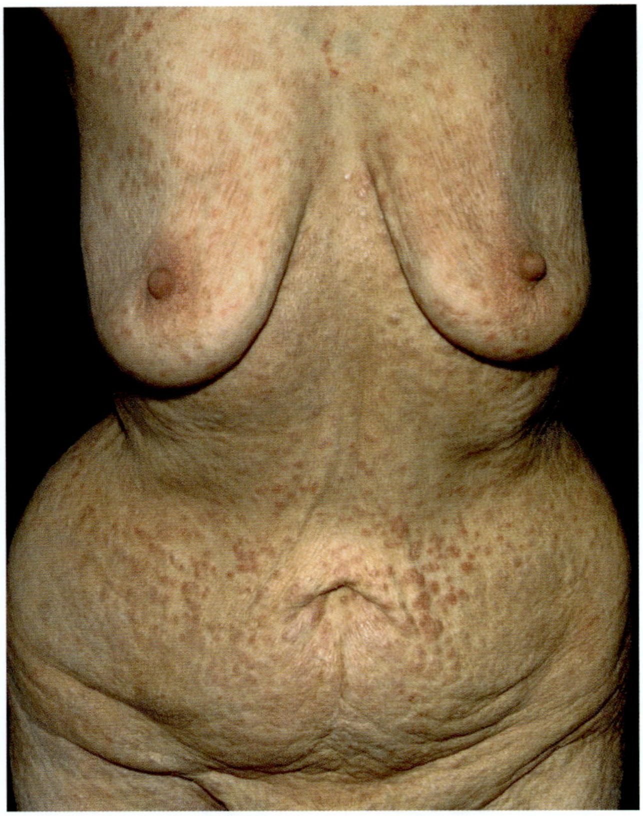

Figure 31.85 Lymphomatoid drug eruption, B-cell type. Generalized papules and small nodules.

features and are usually easily differentiated from malignant follicles of follicular B-cell lymphoma (Fig. 31.89b). Histopathologic criteria for differentiation of reactive germinal centers from malignant lymphoid follicles are summarized in Table 31.4. Cases associated with *Leishmania* infection represent examples of cutaneous leishmaniasis ("oriental sore") [163, 164]. Pseudoepitheliomatous epithelial hyperplasia is a common finding in such cases, and reactive germinal centers are usually found in the deeper portion of the infiltrate (Fig. 31.90). It should be mentioned that cutaneous leishmaniasis may present also with pseudolymphomatous infiltrates devoid of reactive germinal centers, and is characterized by a broad spectrum of histopathologic presentations [166a]. Although cutaneous leishmaniasis is considered to belong to the granulomatous infectious disorders, granulomatous features may be minimal or absent in some cases, and predominance of small and medium-sized lymphocytes may confer to the lesion a pseudolymphomatous appearance (Fig. 31.91). Large cells may be positive for CD30 and mimic a cutaneous $CD30^+$ lymphoproliferative disorder. In all types of cutaneous leishmaniasis, the microorganisms should be searched for in the subepidermal portion of the infiltrate, where they appear within the cytoplasm of histiocytes as 2–4 μm round to oval basophilic structures with an eccentrically located kinetoplast (Fig. 31.91c).

Immunohistology in all types of lymphocytoma cutis reveals a normal phenotype of germinal center cells ($CD20^+$, Bcl-$6^+$, $CD10^+$, Bcl-$2^-$), and a normal (high) proliferation (Fig. 31.92).

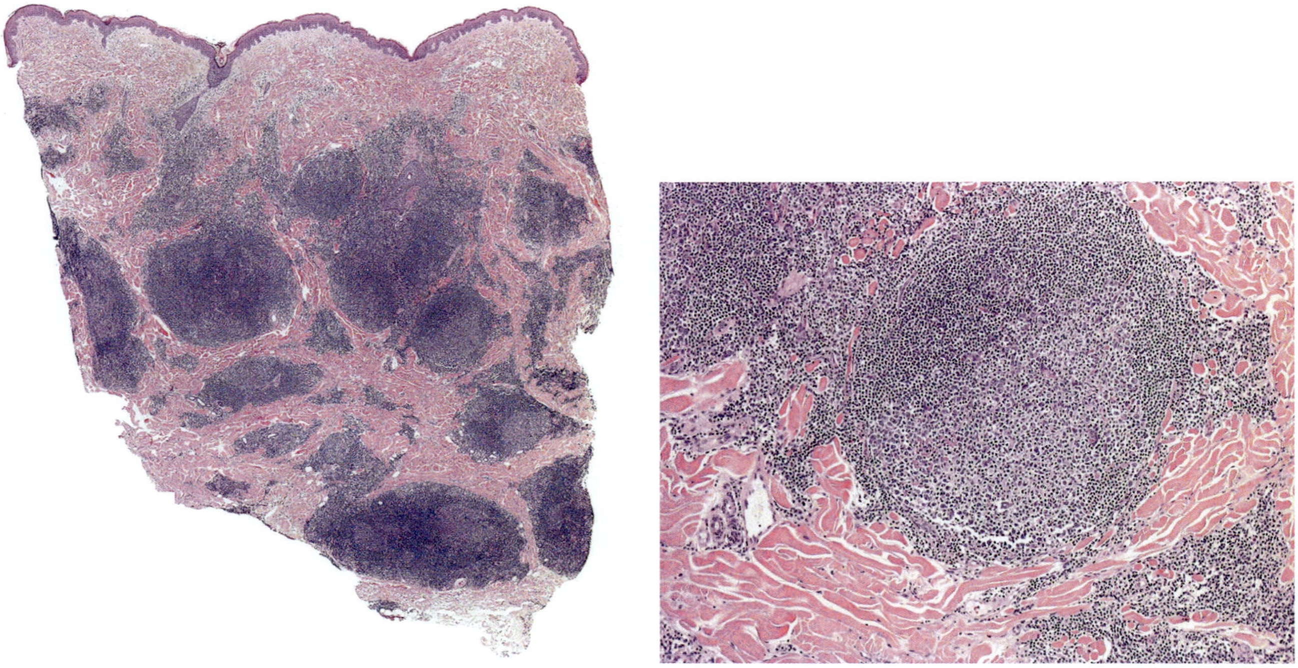

(a) (b)

Figure 31.86 Lymphomatoid drug eruption, B-cell type. (a) Dense infiltrates of lymphocytes within the entire dermis. (b) Detail of a reactive germinal center with normal mantle.

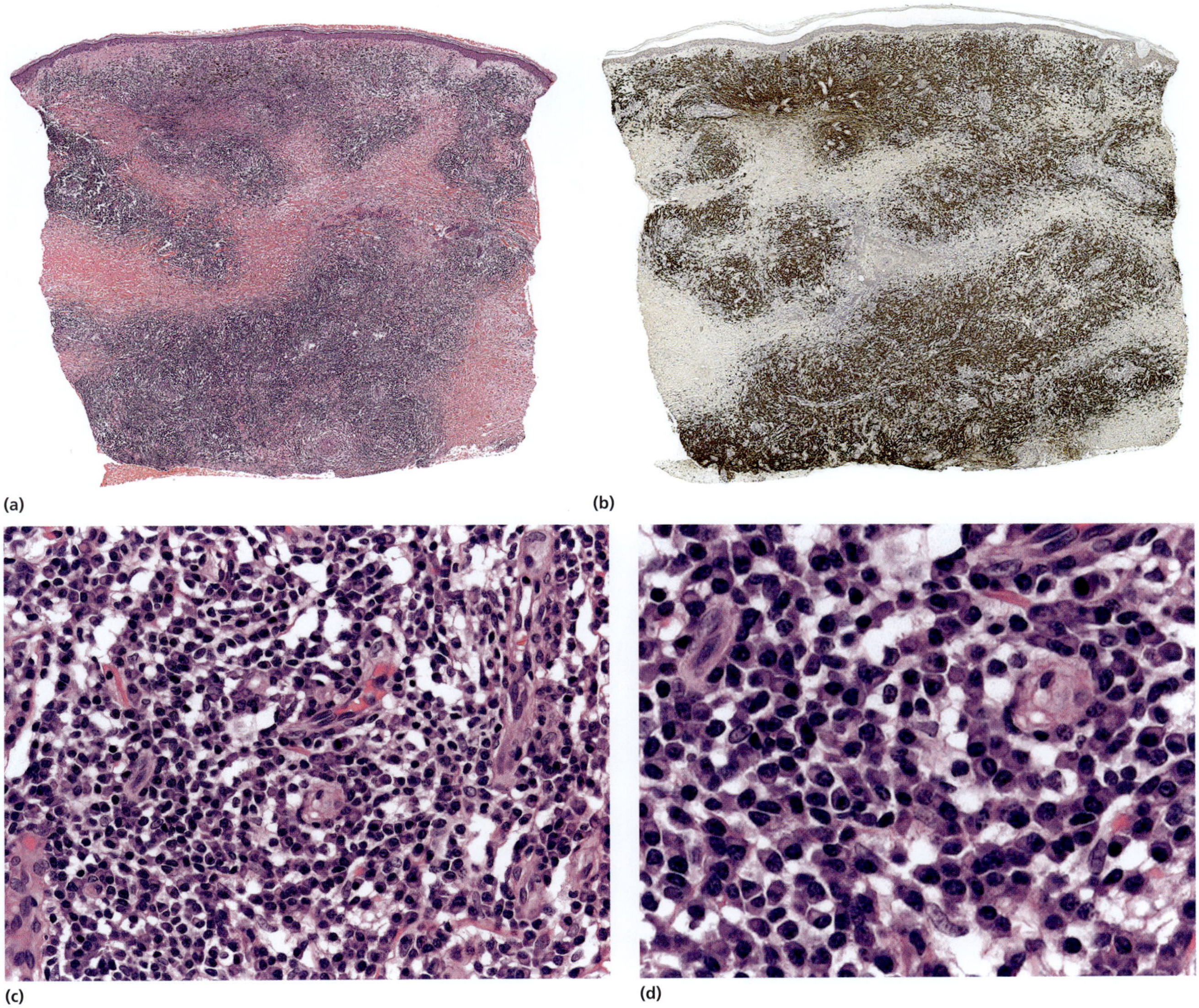

Figure 31.87 Lymphomatoid drug eruption, B-cell type. (a) Dense dermal infiltrates, (b) showing a monoclonal expression of the immunoglobulin light chain kappa. (c, d) The infiltrate is composed almost exclusively of mature plasma cells.

A regular network of follicular dendritic cells can be highlighted with stainings for CD21 or CD35. A prominent population of reactive T lymphocytes is always present. Molecular analysis of the Ig genes rearrangement shows a polyclonal population of B lymphocytes.

Lymphocytoma cutis may resolve spontaneously in several months or years. Small nodules can be removed by surgical excision and local injection of corticosteroids or interferon-α may result in regression. Cryosurgery and topical tacrolimus have also been applied with success. In refractory lesions, a very effective treatment method is local radiotherapy. Ona case was successfully treated with dupilumab [166b].

## Pseudolymphomas associated with infections by *Borrelia* species

***Borrelia lymphocytoma*** represents one of the most typical examples of lymphocytoma cutis, particularly in European countries with endemic *Borrelia* infection [167]. *Borrelia* lymphocytoma is observed in Europe but is very uncommon in other countries with endemic Lyme disease such as the United States, due to the prevalence of different strains of the microorganisms in different areas of the world. In fact, the disease is linked with *Borrelia* species found mostly in Europe, such as *Borrelia afzelii* and occasionally *Borrelia garinii* and *Borrelia*

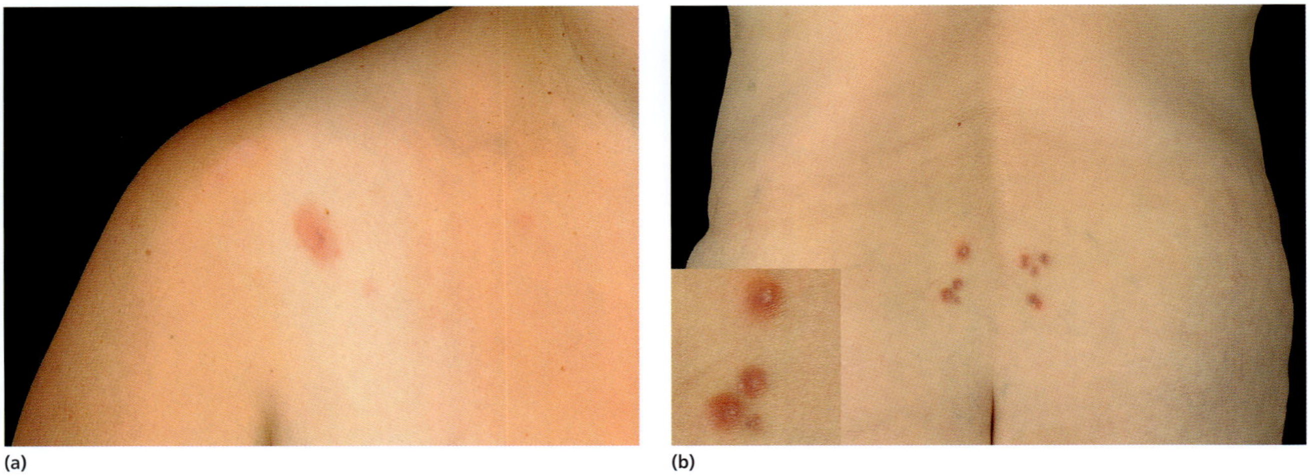

Figure 31.88 Lymphocytoma cutis. (a) Solitary plaque on the shoulder related to an arthropod bite. (b) Localized reddish papules in the lumbal area after local application of leeches (*Hirudo medicinalis*) (detail of the lesions in the inset).

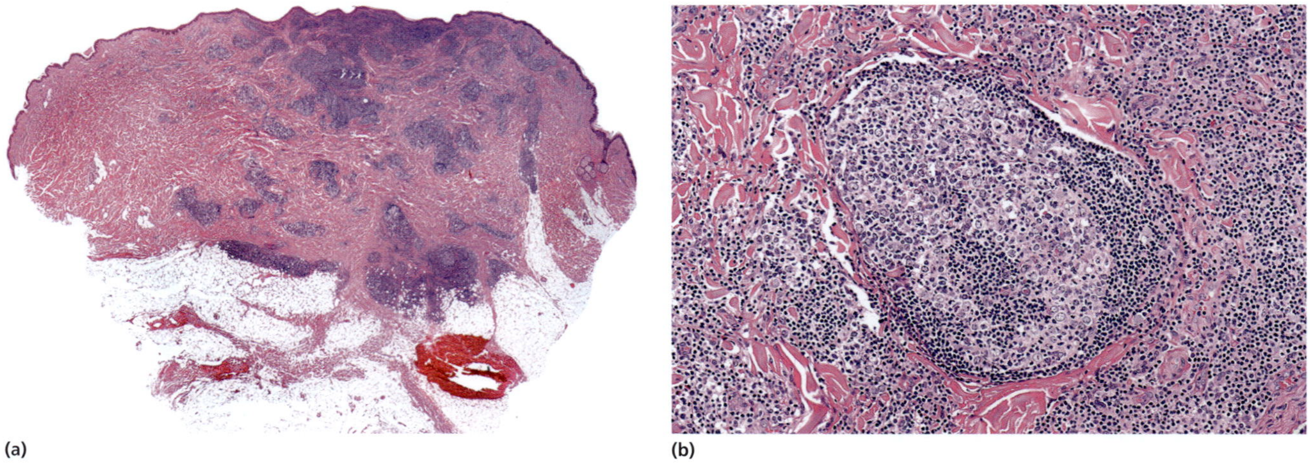

Figure 31.89 Lymphocytoma cutis. (a) Lymphoid infiltrate within the entire dermis. (b) Small germinal center with some tingible body macrophages.

**Table 31.4** Histopathological and immunohistochemical criteria for differentiation of reactive germinal centers in lymphocytoma cutis from malignant lymphoid follicles in cutaneous follicle center lymphoma#

| Lymphocytoma cutis | Follicle center lymphoma |
|---|---|
| Presence of normal mantle zone | Mantle zone absent or markedly reduced |
| Presence of tangible body macrophages | Tingible body macrophages absent |
| Presence of polarization of the lymphoid follicle (i.e., of "dark" and "light" areas) | Monomorphous follicles without polarization |
| Lymphoid follicles do not show confluence, and present as well circumscribed round or oval structures* | Some lymphoid follicles may show confluence in large, irregular structures |
| Complete negativity of the follicle center cells for Bcl-2 | Staining for Bcl-2 shows positivity in a variable proportion (usually a minority) of follicle center cells |
| Clusters of CD20+/Bcl-6+ follicle center cells are confined to well defined germinal centers | Small clusters of CD20+/Bcl-6+ follicle center cells are found outside of the lymphoid follicles§ |
| Strong proliferation in 100% of the cells detected by Ki-67 staining | Reduced proliferation, sometimes <50% of the cells |
| Strong and well circumscribed pattern of staining for CD21 (follicular dendritic cells) | Staining for CD21 shows in some areas "consumption," that is, a faint and not well defined staining |

# Not all features may be present at the same time in all reactive germinal centers or all malignant lymphoid follicles.

§ care should be taken not to misinterpret CD3+/Bcl-6+ T follicular helper cells for cells of the lymphoid follicles; T follicular helper cells are never arranged in large clusters in cutaneous B-cell lymphoproliferative disorders.

* An exception to this rule is represented by lymphocytoma cutis associated with Borrelia infection, in which germinal centers may both lack a distinct mantle and show confluence in large structures, sometimes mimicking the picture of a diffuse large B-cell lymphoma (see section on Borrelia lymphocytoma).

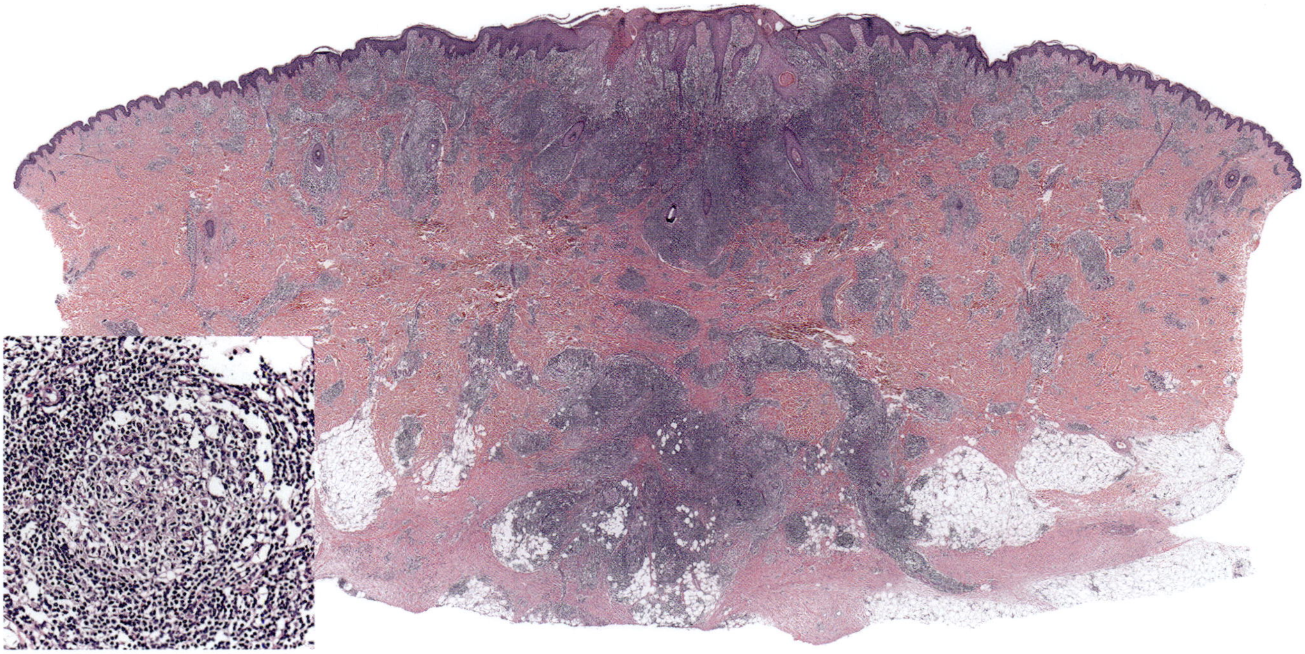

**Figure 31.90** Lymphocytoma cutis associated with infection by *Leishmania* ("oriental sore"). Dense lymphoid infiltrates with small, reactive germinal centers (inset). Note pseudoepitheliomatous hyperplasia of the epidermis in the center of the specimen.

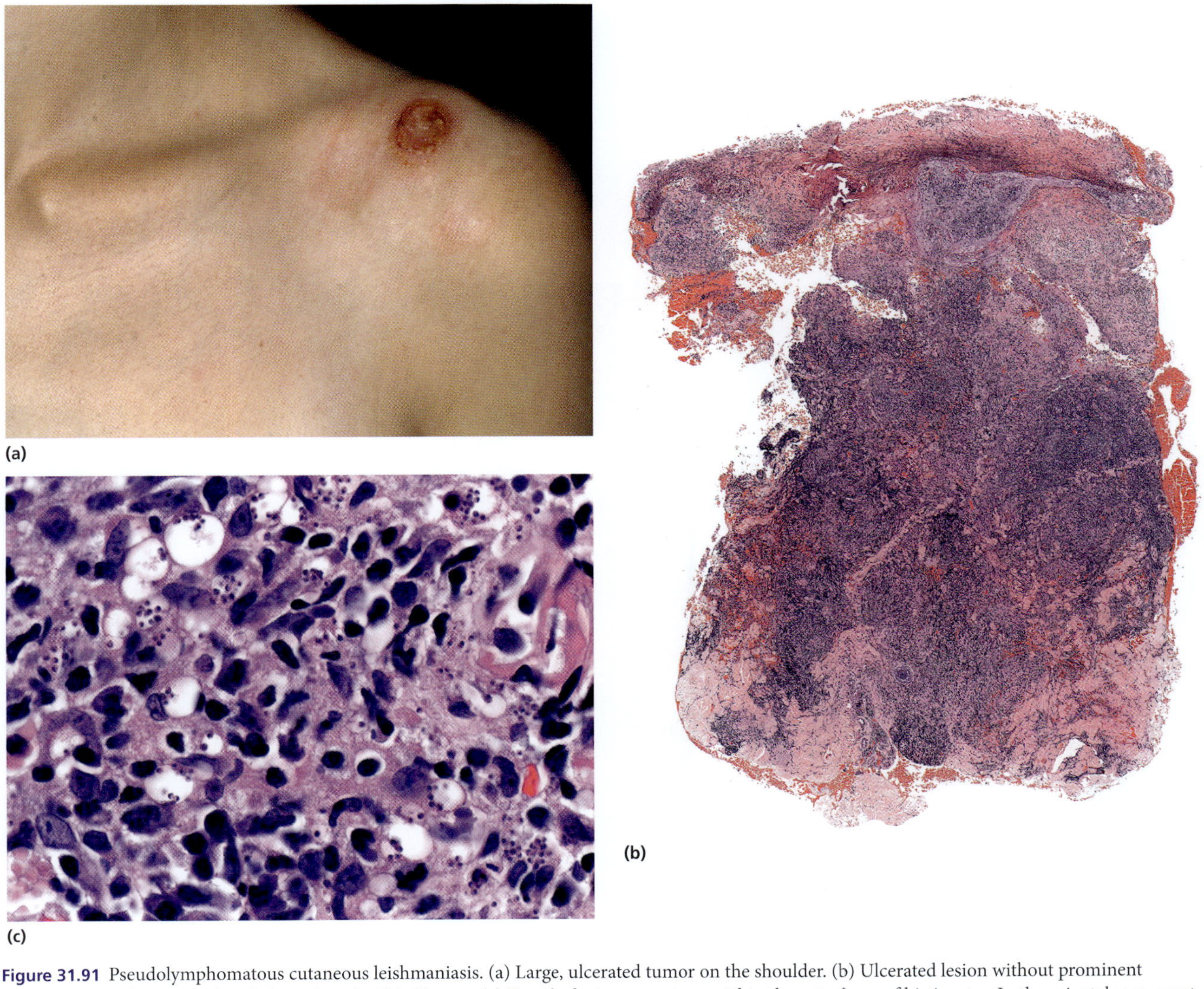

(a)

(b)

(c)

**Figure 31.91** Pseudolymphomatous cutaneous leishmaniasis. (a) Large, ulcerated tumor on the shoulder. (b) Ulcerated lesion without prominent granulomatous features and with dense lymphoid infiltrates. (c) Detail of microorganisms within the cytoplasm of histiocytes. In the oriental sore, most microorganisms are usually located in the superficial part of the lesion.

*bissettii* [168]. Although some cases are due to infection by *B. burgdorferi* sensu strictu, which is found in Europe and is the main strain found in the United States as well, as already mentioned cases of *Borrelia* lymphocytoma are exceedingly rare in the United States.

*Borrelia* lymphocytoma occurs in children as well as in adults, and is the most frequent type of pseudolymphoma in pediatric patients in European regions with endemic *Borrelia* infection. It represents mostly an early manifestation of the disease; thus, the serum antibodies may be negative at first presentation and become positive only over time. The patients usually do not have systemic symptoms of Lyme disease. A solitary nodule is a frequent presentation, located mostly on the earlobe, nipple, or genital area (Fig. 31.93) [167]. A symmetrical distribution has been observed rarely [169, 170]. The color varies from reddish brown to reddish purple. Scaling and ulceration are absent.

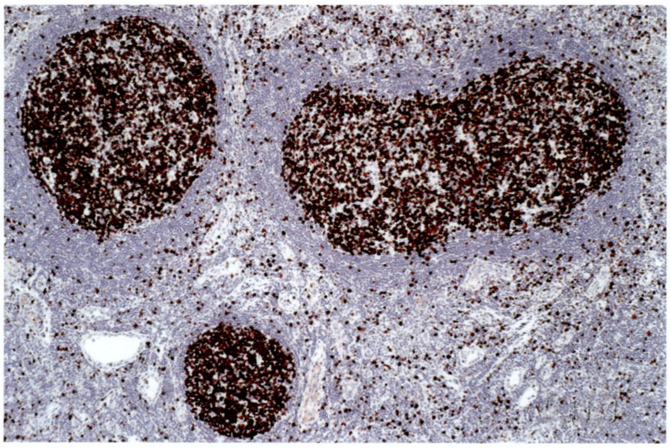

**Figure 31.92** Lymphocytoma cutis. Staining with Ki-67 shows germinal centers with normal (high) proliferation rate. Note normal mantle zone around the Ki-67+ germinal centers.

Histologic examination shows dense, diffuse lymphoid infiltrates involving the entire dermis and superficial subcutaneous fat (Fig. 31.94). In contrast to other variants of lymphocytoma cutis, the reactive germinal centers in *Borrelia*-associated cases are often devoid of mantle zones and commonly show confluence, simulating the histopathologic picture of a diffuse large B-cell lymphoma (Fig. 31.95). A typical feature is the finding of large, confluent germinal centers with indistinct borders and with a "starry sky" pattern due to numerous tingible body macrophages (Fig. 31.95b). Plasma cells, eosinophils, and a distinct population of T lymphocytes are found in almost all cases, features that represent useful clues for the differential diagnosis. It must be underlined that the atypical morphological features of *Borrelia*-associated lymphocytoma cutis have been the cause of severe diagnostic mistakes, as fully benign lesions were diagnosed as aggressive B-cell lymphomas and treated accordingly [171]. For practical purposes, B-cell lymphoid infiltrates arising at sites typical for *Borrelia* infection, namely, the earlobe, nipple, and genital area should be diagnosed as malignant lymphoma only upon compelling evidence (the obvious exception

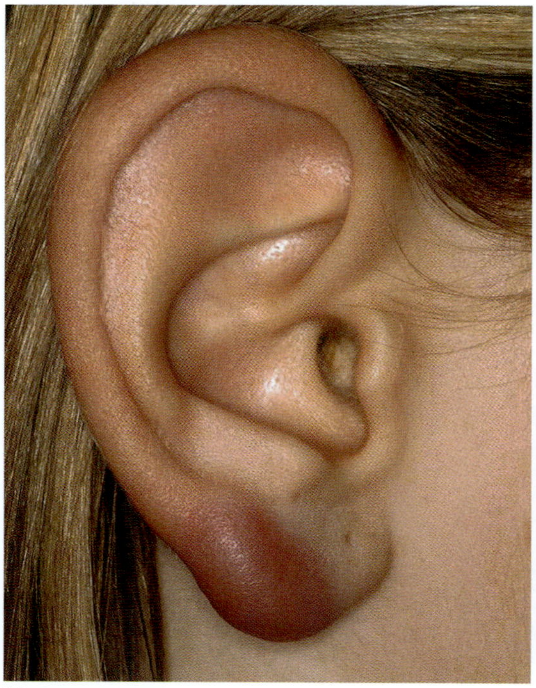

(a)

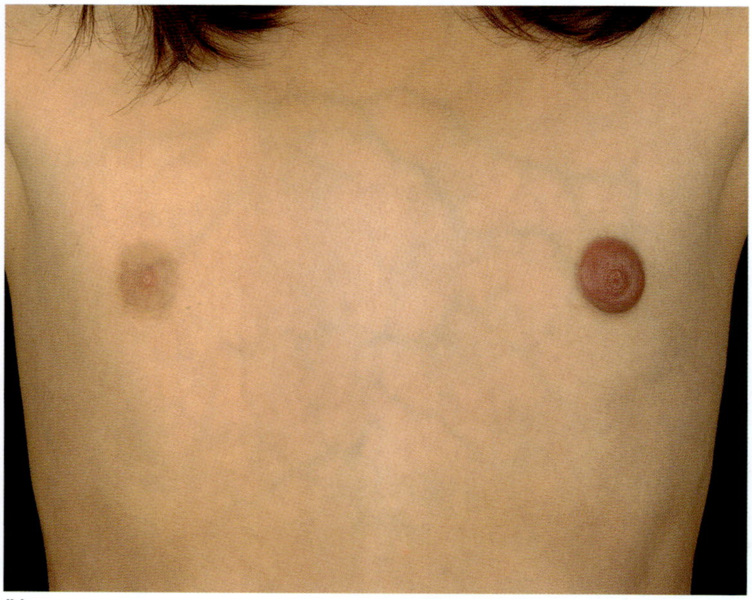

(b)

**Figure 31.93** Lymphocytoma cutis associated with infection by *Borrelia*. (a) Erythematous nodule on the right earlobe. (b) Erythematous nodule on the left nipple. These are two common locations of *Borrelia*-associated lymphocytoma cutis.

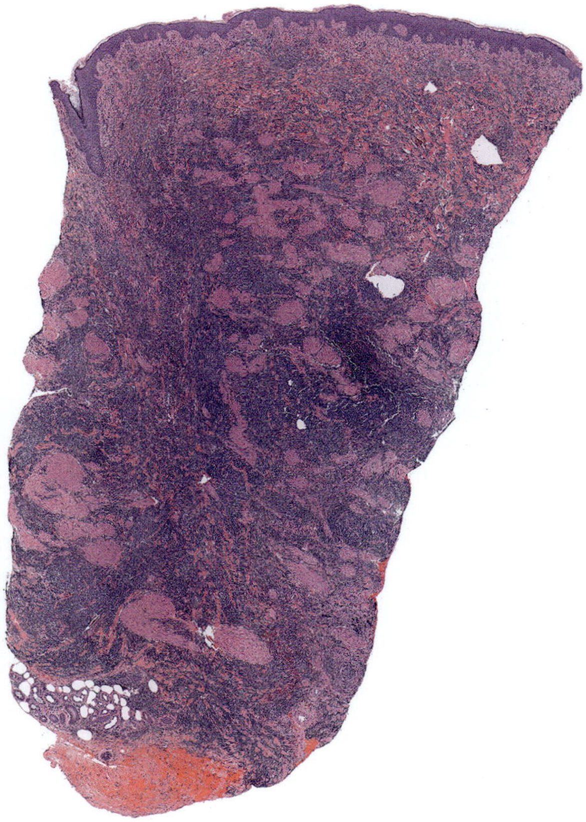

**Figure 31.94** Lymphocytoma cutis associated with infection by *Borrelia*. Dense, diffuse lymphoid infiltrates within the entire dermis. The germinal centers are devoid of well-formed mantles.

to this rule being represented by specific infiltrates of B-CLL arising at sites of and associated with *Borrelia* infection – see Chapter 22).

Immunohistology reveals a pattern similar to that observed in lymphocytoma cutis related to other causes, with reactive features of the germinal centers (see above and Table 31.4). The networks of follicular dendritic cells in cases associated with *Borrelia* infection, however, may be large and irregular, reflecting the atypical features observed histopathologically (Fig. 31.96). Molecular analysis for *Borrelia* species shows the presence of specific DNA sequences. Analysis of the Ig genes rearrangement shows a polyclonal pattern in most (but not all) cases [167].

*Borrelia*-associated lymphocytoma cutis is unrelated to erythema chronicum migrans, which represents the most frequent variant of early cutaneous manifestation in Lyme disease. As a rule, erythema chronicum migrans does not present with clinical or histopathological features of a pseudolymphoma. However, rare cases may show infiltrated lesions clinically, and the picture of *Borrelia*-associated lymphocytoma cutis histopathologically (Fig. 31.97), showing that cutaneous manifestations of Lyme disease are protean and may present with overlapping clinicopathological features. The reason why some patients with *Borrelia* infection develop pseudolymphomas with a T-cell pattern (pseudolymphomatous acrodermatitis chronica atrophicans, see below), while others present with lesions showing a B-cell pattern has not been elucidated yet. However, a different pattern of chemokines has been demonstrated in different manifestations of Lyme disease in Europe: erythema migrans and acrodermatitis chronica atrophicans show high levels of the T-cell-active

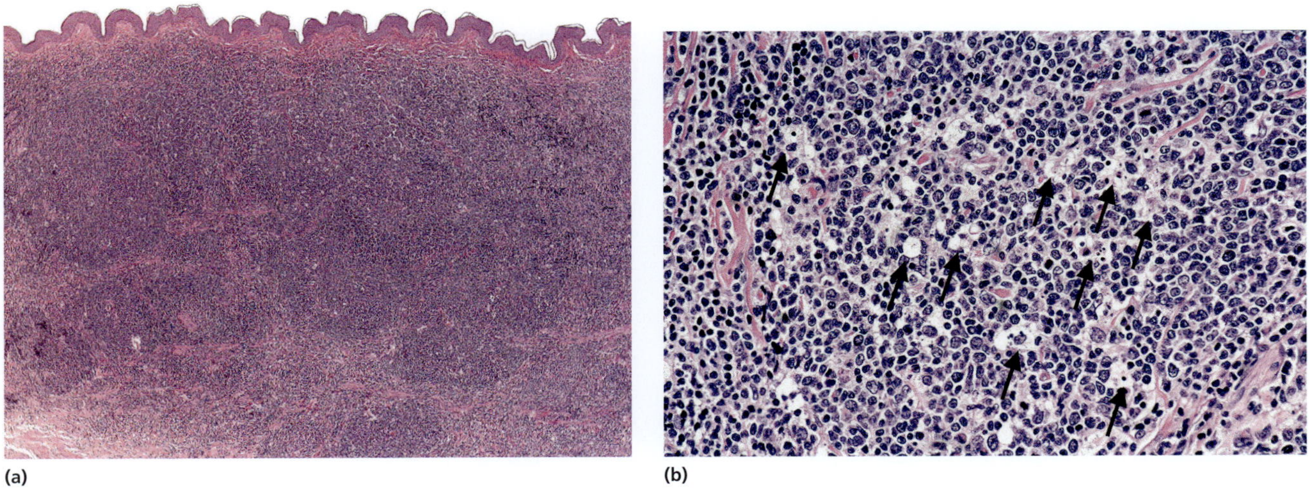

**Figure 31.95** Lymphocytoma cutis associated with infection by *Borrelia*. (a) Several large, confluent germinal centers with many tingible body macrophages but devoid of a mantle zone, conveying the impression of a large cell lymphoma with a "starry sky" pattern. (b) Ill-defined germinal center with large blastic cells (centroblasts, large centrocytes) admixed with several "tingible body" macrophages characterized by large empty spaces with debris of apoptotic cells (arrows).

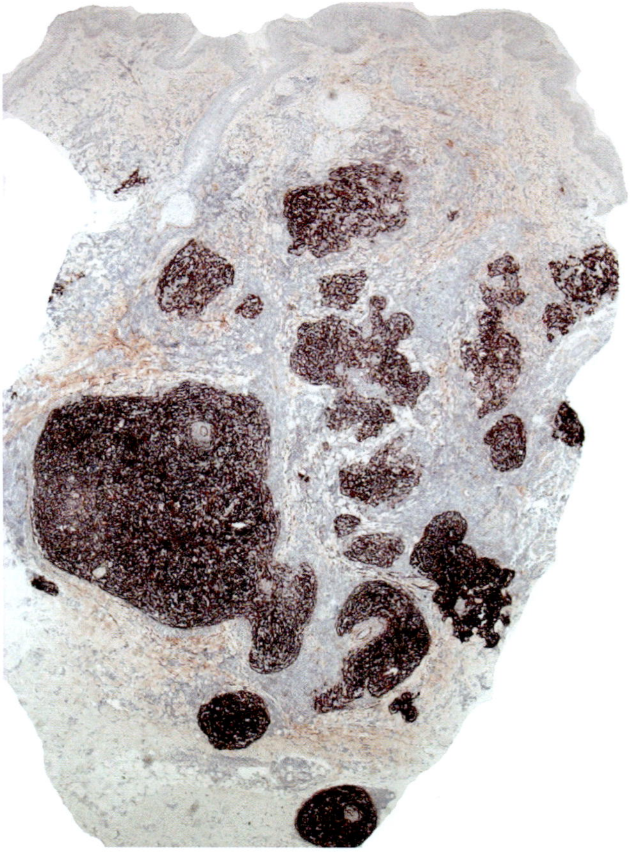

**Figure 31.96** Lymphocytoma cutis associated with infection by *Borrelia*. Large, irregular, partly confluent germinal centers highlighted by a network of CD21+ follicular dendritic cells.

chemokines CXCL9 and CXCL10, whereas *Borrelia*-associated lymphocytoma cutis has high levels of the B-cell-active chemokine CXCL13, thus providing a potential explanation for the histopathological and phenotypic differences [172].

Lesions of lymphocytoma cutis associated with *Borrelia* infection respond to conventional antibiotic treatment with doxycycline, erythromycin, or ceftriaxone.

***Acrodermatitis chronica atrophicans*** is a late cutaneous manifestation of infection by *B. afzelii*. It typically affects elderly individuals, particularly women, usually involving the dorsal surfaces of acral sites. In conventional cases, the infiltrate is moderately dense and does not present differential diagnostic problems with cutaneous lymphomas. Sometimes, however, dense, dermal lymphoid infiltrates may be present [173]. Clinically, patients present with lesions more infiltrated than in conventional acrodermatitis chronica atrophicans (Fig. 31.98). Rarely, cutaneous tumors have been described [174].

Two main histopathological patterns are observed in pseudolymphomatous acrodermatitis chronica atrophicans: one is characterized by dense, band-like infiltrates of T lymphocytes with only a few plasma cells, simulating the histopathologic picture of mycosis fungoides (Fig. 31.99). The benign nature of the infiltrate in these cases is suggested by the small number of intraepidermal lymphocytes, the absence of atypia, and the polyclonal rearrangement of TCR genes. It is important to realize that in cases of acrodermatitis chronica atrophicans with pseudolymphomatous infiltrates this pattern is the most common one, in contrast to the predominance of B-cells observed in other *Borrelia*-associated cutaneous pseudolymphomas and lymphomas.

The second pseudolymphomatous histopathologic pattern of acrodermatitis chronica atrophicans is characterized by large, diffuse aggregates of mature plasma cells (Fig. 31.100), simulating a cutaneous marginal zone lymphoproliferative disorder. The benign nature of the infiltrate in these cases is confirmed by the polyclonal expression of the immunoglobulin light chains kappa and lambda. In both patterns PCR analysis of *Borrelia* DNA demonstrates a positive signal.

Two cases of acrodermatitis chronica atrophicans with monoclonal plasma cells have been reported [175]. However, a diagnosis of marginal zone lymphoproliferative disorder seems to be more appropriate in cases showing monoclonality of the B-cell compartment, as *Borrelia*-associated B-cell lymphomas are well characterized [176], and cutaneous lymphomas arising on the background of chronic *Borrelia* infections have been described [177].

Pseudolymphomatous acrodermatitis chronica atrophicans should be treated like the conventional variant of the disease. The lesions disappear slowly (several weeks or months) after antibiotic treatment.

Besides *Borrelia* lymphocytoma and acrodermatitis chronica atrophicans, I have observed rare cases of cutaneous *Borrelia* infection characterized by a presentation with clustered papular lesions clinically, and ***pseudolymphomatous superficial lymphoid infiltrates*** histopathologically. Such cases show the presence of nodules of B lymphocytes on the background of predominant T cells and of sparse, polytypic plasma cells (Fig. 31.101). Some of these cases most likely represented examples of erythema migrans with papules and small plaques located within the area of the figurate erythema (Fig. 31.102). Other cases were characterized by infiltrated erythematous plaques revealing histopathological features of lymphocytoma cutis, yet in a clinical context different from conventional *Borrelia* lymphocytoma (Fig. 31.97). These cases do not show the typical clinicopathological aspects of erythema migrans, acrodermatitis chronica atrophicans or lymphocytoma, and represent a pitfall in the diagnosis. Cases of ***lobular panniculitis*** associated with infection by *Borrelia* and mimicking subcutaneous panniculitis-like T-cell lymphoma have been reported as well [178, 179]. In endemic countries, as a general rule a dense cutaneous lymphoid infiltrate composed of B- and T-lymphocytes admixed with polytypic plasma cells should always be investigated for association with *Borrelia* infection (syphilis representing a further differential diagnosis).

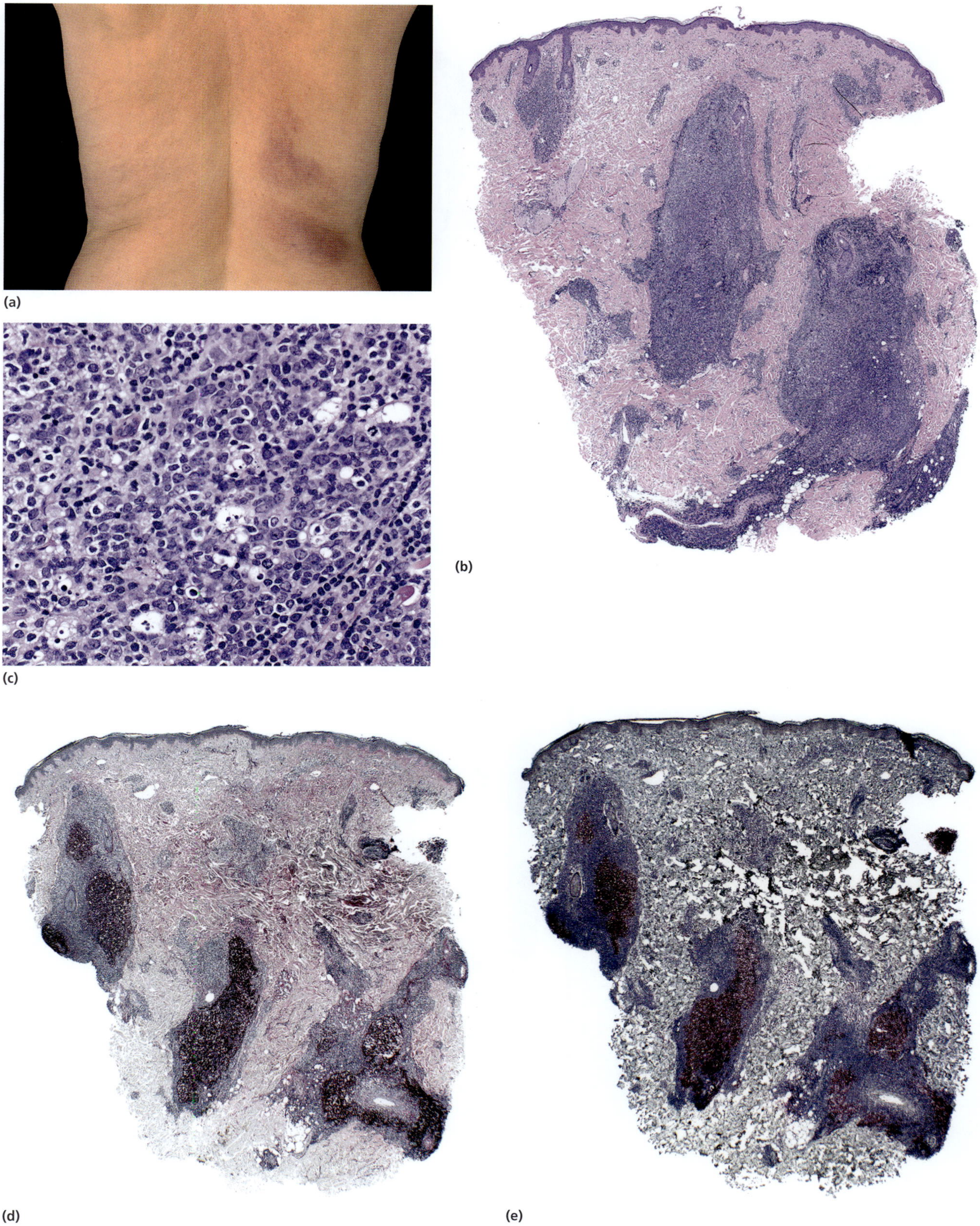


**Figure 31.97** *Borrelia*-associated lymphocytoma cutis in erythema chronicum migrans. (a) Clinical presentation with two large, infiltrated plaques on the back, one showing a central area of clearing. (b) Dense, diffuse infiltrate within the entire dermis with (c) large germinal centers with numerous tingible body macrophages. (d) Large, irregular clusters of CD21+ follicular dendritic cells, and (e) clusters of Bcl-6+ germinal center lymphocytes which are (f) negative for Bcl-2. (g) Staining for Ki-67 reveals a normal (high) proliferation rate of the germinal centers.

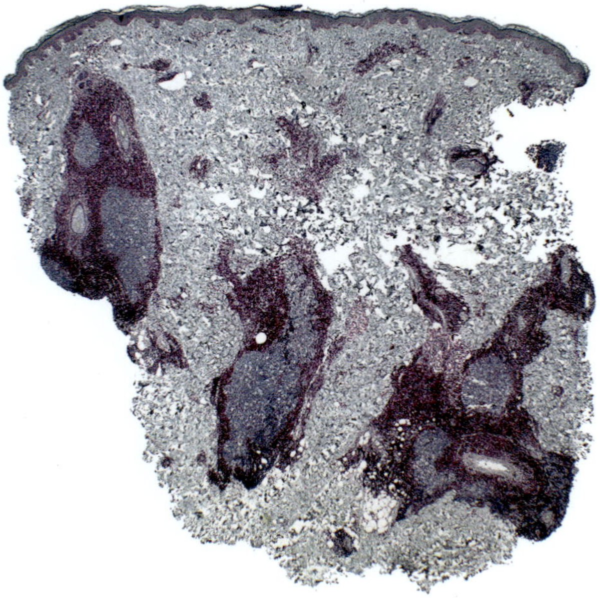

(f)

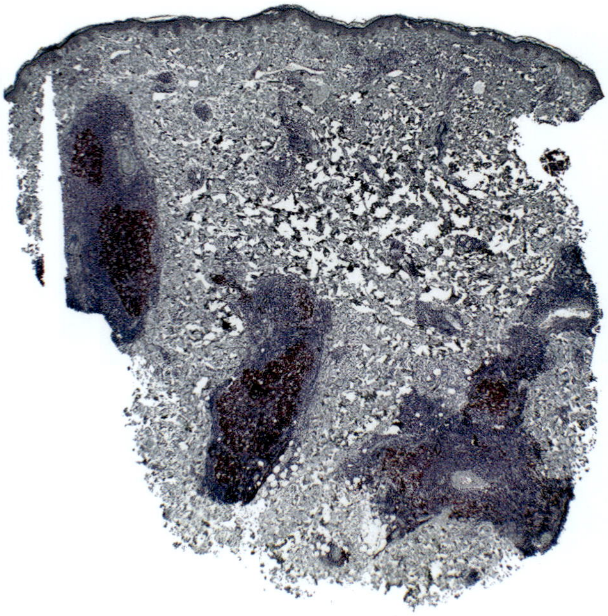

(g)

Figure 31.97 (Continued)

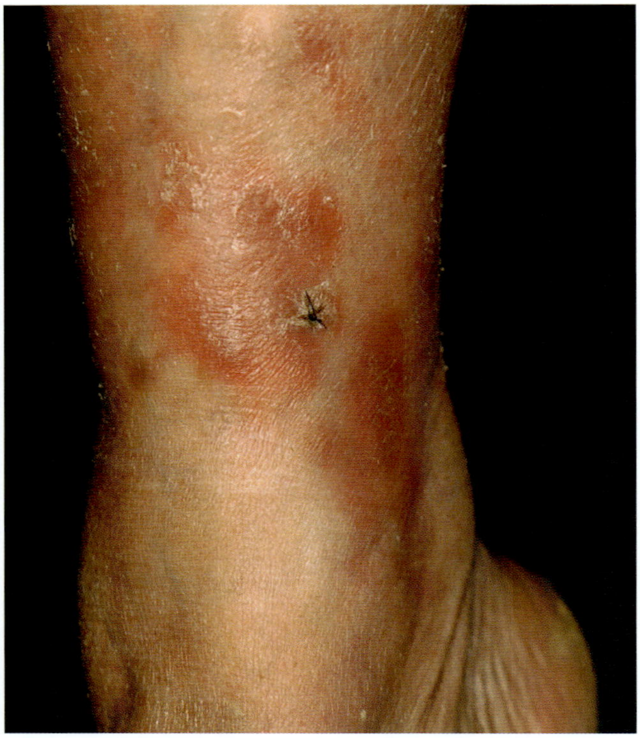

Figure 31.98 Acrodermatitis chronica atrophicans. Irregular, erythematous patches and plaques on the distal portion of one leg.

## Pseudolymphomas at sites of vaccination

Rarely, a florid inflammatory reaction develops at sites of vaccinations [180]. Clinically, lesions may show either superficial papules or nodules, or subcutaneous infiltrations that may result in a panniculitis-like appearance (Fig. 31.103). The histopathologic pattern may be lichenoid, simulating that seen in mycosis fungoides, or nodular with the formation of germinal centers, simulating a follicle center lymphoma and belonging to the group of "lymphocytoma cutis" (Fig. 31.104). The germinal centers display reactive features (well-formed mantle zone, presence of tingible body macrophages and of polarization, high proliferation – see Table 31.4). In contrast to follicle center lymphoma, Bcl-6$^+$ germinal center cells are not observed outside of the germinal centers. Another characteristic histopathologic feature is represented by the presence of areas of degeneration and fibrosis surrounded by a histiocytic reaction characterized by macrophages with granular basophilic cytoplasm (Fig. 31.105) [180]. The presence of macrophages with these peculiar features strongly suggests the causative role of aluminum-adsorbed vaccines in the occurrence of this type of pseudolymphoma [181]. A very good clue for the diagnosis is represented by the positivity of these macrophages for EBER-1, due to a non-specific cross-reaction with the aluminum present in most vaccines (Fig. 31.106) [182].

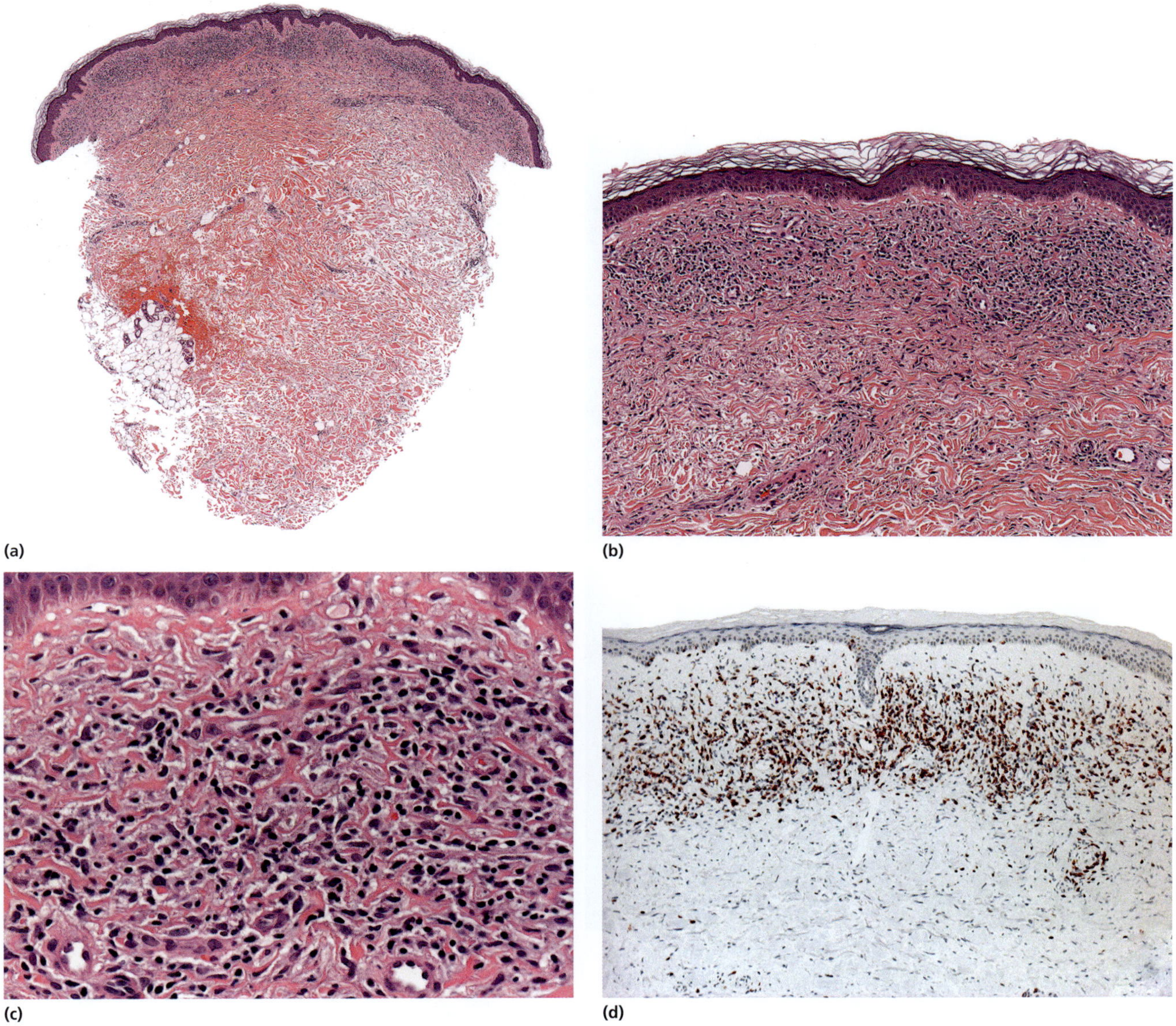

Figure 31.99 Acrodermatitis chronica atrophicans. (a) Band-like infiltrate in the superficial dermis. (b) Detail of the infiltrate composed predominantly of small lymphocytes; (c) note absence of epidermotropism. (d) Staining for CD3 reveals positivity of most lymphocytes.

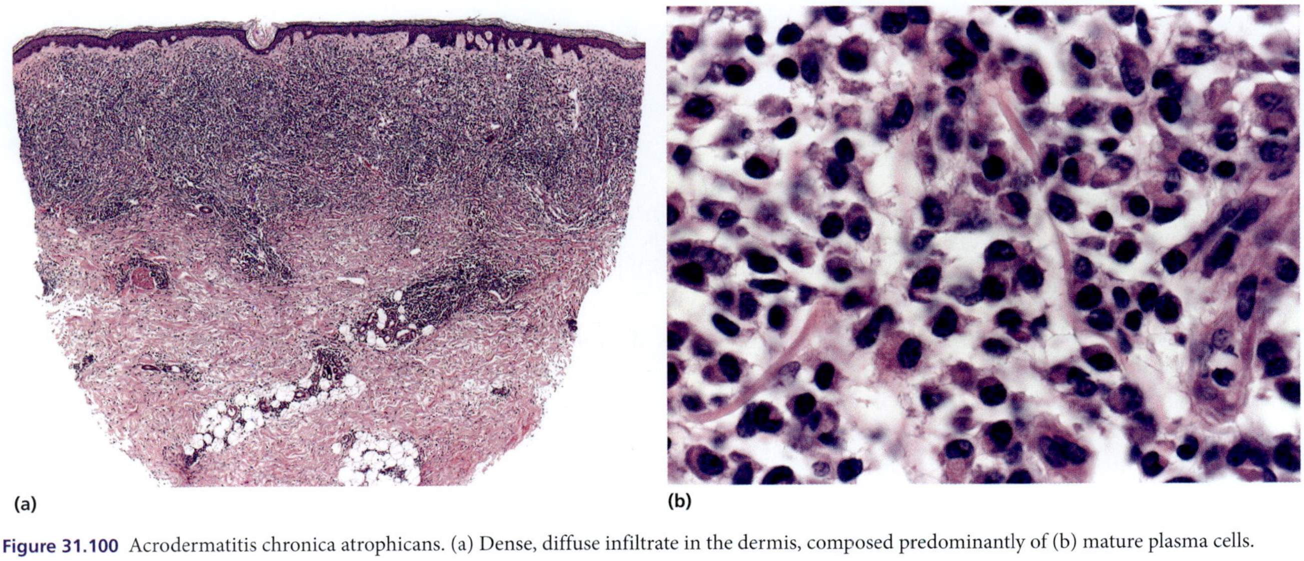

Figure 31.100 Acrodermatitis chronica atrophicans. (a) Dense, diffuse infiltrate in the dermis, composed predominantly of (b) mature plasma cells.

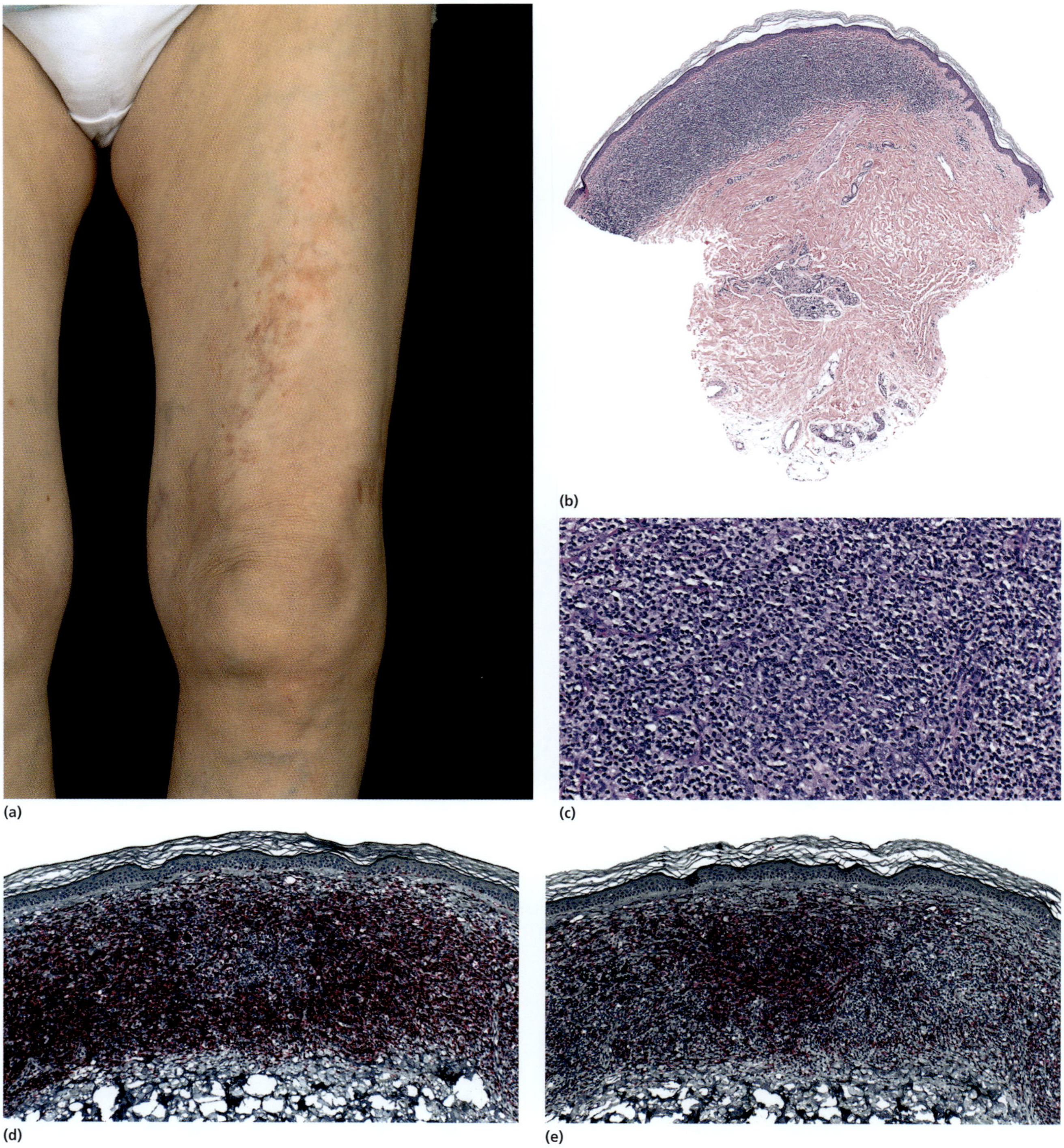

**Figure 31.101** Superficial pseudolymphoma associated with infection by *Borrelia*. (a) Clustered papules on the thigh. (b) Histology reveals dense, band-like lymphoid infiltrates without epidermal involvement. (c) Detail of the infiltrate. Immunohistochemical stainings show (d) positivity for CD3 in the majority of the cells, as well as (e) clusters of B lymphocytes positive for CD19.

It is believed that pseudolymphomas after vaccination represent a form of local reactive hyperplasia or a persisting delayed hypersensitivity reaction to a vaccine constituent, particularly aluminum. Lesions may arise after injection of different vaccines, including those used for allergen hyposensitization and tumor cell vaccines [183]. We have observed the onset of bilateral lesions of lymphocytoma cutis at the skin sites of different injections of vaccine against early summer meningoencephalitis (ESME) performed after an interval of over 1 year [180].

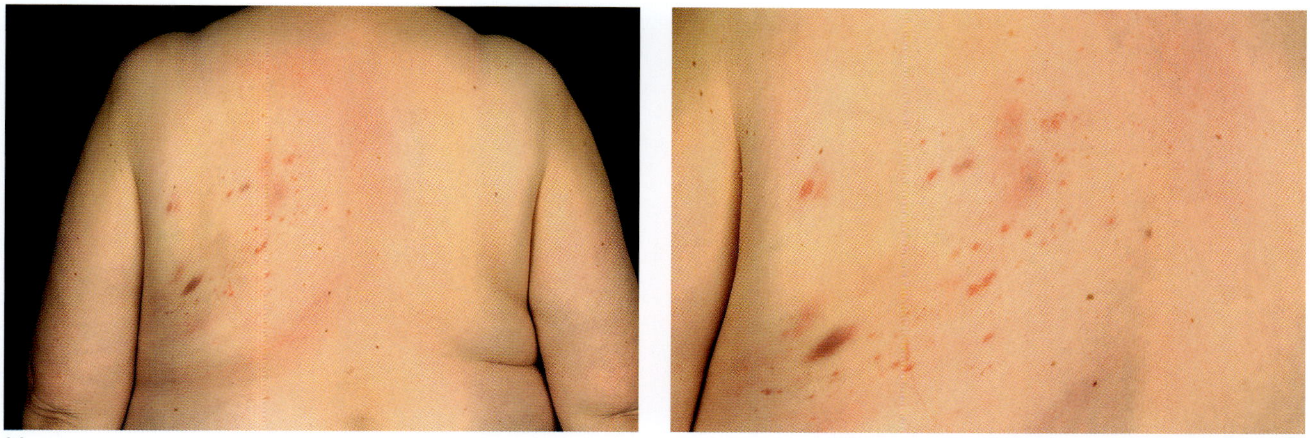

(a) (b)

Figure 31.102 Pseudolymphomatous erythema migrans. (a) Large area of figurate erythema on the left shoulder; (b) In the central part, numerous erythematous macules, papules, and small plaques are visible.

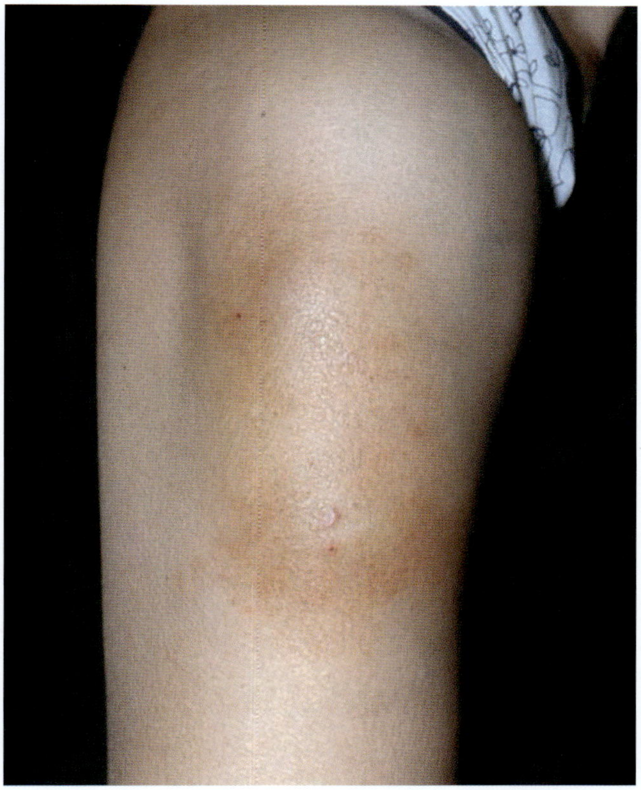

Figure 31.103 Pseudolymphoma after vaccination. Infiltrated (panniculitis-like) subcutaneous plaque at the site of a previous vaccination.

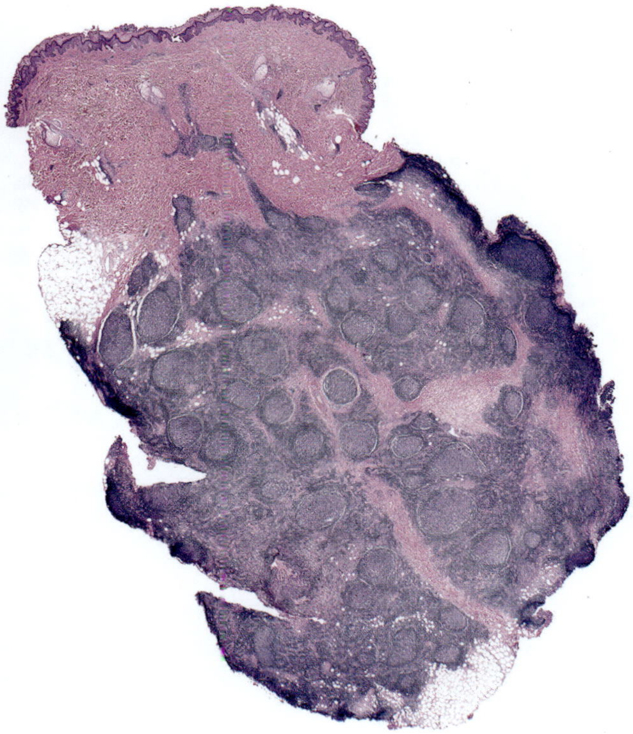

Figure 31.104 Pseudolymphoma after vaccination. Dense nodular infiltrate of lymphocytes within the subcutaneous fat. Note several reactive germinal centers.

Lesions tend to persist unchanged for months or years. Intralesional steroids may be ineffective. I have seen patients with lesions persisting for several years even after local radiotherapy. A case of 12-year persistent cutaneous lymphoid hyperplasia starting at the site of hepatitis B vaccination and spreading to other cutaneous sites has also been reported [184]. The patient was successfully treated by thalidomide.

### Pseudolymphomas in tattoos

Besides granulomatous infiltrates, inflammatory reactions to tattoos may sometimes reveal a pseudolymphomatous pattern [185]. Red tattoo pigment (cinnabar) is most frequently responsible for the pseudolymphomatous infiltrates. Both a band-like and a follicular B-cell pattern may be observed, sometimes in the same patient [186, 187].

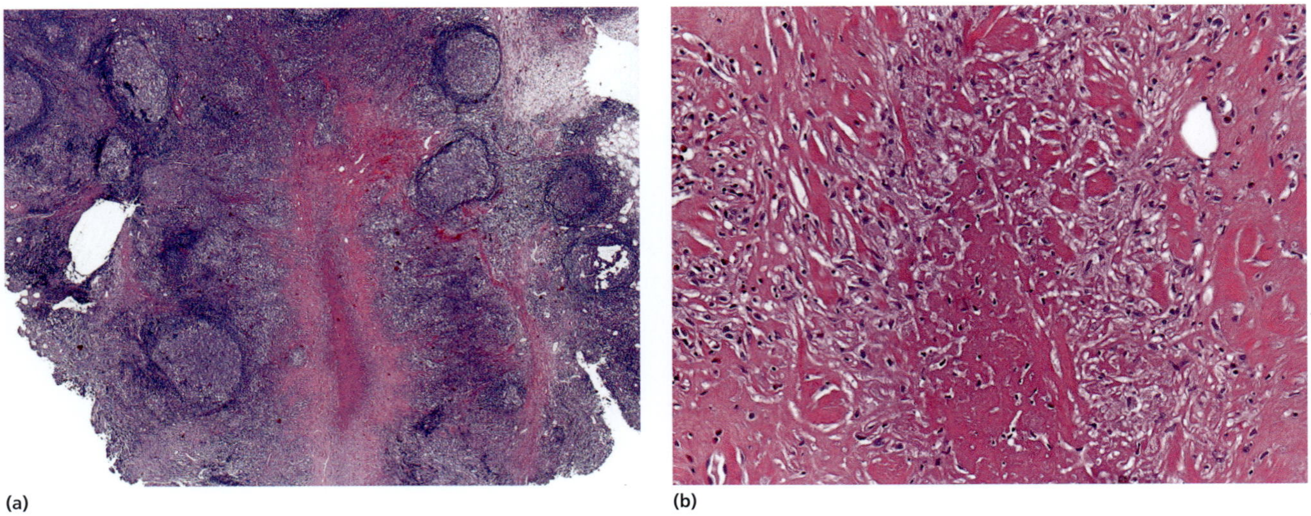

Figure 31.105 Pseudolymphoma after vaccination. (a) Central area of necrosis surrounded by reactive germinal centers. (b) Detail of necrotic area with several macrophages with basophilic granular cytoplasm (see text).

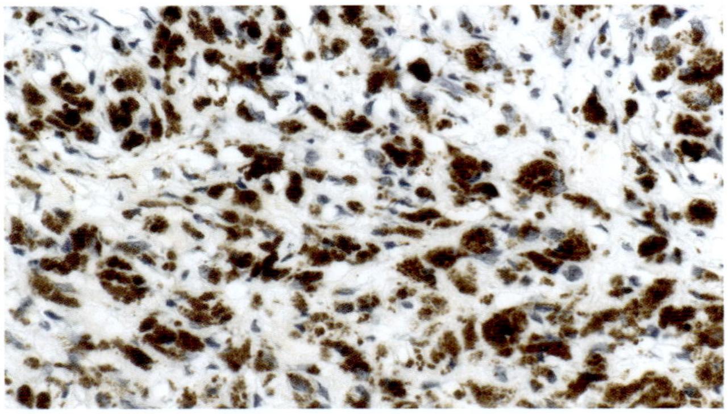

Figure 31.106 Pseudolymphoma after vaccination. Positive in-situ hybridization for EBV (EBER-1) within the histiocytes (see text for explanation).

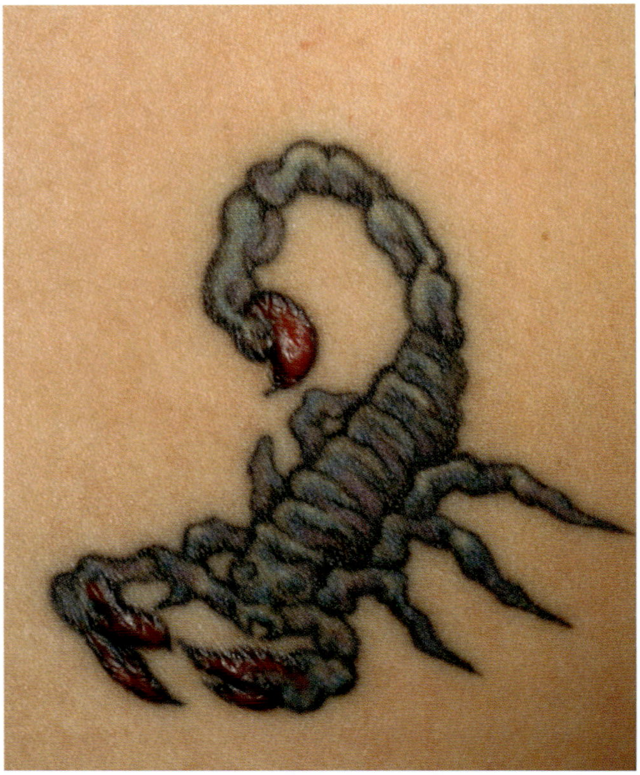

Figure 31.107 Pseudolymphoma within a tattoo. Onset of several papules and small plaques in the red pigmented areas of the tattoo.

Clinically, patients present with erythematous papules, plaques, or small nodules, usually confined to different areas of the tattoo with the same pigment (Fig. 31.107). As already mentioned, histology reveals either a mycosis fungoides-like pattern characterized by dense, band-like lymphoid infiltrates with some large, activated lymphocytes (Fig. 31.108), or a B-cell pattern with prominent germinal centers. $CD30^{+}$ cells are commonly present within the infiltrate, sometimes mimicking the pattern of a $CD30^{+}$ cutaneous lymphoproliferative disorder [188]. The presence of exogenous pigment of the tattoo suggests the correct diagnosis. It should be emphasized that on histopathologic sections the color of the pigment does not always match that of the responsible pigment.

A well-documented case of cutaneous lymphoma arising in a tattoo has been reported, so careful follow-up of these lesions is necessary [189]. In fact, rare cases may harbor a monoclonal population of plasma cells, and the true potential for evolution of these cases is unknown (see also Chapter 17, Fig. 17.6). In this context, it is also interested to note that a study including over 11.000 individuals suggested that tattoos are associated with a higher risk of systemic lymphomas [190].

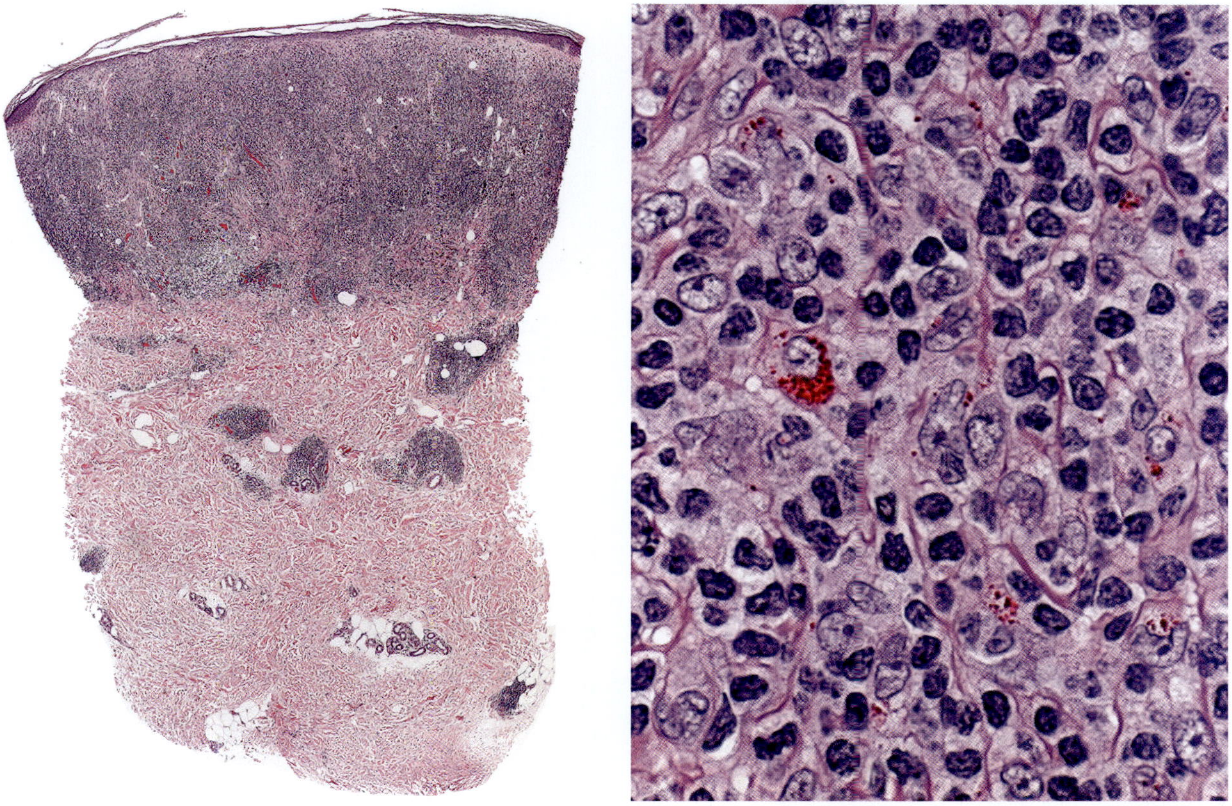

(a) (b)

Figure 31.108 Pseudolymphoma within a tattoo. (a) The clinical appearance is similar to that of conventional amalgama tattoo within the oral mucosa. (b) Histology reveals dense lymphohistiocytic infiltrates with small particles of amalgama within some histiocytes.

The management of pseudolymphomas in tattoos can be very difficult because of the large areas of skin involved in some of the patients. Intralesional steroid injections, laser vaporization, or surgical excision of small lesions may be applied. Conventional laser treatment aimed only at removing the pigment is usually not effective on the pseudolymphomatous infiltrates.

Rarely, pseudolymphomatous features similar to those observed in tattoos may be observed in the oral mucosa at sites of ***amalgama tattoo*** (related to the accidental injection within the oral mucosa of mercury- and silver-containing amalgama during dental procedures). Pseudolymphomatous reactions to amalgama tattoo present clinically with solitary or localized, well-circumscribed, roundish, bluish discolorations of the oral mucosa, and histopathologically with dense lymphoid infiltrates admixed with histiocytes that are engulfing the amalgama (Fig. 31.109). In one reported case, the reaction to amalgama tattoo was characterized by the histopathologic pattern of lymphocytoma cutis, and was possibly related to zinc rather than mercury or silver [191]. Amalgama is being replaced by other compounds in dental procedures, yet it is still being used in many countries because of the low cost, and local reactions may be observed several years after the original procedure, long after replacement of the compound for routine use in dentistry.

## Localized scleroderma/morphea

In the inflammatory stage of connective tissue diseases, especially in localized scleroderma, dense lymphoid infiltrates may be observed, simulating cutaneous lymphomas histopathologically (particularly cutaneous marginal zone lymphoproliferative disorder) (Fig. 31.110) [138, 192, 193]. Plasma cells are almost invariably present and reveal a polyclonal pattern of immunoglobulin light-chain expression. Reactive germinal centers may be observed rarely. Sclerosis of the collagen bundles may not be prominent in the early stages of morphea, thus causing problems in the differential diagnosis. Correlation with the clinical picture confirms the diagnosis. Treatment does not differ from the conventional therapy of the disease.

A report on morphea mimicking histopathologically mycosis fungoides has also been published [194]. However, judging from the pictures published, in my opinion these cases may be better interpreted as lichen sclerosus associated with morphea,

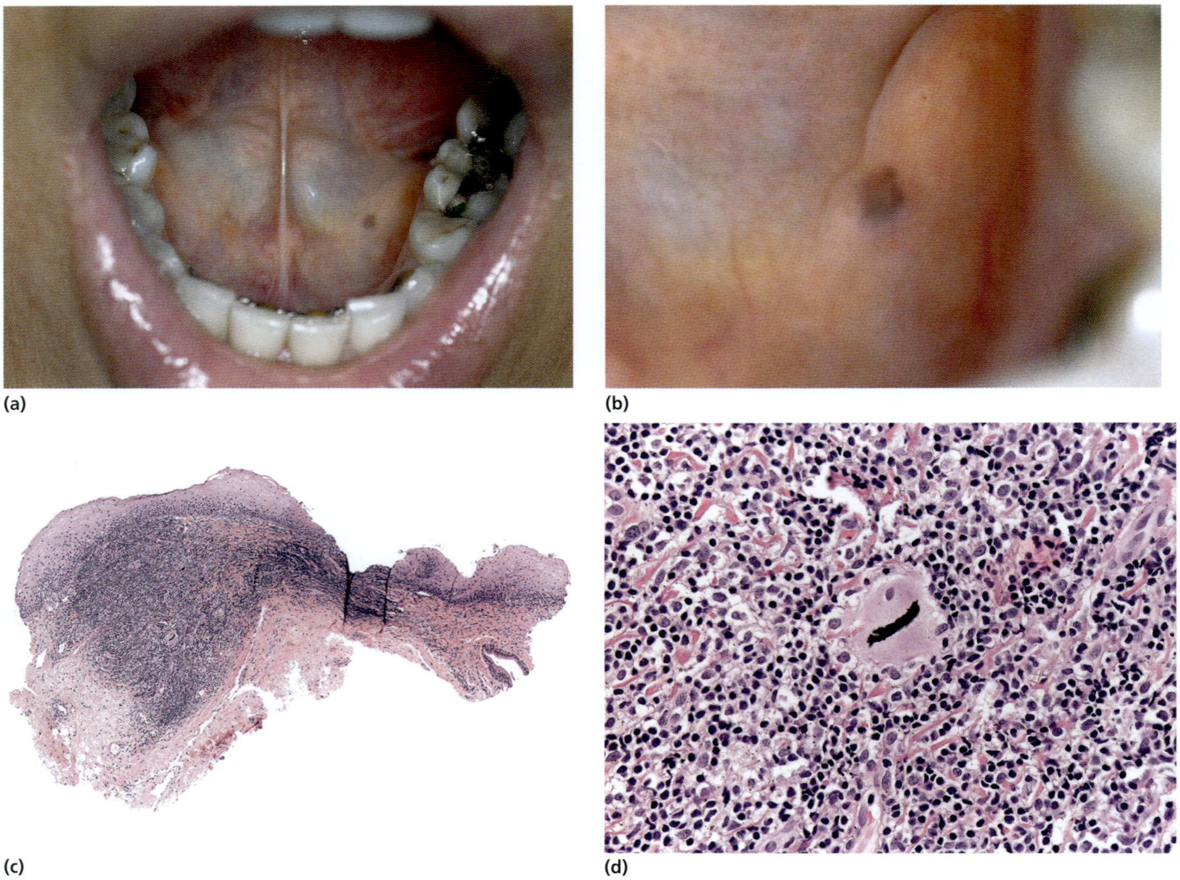

Figure 31.109 Pseudolymphoma due to amalgama tattoo within the oral mucosa. (a, b) Small, regular pigmented macule. (c) Dense dermal infiltrate of lymphocytes. (d) Detail of the infiltrate with some activated lymphocytes and with black pigment of the tattoo within a histiocyte.

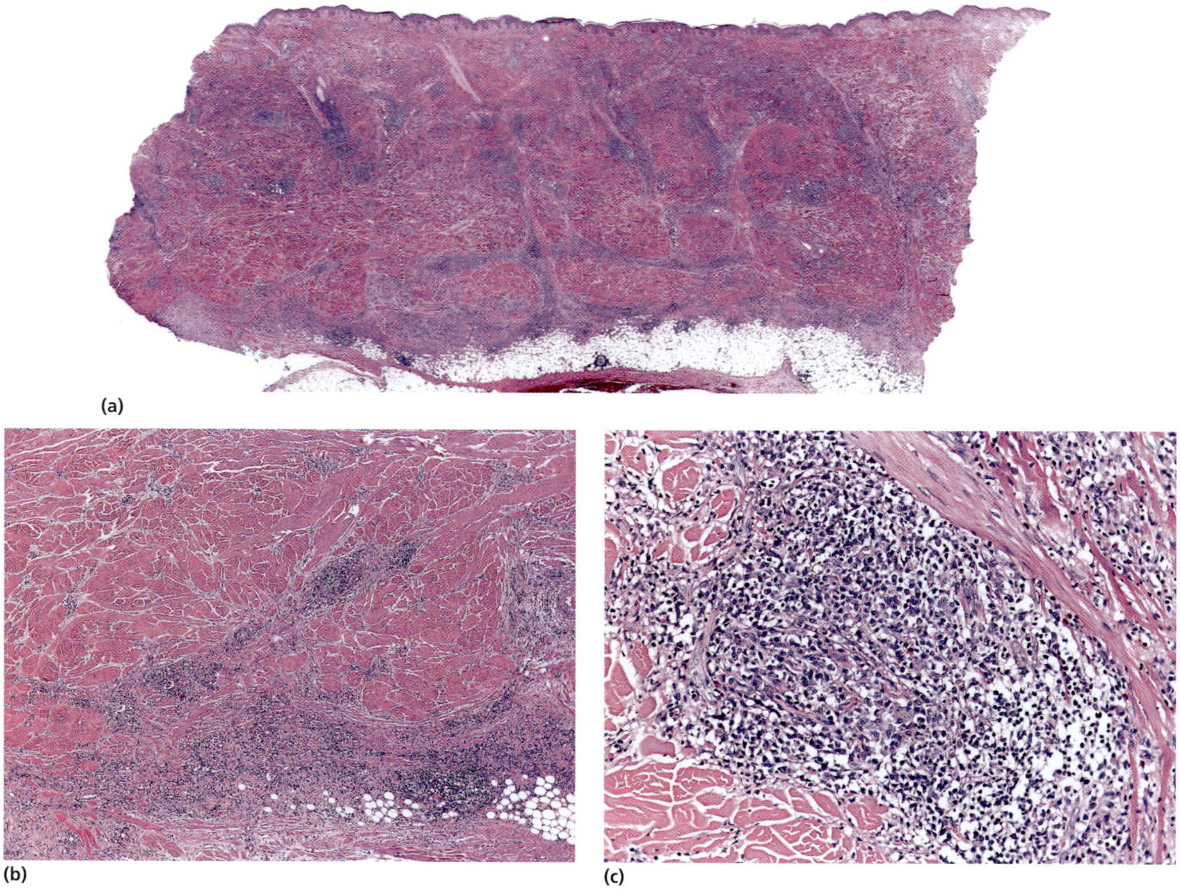

Figure 31.110 Morphea, inflammatory stage. (a) Sclerosis of the collagen fibers and dense lymphoid infiltrates. (b) Details of sclerosing collagen fibers and of (c) lymphoid infiltrates with several plasma cells.

with focal mycosis fungoides-like features related to the lichen sclerosus rather than to the morphea.

## Cutaneous IgG4-related disease

IgG4-related disease is a condition characterized by nodular lesions with lymphoplasmacytic infiltration, increase in the number of $IgG4^+$ cells in affected tissues, and elevation of serum IgG4 levels [195]. Several organs may be affected including the pancreas (autoimmune pancreatitis), lacrimal and salivary glands, retroperitoneal space (fibrosis previously referred to as "idiopathic"), sinonasal tract (angiocentric fibrosis), thyroid (Riedel thyroiditis, fibrous variant of Hashimoto thyroiditis), aorta (aortitis, periaortitis), orbit (pseudotumor, proptosis), lung, pleura, pericardium, kidney (tubulointerstitial nephritis), prostate, stomach (lymphoplasmacytic gastritis), breast (sclerosing mastitis, pseudotumor), and bile duct (sclerosing cholangitis). On histopathological examination, it has been suggested that the presence of a marked lymphoplasmacytic infiltration with fibrosis and of an infiltration of $IgG4^+$ plasma cells with a ratio of IgG4/IgG cells of more than 40% and more than 10 $IgG4^+$ plasma cells/high-power field are needed for the diagnosis [196].

The spectrum of cutaneous presentations varies, with some manifestations related to extracutaneous IgG4-related disease, while others represent purely cutaneous conditions. Cutaneous lesions in extracutaneous IgG4-related disease present mainly on the head and neck region as erythematous plaques and nodules, and are frequently accompanied by regional lymphadenopathy [195]. Histology shows an infiltrate composed by lymphocytes admixed with large numbers of plasma cells and eosinophils located in the dermis and/or subcutis, and accompanied by variable fibrosis. Reactive lymphoid follicles may be observed [197, 198]. The plasma cells produce IgG4 (ratio of $IgG4^+/IgG^+$ plasma cells: minimum of 40%, usually 60–90%). In some cases, the presence of plasma cell-rich infiltrates may prompt a differential diagnosis with marginal zone lymphoproliferative disorder, but plasma cells in cutaneous IgG4-rich infiltrates are invariably polyclonal.

Besides cutaneous manifestations of extracutaneous IgG4-related disease, increased numbers of $IgG4^+$ plasma cells have been observed in different cutaneous conditions, including cutaneous Rosai-Dorfman disease, cutaneous plasmacytosis, Kimura disease, granuloma faciale, and angiolymphoid hyperplasia with eosinophilia [199], suggesting that in the skin the presence of $IgG4^+$ plasma cells is not specific to a given disease. In fact, although dense lymphoplasmacytic infiltrates, storiform pattern of fibrosis, the presence of eosinophils, and obliterative phlebitis are the most important criteria for histopathological diagnosis of IgG4-related diseases at extracutaneous sites [200], even in cutaneous manifestations of extracutaneous IgG4-related disease fibrosis was observed only in a minority of cases, and it did not show a storiform pattern, and obliterative phlebitis was found only in 10% of cases [195]. In addition, the cutaneous disorders with $IgG4^+$ plasma cells do not show sclerosis, and the exact relationship (if any) to the IgG4-related disease is unclear. Furthermore, cases of inflammatory scleroderma with prominent plasma cell infiltrates do not show an increase of $IgG4^+$ cells.

Patients with IgG4-related disease usually have an excellent response to systemic steroid therapy. Thalidomide has also been used with good results [201].

## Pseudolymphomas in syphilis

Syphilis is considered one of the great mimes in dermatology, as it may present with a pronounced variability of clinical manifestations. Sometimes it may simulate a cutaneous lymphoma either clinically, histopathologically, or both. Clinically, patients present with solitary or multiple erythematous papules or small nodules (Figs. 31.111 and 31.112). A patient presenting with so-called "facies leonina," similar to what can be observed in specific manifestations of B-CLL, has also been reported [202]. Clinical presentations simulating a malignant lymphoma with multiple, partly ulcerated plaques and nodules ("lues maligna") are seen mostly in immune-suppressed individuals, particularly in HIV-infected patients (Fig. 31.113), and may harbor monoclonal populations of lymphocytes [203].

Three main histopathological patterns may be observed in pseudolymphomatous syphilis, mainly in the secondary stage of the disease. These patterns can be observed sometimes in different lesions from the same patient. The first pattern is characterized by dense lymphoid infiltrates with epidermotropism, simulating a mycosis fungoides (Fig. 31.114). As plasma cells are rare in early mycosis fungoides, their presence has been considered as a diagnostic clue for syphilis in the histopathologic differential diagnosis between the two diseases [204].

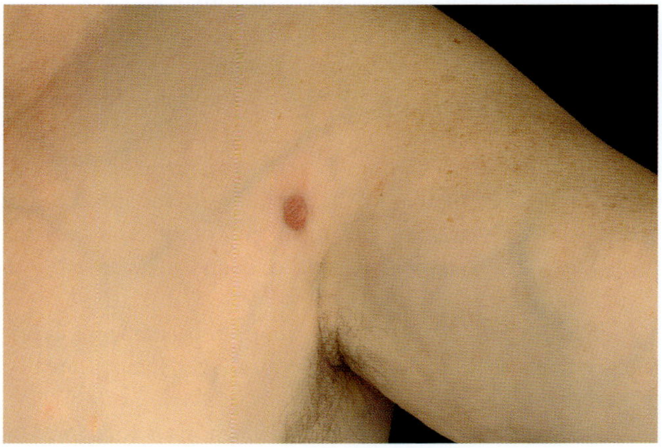

**Figure 31.111** Pseudolymphoma in secondary syphilis. Small, solitary erythematous nodule near the axilla.

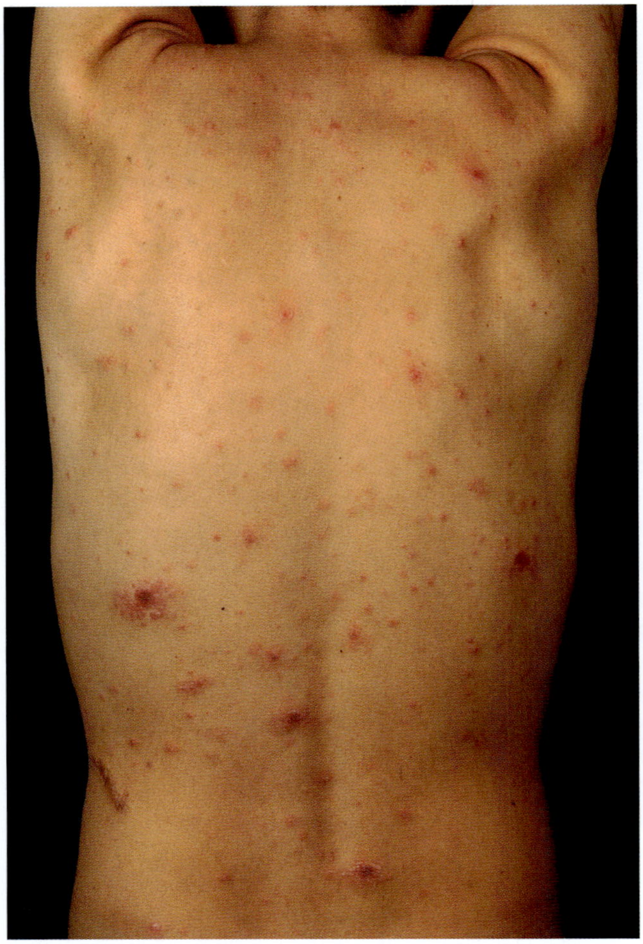

Figure 31.112 Pseudolymphoma in secondary syphilis. Generalized, partly confluent, partly erosive erythematous papules.

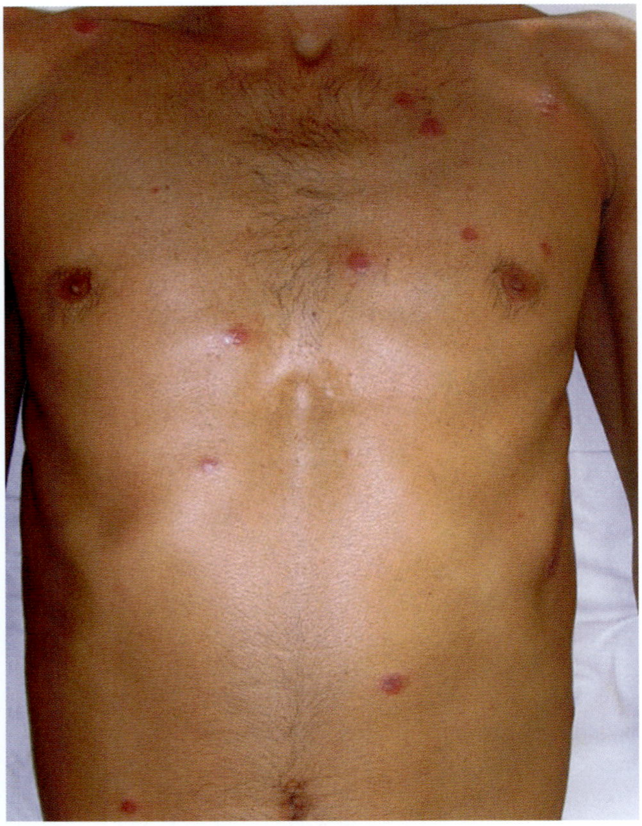

Figure 31.113 Pseudolymphoma in secondary syphilis. Several erythematous plaques in an HIV+ patient. *(Courtesy of Prof. Pablo Umbert, Barcelona, Spain.)*

Particularly in HIV+ patients, however, plasma cells may be sparse or absent and there may be a predominance of $CD8^+$ lymphocytes (Fig. 31.115), making differentiation from cytotoxic mycosis fungoides very difficult. The second pattern shows sheets of plasma cells, often associated with T and B lymphocytes and small granulomas, simulating histopathologically the picture of a cutaneous marginal zone lymphoproliferative disorder (Figs. 31.116a and b). The plasma cells always reveal a polyclonal expression of immunoglobulin light chains (Figs. 31.116c and d). The last pattern is characterized by nodular lymphoid infiltrates in the dermis without involvement of the epidermis and without formation of sheets of plasma cells (Fig. 31.117). Several plasma cells are interspersed with small lymphocytes in this variant.

Pseudolymphomatous infiltrates may be observed also in primary syphilis. Lesions located at typical sites (genital area or oral mucosa) can be identified clinically relatively easily; in general such lesions are not biopsied, and diagnosis is confirmed by serological investigations. However, particularly lesions arising at other sites of the body may be biopsied because the diagnosis has not been made clinically, and pseudolymphomatous infiltrates in this setting may be misleading (Fig. 31.118a). Pseudolymphomatous lesions in primary syphilis are usually ulcerated with involvement of both epidermis and dermis (Fig. 31.118b). The finding of dense infiltrates with a mixed infiltrate containing lymphocytes, histiocytes, plasma cells, and neutrophils should always raise the suspicion of syphilis (Fig. 31.118c), and staining for *Treponema pallidum* confirms the diagnosis (Fig. 31.118d). In primary syphilis, CD30 may be expressed by large, activated lymphocytes. In this context, before making a diagnosis of anaplastic large cell lymphoma or of lymphomatoid papulosis in a biopsy from genital skin, staining for *T. pallidum* should always be carried out.

In the past, pseudolymphomatous infiltrates occurred also in late (tertiary) manifestations of syphilis (gumma syphilitica with dense sheets of lymphocytes admixed with plasma cells), but nowadays this stage is almost never encountered anymore.

In all types of pseudolymphomatous syphilis, immunohistochemical staining for *T. pallidum* reveals variable numbers of microorganisms (Fig. 31.119). *Treponemas* are found at two main locations within the biopsy specimens: within the epidermis, particularly at the dermo-epidermal junction, and

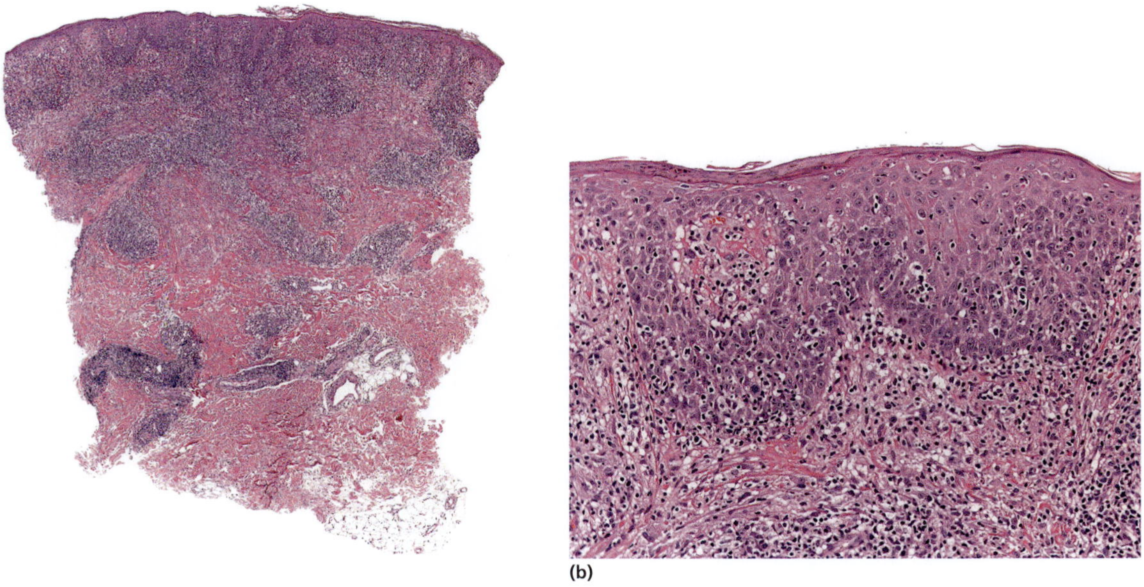

Figure 31.114 Pseudolymphoma in secondary syphilis. (a) Dense lymphoid infiltrates with prominent epidermal involvement. (b) Detail of the superficial part with intraepidermal lymphocytes.

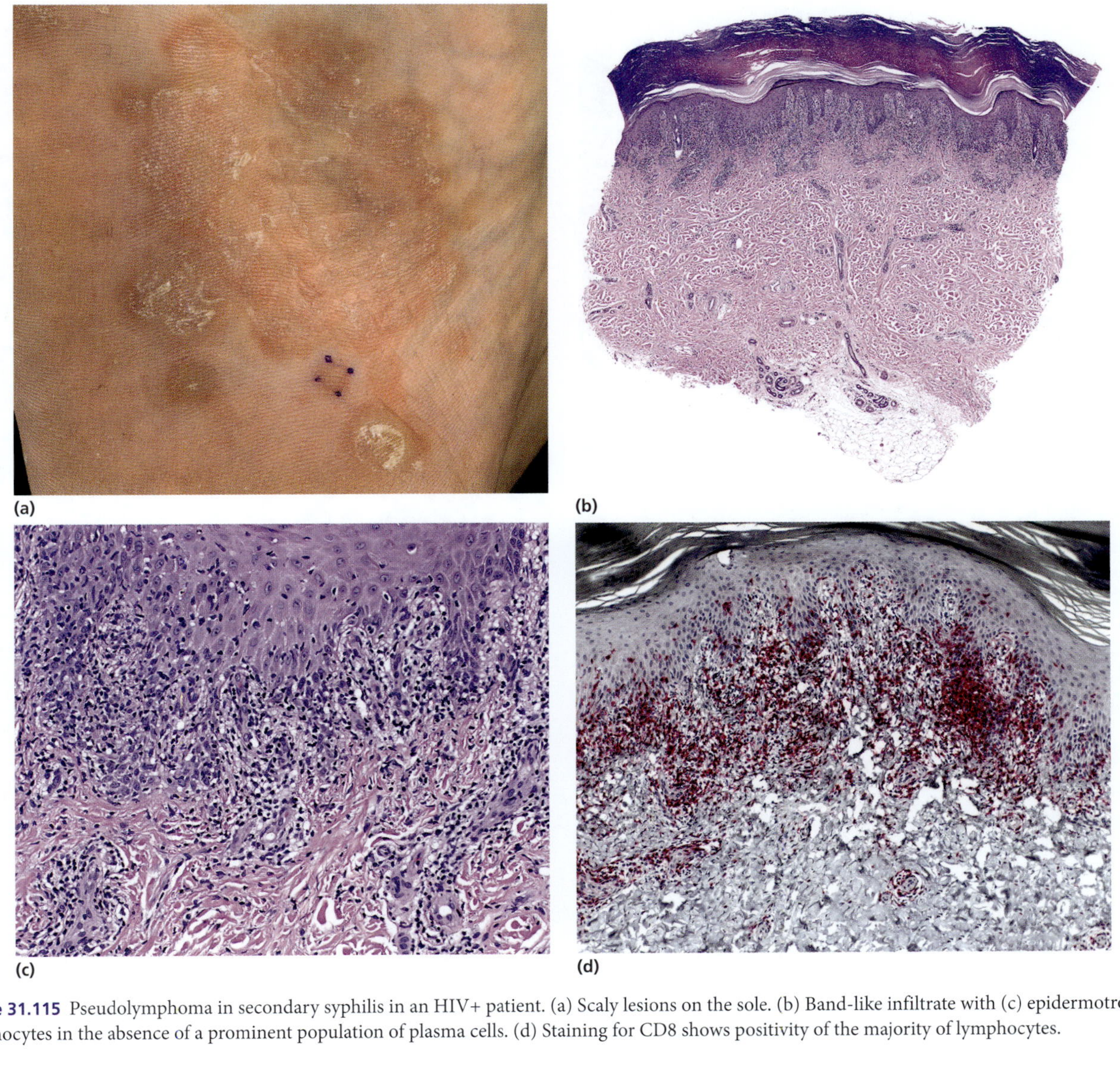

Figure 31.115 Pseudolymphoma in secondary syphilis in an HIV+ patient. (a) Scaly lesions on the sole. (b) Band-like infiltrate with (c) epidermotropic lymphocytes in the absence of a prominent population of plasma cells. (d) Staining for CD8 shows positivity of the majority of lymphocytes.

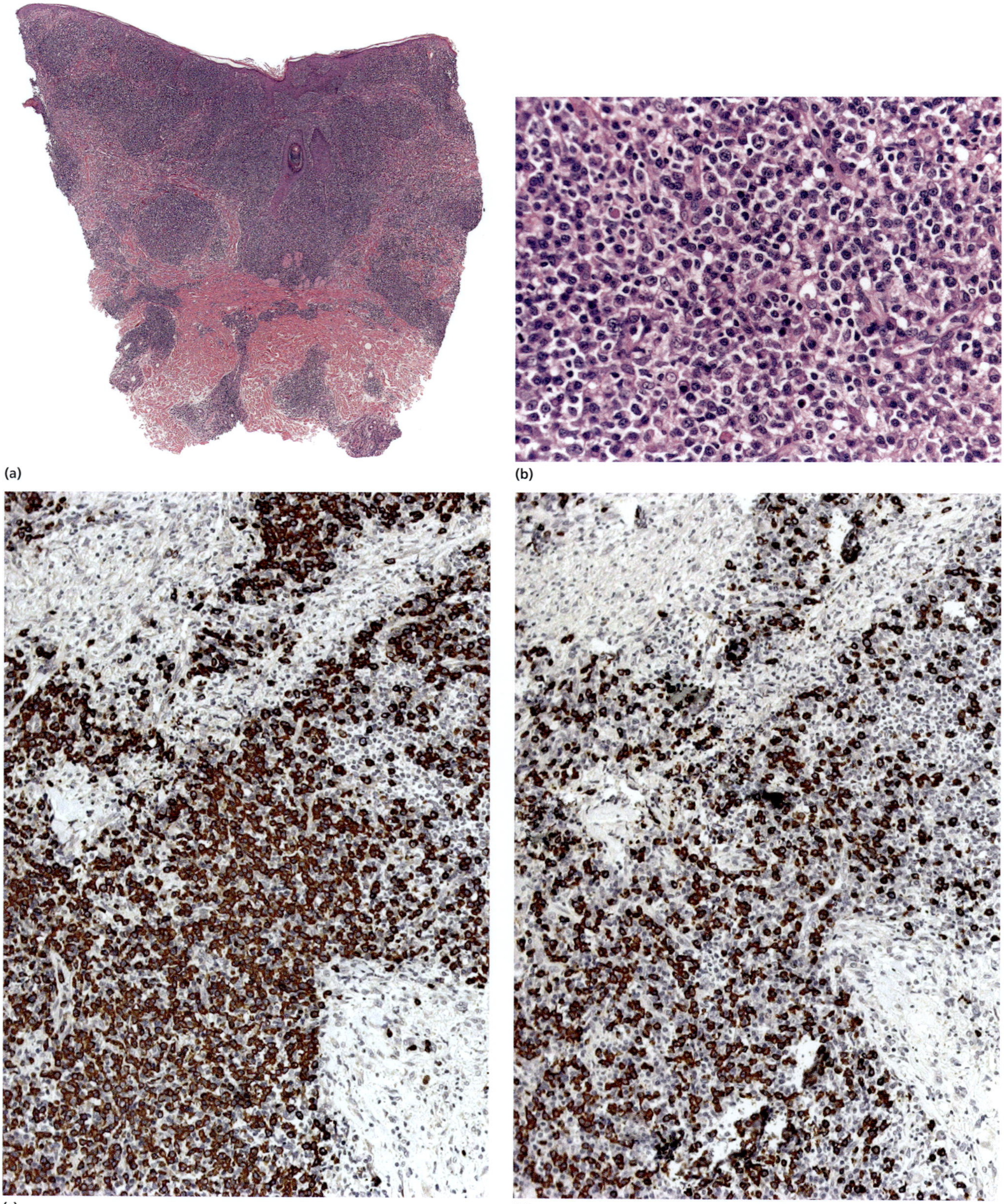

(a) (b) (c) (d)

Figure 31.116 Pseudolymphoma in secondary syphilis. (a) Dense infiltrate of lymphocytes and plasma cells in the entire dermis. (b) Detail of the infiltrate with abundant plasma cells. In situ hybridization for (c) kappa and (d) lambda immunoglobulin light chains reveals a polyclonal pattern.

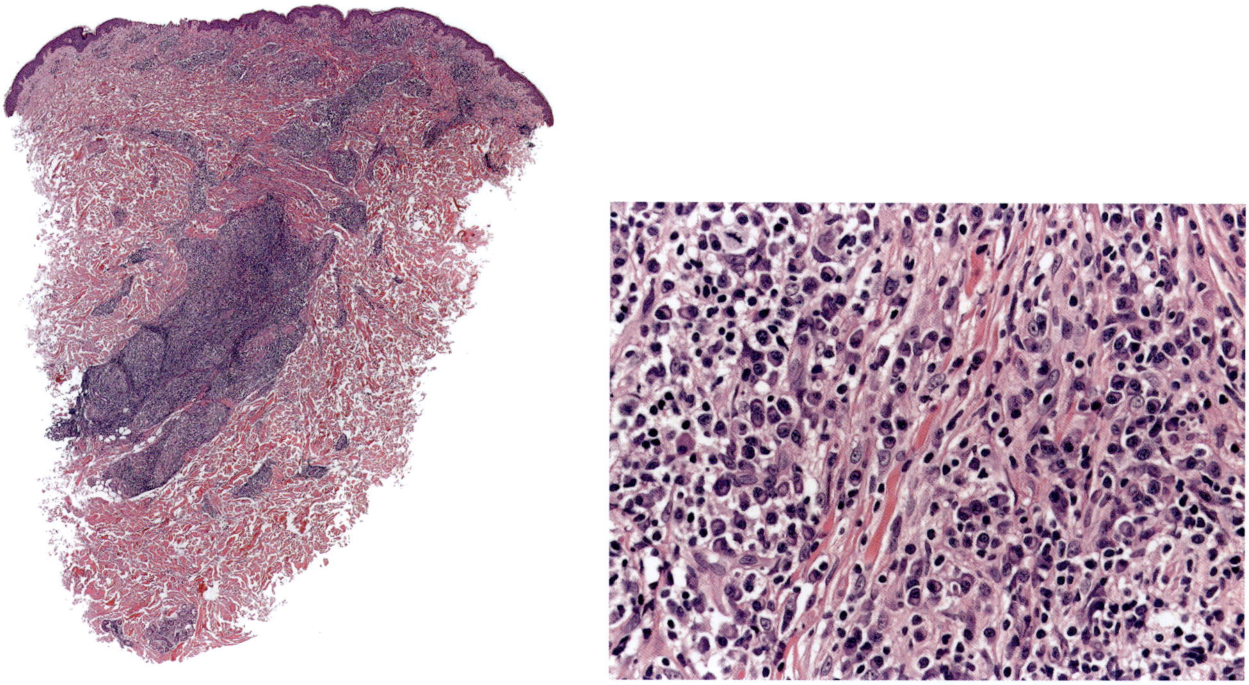

(a) (b)

**Figure 31.117** Pseudolymphoma in secondary syphilis. (a) Nodular dermal infiltrate. (b) Detail of lymphocytes and histiocytes admixed with plasma cells.

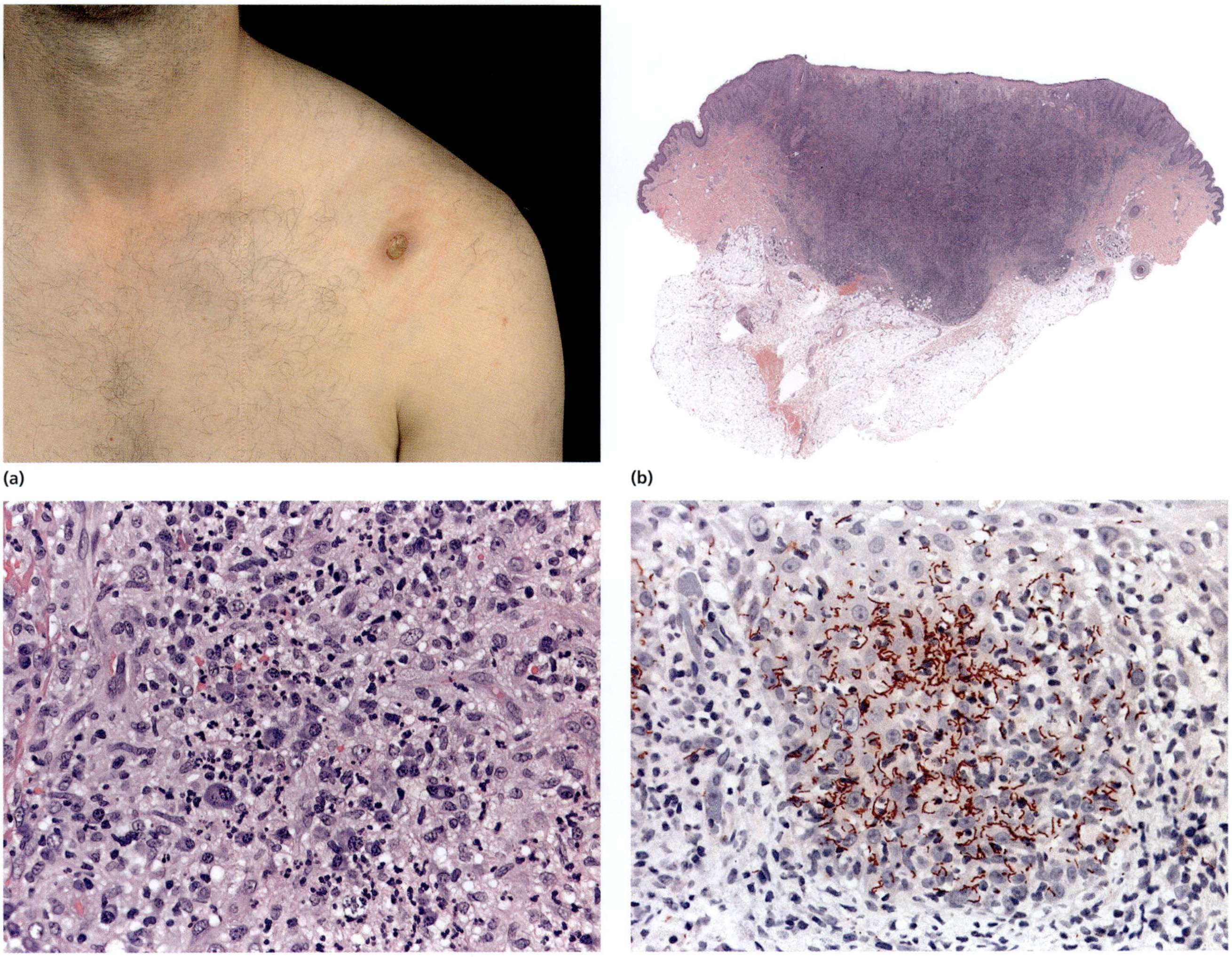

(a) (b) (c) (d)

**Figure 31.118** Pseudolymphoma in primary syphilis. (a) Ulcerated plaque on the shoulder. (b) Large ulcerated nodule with involvement of both the dermis as well as the epidermis at the margins of the ulceration. (c) Several plasma cells and neutrophils admixed with lymphocytes and histiocytes within the infiltrate. (d) Immunohistology shows presence of many microorganisms.

around the dermal vessels, here usually in smaller numbers. In some cases I have observed only a handful of microorganisms within the entire specimen; thus, they should be searched for carefully.

Besides immunohistochemical staining, positivity of serologic tests for syphilis confirms the diagnosis, and antibiotic treatment leads to a rapid resolution of the lesions.

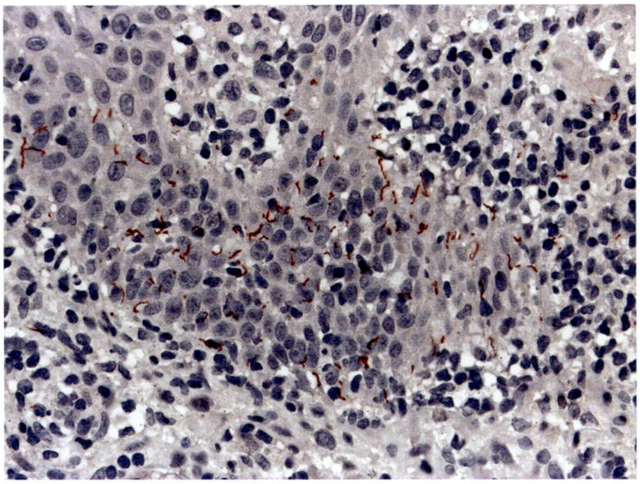

**Figure 31.119** Pseudolymphoma in secondary syphilis. Immunohistological staining for *Treponema pallidum* reveals several intraepidermal microorganisms.

## Cutaneous plasma cell granuloma

Cutaneous inflammatory pseudotumor is a term that in the past encompassed at least two main entities: plasma cell granuloma and inflammatory myofibroblastic tumor. These two diseases are no longer considered related, as inflammatory myofibroblastic tumor is a mesenchymal neoplasm of intermediate biologic potential that frequently recurs and rarely metastasizes, and is not of lymphoid origin, whereas plasma cell granuloma is a fully benign condition. Parenthetically, as cutaneous inflammatory myofibroblastic tumor is positive for anaplastic lymphoma kinase (ALK) [205], care should be taken not to misinterpret this staining for that of an ALK+ anaplastic large cell lymphoma.

Plasma cell granuloma can simulate the histopathologic picture of the plasmacytic variant of marginal zone lymphoproliferative disorder or of secondary skin manifestations of multiple myeloma [206, 207]. Although some cases may represent post-infective reactions to different microorganisms (EBV, mycobacteria, human herpes virus [HHV]-8), definitive proof of an infectious etiology is lacking. A condition called "***juxta-articular fibroid nodule***" represents a rare late manifestation of *Borrelia* infection (related to acrodermatitis chronica atrophicans and *B. afzelii* infection), and is characterized by some morphological resemblance to plasma cell granuloma.

Clinically, patients with plasma cell granuloma present with firm cutaneous or subcutaneous nodules of long duration. On histopathologic examination, circumscribed nodules with

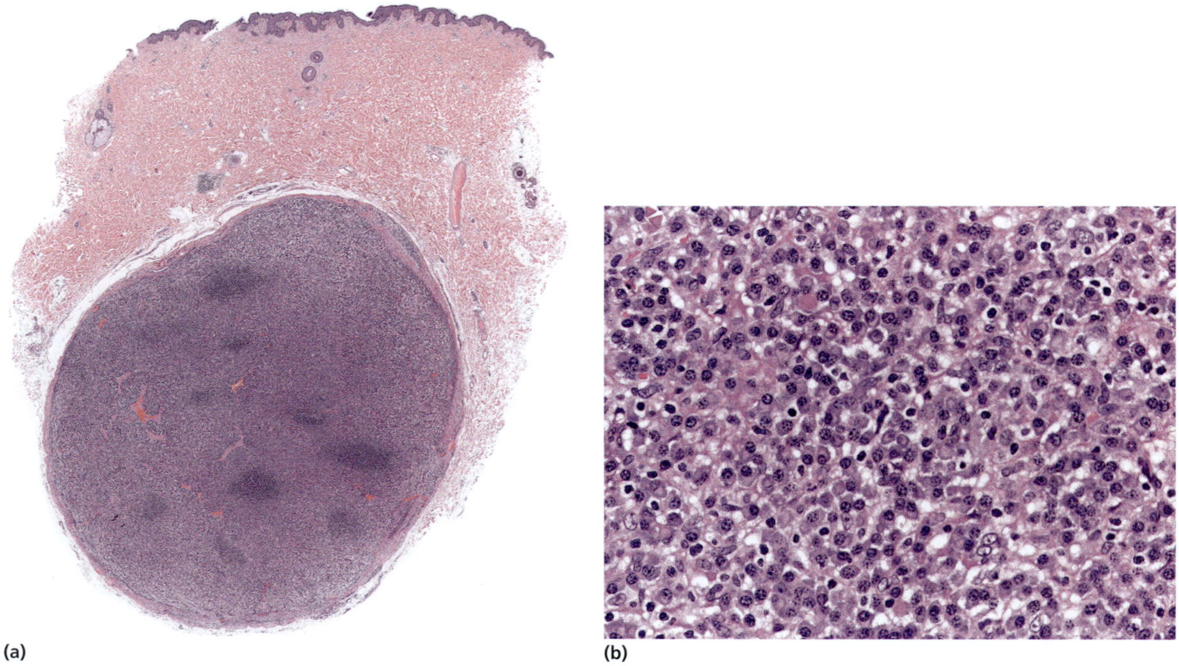

**Figure 31.120** Inflammatory pseudotumor of the skin (plasma cell granuloma). (a) Dermal-subcutaneous nodule composed almost exclusively of (b) mature plasma cells.

thick hyalinized collagen bundles and a dense inflammatory infiltrate composed of lymphocytes, sheets of plasma cells, and occasionally germinal centers are observed (Fig. 31.120). Immunohistology reveals a polyclonal expression of the immunoglobulin light chains. Molecular analyses do not reveal monoclonality of the infiltrate.

Surgical excision of the lesions results in cure.

## Cutaneous and systemic plasmacytosis

Cutaneous plasmacytosis is a condition reported almost exclusively in Japan, or rarely in other Asiatic countries, and is associated with plasma cell infiltrates in the skin [208–211]. Extracutaneous involvement (cutaneous and systemic plasmacytosis) presents with a syndrome characterized by a benign plasma cell proliferation with polyclonal hypogammaglobulinemia, generalized lymphadenopathy, systemic symptoms such as fever, fatigue, and weight loss, and possible involvement of other organs including the spleen, liver, retroperitoneum, and lungs. Clinically, cutaneous plasmacytosis (referred to in the literature also as "cutaneous and systemic plasmacytosis") is characterized by multiple red-brown plaques and nodules located mainly on the trunk (Fig. 31.121). The lesions are asymptomatic.

Histopathologically, cutaneous and systemic plasmacytosis is characterized by variably dense, superficial, and deep infiltrates composed mostly of mature plasma cells without atypical features, usually with a polyclonal pattern of immunoglobulin light chain expression (Fig. 31.122). Germinal centers are present in a distinct proportion of cases [210]. The germinal centers are surrounded by clusters of plasma cells and display reactive features that allow a distinction to be made from cutaneous follicle center lymphoma (Fig. 31.123).

Although the plasma cells in most cases reveal a polyclonal pattern of immunoglobulin light chain expression, some cases of cutaneous and systemic plasmacytosis with otherwise typical clinical presentation were found to harbor a monoclonal population of plasma cells, thus deviating from the conventional presentation of the disease [210]. The existence of such cases may suggest a relationship between cutaneous and systemic plasmacytosis and cutaneous marginal zone lymphoproliferative disorder. However, although there are reports of patients with cutaneous and systemic plasmacytosis developing malignant lymphomas, the relationship (if any) between the disease and malignant lymphomas is not clear. Cutaneous and systemic plasmacytosis has also been linked to the plasma cell type of multicentric Castleman disease (see also the section on Castleman disease in Chapter 21) [212, 213]. However, elevated serum levels of interleukin-6 (IL-6) may be observed only in a minority of patients with cutaneous and systemic plasmacytosis, and the presence of HHV-8 was never demonstrated [209, 210]. Association with *B. burgdorferi* infection has also been ruled out by molecular studies [210].

Treatment of cutaneous plasmacytosis has been described only in anecdotal reports. Successful results have been obtained with topical PUVA therapy, melphalan, a combination of prednisone and cyclophosphamide, intralesional steroids, and topical pimecrolimus.

## Angiomatoid pseudolymphoma (T-cell-rich angiomatoid polypoid pseudolymphoma / Acral pseudolymphomatous angiokeratoma in children / Pre-tibial lymphoplasmacytic plaque in children)

Cases reported as "acral pseudolymphomatous angiokeratoma in children – APACHE" [214], "T-cell-rich angiomatoid polypoid pseudolymphoma" [215], or "pre-tibial lymphoplasmacytic plaque in children" [216–218] show more overlapping than distinguishing clinicopathological features [219]. The term "small papular pseudolymphoma" has been also suggested for similar cases [220], as well as other curious terms such as PALEFACE (papular angiolymphoid proliferation with epithelioid features in adults and children) or TRAPP (T-cell-rich angiomatous polypoid pseudolymphoma). The literature on T-cell-rich angiomatoid polypoid pseudolymphoma, acral pseudolymphomatous angiokeratoma in children, pre-tibial

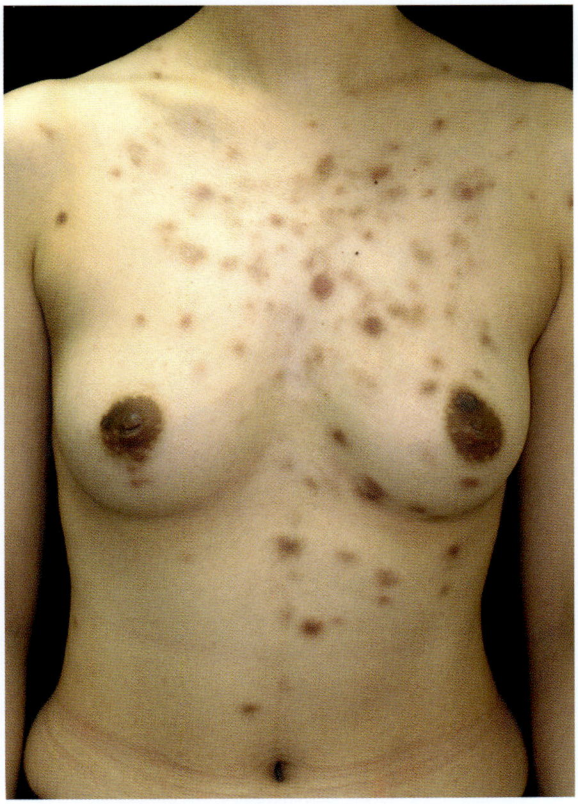

**Figure 31.121** Cutaneous plasmacytosis. Typical clinical appearance with multiple, red-brown plaques and small nodules on the trunk. *(Courtesy of Dr. Akira Ishiko, Tokyo, Japan.)*

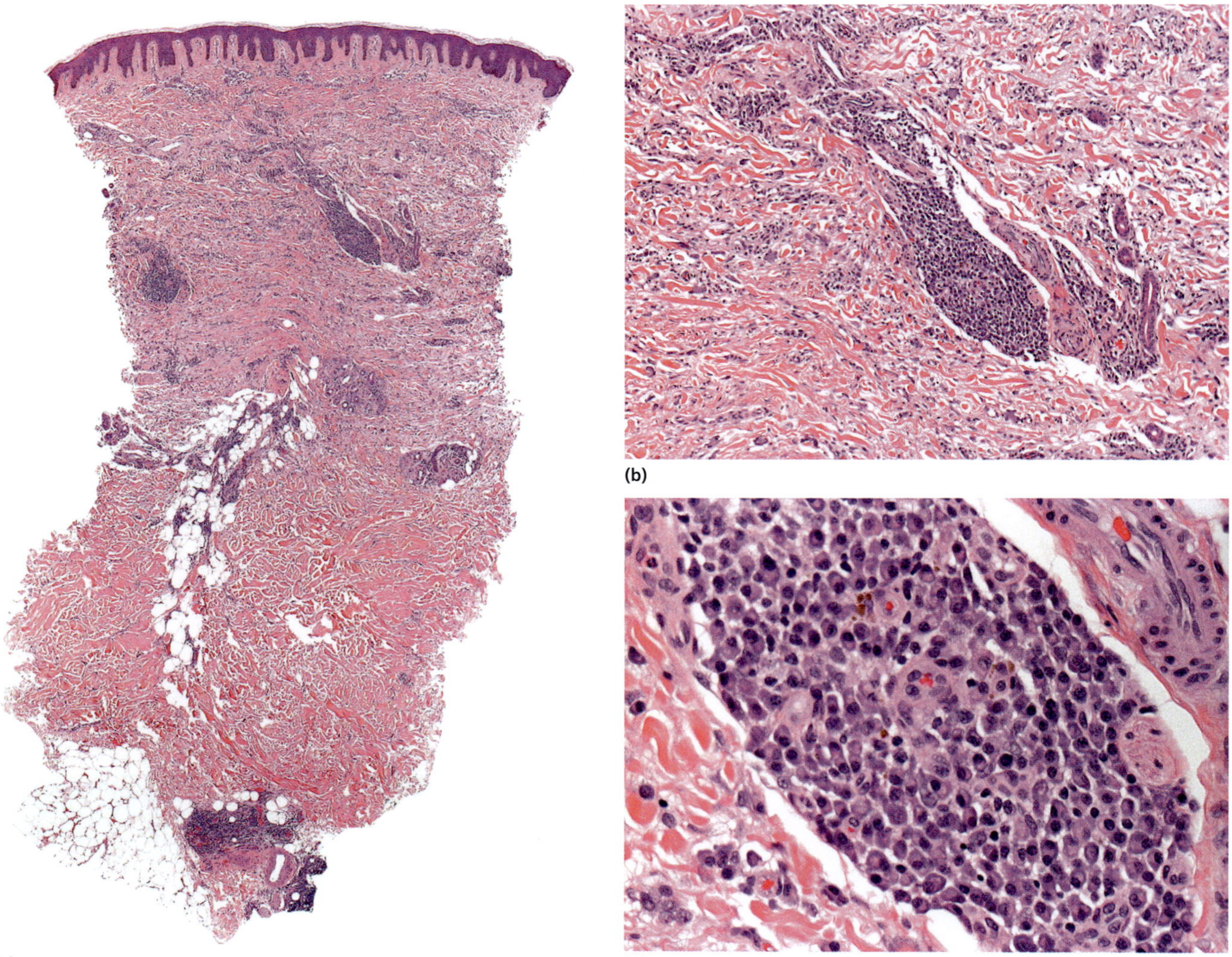


Figure 31.122 Cutaneous plasmacytosis. (a, b) Dense perivascular infiltrates of plasma cells. (c) Normal plasma cells without atypical features.

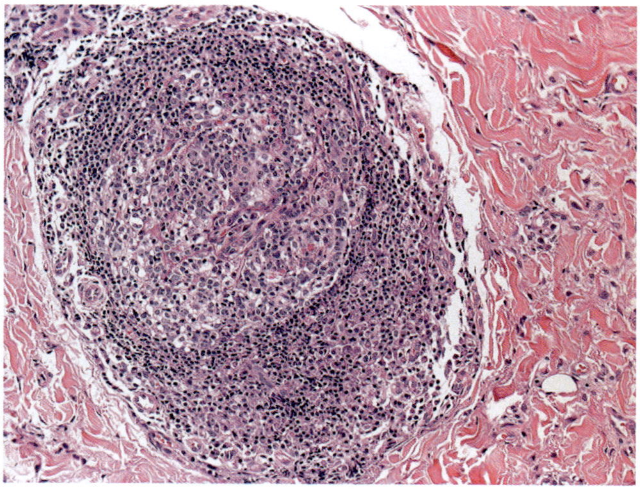

Figure 31.123 Cutaneous plasmacytosis. Reactive germinal center surrounded by mature plasma cells.

lymphoplasmacytic plaque in children, and all other published synonyms / related entities clearly shows the difficulties in classifying these lesions, as new names are regularly introduced for conditions that are most likely variations on the same theme. The best term for this reactive, richly vascularized condition is a matter of discussion, and "angiomatoid pseudolymphoma" is not better than the others, yet it synthesizes in a simple name the least common denominator for describing these lesions.

Lesions described originally as acral pseudolymphomatous angiokeratoma in children are characterized by unilateral, clustered, red-violaceous papules, and small nodules usually located on the hands and feet of children or rarely adults [214, 215, 221]. The etiology is unknown. Histopathologic investigations reveal a dense nodular lymphoid infiltrate with occasional plasma cells and eosinophils, and with increased numbers of capillaries. The infiltrate is usually well circumscribed, sometimes with an epidermal collarette, accentuating the benign

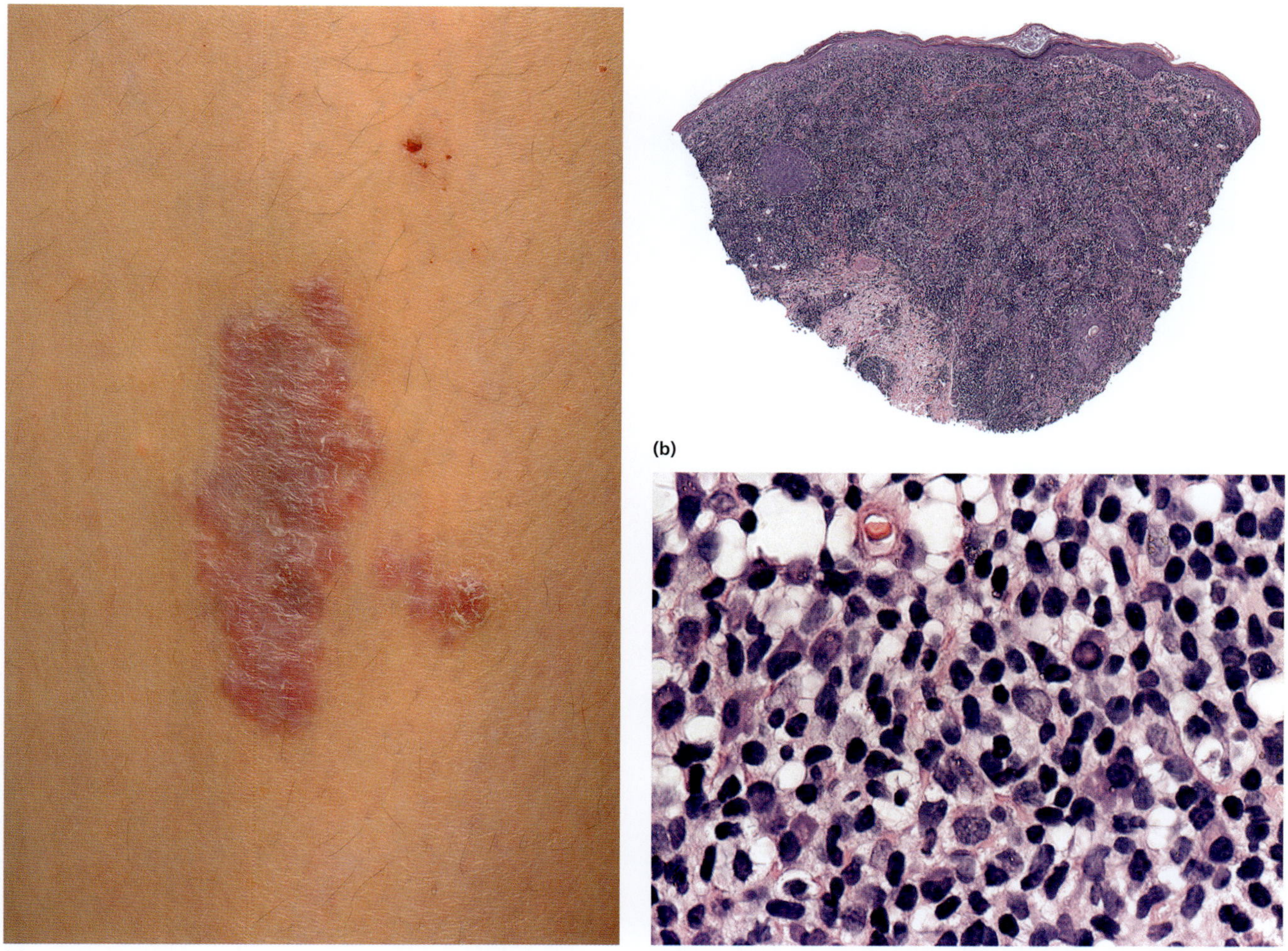

(a) (b) (c)

Figure 31.124 T/B-cell angiomatoid pseudolymphoma ("pre-tibial lymphoplasmacytic plaque in children"). (a) Irregular, infiltrated plaque with small erythematous papules in the surrounding area. (b) Dense inflammatory infiltrates admixed with small granulomas. (c) Details of small lymphocytes admixed with mature plasma cells.

aspect at low power. Histopathological features are similar to those of cases reported as "T-cell-rich angiomatoid polypoid pseudolymphoma" [215]. Features similar to those observed in acral pseudolymphomatous angiokeratoma in children and T-cell-rich angiomatoid polypoid pseudolymphoma were observed also in a case arising in a young girl on the leg, and classified originally as "solitary cutaneous plasmacytosis" [222]. The lesion did not have any clinical resemblance to those of cutaneous and systemic plasmacytosis, and several similar cases characterized by pre-tibial solitary plaques in young patients have been subsequently reported as "pre-tibial lymphoplasmacytic plaque in children" [216–218]. Patients are children or adolescents with erythematous, persistent plaques on the pre-tibial region (Fig. 31.124a). Histology reveals dense lymphoid infiltrates admixed with variable numbers of plasma cells (Figs. 31.124b, c). Small granulomas may be present. In spite of extensive search, microorganisms have not been found in any of the reported cases. The infiltrate contains B as well as T lymphocytes. The density of the infiltrate and the presence of plasma cells convey a resemblance to cutaneous marginal zone lymphoproliferative disorder, but the plasma cells are polyclonal rather than monoclonal.

In all these conditions, a prominent histopathological feature is represented by the presence of increased vessels with similarities to so-called "high endothelial venules," reflected in the original term of "angiokeratoma" (Fig. 31.125). Positivity for WT-1 and negativity for D2–40 (podoplanine) suggest that the vessels in these conditions are proliferative rather than malformative [223]. To my eyes, the main differential diagnosis of angiomatoid pseudolymphoma is represented by epithelioid hemangioma (angiolymphoid hyperplasia with eosinophilia), a benign vascular neoplasm that is characterized by the two main histopathological features of angiomatoid pseudolymphoma, namely, the presence

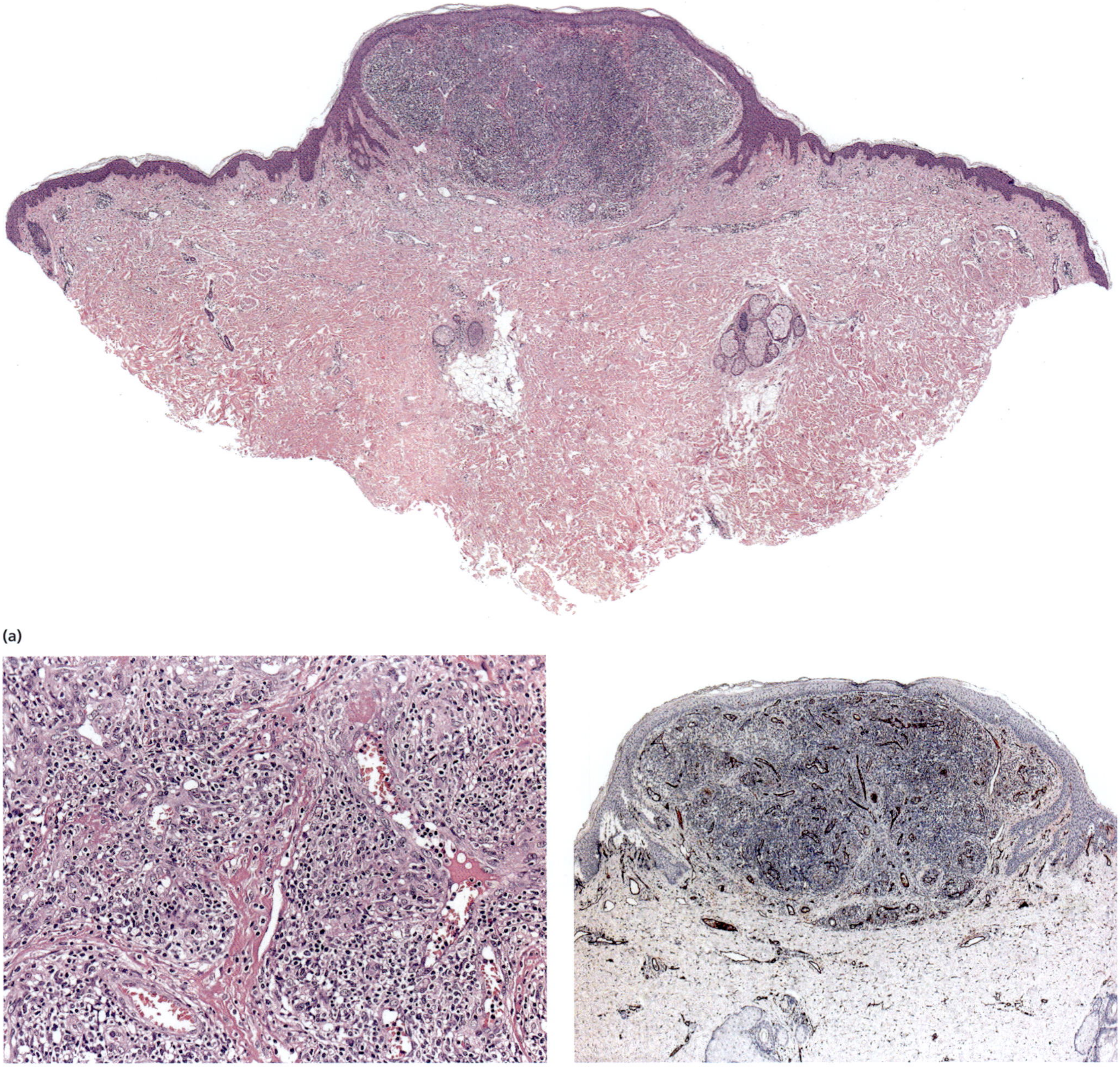

(a) (b) (c)

Figure 31.125 T/B-cell angiomatoid pseudolymphoma ("angiomatoid polypoid pseudolymphoma"). (a) Well circumscribed, exophytic lesion characterized by (b) dense lympho-histiocytic infiltrates admixed with several vessels. (c) Immunohistology for CD31 highlights the numerous vessels.

of increased numbers of vessels with thick endothelial walls, and of a dense lymphoid infiltrate. In this context, cases of angiomatoid pseudolymphoma with many eosinophils should be judged critically, and the differential diagnosis with epithelioid hemangioma should be considered.

These benign lymphoid proliferations do not respond to antibiotic or antimicrobial treatment. Surgical excision is an option for solitary lesions, but it may difficult for cases presenting with multiple lesions. A watchful waiting strategy seems to be the best management for these patients.

## Cutaneous extramedullary hematopoiesis

The skin may rarely be the site of onset of extramedullary hematopoiesis, a disorder caused by abnormal hematopoiesis in the bone marrow often due to chronic myeloproliferative or myelodysplastic disorders, particularly chronic idiopathic myelofibrosis [224]. Both the clinical and the histopathologic presentation may simulate cutaneous manifestations of myeloid leukemia. Clinically there are localized or generalized red-livid papules, plaques, or even tumors (Fig. 31.126).

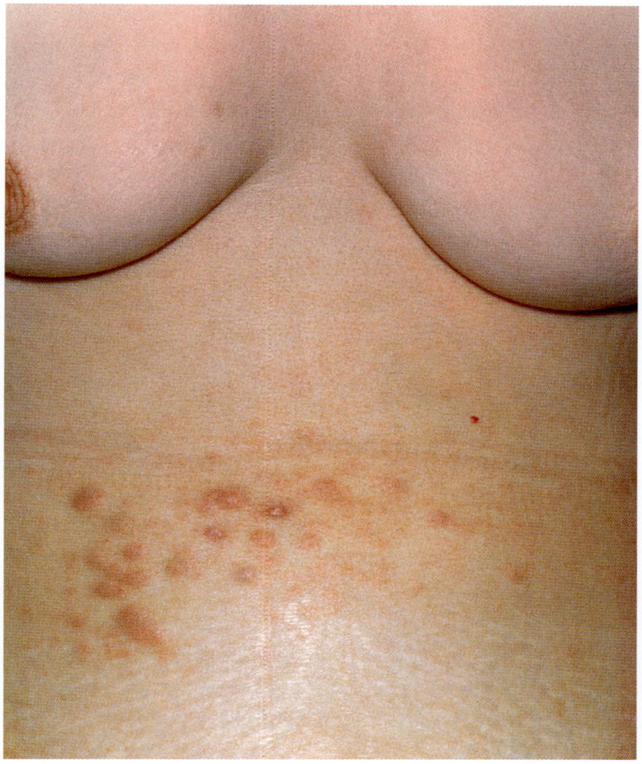

Figure 31.126 Cutaneous extramedullary hematopoiesis. Several erythematous papules and small nodules on the trunk.

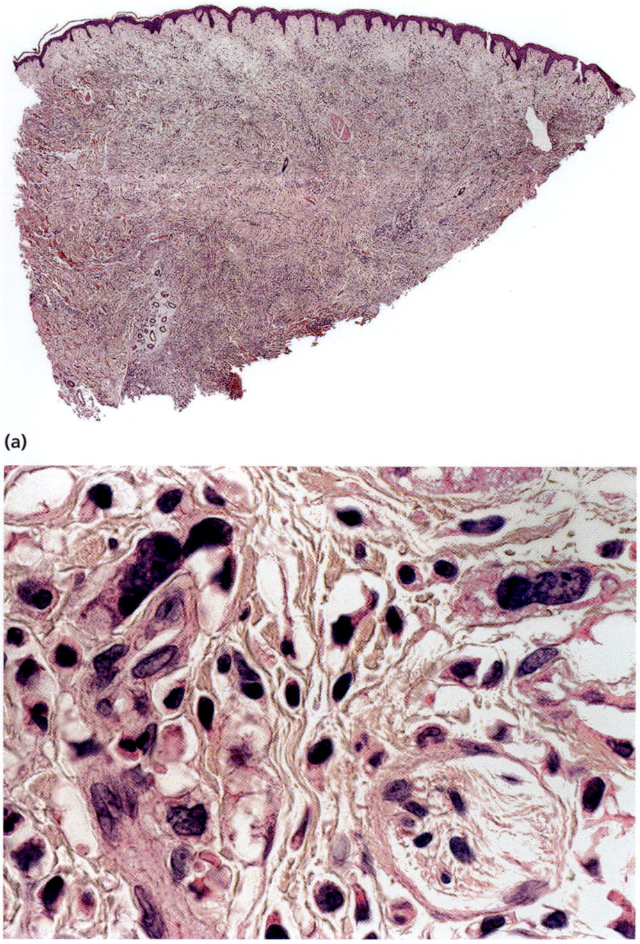

(a)

(b)

Figure 31.127 Cutaneous extramedullary hematopoiesis. (a) Diffuse infiltrate within the entire dermis. (b) Note large megakaryoblast and other immature myeloid cells.

Histology shows in the dermis the presence of bone marrow precursor cells deriving from all three lineages (erythroblasts, megakaryoblasts, and myeloid precursors) (Fig. 31.127). In contrast to leukemic infiltrates, these cells usually do not form sheets or large nodules and are found scattered between the collagen bundles. Immunohistologic stainings for CD41, CD42b, or CD61 allow identification of the megakaryoblasts, whereas erythroblasts may be stained by antibodies against hemoglobin or glycophorin. Myeloid precursors can be identified by markers such as CD68, myeloperoxidase, lysozyme, CD14, CD34, CD117, MNDA, and CD163. Differentiation from myeloid leukemia can be achieved only by comparing the morphology with the phenotype of the cells and integrating it with clinical data, as neoplastic cells of myeloid leukemias may express similar antigens.

Extramedullary hematopoiesis restricted to one lineage only has also been observed in the background of cutaneous pilomatricoma, involuting congenital hemangioma, pyogenic granuloma, and leg ulcers in otherwise healthy individuals, representing a local phenomenon rather than a systemic disorder.

The prognosis of cutaneous trilineage extramedullary hematopoiesis is usually poor. Patients have been managed with chemotherapy or radiation therapy.

## Histiocytoid cells in Sweet syndrome and other conditions

Although ***Sweet syndrome*** (acute febrile neutrophilic dermatosis) is a neutrophilic dermatitis and as such does not represent a simulator of cutaneous lymphomas, an unusual variant of it termed "histiocytoid" Sweet syndrome is characterized histopathologically by the presence of immature myeloid cells, and may be misinterpreted as a specific cutaneous manifestation of a myeloid disorder, particularly myelodysplastic syndrome or myeloid leukemia [225]. It has been suggested that most cases of histiocytoid Sweet syndrome are associated with an underlying myeloid leukemia or with myelodysplastic syndrome [226–229], but other studies did not show a percentage of myeloid leukemia-associated cases higher than expected (see also Chapter 23) [230].

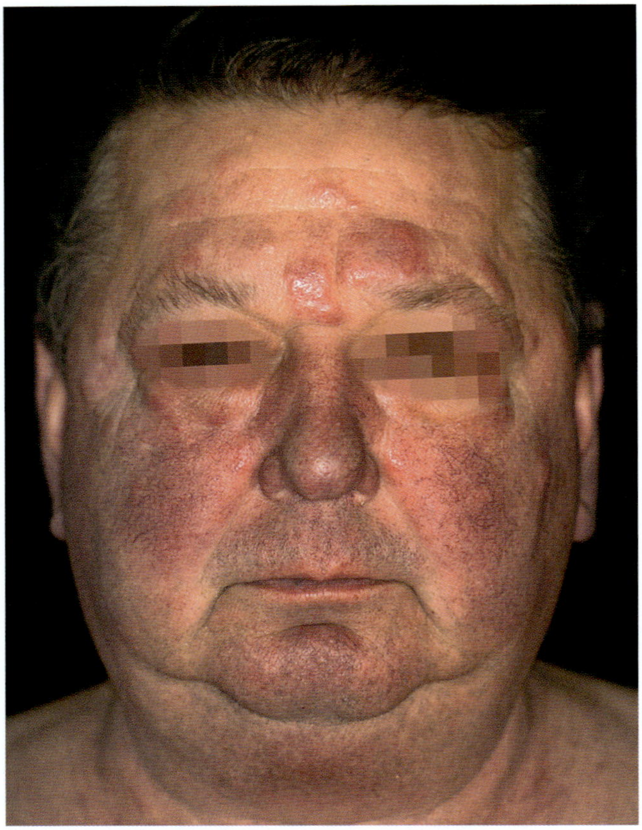

Figure 31.128 Histiocytoid Sweet syndrome. Infiltrated plaques on the face.

Clinically, patients usually present with lesions similar to conventional Sweet syndrome, but in some cases the appearance may be less typical (Fig. 31.128). Histology shows variably dense inflammatory infiltrates of mononuclear cells in the superficial and mid-dermis, admixed with some neutrophils (Fig. 31.129). Papillary dermal edema is frequently present. Immunohistochemical studies reveal that most cells are positive for myeloperoxidase, CD15, CD43, CD68, and lysozyme (Fig. 31.130), raising the suspicion of specific cutaneous involvement by myelogenous leukemia.

The precise classification of histiocytoid Sweet syndrome is made even more difficult by two problems, namely, (i) the fact that Sweet syndrome can arise in patients with myeloid leukemia and (ii) the knowledge that specific cells of myeloid leukemia or of myelodysplastic syndrome may be observed within the infiltrate of Sweet syndrome in some patients [226, 227]. In this context, careful investigations are required in patients with histiocytoid Sweet syndrome. On the other hand, histiocytoid Sweet syndrome is characterized by a benign biological behavior, and lesions respond to low doses of oral corticosteroids or nonsteroidal anti-inflammatory drugs.

Besides Sweet syndrome, I have observed large numbers of "histiocytoid" cells in other conditions characterized histopathologically by mostly neutrophilic infiltrates, such as ***leukocytoclastic vasculitis*** (Fig. 31.131) and ***erysipelas***. Small numbers of "histiocytoid" cells can be observed also in some cases of ***erythema nodosum***. It is conceivable that some of these cases,

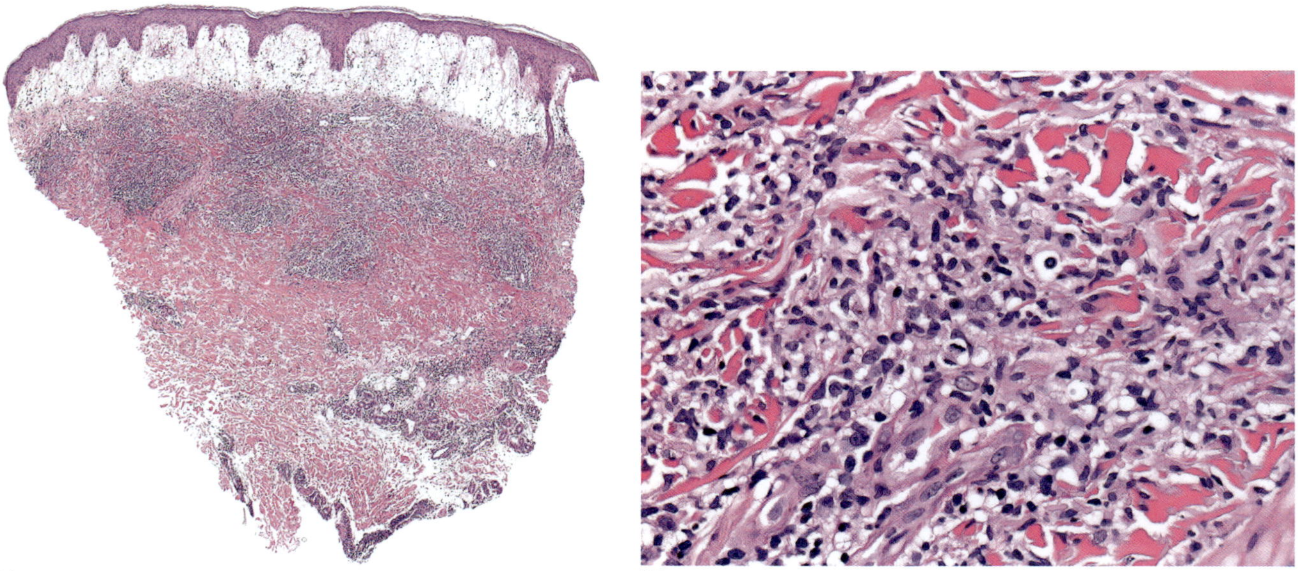

(a) (b)

Figure 31.129 Histiocytoid Sweet syndrome. (a) Subepidermal edema and dense infiltrate in the entire dermis. (b) Detail of "histiocytoid" immature myeloid cells.

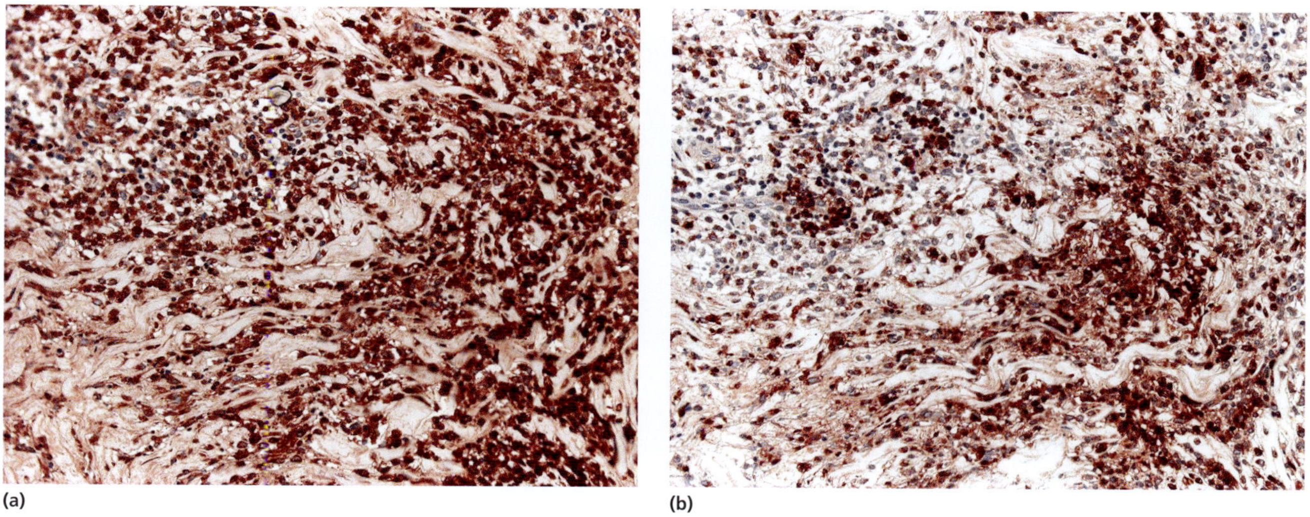

Figure 31.130 Histiocytoid Sweet syndrome. Stainings for (a) lysozyme and (b) myeloperoxidase reveal positivity of the majority of the cells.

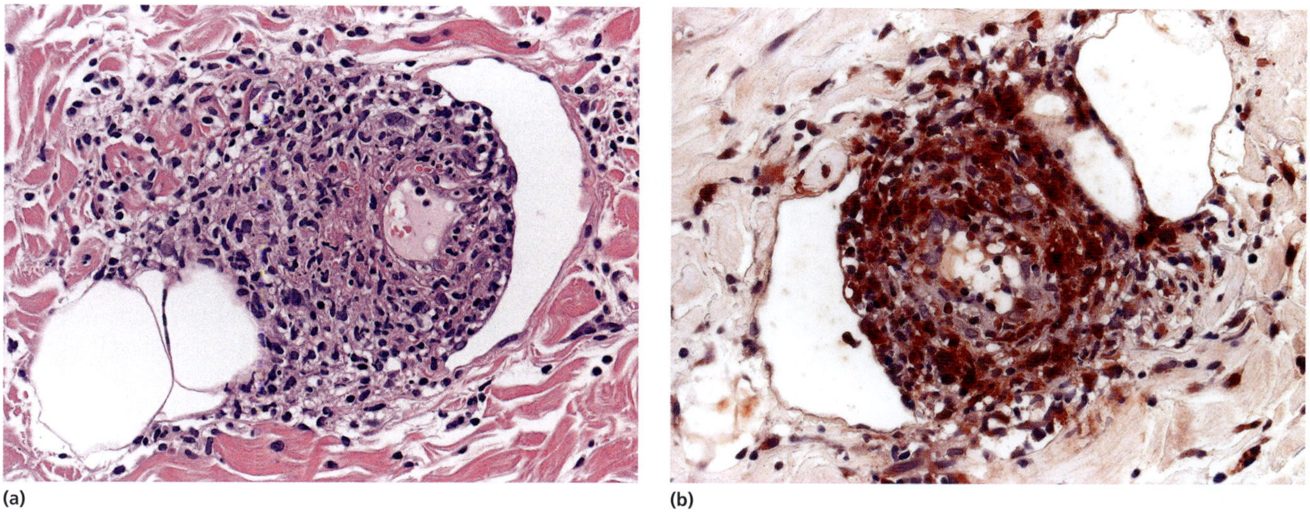

Figure 31.131 Histiocytoid cells in a case of leukocytoclastic vasculitis. (a) Small vessel with vasculitic changes and an inflammatory infiltrate admixed with histiocytoid cells; (b) the histiocytoid cells are positive for myeloperoxidase.

similar to histiocytoid Sweet syndrome, are associated with a myelogenous disorder, and that the histiocytoid cells are clonally related to those of the hematological disease. In fact, in some of the cases that I have observed a myeloid leukemia was known (see Fig. 23.20 in Chapter 23); however, a hematological disease was not known in several other cases, and routine investigations were negative. The histiocytoid cells represent an atypical histopathological feature in these cases, and their presence in large numbers should prompt a careful evaluation of the patient for an underlying hematological condition.

## Intralymphatic histiocytosis

In rare cases, an intralymphatic proliferation of histiocytes may mimic the histopathologic picture of intravascular large cell lymphoma [231]. The disease was formerly termed "intravascular histiocytosis." Lesions may arise on the background of disparate conditions including chronic cutaneous infections, connective tissue disorders (particularly rheumatoid arthritis), or other systemic diseases, and show protean clinical features depending on the original disease. In some cases, they arise near the scar of a previous surgical excision, suggesting that the lymphatic alterations due to the previous intervention may play a role in the etiology of this condition. I have also observed complexes of intralymphatic histiocytosis as a secondary, focal phenomenon in biopsy specimens of mycosis fungoides and of lupus erythematosus. The distinction between a primary form (without associated conditions) and a secondary one (associated with systemic disease) has been proposed [232], but to my eyes it is not necessary for diagnosis and management of patients.

In most cases, patients present clinically with poorly demarcated areas of indurated erythema. A typical presentation is characterized by a "retiform-like," vaguely arciform arrangement of the lesions (Fig. 31.132). Histology reveals clusters of histiocytoid cells within dilated vessels characterized by flat endothelial cell lining (Fig. 31.133a). The cell aggregates usually do not fill the vessels but rather seem to be floating within them (Fig. 31.133b), and are positive for histiocytic markers (CD68, CD163) (Fig. 31.133c). The endothelial cells are positive for CD31, CD34, and podoplanin (D2–40), thus being lymphatic rather than blood vessels (Fig. 31.133d). As CD31 and CD34 stain the endothelial cells of blood vessels as well, a staining for podoplanin should always be added to the phenotypic evaluation of intravascular cell aggregates. The location (intralymphatic versus within blood vessels), the arrangement of the intravascular complexes (usually not filling dilated vessels in intralymphatic histiocytosis as opposed to completely filling small vessels in intravascular large cell lymphoma), and the morphology of the cells (histiocytes with eosinophilic cytoplasm as opposed to large lymphocytes with scant cytoplasm) allow a clear morphologic distinction to be made between the two conditions. However, very rare intravascular (blood vessels) cases of intralymphatic histiocytosis have been documented, which showed otherwise typical features of the condition [233, 234]. Although I was previously skeptical about the existence of true intravascular cases, I have recently observed one biopsy specimen showing intravascular histiocytes restricted to blood vessels (Fig. 31.134).

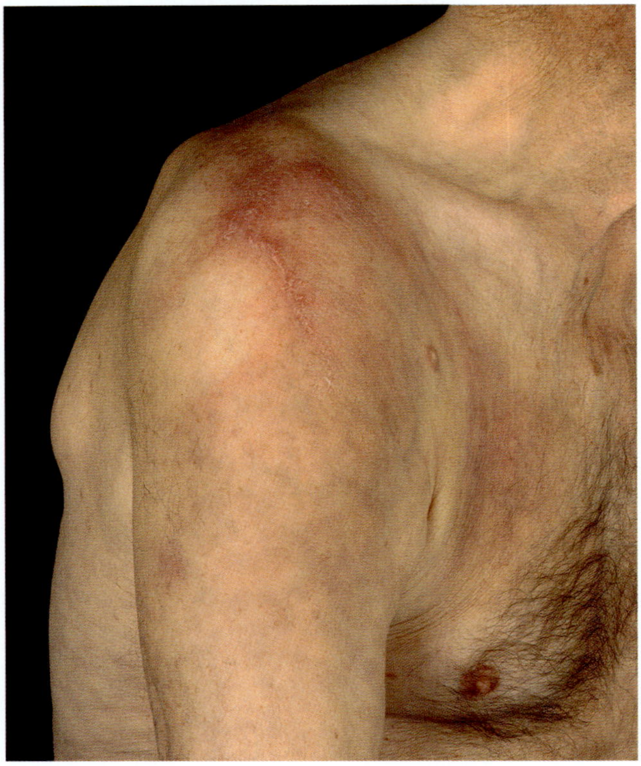

Figure 31.132 Intralymphatic histiocytosis. Erythematous, infiltrated lesions with a vaguely arciform, retiform pattern on the right shoulder of a patient with rheumatoid arthritis.

Molecular analyses do not reveal monoclonality of the Ig or TCR genes rearrangement.

Intralymphatic histiocytosis should be distinguished from intravascular large cell lymphomas (see Chapter 19), intralymphatic $CD30^+$ anaplastic large cell lymphoma and intralymphatic lymphomatoid papulosis (see Chapter 5), and benign intralymphatic proliferation of T-cell lymphoid blasts (see below in this chapter). Immunohistochemical stainings for lymphatic vessels, T- and B-lymphocytes, and histiocytes allow a simple and reliable differentiation of these entities. Intralymphatic histiocytosis should also be distinguished from reactive angioendotheliomatosis, a condition characterized by an intravascular proliferation of endothelial cells that can be encountered also in patients with hematological malignancies (see also Chapter 29) [235]. Although in the past it had been suggested that the two disorders may be related, the location of the cellular aggregates is different (within lymphatic vessels in intralymphatic histiocytosis and within blood vessels in reactive angioendotheliomatosis); thus, they represent distinct entities [231]. CD31, a marker used commonly for endothelial cells, is positive in reactive angioendotheliomatosis, but it may be positive in histiocytes as well; thus, the distinction between the two diseases should be made using a panel of antibodies including podoplanine, CD31, CD68, and CD163.

Management of intralymphatic histiocytosis depends on the associated disorder, but often skin lesions do not show improvement upon successful treatment of the background condition. Partial responses have been described with local radiotherapy, topical corticosteroids, and pentoxifylline, among many others, but there is no evidence that any of the reported treatments were really beneficial.

## Benign intralymphatic proliferation of T-cell lymphoid blasts

Rare cases of a benign intravascular proliferation of large lymphoid cells simulating the picture of intravascular large cell lymphoma have been described in the skin at sites of previous trauma or within hemangiomas, as well as within endometrial polyps and appendicitis [236–241]. An identical case had been described by Ackerman and Tanski in 1977 as "pseudoleukemia cutis" within a molluscum contagiosum [128], and other cases have been reported arising in the context of hidradenitis suppurativa, lichen sclerosus, drug eruption, or regressing keratoacanthoma [242–245]. Reported cases represented always incidental findings

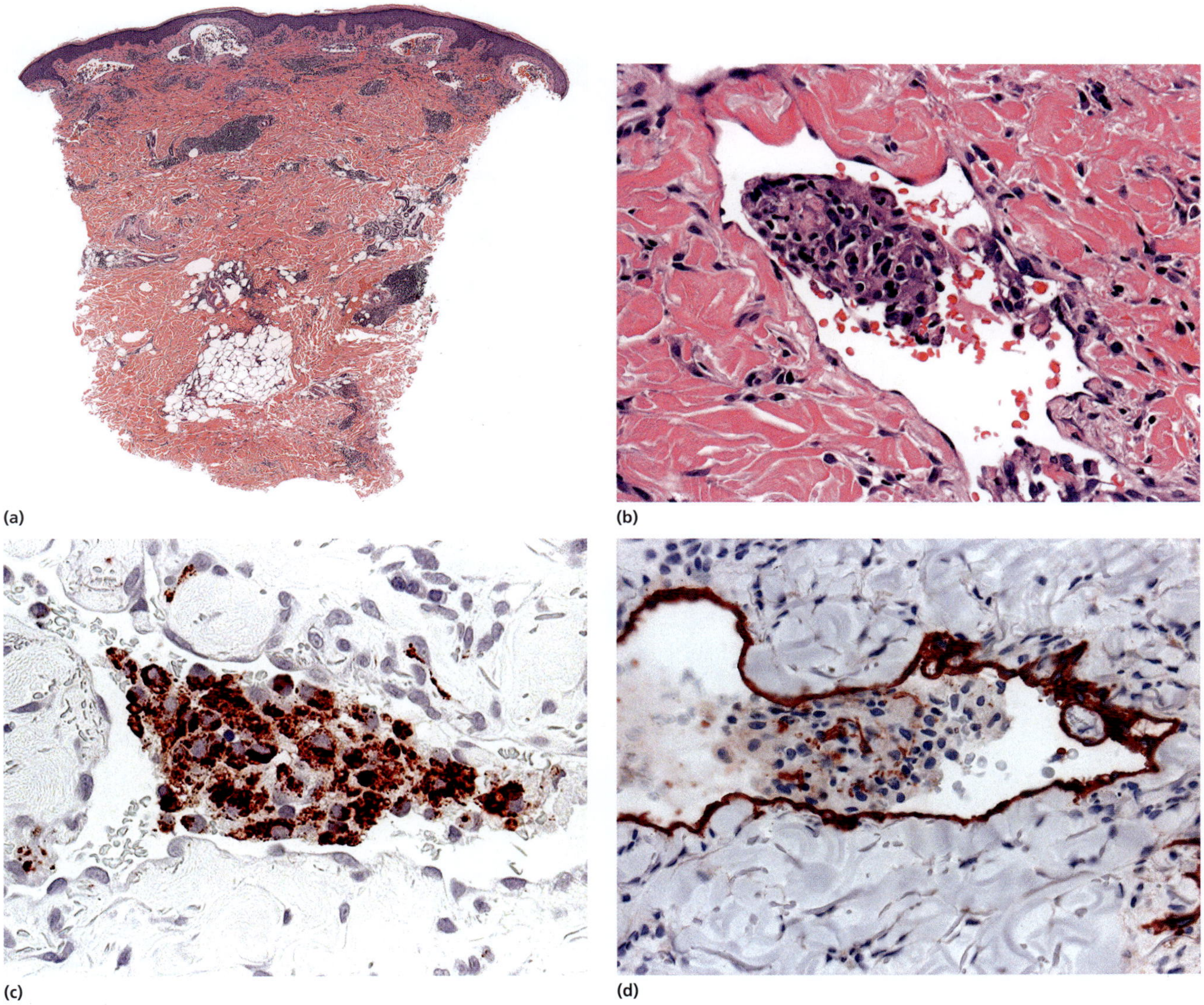

Figure 31.133 Intralymphatic histiocytosis. (a) Large intravascular clusters of cells. (b) Detail showing intravascular mid-sized cells with abundant cytoplasm admixed with small lymphocytes. (c) Positivity of the intravascular cells for CD68 confirms the histiocytic differentiation. (d) Positivity of the endothelial cells for podoplanin confirms the intralymphatic arrangement of the histiocytes.

in biopsies taken for different reasons. Intralymphatic proliferation of T-cell lymphoid blasts is considered to be benign because of the lack of other signs of intravascular large cell lymphoma, the clinical presentation mostly being confined to pre-existing lesions of different conditions, the lack of clonal TCR genes rearrangement, and the favorable course at follow-up. Since experience is limited to a handful of cases, however, care should be taken in the evaluation of these lesions.

Histology shows large, blastoid lymphocytes within and focally outside of the vessels, as opposed to intravascular large cell lymphomas, in which neoplastic lymphocytes are confined within the vessel walls. The blastoid cells fill the vessels, similarly to the picture of intravascular large cell lymphoma and unlike that of intralymphatic histiocytosis, and a background condition is usually the predominating histopathological feature (Fig. 31.135). Immunohistology reveals a T-cell phenotype, often with positivity for CD30. The proliferation rate is usually high, representing a worrying feature (Fig. 31.136a). PCR analysis of the TCR genes rearrangement does not reveal monoclonality in benign intralymphatic proliferation of T-cell lymphoid blasts.

The main differential diagnostic criteria to distinguish this condition from intravascular large cell lymphoma are the following [242]:

1. Presence of histopathological features of an inflammatory skin disorder (e.g., lichen sclerosus, granuloma pyogenicum, etc);
2. Location of the large cells, which are confined to lymphatic vessels (positive for podoplanine) in benign intralymphatic proliferation of T-cell lymphoid blasts, as opposed to blood vessels in intravascular large cell lymphoma (Fig. 31.136b);

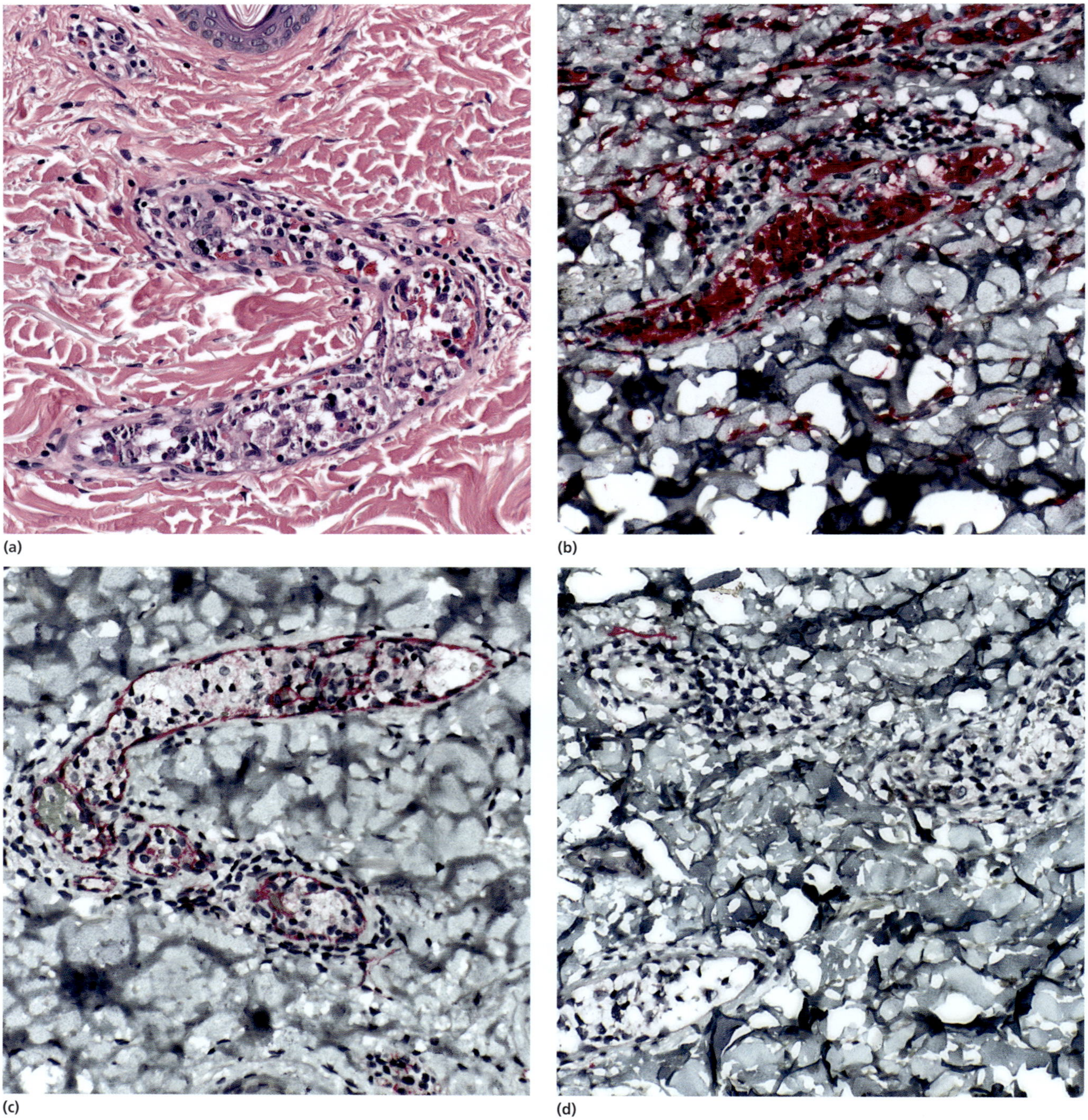

**Figure 31.134** "True" intravascular histiocytosis. (a) Intravascular clusters of mononuclear cells admixed with erythrocytes. (b) Positivity of most cells for CD163, confirming their histiocytic nature. (c) Positivity of the endothelial cells for CD31 and (d) negativity for D2–40, showing that these are indeed blood rather than lymphatic vessels (note a small, D2–40+ lymphatic channel representing an internal control).

3. Common presence of scattered atypical extravascular cells;
4. T-cell phenotype without aberrant features (no loss of pan-T-cell markers, no aberrant double positivity/negativity of CD4 and CD8);
5. Lack of positivity for Epstein–Barr virus (EBER-1 negativity);
6. Lack of monoclonal rearrangement of the TCR genes by polymerase chain reaction or other methods.

Rarely, anaplastic large cell lymphoma may be confined to lymphatic vessels in a given biopsy specimen, thus representing a major differential diagnosis with benign intralymphatic proliferation of T-cell lymphoid blasts (see Chapter 5). In contrast to anaplastic large cell lymphoma, in which neoplastic cells commonly display loss of one or more T-cell markers, the phenotype in the benign form does not show aberrant features. In addition, neoplastic cells in purely intralymphatic anaplastic large cell lymphoma are confined to the affected lymphatic vessels, and no extravascular infiltrate is visible. Distinction from intralymphatic lymphomatoid papulosis is more difficult, as

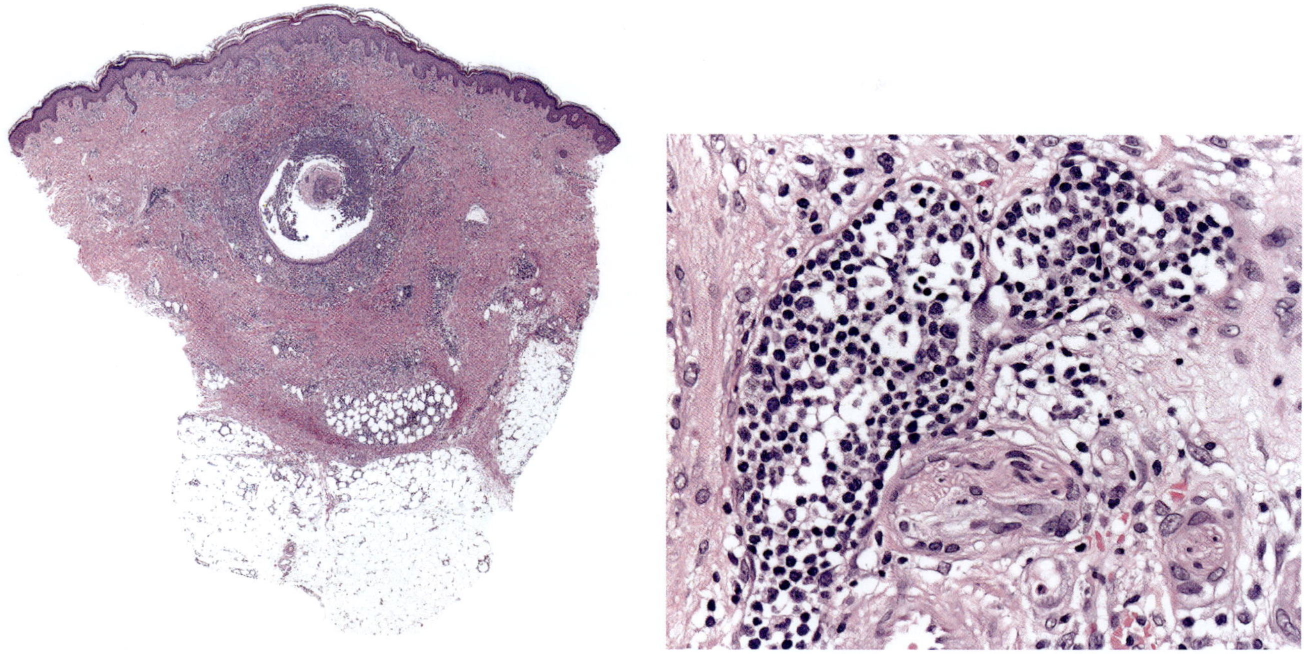

(a) (b)

**Figure 31.135** Benign intralymphatic proliferation of T-cell lymphoid blasts. (a) Ruptured infundibular cyst with dense inflammation; (b) within the inflammatory infiltrate there are clusters of large lymphocytes filling dilated lymphatic vessels.

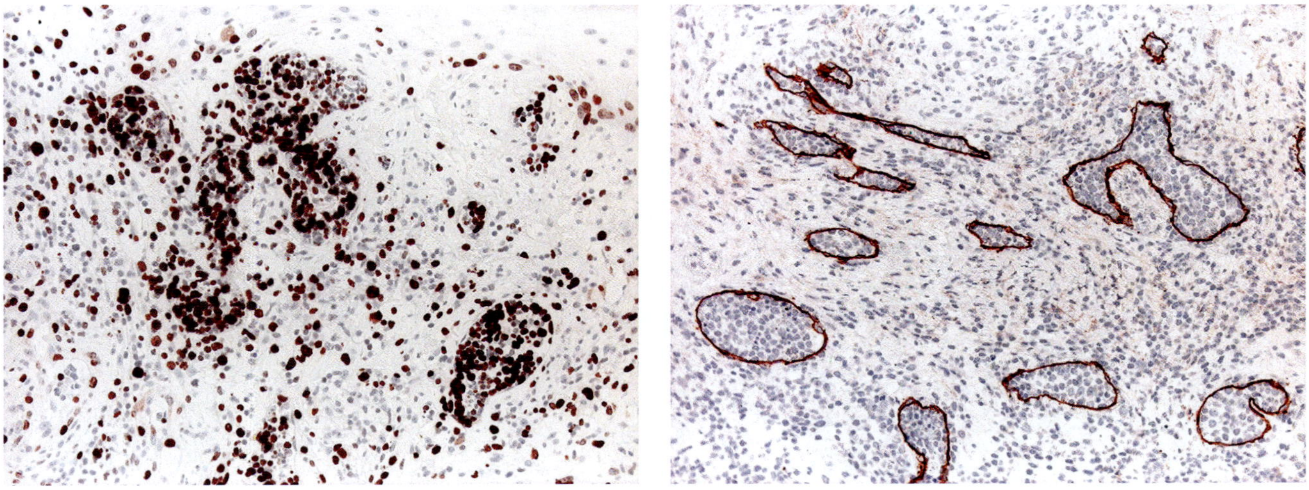

(a) (b)

**Figure 31.136** Benign intralymphatic proliferation of T-cell lymphoid blasts. (a) Staining for Ki-67 shows a high proliferation of the intralymphatic lymphocytes. (b) Staining for podoplanine confirms the intralymphatic arrangement of the cells.

histopathological features of the two conditions may overlap. However, in contrast to intralymphatic lymphomatoid papulosis, in benign intralymphatic proliferation of T-cell lymphoid blasts features of a background condition are invariably present and dominate the histopathological picture.

The etiology of benign intralymphatic proliferation of T-cell lymphoid blasts is unknown. In one reported case, the phenotype of the intralymphatic T-cells corresponded to effector/memory-like T-regulatory cells, suggesting that the process may reflect an immune response to a yet unknown antigen either locally or in the draining lymph nodes [238]. Cesinaro and Luca postulated a role of bacterial infections in the pathogenesis of this condition [239]. In this context, it is interesting to note that large intralymphatic collections of T lymphocytes with normal morphology may be seen in various conditions including cutaneous B-cell lymphomas (Fig. 31.137), possibly representing

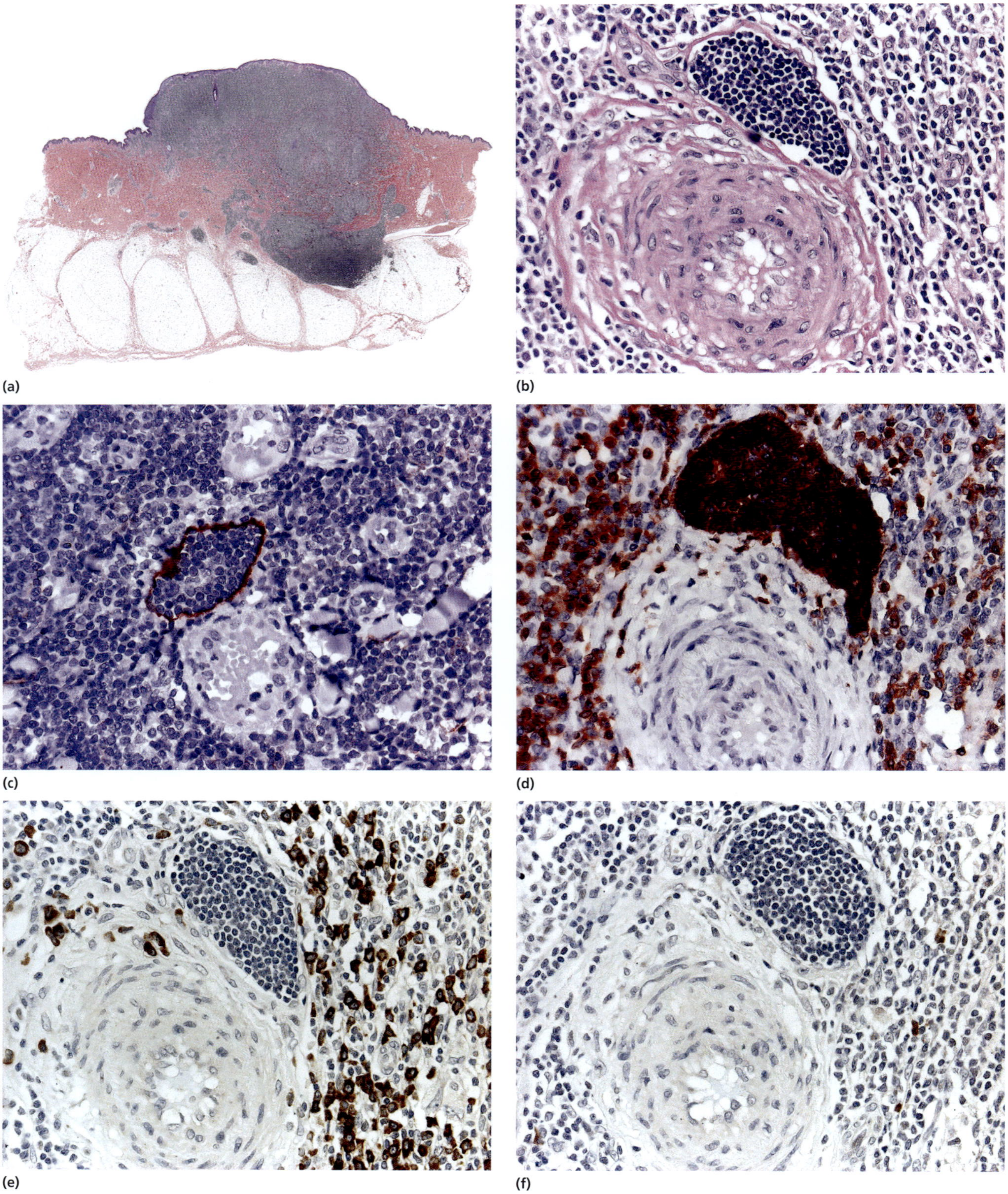


**Figure 31.137** Benign intralymphatic proliferation of T lymphocytes within a cutaneous marginal zone lymphoma. (a) Large, nodular lymphoid infiltrate within the entire dermis and superficial subcutaneous fat. (b) Focal cluster of small lymphoid cells within a dilated vessel. (c) Staining for podoplanine confirms the intralymphatic arrangement of the cells. (d) The intralymphatic cells are positive for CD3; the neoplastic cells of marginal zone lymphoproliferative disorder show positivity for (e) kappa and negativity for (f) lambda immunoglobulin light chain.

a variation on the same theme. It may be hypothesized that these T lymphocytes are trafficking between cutaneous sites of inflammation (including inflammation due to neoplastic processes) and the regional lymph nodes; activated cells may display the atypical morphological features observed in benign intralymphatic proliferation of T-cell lymphoid blasts, as well as CD30 expression.

As already mentioned, benign intralymphatic proliferation of T-cell lymphoid blasts is an incidental finding in biopsies taken for other disorders; thus, no other treatment besides the one planned for the background condition is necessary.

## Other "accidental" pseudolymphomas

In addition to the cutaneous pseudolymphomas discussed in the previous paragraphs, the occurrence of lymphoid infiltrates simulating histopathologically a cutaneous lymphoma has been reported in a wide variety of cutaneous conditions otherwise unrelated to "conventional" pseudolymphomas. The infiltrate in these cases may either be band-like mimicking mycosis fungoides, or nodular with or without the presence of plasma cells mimicking mainly CD4$^+$ small/medium T-cell lymphoproliferative disorder or marginal zone lymphoproliferative disorder, or wedge-shaped with CD30$^+$ cells mimicking lymphomatoid papulosis. A peculiar "pseudolymphomatous" condition is related to the ***immune response to epithelial tumors*** in certain areas of the body, particularly the head and neck. In some cases, the epithelial tumor (usually a superficial lesion such as a carcinoma in situ, superficial basal cell carcinoma, or actinic keratosis) elicits a prominent plasma cell reaction characterized by sheets of mature plasma cells with a polytypic expression of the immunoglobulin light chains kappa and lambda. Occasionally, even reactive germinal centers may be observed, which are easily distinguished morphologically (and if needed phenotypically) from malignant lymphoid follicles of cutaneous follicle center lymphoma.

I have observed "pseudolymphomatous" infiltrates in the most disparate conditions including bullous pemphigoid (Fig. 31.138), inflammatory infiltrates in ruptured infundibular cysts, folliculitis, perniosis, graft-versus-host disease (Fig. 31.139), and lichen striatus, among many others [115, 246]. Interestingly, in ***granuloma annulare*** a florid ("pseudolymphomatous") inflammatory reaction may be observed [247], and a monoclonal population of T-lymphocytes has been detected in a small proportion of cases [248]. Benign clonal T-cell infiltrates may occur in patients with ***hypereosinopilic syndrome***, sometimes showing the presence of several CD30$^+$ cells [243, 249], and have been observed in cases of eruption of lymphocyte recovery as well [250]. Particularly in infectious disorders, the presence of large, activated lymphocytes may be misleading. Many of these cases can be included in one of the categories of pseudolymphoma discussed in this chapter, particularly in the one of CD30$^+$ T-cell pseudolymphomas. In other instances, features of the background disease can be identified, and a specific diagnosis can be made. In one unusual case of cutaneous ***Stenotrophomonas maltophilia infection***, clinicopathological features mimicked that of a gamma/delta T-cell lymphoma [251]. Some cases of ***crystal-storing histiocytosis***, a rare cutaneous condition characterized by the accumulation of immunoglobulin light chain crystals in the cytoplasm of macrophages, usually in the setting of a lymphoplasmacytic light chain-producing lymphoma, may present with dense nodular lymphoid infiltrates besides the typical light chain crystals (see also Chapter 29) [252].

A dermatitis associated with HTLV-1 infection (***HTLV-1-associated infective dermatitis***) is characterized by pruritic, recurrent, severe eczematous lesions mainly affecting seborrheic areas [253]. In some patients, the presence of intraepidermal lymphocytes may mimic the histopathological picture of mycosis fungoides or of cutaneous adult T-cell lymphoma/leukemia. In this context, it must be underlined that patients with HTLV-1-associated infective dermatitis may progress to adult T-cell lymphoma/leukemia or to tropical spastic paraparesis/HTLV-1-associated myelopathy.

As mentioned in Chapter 3, ***nevoid hyperkeratosis of the nipple*** rarely can be characterized histopathologically by the presence of intraepidermal Darier nests, indistinguishable from those observed in mycosis fungoides [254, 255]. The clinical features are identical to those of the conventional variant of the disease and allow to properly classify these cases (see Chapter 3 for a detailed discussion).

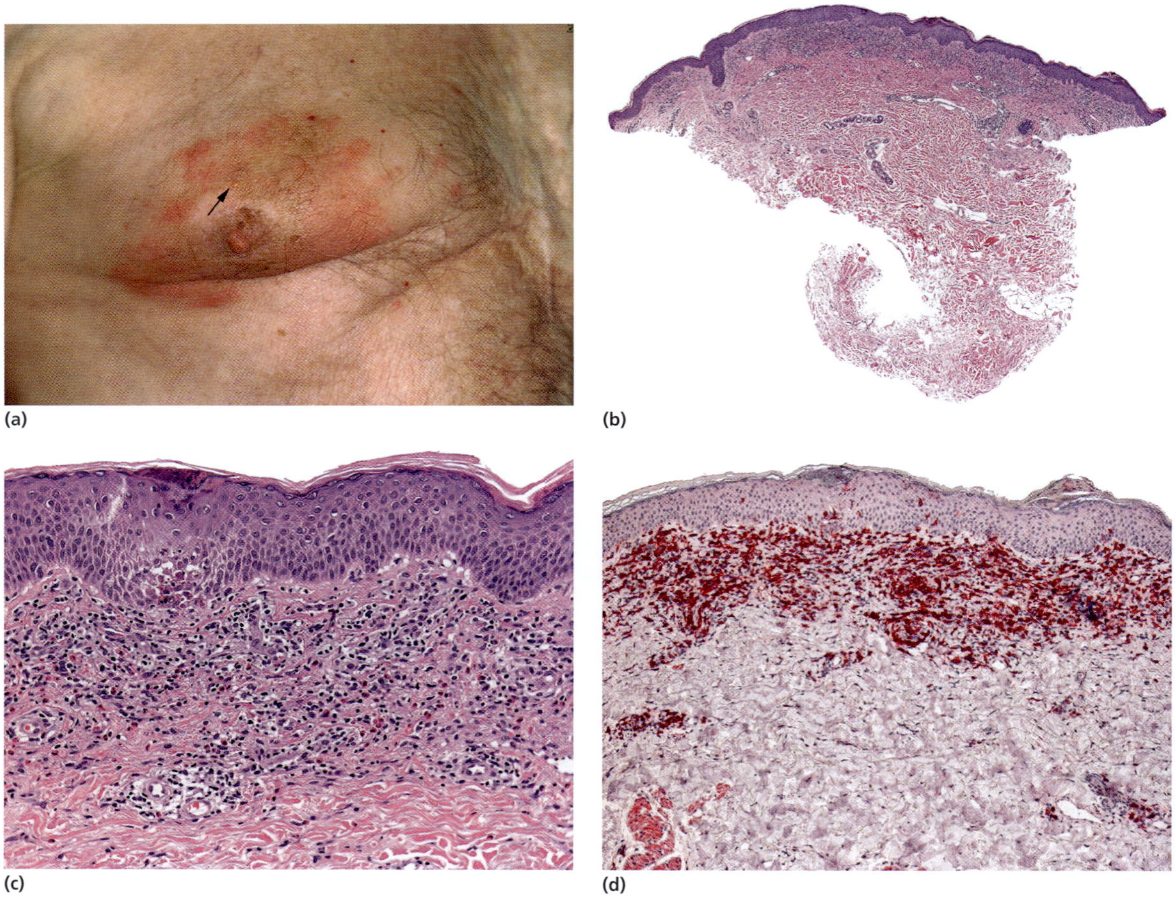

**Figure 31.138** Bullous pemphigoid with an unusually dense, band-like lymphoid infiltrate. (a) Solitary, erythematous, infiltrated plaque on the chest with a small vesicle (arrow) in a patient with history of bullous pemphigoid in remission. (b) Band-like infiltrate composed of (c) lymphocytes admixed with many eosinophils. (d) Staining for CD5 highlights the lymphocytes with some intraepidermal cells. The presence of many eosinophils is very unusual in early mycosis fungoides and should always prompt to consider a differential diagnosis of bullous pemphigoid.

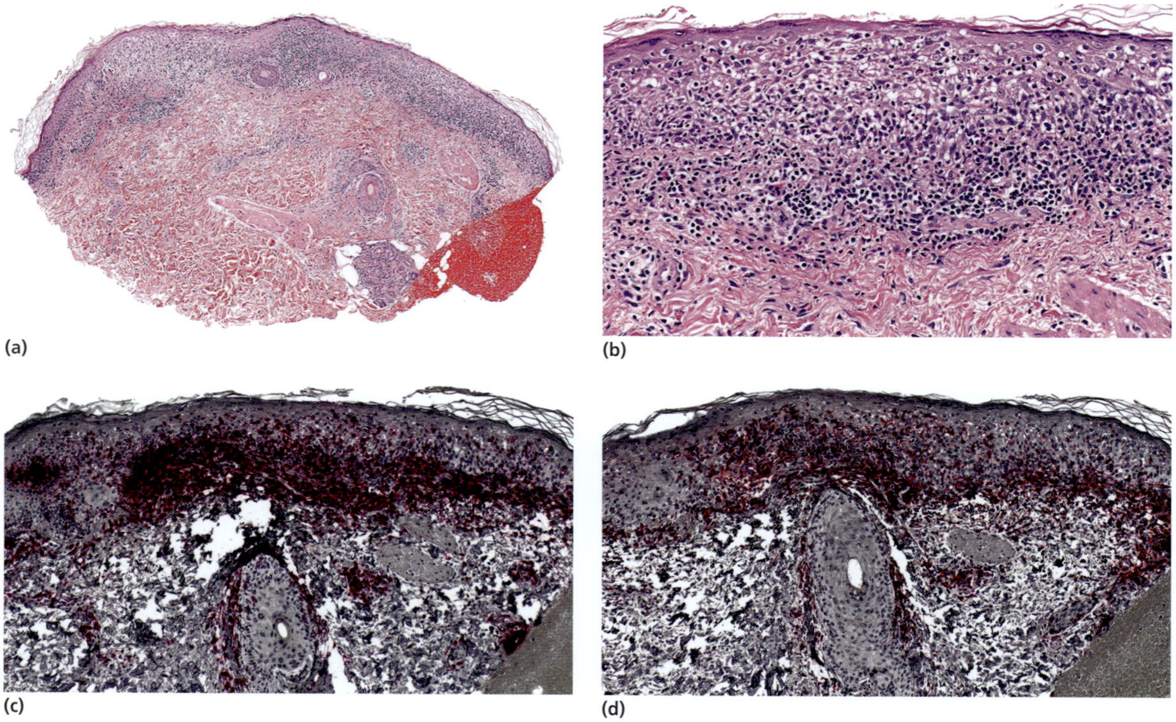

**Figure 31.139** Graft-versus-host disease with a "pseudolymphomatous" band-like lymphoid infiltrate. (a) Band-like infiltrate with (b) epidermotropic lymphocytes and some apoptotic keratinocytes. (c) Staining for CD3 highlights the intraepidermal lymphocytes; (d) staining for CD8 shows positivity of most cells.

## References


1. Mitteldorf C, Kempf W. Cutaneous pseudolymphoma-A review on the spectrum and a proposal for a new classification. *J Cutan Pathol* 2020;**47**:76–97.
2. Böer A, Tirumalae R, Bresch M, Falk TM. Pseudoclonality in cutaneous pseudolymphomas: a pitfall in interpretation of rearrangement studies. *Br J Dermatol* 2008;**159**:394–402.
3. Scherer F, Kurtz DM, Diehn M, Alizadeh AA. High-throughput sequencing for noninvasive disease detection in hematologic malignancies. *Blood* 2017;**130**:440–452.
4. Kirsch IR, Watanabe R, O'Malley JT, *et al.* TCR sequencing facilitates diagnosis and identifies mature T cells as the cell of origin in CTCL. *Sci Transl Med* 2015;**7**:308ra158.
5. Matos TR, de Rie MA, Teunissen MBM. Research techniques made simple: high-throughput sequencing of the T-Cell receptor. *J Invest Dermatol* 2017;**137**:e131–e138.
6. Bilsland D, Crombie IK, Ferguson J. The photosensitivity dermatitis and actinic reticuloid syndrome: no association with lymphoreticular malignancy. *Br J Dermatol* 1994;**131**:209–214.
7. Giannelli F, Botcherby PK, Marimo B, Magnus IA. Cellular hypersensitivity to UV-1: a clue to the aetiology of actinic reticuloid? *Lancet* 1983;**321**:88–91.
8. Toonstra J, Wildschut A, Boer J, *et al.* Actinic reticuloid. *J Am Acad Dermatol* 1989;**21**:205–214.
9. Dawe RS, Crombie IK, Ferguson J. The natural history of chronic actinic dermatitis. *Arch Dermatol* 2000;**136**:1215–1220.
10. Heller P, Wieczorek R, Waldo E, *et al.* Chronic actinic dermatitis: an immunohistochemical study of its T-cell antigenic profile, with comparison to cutaneous T-cell lymphoma. *Am J Dermatopathol* 1994;**16**:510–516.
11. Toonstra J, van der Putte SCJ, van Wichen DF, *et al.* Actinic reticuloid: immunohistochemical analysis of the cutaneous infiltrate in 13 patients. *Br J Dermatol* 1989;**120**:779–786.
12. Neild VS, Hawk JLM, Eady RAJ, Cream JJ. Actinic reticuloid with Sézary cells. *Clin Exp Dermatol* 1982;**7**:143–148.
13. Chu AC, Robinson D, Hawk JLM, *et al.* Immunologic differentiation of the Sezary syndrome due to cutaneous T-cell lymphoma and chronic actinic dermatitis. *J Invest Dermatol* 1986;**86**:134–137.
14. Ferguson J. The management of the photosensitivity dermatitis and actinic reticuloid (PD/AR) syndrome. *J Dermatol Treat* 1990;**1**:143–145.
15. Vesely MD, Imaeda S, King BA. Tofacitinib citrate for the treatment of refractory, severe chronic actinic dermatitis. *JAAD Case Rep* 2016;**3**:4–6.
16. Vanhaecke C, Viguier M. Long-term remission of severe and refractory chronic actinic dermatosis with dupilumab: a case report with review of the literature. *Acta Derm Venereol* 2024 Aug; **23**(104):adv40453.
17. Gomez Orbaneja J, Iglesias Diez L, Sanchez Lozano JL, Conde SL. Lymphomatoid contact dermatitis. *Contact Dermatitis* 1976;**2**:139–143.
18. Ackerman AB, Breza TS, Capland L. Spongiotic simulants of mycosis fungoides. *Arch Dermatol* 1974;**109**:216–220.
19. Smets K, Busschots A, Hauben E, Goossens A. B-cell lymphomatoid contact dermatitis caused by methylisothiazolinone and methylchloroisothiazolinone. *Eur J Dermatol* 2018;**28**:91–93.
20. Wolff-Sneedorff A, Thomsen K, Secher L, Lange VG. Gene rearrangement in positive patch tests. *Exp Dermatol* 1995;**4**:322–326.
21. Stasko T, Van der Ploeg DE, De Villez RL. Hyperkeratotic mycosis fungoides restricted to the palms. *J Am Acad Dermatol* 1982;**7**:792–796.
22. Resnik KS, Kantor GR, Lessin SR, *et al.* Mycosis fungoides palmaris et plantaris. *Arch Dermatol* 1995;**131**:1052–1056.
23. Kim ST, Jeon YS, Sim HJ, *et al.* Clinicopathologic features and T-cell receptor gene rearrangement findings of mycosis fungoides palmaris et plantaris. *J Am Acad Dermatol* 2006;**54**:466–471.
24. Shimomura N, Sugimoto H, Nakayama A, *et al.* Case of mycosis fungoides palmaris et plantaris possibly associated with nail psoriasis. *J Dermatol* 2024;**51**:e13–e15.
25. Cerroni L, Schadelbauer E, Kogler A, Fried I. Clinicopathological spectrum of lichen planus. Skindeep 2025 (in press).
26. Mazzeo M, Saggini A, Rocco T, *et al.* Syringotropic lichen planus: a potential histopathologic mimicker of syringotropic mycosis fungoides. *Am J Dermatopathol* 2019;**41**:e50–e53.
27. Arnold D, Hoffman MB, Onajin O, *et al.* Hypopigmented macules as manifestation of lichen planus and lichen planopilaris. *Am J Dermatopathol* 2019;**41**:514–517.
28. Mir-Bonafé JM, Cañueto J, Fernández-López E, Santos-Briz A. Follicular mucinosis associated with nonlymphoid skin conditions. *Am J Dermatopathol* 2014;**36**:705–709.
29. Geller S, Gomez CJ, Myskowski PL, Pulitzer M. Follicular mucinosis in patients with hematologic malignancies other than mycosis fungoides: a clinicopathologic study. *J Am Acad Dermatol* 2019; **80**:1704–1711.
30. Williams RF, Hoang MP, Kroshinsky D, Smith GP. Infliximab-induced follicular mucinosis of the face. *Int J Dermatol* 2017;**56**:215–217.
31. Heymann WR. Predicting the nature of follicular mucinosis: still a sticky situation. *J Am Acad Dermatol* 2019;**80**:1524–1525.
32. Avitan-Hersh E, Dias-Polak D, Ramon M, *et al.* Follicular eruption with folliculotropic lymphocytic infiltrates associated with iatrogenic immunosuppression: report and study of 3 cases, and review of the literature. *Am J Dermatopathol* 2020;**42**:498–505.
33. Gallo JC, de Wet J, Visser WI, *et al.* Generalized lichen spinulosus and secondary follicular mucinosis. *JAAD Case Rep* 2023; **33**:101–104.
34. Santos-Briz A, Cañueto J, García-Dorado J, *et al.* Pediatric primary follicular mucinosis: further evidence of its relationship with mycosis fungoides. *Pediatr Dermatol* 2013;**30**:e218–e220.
35. Avitan-Hersh E, Dias-Polak D, Ramon M, *et al.* Follicular eruption with folliculotropic lymphocytic infiltrates associated with iatrogenic immunosuppression: report and study of 3 cases, and review of the literature. *Am J Dermatopathol* 2020;**42**: 498–505.
36. Fraitag S, Bodemer C. Neonatal erythroderma. *Curr Opin Pediatr* 2010;**22**:438–444.
37. Ott H. Guidance for assessment of erythroderma in neonates and infants for the pediatric immunologist. *Pediatr Allergy Immunol* 2019;**30**:259–268.
38. Thompson AK, Killian JM, Weaver AL, *et al.* Sézary syndrome without erythroderma: a review of 16 cases at mayo clinic. *J Am Acad Dermatol* 2017;**76**:683–688.
39. Olsen E, Vonderheid E, Pimpinelli N, *et al.* Revisions to the staging and classification of mycosis fungoides and Sezary syndrome: a

proposal of the International Society for Cutaneous Lymphomas (ISCL) and the Cutaneous Lymphoma Task Force of the European Organization of Research and Treatment of Cancer (EORTC). *Blood* 2007;**110**:1713–1722.
40. Klemke CD, Booken N, Weiss C, *et al.* Histopathological and immunophenotypical criteria for the diagnosis of Sézary syndrome in differentiation from other erythrodermic skin diseases: a European Organisation for Research and Treatment of Cancer (EORTC) Cutaneous Lymphoma Task Force Study of 97 cases. *Br J Dermatol* 2015;**173**:93–105.
41. Cetinözman F, Jansen PM, Willemze R. Expression of programmed death-1 in skin biopsies of benign inflammatory vs. lymphomatous erythroderma. *Br J Dermatol* 2014;**171**:499–504.
42. Ram-Wolff C, Martin-Garcia N, Bensussan A, *et al.* Histopathologic diagnosis of lymphomatous versus inflammatory erythroderma: a morphologic and phenotypic study on 47 skin biopsies. *Am J Dermatopathol* 2010;**32**:755–763.
43. Boonk SE, Zoutman WH, Marie-Cardine A, *et al.* Evaluation of immunophenotypic and molecular biomarkers for Sézary syndrome using standard operating procedures: a multicentre study of 59 patients. *J Invest Dermatol* 2016;**136**:1364e1372.
44. Nagler AR, Samimi S, Schaffer A, *et al.* Peripheral blood findings in erythrodermic patients: importance for the differential diagnosis of Sézary syndrome. *J Am Acad Dermatol* 2012;**66**:503–508.
45. Ricci C, Pileri A, Agostinelli C, *et al.* Plaques and tumors in a patient with refractory sézary syndrome treated with mogamulizumab. *J Dtsch Dermatol Ges* 2018;**16**:1263–1265.
46. Hirotsu KE, Neal TM, Khodadoust MS, *et al.* Clinical characterization of mogamulizumab-associated rash during treatment of mycosis fungoides or sézary syndrome. *JAMA Dermatol* 2021;**157**:700–707.
47. Hansen I, Abeck F, Menz A, *et al.* Mogamulizumab-associated rash - case series and review of the literature. *J Dtsch Dermatol Ges* 2024;**22**:1079–1086.
48. Avallone G, Roccuzzo G, Pileri A, *et al.* Clinicopathological definition, management and prognostic value of mogamulizumab-associated rash and other cutaneous events: a systematic review. *J Eur Acad Dermatol Venereol* 2024;**38**:1738–1748.
49. Trum NA, Zain J, Martinez XU, *et al.* Mogamulizumab efficacy is underscored by its associated rash that mimics cutaneous T-cell lymphoma: a retrospective single-centre case series. *Br J Dermatol* 2022;**186**:153–166.
50. Wang JY, Hirotsu KE, Neal TM, *et al.* Histopathologic characterization of mogamulizumab-associated rash. *Am J Surg Pathol* 2020;**44**:1666–1676.
51. Narala S, Saleem A, Brown RA, *et al.* Histopathologic and clinical characterization of brentuximab vedotin-associated rash. *Am J Surg Pathol* 2024;**48**:1131–1137.
52. van der Putte SCJ, Toonstra J, Felten PC, van Vloten WA. Solitary non-epidermotropic T cell pseudolymphoma of the skin. *J Am Acad Dermatol* 1986;**14**:444–453.
53. Arai E, Okubo H, Tsuchida T, *et al.* Pseudolymphomatous folliculitis: a clinicopathologic study of 15 cases of cutaneous pseudolymphoma with follicular invasion. *Am J Surg Pathol* 1999;**23**:1313–1319.
54. Arai E, Shimizu M, Hirose T. A review of 55 cases of cutaneous lymphoid hyperplasia: reassessment of the histopathologic findings leading to reclassification of 4 lesions as cutaneous marginal zone lymphoma and 19 as pseudolymphomatous folliculitis. *Hum Pathol* 2005;**36**:505–511.
55. Beltraminelli H, Leinweber B, Kerl H, *et al.* Primary cutaneous CD4+ small–/medium-sized pleomorphic T-cell lymphoma: a cutaneous nodular proliferation of pleomorphic T lymphocytes of undetermined significance? A study of 136 cases. *Am J Dermatopathol* 2009;**31**:317–322.
56. Willemze R, Cerroni L, Kempf W, *et al.* The 2018 update of the WHO-EORTC classification for primary cutaneous lymphomas. *Blood* 2019;**133**:1703–1714.
57. Kempf W, Mitteldorf C, Cerroni L, *et al.* Classifications of cutaneous lymphomas and lymphoproliferative disorders: An update from the EORTC cutaneous lymphoma histopathology group. *J Eur Acad Dermatol Venereol* 2024;**38**:1491–1503.
58. Rodriguez-Pinilla SM, Cerroni L. Primary cutaneous CD4-positive small/medium T-cell lymphoproliferative disorder. In: Arber DA, Borowitz MJ, Cook JR, *et al.*, eds. *The International Consensus Classification of myeloid and lymphoid neoplasms.* Philadelphia (US): Wolters Kluver, 2025: 695–696.
59. Vergier B, Jansen PM, Mitteldorf C, *et al.* Primary cutaneous CD4-positive small or medium T-cell lymphoproliferative disorder. In: *WHO Classification of Tumours Editorial Board. Haematolymphoid Tumours.* 5th edition. Lyon (France): IARC, 2024: 682–684.
60. Cetinözman F, Jansen PM, Willemze R. Expression of programmed death-1 in primary cutaneous CD4-positive small/medium-sized pleomorphic T-cell lymphoma, cutaneous pseudo-T-cell lymphoma, and other types of cutaneous T-cell lymphoma. *Am J Surg Pathol* 2012;**36**:109–116.
61. Kossard S. Unilesional mycosis fungoides or lymphomatoid keratosis? *Arch Dermatol* 1997;**133**:1312–1313.
62. Arai E, Shimizu M, Tsuchida T, *et al.* Lymphomatoid keratosis. An epidermotropic type of cutaneous lymphoid hyperplasia: clinicopathological, immunohistochemical, and molecular biological study of 6 cases. *Arch Dermatol* 2007;**143**:53–59.
63. Groesser L, Herschberger E, Landthaler M, Hafner C. FGFR3, PIK3CA and RAS mutations in benign lichenoid keratosis. *Br J Dermatol* 2012;**166**:784–788.
64. Cerroni L, Fink-Puches R, El-Shabrawi-Caelen L, *et al.* Solitary skin lesions with histopathologic features of early mycosis fungoides. *Am J Dermatopathol* 1999;**21**:518–524.
65. Mishlab S, Avitan-Hersh E, Zohar Y, *et al.* Immunophenotyping and viral studies in pityriasis lichenoides et varioliformis acuta lesions. *J Cutan Pathol* 2024;**51**:790–798.
66. Kadin ME. T-cell clonality in pityriasis lichenoides. Evidence for a premalignant or reactive immune disorder? *Arch Dermatol* 2002;**138**:1089–1090.
67. Borra T, Custrin A, Saggini A, *et al.* Pityriasis lichenoides, atypical pityriasis lichenoides, and related conditions: a study of 66 cases. *Am J Surg Pathol* 2018;**42**:1101–1112.
68. Tomasini D, Zampatti C, Palmedo G, *et al.* Cytotoxic mycosis fungoides evolving from pityriasis lichenoides chronica in a seventeen-year-old girl. *Dermatology* 2002;**205**:176–179.
69. King RL, Yan AC, Sekiguchi DR, Choi JK. Atypical cutaneous gamma/delta T cell proliferation with morphologic features of lymphoma but with clinical features and course of PLEVA or lymphomatoid papulosis. *J Cutan Pathol* 2015;**42**:1012–1017.
70. Martinez-Escala ME, Sidiropoulos M, DeonizioJ, et al. Gamma/delta T-cell-rich variants of pityriasis lichenoides and lymphomatoid papulosis: benign cutaneous disorders to be distinguished from aggressive cutaneous cd T-cell lymphomas. *Br J Dermatol* 2015;**172**:372–379.

71. Menzinger S, Frassati-Biaggi A, Leclerc-Mercier S, *et al.* Pityriasis lichenoides: a large histopathological case series with a focus on adnexotropism. *Am J Dermatopathol* 2020;**42**:1–10.
72. Raghavan SS, Wang JY, Gru AA, *et al.* Next-generation sequencing confirms T-cell clonality in a subset of pediatric pityriasis lichenoides. *J Cutan Pathol* 2022;**49**:252–260.
73. Zang JB, Coates SJ, Huang J, *et al.* Pityriasis lichenoides: long-term follow-up study. *Pediatr Dermatol* 2018;**35**:213–219.
74. Ersoy-Evans S, Greco MF, Mancini AJ, *et al.* Pityriasis lichenoides in childhood: a retrospective review of 124 patients. *J Am Acad Dermatol* 2007;**56**:205–210.
75. Zaaroura H, Sahar D, Bick T, Bergman R. Relationship between pityriasis lichenoides and mycosis fungoides: a clinicopathological, immunohistochemical, and molecular study. *Am J Dermatopathol* 2018;**40**:409–415.
76. Saggini A, Fink-Puches R, Cota C, *et al.* Papular mycosis fungoides is a distinctive variant of early-stage mycosis fungoides: extended retrospective study with long-term follow-up. *Am J Surg Pathol* 2019;**43**:1129–1134.
77. Rivera R, Ortiz P, Rodriguez-Peralto JL, *et al.* Febrile ulceronecrotic pityriasis lichenoides et varioliformis acuta with atypical cells. *Int J Dermatol* 2003;**42**:26–28
78. Sotiriou E, Patsatsi A, Tsorova C, *et al.* Febrile ulceronecrotic Mucha–Habermann disease: a case report and review of the literature. *Acta Derm Venereol (Stockh)* 2008;**88**:350–355.
79. Marenco F, Fava P, Fierro MT, *et al.* High-dose immunoglobulines and extracorporeal photochemotherapy in the treatment of febrile ulceronecrotic Mucha-Habermann disease. *Dermatol Ther* 2010;**23**:419–422.
80. Miyamoto T, Takayama N, Kitada S, *et al.* Febrile ulceronecrotic Mucha-Habermann disease: a case report and a review of the literature. *J Clin Pathol* 2003;**56**:795–797.
81. Herron MD, Bohnsack JF, Vanderhooft SL. Septic, CD-30 positive febrile ulceronecrotic pityriasis lichenoides et varioliformis acuta. *Ped Dermatol* 2005;**22**:360–365.
82. Kempf W, Kazakov DV, Palmedo G, *et al.* Pityriasis lichenoides et varioliformis acuta with numerous CD30(+) cells: a variant mimicking lymphomatoid papulosis and other cutaneous lymphomas. A clinicopathologic, immunohistochemical, and molecular biological study of 13 cases. *Am J Surg Pathol* 2012;**36**:1021–1029.
83. Fink-Puches R, Wolf P, Kerl H, *et al.* Clinicopathologic features, natural history, and relationship to mycosis fungoides. *Arch Dermatol* 2008;**144**:1169–1173.
84. Kolm I, Buset C, Flury U, *et al.* Lichen aureus with pseudolymphomatous infiltrate. *J Cutan Pathol* 2021;**48**:669–673.
85. (a) Boyd AS, Vnencak-Jones CL. T-cell clonality in lichenoid purpura: a clinical and molecular evaluation of seven patients. *Histopathology* 2003;**43**:302–303.(b) Chang N, Hirsch Y, Nemeth K, Pei S. Pembrolizumab-exacerbated widespread pigmented purpuric dermatosis in an elderly patient, a potential diagnostic pitfall mimicking pigmented purpuric dermatosis-like mycosis fungoides. *J Cutan Pathol* 2025. doi: 10.1111/cup.14841.
86. Barnhill RL, Braverman IM. Progression of pigmented purpuralike eruptions to mycosis fungoides: report of three cases. *J Am Acad Dermatol* 1988;**19**:25–31.
87. Toro JR, Sander CA, LeBoit PE. Persistent pigmented purpuric dermatitis and mycosis fungoides: simulant, precursor, or both? A study by light microscopy and molecular methods. *Am J Dermatopathol* 1997;**19**:108–118.
88. Citarella L, Massone C, Kerl H, Cerroni L. Lichen sclerosus with histopathologic features simulating early mycosis fungoides. *Am J Dermatopathol* 2003;**25**:463–465.
89. Leoni E, Kempf W, Cerroni L. Lichen sclerosus et atrophicus with histopathologic features mimicking mycosis fungoides: a large series of cases comparing genital with extragenital lichen sclerosus. *Am J Surg Pathol* 2022;**46**:83–88.
90. Lukowsky A, Muche JM, Sterry W, Audring H. Detection of expanded T cell clones in skin biopsy samples of patients with lichen sclerosus et atrophicus by T cell receptor-γ polymerase chain reaction assays. *J Invest Dermatol* 2000;**115**:254–259.
91. Suchak R, Verdolini R, Robson A, Stefanato CM. Extragenital lichen sclerosus et atrophicus mimicking cutaneous T-cell lymphoma: report of a case. *J Cutan Pathol* 2010;**37**: 982–986.
92. Coleman E, Bhawan J. Baby wet wipes: an unusual culprit of lymphomatoid contact dermatitis mimicking mycosis fungoides. *Am J Dermatopathol* 2022;**44**:205–206.
93. Petit T, Cribier B, Bagot M, Wechsler J. Inflammatory vitiligo-like macules that simulate hypopigmented mycosis fungoides. *Eur J Dermatol* 2003;**13**:410–412.
94. El-Darouti MA1, Marzouk SA, Azzam O, et al. Vitiligo vs. hypopigmented mycosis fungoides (histopathological and immunohistochemical study, univariate analysis). *Eur J Dermatol* 2006;**16**:17–22.
95. Furlan FC, Pereira BAP, da Silva LF, Sanches JA. Loss of melanocytes in hypopigmented mycosis fungoides: a study of 18 patients. *J Cutan Pathol* 2014;**41**:101–107.
96. Annessi G, Paradisi M, Angelo C, *et al.* Annular lichenoid dermatitis of youth. *J Am Acad Dermatol* 2003;**49**:1029–1036.
97. Fabroni C, Salvini C, Piana S, Lo SG. Annular lichenoid dermatitis. *Clin Exp Dermatol* 2010;**35**:921–923.
98. Cesinaro AM, Sighinolfi P, Greco A, *et al.* Annular lichenoid dermatitis of youth … and beyond: a series of 6 cases. *Am J Dermatopathol* 2009;**31**:263–267.
99. Mahmoudi H, Ghanadan A, Fahim S, *et al.* Annular lichenoid dermatitis of youth: report on two adult cases and one child. *J Dtsch Dermatol Ges* 2019;**17**:1173–1176.
100. Di Mercurio M, Gisondi P, Colato C, *et al.* Annular lichenoid dermatitis of youth: report of six new cases with review of the literature. *Dermatology* 2015;**231**:195–200.
101. Kazlouskaya V, Trager JDK, Junkins-Hopkins JM. Annular lichenoid dermatitis of youth: a separate entity or on the spectrum of mycosis fungoides? Case report and review of the literature. *J Cutan Pathol* 2015;**42**:420–426.
102. Cesinaro AM. Annular lichenoid dermatitis (of youth): report of a case with lichen planus-like features. *Am J Dermatopathol* 2017;**39**:914–915.
103. Wilk M, Zelger BG, Emberger M, *et al.* Annular lichenoid dermatitis (of youth) immunohistochemical and serological evidence for another clinical presentation of borrelia infection in patients of Western Austria. *Am J Dermatopathol* 2017;**39**:177–180.
104. Cogrel O, Boralevi F, Lepreux S, *et al.* Lymphomatoid annular erythema: a new form of juvenile mycosis fungoides. *Br J Dermatol* 2005;**152**:565–566.
105. Guitart J, Variakojis D, Kuzel T, Rosen S. Cutaneous $CD8^+$ T cell infiltrates in advanced HIV infection. *J Am Acad Dermatol* 1999;**41**:722–727.

106. Zhang P, Chiriboga L, Jacobson M, *et al.* Mycosis fungoideslike T-cell cutaneous lymphoid infiltrates in patients with HIV infection. *Am J Dermatopathol* 1995;**17**:29–35.
107. Fernández-Morano T, Aguilar-Bernier M, del Boz J, Fúnez-Liébanab R. Cutaneous CD8+ T-cell infiltrates associated with human immunodeficiency virus. *Actas Dermosifiliogr* 2012;**103**: 638–640.
108. Bachelez H, Hadida F, Gorochov G. Massive infiltration of the skin by HIV-specific cytotoxic CD8+ T cells. *N Engl J Med* 1996; **335**:61–62.
109. Sbidian E, Battistella M, Rivet J, *et al.* Remission of severe CD8 (+) cytotoxic T cell skin infiltrative disease in human immunodeficiency virus-infected patients receiving highly active antiretroviral therapy. *Clin Infect Dis* 2010;**51**:741–748.
110. Schartz NEC, De la Blanchardiere A, Alaoui S, *et al.* Regression of CD8+ pseudolymphoma after HIV antiviral triple therapy. *J Am Acad Dermatol* 2003;**49**:139–141.
111. Simonitsch I, Geusau A, Chott A, Jurecka W. Cutaneous dendritic cells are main targets in acute HIV-1-Infection. *Mod Pathol* 2000; **13**:1232–1237.
112. Baykal C, Büyükbabani N, Seçkin D, *et al.* Cutaneous atypical papular CD8+ lymphoproliferative disorder at acral sites in a renal transplant patient. *Clin Exp Dermatol* 2017;**42**:902–905.
113. Gammon B, Robson A, Deonizio J, *et al.* CD8(+) granulomatous cutaneous T-cell lymphoma: a potential association with immunodeficiency. *J Am Acad Dermatol* 2014;**71**:555–560.
114. Olsen SH, Ma L, Schnitzer B, *et al.* Clusterin expression in cutaneous CD30-positive lymphoproliferative disorders and their histologic simulants. *J Cut Pathol* 2009;**36**:302–307.
115. Werner B, Massone C, Kerl H, Cerroni L. Large CD30-positive cells in benign, atypical lymphoid infiltrates of the skin. *J Cutan Pathol* 2008;**35**:1100–1107.
116. Magro CM, Olson LC, Nguyen GH, *et al.* CD30 positive lymphomatoid angiocentric drug reactions: characterization of a series of 20 cases. *Am J Dermatopathol* 2017;**39**:508–517.
117. Massey PR, Wanat KA, Stewart CL, *et al.* CD30 positive atypical lymphocytes in perniosis: a potential histopathologic pitfall in a benign condition. *Am J Dermatopathol* 2014;**36**:730–733.
118. Kash N, Ginter-Hanselmayer G, Cerroni L. Cutaneous mycotic infections with pseudolymphomatous infiltrates. *Am J Dermatopathol* 2010;**32**:514–517.
119. Kempf W, Kazakov DV, Szep Z, Vanecek T. CD30+ clonal T-cell lymphoid proliferation of the skin in a patient with hypereosinophilic syndrome. *J Cutan Pathol* 2015;**42**:130–135.
120. Martin SM, Flowers R, Saavedra AP, Gru AA. A reactive peripheral Gamma-Delta T-cell lymphoid proliferation after a tick bite. *Am J Dermatopathol* 2019;**41**:e73–e75.
121. Hata DJ, Powell EA, Starolis MW, Realegeno SE. What the pox? Review of poxviruses affecting humans. *J Clin Virol* 2024; **174**:105719.
122. de Diego J, Berridi D, Saracibar N, Requena L. Cutaneous pseudolymphoma in association with molluscum contagiosum. *Am J Dermatopathol* 1998;**20**:518–521.
123. Kim MS, Noh TK, Won CH, *et al.* Atypical molluscum contagiosum accompanied by CD30-positive lymphoid infiltrates. *Pediatr Dermatol* 2013;**30**:141–142.
124. Moreno-Ramirez D, Garcia-Escudero A, Rios-Martin JJ, *et al.* Cutaneous pseudolymphoma in association with molluscum contagiosum in an elderly patient. *J Cutan Pathol* 2003;**30**:473–475.
125. Guitart J, Hurt MA. Pleomorphic T-cell infiltrate associated with molluscum contagiosum. *Am J Dermatopathol* 1999;**21**: 178–180.
126. Shalabi D, Ringe J, Lee JB, Nikbakht N. Molluscum contagiosum infection with features of primary cutaneous anaplastic large cell lymphoma. *Dermatol Online J* 2019;**25**:13030/qt7vp863hz.
127. Cribier B, Scrivener Y, Grosshans E. Molluscum contagiosum: histologic patterns and associated lesions. A study of 578 cases. *Am J Dermatopathol* 2001;**23**:99–103.
128. Ackerman AB, Tanski EV. Pseudoleukemia cutis. Report of a case in association with molluscum contagiosum. *Cancer* 1977;**40**: 813–817.
129. Espósito ACC, Jorge MFS, Marques MEA, Abbade LPF. Milker's nodules: classic histological findings. *An Bras Dermatol* 2017;**92**:838–840.
130. Leinweber B, Kerl H, Cerroni L. Histopathologic features of cutaneous herpes virus infections (herpes simplex, herpes varicella/zoster). A broad spectrum of presentations with common pseudolymphomatous aspects. *Am J Surg Pathol* 2006;**30**:50–58.
131. Wain EM, Antony F, Appleton MAC, *et al.* Genital herpes masquerading as a cutaneous T-cell lymphoma: a report of two cases. *J Cutan Pathol* 2008;**35**:770–773.
132. Aram G, Rohwedder A, Nazeer T, *et al.* Varicella-zoster-virus folliculitis promoted clonal cutaneous lymphoid hyperplasia. *Am J Dermatopathol* 2005;**27**:411–417.
133. Salem A, Loghavi S, Khoury JD, *et al.* Herpes simplex infection simulating Richter transformation: a series of four cases and review of the literature. *Histopathology* 2017;**70**:821–831.
134. Cerroni L, Zenahlik P, Kerl H. Specific infiltrates of B-cell chronic lymphocytic leukemia (B-CLL) arising at sites of herpes simplex and herpes zoster scars. *Cancer* 1995;**76**:26–31.
135. Mitteldorf C, Geissinger E, Pleimes M, *et al.* T-cell pseudolymphoma in recurrent herpes simplex virus infection. *J Cutan Pathol* 2019;**46**:717–722.
136. Böer A, Herder N, Winter K, Falk T. Herpes folliculitis: clinical, histopathological, and molecular pathologic observations. *Br J Dermatol* 2006;**154**:743–746.
137. Pereira A, Ferrara G, Calamaro P, *et al.* The histopathological spectrum of pseudolymphomatous infiltrates in cutaneous lupus erythematosus. *Am J Dermatopathol* 2018;**40**:247–253.
138. Magro CM, Crowson AN, Harrist TJ. Atypical lymphoid infiltrates arising in cutaneous lesions of connective tissue disease. *Am J Dermatopathol* 1997;**19**:446–455.
139. Tallon B, Kaddu S, Cerroni L, *et al.* Pseudolymphomatous tumid lupus erythematosus of the oral mucosa. *Am J Dermatopathol* 2010;**32**:704–707.
140. Weber F, Schmuth M, Fritsch P, Sepp N. Lymphocytic infiltration of the skin is a photosensitive variant of lupus erythematosus: evidence by phototesting. *Br J Dermatol* 2001;**144**:292–296.
141. Massone C, Kodama K, Salmhofer W, *et al.* Lupus erythematosus panniculitis (lupus profundus): clinical, histopathological, and molecular analysis of nine cases. *J Cutan Pathol* 2005;**32**:396–404.
142. Walsh NM, Lai J, Hanly JG, *et al.* Plasmacytoid dendritic cells in hypertrophic discoid lupus erythematosus: an objective evaluation of their diagnostic value. *J Cutan Pathol* 2015;**42**:32–38.
143. LeBlanc RE, Tavallaee M, Kim YH, Kim J. Useful parameters for distinguishing subcutaneous panniculitis-like T-Cell lymphoma from lupus erythematosus panniculitis. *Am J Surg Pathol* 2016;**40**:745–754.

144. Chen SJT, Tse JY, Harms PW, *et al.* Utility of CD123 immunohistochemistry in differentiating lupus erythematosus from cutaneous T cell lymphoma. *Histopathology* 2019;**74**:908–916.
145. Sitthinamsuwan P, Pattanaprichakul P, Treetipsatit J, *et al.* Subcutaneous panniculitis-like T-Cell lymphoma versus lupus erythematosus panniculitis: distinction by means of the periadipocytic cell proliferation index. *Am J Dermatopathol* 2018;**40**:567–574.
146. Fernandez-Pol S, De Stefano D, Kim J. Immunohistochemistry reveals an increased proportion of MYC-positive cells in subcutaneous panniculitis-like T-cell lymphoma compared with lupus panniculitis. *J Cutan Pathol* 2017;**44**:925–930.
147. Pincus L, LeBoit PE, McCalmont TH, *et al.* Subcutaneous panniculitis-like T-cell lymphoma with overlapping clinicopathologic features of lupus erythematosus: coexistence of 2 entities? *Am J Dermatopathol* 2009;**31**:520–526.
148. Bosisio F, Boi S, Caputo V, *et al.* Lobular Panniculitic Infiltrates With Overlapping Histopathologic Features of Lupus Panniculitis (Lupus Profundus) and Subcutaneous T-cell Lymphoma A Conceptual and Practical Dilemma. *Am J Surg Pathol* 2015;**39**:206–211.
149. Santonja C, Gonzalo I, Feito M, *et al.* Lipoatrophic panniculitis of the ankles in childhood: differential diagnosis with subcutaneous panniculitis-like T-cell lymphoma. *Am J Dermatopathol* 2012;**34**:295–300.
150. Roda Â, Travassos AR, Soares-de-Almeida L, Kutzner H. Lupus erythematosus mimicking mycosis fungoides: CD123+ plasmacytoid dendritic cells as a useful diagnostic clue. *J Cutan Pathol* 2019;**46**:167–170.
151. Boehm I, Schupp G, Bauer R. Milia en plaque arising in discoid lupus erythematosus. *Br J Dermatol* 1997;**137**:649–651.
152. Schreiber MM, McGregor JG. Pseudolymphoma syndrome: a sensitivity to anticonvulsant drugs. *Arch Dermatol* 1968;**97**:297–300.
153. Magro CM, Crowson AN, Kovatich AJ, Burns F. Drug-induced reversible lymphoid dyscrasia: a clonal lymphomatoid dermatitis of memory and activated T cells. *Hum Pathol* 2003;**34**:119–129.
154. Kardaun SH, Scheffer E, Vermeer BJ. Drug-induced pseudolymphomatous skin reactions. *Br J Dermatol* 1988;**118**:545–552.
155. Rosenthal CJ, Noguera CA, Coppola A, Kapelner SN. Pseudolymphoma with mycosis fungoides manifestations, hyper responsiveness to diphenylhydantoin, and lymphocyte dysregulation. *Cancer* 1982;**49**:2305–2314.
156. Pulitzer MP, Nolan KA, Oshman RC, *et al.* CD30+ lymphomatoid drug eruption. *Am J Dermatopathol* 2013;**35**:343–350.
157. Nathan DL, Belsito DV. Carbamazepine-induced pseudolymphoma with CD-30 positive cells. *J Am Acad Dermatol* 1998; **38**:806–809.
158. Shalin SC, Brantley J, Diwan AH. Follicular mucinosis and mycosis-fungoides-like drug eruption due to leuprolide acetate: a case report and review. *J Cut Pathol* 2012;**39**:1022–1025.
159. Richtig G, Cerroni L, Schmidt H, *et al.* Talimogene laherparepvec can initiate plasma cell invasion into infiltrated melanoma lesions - a case series. *J Eur Acad Dermatol Venereol* 2021;**35**:e209–e211.
160. Sweeney KJ, Tetzlaff MT, Vega F, *et al.* Tertiary lymphoid structures with overlapping histopathologic features of cutaneous marginal zone lymphoma during neoadjuvant cemiplimab therapy are associated with antitumor response. *J Cutan Pathol* 2021;**48**:674–679.
161. Siref A, Kitahara S, Balzer B. Proliferative clonal T-Cell infiltrate mimicking a cutaneous T-Cell lymphoma arising in active regression of melanoma. *Am J Dermatopathol* 2022;**44**:141–144.
162. Sangueza OP, Cohen DE, Calciano A, *et al.* Mycosis fungoides induced by phenytoin. *Eur J Dermatol* 1993;**3**:474–477.
163. Flaig MJ, Rupec RA. Cutaneous pseudolymphoma in association with Leishmania donovani. *Br J Dermatol* 2007;**157**:1042–1043.
164. Recalcati S, Vezzoli P, Girgenti V, *et al.* Cutaneous lymphoid hyperplasia associated with Leishmania panamensis infection. *Acta Derm Venereol (Stockh)* 2010;**90**:418–419.
165. Moulonguet I, Ghnassia M, Molina T, Fraitag S. Miliarial-type perifollicular B-cell pseudolymphoma (lymphocytoma cutis): a misleading eruption in two women. *J Cutan Pathol* 2012;**39**: 1016–1021.
166. (a)Saab J, Fedda F, Khattab R, *et al.* Cutaneous leishmaniasis mimicking inflammatory and neoplastic processes: a clinical, histopathological and molecular study of57 cases. *J Cut Pathol* 2012;**39**:251–262.(b) Mishlab S, Horowitz N, Bergman R. Refractory facial cutaneous B-cell pseudolymphoma in an atopic patient responsive to dupilumab. *J Dermatol* 2025;**52**:e843–e845.
167. Colli C, Leinweber B, Müllegger R, *et al.* Borrelia burgdorferi associated lymphocytoma cutis: clinicopathologic, immunophenotypic, and molecular study of 106 cases. *J Cutan Pathol* 2004; **31**:232–240.
168. Maraspin V, Nahtigal Klevišar M, Ružić-Sabljić E, *et al.* Borrelial lymphocytoma in adult patients. *Clin Infect Dis* 2016;**63**:914–921.
169. Emberger M, Laimer M, Lanschuetzer CM, *et al.* Symmetrical reddish swelling of the eyebrows in a 12-year-old girl – symmetrical Borrelia burgdorferi-associated lymphocytoma cutis of the eyebrows. *Arch Dermatol* 2008;**144**:673–678.
170. Laftah Z, Benton E, Bhargavat K, *et al.* Two cases of bilateral earlobe cutaneous pseudolymphoma. *Br J Dermatol* 2014; **171**:1567–1570.
171. Grange F, Wechsler J, Guillaume JC, *et al.* Borrelia burgdorferi associated lymphocytoma cutis simulating a primary cutaneous large B-cell lymphoma. *J Am Acad Dermatol* 2002;**47**:530–534.
172. Müllegger RR, Means TK, Shin JJ, *et al.* Chemokine signatures in the skin disorders of Lyme borreliosis in Europe: predominance of CXCL9 and CXCL10 in erythema migrans and acrodermatitis and CXCL13 in lymphocytoma. *Infect Immun* 2007;**75**:4621–4628.
173. Tee SI, Martínez-Escanamé M, Zuriel D, *et al.* Acrodermatitis chronica atrophicans with pseudolymphomatous infiltrates. *Am J Dermatopathol* 2013;**35**:338–342.
174. Bauvin O, Schmutz JL, De Martino S, *et al.* A foot tumour as late cutaneous Lyme borreliosis: a new entity? *Br J Dermatol* 2017;**177**:1127–1130.
175. Bertolotti A, Pham-Ledard A, Petrot D, *et al.* Two cases of proliferation of monoclonal and monotypic lymphocytes and plasma cells corresponding to acrodermatitis chronica atrophicans. *Ann Dermatol Venereol* 2014;**141**:452–457.
176. Cerroni L, Zöchling N, Pütz B, Kerl H. Infection by Borrelia burgdorferi and cutaneous B-cell lymphoma. *J Cutan Pathol* 1997;**24**:457–461.
177. Goos N. Acrodermatitis chronica atrophicans and malignant lymphoma. *Acta Derm Venereol (Stockh)* 1971;**51**:457–459.
178. Kempf W, Kazakov DV, Kutzner H. Lobular panniculitis due to Borrelia burgdorferi infection mimicking subcutaneous panniculitis-like T-cell lymphoma. *Am J Dermatopathol* 2013;**35**: e30–e33.

179. Dittmer MR, Willis MS, Selby JC, Liu V. Septolobular panniculitis in disseminated Lyme borreliosis. *J Cutan Pathol* 2018; **45**:274–277.
180. Cerroni L, Borroni RG, Massone C, *et al.* Cutaneous B-cell pseudolymphoma at the site of vaccination. *Am J Dermatopathol* 2007;**29**:538–542.
181. Chong H, Brady K, Metze D, Calonje E. Persistent nodules at injection sites (aluminium granuloma)-clinicopathological study of 14 cases with a diverse range of histological reaction patterns. *Histopathology* 2006;**48**:182–188.
182. Frings VG, Roth S, Rosenwald A, *et al.* EBER in situ hybridization in subcutaneous aluminum granulomas/lymphoid hyperplasia: a diagnostic clue to differentiate injection-associated lymphoid hyperplasia from other forms of pseudolymphomas and cutaneous lymphomas. *J Cutan Pathol* 2021;**48**:625–631.
183. Staser K, Abner S, Anadkat M, *et al.* Injection-site cutaneous pseudolymphoma induced by a GM-CSF–Producing tumor cell vaccine. *JAMA Dermatol* 2017;**153**:332–334.
184. Pham-Ledard A, Vergier B, Doutre MS, Beylot-Barry M. Disseminated cutaneous lymphoid hyperplasia of 12 years' duration triggered by vaccination. *Dermatology* 2010;**220**:176–179.
185. Kluger N, Vermeulen C, Mouguelet P, *et al.* Cutaneous lymphoid hyperplasia (pseudolymphoma) in tattoos: a case series of seven patients. *J Eur Acad Dermatol Venereol* 2010;**24**:206–213.
186. King BJ, Lehman JS, Macon WR, *et al.* Red tattoo-related mycosis fungoides-like CD8+ pseudolymphoma. *J Cutan Pathol* 2018;**45**: 226–228.
187. Zaaroura H, Bergman R. Mixed Lichenoid and follicular T- and B-Cell lymphoid reaction to red tattoos with monoclonal T cells. *Am J Dermatopathol* 2018;**40**:438–441.
188. Haus G, Utikal J, Geraud C, *et al.* CD30-positive lymphoproliferative disorder in a red tattoo: regional lymphomatoid papulosis type C or pseudolymphoma? *Br J Dermatol* 2014;**171**:668–670.
189. Sangueza OP, Yadav S, White CR Jr, Braziel RM. Evolution of B-cell lymphoma from pseudolymphoma: a multidisciplinary approach using histology, immunohistochemistry, and Southern blot analysis. *Am J Dermatopathol* 1992;**14**:408–413.
190. Nielsen C, Jerkeman M, Jöud AS. Tattoos as a risk factor for malignant lymphoma: a population-based case–control study. *EClin Med* 2024;**72**:102649. doi: 10.1016/j.eclinm.2024.102649.
191. Komatsu H, Aiba S, Mori S, *et al.* Lymphocytoma cutis involving the lower lip. *Contact Dermatitis* 1997;**36**:167–169.
192. Brazzelli V, Vassallo C, Ardigo M, *et al.* Unusual histologic presentation of morphea. *Am J Dermatopathol* 2000;**22**:359.
193. Aragon Sierra AM, Hwang AS, Kechter J, *et al.* Systemic sclerosis with morphea-like plaques histopathologically mimicking cutaneous B-cell lymphoma. *JAAD case rep* 2024;**47**:32–34.
194. Kazmi A, Feuerhake T, Zidan A, *et al.* Morphoea presenting histopathologically as mycosis fungoides: an illustrative series of four cases. *Histopathology* 2024;**85**:353–358.
195. Sato Y, Takeuchi M, Takata K, *et al.* Clinicopathologic analysis of IgG4-related skin disease. *Mod Pathol* 2013;**26**:523–532.
196. Umehara H, Okazaki K, Masaki Y, *et al.* Comprehensive diagnostic criteria for IgG4-related disease (IgG4-RD), 2011. *Mod Rheumatol* 2012;**22**:21–30.
197. Cheuk W, Lee KC, Chong LY, *et al.* IgG4-related sclerosing disease: a potential new etiology of cutaneous pseudolymphoma. *Am J Surg Pathol* 2009;**33**:1713–1719.
198. Shakeri A, Kindley KJ, Noland MM, Gru AA. IgG4-Related skin disease presenting as a pseudolymphoma in a white adolescent girl. *Am J Dermatopathol* 2019;**41**:675–679.
199. Cesinaro AM, Lonardi S, Facchetti F. Granuloma faciale: a cutaneous lesion sharing features with IgG4-associated sclerosing diseases. *Am J Surg Pathol* 2013;**37**:66–73.
200. Deshpande V, Zen Y, Chan JK, *et al.* Consensus statement on the pathology of IgG4-related disease. *Mod Pathol* 2012;**25**:1181–1192.
201. Ingen-Housz-Oro S, Ortonne N, Elhai M, *et al.* IgG4-related skin disease successfully treated by thalidomide: a report of 2 cases with emphasis on pathological aspects. *JAMA Dermatol* 2013;**149**: 742–747.
202. Battistella M, Le Cleach L, Lacert A, Perrin P. Extensive nodular secondary syphilis with prozone phenomenon. *Arch Dermatol* 2008;**144**:1078–1079.
203. Mitteldorf C, Plumbaum H, Zutt M, *et al.* CD8-positive pseudolymphoma in lues maligna and human immunodeficiency virus with monoclonal T-cell receptor-beta rearrangement. *J Cutan Pathol* 2019;**46**:204–210.
204. Flamm A, Alcocer VM, Kazlouskaya V, *et al.* Histopathological features distinguishing secondary syphilis from its mimickers. *J Am Acad Dermatol* 2020;**82**:156–160.
205. Leguellec S, Tournier E, Karanian M, *et al.* Cutaneous inflammatory myofibroblastic tumours can be anaplastic lymphoma kinase-positive: report of the first four cases. *Histopathology* 2016;**68**:297–302.
206. Hurt MA, Santa Cruz DJ. Cutaneous inflammatory pseudotumor: lesions resembling "inflammatory pseudotumors" or "plasma cell granulomas" of extracutaneous sites. *Am J Surg Pathol* 1990;**14**: 764–773.
207. El Shabrawi-Caelen L, Kerl K, Cerroni L, *et al.* Cutaneous inflammatory pseudotumor – a spectrum of various diseases? *J Cutan Pathol* 2004;**31**:605–611.
208. Uhara H, Saida T, Ikegawa S, *et al.* Primary cutaneous plasmacytosis: report of three cases and review of the literature. *Dermatology* 1994;**189**:251–255.
209. Jayaraman AG, Cesca C, Kohler S, Cutaneous plasmacytosis. A report of five cases with immunohistochemical evaluation for HHV-8 expression. *Am J Dermatopathol* 2006;**28**:93–98.
210. Honda R, Cerroni L, Tanikawa A, *et al.* Cutaneous plasmacytosis: report of 6 cases with or without systemic involvement. *J Am Acad Dermatol* 2013;**68**:978–985.
211. Han XD, Lee SSJ, Tan SH, *et al.* Cutaneous plasmacytosis: a clinicopathologic study of a series of cases and their treatment outcomes. *Am J Dermatopathol* 2018;**40**:36–42.
212. Haque M, Hou JS, Hisamichi K, *et al.* Cutaneous and systemic plasmacytosis vs. cutaneous plasmacytic Castleman disease: review and speculations about pathogenesis. *Clin Lymphoma Myeloma Leuk* 2011;**11**:453–461.
213. Shimizu S, Tanaka M, Shimizu H, Hanyaku H. Is cutaneous plasmacytosis a distinct clinical entity? *J Am Acad Dermatol* 1997;**36**:876–880.

214. Hara M, Matsunaga J, Tagami H. Acral pseudolymphomatous angiokeratoma of children (APACHE): a case report and immunohistologic study. *Br J Dermatol* 1991;**124**:387–388.
215. Dayrit JF, Wang WL, Goh SGN, *et al.* T-cell-rich angiomatoid polypoid pseudolymphoma of the skin: a clinicopathologic study of 17 cases and a proposed nomenclature. *J Cut Pathol* 2011;**38**:475–482.
216. Fried I, Wiesner T, Cerroni L. Pretibial lymphoplasmacytic plaque in children. *Arch Dermatol* 2010;**146**:95–96.
217. Moulonguet I, Hadj-Rabia S, Gounod N, *et al.* Tibial lymphoplasmacytic plaque: a new, illustrative case of a recently and poorly recognized benign lesion in children. *Dermatology* 2012;**225**: 27–30.
218. Porto DA, Sutton S, Wilson JB, *et al.* Lymphoplasmacytic plaque in children: a report of two new cases with review of the literature. *J Cutan Pathol* 2013;**40**:50–55.
219. Harkemanne E, Dargent JL, Roquet-Gravy PP, Bulinckx A. Lymphoplasmacytic plaque in children: case report and literature review. *Pediatr Dermatol* 2019;**36**:365–367.
220. Kaddu S, Cerroni L, Pilatti A, *et al.* Acral pseudolymphomatous angiokeratoma. *Am J Dermatopathol* 1994;**16**:130–133.
221. Geller S, Markova A, Pulitzer M, *et al.* Acral angiokeratoma-like pseudolymphoma in a middle-aged woman. *J Cutan Pathol* 2017;**44**:878–881.
222. Gilliam AC, Mullen RH, Oviedo G, *et al.* Isolated benign primary cutaneous plasmacytosis in children: two illustrative cases. *Arch Dermatol* 2009;**145**:299–302.
223. Fernandez-Flores A, Fierro S, Larralde M. Expression of WT-1 by the vascular component of acral pseudolymphomatous angiokeratoma of children. *J Cutan Pathol* 2015;**42**:50–55.
224. Haniffa MA, Wilkins BS, Blasdale C, Simpson NB. Cutaneous extramedullary hemopoiesis in chronic myeloproliferative and myelodysplastic disorders. *J Am Acad Dermatol* 2006;**55**:s28–s31.
225. Requena L, Kutzner H, Palmedo G, *et al.* Histiocytoid sweet syndrome: a dermal infiltration of immature neutrophilic granulocytes. *Arch Dermatol* 2005;**141**:834–842.
226. Chavan RN, Cappel MA, Ketterling RP, *et al.* Histiocytoid sweet syndrome may indicate leukemia cutis: a novel application of fluorescence In situ hybridization. *J Am Acad Dermatol* 2014; **70**:1021–1027.
227. Magro CM, Momtahen S, Nguyen GH, Wang X. Histiocytoid sweet's syndrome: a localized cutaneous proliferation of macrophages frequently associated with chronic myeloproliferative disease. *Eur J Dermatol* 2015;**25**:335–341.
228. Calvo KR. Skin in the game: the emergence of myelodysplasia cutis. *Blood* 2022;**139**:1132–1134.
229. Delaleu J, Kim R, Zhao LP, *et al.* Clinical, pathological, and molecular features of myelodysplasia cutis. *Blood* 2022;**139**:1251–1253.
230. Alegría-Landa V, Rodríguez-Pinilla SM, Santos-Briz A, *et al.* Clinicopathologic, immunohistochemical, and molecular features of histiocytoid sweet syndrome. *JAMA Dermatol* 2017; **153**:651–659.
231. Requena L, El-Shabrawi-Caelen L, Walsh SN, *et al.* Intralymphatic histiocytosis. a clinicopathologic study of 16 cases. *Am J Dermatopathol* 2009;**31**:140–151.
232. Bakr F, Webber N, Fassihi H, *et al.* Primary and secondary intralymphatic histiocytosis. *J Am Acad Dermatol* 2014;**70**:927–933.
233. Demirkesen C, Kıran T, Leblebici C, *et al.* Intravascular/Intralymphatic histiocytosis: a report of 3 cases. *Am J Dermatopathol* 2015;**37**:783–789.
234. Fernández-Figueras MT, Martín-Urdà MT, Plana A, *et al.* Intravascular (blood vessel) histiocytosis with haemophagocytosis. *Histopathology* 2016;**69**:1077–1081.
235. Mazloom SE, Stallings A, Kyei A. Differentiating intralymphatic histiocytosis, intravascular histiocytosis, and subtypes of reactive angioendotheliomatosis: review of clinical and histologic features of all cases reported to date. *Am J Dermatopathol* 2017;**39**:33–39.
236. Bryant A, Lawton H, Al-Talib R, *et al.* Intravascular proliferation of reactive lymphoid blasts mimicking intravascular lymphoma – a diagnostic pitfall. *Histopathology* 2007;**51**:401–402.
237. Baum CL, Stone MS, Liu V. Atypical intravascular CD30+ T-cell proliferation following trauma in a healthy 17-year-old male: first reported case of a potential diagnostic pitfall and literature review. *J Cut Pathol* 2009;**36**:350–354.
238. Ardighieri L, Lonardi S, Vermi W, *et al.* Intralymphatic atypical T-cell proliferation in a cutaneous hemangioma. *J Cut Pathol* 2010;**37**:497–503.
239. Cesinaro AM, Luca RB. Atypical lymphoid proliferation in capillary hemangioma: a finding related to bacterial infection? *J Cutan Pathol* 2010;**37**:1021–1022.
240. Riveiro-Falkenbach E, Fernandez-Figueras MT, Rodriguez-Peralto JL. Benign atypical intravascular CD30+ T-cell proliferation: a reactive condition mimicking intravascular lymphoma. *Am J Dermatopathol* 2013;**35**:143–150.
241. Lee S, Ogilvie RT, Dupre M, *et al.* Intravascular lymphocytosis in acute appendicitis: potential mimicry of chronic lymphocytic leukaemia. *Histopathology* 2009;**55**:660–664.
242. Calamaro P, Cerroni L. Intralymphatic proliferation of T-cell lymphoid blasts in the setting of hidradenitis suppurativa. *Am J Dermatopathol* 2016;**38**:536–540.
243. Kempf W, Keller K, John H, Dommann-Scherrer C. Benign atypical intravascular CD30+ T-Cell proliferation: a recently described reactive lymphoproliferative process and simulator of intravascular lymphoma report of a case associated with lichen sclerosus and review of the literature. *Am J Clin Pathol* 2014;**142**:694–699.
244. Weingertner N, Mitcov M, Chenard M-P, Cribier B. Intralymphatic CD30+ T-cell proliferation during DRESS: a mimic of intravascular lymphoma. *J Cutan Pathol* 2016;**43**:1036–1040.
245. Kailas A, Elston DM, Crater SE, *et al.* Cutaneous intravascular CD30+ T-cell pseudolymphoma occurring in a regressing keratoacanthoma. *J Cutan Pathol* 2018;**45**:296–298.
246. Mascolo M, Russo D, Scalvenzi M, *et al.* Lichen striatus mit histopathologischer Imitation einer Mycosis fungoides. *J Deutsch Dermatol Gesell* 2014;**12**:1048–1050.
247. Cota C, Ferrara G, Cerroni L. Granuloma annulare with prominent lymphoid infiltrates ("pseudolymphomatous" granuloma annulare). *Am J Dermatopathol* 2012;**34**:259–262.
248. Pfaltz K, Kerl K, Palmedo G, *et al.* Clonality in sarcoidosis, granuloma annulare, and granulomatous mycosis fungoides. *Am J Dermatopathol* 2011;**33**:659–662.

249. González Delgado P, de la Sen Fernández ML, Soriano Gomis V, *et al.* Cyclical hypereosinophilia with skin manifestations and a clonal T cell population. *J Investig Allergol Clin Immunol* 2008; **18**:401–403.
250. Hurabielle C, Sbidian E, Beltraminelli H, *et al.* Eruption of lymphocyte recovery with atypical lymphocytes mimicking a primary cutaneous T-cell lymphoma: a series of 12 patients. *Hum Pathol* 2018;**71**:100–108.
251. Kash N, Vin H, Danialan R, *et al.* Stenotrophomonas maltophilia with histopathological features mimicking cutaneous gamma/delta T-cell lymphoma. *Int J Infect Dis* 2014;**30**:e7–e9.
252. Li JJ, Henderson C. Cutaneous crystal storing histiocytosis: a report of two cases. *J Cutan Pathol* 2015;**42**:136–143.
253. McGill NK, Vyas J, Shimauchi T, *et al.* HTLV-1-associated infective dermatitis: updates on the pathogenesis. *Exper Dermatol* 2012;**21**:815–821.
254. Roustan G, Yus ES, Simón A. Nevoid hyperkeratosis of the areola with histopathological features mimicking mycosis fungoides. *Eur J Dermatol* 2002;**12**:79–81.
255. Rosman IS, Hepper DM, Lind AC, Anadkat MJ. Nevoid hyperkeratosis of the areola misinterpreted as mycosis fungoides. *J Cutan Pathol* 2012;**39**:545–548.

## CHAPTER 32

# Nonlymphoid malignant neoplasms of the skin mimicking histopathologically cutaneous lymphomas ("malignant pseudolymphomas")

Although the definition of cutaneous pseudolymphoma is that of a benign condition that simulates a malignant lymphoma clinically and/or histopathologically, there are rare examples of nonlymphoid malignancies that may be misinterpreted as malignant lymphomas, with consequences as catastrophic as those of an erroneous diagnosis of lymphoma in a reactive infiltrate. I refer to these conditions as "malignant" pseudolymphomas, although I am well aware of the semantic contradiction related to the use of this term. On the other hand, this oxymoron helps to remind us that not all simulators of cutaneous lymphomas are benign disorders. A detailed discussion of these entities is beyond the scope of this book; in what follows, I will only summarize the clinicopathological features that may be misinterpreted as those of a cutaneous lymphoproliferative disorder.

***Lymphoepithelial-like carcinoma of the skin*** represents a cutaneous carcinoma of unknown histogenesis and with prominent lymphoid infiltrates [1, 2]. I have seen cases characterized by prominent germinal centers that, together with the nodules of large keratinocytes surrounded by lymphoid infiltrates, simulated the picture of a cutaneous follicle center lymphoma (Fig. 32.1). Complete phenotypic analyses, of course, reveal the epithelial origin of the neoplastic cells, thus allowing a precise diagnosis. Plasma cells, when present, are polytypic, but at a dermatopathology meeting Dr. Ed Rytina (Cambridge, UK) showed a case of cutaneous lymphoepithelial-like carcinoma with monotypic plasma cells, thus further complicating the differential diagnosis. Cutaneous cases of lymphoepithelial-like carcinoma are not associated with Epstein-Barr virus (EBV) infection and are not related to the true lymphoepithelial carcinoma. The treatment and prognosis are similar to those of other cutaneous squamous cell carcinomas.

Cutaneous angiosarcomas may present with heavy inflammatory infiltrates, simulating the picture of a cutaneous T- or B-cell lymphoma ("***pseudolymphomatous angiosarcoma***") [3, 4]. The clinical presentation is usually that of a conventional cutaneous angiosarcoma, but histology shows dense lymphoid infiltrates intermingled with sheets of atypical endothelial cells that resemble the diffuse areas of a large cell lymphoma (Figs. 32.2a and b). As germinal centers are often present as well, the erroneous diagnosis of cutaneous follicle center lymphoma may be made. Again, complete phenotypic investigations allow the correct diagnosis to be made (Figs. 32.2c, d and e). It has been suggested that the presence of a pseudolymphomatous reaction is related to a better prognosis in cutaneous angiosarcoma [3].

Besides these two malignant tumors, typical mimickers of a cutaneous lymphoma are represented by ***histiocytic sarcoma*** and related entities. Before immunohistological analyses became routine, many cases of lymphoma with "immunoblastic" morphology were classified as histiocytic sarcoma. Reclassification of these cases thanks to monoclonal antibodies led to the suggestion that a "true" histiocytic sarcoma does not exist at all. However, today histiocytic sarcoma is a well-defined (albeit rare) entity [5] that can be classified with confidence according to histopathological and phenotypic criteria. Histiocytic sarcoma can occur at any age, and cutaneous lesions are characterized by large, ulcerated tumors, mostly solitary at outset (Fig. 32.3a). The neoplasm is aggressive with poor response to therapy. Histology shows a diffuse proliferation of large cells with morphological features that may resemble immunoblasts (Figs. 32.3b and c). A variable number of reactive cells may be observed, but usually the picture is dominated by the atypical cells (Fig. 32.4). Neoplastic cells are positive for CD163 (Fig. 32.3d), CD68 (KP1 and PGM1), and lysozyme, and negative for markers of T- and B-lymphocytes, Langerhans cells (CD1a and CD207; S100 may be weakly positive in some cells), follicular dendritic cells (CD21, CD35, CXCL13, CD23, podoplanine), and myeloid cells (CD13, myeloperoxidase). Undifferentiated carcinomas and melanoma represent further differential diagnoses, and should be excluded by appropriate immunohistochemical stainings (i.e., cytokeratins, Melan-A, HMB45, SOX10).

***Follicular dendritic cell sarcoma*** is another malignant tumor that may simulate a lymphoma by showing tissue infiltration by

*Skin Lymphoma: The Illustrated Guide*, Sixth Edition. Lorenzo Cerroni.

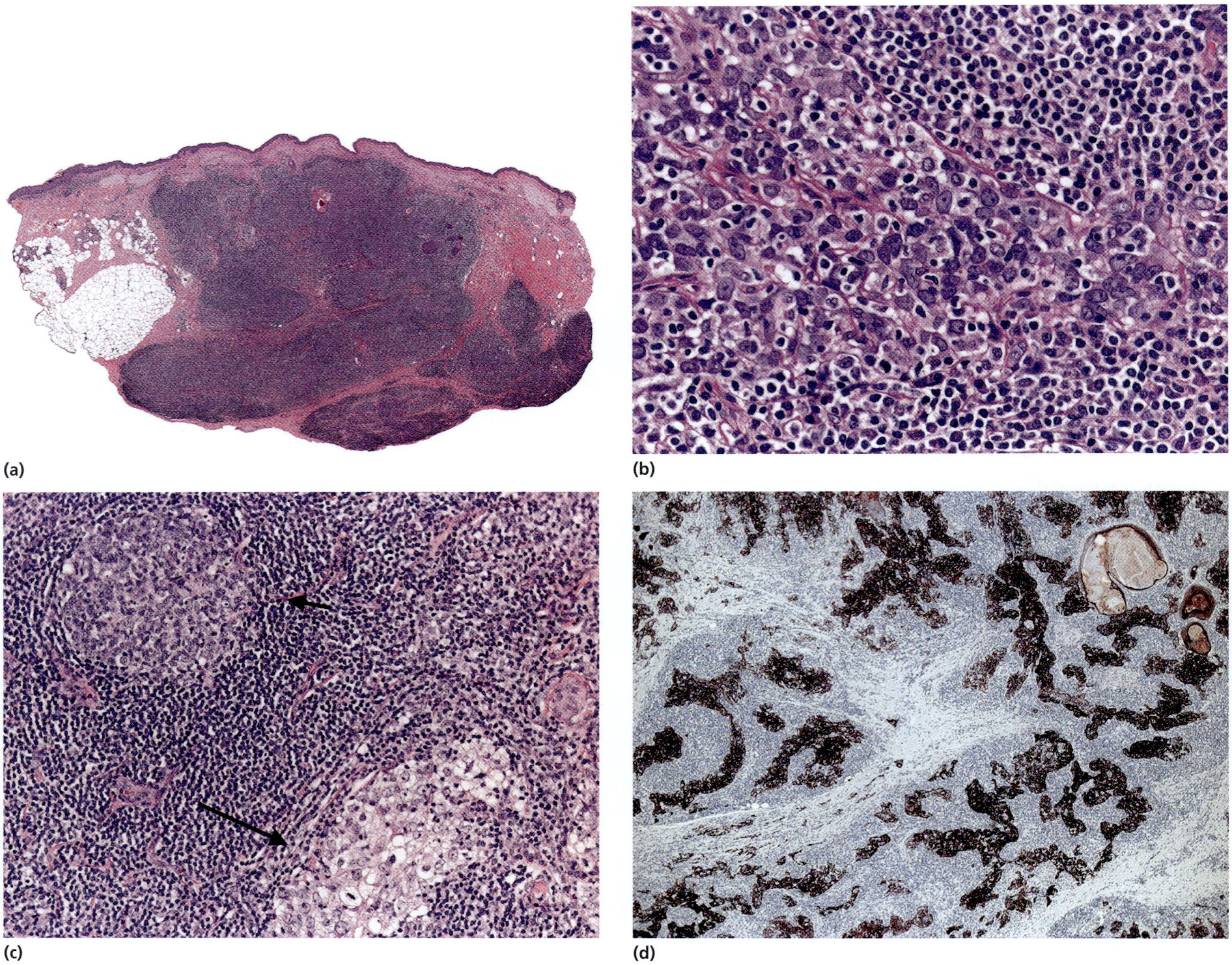

Figure 32.1 Lymphoepithelial-like carcinoma. (a) At scanning magnification the epithelial complexes are not recognizable on the background of dense lymphoid infiltrates. (b) Cluster of atypical epithelial cells showing morphologic similarities to blastoid lymphocytes. (c) In another case, a cluster of pale epithelial cells (long arrow) admixed with a heavy inflammatory infiltrate. Note the reactive germinal center (short arrow). (d) Staining for pan-cytokeratin highlights the epithelial complexes.

oval, blastoid-like cells [6]. It occurs only rarely in the skin. The neoplasm is relatively indolent, with local recurrences and distant metastases in about one-fourth of patients. Clinical presentation is usually with subcutaneous masses. Histology is characterized by large, oval cells with vesicular chromatin and distinct nucleoli. Pleomorphism is variable. Immunohistology shows positivity for CD21, CXCL13, CD23, CD35, FDCSP, SRGN, and podoplanine, as well as for PD-L1. A panel of antibodies including CXCL13, CD21, CD35, FDCSP, and SRGN could discriminate >95% of cases of follicular dendritic cell sarcoma from other mesenchymal tumors in one study [7]. There is a variable positivity for CD68, whereas markers of Langerhans cells and myeloid cells are negative.

***Cutaneous mastocytoses*** usually do not represent a mimicker of cutaneous lymphomas. In addition, most cases of cutaneous mastocytosis are not "malignant," and the prognosis is excellent. In adults, however, cases of urticaria pigmentosa (maculopapular cutaneous mastocytosis) that resemble mycosis fungoides histopathologically are characterized by dense infiltrates, usually corresponding to systemic mastocytosis, and sometimes showing an aggressive course. For this reason I decided to include the cutaneous mastocytoses in this chapter rather than in the one on conventional ("benign") pseudolymphomas.

Tumoral lesions (mastocytoma) are composed of sheets of mast cells, which can be easily recognized morphologically and with stain for CD117. Urticaria pigmentosa in most instances represents an example of the "invisible" dermatoses, that is, of those conditions characterized by histopathological features that are so subtle that they can be misinterpreted as "normal" skin. In short, mastocytoma and urticaria pigmentosa do not

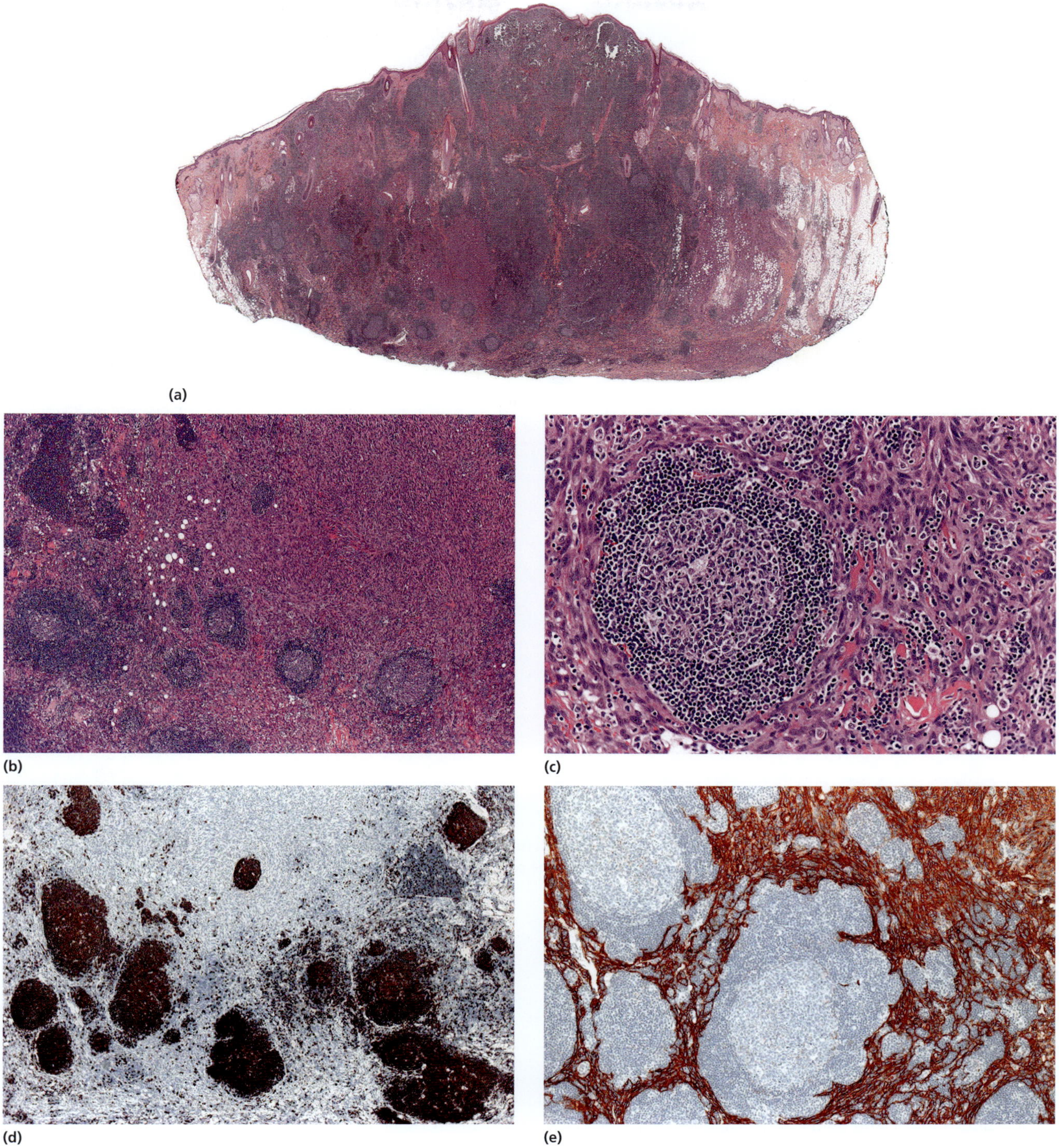


**Figure 32.2** Pseudolymphomatous angiosarcoma. (a) At low power, the tumor shows similarities to a lymphoma. (b) Sheets of cells with reactive germinal centers. (c) Detail of sheets of large epithelioid cells admixed with small lymphocytes; note a reactive germinal center. (d) Staining for CD20 shows many large nodules of B cells, some representing lymphatic follicles. (e) Staining for podoplanine confirms that the large cells outside of the germinal centers are endothelial cells with lymphatic differentiation.

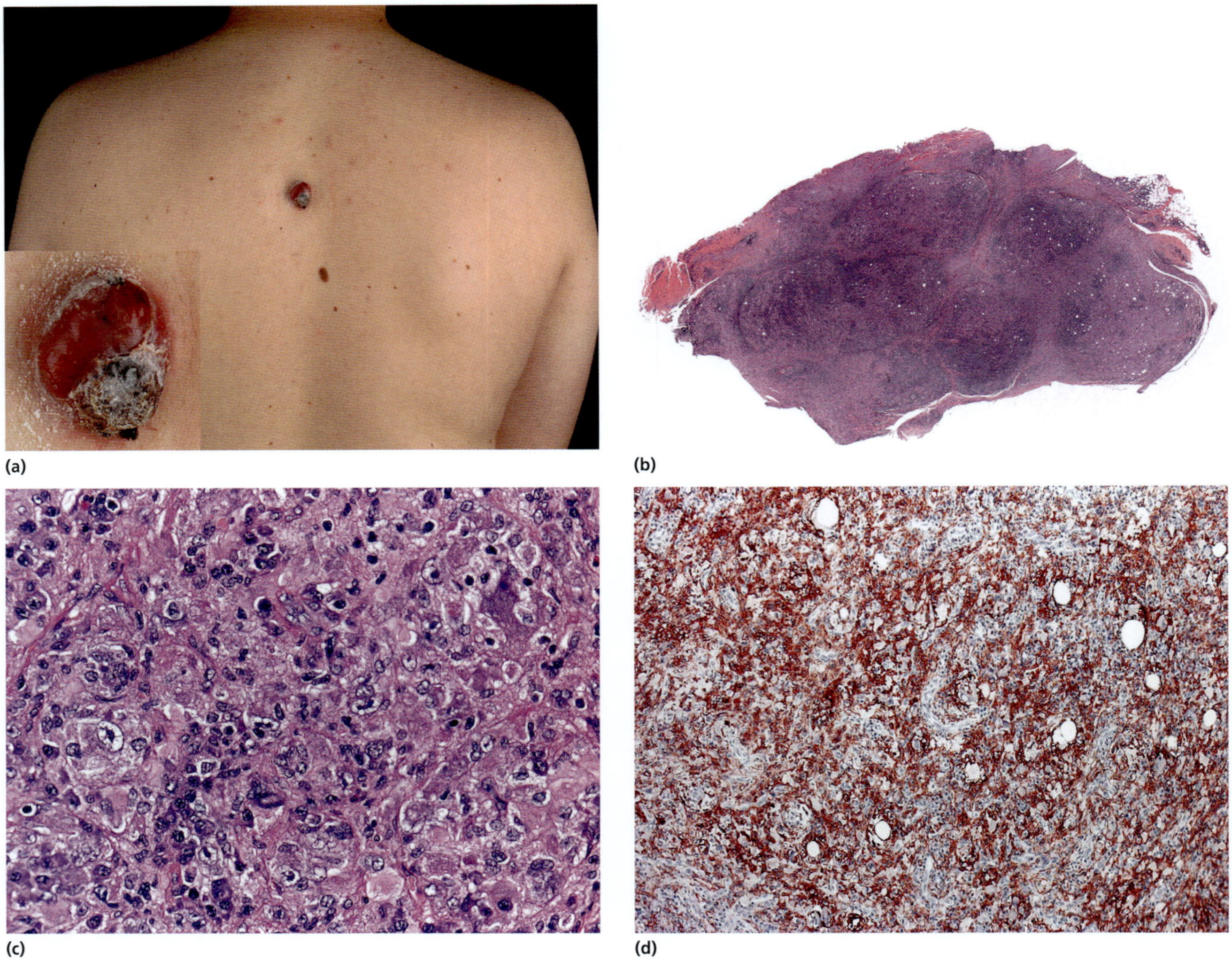

Figure 32.3 Cutaneous histiocytic sarcoma. (a) Ulcerated tumor on the back (inset with detail). (b) Histology shows diffuse infiltrates composed of (c) large, atypical cells, some resembling blastoid lymphocytes. (d) Neoplastic cells are positive for CD163 (T- and B-cell markers were negative).

represent a mimicker of cutaneous lymphomas. However, in some cases of urticaria pigmentosa, the lesions are characterized histopathologically by dense, band-like infiltrates of mast cells admixed with many lymphocytes, thus potentially mimicking a lymphoproliferative disorder, and particularly mycosis fungoides (Fig. 32.5) [8, 9]. As mast cells may be positive for CD4 and CD30, and other lymphoid-related antigens can also be expressed in systemic mast cell diseases [10], such cases represent a pitfall in the diagnosis. Careful clinicopathological correlation as well as staining for CD117 reveal the typical features of the disease, and allows to distinguish it from cutaneous lymphoproliferative disorders. Positivity for CD4 and CD30 is usually a feature of systemic mastocytosis with aggressive behavior or of mast cell leukemia [11], and patients with such lesions should undergo careful staging investigations. Only a few mast cells are positive for CD30 in indolent systemic mastocytoses (including "conventional" urticaria pigmentosa) [11]. The role of CD30 expression in mastocytosis is poorly understood, and it seems that CD30$^+$ mast cells are activated independently from the IgE pathway [12].

Cutaneous mastocytosis is included in the International Consensus Classification (ICC) *of Myeloid and Lymphoid Neoplasms* and in the 5th edition of the World Health Organization (WHO) *Classification of Haematolymphoid Tumours* [13, 14]. In the WHO classification, the traditional terms "urticaria pigmentosa" and "telangiectasia macularis eruptiva perstans" are discouraged, and the term "maculopapular cutaneous mastocytosis" is used instead, a change in nomenclature that in my opinion does not introduce any significant improvement. In fact, the term "urticaria pigmentosa" is used together with "maculopapular cutaneous mastocytosis" in the ICC terminology.

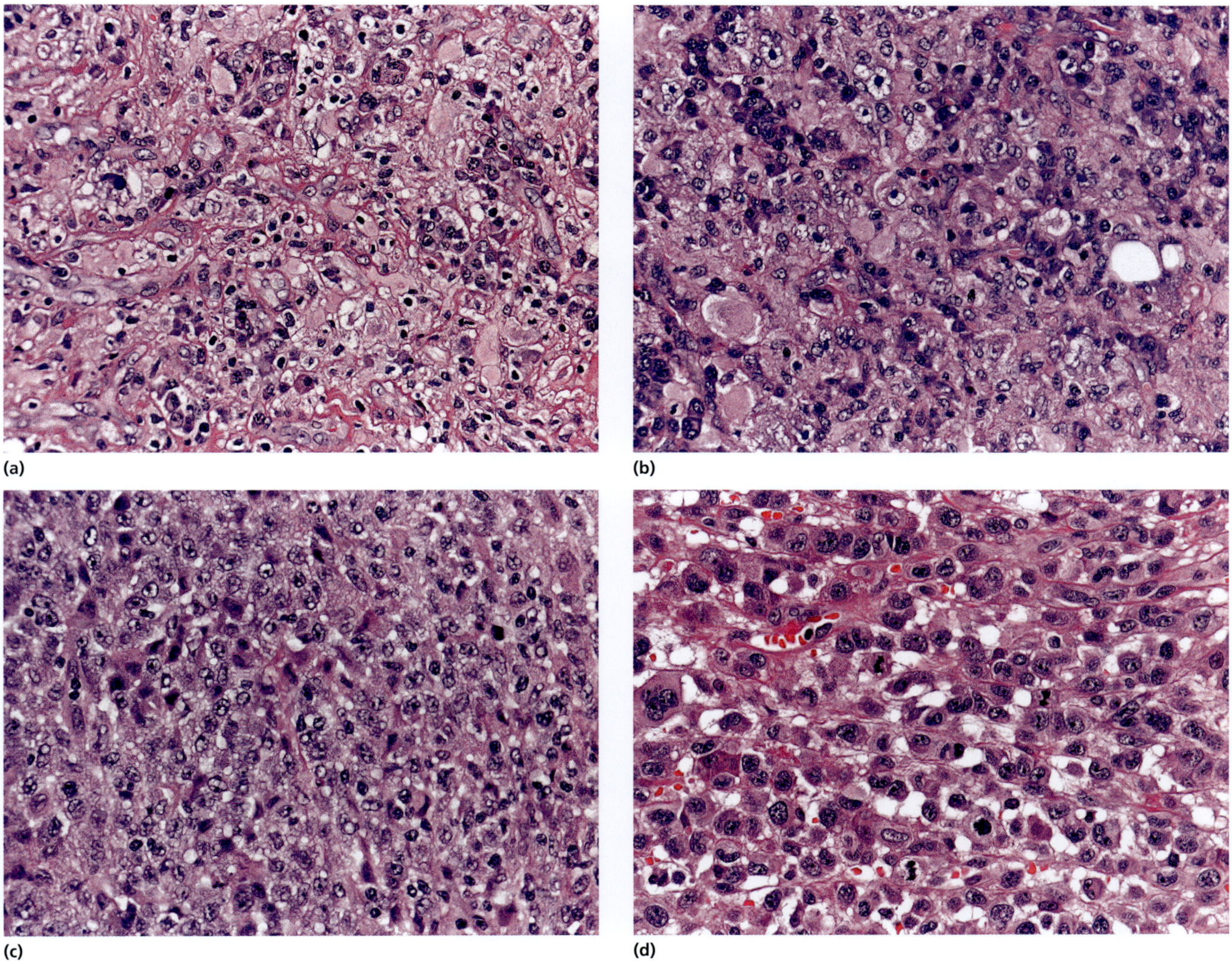


**Figure 32.4** Cutaneous histiocytic sarcoma. Morphologic variations of neoplastic cells in different cases with features that resemble (a, b) histiocytes, (c) pleomorphic lymphocytes, or (d) even plasmablasts.

Cutaneous lesions of ***Langerhans cell histiocytosis*** may show clusters of epidermotropic neoplastic cells, sometimes mimicking the Darier nests of mycosis fungoides (Fig. 32.6). In contrast to the normal Langerhans cells that are resident within the epidermis, neoplastic ones are rounded rather than dendritic, thus being possibly mistaken for large lymphocytes. Neoplastic cells in Langerhans cell histiocytosis are positive for CD1a, langerin (CD207), and S100, as well as for CD4, and these markers allow to clearly differentiate them from lymphocytes of epidermotropic lymphomas.

It should be reminded that Langerhans cells may be present in large amounts in several cutaneous lymphomas, particularly in mycosis fungoides, sometimes arranged in large clusters in the dermis. I have seen many cases sent in consultation with the diagnosis of "coexistent mycosis fungoides and Langerhans cell histiocytosis" that, in truth, represented examples of mycosis fungoides with Langerhans cell hyperplasia. As already mentioned, neoplastic Langerhans cells are rounded rather than dendritic, and are usually epidermotropic, thus allowing an easy distinction from hyperplastic Langerhans cells.

Finally, a ***"pagetoid" distribution of intraepidermal neoplastic cells*** may be observed in different conditions including, among others, melanoma, mammary and extramammary Paget disease, and Bowen disease (carcinoma in situ). However, the histopathological context in these conditions is completely different, and they do not represent a differential diagnostic concern with epidermotropic lymphomas. In the unlikely case that doubts should arise concerning a specific biopsy specimen, besides clinicopathological correlation, appropriate immunohistochemical stains allow to separate these entities from lymphomas (and from one another).

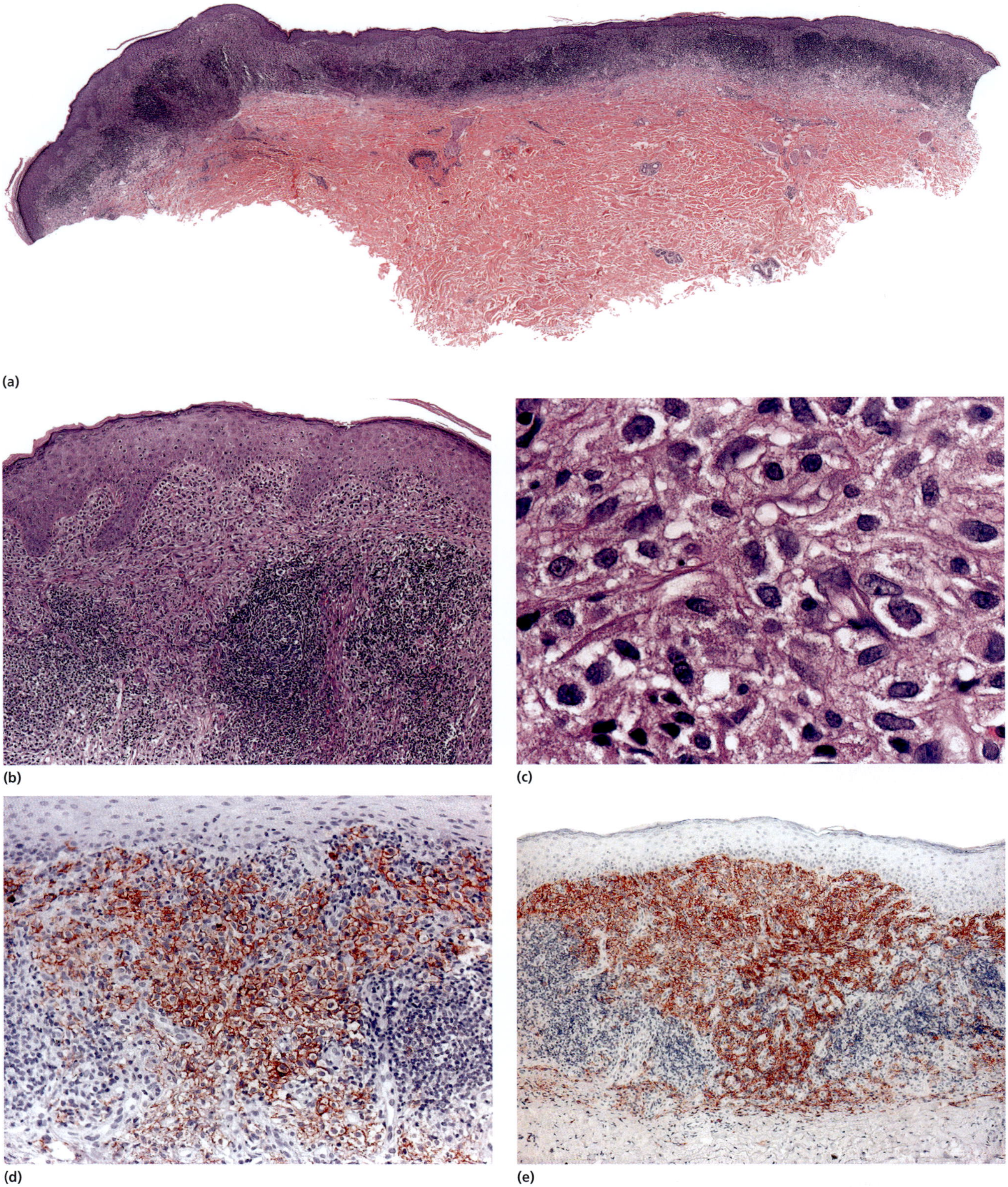

**Figure 32.5** An 81-year-old man presented with generalized, infiltrated, brownish lesions thought clinically to represent urticaria pigmentosa. No relevant history was known. A biopsy showed a dense, band-like infiltrate (a) composed of two different cell types, namely, small lymphocytes admixed with aggregates of large cells with granular cytoplasm (b, c). Immunohistology revealed that the small lymphocytes were partly of B- and partly of T-cell phenotype without aberrant phenotypic features. The large cells were positive for CD4, CD30 (d) and CD117 (e), and negative for other T- and B-cell antigens. A diagnosis of mastocytosis (highly suspicious for systemic mastocytosis) with CD4 and CD30 positivity was made. The patient was lost to follow-up.

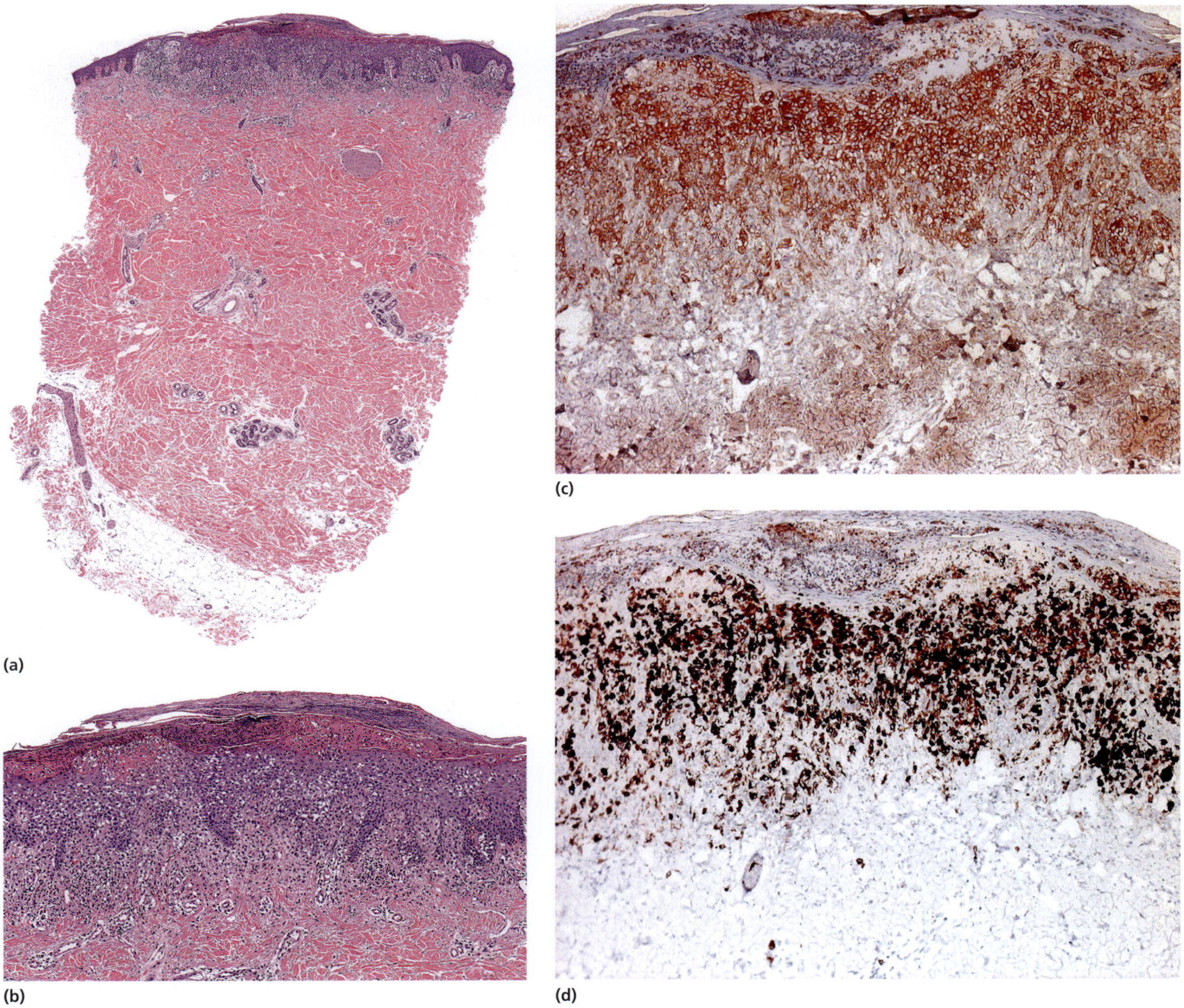


**Figure 32.6** Cutaneous Langerhans cell histiocytosis. (a) Band-like infiltrate with (b) epidermotropic cells resembling large lymphocytes. Immunohistology shows positivity for (c) CD1a and (d) Langerin (CD207).

## References

1. Requena L, Sánchez Yus E, Jiménez E, Roo E. Lymphoepithelioma-like carcinoma of the skin: a light-microscopic and immunohistochemical study. *J Cutan Pathol* 1994;**21**:541–548.
2. Kazakov DV, Nemcova J, Mikyskova I, Michal M. Absence of Epstein-Barr virus, human papillomavirus, and simian virus 40 in patients of central European origin with lymphoepithelioma-like carcinoma of the skin. *Am J Dermatopathol* 2007;**29**:365–369.
3. Requena L, Santonja C, Stutz N, *et al.* Pseudolymphomatous cutaneous angiosarcoma: a rare variant of cutaneous angiosarcoma readily mistaken for cutaneous lymphoma. *Am J Dermatopathol* 2007;**29**:342–350.
4. Rongioletti F, Albertini AF, Fausti V, *et al.* Pseudolymphomatous cutaneous angiosarcoma: a report of 2 new cases arising in an unusual setting. *J Cutan Pathol* 2013;**40**:848–854.
5. Takahashi E, Hung YP. Histiocytic sarcoma. In: *WHO Classification of Tumours Editorial Board. Haematolymphoid Tumours.* 5th edition. Lyon: IARC, 2024: 255–257.
6. Rech KL, Picarsic J, Demicco EG, *et al.* Follicular dendritic cell sarcoma. In: *WHO Classification of Tumours Editorial Board. Haematolymphoid Tumours.* 5th edition. Lyon: IARC, 2024: 787–790.
7. Lorenzi L, Döring C, Rausch T, *et al.* Identification of novel follicular dendritic cell sarcoma markers, FDCSP and SRGN, by whole transcriptome sequencing. *Oncotarget* 2017;**8**:16463–16472.

8. Kulberg A, Mitteldorf C. CD4 and CD30 coexpression in a cutaneous manifestation of systemic mastocytosis—A pitfall. *Am J Dermatopathol* 2018;**40**:628–630.
9. Soilleux EJ, Bowling J, Hollowood K. CD4 expression by mast cells in mastocytosis: a case report. *J Clin Pathol* 2009;**62**:564–566.
10. Escribano L, Orfao A, Villarrubia J, *et al.* Expression of lymphoid-associated antigens in mast cells: report of a case of systemic mast cell disease. *Br J Haematol* 1995;**91**:941–943.
11. Sotlar K, Cerny-Reiterer S, Petat-Dutter K, *et al.* Aberrant expression of CD30 in neoplastic mast cells in high-grade mastocytosis. *Mod Pathol* 2011;**24**:585–595.
12. Fischer M, Harvima IT, Carvalho RF, *et al.* Mast cell CD30 ligand is upregulated in cutaneous inflammation and mediates degranulation-independent chemokine secretion. *J Clin Invest* 2006;**116**:2748–2756.
13. Reichard K, George TI, Leguit R, *et al.* Mastocytosis. In: Arber DA, Borowitz MJ, Cook JR, *et al.*, eds. *The International Consensus Classification of Myeloid and Lymphoid Neoplasms*. Philadelphia, PA: Wolters Kluwer, 2025: 84–100.
14. Colmenero I, Alvarez-Twose I, Sotlar K, Torrelo A. Cutaneous mastocytosis. In: *WHO Classification of Tumours Editorial Board. Haematolymphoid Tumours*. 5th edition. Lyon: IARC, 2024: 61–63.

SECTION 8

# The cutaneous "atypical lymphoid proliferation"

# CHAPTER 33

# The cutaneous "atypical lymphoid proliferation"

In spite of refined diagnostic criteria, better and powerful ancillary techniques, and adequate clinicopathologic correlation, some cutaneous lymphoid proliferations defy precise diagnosis and classification. Sometimes this may be due to the submission by surgeons of inadequate material (e.g., crushed specimens, superficial biopsies, or specimens that show drying artifacts – see Chapter 1), and a repeat biopsy may allow the correct diagnosis. Other times, however, an individual case cannot be classified unambiguously into a given category of cutaneous lymphoma, lymphoproliferative disorder, or pseudolymphoma. I use for such cases the working term "cutaneous atypical lymphoid proliferation" (Fig. 33.1). Some of these cases show an overlap with those published in the literature as "borderline" between cutaneous lymphomas and pseudolymphomas, and are reported under various names including cutaneous lymphoid dyscrasia and clonal dermatitis, among others. It must be clearly underlined that the term "cutaneous atypical lymphoid proliferation" does not refer to cases of clear-cut cutaneous lymphoma that cannot be classified with precision. For such cases, the term "unclassifiable cutaneous (B- or T-cell) lymphoma" should be used instead, and staging investigations should be carried out.

The term "cutaneous atypical lymphoid proliferation" is essentially a histopathologic one and encompasses four main patterns:

1. The first is characterized by *superficial infiltrates of lymphocytes* (main differential diagnosis: mycosis fungoides versus simulators). In general, conventional molecular analyses of the T-cell receptor (TCR) genes are not diriment in such cases, but better information may be gathered by next-generation sequencing of the TCR genes [1–3]. If epidermotropism of pleomorphic lymphocytes is striking, then the term "atypical lymphoid proliferation" should be avoided and the specimen should be properly classified within one of the epidermotropic lymphomas or, if not possible, reported as "unclassifiable epidermotropic lymphoma." Benign conditions do not show Darier's nests or prominent ("pagetoid") epidermotropism of pleomorphic lymphocytes as a rule, but I have encountered exceptional cases that defy this rule (see Chapter 31, Figs. 31.26 and 31.45).
2. The second pattern is characterized by *nodular proliferations of small lymphocytes admixed with reactive cells, without formation of lymphoid follicles* (main differential diagnosis: pseudolymphoma versus cutaneous low-grade B- or T-cell lymphoma). A typical example of the second pattern is represented by lesions that are suggestive of cutaneous marginal zone lymphoproliferative disorder on clinicopathologic grounds, but in which monoclonal expression of the immunoglobulin (Ig) light chains is lacking. Complete phenotypic analyses should always be carried out in these cases. If medium–large cells predominate, then the term "cutaneous atypical lymphoid proliferation" should not be used and a report of "unclassifiable (B- or T-cell) lymphoma" should be made instead. Molecular analyses of the TCR and immunoglobulin genes provide useful information in such cases.
3. The third pattern is characterized by *nodular proliferations of small lymphocytes admixed with reactive cells, with the formation of lymphoid follicles* (main differential diagnosis: pseudolymphoma versus cutaneous low-grade B-cell lymphoma). The lymphoid follicles should be checked for reactive or malignant features (see Chapters 16 and 31). It should be remembered that reactive germinal centers may be encountered in B-cell lymphomas other than follicle center lymphoma, as well as in T-cell lymphomas and other hematological disorders. Stainings for kappa and lambda should always be performed. Molecular analyses of the TCR and Ig genes may provide useful information in these cases.
4. Finally, the last pattern is represented by *predominant involvement of the subcutaneous fat* (main differential diagnosis: lobular panniculitis versus subcutaneous panniculitis-like T-cell lymphoma). If the infiltrate is limited to the septa or shows clear-cut involvement of the dermis, then subcutaneous panniculitis-like T-cell lymphoma can be ruled out. However, other T- and also B-cell lymphomas can present with prominent involvement of the subcutaneous fat (e.g., cutaneous gamma/delta T-cell lymphoma). Complete phenotypic analyses should be carried out, keeping in mind that reactive changes (e.g., granulomatous infiltrates, degenerative changes) can be observed in old lesions of subcutaneous panniculitis-like T-cell lymphoma. Subcutaneous infiltrates composed entirely of B lymphocytes are never reactive, and phenotypic analyses should be carried out in order to classify

*Skin Lymphoma: The Illustrated Guide*, Sixth Edition. Lorenzo Cerroni.

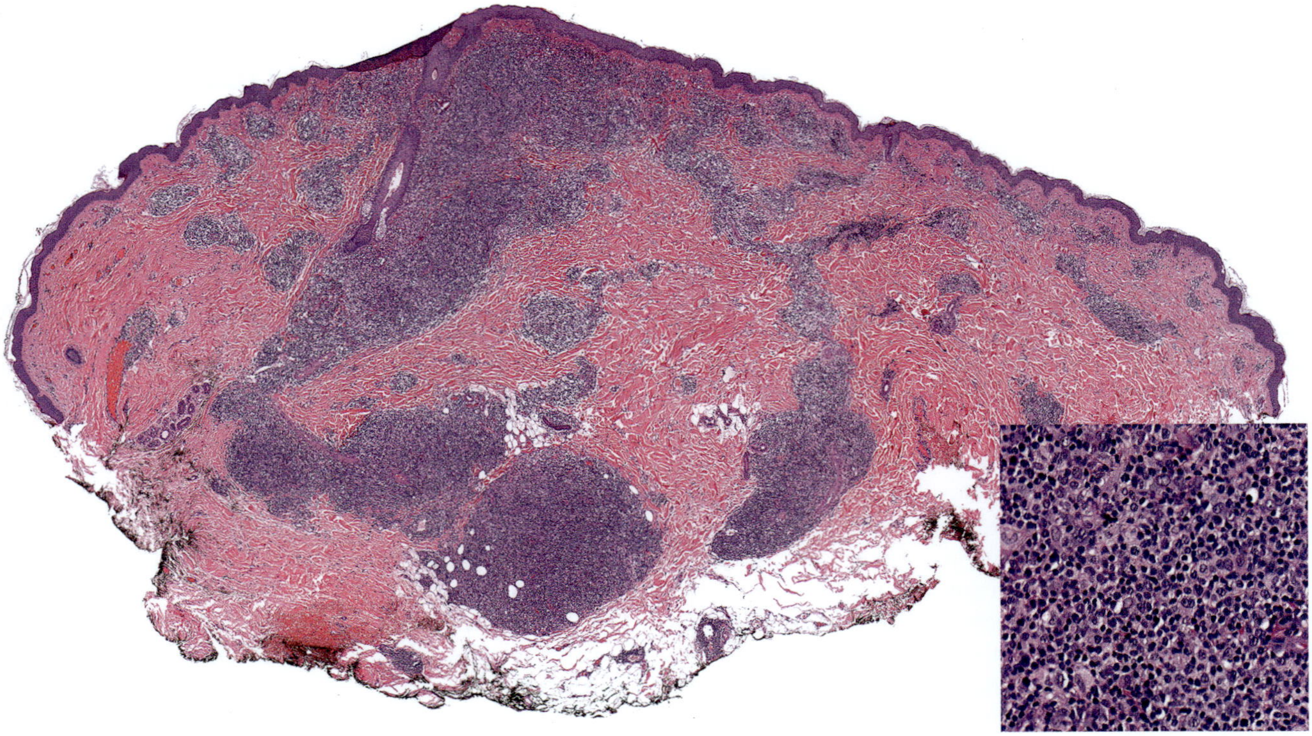

(a)

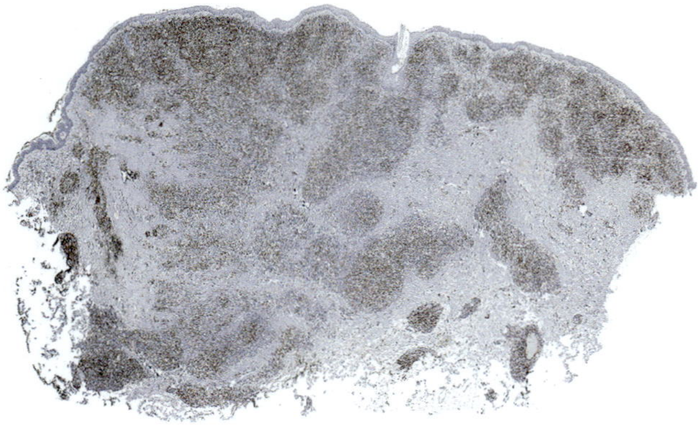

(b)

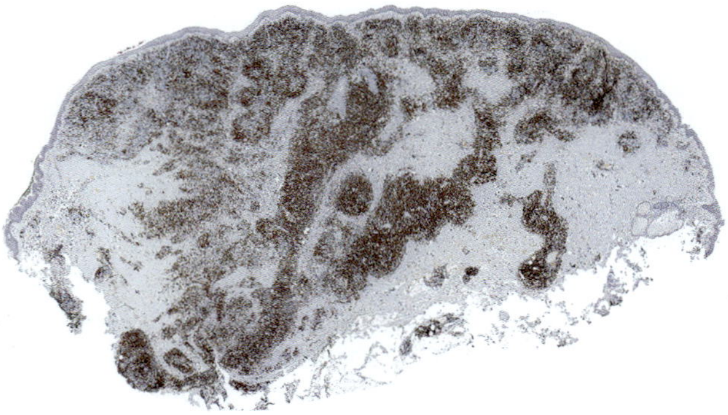

(c)

Figure 33.1 Example of a cutaneous atypical lymphoid proliferation. This solitary lesion on the neck of a 59-year-old woman shows (a) a bottom heavy infiltrate composed predominantly of small lymphocytes (inset) that are (b) partly positive for CD3 and (c) partly for CD20. The lesion is not unequivocally benign because it is bottom-heavy, and it is not unequivocally malignant because the morphology is not atypical. Although the predominance of B lymphocytes may suggest a low-grade cutaneous B-cell lymphoma, the lack of a specific pattern is not consistent with either cutaneous marginal zone lymphoproliferative disorder or cutaneous follicle center lymphoma, thus not allowing a clear-cut diagnosis to be made.

these cases properly. In cases with a predominance of T lymphocytes, molecular analysis of the TCR genes provides useful diagnostic information.

Combining clinical, histopathologic, phenotypic, and molecular features, the number of "cutaneous atypical lymphoid proliferations" will be reduced to a minimum, but such cases nonetheless exist and represent a problem in daily routine. Many colleagues who send me biopsy specimens in consultation know this problem very well, as well as the frustration of receiving back a diagnosis of "cutaneous atypical lymphoid proliferation." In cases of cutaneous lymphoid infiltrates that cannot be classified accurately, the following guidelines may be used.

**(a)** As already mentioned, cases with obvious malignant features, but which cannot be classified precisely, should not be included in the group of the "cutaneous atypical lymphoid proliferations" but rather be termed "cutaneous lymphoma, unclassifiable." In such cases, repeat biopsies should be obtained, and all available ancillary techniques should be used. Complete staging investigations should be performed as well.

**(b)** If there are no features of an aggressive cutaneous lymphoma (both clinically and histopathologically), a general term such as "cutaneous atypical lymphoid proliferation" may be better than a more specific diagnosis that may prove to be wrong. Repeat and follow-up biopsies are often diriment for the final classification of such cases.

**(c)** In most cases with ambiguous histopathologic features (particularly in those with mycosis fungoides-like aspects), correlation with the clinical picture allows a precise diagnosis.

**(d)** A staining for Ki-67 is useful, as it highlights the "proliferation pattern" of the infiltrate, allowing to evaluate eventual "hot spots" both morphologically and phenotypically.

**(e)** In-situ hybridization for Epstein–Barr virus (EBV) may be of relevance, and should always be performed in cases arising in the setting of known immune deficiency/dysregulation (regardless of the type of immune deficiency), as it may show the pattern of post-transplant lymphoproliferative disorders (which is not restricted to patients who received a solid organ transplantation).

**(f)** If a precise diagnosis is not possible, the histopathologic report should mention all differential diagnoses applicable to a given case (e.g., inflammatory dermatosis versus early mycosis fungoides).

**(g)** If possible, obtain a second expert opinion. In this context, it should be clearly underlined that a second meaningful opinion can be given only when complete information and sufficient histopathologic material are available. Superficial biopsies and/or biopsies with artifacts are not adequate for diagnosis and classification of cutaneous lymphoproliferative disorders, regardless of the experience of the person looking at them. Particularly in ambiguous cases, diagnosis of cutaneous lymphoid infiltrates requires the integration of accurate and complete clinical data with histopathological features studied on a representative biopsy specimen, pertinent immunohistochemical stainings, and molecular analyses.

**(h)** Finally, a diagnosis of "cutaneous atypical lymphoid proliferation" does not imply the need to perform staging investigations; short-term follow-up controls suffice. In fact, management of patients with low-grade cutaneous lymphomas includes for many entities the option of a "watchful waiting" strategy, thus implying that a delay in the diagnosis is not crucial in these cases.

In cases without clear-cut clinicopathological features, the term "cutaneous atypical lymphoid proliferation" may be useful to prevent a potentially incorrect diagnosis as well as the psychological and economic burden of staging investigations, at the same time avoiding dismissal of the patient from follow-up programs.

## References

1. Scherer F, Kurtz DM, Diehn M, Alizadeh AA. High-throughput sequencing for noninvasive disease detection in hematologic malignancies. *Blood* 2017;**130**:440–452.
2. Kirsch IR, Watanabe R, O'Malley JT, *et al.* TCR sequencing facilitates diagnosis and identifies mature T cells as the cell of origin in CTCL. *Sci Transl Med* 2015;**7**:308ra158.
3. Matos TR, de Rie MA, Teunissen MBM. Research techniques made simple: high-throughput sequencing of the T-cell receptor. *J Invest Dermatol* 2017;**137**:e131–e138.

# Index



*Skin Lymphoma: The Illustrated Guide*, Sixth Edition. Lorenzo Cerroni.